# Management of
# HIGH-RISK PREGNANCY
## A Practical Approach

## DISCLAIMER

It is often said that knowledge has a beginning but no end. This is particularly relevant to the field of medicine which is ever changing. Guidelines and recommendations are updated on regular basis, backed by recent developments in medical literature. The authors, editors and publishers of this book have done a meticulous check of all the available evidence with reliable sources, at the time of publication, which is in accordance with the acceptable standards. However, there is always a possibility of human error as well as error in view of nonincorporation of emerging evidence. The authors, editors, publisher or any other party involved with this book do not claim that the information contained in this book is complete or accurate in all aspects. Thus, they shall not be held accountable for any errors or deficiencies in the book as well as for any outcome obtained from the use of information contained in the book. It is the responsibility of the practitioner to take all safety precautions. It is suggested that the readers should check the most current information available on procedures before practical application. Before prescribing a drug, complete, most recent information about recommended dose, side effects and contraindications should always be checked with manufacturer's product information of each drug.

# Management of HIGH-RISK PREGNANCY
## A Practical Approach

**Third Edition**

*Editors*

**Shubha Sagar Trivedi**
MS FRCOG (Hon. Causa) FIMSA FICOG
Former Director Professor and Head
Department of Obstetrics and Gynecology
Lady Hardinge Medical College and Smt Sucheta Kriplani Hospital
New Delhi
Former Professor and Head, Department of Obstetrics and Gynecology
SGT University, Gurugram, Haryana, India

**Manju Puri**
MD FICOG
Director Professor and Former Head
Department of Obstetrics and Gynecology
Lady Hardinge Medical College and Smt Sucheta Kriplani Hospital
New Delhi, India

**Swati Agrawal**
MD FICOG FMAS
Professor
Department of Obstetrics and Gynecology
Lady Hardinge Medical College and Smt Sucheta Kriplani Hospital
New Delhi, India

*Foreword*
**Sir Sabaratnam Arulkumaran**

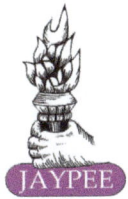

# JAYPEE BROTHERS MEDICAL PUBLISHERS
*The Health Sciences Publisher*

**New Delhi | London**

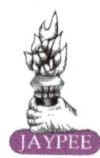
**Jaypee Brothers Medical Publishers (P) Ltd**

**Headquarters**
Jaypee Brothers Medical Publishers (P) Ltd
EMCA House, 23/23-B
Ansari Road, Daryaganj
New Delhi 110 002, India
Landline: +91-11-23272143, +91-11-23272703
+91-11-23282021, +91-11-23245672
Email: jaypee@jaypeebrothers.com

**Corporate Office**
Jaypee Brothers Medical Publishers (P) Ltd
4838/24, Ansari Road, Daryaganj
New Delhi 110 002, India
Phone: +91-11-43574357
Fax: +91-11-43574314
Email: jaypee@jaypeebrothers.com

**Overseas Office**
JP Medical Ltd
83 Victoria Street, London
SW1H 0HW (UK)
Phone: +44 20 3170 8910
Fax: +44 (0)20 3008 6180
Email: info@jpmedpub.com

Website: www.jaypeebrothers.com
Website: www.jaypeedigital.com

© 2022, Jaypee Brothers Medical Publishers

The views and opinions expressed in this book are solely those of the original contributor(s)/author(s) and do not necessarily represent those of editor(s) of the book.

All rights reserved. No part of this publication may be reproduced, stored or transmitted in any form or by any means, electronic, mechanical, photocopying, recording or otherwise, without the prior permission in writing of the publishers.

All brand names and product names used in this book are trade names, service marks, trademarks or registered trademarks of their respective owners. The publisher is not associated with any product or vendor mentioned in this book.

Medical knowledge and practice change constantly. This book is designed to provide accurate, authoritative information about the subject matter in question. However, readers are advised to check the most current information available on procedures included and check information from the manufacturer of each product to be administered, to verify the recommended dose, formula, method and duration of administration, adverse effects and contraindications. It is the responsibility of the practitioner to take all appropriate safety precautions. Neither the publisher nor the author(s)/editor(s) assume any liability for any injury and/or damage to persons or property arising from or related to use of material in this book.

This book is sold on the understanding that the publisher is not engaged in providing professional medical services. If such advice or services are required, the services of a competent medical professional should be sought.

Every effort has been made where necessary to contact holders of copyright to obtain permission to reproduce copyright material. If any have been inadvertently overlooked, the publisher will be pleased to make the necessary arrangements at the first opportunity. The **CD/DVD-ROM** (if any) provided in the sealed envelope with this book is complimentary and free of cost. **Not meant for sale.**

**Inquiries for bulk sales may be solicited at**: jaypee@jaypeebrothers.com

*Management of High-Risk Pregnancy: A Practical Approach*

*First Edition*: 2010

*Second Edition*: 2016

*Third Edition*: **2022**

ISBN: 978-93-5465-129-8

**Dedicated to**

*Our Parents*
*Mrs Saubhagya Wati and Mr Keshav Sagar*
*Mrs Sushila and Mr Santlal*
*Mrs Jyoti and Dr Narayan Prasad Agrawal*

# Contributors

**Abha Singh** MS FICOG FIMCH
Director Professor and Former Head
Department of Obstetrics and Gynecology
Lady Hardinge Medical College and
Smt Sucheta Kriplani Hospital
New Delhi, India

**Amita Suneja** MD
Director Professor and Head
Department of Obstetrics and Gynecology
University College of Medical Sciences
and GTB Hospital
New Delhi, India

**Anju Bhatia** MBBS MD MRCOG (UK)
Masters Fetal Medicine (Barcelona)
Staff Physician
Department of Maternal Fetal Medicine
Clinical Lecturer Yong Loo Lin Medical
School, Duke NUS Medical School
KK Women's and Children's Hospital
Thomson, Singapore

**Anubhuti Rana** MBBS MS Fellowship in
Maternal Fetal Medicine
Assistant Professor
Department of Obstetrics and
Gynecology
All India Institute of Medical Sciences
New Delhi, India

**Aruna Nigam** MS MNAMS FMAS FICOG
Professor and Unit Head
Department of Obstetrics and Gynecology
Hamdard Institute of Medical Sciences
and Research, Jamia Hamdard
New Delhi, India

**Bhawani Singh** MD DM (Pulm Medicine)
Visiting Senior Consultant
Pulmonologist
Department of Pulmonary Medicine
National Heart Institute
New Delhi, India

**Bindiya Gupta** MD MAMS FICOG
Associate Professor
Department of Obstetrics and Gynecology
University College of Medical Sciences
and GTB Hospital
New Delhi, India

**Chitra Raghunandan** MBBS MD FICOG
Former Director Professor and Head
Department of Obstetrics and Gynecology
Lady Hardinge Medical College and
Smt Sucheta Kriplani Hospital
New Delhi, India

**Deepika Deka** MD Fellowship Fetal Medicine
Former Professor
Department of Obstetrics and
Gynecology
All India Institute of Medical Sciences
New Delhi
Consultant
Division of Fetal Medicine
Department of Fetal Medicine and Genetics
CloudNine Hospital
Gurugram, Haryana, India

**Divya Verma** MBBS MS DNB MNAMS
Consultant
Department of Obstetrics and Gynecology
Shree Balaji Hospital and Nursing College
Kangra, Himachal Pradesh, India

**K Aparna Sharma** MD DNB
Additional Professor
Department of Obstetrics and Gynecology
All India Institute of Medical Sciences
New Delhi, India

**Kanika Chopra** MBBS MS
Assistant Professor
Department of Obstetrics and Gynecology
Lady Hardinge Medical College
New Delhi, India

**Kanti Gombar** MD (Anesthesia)
Former Professor and Head
Department of Anesthesia
Government Medical College and
Hospital, Chandigarh
Senior Consultant and Head
Department of Critical Care
Healing Hospital
Chandigarh, India

**Kanwal Gujral** DGO MS FICOG FIMSA
FICMCH
Chairperson and Head
Institute of Obstetrics and Gynecology
Sir Ganga Ram Hospital
New Delhi, India

**Kazila Bhutia** MBBS MD MRCOG (UK)
FAMS (Singapore)
Consultant
Division of Obstetrics and Gynecology
KK Women's and Children's Hospital
Singapore

**Kiran Aggarwal** MD FICOG
Director Professor
Department of Obstetrics and Gynecology
Lady Hardinge Medical College and
Smt Sucheta Kriplani Hospital
New Delhi, India

**Kiran Guleria** MD DNB FICOG FICMCH
FNAMS FRCOG
Director Professor and Unit Head
Department of Obstetrics and Gynecology
University College of Medical Sciences
and GTB Hospital, New Delhi, India

**Madhavi Puri** MBBS
Junior Resident
NIMHANS
Bengaluru, Karnataka, India

**Madhu Goel** MD DNB MNAMS FICOG
Associate Director
Department of Obstetrics and Gynecology
Fortis La Femme Hospital
New Delhi, India

**Mandakini Pradhan** MD DNB MNAMS
DM (Medical Genetics)
Professor and Head
Department of Maternal and
Reproductive Health
Sanjay Gandhi Postgraduate Institute of
Medical Sciences
Lucknow, Uttar Pradesh, India

**Manisha Kumar** MBBS MS FICOG
Director Professor
Department of Obstetrics and Gynecology
Lady Hardinge Medical College
New Delhi, India

**Manju Puri** MD FICOG
Director Professor and Former Head
Department of Obstetrics and Gynecology
Lady Hardinge Medical College and
Smt Sucheta Kriplani Hospital
New Delhi, India

**Manju Saini** MBBS MS
Assistant Professor
Department of Obstetrics and
Gynecology
Sawai Man Singh Medical College
Jaipur, Rajasthan, India

**Manoj Kumar Sharma** MBBS MD DM
Professor, Department of Hepatology
Institute of Liver and Biliary Sciences
New Delhi, India

**Monika Bhatia** MBBS DCH MS DNB
MRCOG (UK, Gold Medallist) DIP
in Laparoscopy (Germany)
Senior Consultant and Head
Department of Obstetrics and Gynecology
Venkateshwar Hospital, New Delhi, India

**Monika Madaan** MD DNB FICOG FMAS
Specialist and Head
Department of Obstetrics and Gynecology
ESIC Hospital, Manesar, Haryana, India

**Neeta Singh** MBBS MS
Additional Professor
Department of Maternal and
Reproductive Health
Sanjay Gandhi Postgraduate Institute of
Medical Sciences
Lucknow, Uttar Pradesh, India

**Nidhi Bhatia** MD (Anesthesia) DNB MAMS
Additional Professor
Department of Anesthesia and Intensive
Care, Postgraduate Institute of Medical
Education and Research
Chandigarh, India

**Nidhi Malhotra** MBBS MS
Consultant
Department of Obstetrics and Gynecology
Shri Krishna Hospital
Ludhiana, Punjab, India

**Pakhee Aggarwal** MS MRCOG MICOG
MIPHA PGDMRCH
Senior Consultant
Department of Obstetrics and Gynecology
Fortis Memorial Research Institute
Gurugram, Haryana, India

**Pikee Saxena** MD FICOG MNAMS FMAS
FIMCH PGCC (Hospital Management) PGDCR
(Clinical Research)
Director Professor
Department of Obstetrics and Gynecology
Lady Hardinge Medical College and Smt
Sucheta Kriplani Hospital
New Delhi, India

**Prabha Lal** MBBS MD FMAS FICOG
Professor
Department of Obstetrics and Gynecology
Lady Hardinge Medical College and
Smt Sucheta Kriplani Hospital
New Delhi, India

**Prerna Kukreti** MBBS MD
Associate Professor
Department of Psychiatry
Lady Hardinge Medical College
New Delhi, India

**Qiu Ju Ng** MBBS MRCS (Edin) MRCOG (UK)
MMed (Obs & Gynec)
Associate Consultant
Division of Obstetrics and Gynecology
KK Women's and Children's Hospital
Singapore

**Raksha Soni** MD
Senior Resident
Department of Obstetrics and Gynecology
University College of Medical Sciences
and GTB Hospital, New Delhi, India

**Ratna Biswas** MBBS MD
Director Professor
Department of Obstetrics and Gynecology
Lady Hardinge Medical College and
Smt Sucheta Kriplani Hospital
New Delhi, India

**Reena Jain** MBBS MD
Senior Consultant
Department of Obstetrics and Gynecology
Batra Hospital and Medical
Research Centre, New Delhi, India

**Reena Yadav** MBBS DGO MD FICOG
Director Professor and Head
Department of Obstetrics and Gynecology
Lady Hardinge Medical College and
Smt Sucheta Kriplani Hospital
New Delhi, India

**Reva Tripathi** DGO MD FICOG
Professor and Head
Department of Obstetrics and Gynecology
Hamdard Institute of Medical Sciences
and Research
Former Director Professor and Head
Department of Obstetrics and Gynecology
Maulana Azad Medical College
New Delhi, India

**Ritu Rana** MD FRCOG European Diploma
in Gynecology Endoscopy (France) DFFP
Consultant
Darent Valley Hospital, BMI Sloane and
Chelsfield, Orpington/Kent/
Beckenham, London, UK

**Sakshi Nayar** MBBS MS Diploma in
Gynec endoscopy (KIEL)
Associate Consultant
Institute of Obstetrics and Gynecology
Sir Ganga Ram Hospital
New Delhi, India

**Sandhya Jain** MD DNB MNAMS MRCOG
Professor
Department of Obstetrics and Gynecology
University College of Medical Sciences
and GTB Hospital, New Delhi, India

**Sangeeta Gupta** MD FRCOG (UK)
Director Professor
Department of Obstetrics and Gynecology
Maulana Azad Medical College
New Delhi, India

**Sarita Singh** MD
Associate Professor
Department of Obstetrics and Gynecology
Vardhman Mahavir Medical College and
Safdarjung Hospital
New Delhi, India

**Saritha Shamsunder** MD FRCOG
Consultant and Professor
Department of Obstetrics and Gynecology
Vardhman Mahavir Medical College and
Safdarjung Hospital
New Delhi, India

**Satinder Gombar** MD (Anesthesia)
Former Professor and Head
Department of Anesthesia and
Intensive Care
Government Medical College and Hospital
Chandigarh, India

**Seema Singhal** MS MCh (Gynec-Onco)
Additional Professor
Department of Obstetrics and Gynecology
All India Institute of Medical Sciences
New Delhi, India

**Shalini Malhotra** MS DNB MNAMA
MRCOG
Console Surgeon, Da Vinci Robot
Consultant
Department of Obstetrics and Gynecology
Al Qassimi Women and Children
Hospital, Sharjah, UAE

**Sharda Patra** MD DNB Fellow in Gynec
Oncology
Professor
Department of Obstetrics and Gynecology
Lady Hardinge Medical College and Smt
Sucheta Kriplani Hospital
New Delhi, India

**Shivangi Shanker Srivastava** MBBS
Junior Resident
Department of Obstetrics and Gynecology
Lady Hardinge Medical Hospital and
Smt Sucheta Kriplani Hospital
New Delhi, India

**Shivangini Rana** MBBS MD
Attending Consultant
Department of Obstetrics and
Gynecology
Fortis Flt. Lt. Rajan Dhall Hospital
New Delhi, India

**Shubha Sagar Trivedi** MS FRCOG (Hon. Causa) FIMSA FICOG
Former Director Professor and Head
Department of Obstetrics and Gynecology
Lady Hardinge Medical College and Smt Sucheta Kriplani Hospital
New Delhi
Former Professor and Head Department of Obstetrics and Gynecology
SGT University
Gurugram, Haryana, India

**Shubham Bidhuri** MS
Senior Resident
Department of Obstetrics and Gynecology
Vardhman Mahavir Medical College and Safdarjung Hospital
New Delhi, India

**Sirisha Rao Gundabattula** MD
Consultant
Department of Obstetrics and Gynecology
Fernandez Hospital
Hyderabad, Telangana, India

**Smiti Nanda** MD
Senior Professor and Head
Department of Obstetrics and Gynecology
Postgraduate Institute of Medical Sciences
Rohtak, Haryana, India

**Sneha Shree** MBBS MD
Consultant
Department of Obstetrics and Gynecology
Tulsi Multispecialty Hospital and
Shanti Nursing Home
New Delhi, India

**Sudha Salhan** MD FICMCH MICOG PGCHA CIC
Former Professor and Head
Department of Obstetrics and Gynecology
Vardhman Mahavir Medical College and Safdarjung Hospital
New Delhi, India

**Sumedha Sharma** MS
Assistant Professor
Department of Obstetrics and Gynecology
Hamdard Institute of Medical Science and Research, New Delhi, India

**Suneeta Mittal** MD FRCOG FICOG FAMS FICMCH FIMSA FICLS
Director and Head
Department of Obstetrics and Gynecology
Fortis Memorial Research Institute
Gurugram
Former Professor and Head
Department of Obstetrics and Gynecology
All India Institute of Medical Sciences
New Delhi, India

**Swaraj Batra** MS (Obs & Gynec)
Former Director Professor and Head
Department of Obstetrics and Gynecology
Maulana Azad Medical College, New Delhi
Former Professor and Head
Department of Obstetrics and Gynecology
Hamdard Institute of Medical Sciences and Research
New Delhi, India

**Swati Agrawal** MD FICOG FMAS
Professor
Department of Obstetrics and Gynecology
Lady Hardinge Medical College and
Smt Sucheta Kriplani Hospital
New Delhi, India

**Usha Gupta** MD
Former Director Professor
Department of Obstetrics and Gynecology
Lady Hardinge Medical College
New Delhi, India

**Vani Malhotra** MBBS MD
Professor
Department of Obstetrics and Gynecology
Pt BD Sharma Postgraduate Institute of Medical Sciences
Rohtak, Haryana, India

# Foreword

*Management of High-Risk Pregnancy: A Practical Approach* edited by Professors Shubha Sagar Trivedi, Manju Puri and Swati Agrawal covers the entire spectrum of high-risk pregnancy related conditions that affect the materno-fetal-neonatal and long-term health. The book consists of 34 chapters (424 pages) authored by internationally renowned clinical academics and scientists who are well recognized for their area of expertise.

The book covers obstetric disorders like placental, hypertensive, bleeding, multiple pregnancy, thromboembolism and others that affect the mother, the fetus and the newborn. The chapters, on the medical disorders explain on "one side of the coin" how the medical disorders and medications given for treatment of these medical conditions affect the maternal and fetal/neonatal health and on the "other-side of the coin" how the pregnancy affects the medical disorders. The chapters on infectious disorders that affect the pregnancy provide information of how the infections affect the fetus, the newborn and the mother. Most frequently encountered issues of obesity in pregnancy, gynecological diseases in pregnancy, critical care in obstetrics and drugs in pregnancy are dealt in detail in different chapters. The chapters are well written, easy to read and provide comprehensive information on clinical presentation, diagnosis and management.

The popularity of this book is reflected by the current 3rd edition; each edition being published every sixth year—this is commendable. I would recommend this book as essential reading for trainee obstetricians and gynecologists, midwives, consultant obstetricians, physicians and anesthetists. It will be good to have a copy of the book in every medical library and wards in maternity hospitals and medical schools for easy reference.

My sincere congratulations and best wishes to the editors, authors and publisher of the book *Management of High-Risk Pregnancy: A Practical Approach*.

**Sir Sabaratnam Arulkumaran**
Past President of the Royal College of Obstetricians
and Gynaecologists (RCOG)
International Federation of Obstetrics and
Gynaecology (FIGO) and the
British Medical Association (BMA)

# Preface to the Third Edition

*'An investment in knowledge pays the best interest'*
—**Benjamin Franklin**

The rapidly emerging new evidence based on the ongoing research makes it mandatory for the editors to continue the process of revising the previous version of the book. It was in 2010 that the first edition of the book *Management of High-Risk Pregnancy: A Practical Approach* was published, followed by the 2nd edition in 2016. This is the 3rd edition, updated with the latest available evidence and guidelines. The profile of pregnant women is changing, expanding the spectrum of high-risk pregnancies. The advances in the field of medicine have made it possible for women with certain medical conditions, in which pregnancy was not advisable in the past, to experience motherhood. Practical aspects of managing pregnancy in cancer survivors, in women with renal or cardiac transplant have been described. These and many other evolving issues in maternal care, including pregnancy preserving management of the early cancer cervix, staging lymphadenectomy and neoadjuvant chemotherapy during pregnancy have been addressed in this new edition. Some of the chapters are not exhaustive, but will stimulate the reader to further reading of recent literature given as references at the end of each chapter. In recent times, attention has also been focused on the association between high-risk pregnancies and cardiometabolic disorders later in life. A new chapter High-risk Pregnancy: Before, After and Beyond has been included to address this. Dedicated new chapters on recurrent pregnancy loss, psychiatric disorders and malaria in pregnancy have been added. The content of the new edition has been thoroughly researched and revised by the authors and presented in a clinically relevant and easy to understand format. Some of the senior most teachers of the major teaching hospitals, actively involved in academics and with vast experience of managing high-risk pregnancies, have very kindly contributed the various chapters. We are thankful to them for their efforts and sharing their expertise and wisdom. We also wish to thank Jaypee Brothers Medical Publishers for initiating, providing technical and logistic support and bringing out this revised edition. We hope that this book will serve as a 'go-to' book for the students, residents, teachers as well as for the practicing obstetricians. Any suggestions or comments from the readers are most welcome.

**Shubha Sagar Trivedi**
**Manju Puri**
**Swati Agrawal**

# Preface to the First Edition

Management of high-risk pregnancy is a challenge for all practicing obstetricians. True to its title, *Management of High-Risk Pregnancy: A Practical Approach*, this book focuses mainly on the practical aspects of the management of high-risk pregnancies. The various chapters have been contributed by clinicians with vast academic and clinical experience. The text is presented in an easy-to-read and user-friendly manner. The material is essentially evidence based and derived from the personal experience of the contributors. A number of flowcharts have been included to serve as ready reckoners. This book includes most of the high-risk pregnancy situations and will be valuable to practicing clinicians, residents and faculty. A dedicated chapter on critical care in obstetrics—what an obstetrician should know, provides useful information which needs to be known to clinicians taking care of critically ill obstetric patients. Topics like prenatal screening and diagnosis, diagnosis and management of congenital malformations and antepartum fetal surveillance have been included to guide the clinicians in screening and monitoring of high-risk pregnancy situations. We have also included a chapter on drugs in pregnancy which discusses the safety profile of drugs used in the management of at-risk pregnancies. This is not a complete textbook of obstetrics but will serve as a useful complement to the already existing textbooks with special emphasis on the management of high-risk pregnancies.

We are thankful to our Director, GK Sharma who encouraged us to take up the task of writing this book and gave his constant support. Our thanks are due to all the contributors who spared their valuable time to write the various chapters of this book. Efforts of Dr Shalini Singh deserve special mention as she tirelessly assisted us in giving the final shape to the book. Finally, this book would not have been possible without the expert and organized support and cooperation of our publishers M/s Jaypee Brothers Medical Publishers (P) Ltd.

We hope that all practicing obstetricians, residents and teachers will benefit from this book and we would welcome any comments and suggestions from them.

**Shubha Sagar Trivedi**
**Manju Puri**

# Acknowledgments

I owe a deep debt of gratitude to my parents who always supported us, my siblings and me, in all our endeavors, provided us with a conducive learning environment and encouraged us to achieve the best in us. They gave us confidence, made us believe in ourselves, our capabilities and strengths.

I am thankful to my aunts, Mrs Laj Chawla, Dr VK Bhasin, Dr VV Saiyed and Mrs Usha Nayer, who were my inspiration and role models from my early childhood and were always there for me.

This book would not have seen the light of the day if it was not for Dr Manju Puri, who from day one said, "yes we will do it"! Her contribution to this book has been immense. Her commitment and dedication, eye for detail, and deep knowledge of the subject has added great value to this book.

Dr Swati Agrawal, enthusiastic, diligent and ever ready to meticulously check, recheck, write and rewrite, has been a great co-editor to work with. Her proficiency as an editor has helped greatly in bringing out this edition.

I am highly obliged to all the authors, who despite their hectic schedules, especially during these tiring COVID pandemic times, worked tirelessly to write the chapters, sharing their vast knowledge and experience through their contribution to this book.

It was a moment of pride for me when Professor Arulkumaran graciously wrote the foreword for this book. He is an accomplished academician and a source of inspiration for us all. I will always remain grateful to him.

I am thankful to all my teachers, my seniors, my colleagues, my students and especially to my patients who helped me learn at every step of my professional life and enabled me to bring out this book.

I am grateful for the constant, invaluable support of my husband, Dr RK Trivedi, who has been patient and always available throughout the arduous process of writing this book.

I immensely appreciate the encouragement received from my brother, my sisters, my daughter-in-law, Aprajita, and above all from my son, Rohan, who has also been my day and night "technical problem solver" during the course of writing this book on the computer.

It is a genuine pleasure to acknowledge the contribution of Jaypee Brothers Medical Publishers from the initiation to the publication of this book. I am thankful to the entire team, especially to Ms Chetna Malhotra and Ms Kritika Dua who have put in great efforts to bring out this edition in the present form.

Last but not the least, I am most obliged to all the readers of the book, who stimulated me to update it and bring out the new edition of *Management of High-Risk Pregnancy: A Practical Approach*.

**Shubha Sagar Trivedi**

# Contents

1. **High-risk Pregnancy: Before, After, and Beyond** .......... 1
   *Anju Bhatia*

2. **Prenatal Diagnosis** .......... 10
   *Mandakini Pradhan, Ratna Biswas, Neeta Singh*

3. **Screening and Management of Congenital Anomalies** .......... 25
   *Manisha Kumar, Shivangi Shanker Srivastava*

4. **Recurrent Pregnancy Loss** .......... 43
   *Sangeeta Gupta, Shivangini Rana*

5. **Antepartum Hemorrhage** .......... 51
   *Madhu Goel, Monika Bhatia, Shubha Sagar Trivedi*

6. **Multifetal Pregnancy** .......... 64
   *Reena Yadav*

7. **Fetal Growth Restriction** .......... 80
   *Kanwal Gujral, Sakshi Nayar*

8. **Antepartum Fetal Surveillance** .......... 90
   *Anubhuti Rana, Seema Singhal*

9. **Polyhydramnios Oligohydramnios** .......... 102
   *Prabha Lal*

10. **Preterm Labor** .......... 110
    *Kanika Chopra, Monika Bhatia, Shubha Sagar Trivedi*

11. **Premature Rupture of Membranes** .......... 124
    *Sharda Patra*

12. **Prolonged Pregnancy** .......... 136
    *Amita Suneja, Sandhya Jain, Raksha Soni*

13. **Rh Negative Pregnancy** .......... 142
    *Aruna Nigam, Sumedha Sharma*

14. **Pregnancy in Previous Cesarean Section** .......... 152
    *Shubham Bidhuri, Ritu Rana, Saritha Shamsunder*

15. **Malpresentations** .......... 166
    *Usha Gupta, Swati Agrawal*

16. **Anemia in Pregnancy** .......... 186
    *Manju Puri, Nidhi Malhotra*

17. **Hypertensive Disorders of Pregnancy** .......... 202
    *Swati Agrawal, Monika Bhatia, Shubha Sagar Trivedi*

18. **Diabetes Mellitus in Pregnancy** .......... 218
    *Kazila Bhutia, Qiu Ju Ng, Manju Puri*

19. **Thyroid Disorders in Pregnancy** .......... 236
    *Kiran Aggarwal*

20. **Heart Disease in Pregnancy** .......... 249
    *Shalini Malhotra, Reva Tripathi, Monika Bhatia, Divya Verma*

21. **Jaundice in Pregnancy** ............................................................................................................263
    *Chitra Raghunandan, Swati Agrawal, Manoj Kumar Sharma*

22. **Renal Disease in Pregnancy** ...................................................................................................281
    *Pakhee Aggarwal, Suneeta Mittal*

23. **Pregnancy with Epilepsy** ........................................................................................................290
    *Monika Madaan*

24. **Autoimmune Disorders in Pregnancy** ...................................................................................297
    *Kiran Guleria, Bindiya Gupta, Sneha Shree*

25. **Thromboembolism in Pregnancy** ..........................................................................................306
    *Sarita Singh, Swaraj Batra, Reena Jain*

26. **Psychiatric Disorders in Pregnancy** ......................................................................................318
    *Prerna Kukreti, Madhavi Puri*

27. **Tuberculosis in Pregnancy** .....................................................................................................329
    *Abha Singh, Bhawani Singh*

28. **Malaria in Pregnancy** .............................................................................................................334
    *Abha Singh, Bhawani Singh*

29. **HIV Infection in Pregnancy** ....................................................................................................338
    *Sudha Salhan*

30. **TORCH Infections in Pregnancy** ............................................................................................347
    *K Aparna Sharma, Deepika Deka*

31. **Obesity and Pregnancy** .........................................................................................................356
    *Sirisha Rao Gundabattula*

32. **Gynecological Diseases in Pregnancy** ...................................................................................365
    *Smiti Nanda, Vani Malhotra*

33. **Critical Care in Obstetrics** .....................................................................................................378
    *Nidhi Bhatia, Satinder Gombar, Kanti Gombar*

34. **Drugs in Pregnancy** ...............................................................................................................393
    *Pikee Saxena, Manju Saini*

    *Index* ..........................................................................................................................................411

# CHAPTER 1

# High-risk Pregnancy: Before, After, and Beyond

*Anju Bhatia*

## INTRODUCTION

*"Pregnancy is special. Let's make it safe"* —WHO

Pregnancy and childbirth are unique physiological events in women's life journey in which she undergoes multisystem changes to nurture the developing fetus and prepare herself for labor and delivery. Obstetrics is commonly believed to be simply, "stand by, stay near" discipline. However, it is not; an unexpected medical condition of the mother or fetus can complicate any pregnancy. In obstetrics, predicting when a patient will require additional interventions beyond routine obstetric and neonatal care, is difficult. A pregnancy is defined as *high risk* when the probability of an adverse outcome for the mother or child is increased over and above the baseline risk of that outcome among the general pregnant population (or reference population) by the presence of one or more ascertainable risk factors, or indicators.[1] Risk assessment in pregnancy helps to stratify the women who are likely to experience adverse health events and enables providers to administer risk-appropriate perinatal care. However, low-risk pregnancy is also a dynamic situation, subject to change throughout the antepartum, intrapartum, and postpartum periods. The change can be acute and unexpected. Hence, women without prenatal risk factors and their newborns may experience unexpected complications during delivery or postpartum.

The prenatal care of a high-risk pregnancy does not end with delivery but rather includes both postpartum and interconception care. International societies have recognized the importance of the continuum of preconception, antenatal, and interconception care as a comprehensive public health priority. Obstetricians need to be aware to assess the risk at every interaction with reproductive-age couples; promote healthy lifestyle behaviors; and identify, treat, and optimize medical and psychosocial issues that could impact pregnancy and the lifetime health of the mother and child.

## WHAT MAKES A PREGNANCY HIGH RISK?

### Age

*Teenage Pregnancy*

The median age of menarche has shown a downward trend with an improvement of socioeconomic conditions and teenage pregnancies are common. Estimates suggest adolescent pregnancy occurs in 13% of the US population and 25% worldwide, although, its true prevalence is difficult to determine.[2] These pregnancies are often unintended in the majority of girls and approximately half of them end up in abortions.[3] Chief risk factors for adverse outcomes include a maternal history of adverse childhood experiences including emotional, physical, or sexual abuse; living with someone with substance abuse or mental illness or involvement in criminal activity; broken families; socioeconomic deprivation, low educational achievement, and having teenage parents. These experiences are associated with subsequent sexual risk behaviors, smoking, alcohol consumption, and depression.[4] In developing countries such as India, situation is different where 26.8% of girls (17.5% in urban and 31.5% in rural areas) were married before 18 years of age in 2015–16, predisposing them to teenage pregnancy.[5] Early marriage of girls impacts their social and health rights, they are less likely to use contraceptives and are more vulnerable to social isolation, domestic violence, etc.[6]

Pregnant adolescents may have unsupervised pregnancies or suboptimal late prenatal care. They are at a significantly higher risk for development of severe anemia (RR 1.61, $p < 0.02$), eclampsia (RR 1.95, $p < 0.05$), preterm birth (PTB) (RR 1.25, $p < 0.001$), intrauterine growth restriction (RR 2.29, $p < 0.001$), and low birth weight (LBW) (RR 1.24, $p < 0.001$). Assisted delivery (11.78% vs. 2.23%, $p < 0.001$) was significantly more common and cesarean section (CS) delivery (9.64% vs. 17.18%, $p < 0.001$) was significantly less common in teenagers[7] **(Box 1)**.

Pregnant adolescents should be encouraged to seek early adequate prenatal care and to discuss options such as termination or continuation of pregnancy, adoption, etc. The legal guardian should be involved with the girl's consent. They should preferably be seen in specially designated teenage care clinics along with medical social workers. Adequate psychological support should be provided throughout pregnancy and labor. Information on pregnancy, delivery, vaccinations, breastfeeding, contraception, and child-rearing should be made available. Social and financial concerns should be addressed.

> **BOX 1:** Risks of teenage pregnancy.[8]
> - Anemia
> - Pregnancy induced hypertension
> - Preterm birth
> - Small for gestational age babies
> - Low birth weight babies
> - Increased neonatal mortality
> - Postnatal depression
> - Sexually transmitted infections
> - Children of adolescent mothers are at risk of
>   – Poorer cognitive development
>   – Lower educational attainment
>   – Higher risks of abuse, neglect, and behavioral problems

The obstetrician providing care for these young girls should be aware of the potential challenges, while there is no evidence to date of any medical interventions that can specifically reduce associated adverse outcomes. Prenatal care should be tailored to the individual needs of every client, particularly about encouraging compliance with the antenatal visits, smoking cessation programs, counseling regarding the risk of sexually transmitted infections, and future contraception.

## Advanced Maternal Age

The average maternal age at first birth has increased steadily over the last four decades across the globe secondary to late marriage, wider opportunities for further education and career advancement, and the availability of better contraceptive options.

Older women experience an increased rate of spontaneous miscarriages, losses include both aneuploid and euploid fetuses. There is a steady increase in the risk of aneuploidy, as a woman ages, secondary to aging oocytes, the most common being autosomal trisomy due to increased risk of nondisjunction leading to unequal chromosome products after cell division.[9] The calculated risk of spontaneous loss in each age group was: < 30 years of age (12%), 30–34 years (15%), 35–39 years (25%), 40–44 years (51%), and ≥ 45 years (93%). Maternal age above 35 years is associated with a four- to eightfold increased risk of ectopic pregnancy compared with younger women.[10] Several studies have suggested that the risk of structural anomalies in the fetus also increase as women age. Offspring of women ≥40 years of age compared with the reference group of women 25–29 years of age were at increased risk of cardiac defects (aOR 2.2–2.9), as well as for esophageal atresia (aOR 2.9, 95% CI 1.7–4.9), hypospadias (aOR 2.0; 95% CI 1.4–3.0), and craniosynostosis (aOR 1.6, 95% CI 1.1–2.4).[11]

The prevalence of preexisting medical and surgical illnesses such as cardiovascular, renal, autoimmune disease; obesity, fibroids, and cancer increases with advancing age. A recent systematic review and meta-analysis found that women over 35 years of age can expect to experience two- to threefold higher rate of hospitalization, CS, and pregnancy-related complications than their younger counterparts. They are at increased risk of stillbirth (OR, 1.75; 95% CI, 1.62–1.89), preeclampsia (OR 1.99; 95% CI, 1.65–2.36), neonatal death (OR, 1.48; 95% CI, 1.30–1.67), NICU admission (OR, 1.49; 95% CI, 1.34–1.66), and gestational diabetes mellitus (GDM) (OR, 2.85; 95% CI, 2.46–3.32).[12] The prevalence of placental problems, such as abruptio placenta and placenta previa, is higher among older women. Multiple gestations are also more prevalent, which is related to both a higher risk of naturally-conceived twins and higher use of assisted reproductive techniques (ART). Population-based studies consistently report that women ≥35 years of age are more likely to experience labor dystocia, operative delivery, perinatal and maternal mortality.[13]

Medical and obstetric complications tend to be more common in older women, in practice, however, normal prenatal care is not modified unless specific complications or another risk factor is identified. Benefits and limitations of screening and prenatal diagnosis for chromosomal and structural anomalies including invasive testing need to be discussed. Elderly women are usually advised to be delivered in tertiary care facility. The woman's age often contributes strongly to decisions to intervene. Optimal antenatal surveillance remains unclear in this group in the absence of any additional risk factors. It is recommended that they undergo induction at 39 weeks of gestation (Grade 2C).

A category of "very advanced maternal age" has been proposed for women ≥45 years or ≥50 years. Fitzpatrick et al.[14] reported women giving birth at advanced maternal age (≥ 48 years) are more likely to be overweight (33% vs. 23%, $p = 0.0011$) or obese (23% vs. 19%, $p = 0.0318$), nulliparous (53% vs. 44%, $p = 0.0299$), have preexisting medical conditions (44% vs. 28%, $p < 0.0001$), multiple pregnancy (18% vs. 2%, $p < 0.0001$), and conceived following assisted conception (78% vs. 4%, $p < 0.0001$) compared to younger cohort. Accordingly pregnancy complications including gestational hypertensive disorders, GDM, postpartum hemorrhage (PPH), CS, iatrogenic and spontaneous PTB on univariable analysis are also more frequent even after adjustment for demographic and medical factors.

## Ethnicity

Racial and ethnic disparities exist in specific congenital malformations, pregnancy complications, and birth outcomes. Many diseases and obstetric problems have both ethnic and geographic distributions. For example, alpha ($\alpha$)-thalassemia is the most common cause of fetal nonimmune hydrops in Southeast Asia with up to 40% of the regional population being carriers, and sickle cell anemia prevalent in Afro-Caribbean, Mediterranean, Middle East countries with consequent maternal infection, sickling crises, preeclampsia, renal compromise, jaundice and fetuses at risk of inheriting these diseases. Prenatal diagnosis of these single gene conditions is possible with invasive genetic testing so should be offered in these populations if parents are carriers. Risk of symptomatic HIV infection, malaria, etc., are well-known in women from Africa and the Caribbean islands. These communities also practice female circumcision which poses problems with vaginal delivery including dystocia, trauma, hemorrhage.

In present times, when expectant women often travel for work and leisure and increasing medical tourism, obstetricians should be aware of these race-specific issues while taking care of such women. Communication may be a problem because of language barriers. Information, screening, and appropriate counseling services should be made available for communities that are considered at risk for specific diseases.

## Parity

Parity is the number of times a woman has given birth to an infant, dead or alive. However, the gestational threshold for defining may vary between countries (e.g., 23 completed weeks' gestation vs. 27 completed weeks' gestation).[1]

The relationship between parity and birth outcomes is not consistent due to a discrepancy in the definition of parity. Cross-sectional analysis of births between 1992 and 1997 to women of parity 0–8 in Australia, showed that the risk of obstetric complications was highest in nulliparas, lowest in multiparas who had one to three deliveries, and intermediate in multiparas with four or more deliveries and hence, following a bimodal pattern (for any obstetric complication: nulliparas OR 1.75, para 1 to 3 OR 0.96–1.03, para 4 to 8 OR 1.19–1.35).[15] Most of the complications associated with grand multiparity may be confounded by advanced maternal age.

Nulliparity is associated with an increased risk of hypertensive disorders of pregnancy, LBW, birth trauma. Grand multiparity probably increases the risk of the placental abnormalities, such as placenta previa and abruption, abnormal fetal presentation, precipitate labor, postpartum hemorrhage (PPH), macrosomia, cord prolapse, venous thromboembolic events etc.,[16-18] although findings are conflicting across various observational studies. Women who undergo multiple repeat CSs are at increased risk of maternal morbidity and mortality, secondary to placenta accreta.

Antepartum clinical care is similar for all multiparous women, regardless of the number of previous deliveries. During labor, obstetrician caring for grand multiparas should anticipate and be prepared to manage macrosomia, shoulder dystocia, labor complications related to malposition, and PPH.

## Maternal Weight

Abnormal maternal weight is an increasingly common global obstetric complication. Approximately 40–50% of reproductive age women are overweight or obese. Underweight pregnant women are also frequently encountered in obstetric clinics because of cultural pressure on the drive for thinness. Anorexia nervosa, and bulimia, are no longer rare eating disorders in developed countries. Undernourished pregnant women are also encountered because of actual food deprivation in certain parts of the world secondary to poverty or natural disasters as droughts and famines. Pregestational obesity and excessive gestational weight gain are independent risk factors for maternal-fetal complications and long-term risks in adult life for the child. The risks include increase in miscarriage, structural anomalies, hypertensive disorders, GDM, macrosomia, and intrapartum complications including instrumental delivery, shoulder dystocia, emergency CS, PPH, venous thromboembolism, anesthetic complications, and wound sepsis.[19-22]

Women who become pregnant after bariatric surgery constitute a unique obstetric population. A recent systematic review and meta-analysis of 20 cohort studies including 8,364 women, postbariatric surgery conception was associated with reduced rates of GDM, macrosomia, pregnancy-induced hypertension (PIH), PPH, and CS rates.[23] A group of this cohort showed an increase in SGA and PTB when compared with controls matched for presurgery body mass index. These women are at an increased risk of severe micronutrient deficiencies. Screening for micronutrients levels should be considered in the preconception period or at the first prenatal visit including complete blood count, iron, ferritin, folate, calcium, zinc, magnesium, iodine, and vitamins A, $B_{12}$, D, and K.[24] Additional screening and supplementation is desirable in every trimester and postpartum.

Mothers who are underweight before pregnancy, or have suboptimal gestational weight gain are more likely to have SGA babies (OR, 1.53; 95% CI, 1.44–1.64) and may deliver preterm (OR, 1.70; 95% CI, 1.32–2.20).[20] Perinatal complications such as neonatal hypoglycemia, hypothermia and mortality are increased in their babies. Women with anorexia and bulimia can have variable obstetric outcomes. Pregnancy is likely to be uneventful if their eating disorder is in remission. However, in the case of active disorder at the time of conception, severe implications including nutritional deficiencies, dehydration, depression, fetal growth restriction (FGR), etc., can be anticipated and need to be managed by a multidisciplinary approach involving psychiatrists, dietitian, maternal-fetal medicine specialist, and neonatologists.

## Intimate Partner Violence

Intimate partner violence (IPV)—also called domestic violence, battering, or domestic abuse is a pervasive problem that cuts across racial, ethnic, and socioeconomic boundaries.

"Domestic abuse" is defined by the UK Home Office as "Any incident of threatening behavior, violence, or abuse (psychological, physical, sexual, financial, or emotional) between adults who are or have been intimate partners or family members, regardless of gender or sexuality".[25] The prevalence of domestic violence in pregnancy is reported to be between 3[26] and 33.7%,[27] with the greatest risk occurring during the postpartum period. Mostly there is preexisting violence that continues but may begin during the pregnancy as well. It may also contribute either directly or indirectly to maternal mortality, by grievous injury or impeding access to prenatal care.[28]

Irrational explanations of visible injuries, distress, or hostility at the time of pelvic examination, over-possessive partner, noncompliance with treatment regimens, lack of independent transportation, and difficulties in communicating by telephone may raise a clinician's index of suspicion about domestic abuse. These women may have physical and mental complications such as injuries to breast, abdomen or genitals, dizziness, vaginal bleeding, chronic pains (e.g., headaches, backaches, pelvic pain), hearing or vision problems, sleep disturbance, poor appetite, depression, anxiety, increased risk for suicide, poor maternal bonding, substance abuse, smoking, late entry into prenatal care, and preterm delivery.[29,30]

Infants of the abused mother may have lifelong impacts ranging from LBW to developmental delay, emotional problems, sleep problems, and the potential to perpetrate IPV.[31]

As there are serious health implications of domestic violence, guidelines have been published for the identification and support of affected women.[32] Five key steps to the clinical management of domestic violence include increasing awareness and recognition of domestic violence and its health effects through training and education; providing the woman with a safe and private environment away from abusive partners, family, or friends; identification and aiding disclosure of abuse; documentation; as well as safety assessment and ongoing support.[33,34]

Intimate partner violence is a complex issue, obstetrician should equip themselves with the skills and knowledge necessary to provide an informed response to the affected women and involve medical social workers, psychologists, psychiatrist, and neonatologists as per the need for the optimal management of this condition.

## Substance Abuse and Other Hazards

Lifestyle choices such as smoking, use of alcohol and drugs by pregnant women are all harmful to the developing fetus besides long term implications on maternal health. Smoking is an established risk factor for PTB, FGR, and sudden infant death syndrome.[35]

Despite well-known negative consequences, epidemiologic studies have shown that 20–50% of pregnant women smoke or are exposed to passive smoking. Cigarette smoke exerts a direct toxic effect on placental and fetal cell proliferation and differentiation. It is associated with placenta previa, placental abruption, and preterm premature rupture of membranes. Smoking during pregnancy has been recognized as the most important modifiable risk factor associated with adverse perinatal outcomes. As most of the placental and fetal damage happens in the first trimester of pregnancy, preconception visit or booking visit should include guidance regarding smoking cessation.

Alcohol use in pregnancy is a major public health problem worldwide. According to WHO, alcohol consumption in India has increased by 38% between 2010 and 2017. Rising affluence, societal pressure, and exposure to different lifestyles have driven women to alcohol as well. Alcohol is an identified teratogen since the 19th century, 15–20% of pregnant women consume alcohol. Alcohol during early pregnancy can lead to miscarriage, PTB.[36,37] Overall incidence of fetal alcohol syndrome (FAS) is 1 in 300 to 1 in 1,000, which includes specific morphologic features such as microcephaly, midface hypoplasia, FGR, and long-term abnormal neuropsychologic outcomes as developmental delay, increased rates of attention-deficit/hyperactivity disorder, and mild cognitive impairment.

Substance abuse in pregnancy has increased over the past few decades. *Cannabis* is the most commonly used illicit substance, predominantly for its pleasurable physical and psychotropic effects. Use during pregnancy is associated with increased risk for PTB, FGR, increased perinatal morbidity and mortality, withdrawal symptoms in the neonate,[38] as well as negative effects on the intellectual outcome. *Cocaine* use in pregnancy can lead to spontaneous miscarriages, PTB, placental abruption, and preeclampsia. Neonatal issues include poor feeding, lethargy, and seizures and it may impact attention span, neurophysiologic function. *Opiate abuse* such as heroin and methadone is associated with six times higher poor obstetric outcomes. Withdrawal syndrome that affects central nervous, autonomic, and gastrointestinal systems has been well described.

Mothers with substance abuse require specialized prenatal care, and the neonate may need extra supportive care. Once recognized, a specialized multidisciplinary approach that includes access to rehabilitation centers can lead to improved maternal and neonatal outcomes.

## Preexisting Medical Illness

Optimizing medical disease management before conception can positively influence obstetric outcomes. There is clear evidence of improved outcome for conditions—such as diabetes mellitus, hypertension, inflammatory bowel disease, asthma, epilepsy, depression, chronic renal disease, autoimmune disorders like systemic lupus erythematosus (SLE), Grave's disease, etc. Medical management to normalize the intrauterine environment, switching to monotherapy, avoiding teratogen exposure should be discussed with the patient, and appropriate management plans should be outlined before conception. Women planning to conceive should be advised about avoiding specific medications in the first trimester (e.g., isotretinoin) **(Table 1)**.

## PREGNANCY AMONG CANCER SURVIVORS

Cancer survivors are increasing following the improvements in cancer diagnosis and treatment. Many childhood cancers such as lymphoma, testicular, and breast cancers, are also associated with good survival outcomes.[39] As young survivors reach adulthood and contemplate pregnancy, it is important to understand the impact of cancer and its treatment on fertility and pregnancy outcomes **(Table 2)**.

Pregnancy is particularly complex for women treated with breast cancer before completing their families, as the hormone receptor positive breast cancer can recur even after a decade or longer after diagnosis, and treatment can continue with years of extended adjuvant hormonal therapy. Hormonal changes associated with pregnancy may increase the risk of recurrence and compromise patients' long-term survival and further complicate management decisions. Azim et al. conducted a meta-analysis of 14 studies, which showed that breast cancer survivor women who became

**TABLE 1:** Chronic medical illness and preconception care.

| Clinical condition | Preconception care |
|---|---|
| *Cardiac:* Congenital cardiac disease or valve disease, Ischemic heart disease<br>• Hypertension | • Coordinate with cardiologist; pregnancy may be contraindicated with some conditions depending on severity or medications needed; evaluate current cardiac status; discuss maternal and fetal risks<br>• Establish the cause and severity of hypertension; evaluate renal function; adjust medications to optimize blood pressure. Discontinue ACE inhibitors and ARBs; these drugs are associated with congenital abnormalities |
| *Respiratory:* Asthma | Optimize treatment regimen as per stepped protocol; counsel regarding increased risk for GDM on long-term steroids; emphasize the safety of medications |
| *Gastrointestinal:* Inflammatory bowel disease | • Optimize treatment regimen<br>• Ideal to conceive while in remission<br>• Ensure folate supplementation 5 mg/day |
| *Metabolic/Endocrine:* Diabetes<br><br>• Thyroid disorders | • Achieve euglycemia before conception (HbA1c < 7%). Explain dose-dependent risk of congenital anomalies with medications<br>• For type 1 DM and long-standing type 2 DM, insulin therapy is best<br>• Obtain baseline thyroid function tests; optimize medical therapy; delay pregnancy until good control |
| *Psychiatric/Neurologic:* Migraines<br>• Depression, anxiety<br><br>• Seizure disorders | • Migraine pattern can change with pregnancy<br>• Adjust medications at the lowest possible dose; counsel about fetal echocardiography and neonatal withdrawal syndrome for some medications<br>• Adjust medications to those most favorable to pregnancy to avoid risk of dysmorphic structural malformation syndromes; close serum monitoring is required during pregnancy; if no seizure in 2 years, consider trial "off medication"; start folic acid 5 mg/day when considering pregnancy to decrease risk of NTD |
| *Hematologic:* Sickle cell/thalassemia | • Genetic counseling<br>• Risks of inheritance and modes of prenatal testing should be discussed |
| *Rheumatologic:* SLE | • Ideal to conceive while SLE is in remission<br>• Assess for organ damage (renal) or cardiac insufficiency and asses for clinical activity<br>• Check antibodies profile<br>• Some medications may be contraindicated<br>• Pregnancy not advisable in case of severe pulmonary hypertension, severe restrictive lung disease, heart failure, chronic renal failure, history of stroke or severe lupus flare in past 6 months |
| Pregnancy after transplantation | • Patients should defer conception for at least 1 year after transplantation, with adequate contraception<br>• Graft function to be assessed with recent biopsy, proteinuria, and infection serology<br>• Maintenance immunosuppression to continue, with azathioprine, tacrolimus<br>• Methotrexate, cyclophosphamide, mycophenolate to be suspended while planning as these are teratogenic<br>• The effect of comorbid conditions (e.g., DM, hypertension) should be considered and their management optimized; nonrenal recipients should have their baseline kidney function assessed<br>• Vaccinations should be given, if needed (e.g., rubella)<br>• Explore the etiology of the original disease; discuss genetic issues, if relevant<br>• Discuss the risks of intrauterine growth restriction, PTB and LBW<br>• Discuss the effect of pregnancy on renal allograft function |

(ACE: angiotensin converting enzyme; ARBs: angiotensin-receptor blockers; DM: diabetes mellitus; GDM: gestational diabetes mellitus; LBW: low birthweight; NTD: neural tube defect; PTB: preterm birth; SLE: systemic lupus erythematosus)

**TABLE 2:** Fertility and pregnancy-related problems in cancer survivors.[40]

| Problem | Mechanism | |
|---|---|---|
| *Fertility-related problems* | | |
| Loss of ovarian function | Cytotoxic chemotherapy accelerates oocyte depletion, causing loss of hormone production and premature menopause | Alkylating agents are most likely to affect ovarian function |
| | Pelvic radiotherapy or total body irradiation causes accelerated oocyte depletion and premature ovarian failure | More common in patients with older age at diagnosis and receiving high dose chemotherapy |
| Hypothalamic-pituitary axis dysfunction (HPA) | Cranial irradiation causes HPA dysfunction and hypogonadism through GnRH deficiency | |
| *Pregnancy-related problems* | | |
| Metabolic syndrome and GDM | Possibly related to hyperinsulinemia associated with TBI, and/or growth hormone treatment for radiotherapy-related GnRH deficiency | |
| Cardiac dysfunction | Anthracycline chemotherapy may cause cardiac dysfunction, which may worsen during pregnancy | Risk of cardiotoxicity increases with higher total cumulative dose of anthracycline |
| Preterm delivery and LBW | Uterine irradiation may reduce uterine volume and blood supply | Degree of uterine damage depends on total radiation dose, site of irradiation and patient age |
| Diminished or failed lactation | • Cranial irradiation causes HPA dysfunction<br>• Breast irradiation affects lactational capacity of treated breast | |
| *Family cancer syndromes* | • Identification of a number of germline genetic mutations that increase the risk of developing certain cancers and may be passed onto offspring, e.g., *BRCA1* and *BRCA2* | Genetic counseling<br>Offer IVF with preimplantation screening |

(GDM: gestational diabetes mellitus; GnRH: gonadotropin-releasing hormone; IVF: in vitro fertilization; LBW: low birth weight; TBI: total body irradiation)

pregnant had a 41% reduced risk of death compared to women who did not become pregnant. Subgroup analysis revealed no difference in survival and relapse rate between pregnant and those who did not become pregnant. Probably women who remained well and relapse-free were more likely to choose pregnancy.[41] One can reassure, women with previous breast cancer that pregnancy is safe and does not compromise overall survival.

Cancer cervix is one of the most common cancers affecting women in developing countries including India. Fertility preservation is possible in early cervical cancer including cancer in situ, microinvasive cancer, and stage IB cancers less than 2 cm in size. Radical trachelectomy is usually performed vaginally with laparoscopic pelvic lymphadenectomy. Of those attempting to conceive, 41–79% were able to conceive. The rate of miscarriage in the 1st trimester was similar to the background population at 16–20% but there was an increase to 8–10% in the risk of 2nd trimester miscarriage. Only 70–75% of pregnancies delivered at term (>37 weeks of gestation), the risk of significant prematurity was 12%.[42] The higher rate of second trimester miscarriage was due to ascending infection with premature rupture of membranes. The lack of cervix and cervical mucus during pregnancy causes cervical incompetence and ascending infections. These women need careful evaluation for cervical incompetence and antepartum management with prophylactic antibiotics.

Ovarian cancer is another common malignancy of the female reproductive system. Fertility preservation is possible in germ cell cancers, borderline tumors, sex cord stromal tumors, and even early epithelial ovarian cancers. Assisted reproductive techniques are safe in borderline and germ cell tumors but there is limited evidence of their use in epithelial cancers. Completion surgery after child bearing is usually not performed in germ cell and borderline tumors but in early epithelial cancers the women is given the option of close follow up or completion surgery.

Patients should be offered timely discussions, information, and counseling regarding the impact of gynecological cancer treatment on a patient's pregnancy and managed by multidisciplinary teams including maternal fetal specialists, obstetric physicians, medical oncologist, neonatologists and psychologists.

# HIGH-RISK PREGNANCY: MANAGEMENT IN POSTPARTUM PERIOD AND BEYOND

Optimal pregnancy outcomes require vast maternal vascular, immune, and metabolic adaptations to support placentation and fetal growth. Adverse pregnancy outcomes such as preeclampsia, PTB, FGR, stillbirth, and GDM may result due to an impaired ability to mount these adaptations. Pregnancy has been described basically as a physiologic stress test where these adverse outcomes reveal women's vulnerability to excess cardiometabolic risk. Hence, once pregnancy is over, the postpartum period may provide a window of opportunity to identify risk factors and offer interventions to improve long-term health of the woman.

## Hypertensive Disorders of Pregnancy

Hypertensive disorders of pregnancy (preeclampsia, PIH) are the most common medical pregnancy complications, affecting 5–7% of births, with long-term health implications. Exact mechanism is not clear, probably preeclampsia unmasks the vascular dysfunction phenotype among women which is associated with high cardiometabolic risks. Epidemiological studies show double the elevated risk for chronic hypertension, cardiovascular disease, and renal disease later in life, and it can be as high as eightfold for early-onset preeclampsia requiring delivery before 34 weeks' gestation.[43]

Chronic hypertension rates in women with normotensive term births are very low (1%) 2–5 years after delivery[44] whereas following early-onset preeclampsia, risks are as high as 50%, 39% after PIH, and 25% following late-onset preeclampsia. American Heart Association since 2011 identifies a history of hypertension in pregnancy to be an established risk factor for the cardiovascular disease.[45]

The American College of Obstetricians and Gynecologists (ACOG) recommends annual screening for hypertension, diabetes, and dyslipidemia among women with a history of recurrent hypertensive disease of pregnancy or preterm delivery complicated by hypertensive disease of pregnancy, although based primarily on expert opinion.

## Gestational Diabetes Mellitus

Gestational diabetes mellitus affects roughly 5% of pregnancies. It is a condition, in which carbohydrate intolerance develops or is first diagnosed during pregnancy.

A meta-analysis of 675,455 women reported that women with a history of GDM have a 7.4-fold increased lifetime risk for type 2 DM later in life compared with women without GDM.[46] These women are also at increased risks of either having or acquiring the components of the metabolic syndrome, hence, are at increased risk for cardiovascular disease. This is likely due to ongoing subclinical inflammation and vascular dysfunction.[47] Approximately, one-third of women with a history of GDM will have developed metabolic syndrome within 5–10 years of delivery.[48]

Current ACOG guidelines[49] and the American Diabetes Association[50] recommendations for all women with GDM include nutritional modification, exercise, glucose testing after delivery, and referral for ongoing primary care.

Infants delivered following pregnancies complicated by GDM are at increased risk for perinatal complications, birth trauma, neonatal hypoglycemia, hyperbilirubinemia, hypocalcemia, polycythemia, and hypertrophic cardiomyopathy. Children are also at risk for chronic diseases later in life, including obesity and metabolic disease.[51]

## Preterm Birth

Consistent epidemiologic evidence shows that women with PTBs have a two-fold excess risk for cardiovascular disease compared with women with term births.[52,53] The reported risks for heart disease and stroke were highest among women who had medically indicated PTB. Women with spontaneous PTBs also had significantly increased risks for cardiovascular disease, and stroke. Possibly inflammation and placental senescence responsible for early delivery predisposes to systemic inflammation and vascular senescence associated with cardiovascular disease.

Preterm infants have long been recognized to be at risk of various complications including chronic lung disease, cerebral palsy, mental retardation, visual and hearing impairments, behavioral and social-emotional problems, learning difficulties and poor health and growth. Children who are born even early-term remain at risk for the development of obesity, diabetes, and cardiovascular disease later in life as compared with offspring of pregnancies delivered at term.[54]

## Fetal Growth Abnormalities

Fetal growth restriction and placental insufficiency share pathophysiologic changes with other ischemic placental diseases such as hypertensive disorders of pregnancy. FGR is related to about two-fold excess cardiovascular disease risk in mothers.[55]

Fetal growth restriction is also associated with adverse long-term health outcomes for the affected offspring. Barker, an epidemiologist, hypothesized that impaired prenatal and early postnatal growth were important risk factors for ischemic heart disease later in life. The "Barker hypothesis", that there are fetal origins of adult disease, has since been tested for a multitude of prenatal exposures and adult outcomes, with substantial observational evidence supporting it.[56]

Pregnancy has been described as a window that provides potential insight into women's own as well as her baby's future health. Certain common pregnancy complications are associated with adverse long-term health outcomes for both the affected mother and their offspring. Although the evidence is largely from observational studies, and there are knowledge gaps regarding pathophysiology, obstetricians need to be aware of these associations. Early screening and interventions may improve women's continuity of care across the life span.

## KEY POINTS

- Risk stratification of pregnancy into low-risk and high-risk categories allows appropriate allocation and utilization of resources.
- Prenatal care is the systematic assessment intended to ensure the best possible health of the mother and her fetus. It is a preventive service and can identify, prevent, or minimize many social, behavioral, environmental, and biomedical risks to a woman's pregnancy through education, counseling, and appropriate intervention.
- Age, parity, ethnicity, weight (BMI), and gestational weight gain impact pregnancy outcome, long-term maternal health, and health of the child.
- Smoking, alcohol, and illicit drug use by pregnant women are all harmful to the developing fetus. Identification and appropriate prenatal care of these women is complex and requires teamwork.
- Clear evidence shows that optimizing disease management for some conditions such as DM, phenylketonuria, inflammatory bowel disease, etc., before conception can positively influence pregnancy outcome. Many women with complex medical issues, who are advised against unplanned pregnancy, conceive unintentionally and need multidisciplinary team management.
- Psychosocial issues such as domestic violence, substance abuse have major impact on health of the woman and her unborn fetus, systematic evaluation during antenatal visits and referral to psychologist, medical social worker, etc., may mitigate associated short- and long-term adverse outcomes.
- The prenatal care does not end with delivery but rather includes postpartum, inter-conception and preconception care.
- All healthcare interactions during the course of pregnancy with reproductive-age couples offer opportunities to assess the risk, promote healthy lifestyle behaviors, and identify and treat medical and psychosocial issues.
- Pregnancy offers a glimpse into women's own as well as her baby's future health where appropriate preventive actions can minimize the possible risks.

## REFERENCES

1. Wildschut HIJ. Constitutional and environmental factors leading to a high-risk pregnancy. In: James D, Steer P, Weiner C, Gonik B (Eds). High Risk Pregnancy Management Options, 4th edition. Cambridge: Cambridge University Press; 2011; pp. 11-28.
2. Leftwich HK, Alves MV. Adolescent pregnancy. Pediatr Clin North Am. 2017;64:381-8.
3. Falk G, Ostlund I, Magnuson A, Schollin J, Nilsson K. Teenage mothers—a high risk group for new unintended pregnancies. Contraception. 2006;74:471-5.
4. Hillis SD, Anda RF, Dube SR, Felitti VJ, Marchbanks PA, Marks JS. The association between adverse childhood experiences and adolescent pregnancy, long-term psychosocial consequences, and fetal death. Pediatrics. 2004;113:320-7.
5. International Institute for Population Sciences (IIPS) and ICF. National Family Health Survey (NFHS-4) 2015-16. Mumbai: International Institute for Population Sciences; 2017.
6. Bhan N. Preventing teenage pregnancy in India to end the cycle of undernutrition. Lancet Child Adolesc Health. 2019;3(7):439-40.
7. Trivedi SS, Pasrija S. Teenage pregnancies and their obstetric outcomes. Trop Doc. 2007;37(2):85-8.
8. Richard HP, Louise KC. Management of teenage pregnancy. Obstet Gynaecol. 2011;9(3):153-8.
9. Hook EB, Cross PK, Schreinemachers DM. Chromosomal abnormality rates at amniocentesis and in live born infants. JAMA. 1983;249:2034.
10. Nybo Andersen AM, Wohlfahrt J, Christens P, Olsen J, Melbye M. Maternal age and fetal loss: population based register linkage study. BMJ. 2000;320(7251):1708.
11. Gill SK, Broussard C, Devine O, Green RF, Rasmussen SA, Reefhuis J. Association between maternal age and birth defects of unknown etiology; United States, 1997-2007. Birth Defects Res A Clin Mol Teratol. 2012;94(12):1010.
12. Lean SC, Derricott H, Jones RL, Heazell AEP. Advanced maternal age and adverse pregnancy outcomes: a systematic review and meta-analysis. PLoS One. 2017;12:e0186287.
13. Waldenström U, Ekéus C. Risk of labor dystocia increases with maternal age irrespective of parity: a population-based register study. Acta Obstet Gynecol Scand. 2017;96:1063.
14. Fitzpatrick KE, Tuffnell D, Kurinczuk JJ, Knight M. Pregnancy at very advanced maternal age: a UK population-based cohort study. BJOG. 2017;124(7):1097-106.
15. Bai J, Wong FW, Bauman A, Mohsin M. Parity and pregnancy outcomes. Am J Obstet Gynecol. 2002;186:274.
16. Agarwal S, Agarwal A, Das V. Impact of grandmultiparity on obstetric outcome in low resource setting. J Obstet Gynaecol Res. 2011;37:1015.
17. Al-Shaikh GK, Ibrahim GH, Fayed AA, Al-Mandeel H. Grand multiparity and the possible risk of adverse maternal and neonatal outcomes: a dilemma to be deciphered. BMC Pregnancy Childbirth. 2017;17:310.
18. Alsammani MA, Ahmed SR. Grand multiparity: risk factors and outcome in a tertiary hospital: a comparative study. Med Arch. 2015;69:38.
19. Athukorala C, Rumbold AR, Willson KJ, Crowther CA. The risk of adverse pregnancy outcomes in women who are overweight or obese. BMC Pregnancy Childbirth. 2010;10:56.
20. Goldstein RF, Abell SK, Ranasinha S, Misso M, Boyle JA, Black MH, et al. Association of gestational weight gain with maternal and infant outcomes: a systematic review and meta-analysis. JAMA. 2017;317:2207-25.
21. Gaskins AJ, Rich-Edwards JW, Colaci DS, Afeiche MC, Toth TL, Gillman MW, et al. Prepregnancy and early adulthood body mass index and adult weight change in relation to fetal loss. Obstet Gynecol. 2014;124:662-9.
22. Forno E, Young OM, Kumar R, Simhan H, Celedón JC. Maternal obesity in pregnancy, gestational weight gain, and risk of childhood asthma. Pediatrics. 2014;134:e535-46.
23. Kwong W, Tomlinson G, Feig DS. Maternal and neonatal outcomes after bariatric surgery; a systematic review and meta-analysis: do the benefits outweigh the risks? Am J Obstet Gynecol. 2018;218:573-80.

24. Dolin C, Akuezunkpa O, Welcome U, Caughey AB. Management of pregnancy in women who have undergone bariatric surgery. Obstet Gynecol Surv. 2016;71:734-40.
25. Domestic Violence: A National Report. London: Home Office; 2005. p. 7.
26. Bacchus L, Mezey G, Bewley S. Domestic violence: prevalence in pregnant women and associations with physical and psychological health. Eur J Obstet Gynecol Reprod Biol. 2004;113:6-11.
27. Huth-Bocks AC, Levendosky AA, Bogat GA. The effects of domestic violence during pregnancy on maternal and infant health. Violence Vict. 2002;17:169-85.
28. Lewis G, Clutton-Brock T, Cooper G, Drife J, Edwards G, Harper N, et al. Saving Mother's Lives: Reviewing Maternal Deaths to Make Motherhood Safer—2003 to 2005. The Seventh Report of the Confidential Enquiries into Maternal Deaths in the United Kingdom. London: CEMACH; 2007. pp. 173-9.
29. Silverman JG, Decker MR, Reed E, Raj A. Intimate partner violence victimization prior to and during pregnancy among women residing in 26 U.S. states: associations with maternal and neonatal health. Am J Obstet Gynecol. 2006;195(1):140.
30. Ludermir AB, Lewis G, Valongueiro SA, de Araújo TV, Araya RS. Violence against women by their intimate partner during pregnancy and postnatal depression: a prospective cohort study. Lancet. 2010;376(9744):903.
31. Levendosky AA, Lannert B, Yalch M. The effects of intimate partner violence in women and child survivors: an attachment perspective. Psychodyn Psychiatry. 2012;40:397-433.
32. American College of Obstetricians and Gynecologists. ACOG Technical Bulletin 209. Domestic Violence. Washington DC: ACOG; 1995.
33. Royal College of Midwives. Domestic Abuse: Pregnancy, Birth and the Puerperium. Guidance Paper No. 5. London: RCM; 2006.
34. Department of Health. Responding to Domestic Abuse. A Handbook for Health Professionals. London: DOH; 2006.
35. Cnattingius S. The epidemiology of smoking during pregnancy: smoking prevalence, maternal characteristics, and pregnancy outcomes. Nicotine Tob Res. 2004;6(Suppl 2):S125-40.
36. Rasch V. Cigarette, alcohol, and caffeine consumption: risk factors for spontaneous abortion. Acta Obstet Gynecol Scand. 2003;82:182-8.
37. Flynn HA, Marcus SM, Barry KL, Blow FC. Rates and correlates of alcohol use among pregnant women in obstetrics clinics. Alcohol Clin Exp Res. 2003;27:81-7.
38. Metz TD, Allshouse AA, Hogue CJ. Maternal marijuana use, adverse pregnancy outcomes, and neonatal morbidity. Am J Obstet Gynecol. 2017;217(4):478.e1-8.
39. Australian Institute of Health and Welfare. Cancer in Australia: an overview 2014 (Cancer series no. 90. Cat no. CAN 88). Canberra: AIHW; 2014.
40. Tang M, Webber K. Fertility and pregnancy in cancer survivors. Obstet Med. 2018;11(3):110-5.
41. Azim HA, Santoro L, Pavlidis N, Gelber S, Kroman N, Azim H, et al. Safety of pregnancy following breast cancer diagnosis: a meta-analysis of 14 studies. Eur J Cancer. 2011;47:74-83.
42. Gien LT, Covens A. Fertility-sparing options for early stage cervical cancer. Gynecologic Oncol. 2010;117:350-7.
43. Bellamy L, Casas JP, Hingorani AD, Williams DJ. Preeclampsia and risk of cardiovascular disease and cancer in later life: systematic review and meta-analysis. BMJ. 2007;335:974.
44. Hermes W, Franx A, van Pampus MG, Bloemenkamp KW, Bots ML, van der Post JA, et al. Cardiovascular risk factors in women who had hypertensive disorders late in pregnancy: a cohort study. Am J Obstet Gynecol. 2013;208(6):474e1-8.
45. Mosca L, Benjamin EJ, Berra K, Bezanson JL, Dolor RJ, Lloyd-Jones DM, et al. Effectiveness-based guidelines for the prevention of cardiovascular disease in women–2011 update: a guideline from the American Heart Association. Circulation. 2011;123:1243-62.
46. Bellamy L, Casas JP, Hingorani AD, Williams D. Type 2 diabetes mellitus after gestational diabetes: a systematic review and meta-analysis. Lancet. 2009;373:1773-9.
47. Heitritter SM, Solomon CG, Mitchell GF, Skali-Ounis N, Seely EW. Subclinical inflammation and vascular dysfunction in women with previous gestational diabetes mellitus. J Clin Endocrinol Metab. 2005;90(7):3983-8.
48. Varner MW, Rice MM, Landon MB, Casey BM, Reddy UM, Wapner RJ, et al. Pregnancies after the diagnosis of mild gestational diabetes mellitus and risk of cardiometabolic disorders. Obstet Gynecol. 2017;129(2):273-80.
49. Committee on Practice Bulletins—Obstetrics. ACOG Practice Bulletin No. 190: Gestational diabetes mellitus. Obstet Gynecol. 2018;131(2):e49-64.
50. American Diabetes Association. Standards of medical care in diabetes–2017 abridged for primary care providers. Clin Diabetes. 2017;35(1):5-26.
51. Durnwald C, Landon M. Fetal links to chronic disease: the role of gestational diabetes mellitus. Am J Perinatol. 2013;30(5):343-6.
52. Robbins CL, Hutchings Y, Dietz PM, Kuklina EV, Callaghan WM. History of preterm birth and subsequent cardiovascular disease: a systematic review. Am J Obstet Gynecol. 2014;210:285-97.
53. Wu P, Gulati M, Kwok CS, Wong CW, Narain A, O'Brien S, et al. Preterm delivery and future risk of maternal cardiovascular disease: a systematic review and meta-analysis. J Am Heart Assoc. 2018;7(2):e007809.
54. Paz Levy D, Sheiner E, Wainstock T, Sergienko R, Landau D, Walfisch A. Evidence that children born at early term (37-38 6/7 weeks) are at increased risk for diabetes and obesity-related disorders. Am J Obstet Gynecol. 2017;217(5):588.e1-11.
55. Bonamy A-KE, Parikh NI, Cnattingius S, Ludvigsson JF, Ingelsson E. Birth characteristics and subsequent risks of maternal cardiovascular disease: clinical perspective. Circulation. 2011;124:2839-46.
56. Barker DJ, Winter PD, Osmond C, Margetts B, Simmonds SJ. Weight in infancy and death from ischaemic heart disease. Lancet. 1989;2(8663):577-80.

# CHAPTER 2

# Prenatal Diagnosis

*Mandakini Pradhan, Ratna Biswas, Neeta Singh*

## INTRODUCTION

Congenital disorder is one of the leading causes of mortality and morbidity in the newborn. The magnitude of problem is particularly significant in the developing world, where congenital disorders are common because of high birth rate, consanguineous marriages, and nutritional deficiency. In the absence of curative treatment, the financial and social burden on the family and country is enormous. Hence, lies the importance of prenatal diagnosis and prevention of birth of affected newborn or prenatal therapy as the case may be.

Prenatal diagnosis involves initial screening to detect couples at higher risk followed by definite diagnosis. It could be structural defects in fetus or may be without any structural defect. It could be due to chromosomal abnormalities, genetic diseases or metabolic abnormality. The procedure can be invasive or noninvasive. The aim of the diagnostic procedures is to provide an accurate and early diagnosis of the fetal disease, so as to enable the couple to make an informed choice on the management options. The modalities of management are either termination of pregnancy, fetal therapy wherever applicable or to prepare the couple for birth of an affected child. Preimplantation diagnosis, too, is a management option whereby an unaffected embryo is chosen for implantation. Thorough genetic counseling is essential and ethical issues need to be considered when opting for this method.

## SCREENING METHODS

These are methods which can identify fetus at high-risk of having malformations, genetic disorders, chromosomal abnormalities, etc. Though the screening methods widely discussed are for detection of fetal chromosomal aneuploidy, other fetal conditions which can affect the pregnancy outcome need to be kept in mind. For a screening method to be effective it needs to have a high detection rate with an acceptable false-positive rate. The couples at high-risk of fetal disorder can be identified based on history, examination, and investigations.

### History

- *During present pregnancy:* Certain history during ongoing pregnancy may indicate a high-risk fetus.
    - Exposure to teratogens like anticancer drugs, anti-epileptics especially sodium valproate, anticoagulant like warfarin, and radioactive iodine therapy for thyroid cancer, etc.
    - Contact with patients suffering from infectious diseases like rubella.
    - History of infectious diseases such as chickenpox or fever with rash may indicate likelihood of fetus being infected.
    - Anemia in the women not due to iron deficiency or not improving after iron therapy may need further evaluation to detect carrier of hemoglobinopathies. Such woman may be at risk of having an affected fetus.
- *Past history:* Previous history of fetus being affected with a specific disease warrants a prenatal diagnosis in subsequent pregnancy. The method of prenatal diagnosis differs depending upon the diagnosis in the previous child. **Table 1** delineates few of the common disorders, their risk of recurrence, and method of prenatal diagnosis.
- *Family history:* A minimum three generation pedigree should be drawn to find out any significant risk to the couple of having an affected baby. For example, a history of maternal brother being affected with Duchenne muscular dystrophy may indicate a possibility of the woman being carrier and hence having 25% risk of affected child. A history of consanguinity may suggest investigating parents for carrier of a common autosomal recessive disease like β-thalassemia.

### Examination

As in any clinical setting, detailed examination of a pregnant woman is important. It is important because many of them visit a doctor for the first time and asymptomatic conditions can be picked-up. Examination of the couple becomes more important to detect single incisor teeth in holoprosencephaly, features of myotonia in recurrent polyhydramnios, spinal abnormality in spondylocostal dysplasia, etc.

**TABLE 1:** Common disorders, their risk of recurrence, and method of prenatal diagnosis.

| Single gene disorder | Mode of inheritance | Recurrence risk | Method of prenatal diagnosis |
|---|---|---|---|
| β-thalassemia | Autosomal recessive | 25% | Carrier screening of both parents and subsequently in the fetal sample obtained after invasive method |
| Cystic fibrosis | Autosomal recessive | 25% | Mutation detection in both parents and subsequently in the fetal sample obtained after invasive method |
| Sickle cell disease | Autosomal recessive | 25% | Direct detection of mutation by molecular method in the fetal sample obtained after invasive method if both parents are carrier |
| Duchenne muscular dystrophy (DMD) | X-linked recessive | 25% of all children or 50% of male children | Mutation detection in the previous affected child |
| Spinal muscular atrophy (SMA) | Autosomal recessive | 25% | Mutation detection in the fetal sample obtained after invasive method |
| Achondroplasia | Autosomal dominant | 50% if one of the parents is affected; 1% if both parents are normal as it is usually due to new mutation | Mutation detection in the fetal sample if couple is willing after counseling |
| Multifactorial disease neural tube defect (NTD) | Unknown | 3–5% after one affected pregnancy; 10% after two affected pregnancies | Detection of spinal defect in fetus by ultrasound |

## Investigations

The noninvasive procedures are generally used for screening whereas the invasive procedures give a definite diagnosis. Various screening and diagnostic procedures for prenatal diagnosis are tabulated in **Table 2**.

Fetal aneuploidy is the most common indication for prenatal screening and diagnostic test. Aneuploidy is defined as an abnormal number of chromosomes in place of the usual diploid complement. Down syndrome (trisomy 21), Edward syndrome (trisomy 18), and Patau syndrome (trisomy 13) are the most common trisomies. Down syndrome occurs in 1:800 to 1:900 live births. It is compatible with life. Edward syndrome occurs in 1:3,000 live births and Patau syndrome occurs in 1:5,000 live births. Both are lethal anomalies.[1] The age-related risk of Down syndrome in a pregnant woman at mid-trimester is 1:417 at 33 years, 1:250 at 35 years, 1:149 at 37 years, 1:69 at 40 years, and 1:19 at 45 years.[1]

Women should be given information on the screening process and be provided with an opportunity to discuss this with a health professional before making a decision to accept or decline screening. Following the screening test, results should be explained in the context of the hazards and benefits of definitive diagnosis through amniocentesis or chorionic villus sampling (CVS). Information must be provided through nondirective counseling. Each couple make their own decision whether they wish to receive these services. Respect for ethical values, sensitivities, and the decisions made by each patient are of key importance in the delivery of these services. Prenatal aneuploidy risk assessment services often vary according to the healthcare systems that are present in different countries. Furthermore, service delivery may be modified to reflect individual women's clinical conditions such as infertility, co-existing risk for other genetic disorders or their moral and ethical values.

**TABLE 2:** Screening and diagnostic procedures for prenatal diagnosis.

*Noninvasive screening procedures for*
- Carrier of hemoglobinopathy,
- Single gene disorder if at higher risk and
- Fetal aneuploidy

First trimester screening
- Double marker test along with ultrasound
- Cell free fetal DNA

Second trimester screening
- Quadruple test along with ultrasound soft marker

Integrated screening
Serum integrated screening
Sequential stepwise screening
Contingent screening

- Fetal imaging
  – Ultrasonography
  – Doppler sonography
  – Magnetic resonance imaging

*Invasive diagnostic procedures*
- Amniocentesis
  – Second trimester amniocentesis
- Chorionic villous sampling (CVS)
  – Transcervical CVS
  – Transabdominal CVS
- Fetal blood sampling
  – Percutaneous umbilical blood sampling or cordocentesis
  – Fetal intrahepatic vessel sampling
  – Fetal cardiac sampling
- Fetal tissue biopsy
- Fetoscopy

*Preimplantation diagnosis*

(DNA: deoxyribonucleic acid)

Guidelines from American College of Obstetricians and Gynecologists (ACOG) and American College of Medical Genetics (ACMG) recommend screening of all pregnant women regardless of maternal age.[2,3] The screening strategy chosen depends on the gestational age at which the woman attends the antenatal clinic and availability of expertise in ultrasound.

## First Trimester Screening

The methods used are:
- Nuchal translucency (NT) sonography
- Nasal bone sonography
- Doppler sonography of ductus venosus (DV)
- Pregnancy associated plasma protein A (PAPP-A) in maternal serum
- Free β–subunit of human chorionic gonadotropin (hCG) in maternal serum.

### Nuchal Translucency

It refers to the space between spine and overlying skin at the back of fetal neck. Measurement is done between 11 weeks and 13 weeks + 6 days of gestation. Increased NT is a strong marker of Down syndrome.[4] Possible mechanisms leading to increased NT are fluid accumulation secondary to heart failure caused by structural anomalies of heart, abnormal extracellular matrix or abnormal lymphatic development.[5]

Nuchal translucency can be obtained by transabdominal or transvaginal route. By transabdominal route it is possible to obtain 95% of NT measurements and combining the two routes results in almost 100% chance of obtaining the NT measurement. Correct technique for measurement of NT is to obtain a view of the midsagittal plane with the fetal head in neutral position and fetal image occupying 75% of viewable screen. The fetal image to be obtained consists of fetal head, neck, and upper part of thorax. Crown-rump length (CRL) measurement is mandatory to accurately estimate the period of gestation since NT varies with gestational age. A CRL of 45–84 mm is required to have accurate NT measurements. Distinction between amnion and overlying fetal skin should be confirmed on fetal movement. Calipers are placed at inner borders of the NT space.[4,6,7] Three NT measurements are obtained, and the largest value taken.

Nuchal translucency measurement requires considerable skill which can be acquired with training. The accuracy of NT measurement is said to be reached when the difference in intra- and interobserver variation is <0.5 mm in 95% of the measurements. Approximately 100 scans must be performed to attain such level of perfection. A good quality ultrasound machine with video loop function and an ability to measure up to a 10th of a millimeter is needed for measuring NT.[7] Adequate time should be spared for proper measurement and at least 20 minutes time should be given before labeling an attempt unsuccessful.[1] In such a situation a rescan should be scheduled after a week's time or earlier depending on the period of gestation. Quality control measures need to be instituted for maintaining high standards of performance. The rate of detection of Down syndrome based on NT in high-risk women ranges from 46 to 62%, whereas the detection rate in low-risk women varies from 29 to 91%.[6] The average detection rate with NT is 77% at false-positive rate of 5%.[6]

Specific cutoff values (2.5 or 3 mm) are inappropriate because of gestational age dependent variations in NT. Gestational age specific thresholds are available for NT measurement which is combined with maternal age to arrive at a risk estimate.[7] Alternatively, it can be expressed as, multiple of median (MOM) and combined with PAPP-A and β-hCG to give a risk estimate.

Detection of cystic hygroma during first trimester sonography for evaluation of NT is the most powerful predictor for trisomy 21 with 50% risk of fetal aneuploidy. This finding is an indication for a CVS.[5]

### Nasal Bone Sonography

To obtain accurate measurement, the mid-sagittal plane is viewed with the neck in slight flexion position and the fetal profile facing upwards. In normal pregnancy two echogenic lines, one representing the fetal skin and the other the fetal nasal bone is visualized. Failure to visualize the nasal bone is an independent risk factor for Down syndrome.[4] However, accurate imaging of fetal nasal bone in first trimester is technically challenging with a significant intra- and interobserver variation.

The ultrasound beam should strike at right angles to the nasal skin for visualization of the nasal bone. The normal ossification of nasal bone develops on both sides of the cartilaginous septum from 10 weeks onwards. New ossification appears as less echogenic lines on both sides of bone. Only the echogenic part should be measured. Difference in timing of appearance and ossification of both nasal bones may cause technical difficulty in measurement leading to intra- and interobserver variation.[8,9] Hence, its routine use in clinical setting is not recommended.

### Doppler Sonography

*Ductus venosus:* DV is a small vessel that shunts 30% of the blood flow from the umbilical vein directly to the right atrium. The blood flow in this vessel on color Doppler ultrasonography (USG) has a typical triphasic pattern. Absence or reversal of "a" wave in DV is associated with fetal cardiac defects and Down syndrome. Perfumo et al. have described a positive likelihood ratio of 7.05 for Down syndrome in the presence of abnormal DV flow.[8] In chromosomally normal fetuses with normal DV, abnormal DV blood flow in first trimester has been associated with fetal cardiac defects and fetal growth restriction.

Absence of DV or aberrations in the anatomy of DV is an independent marker of fetal chromosomal abnormalities. It is known to be associated with various hepatic vascular malformations and is associated with poor fetal prognosis.

*Tricuspid regurgitation (TR):* TR is another potential ultrasound marker determined by pulse wave Doppler USG. In the apical 4 chamber view of the fetal heart with insonation parallel to the ventricular septum, with a gate of 3 mm, pulse wave Doppler is taken. A regurgitant jet should be present over at least half of the systole with a velocity of 60–80 cm/sec for the diagnosis of TR to be met. Approximately 75% of Down syndrome fetuses have TR as compared to 7% of normal fetuses.

In addition to presence of soft markers for fetal aneuploidy there are multiple fetal congenital malformations which can be detected in the first trimester with variable sensitivity and are associated with increased risk of fetal genetic abnormalities. For example, presence of increased NT in first trimester is associated with fetal aneuploidy in 60–70% of cases whereas anencephaly, a lethal malformation, though associated with decreased risk of chromosomal abnormality, can be detected as early as 10–11 weeks of gestation. Hence, a targeted ultrasound for fetal malformations should be offered to the patient where possible and if detected, depending on the anomaly, invasive prenatal diagnostic test for chromosomal analysis may be offered or on the other hand, if anomaly is incompatible with life, medical termination of pregnancy with subsequent evaluation of the fetus and placenta for genetic and molecular study may be offered.

The use of ultrasound needs to be consistent with fetal safety recommendations, i.e., with an ultrasound exposure that is as low as reasonably achievable (ALARA) [American Institute of Ultrasound in Medicine (AIUM) Practice Guideline, 2007].

### Biochemical Markers in Maternal Serum

Double marker test consists of two serum markers, PAPP-A and β-hCG. Along with maternal age, gestational age, and maternal medical and obstetric history, a risk of fetal aneuploidy for that gestational age is calculated by the software.

### Combined First Trimester Screening (Flowchart 1)

Combined NT, PAPP-A, and β-hCG in association with maternal age detects 85% of trisomy 21 with the false-positive rate of 5%. The earlier in first trimester the measurements are taken the higher is the detection rate, 87% at 11 weeks as compared to 82% at 13 weeks.[4]

A National Institute of Health (NIH) sponsored study called the blood, ultrasound and nuchal translucency (BUN) trial evaluating the results of first trimester screening in 8,500 high-risk cases detected 79% of all Down syndrome cases with 5% false-positive rate.[10] The FASTER (First and second trimester evaluation of risk) study with 36,000 pregnancies detected 85% of Down syndrome with a false-positive rate of 5%.[11]

The one stop clinic to assess risk (OSCAR) study involving 12,000 pregnancies had a 90% detection rate at a false-positive rate of 5%.[10] The Serum, Urine and Ultrasound Screening (SURUSS) study involving 48,000 pregnancies had an 86% detection rate for a 5% false-positive rate.[12] The average derived from these four large trials is 85% which is better than quadruple screening in second trimester. Both BUN and FASTER study support the efficacy of free β-hCG over total β-hCG. However, the recent guidelines from the ACMG state that free β-hCG, total hCG or hyperglycosylated hCG should be interchangeable.[3] As individual marker, NT is most informative followed by PAPP-A.

### Second Trimester Screening (Flowchart 2)

It is indicated in pregnant women who present for the first time in second trimester or when expertise in first trimester screening, like measurement of NT is not available. Methods of second trimester screening are:

- Biochemical serum markers
- Sonographic detection of major structural malformation
- Sonographic evaluation of minor markers.

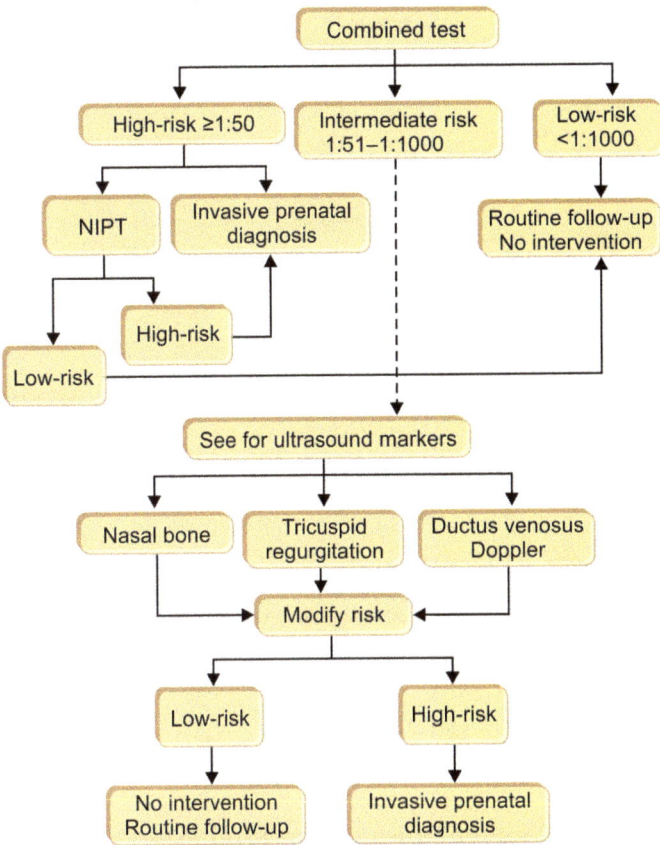

**Flowchart 1:** Management based on combined test and USG results.

(NITP: noninvasive prenatal testing)

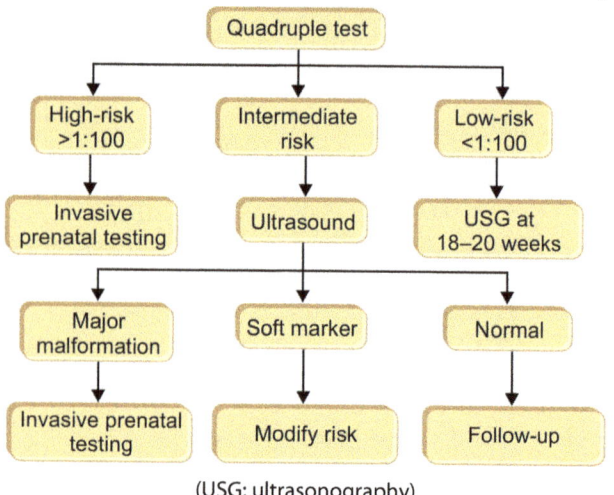

**Flowchart 2:** Interpretation of second trimester serum screening.

(USG: ultrasonography)

## Biochemical Serum Markers

Quadruple test—have the following components:
- Maternal serum alpha-fetoprotein (MSAFP)
- β-hCG
- Unconjugated estriol (uE3)
- Inhibin A.

## Maternal Serum Assay in Second Trimester

Maternal serum assay in second trimester screening is most accurate when performed between 16 and 18 weeks of gestation.[10] Low MSAFP has been associated with Down syndrome. One-third to one-fifth of Down syndrome pregnancies present with low MSAFP levels with the median MSAFP level of 0.7.[10] MSAFP values need correction for weight, race, diabetes, and multiple gestation.[2] In insulin dependent diabetics, MSAFP levels are 60% of nondiabetics.[13] In twin pregnancy, the median MSAFP levels from 16 to 20 weeks of gestation is 2.5 MoM for single pregnancy. Combined biochemical screening procedures are as given here.

*Quadruple test:* Maternal serum assay in second trimester, uE3, MSFP, hCG, and inhibin-A are the components of quadruple test. Maternal serum levels of AFP and uE3 are 25% lower in Down syndrome as compared to normal pregnancy. Serum hCG is twice as high in Down syndrome as compared to normal pregnancy. Maternal serum inhibin A levels are increased to 2.1 times the median value of control in Down syndrome. It is usually performed between 16 and 20 weeks of gestation. The serum levels of each of the proteins is expressed as MoM for gestational age. The composite estimate of the risk of trisomy 21 is calculated. Standard cut off is 1/270 which is equal to the second trimester risk of Down syndrome in a 35-year-old woman.[2,14] It has a 67–76% detection rate of trisomy 21 in women younger than 35 years.[15] Some studies have quoted a detection rate of 80%.[15,16]

*Ultrasound:* Ultrasound examination done between 18 and 20 weeks helps in diagnosis of major congenital malformations and various soft markers for Down syndrome. Trisomy 18 and 13 are associated with fetal congenital malformation and fetal growth restriction in approximately 90–95% of cases and are likely to be picked up by ultrasound alone. However, only 60% of Down syndrome fetuses have abnormalities on ultrasound and can be missed if only ultrasound is used for diagnosis of Down syndrome. Hence, it is important to offer a pregnant women biochemical screening for Down syndrome in the second trimester if she has missed the chance in the first trimester. This is especially useful in India as women commonly present late for antenatal booking.

Physical characteristics which are on their own not malformations or anomalies, but they are found more commonly in fetuses with Down syndrome are called as soft markers. The ratio of the prevalence of these markers in trisomy 21 fetuses to their prevalence in the normal population is the likelihood ratio for that particular soft marker. This can be used to modify a priori risk or serum screening risk for Down syndrome. Each soft marker as mentioned in **Table 3**, is associated with a definite likelihood ratio for Down syndrome.

## Sonographic Evaluation of Minor Markers

These are specific ultrasound findings that have been associated with increased risk of fetal aneuploidy. The minor markers are:
- *Absent or hypoplastic nasal bone:* Hypoplastic or absent nasal bones on second trimester sonography is associated with increased risk of Down syndrome. As indicated in the table above it is the soft marker associated with highest risk of fetal aneuploidy. The measurements of the length of the nasal bone is to be plotted against a nomogram for determining if it is hypoplastic.
- *Aberrant right subclavian artery:* Aberrant right subclavian artery (ARSA) is a rare anomaly, in which

**TABLE 3:** Soft marker associated with a definite likelihood ratio for Down syndrome.

| S. No. | Soft marker | Likelihood ratio (for presence of only one soft marker) |
|---|---|---|
| 1. | Absent/hypoplastic nasal bone | 6.58 |
| 2. | Aberrant right subclavian artery | 3.94 |
| 3. | Ventriculomegaly | 3.81 |
| 4. | Nuchal fold thickness | 3.79 |
| 5. | Echogenic bowel | 1.65 |
| 6. | Pyelectasis/mild hydronephrosis | 1.08 |
| 7. | Echogenic intracardiac focus | 0.95 |
| 8. | Short humerus | 0.78 |
| 9. | Short femur | 0.61 |

the right subclavian artery arises directly from the aortic arch instead of originating from the brachiocephalic artery. Postnatal radiographic studies have shown that an ARSA is present in 16–35%[17,18] of infants or adults with Down syndrome, and in 0.4–2.3% of the general population.[19,20-23] Chaoui et al. reported a prenatal incidence of ARSA in Down syndrome fetuses of 35.7%.[24]

- *Ventriculomegaly:* Lateral atrial width of >10 mm increased the risk of fetal aneuploidy especially when it is between 10 and 15 mm.
- *Nuchal fold thickness:* This measures the area between the outer aspect of occipital bone and outer aspect of skin in the axial plane passing through the posterior fossa in the midline. It is measured between 15 and 20 weeks. In normal pregnancy it is <5 mm, if it is >6 mm then the risk of Down syndrome increases by 11 fold.[4] It is also increased in Noonan's syndrome and in congenital cardiac defects.
- *Echogenic bowel:* A very bright bowel in the fetal abdomen is associated with a 6–7 fold increased risk of Down syndrome. While performing ultrasound, it is important to check the gain settings as false-positive results will occur if the gain settings are high. The echogenicity of bowel should be comparable to that of fetal bone.[4] It is also seen in association with disorders such as cystic fibrosis, cytomegalovirus (CMV) infection, and other aneuploidies. Structural malformations such as small bowel obstruction, malrotation of gut, meconium ileus, and peritonitis are also associated with this observation.[8] In its presence, a maternal screening for cystic fibrosis, CMV infection, and aneuploidy should be done. On the other hand, amniocentesis can be done for fetal karyotyping, detection of cystic fibrosis mutation, and deoxyribonucleic acid (DNA) analysis of CMV infection.
- *Pyelectasis:* A renal pelvis measurement in the anteroposterior diameter of >4 mm is abnormal when measured between 14 and 20 weeks. Pyelectasis is associated with 1.5 fold increased risk of Down syndrome.
- *Echogenic intracardiac focus:* This is caused by calcification of papillary muscles of ventricle. It is mainly seen in the left ventricle. To prevent over diagnosis, multiple angles are visualized to rule out specular reflections. The presence of echogenic intracardiac focus does not increase the risk of Down syndrome. The point to be noted is that it may be present in 30% of normal Asian fetuses and hence it is not a marker for aneuploidies. Therefore, other ultrasound findings or positive serum screening should be present to justify invasive testing.[4,8]
- *Short humerus and femur:* In normal fetus, the ratio of expected to observed length of these two bones should not be <2SD for that gestational age corrected for the ethnicity. The presence of short humerus increases the risk of Down syndrome by 5 fold, whereas short femur increases the risk by 1.5 fold. However, racial difference in biometry exists and Asian fetuses have shorter biometric measurements. Hence, nomogram for individual population should be available to prevent overdiagnosis. The sensitivity and specificity of this marker is not high and hence its isolated presence does not justify an invasive diagnosis.[4]

It is important to remember that a pregnancy should never be terminated based on the risk of serum screening in the first or second trimester as this is only a screening test and not a diagnostic test. This screening test is followed by a diagnostic test, if the women are at a high risk. There can be two scenarios in second trimester when a woman presents with a report of quadruple screen. This can either be a high risk or it can be a low-risk. An ultrasound is done and findings incorporated into a serum screening will give the modified risk which will be the final risk of Down syndrome for the fetus. For example, if a patient comes with a high risk of one in 100 and her ultrasound does not show any congenital malformation or any soft marker, the likelihood of Down syndrome in the fetus is reduced by 0.09 times and hence her modified risk is one in 900 which is a low risk and does not mandate an invasive testing **(Flowchart 3)**. But it is important to counsel the patient that the sensitivity of quadruple screen is 70–80% and not 100%. She can be given an option of a more sensitive screening test like cell free fetal DNA analysis at this point of time.

In another clinical scenario a woman can come with a low risk and presence of an ultrasound soft marker can modify the risk and make it a high risk. For example, a woman comes with a low risk of one in 600 in quadruple screening. Ultrasound shows presence of absent nasal bone whose likelihood ratio is 6.5. On multiplying the risk of 1:600 with 6.5, the final risk is 1:92 which is a high risk and hence mandates an invasive testing **(Flowchart 4)**.

It is important to remember that there is a class of patients who should not be offered serum screening or biochemical screening during pregnancy because they warrant an invasive testing otherwise also. They are the

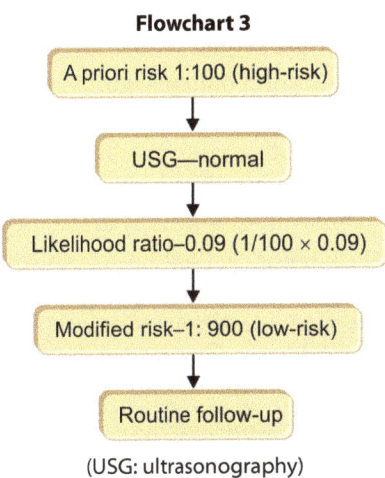

**Flowchart 3**

(USG: ultrasonography)

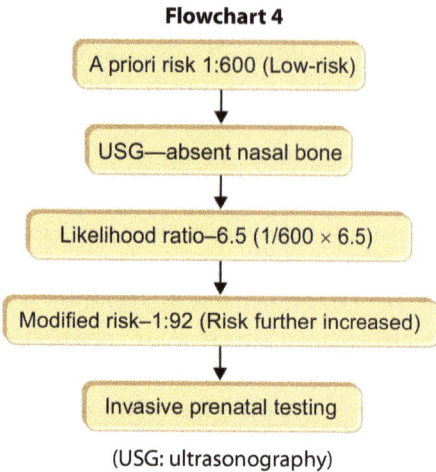

**Flowchart 4**

(USG: ultrasonography)

couple with previous baby with trisomy 21 where a priori risk is high and they can be offered a more sensitive screening such as noninvasive prenatal testing by cell free fetal DNA or invasive prenatal testing, where either of the couple is a carrier of balance translocation and in fetus having major congenital malformation.

## Combined First and Second Trimester Screening

It maximizes the performance of these screening modalities. It is of two types—(1) integrated screening and (2) sequential or contingent screening.

1. *Integrated screening:* This is a type of noninformative sequential screening in which the first trimester screening (NT and PAPP-A) is incorporated with second trimester screening (Quadruple screening) and a combined risk is then calculated. The sensitivity of integrated screening is 95% for a 5% false-positive rate. However, the disadvantage of this test is that the results of first trimester screening is withheld and the patients who are high-risk for trisomy 21 do not get a chance for early prenatal diagnosis.
2. *Sequential and contingent screening:* In an attempt to maximize the screen performance by combining the first and the second trimester serum analytes, sequential testing was introduced. In the most commonly used sequential testing, which is also called as contingent sequential testing, the patients with a high risk cut-off in the first trimester are subjected to invasive testing and the patients with low risk cut-off are advised routine follow-up. The patients who are at intermediate risk are subjected to quadruple screening in the second trimester. However in stepwise sequential screening, both the low risk and the intermediate risk patients are subjected to second trimester quadruple screening. The detection rate of contingent testing is 92–94% and that of stepwise sequential testing is 95% for a 5% false-positive rate.

Pretest counseling of the parents is particularly important before advising a serum screening test. This will help them to understand the test, its implications, interpretation of results, and further line of management if the result shows the fetus to be at high risk for trisomy 21/18/13. In cases of pregnancy following in vitro fertilization with a donor ovum, the age of the donor is used for risk assessment.

The first trimester serum markers are also abnormal in trisomy 18. Levels of PAPP-A and β-hCG are low and NT is increased. In the second trimester, α-fetoprotein, β-hCG, and estriol are all low in trisomy 18. Algorithms are available to detect risk of trisomy 18 based on first trimester and integrated screening.

## Fetal Imaging

### Sonographic Detection of Major Fetal Structural Malformation

This is done between 16 and 20 weeks of gestation to maximize fetal anatomic evaluation. The major structural malformations associated with aneuploidy are as follows:[4,8]

- *Cardiac defects:* Atrial septal defect (ASD), ventricular septal defects (VSD), tetralogy of Fallot (TOF), double outlet right ventricle, hypoplastic left heart, septal and endocardial cushion defects, valvular defects, and coarctation of aorta.
- *Gastrointestinal malformations:* Duodenal atresia, esophageal atresia, omphalocele, tracheoesophageal fistula, annular pancreas, imperforate anus, and diaphragmatic hernia.
- *Central nervous system malformations:* Meningomyelocele, holoprosencephaly, agenesis of corpus callosum, ventriculomegaly, microcephaly, posterior fossa defects, etc.
- *Skeletal malformations:* Clubfoot, rocker bottom feet, and polydactyly.
- *Renal malformations:* Horseshoe kidney, polycystic kidney, and hydronephrosis.
- *Facial anomalies:* Cleft lip and palate, microphthalmia, anophthalmia, macroglossia, and cyclopia.

Nicolaides and colleagues observed that detection of aneuploidy on sonography was related to the number of defects identified.[8,25,26] They assigned points to specific markers. Structural malformation and thickened nuchal fold were assigned two points each and shortened femur, shortened humerus, echogenic intracardiac focus, hyperechoic bowel, and pyelectasis were given one point each. An invasive test is recommended in high-risk women with one or more points or in low-risk women with two or more points based on his scoring system.

### Genetic Sonography

It is a targeted sonography which is done for fetal aneuploidy. It is done between 18 and 20 weeks of gestation and special attention is given to detect abnormal fetal biometry, fetal structural anomalies, and minor (soft) markers of fetal aneuploidy.[15]

In Down syndrome the following sonographic findings should be looked for:

Skeletal abnormalities such as sandal gap toes, 11 pairs of ribs, short fingers, brachymesophalangia, etc. Facial abnormalities such as flattened face and occiput, oblique palpebral fissure, high arch palate, low nasal bridge, low set ears, nasal hypoplasia, macroglossia, and epicanthic fold. Central nervous system (CNS) abnormalities which are frequently associated with Down syndrome are ventriculomegaly, microcephaly, and brachycephaly. Cardiovascular defects include ASD, VSD, TOF, endocardial cushion defects, echogenic cardiac focus, and pericardial effusion. Gastrointestinal and genitourinary abnormalities such as duodenal atresia, tracheoesophageal fistula, omphalocele, annular pancreas, imperforate anus, hyperechogenic bowel, and mild pyelectasis. Hypotonia and goiter are other findings seen in trisomy 21. Fetal growth restriction (FGR) may or may not be an associated finding.[8]

In trisomy 18, growth is usually restricted. CNS abnormalities associated with Edward syndrome are choroid plexus cyst, abnormal cisterna magna, absent corpus callosum, cerebellar hypoplasia, ventriculomegaly, strawberry-shaped calvarium, and neural tube defects. Skeletal abnormalities include limb reduction defects, overlapping index finger, clubbed feet, rocker bottom feet, and polydactyly. Facial defects seen are cleft lip and palate, micrognathia, low set ears, and microphthalmos. Cardiovascular abnormalities such as septal and valvular defects may be present. Gastrointestinal and genitourinary anomalies associated with this syndrome are omphalocele, diaphragmatic hernia, hydronephrosis, and horseshoe kidney. Umbilical cord cysts and double vessel umbilical cord may also be observed.[8]

Trisomy 13 is associated with growth restriction. CNS malformations such as holoprosencephaly, posterior fossa abnormalities, corpus callosum agenesis, ventriculomegaly, and neural tube defects may be seen. Skeletal abnormalities such as polydactyly and facial malformations such as cyclopia, midline facial clefts, anophthalmia, and hypoplastic nose are associated with Patau syndrome. CVS abnormalities such as septal defects, TOF, hypoplastic left ventricle, coarctation of aorta, echogenic intracardiac focus, and gastrointestinal malformations like omphalocele and genitourinary abnormalities such as polycystic kidneys, horseshoe kidney, enlarged echogenic kidney, and nuchal thickening may be observed.[8]

## Other Imaging Studies

- *3D ultrasound:* Other than the standard 2D ultrasound, 3D ultrasound allows multiplanar imaging and is an adjunct to the 2D ultrasound. In special situations such as fetal echocardiography, detection of cleft lip and cleft palate, and in skeletal abnormalities, its role is more certain.[2] Because of multiplanar imaging and rapid acquisition of volume data, more accurate information is possible like, for example, in the evaluation of the extent and size of anomaly.[15] It provides better comprehension of fetal anatomy especially for the patient. It is semimanual and partly dependent on operator skill, hence adequate training is required.
- *Magnetic resonance imaging (MRI):* It was first used in obstetrics in 1983. Its advantage lies in its ability to use multiple planes for reconstruction and a large field of view making the visualization of complicated anomalies easier. The development of single shot rapid acquisition sequence with refocused echoes and high quality $T_2$ weighted image provides excellent fetal imaging. This has obviated the need to sedate the mother or fetus. It is especially useful when ultrasound findings are inconclusive as in oligohydramnios, maternal obesity or when posterior cranial fossa is to be visualized where bone calcification hampers the ultrasonographic study. MRI has been used extensively in the diagnosis of ventriculomegaly, corpus callosum agenesis, posterior fossa abnormalities, cortical gyral malformation, hemorrhage, holoprosencephaly, arachnoid cyst, neural tube defects, and vascular malformations.[2]

## Detection of Fetal Deoxyribonucleic Acid and Fetal Cells in Maternal Circulation

A new area of research developed following the discovery of large amounts of circulating cell-free tumor DNA in plasma and serum from cancer patients. Reasoning that the rapidly growing fetus and placenta possessed tumor-like qualities, Lo et al. first demonstrated the presence of male fetal DNA sequences in maternal plasma and serum.[27] The results of subsequent studies by the same group showed surprisingly high mean concentrations of fetal DNA in maternal plasma. Significantly, more fetal DNA is present in the cell-free plasma (or serum) of pregnant women as compared with the fetal DNA extracted from the cellular fraction of maternal blood. Further investigations have focused on the clinical implications of this technique, specifically using real-time polymerase chain reaction (PCR) amplification assays for prenatal screening and diagnosis of pregnancy complications, and genetic disorders.

Fetal DNA analysis has the advantage of being rapid, reliable, reproducible, and easily carried out for a large number of samples. The majority of the cell-free fetal DNA in the maternal circulation probably originates from the placenta with an additional (minor) contribution from hematopoietic cells and possibly from the fetus itself via direct transfer. It comprises approximately 3–13% of the total cell-free DNA in maternal circulation and is cleared from maternal blood within hours of childbirth.

In countries where permissible, it is useful in fetal gender determination in women at high-risk of X-linked recessive disorders such as Duchenne muscular dystrophy, hemophilia, etc. or to decide continuation of steroid administration in women at risk of having fetus affected with congenital adrenal hyperplasia. Fetal RhD blood group is routinely being determined in pregnant women with RhD negative blood group. Detection of RhD gene in cell-free DNA from maternal plasma indicates fetal blood group to be RhD positive as RhD negative individual does not carry that gene.[28]

Recently, cell-free fetal DNA analysis has become clinically available to women at high-risk for fetal aneuploidy by technology known as massively parallel genomic sequencing.[29] It uses a highly sensitive assay to quantify millions of DNA fragments in biological samples in a span of days and has been reported to accurately detect trisomy 13, trisomy 18, and trisomy 21 as early as 10th week of pregnancy with results available approximately 1 week after maternal sampling. Several large-scale validation studies have demonstrated detection rates for fetal trisomy 13, trisomy 18, and trisomy 21 of >98% with very low false-positive rates (<0.5%). The American College of Obstetricians and Gynecologists has recommended that cell-free fetal DNA is one option that can be used as a primary screening test in women at increased risk of aneuploidy.[30] This includes women aged 35 years or older, fetuses with ultrasonographic findings that indicate an increased risk of aneuploidy, women with a history of a child affected with a trisomy, or a parent carrying a balanced Robertsonian translocation with increased risk of trisomy 13 or trisomy 21. It can also be used as a follow-up test for women with a positive first trimester or second trimester screening test result. Counseling regarding the limitation of cell-free fetal DNA testing should include a discussion that the screening test provides information regarding only trisomy 21 and trisomy 18 and in some laboratories trisomy 13.[31] It does not replace the precision obtained with diagnostic tests such as CVS and amniocentesis and currently does not offer other genetic information.[32] Other limitation of cell-free fetal DNA includes the lack of data for low-risk population and currently not recommended for low-risk women as well as in multifetal gestation.[33] In a small percentage of cases, a cell-free fetal DNA result will not be able to be obtained.

## SCREENING FOR FETAL CHROMOSOMAL ABNORMALITIES

On the basis of both observational studies and interventional projects, important recommendations as regards screening for fetal chromosomal abnormality are summarized as below:[31]

These recommendations and conclusions are based on good and consistent scientific evidence (Level A):

- Prenatal genetic screening (serum screening with or without NT ultrasound or cell-free DNA screening) and diagnostic testing (CVS or amniocentesis) options should be discussed and offered to all pregnant women regardless of maternal age or risk of chromosomal abnormality. After review and discussion, every patient has the right to pursue or decline prenatal genetic screening and diagnostic testing.
- If screening is accepted, pregnant women should have one prenatal screening approach, and should not have multiple screening tests performed simultaneously.
- Cell-free DNA is the most sensitive and specific screening test for the common fetal aneuploidies. Nevertheless, it has the potential for false-positive and false-negative results. Furthermore, cell-free DNA testing is not equivalent to diagnostic testing.
- All pregnant women should be offered a second-trimester ultrasound for fetal structural defects, since these may occur with or without fetal aneuploidy; ideally this is performed between 18 and 20 weeks of gestation.
- Pregnant women with a positive screening test result for fetal aneuploidy should undergo counseling and a comprehensive ultrasound evaluation with an opportunity for diagnostic testing to confirm results.
- Pregnant women with a negative screening test result should be made aware that this substantially decreases their risk of the targeted aneuploidy but does not ensure that the fetus is unaffected. The potential for a fetus to be affected by genetic disorders that are not evaluated by the screening or diagnostic test should also be reviewed. Even if women have a negative screening test result, they may choose diagnostic testing later in pregnancy, particularly if additional findings become evident such as fetal anomalies identified on ultrasound examination.
- Women whose cell-free DNA screening test results are not reported by the laboratory or are uninterpretable (a no-call test result) should be informed that test failure is associated with an increased risk of aneuploidy, receive further counseling and be offered comprehensive ultrasound evaluation and diagnostic testing.
- If an enlarged NT or an anomaly is identified on ultrasound examination, the patient should be offered counseling and diagnostic testing for genetic conditions as well as a comprehensive ultrasound evaluation including detailed USG at 18–20 weeks of gestation to assess for structural abnormalities.

## INVASIVE PRENATAL DIAGNOSTIC PROCEDURES

These are techniques to obtain samples which are of fetal origin and can be used for analysis to make a definite fetal diagnosis.

In presence of indications, the couple have to be counseled for an invasive test. Counseling has to encompass all aspects of the procedure such as the technique, the rate of complications especially that of pregnancy loss, the timing of results, and the management options available. The decision of going for the procedure is absolutely voluntary and written consent is mandatory. All the forms, i.e., Form D, E, F, and G need to be filled up duly as per Preconception and Prenatal Diagnostic Techniques (PCPNDT) Act.

## Amniocentesis

It is an invasive procedure where a needle is introduced into the amniotic cavity under sonographic guidance and amniotic fluid is withdrawn for analysis. The indications for amniocentesis are:

- Mother at high-risk of fetal aneuploidy:
  - Increased risk on first or second trimester screening for Down syndrome.
  - Ultrasound finding suggestive of major structural malformation.
  - One of the parents is a carrier of balanced chromosomal translocation.
- Fetus at high-risk of metabolic disorder:
  - A definite diagnosis was made in previous affected child.
  - Previous affected child may have a typical clinical presentation/investigations without a definite diagnosis.
- Fetus at risk of single gene disorder (autosomal recessive, autosomal dominant, and X-linked recessive disorder) where amniotic fluid can also be used for extracting DNA for diagnosis.
- RhD isoimmunized pregnancy management by spectrophotometric analysis of bilirubin in amniotic fluid and plotting of Liley's curve. Though, this is rarely practiced today in the light of availability of noninvasive technique like middle cerebral artery peak systolic velocity by Doppler flow.

Amniocentesis is done between 16 and 20 weeks of gestation. Technically, the procedure is easier to perform at this period of gestation since the uterus is accessible per abdomen and sufficient amount of amniotic fluid is available for withdrawing.

It is performed under aseptic precaution using a 20 G spinal needle. A preliminary sonography is performed to document the number of fetuses, the viability of the fetus, gestational age, placental localization, and liquor volume. A site which has sufficient liquor volume, and which is free of placenta or cord is chosen for needle insertion. Local anesthesia at puncture site is optional. A sterile transducer cover is put over the transducer and under sonographic vision, 20G needle is inserted into the amniotic cavity. The stylet is removed and fluid is aspirated by syringe **(Fig. 1)**.[16]

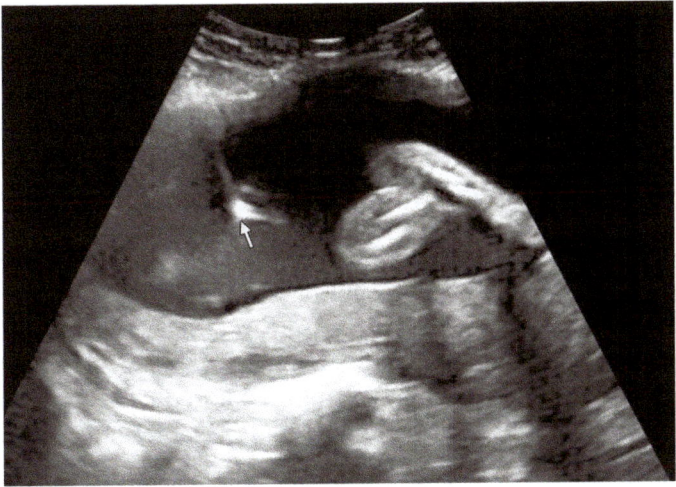

**Fig. 1:** Amniocentesis.

Initial 1–2 mL of fluid is discarded to prevent contamination of maternal cells. Using separate syringe of 10 mL volume, amniotic fluid is aspirated–1 mL/week of gestation being the upper limit of fluid aspirated and is transferred into centrifugation tubes.

Dry tap during amniocentesis is due to tenting of membranes. In such a situation needle should be withdrawn into the myometrium and reinserted with a forceful thrust to penetrate the membranes. The use of stylet with needle also helps to overcome the problem of tenting of membranes. The stylet is longer than the needle and by advancing the stylet 10 mm beyond the needle tip the membranes can be entered.[34] Following the procedure the fetal heart rate is checked and injection anti-D is given to Rh negative mothers. Postprocedure amniotic fluid leakage occurs in 0.2% cases but is usually self-limiting. Chorioamnionitis occurs in 1 in 1,000 procedures. The rate of pregnancy loss is as low as 0.3% in experienced hands.[13]

Early amniocentesis is performed between 11 and 14 weeks of gestation. The incidence of limb deformities, like talipes equinovarus is significantly high in early amniocentesis. It is seen in 0.75–1.7% cases. The miscarriage rate is 1.5%.[3] Hence, this procedure is not preferred. The Canadian Early and Mid-trimester Amniocentesis Trial (CEMAT) randomized 4,000 pregnant women for early and mid-trimester amniocentesis. The success rate of culture was 97.7% with an accuracy of 99.8% for early amniocentesis but there was higher rate of complications in form of fetal loss, increased incidence of talipes equinovarus, and postprocedural amniotic fluid leakage.[35-37]

Fetal cells obtained from amniotic fluid or CVS are cultured for chromosomal analysis called karyotype and DNA study. Rapid diagnosis of common fetal aneuploidies such as trisomy 13, 18, 21, and sex chromosomes is possible by techniques such as fluorescent in situ hybridization (FISH) and quantitative fluorescent-polymerase chain reaction (QF-PCR). Specific probes for FISH technique have been developed to detect numerical aberrations of metaphase chromosomes and interphase nuclei of nonmitotic cell.[16,38]

The limitations of rapid diagnostic techniques are that they fail to detect structural chromosomal aberrations such as translocation and inversion and in addition they miss out nearly half (47.4%) of the aneuploidies when compared to karyotyping.[39] However, more recent studies involving more than 2,000 women, both the sensitivity and specificity of FISH on uncultured amniocytes for detecting these chromosomal abnormalities were more than 99%. But there were both false-positive and negative reports. Further maternal cell contamination on uncultured cells remains a problem. Mosaicism and confined placental mosaicism (CPM) in chorionic villus samples are not identified accurately by FISH. The ACMG does not recommend management on basis of result of FISH alone. QF-PCR amplifies highly polymorphic short tandem repeats on chromosomes 13, 18, 21, X, and Y using fluorescent primers and PCR. This method is comparable to FISH in sensitivity but maternal cell contamination is more easily identified. Hence, it has replaced FISH for rapid aneuploidy screening in European countries.[38] Newer technologies are being developed like the array-based comparative genome hybridization (aCGH) or called chromosomal microarray. It has a high resolution, genome wide screening strategy for obtaining DNA copy number information in a single measurement. It is readily amendable to automation and is less labor intensive. It can identify deletion or duplication in the submicroscopic level. It fails to detect balanced chromosome rearrangements, alteration in ploidy levels such as triploidy and tetraploidy, and mosaicism necessitating further diagnostic tests like karyotyping.[39] Increasing role of aCGH in prenatal diagnosis has been realized and recommended especially in case of fetal abnormality detected on ultrasound with normal chromosomal study.

## Chorionic Villus Sampling

This procedure is carried out between 11 and 14 weeks of gestation. It can be performed by transabdominal or transvaginal route. The indication of CVS is essentially the same as amniocentesis except for a few conditions which require either amniotic fluid or placental tissue for analysis.[3] The advantage of CVS is that the results are available earlier hence providing enough time for medical termination of pregnancy if needed. The complications of these two procedures are similar.

### Transcervical Chorionic Villus Sampling

This procedure is performed using a polyethylene catheter of 5.7 F diameter and 27 cm length. The cervix and placenta are visualized by transabdominal sonography and the catheter is introduced through the cervix along the uterine wall to reach the placental tissue till its distal end. The stylet is removed and 20 cc syringe containing 5 mL tissue culture fluid is attached to the catheter. Suction is applied as the catheter is gradually withdrawn.[40] This allows placental tissue aspiration into the syringe. If material obtained is inadequate, then another two attempts are permitted with fresh catheters.[41] This route is rarely used because of higher miscarriage rate of 3.7% compared to mid-trimester amniocentesis.[16]

### Transabdominal Chorionic Villus Sampling

There are two techniques of transabdominal CVS. The two needle method recommended by Smidt Jensen and Hahnemann utilizes an outer needle as trocar to pierce the maternal skin, uterine myometrium, and the placenta. A thinner needle is passed through it into the placental tissue. This technique allows reinsertion in case the tissue sample is inadequate and also prevents maternal contamination.[42]

The single needle technique proposed by Brambati[43] is the commonly preferred method for CVS. An 18 G spinal needle is inserted percutaneously into the placenta under sonographic vision. The stylet is removed, and contents are aspirated into a 20 mL syringe containing 5 mL of media. The needle is moved backward and forward in the placental tissue for a few times to obtain adequate amount of tissue **(Fig. 2)**. Skin infiltration with local anesthetic is required to be given at the needle insertion site.

The cytogenetic analysis is similar to amniocentesis. Chorionic villus has four different type of tissues— (1) cytotrophoblast, (2) mesenchyme, (3) fetal blood vessels, and (4) fetal blood. Cytotrophoblast can be analyzed by "rapid prep" between 24 and 48 hours because of presence of spontaneous mitosis in these cells. Mesenchymal cells need culturing and hence tissue analysis takes 5–10 days' time, but the result is more reliable. Sometimes, there is a discrepancy between the placental and fetal tissue which could be either due to contamination by maternal cells or due to CPM. In CPM, the normal euploid chromosome is found along with abnormal cell line in the placental tissue, although the fetus may have normal karyotype. In such a situation amniocentesis is done to confirm fetal karyotype.

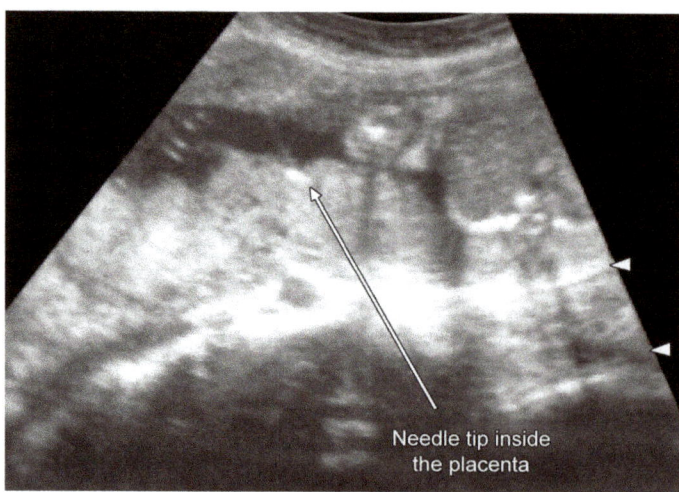

**Fig. 2:** Chorionic villus sampling.

Mosaicism is identified in 1% of CVS samples and the abnormal cell line is confirmed in 10–40% of these fetuses.[40] The complication of these procedures is vaginal spotting, bleeding or leakage of fluid which occurs in 7–10% of cases performed transvaginally and 1% of cases performed transabdominally. Miscarriage rate is 0.5%. Procedure related fetal malformations such as limb reduction defects and oromandibular hypoplasia is seen if CVS is performed below 9 weeks. Hence early CVS has been abandoned now.[40]

## Fetal Blood Sampling

- Percutaneous umbilical blood sampling or cordocentesis.
- Intrahepatic vessel sampling.
- Fetal cardiac sampling.

### Percutaneous Umbilical Blood Sampling or Cordocentesis

This procedure is done under real time ultrasonographic guidance. Preprocedure antibiotics prophylaxis may be given, and antenatal corticosteroid is administered in preterm fetuses 24 hours prior to the procedure. The free-hand technique of sampling uses a 20–22 G spinal needle of length around 15 cm to pierce the umbilical vein at relatively fixed segment of the cord near its insertion into the placenta **(Fig. 3)**. In this method, the needle is free to move in all directions and hence the chances of injury to cord and other structures are more. In the other technique, a fixed needle guide is attached to the ultrasound transducer through which a 22–25 G needle is introduced. The predicted path of needle appears on screen and allows prior selection of sample site. Lateral movement of the needle is not possible.[44,45] In both methods umbilical vein is punctured, and the blood obtained is tested for its fetal origin. The acid dilution test of Loendersloot distinguishes maternal from fetal blood. When fetal blood is added to 0.1 M potassium hydroxide it turns pink, while if maternal blood is added it turns brown. In addition, the mean corpuscular volume of fetal blood can be measured which is >100 fl and are larger than maternal red blood cell (RBC).[45] After confirming the fetal origin of blood, the sample collected in sterile heparin tube is sent for karyotyping. Postprocedure the puncture site is monitored for bleeding.

### Fetal Intrahepatic Vessel Sampling

In this procedure intrahepatic vessels are sampled. This procedure is opted when cordocentesis is difficult to perform or is unsuccessful **(Fig. 4)**. It is rarely used nowadays. Fetal hepatic necrosis is a known complication.[46]

### Fetal Cardiac Blood Sampling

Fetal blood sampling by cardiac puncture is used when other methods fail to provide a sample. It is an easy procedure and

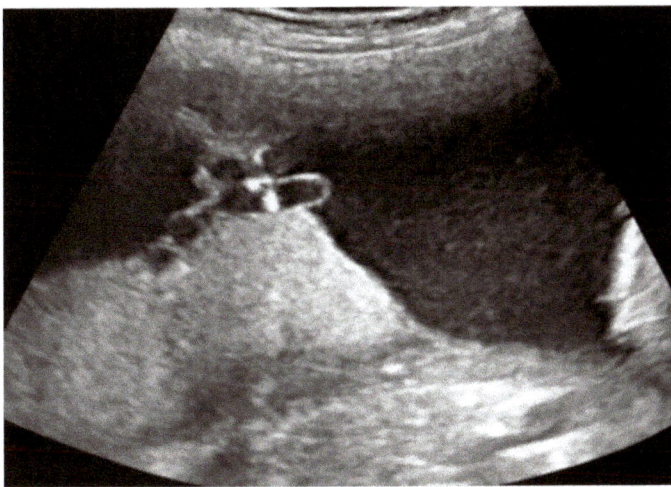

**Fig. 3:** Cordocentesis.

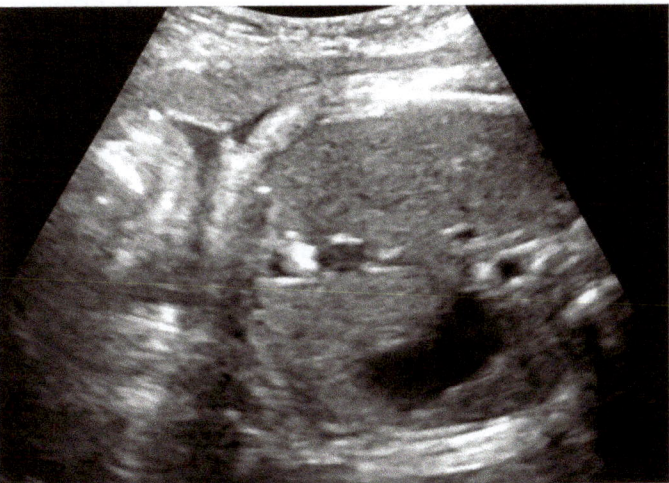

**Fig. 4:** Intrahepatic cordocentesis.

is quite safe. This route can also be utilized for emergency fetal blood transfusion like in case of postprocedural fetal bleed or for performing feticide.[46]

The results of karyotype analysis from fetal blood is available earlier than any other fetal sample. Blood obtained from cordocentesis can also be analyzed for fetal single gene disorder, fetal infection, fetal RhD analysis, for assessment of fetal anemia and need for transfusion in Rh incompatibility, immunologic thrombocytopenias, and coagulopathies.[45,46] The complications are cord vessel bleeding (50%), cord hematoma (17%), fetomaternal hemorrhage (66%), intrauterine death (1.4%).[45,46] Fetal loss is more when concurrent fetal pathology such as growth restriction and hydrops fetalis is present.

## Fetal Tissue Biopsy

Biopsy of fetal skin, liver, and muscle is performed under sonographic or fetoscopic visualization. Tissue is analyzed by electron microscopy or by biochemical analysis. Conditions such as muscular dystrophy, mitochondrial myopathy and skin disorders like epidermolysis bullosa can be diagnosed by this procedure.[46] With availability of molecular testing fetal tissue sampling is abandoned now.

## Fetoscopy

It is done through an endoscope which allows fetal inspection for structural anomalies and allows fetal blood sampling and tissue biopsy.

It is a technique of direct visualization of the fetus using a small bore fiberoptic endoscope. The trocar of the fetoscope measures 2.2 mm in diameter and the scope measures 1.7 mm in diameter.[13] In the first trimester embryofetoscopy, a 0.8 mm fiberoptic endoscope, and a 27 G needle are passed through a 16 G double barrel instrument sheath. It is passed transabdominally into the extracelomic or amniotic cavity. Study of morphology of the embryo-fetus and fetal blood sampling are its major clinical applications.[47] The drawback of fetoscopy is narrow field of vision and limited view of the small parts of the fetus because of short focal length. Scopes small enough to go through the shaft of a 20 G needle have been developed but vision is hampered because of diminished intensity of light.[13]

## Summary of Recommendations and Conclusions of ACOG Practice Bulletin No. 88[48]

### Invasive Prenatal Testing for Aneuploidy

The following recommendation is based on good and consistent scientific evidence (Level A):
- Early amniocentesis (at <15 weeks of gestation) should not be performed because of the higher risk of pregnancy loss and complications compared with traditional amniocentesis (15 weeks of gestation or later).

The following conclusions are based on limited or inconsistent scientific evidence (Level B):
- Amniocentesis at 15 weeks of gestation or later is safe procedure. The procedure-related loss rate after mid-trimester amniocentesis is <1 in 300–500.
- In experienced hands and centers, CVS procedure-related loss rates may be the same as those for amniocentesis.

The following recommendations and conclusions are based primarily on consensus and expert opinion (Level C):
- Invasive diagnostic testing for aneuploidy should be available to all women, regardless of maternal age.
- Patients with an increased risk of fetal aneuploidy include women with a previous fetus or child with an autosomal trisomy or sex chromosome abnormality, one major or at least two minor fetal structural defects identified by USG, either parent with a chromosomal translocation or chromosomal inversion or parental aneuploidy.
- Nondirective counseling before prenatal diagnostic testing does not require a patient to commit to pregnancy termination if the result is abnormal.[47]

## Preimplantation Diagnosis

It is a technique of diagnosing genetic abnormalities before the pregnancy is formally established. It has been used in couples who are carriers of balanced translocations. It has also been used for diagnosis of X-linked disorder or single gene disorder.

Preimplantation diagnosis is done during in vitro fertilization procedures wherein the gametes or the cells from an embryo are biopsied for genetic analysis. The oocyte is tested indirectly by analyzing the first polar body. It is removed by micromanipulation technique and subjected to DNA analysis or chromosomal study. The disadvantage of this procedure is that it is an indirect analysis and it can be used only for maternal carriers. Furthermore recombination will occur if defective gene lies away from the centromere making result indeterminate. Contamination with the cumulus cells can lead to error in diagnosis.

Sperm sorting techniques using molecular probes tagged with laser activated dye has been used followed by separation techniques like flow cytometry. But, this method can cause considerable damage to the sperm.[13]

The most successful method of preimplantation diagnosis is biopsy of single cell from embryo at the eight-cell stage or blastocyst stage. The eight-cell stage embryo have independent cells and a single cell can be removed without damage to the neighboring cells because at this stage, cells do not develop gap junctions and are less adherent. But the drawback of this technique is that the cells are large hence difficult to remove, contamination can occur by sperm or cumulus cells and there is short-time for analysis of results since successful implantation depends on early transfer of embryo.[13]

Blastomere biopsy is performed 5 days following fertilization at the 120-cell stage. It contains mainly trophoblastic cells but the inner cell mass that forms the embryo is clearly demarcated at this stage. The cells are biopsied after mechanical disruption of the zona or after spontaneous hatching. The advantages are that more number of cells are available for analysis and they are well-differentiated. The disadvantage is that there is increased risk of damage to the inner cell mass due to greater adherence of the cells to each other and there is limited incubation time. The trophectoderm may not always be similar to the fetus in karyotype and biochemical status. The role of preimplantation diagnosis at present is limited.[13]

## KEY POINTS

- Prenatal screening procedures are noninvasive methods whereas the diagnostic procedures are usually invasive. The ACOG and ACMG guidelines recommend all pregnant women should be informed for fetal chromosomal aneuploidy.

- The noninvasive prenatal screening procedures are a combination of maternal serum assays and fetal sonographic evaluation.
- The first trimester combined screening measures fetal NT and maternal serum markers PAPP-A and β-hCG and in association with maternal age provides a risk estimate.
- The second trimester screening traditionally called the quadruple screening measures MSAFP, hCG, uE3, and inhibin-A; and calculates relative risk of trisomy 18 and 21 in association with maternal age.
- Combined first and second trimester screening has higher detection rate than individual screening. A positive result has to be confirmed by a diagnostic invasive procedure. If a pregnant woman presents early in pregnancy for antenatal care, that is before 14 weeks of gestation then integrated or sequential or contingent screening should be offered while if she presents after 14 weeks, then second trimester screening procedures should be recommended.
- Detection of cell free fetal DNA in maternal circulation has revolutionized prenatal screening with a very high detection rate and a low false-positive rate for common trisomies and is recommended for high-risk women. Its use in low-risk population is still debatable.
- Invasive methods of prenatal diagnosis such as CVS, amniocentesis, percutaneous umbilical blood sampling, etc. provide embryonic or extraembryonic tissue for chromosomal, genetic, or biochemical analysis. The techniques used for analysis of fetal material are PCR, FISH, aCGH or karyotyping of cultured fetal cells. Mutation study on DNA and biochemical analysis is also possible. While rapid aneuploidy tests such as FISH and QF-PCR provide an early report, they have higher rate of false-positive and negative results. Traditional karyotyping gives more accurate results.
- Preimplantation diagnosis is an invasive method of diagnosis of fetal disease before the formal establishment of pregnancy. Hence, it offers a choice to differentiate the healthy embryos from unhealthy ones and pick up the healthy embryos for embryo transfer.

## REFERENCES

1. Cunningham GF, Gant FN, Levino KJ, Gillstrap LC, Hauth GC, Welstrom KD. Prenatal diagnosis and fetal therapy. In: William's Obstetrics, 22nd edition. New York: McGraw Hill; 2005. pp. 313-39.
2. ACOG Committee on Practice Bulletins. ACOG Practice Bulletin No. 77: screening for fetal chromosomal abnormalities. Obstet Gynecol. 2007;109(1):217-27.
3. Palomaki GE, Lee JE, Canick JA, McDowell GA, Donnenfeld AE. Technical standards and guidelines: prenatal screening for Down syndrome that includes first-trimester biochemistry and/or ultrasound measurements. Genet Med. 2009;11(9):669-81.
4. Melon FD. Sonographic and first trimester detection of aneuploidy. In: Queenan JT, Hopkins JC, Spong CY (Eds). Protocol for High Risk Pregnancy, 4th edition. New Jersey: Blackwell publishing; 2005. pp. 75-88.
5. Nicolaides KH. Nuchal translucency and other first trimester sonographic markers of chromosomal abnormalities. Am J Obstet Gynecol. 2004;191(1):45-67.
6. Said S, Malone FD. The use of nuchal translucency in contemporary obstetric practice. Clin Obstet Gynecol. 2008;51(1):37-47.
7. Robyr R, Ville Y. First-trimester screening for fetal abnormalities. In: James DK, Weiner CP, Steer PJ, Gonik B (Eds). High Risk Pregnancy—Management Options, 3rd edition. Netherlands: Elsiever 2006. pp. 138-56.
8. Holmgren C, Lacoursiere DY. The use of prenatal ultrasound in the detection of fetal aneuploidy. Clin Obstet Gynecol. 2008;51(1):48-61.
9. Bekker MN, Twist JW, van Vugt JM. Reproducibility of fetal nasal bone length measurement. J Ultrasound Med. 2004;23(12):1613-8.
10. Spencer K, Spencer CE, Power M, Dawson C, Nicolaides KH. Screening for chromosomal abnormalities in the first trimester using ultrasound and maternal serum biochemistry in a one-stop clinic: a review of three years prospective experience. BJOG. 2003;110(3):281-6.
11. Malone F, Wald NJ, Canick JA, Ball RH. First and second trimester evaluation of risk (FASTER) trial principle result of the NICHD multicenter down syndrome screening study. Am J Obstet Gynecol. 2003;189(6):S56.
12. Wald NJ, Rodeck C, Hackshaw AK, Walters J, Chitty L, Mackinson AM. First and second trimester antenatal screening for Down syndrome: the result of Serum, Urine, Ultrasound screening study (SURUSS). J Med Screen. 2003;10(2):56-104.
13. Ward K. Genetics and Prenatal diagnosis. In: Scott JR, Gibbs RS, Karlan BY, Haney AF (Eds). Danforth's Obstetrics and Gynaecology, 9th edition. Philadelphia: Lippincott Williams and Wilkins; 2003. pp. 105-28.
14. Wapner R, Thom E, Simpson JL, Pergament E, Silver R, Filkins K, et al. First trimester screening of trisomy 21 and 18. N Engl J Med. 2003;349(15):1405-13.
15. Yeo L, Vintzileous AM. Second trimester screening for fetal abnormalities. In: James PK, Weiner CP, Steer PJ, Gonik B (Eds). High Risk Pregnancy—Management Options, 3rd edition. Netherlands: Elsiever; 2006. pp. 157-89.
16. Wimalasundera RC. Fetal medicine in clinical practice. In: Edmonds KD (Ed). Dewhurst's Textbook of Obstetrics and Gynaecology, 7th edition. New Jersey: Blackwell publishing; 2007. pp. 132-44.
17. Lo NS, Leung PM, Lau KC, Yeung CY. Congenital cardiovascular malformations in Chinese children with Down's syndrome. Chin Med J (Engl). 1989;102(5):382-6.
18. Goldstein WB. Aberrant right subclavian artery in mongolism. Am J Roentgenol Radium Ther Nucl Med. 1965;95:131-4.
19. Edwards JE. Malformations of the aortic arch system manifested as vascular rings. Lab Invest. 1953;2(1):56-75.
20. Zapata H, Edwards JE, Titus JL. Aberrant right subclavian artery with left aortic-arch: associated cardiac anomalies. Pediatr Cardiol. 1993;14(3):159-61.
21. Raider L. Aberrant right subclavian artery. South Med J. 1967;60(2):145-51.

22. Nguyen KT, Vas W, Zylak CJ. Diagnosis of an aberrant right subclavian artery on CT. J Comput Tomogr. 1981;5(1):38-40.
23. Hara M, Satake M, Itoh M, Ogino H, Shiraki N, Taniguchi H, Shibamoto Y. Radiographic findings of aberrant right subclavian artery initially depicted on CT. Radiat Med. 2003;21(4):161-5.
24. Chaoui R, Heling KS, Sarioglu N, Schwabe M, Dankof A, Bollmann R. Aberrant right subclavian artery as a new cardiac sign in second- and third-trimester fetuses with Down syndrome. Am J Obstet Gynecol. 2005;192(1):257-63.
25. Saller DN Jr, Canick JA. Current methods of prenatal screening for Down syndrome and other fetal abnormalities. Clin Obstet Gynecol. 2008;51(1):24-36.
26. Nicolaides KH, Snijders RJ, Gosden C, Berry C, Campbell S. Ultrasonographically detectable markers of fetal chromosomal abnormalities. Lancet. 1992;340(8821):704-7.
27. Lo YM, Corbetta N, Chamberlain PF, Rai V, Sargent IL, Redman CW, et al. Presence of fetal DNA in maternal plasma and serum. Lancet. 1997;350(9076):485-7.
28. Lo YM, Hjelm NM, Fidler C, Sargent IL, Murphy MF, Chamberlain PF, et al. Prenatal diagnosis of fetal RhD status by molecular analysis of maternal plasma. N Engl J Med. 1998;339(24):1734-8.
29. Palomaki GE, Kloza EM, Lambert-Messerlian GM, Haddow JE, Neveux LM, Ehrich M, et al. DNA sequencing of maternal plasma to detect Down syndrome: an international clinical validation study. Genet Med. 2011;13(11):913-20.
30. American College of Obstetricians and Gynecologists Committee on Genetics. Committee Opinion No. 545: Noninvasive prenatal testing for fetal aneuploidy. Obstet Gynecol. 2012;120(6):1532-4.
31. American College of Obstetricians and Gynecologists' Committee on Practice Bulletins—Obstetrics; Committee on Genetics; Society for Maternal-Fetal Medicine. Screening for fetal chromosomal abnormalities: ACOG Practice Bulletin, number 226. Obstet Gynecol. 2020;136(4):e48-69.
32. Wilson KL, Czerwinski JL, Hoskovec JM, Noblin SJ, Sullivan CM, Harbison A, et al. NSGC practice guideline: prenatal screening and diagnostic testing options for chromosome aneuploidy. J Genet Couns. 2013;22(1):4-15.
33. Bianchi DW, Parker RL, Wentworth J, Madankumar R, Saffer C, Das AF, et al. DNA sequencing versus standard prenatal aneuploidy screening. N Engl J Med. 2014;370(9):799-808.
34. Perni CS, Chervenak FA. Amniocentesis. Apuzzio JJ, Vintzeleous AM, Iffy L (Eds). Operative Obstetrics, 3rd edition. UK: Taylor Francis; 2006. pp. 57-63.
35. Randomised trial to assess safety and fetal outcome of early and midtrimester amniocentesis. The Canadian Early and Midtrimester Amniocentesis Trial Group (CEMAT). Lancet. 1998;351(9098):242-47.
36. Winsor EJ, Tomkins DJ, Kalousek D, Farrell S, Wyatt P, Fan YS, et al. Cytogenetic aspects of the Canadian Early and Mid-trimester Amniocentesis Trial (CEMAT). Prenat Diagn. 1999;19(7):620-7.
37. Johnson JM, Wilson RD, Singer J, Winsor E, Harman C, Armson BA, et al. Technical factors in amniocentesis predict worse outcome. Results of the Canadian Early (EA) versus Mid-trimester Amniocentesis Trial. Prenat Diagn. 1999;19(8):732-8.
38. South ST, Chen Z, Brothman AR. Genomic medicine in prenatal diagnosis. Clin Obstet Gynecol. 2008;51(1):62-73.
39. Leung WC, Lau ET, Lau WL, Tang R, Wong SF, Lau TK, et al. Rapid aneuploidy testing (knowing less) versus traditional karyotyping (knowing more) for advanced maternal age: What would be missed, who should decide? Hong Kong Med J. 2008;14(1):6-13.
40. Wapner RJ. Chorionic villus sampling. In: Queenan JT, Hopkins JC, Spong CY (Eds). Protocol for High Risk Pregnancy, 4th edition. New Jersey: Blackwell Publishing; 2005. pp. 119-24.
41. Trauffer PML, Silverman NS, Wapner RJ. Chorionic villus sampling. In: Apuzzio JJ, Vintzeleous AM, Iffy L (Eds). Operative Obstetrics, 3rd edition. UK: Taylor & Francis Books India Pvt Ltd; 2006;41-5.
42. Smidt Jensen S, Hahnemann N, Jensen PKA. Experience with the needle biopsy in first trimester: an alternative to amniocentesis. Clin Genet. 1984;26;272.
43. Brambati B, Oldrini A, Lanzani A. Transabdominal chorionic villus sampling: a free hand ultrasound–guided technique. Am J Obstet Gynecol. 1987;157(1):134-7.
44. Ghidini A, Locatelli A. Fetal blood sampling. In: Queenan JT, Hopkins JC, Spong CY (Eds). Protocol for High Risk Pregnancy, 4th edition. New Jersey: Blackwell Publishing; 2005. pp. 134-39.
45. Weiner CP. Cordocentesis. In: Apuzzio JJ, Vintzeleous AM, Iffy L (Eds). Operative Obstetrics, 3rd edition. UK: Taylor & Francis; 2006. pp. 121-35.
46. Hunter A, Soothill P. Invasive procedure for antenatal diagnosis. In: James PK, Weiner CP, Steer PJ, Gonik B (Eds). High Risk Pregnancy—Management Options, 3rd edition. Netherland: Elseiver; 2006. pp. 209-24.
47. Reece EA, Vintzileous AM. First trimester embryofetoscopy. In: Apuzzio JJ, Vintzeleous AM, Iffy L (Eds). Operative Obstetrics, 3rd edition. UK: Taylor & Francis; 2006. pp. 33-39.
48. American College of Obstetricians and Gynecologists. ACOG Practice Bulletin No. 88, December 2007. Invasive prenatal testing for aneuploidy. Obstet Gynecol. 2007;110(6):1459-67.

# CHAPTER 3

# Screening and Management of Congenital Anomalies

*Manisha Kumar, Shivangi Shanker Srivastava*

## INTRODUCTION

An expecting mother always expects a normal child at birth, however, 15% of conceptuses abort spontaneously, 1% are stillborn; 3% of live births, and 20-30% of stillbirths have a major congenital malformation, about 10% have minor defects and 0.7% of neonates have multiple congenital malformations. Cardiovascular defects are the most common birth defects with an incidence of 10/1,000 births. Central nervous system defects are next common and seen in 8-10/1,000 births. Gastrointestinal and renal anomalies are seen in 4/1,000 births each. The causes of congenital malformation are listed in **Table 1**.[1]

Majority of birth defects occur in families with no prior history of birth defect. Prenatal screening for only high-risk women fails to recognize most of the affected fetuses. Therefore, all antenatal women should be counseled and offered screening tests to identify fetal anomalies.

## FIRST TRIMESTER SCREENING

### Ultrasonography

Most fetal structures can be visualized at 12-13 weeks and this gestational age offers earliest opportunity to screen for fetal anomaly.

### Objectives of First Trimester Screening

- *Identification of viable pregnancy:* Chances of miscarriage are around 2% after 14 weeks, if a viable pregnancy is identified at this stage.[2]
- *Dating:* In a normal pregnancy, gestational sac is always visible by 5 weeks by transvaginal sonography. Fetal heart is present by 7 weeks. Gestational age should not be altered, if discrepancy between the last menstrual period and crown rump length (CRL) measurement is less than 7 days.
- *Detecting multiple pregnancies and determining chorionicity:* Twin pregnancy comprises 2% of all pregnancies. The first trimester is the best time to determine chorionicity. Characteristic USG finding in dichorionic twin is lambda sign[3] **(Fig. 1)**, which is most accurately determined at 11-14 weeks as amnion and chorion have not fused yet.[4] In monochorionic twin pregnancy, there is no layer of chorion between the two layers of amnion therefore 'T' sign is seen instead of lambda sign **(Fig. 2)**.
- *Assessment of general fetal anatomy:*
  - *Central nervous system:* From 9 weeks onward the falx, lateral ventricles, and echogenic choroid plexus are visible. From 14 weeks cerebellum and thalami are seen. Choroid plexus cysts, if present in isolation are not known to be associated with fetal chromosomal anomalies.[3]
  - *Heart:* The position, axis, and four chamber view can be appreciated at 12-14 weeks. Women with increased nuchal translucency (NT) are at increased

| TABLE 1: Causes of congenital malformations.[1] | |
| --- | --- |
| Malformations | Percentage |
| Unknown | 51% |
| Multifactorial/familial | 20.8% |
| Chromosomal abnormalities | 11% |
| Environmental | 3.4% |
| Single gene defect | 1.6% |

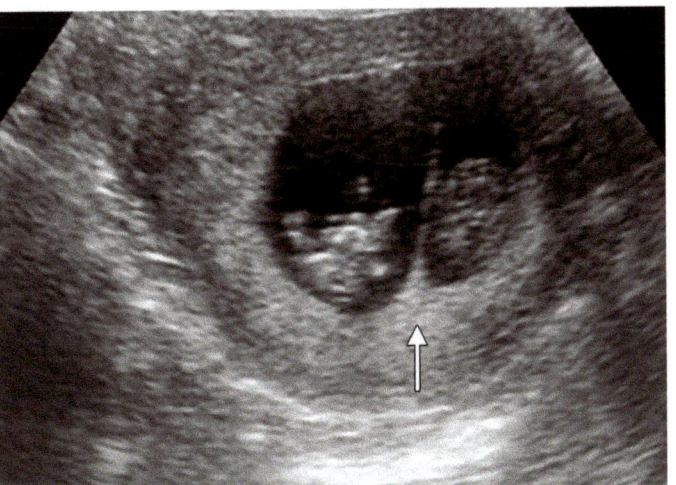

**Fig. 1:** Dichorionic twin pregnancy showing "lambda" sign.

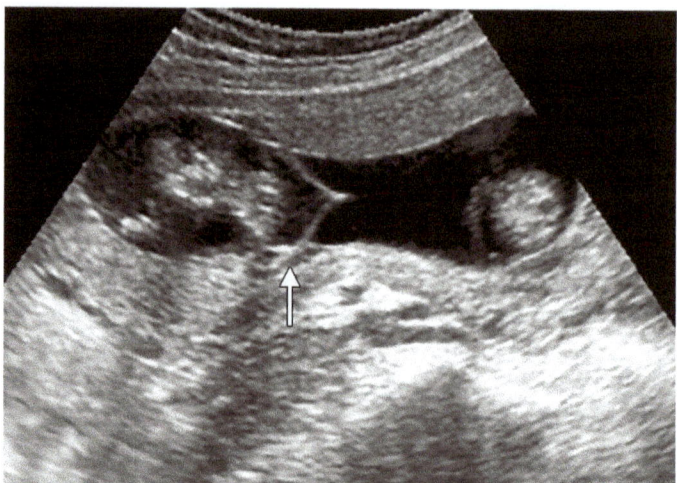

Fig. 2: Monochorionic twin pregnancy showing "T" sign.

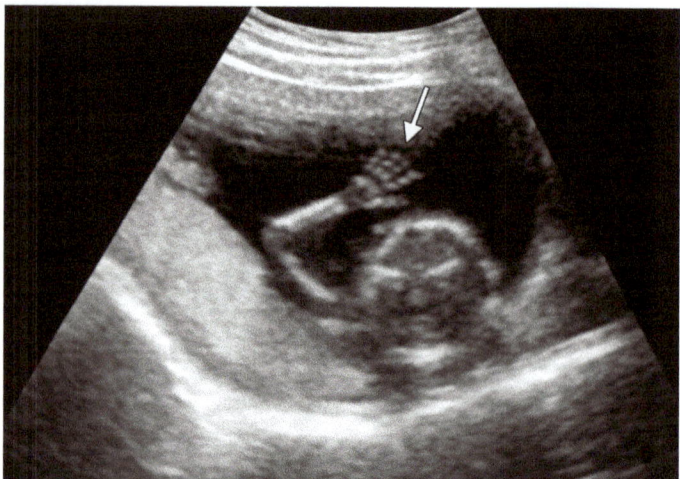

Fig. 3: All five digits are clearly visible.

risk for cardiac anomaly.[5] Hypoplastic left heart can be diagnosed in the first trimester.
- *Stomach*: Stomach bubble can be seen in all cases by 12–13 weeks.
- *Abdominal wall*: Physiologic hernia of midgut into umbilical cord is a normal feature in early pregnancy but is not normal after 12 weeks.
- *Kidneys and bladder*: In sagittal section, the long axis of bladder is less than 6 mm in the first trimester. Kidneys appear as echogenic structure in the first trimester.
- *Skeleton*: All long bones are similar in size at 11–14 weeks, ranging from 6 mm at 11 weeks to 13 mm at 14 weeks. Lethal defects, such as anencephaly, can be diagnosed in the first trimester. Digits can be clearly visualized **(Fig. 3)**.
- *Nuchal translucency*: It is the USG visualization of physiologic collection of fluid in the skin behind the fetal neck at 11–14 weeks **(Fig. 4)**.
  Nuchal translucency normally increases with CRL.[6] It is important to consider gestational age while deciding whether NT is normal or increased. The chance of cardiac defects increases with increase in NT (see Chapter 1 for details of NT measurement).
- *Fetal nasal bone*: Nasal bone is not visualized on USG between 11 and 14 weeks in 60% of fetuses with trisomy 21 and in only 3% of chromosomally normal fetus.[5]

### Three-dimensional USG

It has the advantage of minimizing the actual scanning time for diagnosing anomalies in the first trimester. As it is easy to get the sagittal view, therefore NT can be measured easily.

### ■ SECOND TRIMESTER SCREENING

### Biochemical Screening

*Maternal serum alpha-fetoprotein for neural tube defects:* It was recognized in 1972 that in many pregnancies the open

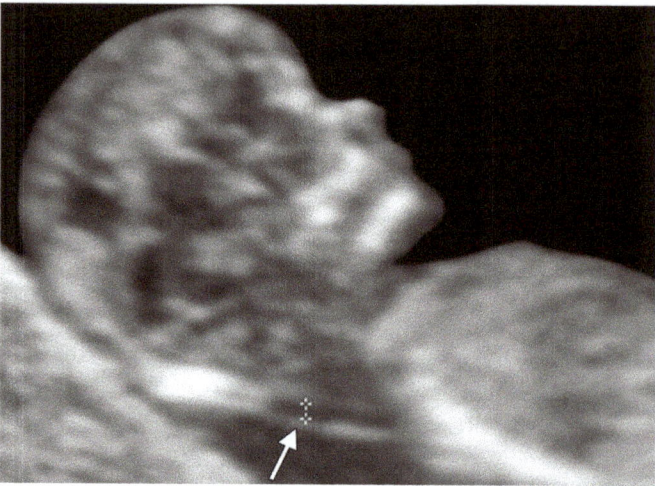

Fig. 4: Sagittal view of a 12-week fetus, showing nuchal translucency and nasal bone.

neural tube defects (NTD) could be detected at 16 weeks gestation by assay of a protein in maternal serum known as alpha-fetoprotein (AFP). The AFP is the fetal equivalent of albumin and is the major protein in fetal blood. If the fetus has an open NTD, the level of AFP is elevated in both amniotic fluid and maternal serum as a result of leakage from the open defect.

Unfortunately, maternal serum AFP is neither 100% sensitive nor specific. The curves for the levels of AFP in normal and affected pregnancies overlap so that in practice an arbitrary cutoff level is introduced below which no further action needs to be taken. This is usually either 95th centile or 2.5 multiples of median and as a result 75% of screened open spina bifida cases are detected. The pregnant women with AFP level above this arbitrary cut-off levels are offered detailed USG. AFP levels might be raised in conditions other than NTD; which are enumerated in **Table 2**.

Despite these limitations prenatal maternal serum AFP screening has been implemented widely and is one of the main factors, which has led to striking decline in incidence of open NTD.

**TABLE 2:** Conditions other than neural tube defects (NTD) associated with increased and decreased levels of AFP.

| Increased levels of AFP | Decreased levels of AFP |
| --- | --- |
| • Multifetal gestation<br>• Oligohydramnios<br>• Chorioangioma of placenta<br>• Renal anomalies—polycystic kidney<br>• Separate sacrococcygeal teratoma with fetal death<br>• Abdominal wall defects<br>• Underestimated gestational age<br>• Urinary obstruction<br>• Cystic hygroma<br>• Chromosomal trisomies | • Gestational trophoblastic disease<br>• Increased maternal weight |

**BOX 1:** Soft markers.[7,8]
- Nuchal thickening
- Echogenic cardiac focus
- Pyelectasis
- Echogenic bowel
- Short long bones
- Absent/hypoplastic nasal bones
- Single umbilical artery
- Ventriculomegaly
- Choroid plexus cyst
- Aberrant right subclavian artery

## Second Trimester USG Scan

The sensitivity and detection of the anomaly depends upon the skill of the observer and the gestational age at the time of scan, as many abnormalities appear later in the gestational age and some disappear with advancing gestation. In the low-risk women, the USG helps in excluding anomaly and detecting normal features. Genetic sonography is offered to high-risk women and has a sensitivity of 50–93%.

There are two types of sonographic markers that are suggestive of aneuploidy:
1. Major structural abnormalities.
2. *Soft markers:* These are nonspecific, transient, easily detectable, and nonpathological markers which may be associated with chromosomal anomalies although these may be present normally also. Various ultrasonographic soft markers are enumerated in **Box 1**.

The examination starts with the examination of fetal head.

### Intracranial Anatomy

- *Transventricular view:* This plane includes visualization of anterior and posterior portion of lateral ventricle and cavum septum pellucidum (CSP). Lateral ventricle is measured through atrium and is normally < 10 mm. CSP is visible at around 16 weeks and obliterates near term.
- *Transthalamic view:* Biparietal diameter is taken at this level, measured from outer margin to inner margin.

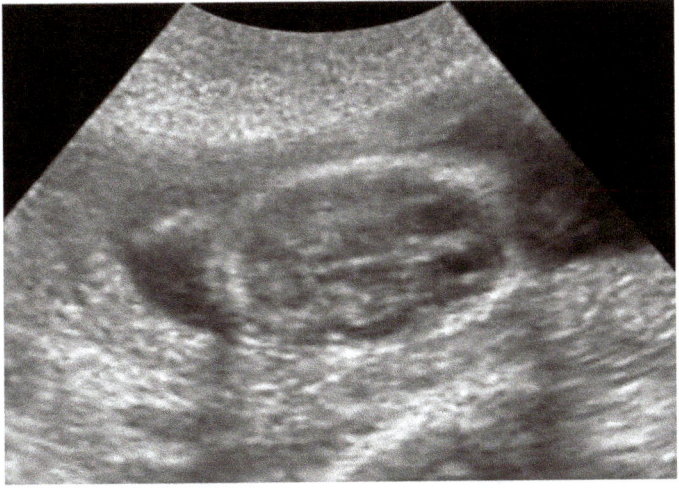

**Fig. 5:** Intracranial anatomy in transcerebellar view.

Head circumference is measured at the outer margin. Observation about mineralization is made whether adequate or not, and about the shape whether elliptical or otherwise.

- *Transcerebellar view:* Cerebellum is visualized and measured. Its measurement is not affected by fetal growth restriction and can be used to assess the exact gestational age. Cisterna magna is seen behind the cerebellum **(Fig. 5)**.

*Nuchal fold:* It is the skin thickness in the posterior aspect of fetal neck. A nuchal fold is measured in transverse section of fetal head at the level of CSP and thalami and angled posterior to include the cerebellum. The measurement is taken from outer edge of occipital bone to outer skin limit directly in the midline. The nuchal fold thickness of more than 6 mm is considered significant between 18 and 24 weeks and a measurement of more than 5 mm considered significant at 16–18 weeks. A thickened nuchal fold should be distinguished from cystic hygroma in which the skin in this area is filled with fluid-filled locculations. A thickened nuchal fold should not be confused with NT, which is a specific measurement of fluid in the posterior aspect of neck at 11–14 weeks of gestation. Increased nuchal fold thickness signifies increased risk of aneuploidy, single gene disorders, and congenital cardiac defects in the fetus.

*Face:* It is important in the diagnosis of genetic disorders and syndromes. Important structures visualized are the orbits, its diameter and distance between them, nose, lips, palate, chin and the ears.

*Spine:* It is imaged in coronal, transverse, and sagittal views. In transverse view, the vertebral segment normally consists of three echogenic ossification centers, two posterolateral and one in midline anteriorly. Normally, they lie in symmetrical triangular configuration. Splaying of these ossifications centers indicate NTD.

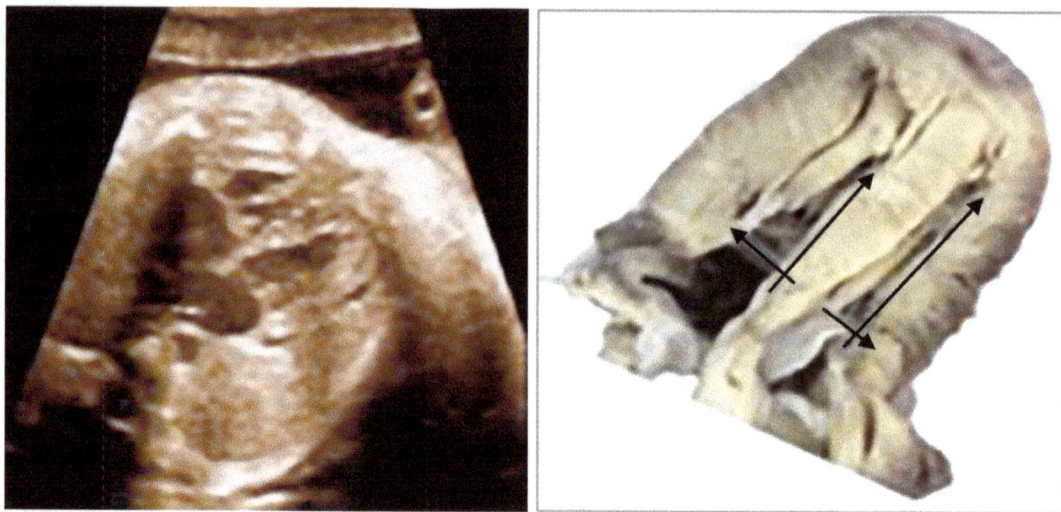

**Fig. 6:** Four chamber view of the fetal heart on ultrasound and autopsy.

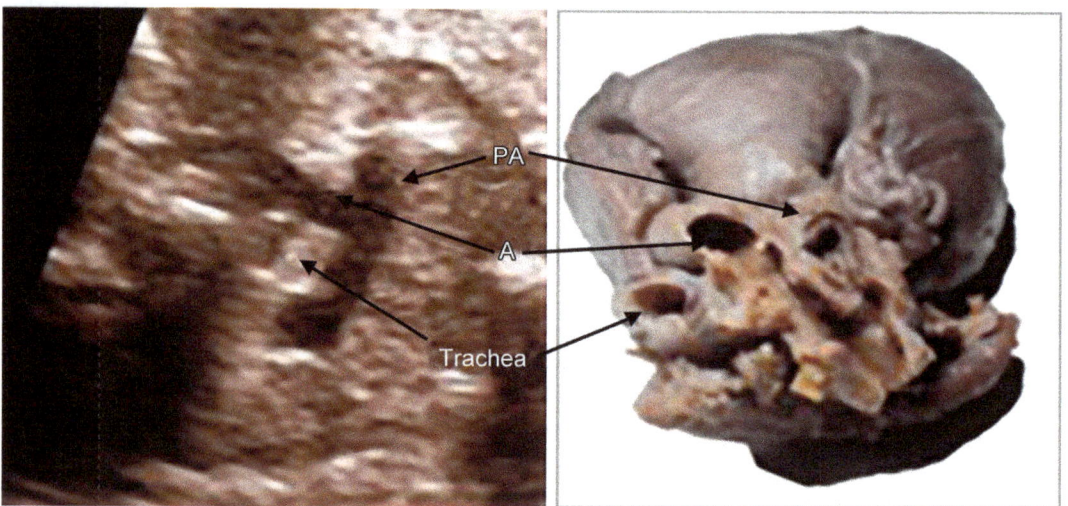

**Fig. 7:** Three vessel and trachea (3VT) view of fetal heart on ultrasound and autopsy.

*Heart:* Cardiac rate and rhythm is observed in M-mode. The size of heart normally is one-third of fetal thorax at 16–20 weeks and cardiothoracic ratio increases with gestation to be 0.5 at 40 weeks. The axis of heart is said to be normal, if the apex points toward left with an angle of 45 ± 20° to midline. Demonstration of four chamber view allows detection of 40% of congenital heart defects and with visualization of outflow tracts; the anomaly detection rate reaches 70% **(Figs. 6 and 7)**. Echogenic focus, if seen in the ventricle, is a soft marker for detection of Down syndrome. Doppler sonography assists in visualization and confirmation of heart abnormality. Indications for fetal echocardiography are enumerated in **Box 2**.

*Echogenic intracardiac focus (ECIF):* It is defined as focus of echogenicity comparable to bone in the region of papillary muscle in either or both ventricles of the fetal heart. Studies suggest that the less frequent right sided, biventricular or particularly conspicuous echogenic intracardiac focus are associated with higher risk of fetal aneuploidy.

> **BOX 2:** Indications for fetal echocardiography.
> - Family history of congenital heart disease
> - Maternal diabetes
> - Maternal drug exposure or infections during pregnancy
> - Maternal systemic lupus erythematosus
> - Maternal phenylketonuria
> - Polyhydramnios
> - Nonimmune hydrops
> - Fetal dysrhythmias
> - Fetal extracardiac abnormalities
> - Fetal chromosomal abnormalities
> - Symmetrical intrauterine growth restriction

*Abdomen:* Abdominal circumference is measured at the transverse level where the umbilical vein joins the portal vein. It is the most sensitive indicator of intrauterine growth restriction. Stomach bubble is visualized in the transverse plane, located to the left of the diaphragm **(Fig. 8)**. Normally, bowel appears as midlevel echogenicity filling the abdomen.

*Genitourinary tract:* Kidneys are bilaterally hypoechoic paraspinal structures. Renal pelvis is measured in

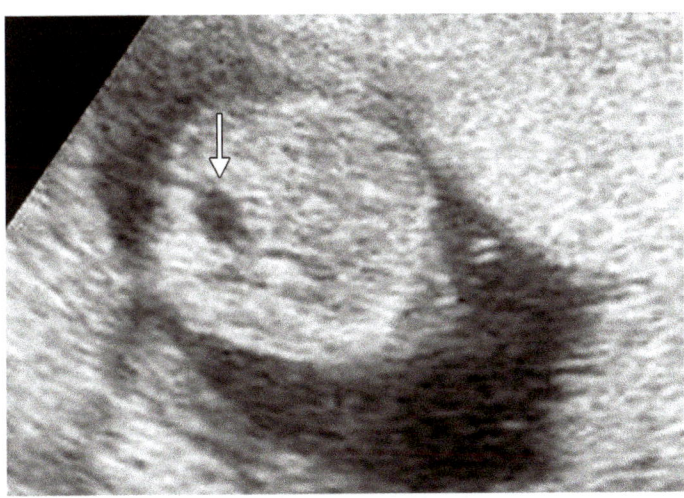

**Fig. 8:** Fetal abdomen in transverse plane showing stomach bubble.

anteroposterior diameter. Abnormal findings are presence of cysts and dilatation of calyces. Doppler imaging is useful in identifying the renal artery especially when kidneys cannot be visualized on USG. Gender is assigned by the visualization of genitalia and not by lack of the image.

*Fetal extremity:* Survey of all long bones provides diagnostic information. Digits are visualized and counted in extension. Movement and tone of the extremities is observed. Absence, fractures, contractures, and bowing of long bones is abnormal.

## INDIVIDUAL CONGENITAL MALFORMATIONS
## Cardiac Defects
### Fetal Cardiac Arrhythmia

Normal fetal heart rate is 100–160/min. Frequency of arrhythmia is 1–3% of all pregnancies.[6] Tachycardia is twice more common than bradycardia. Maternal causes of arrhythmia are connective tissue disorders, drugs, hyperthyroidism, infections, and heritable diseases such as prolonged QT interval syndrome and tuberous sclerosis.

The fetal causes leading to arrhythmia are hydrops fetalis, fetal compromise, and structural cardiac disease. Currently, methods for detection of fetal arrhythmia include electrocardiography, cardiotocography, echocardiography, and magnetocardiography.

Fetal echocardiography and Doppler are indicated to rule out structural cardiac disease.

*Irregular heart rate:*
- *Premature atrial contractions:* It is the most common cause of dysrhythmia. It generally requires no treatment. Patient is asked to avoid caffeine. Investigations to rule out illicit drug use, hyperthyroidism should be done.
- *Premature ventricular contractions:* This also does not require any treatment.

*Tachycardia:* It is diagnosed when the fetal heart beat is >160/minute.

- *Supraventricular tachycardia:* It is the most common cause of fetal tachycardia. Supraventricular tachycardia is diagnosed, if there is 1:1 atrioventricular conduction. As it is difficult to predict, which fetus with tachycardia will eventually develop hydrops most centers initiate treatment as soon as the diagnosis of fetal tachycardia is established.[9]
  The primary form of pharmacological intervention is maternal transplacental therapy. Other routes of treatment are intravascular and intramuscular treatment of fetus, which is mainly used in refractory cases. Digoxin is the most common drug used to treat fetal tachycardia.[9] In a meta-analysis comparing transplacental medications with digoxin, flecainide and sotalol as first line therapy for fetal tachycardias, flecainide, and sotalol were superior to digoxin for the conversion of tachycardia to sinus rhythm. In hydrops fetalis, flecainide and sotalol were more effective than digoxin.[10]
- *Atrial flutter:* It is associated with atrial rates 400–450 beats/min. Most common form is 2:1 AV block. Structural heart defect is ruled out in all cases. Common structural defects causing flutter are Ebstein anomaly, atrial septal defect; hypoplastic left heart syndrome, and cardiomyopathy.

*Bradycardia:* Fetal bradycardia is defined as persistent heart rate below 100 beats/min not associated with uterine contractions or periodic decelerations. Bradycardia once detected, extrinsic causes are ruled out. These are drugs, maternal hypothermia, and cord compression. Type of bradycardia is determined whether it is sinus bradycardia or partial or complete AV block. Maternal testing for connective tissue disorders, screening for anti-Ro, anti-La antibodies is done. Family history of arrhythmia or structural cardiac defect is also inquired.

### Structural Cardiac Defects

Cardiac malformations are the most common birth defect. Incidence of structural cardiac defects is 4–5 per 1,000 live births. It can be present in the form of septal defects, outflow tract obstruction or conotruncal malformations.

*Septal defects:*
- *Atrial septal defect (ASD):*
  - *Incidence:* 1 per 1,000 live births.
  - *Diagnosis:* Demonstration of either the absence or reduction in the dimension of foramen ovale flap.
  - *Prognosis:* ASD does not impair cardiac function in utero. Associated defects, chromosomal abnormality or syndrome may be present and has to be ruled out.
- *Ventricular septal defect:*
  - *Incidence:* 2.5 per 1,000 live births.
  - *Diagnosis:* Classified by the location of septum, may be perimembranous, inlet, trabecular and outlet VSD.

Diagnosis is made only when demonstrated while the USG beam is perpendicular to the septum.
- *Prognosis:* It is good but the extracardiac anomaly and karyotypic abnormality has to be ruled out.

- *Hypoplastic left ventricle:*
  - *Incidence*: 0.16 per 1,000 live births.
  - *Diagnosis*: A small left ventricle and hypoplastic ascending aorta with relatively enlarged right atrium, right ventricle and pulmonary artery point toward hypoplastic left ventricle. Color Doppler shows absence of flow from left atrium to ventricle.
  - *Prognosis:* Postnatal prognosis is poor. In 25% cases, death occurs during 1st week of life. Survival rate is 60% after surgery.

*Outflow tract obstruction:*
- *Aortic stenosis:*
  - *Incidence:* 0.04 per 1,000 live births. It may be supravalvular, valvular, or subvalvular.
  - *Prognosis and treatment*: In utero treatment in the form of balloon dilatation of stenotic aortic valve by transverse puncture has been tried with technical success.[11] None of the babies survived past neonatal period.
- *Coarctation of aorta:* There is narrowing of the portion of ascending aorta between subclavian artery and ductus arteriosus. Echocardiographic findings are an enlarged right ventricle and hypoplastic aortic arch.
  - *Incidence:* 0.18 per 1,000 live births. It is frequently associated with other cardiac anomalies such as VSD (in 90% cases), aortic stenosis, and transposition of great vessels. Extracardiac anomalies are also common.
  - *Prognosis:* There is no significant impact on intrauterine hemodynamics. Surgery is required after birth.
- *Pulmonary stenosis:*
  - *Incidence:* 0.9 per 1,000 live births. Associated anomalies are ASD, Noonan syndrome and tricuspid regurgitation.
  - *Prognosis* is good. Postnatal balloon valvoplasty is required.

## Conotruncal Malformation

These anomalies are commonly missed when the routine USG of heart only involves the four chamber view. It includes malformations such as:
- Transposition of great vessels
- Tetralogy of Fallot
- Double outlet right ventricle
- Truncus arteriosus.

*Transposition of great vessels:*
- *Incidence:* 0.2 per 1,000 live births.
- *Prognosis*: Rarely associated with other cardiac malformations or abnormal karyotype. In utero, the fetus shows no signs of compromise but becomes cyanotic at birth and deteriorates rapidly. Survival after neonatal surgery is 85–90%.

*Tetralogy of Fallot:* It includes stenosis of pulmonary artery, ventricular septal defect, overriding of aorta and hypertrophy of right ventricle.
- *Incidence*: It is 0.4 per 1,000 live births.
- *Prognosis*: Other cardiac defects should be ruled out. Karyotypic abnormalities are common. Survival rate after corrective surgery is 95%.

# HEAD, NECK, AND SPINE

## Open Neural Tube Defect

Neural tube defect comprises anencephaly, spina bifida, and encephalocele.

*Incidence:* The incidence of neural tube defect is 4 per 1,000 live births. They are most commonly multifactorial but can occur as a Mendelian syndrome, chromosomal abnormality, or might result from teratogenic exposure. Only 5% of the children with NTD are born in the families with other affected members. So, screening is required for all pregnant women.

### Anencephaly

*Diagnosis:* Can be made as early as 10 weeks. It is diagnosed by ultrasound finding of absence of calvarium.

*Prognosis:* Pregnancy can be terminated after diagnosis at any period of gestation as it is lethal.

### Encephalocele

*Prognosis:* Additional congenital anomalies are present in 50–65% of cases. Mortality rate is high, only 50% survive after surgery. Prognosis is better if encephalocele is frontal, microcephaly secondary to brain herniation shows poor prognosis **(Fig. 9)**.

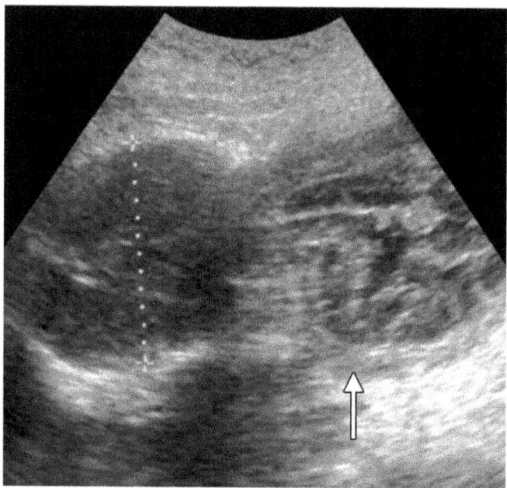

**Fig. 9:** Transcerebral view showing microcephaly with encephalocele (arrow).

## Spina Bifida

*Diagnosis:* It appears on USG as splaying of the posterior ossification centers **(Fig. 10)**. The intracranial signs, which aid in diagnosis, are:
- Lemon sign: Frontal notching **(Figs. 11A to C)**
- Ventriculomegaly (>10 mm)
- Obliteration of cisterna magna
- Small BPD

- Banana sign: It is due to abnormal shape of cerebellum as it is displaced into foramen magnum (Banana sign disappears after 24 weeks).

About 90% of fetuses with NTD have one of the above-mentioned five specific cranial abnormalities.

The entire anatomical survey should be done to exclude other anomalies; ventriculomegaly is present in majority of them. Fetal karyotype is recommended in all instances.

*Prognosis:* Prognosis depends upon the extent of defect. Lower extremity paralysis and incontinence of bowel and bladder are common. 75% of the fetuses have a long-term survival.[12] Neurologic state varies from normal to severe disability, late deterioration is common. On the whole about 75% will have mild-to-severe paralysis with only 17% having normal continence on late follow-up.

It is difficult to predict the prognosis in the first half of pregnancy, option for termination is to be given if diagnosis is made before 20 weeks.

*In utero treatment:* The in utero closure of spinal defect has been tried on experimental basis.[13] If the diagnosis is made after viability, monitoring of fetal growth, head size, and enlargement of ventricles is noted. Delivery is done at term. There is no clear evidence that the lower segment cesarean section (LSCS) improves the outcome thus LSCS for fetal

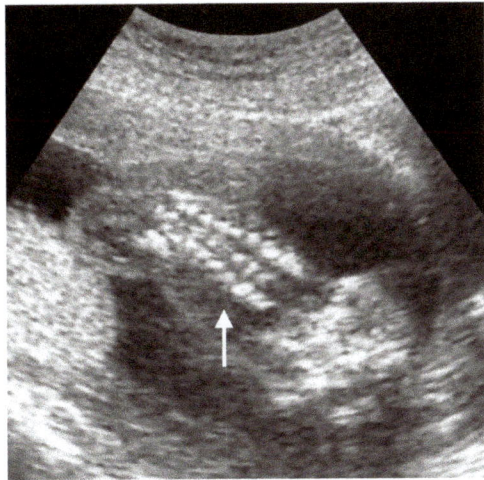

**Fig. 10:** Splaying of lateral vertebral lamina in coronal view suggesting spina bifida (arrow).

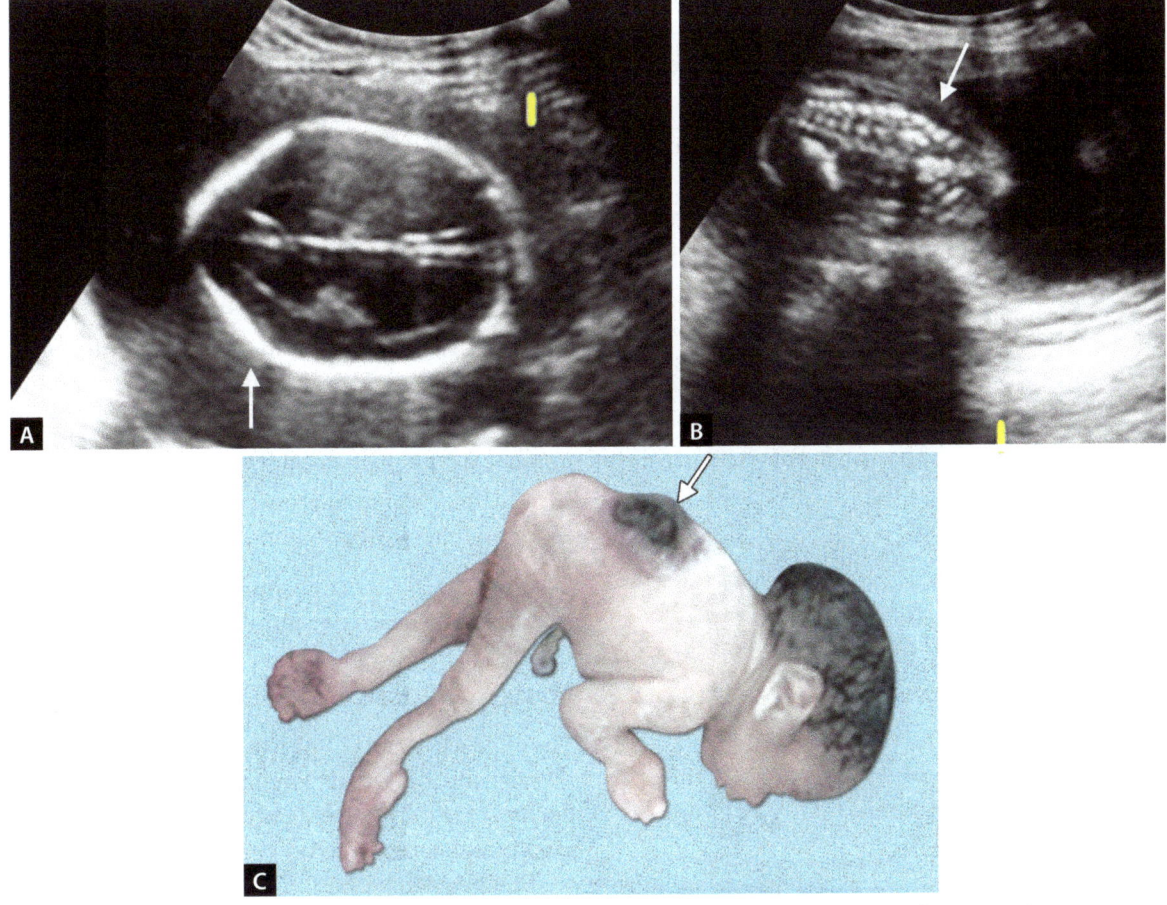

**Figs. 11A to C:** Transcerebral view showing "lemon sign"; baby with neural tube defect (arrows).

indication is avoided. Examination of fetus after delivery is advised.

*Recurrence risk:* The risk in the next pregnancy is 4%, if it is due to a multifactorial cause. If it occurs as a part of genetic syndrome it depends upon the mode of inheritance of the syndrome associated, e.g., there is 25% recurrence risk in Meckel-Gruber syndrome and Robert syndrome both of which show autosomal recessive inheritance.

Periconceptional administration of folic acid after birth of one affected child can reduce recurrence of the disease in the next baby in up to 70% cases.

## Hydrocephalus

*Diagnosis:* It is a pathological increase in CSF usually within the lateral ventricles **(Fig. 12)**. The mean value of atrial diameter is 7 mm; it remains constant from 14 to 38 weeks. Hydrocephalus is diagnosed when the atrial diameter is >10 mm. Choroid plexus appears as a dangling structure as it assumes a dependent posture.

*Prognosis:* If hydrocephalus is detected, general structural survey to look for other anomaly is done as other abnormalities are associated in 90% of the cases. Fetal echocardiography is advised and possible causes need to be investigated. Amniocentesis for karyotyping is done as abnormal karyotype may be associated in up to 10% of the affected fetus. Pregnancy termination is offered if diagnosis is made before viability. If pregnancy is continued serial ultrasound to identify progressive ventricular enlargement is done.

Borderline ventriculomegaly (atrial width 10-15 mm): Isolated borderline ventriculomegaly in most of the cases it is of no consequence. In a distinct minority, it may be an early manifestation of increasing severity later on in gestation. Abnormal outcome is seen in nearly 25% cases. Ventriculomegaly if unilateral is a benign finding.

Overt enlargement (Atrial width > 15 mm): Overall mortality rate ranges from 15 to 70%. Cognitive impairment may be seen in up to 70%. Cortical mantle thickness if less than 1 cm is a poor prognostic sign but if more does not definitely indicate good prognosis.

*Parental counseling:* Parents need to be informed about the problem and its prognosis. Consultation of both neonatologist and neurosurgeon is required. If the abnormality is detected before viability, option for termination should be offered.

*In utero treatment:* In utero placement of shunt did not yield encouraging results as there was increase in survival but the survivors still had varying degree of neurological impairment.[14] Most fetal medicine practitioners are not routinely placing intra-amniotic shunts. At present shunting is being done only on experimental basis.[15]

*Mode of delivery:* LSCS is indicated for obstetric reasons only. Cephalocentesis can be done if the biparietal diameter is large and is indicated only in those cases which have a dismal prognosis.

*Recurrence risk:* Empiric recurrence risk is 2%. Precise risk depends upon the underlying cause.

## Holoprosencephaly

*Incidence:* 1 in 10,000 live births. It can be alobar, semilobar, and lobar. These categories are based on degree of separation of cerebral hemispheres. Alobar is most severe with no evidence of cerebrocortical division. On ultrasound examination, falx cerebri and interhemispheric fissure is absent and the thalami appear fused. Examination of face is necessary whenever we suspect holoprosencephaly.

*Prognosis:* Prognosis is uniformly poor. Most die shortly after birth. Survivors have profound mental retardation.[16] Karyotyping should be offered. Maternal diabetes is to be ruled out. A close look at the parents for minor signs should be done as it can be familial with autosomal recessive or dominant inheritance.

*Labor and delivery:* Option for termination before viability should be given. Macrocephaly may obstruct labor and cephalocentesis can be done.

*Recurrence risk:* In the absence of chromosomal abnormality empiric recurrence risk is 6-14%.

## Posterior Fossa Cystic Defects (Figs. 13A to C)

There is abnormal collection of fluid in these defects. Ultrasound diagnosis is challenging as it can range from normal variant to severe anomalies. It includes:
- Megacisterna magna
- Blake's pouch cyst
- Dandy-walker malformation

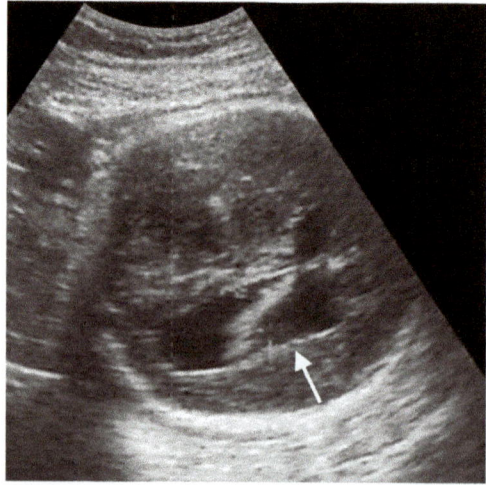

**Fig. 12:** Axial scan showing dilated lateral ventricles (arrow).

# Screening and Management of Congenital Anomalies

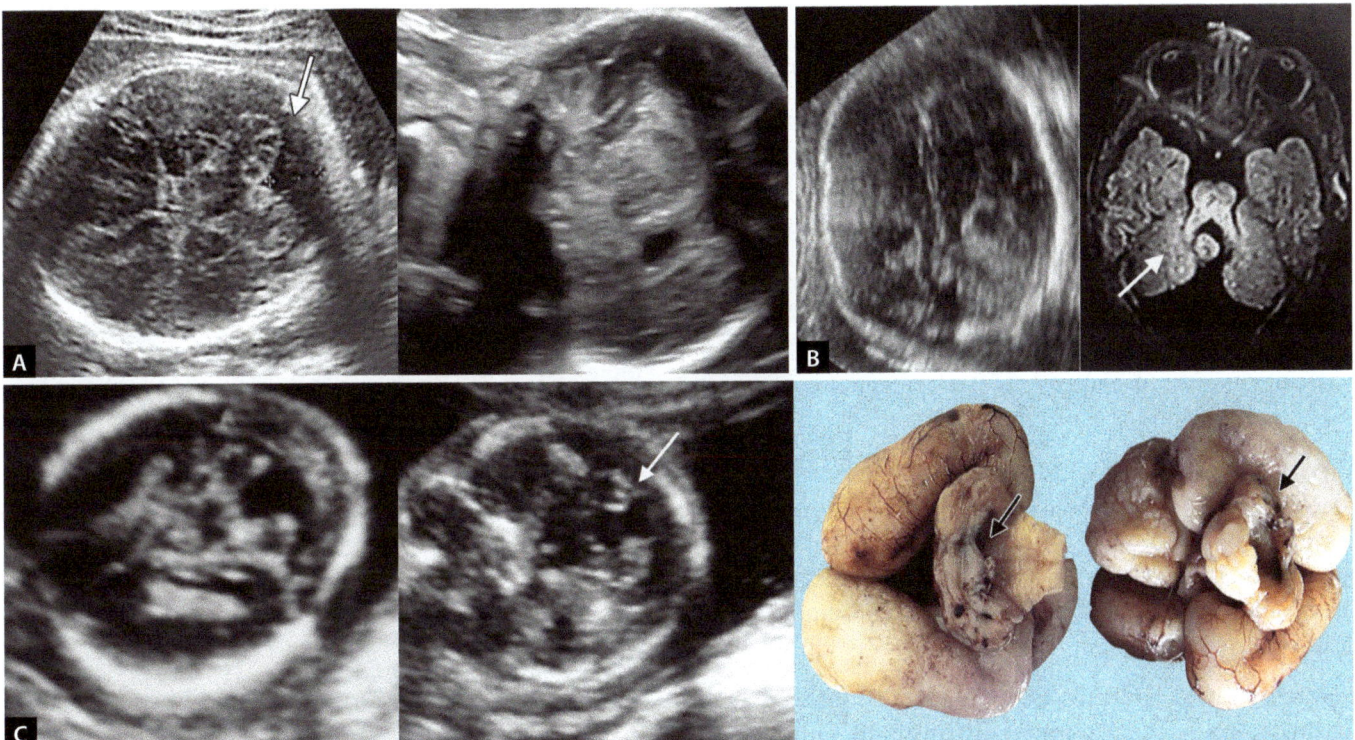

**Figs 13A to C:** Posterior fossa defects: (A) Megacisterna magna; (B) Joubert syndrome showing molar tooth sign on ultrasound and post natal MRI; (C) Dandy–Walker malformation on ultrasound and autopsy (arrows).

- Vermian hypoplasia
- Joubert syndrome
- Arachnoid cyst.

## Dandy–Walker Malformation

*Incidence:* 1 in 30,000 live births.

*Diagnosis:* It is characterized by complete or partial absence of cerebellar vermis with enlarged posterior fossa cyst. There is associated hydrocephalus. In Dandy-Walker variant there is variable hypoplasia of cerebellar vermis with or without enlargement of posterior fossa. After diagnosis is made, other anomalies are looked for, which are seen in up to 85% of cases. There is increased risk of chromosomal abnormality also.

## Cystic Hygroma

*Diagnosis:* Cystic hygroma appears as simple loculated fluid-filled cavities located postero-laterally in neck region. It is often associated with hydrops **(Figs. 14 and 15)**. Therefore, whenever cystic hygroma is detected careful search for fluid accumulation in other cavities is noted. Fetal karyotype is essential.

*Prognosis:* It depends upon associated anomalies. Prognosis is poor when there is associated hydrops. Careful postmortem examination is required.

## Facial Cleft

Careful search for other anomalies is done if facial cleft is suspected. Fetal karyotype should be offered.

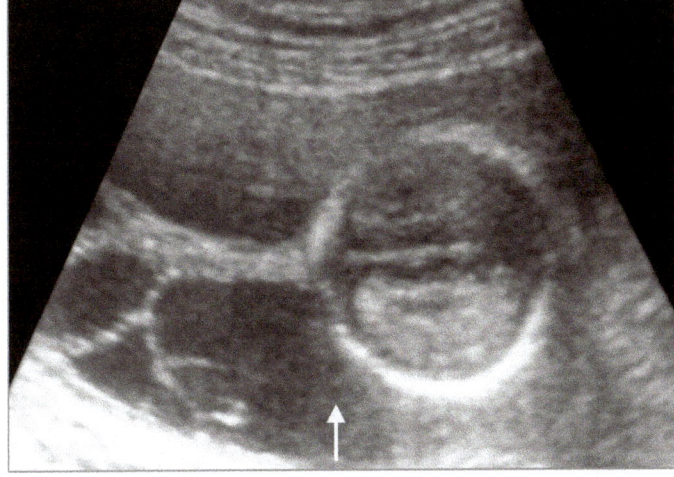

**Fig. 14:** Axial scan at the level of BPD shows soft tissue swelling behind the neck with septae suggestive of cystic hygroma (arrow).

*Prognosis:* It depends upon presence of associated anomalies and the severity of the defect. Prenatal diagnosis of cleft lip helps parents to prepare for a visibly disturbing deformity which is correctable. Prior to corrective surgery there is difficulty in feeding.

## ▌ GENITOURINARY SYSTEM

### Kidney Abnormalities

*Renal Agenesis*

Bilateral renal agenesis is found in 1 in 5,000 live births and unilateral agenesis is seen in 1 in 2,000 live births. It is

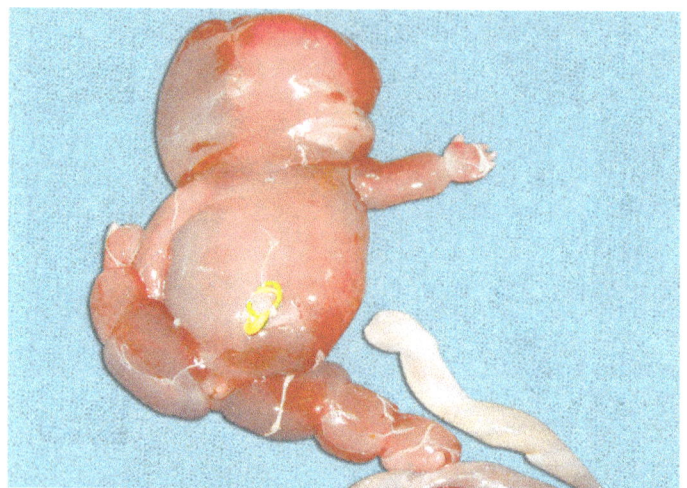

Fig. 15: Cystic hygroma and hydrops in the same fetus.

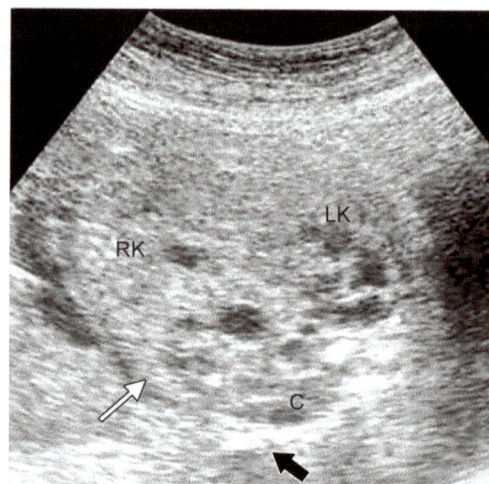

Fig. 16: Transverse scan of the fetus with multicystic kidney disease involving right and left kidneys (RK and LK). Note the multiple cystic structures (C).

usually sporadic in occurrence but may be associated with chromosomal abnormality or with some syndrome such as Fraser syndrome.

*Diagnosis:* The condition is suspected by presence of oligohydramnios and nonvisualization of kidneys on ultrasound usually around 16–18 weeks. Failure to visualize renal arteries on Doppler is another important clue.

*Prognosis:* Bilateral renal agenesis is lethal, however, unilateral agenesis has good prognosis. Associated oligohydramnios leads to pulmonary hypoplasia.

*Recurrence risk:* In non-syndromic cases, the risk of recurrence is 3%.

## Multicystic Dysplasia

*Incidence*: 1 in 1,000 live births.

*Diagnosis:* Appears antenatally as kidneys that have lost the normal shape and appears as collection of cysts that are of variable size (0.5–3 cm) not connected to the urinary tract **(Figs. 16 and 17)**. It is usually a sporadic abnormality but chromosomal defect or other abnormality may be associated in 50% cases.

*Prognosis:* It is good when unilateral but is uniformly bad in bilateral affection and when associated oligohydramnios is present.

## Infantile Polycystic Kidney Disease

*Diagnosis:* It appears as bilaterally enlarged, homogeneously hyperechoic kidneys that retain their shape. There is often associated oligohydramnios. The dilated cysts are dilated collecting ducts. The liver is always involved with portal fibrosis and proliferation of bile ducts.

*Prognosis:* The prognosis depends upon clinical variety of disease. The perinatal type has severe renal involvement and leads to stillbirth. The gene of infantile polycystic kidney

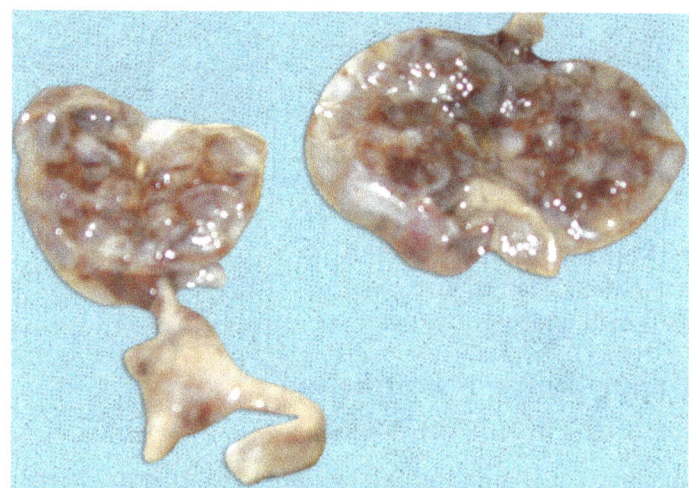

Fig. 17: Bilateral multicystic kidney at autopsy.

disease (IPKD) has been mapped. Fetal blood can be saved for genetic analysis **(Figs. 18 and 19)**.

*Recurrence risk:* Since, the disease is autosomal recessive the risk of recurrence is 25%.

## Adult Polycystic Disease

*Diagnosis:* The ultrasound appearance is of enlarged kidneys with increased parenchymal echogenicity or multiple cysts. The liquor amount may be normal or decreased. Diagnosis is usually done in late second and third trimester. The diagnosis is easy when cyst is present in one of the parents.

*Prognosis:* The prognosis is not good in fetuses who present in utero. In counseling the affected parents, it is necessary to emphasize that in many cases the cysts develop later in life so the absence of cyst does not rule out the disease. The prenatal diagnosis can be made by chorionic villus sampling as the gene responsible has been identified.

# Screening and Management of Congenital Anomalies

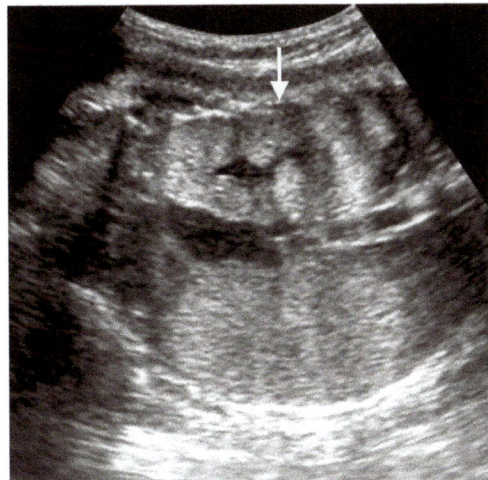

Fig. 18: Transverse scan of fetus with infantile polycystic kidney disease. Multiple small cysts are visualized.

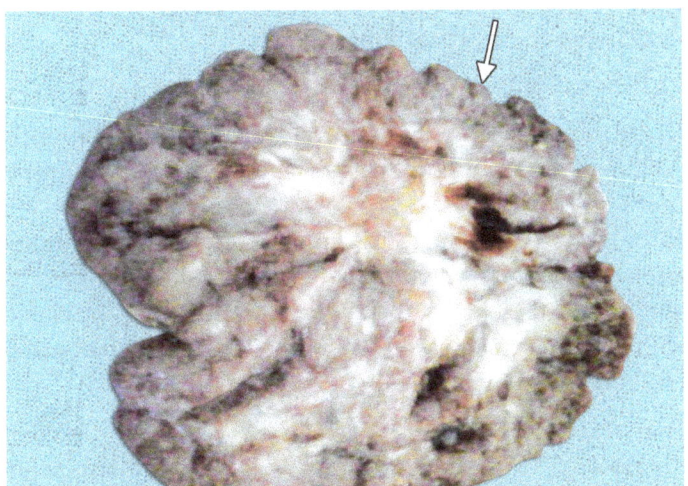

Fig. 19: Cut section of same kidney showing multiple tiny cysts.

*Recurrence risk:* It is 50% as the disease is autosomal dominant.

## Obstructive Uropathies

### Pylectasis

Pylectasis is said to be present when anteroposterior diameter of the renal pelvis is more than 4–6 mm in second trimester and more than 10 mm in the third trimester.[17] It can be physiologic.

*Incidence:* 1–3% of pregnancies.

### Hydronephrosis

*Diagnosis:* It is the dilatation of renal pelvis with calyceal system. It is diagnosed as severe when the anteroposterior diameter of renal pelvis is >1.5 cm with calyceal dilatation. The classification of antenatal hydronephrosis is listed in **Table 3**. Fetal uropathies are classified by the level of dilatation. In upper obstruction only the kidneys are dilated. In midlevel obstructions, ureters are also dilated. Upper and

**TABLE 3:** Classification of antenatal hydronephrosis based on renal pelvic anteroposterior diameter.

| Classification | Second trimester | Third trimester |
| --- | --- | --- |
| Mild | 4–6 mm | 7–9 mm |
| Moderate | 7–10 mm | 10–15 mm |
| Severe | >10 mm | >15 mm |

midlevel dilatation can be unilateral and bilateral. It may be due to obstruction of ureteropelvic junction, ureterovesical junction or due to ureteropelvic reflux.

*Prognosis:* It is good in unilateral dilatation. Corticomedullary differentiation is more important than cortical thickness in deciding the prognosis.

### Lower Urinary Tract Obstruction

Posterior urethral valve is seen almost exclusively in males. It may be seen in females with complex pelvic floor malformations.

## ABDOMINAL WALL AND GASTROINTESTINAL SYSTEM

### Omphalocele

*Incidence:* 1 in 4,000 births.

*Diagnosis:* The diagnosis is made after 11 weeks (as normal physiological herniation process occurs before this) when on USG an anterior extra-abdominal mass is detected upon which the umbilical cord inserts **(Figs. 20 and 21)**.

*Prognosis:* Other malformations are associated in 60% of the cases. Karyotypic abnormality is seen in up to 50%. We must look for other abnormalities on USG. Fetal echocardiography and karyotyping is advised. The survival rate in absence of any other abnormality is 75%.[18]

*Labor and delivery:* Elective cesarean section does not offer any benefit over vaginal delivery. Care of fetus immediately after delivery is required. Long-term prognosis is usually good.

*Recurrence risk:* It is low in subsequent pregnancy.

### Gastroschisis

It is an anterior abdominal wall defect. It occurs usually on the right side **(Figs. 22A and B)**.

*Incidence:* 1 in 3,000 live births.

*Diagnosis:* The loops of bowel appear floating freely in the amniotic fluid on USG giving appearance of a bunch of grapes.

*Prognosis:* The chance of presence of associated anomaly is less than 10%. The probability of associated chromosomal abnormality is <1%. The prognosis of affected fetus is good with over 80% survival after surgical treatment. There is no

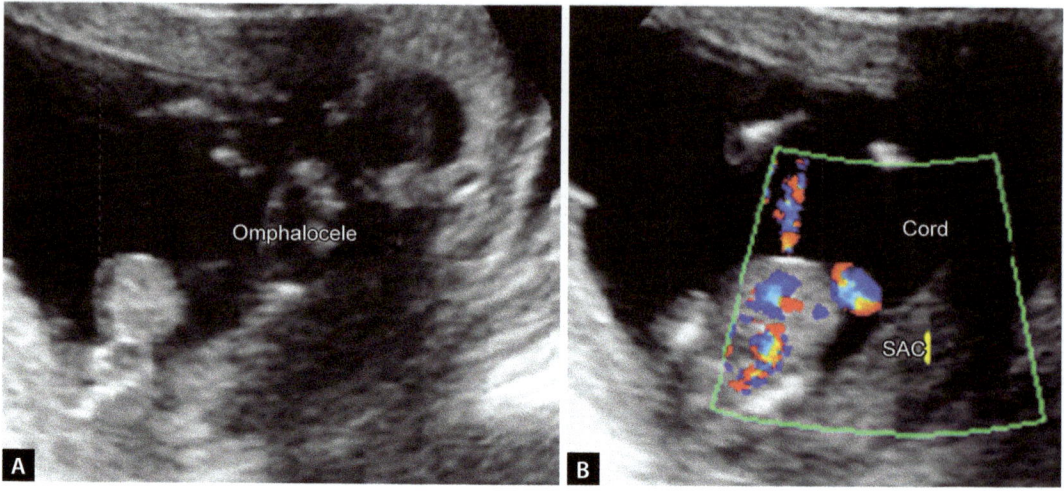

**Figs. 20A and B:** Transverse scan of fetal abdomen at the level of umbilicus demonstrating omphalocele.

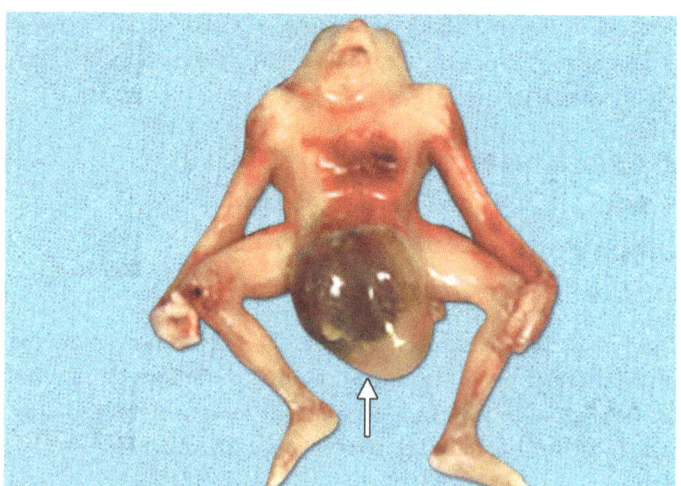

**Fig. 21:** Typical omphalocele with lesion in midline covered by membrane.

evidence that cesarean delivery improves outcome. Primary surgical closure can be achieved in 52–85% cases.[19]

*Recurrence risk:* It is very low. Very few cases with familial occurrence have been noted.

## Congenital Diaphragmatic Hernia

It is the herniation of the gastrointestinal contents into the thoracic cavity.

*Incidence:* 1 in 3,500 live births.[20]

*Diagnosis:* Antenatal sonographic diagnosis is done by presence of abnormal position of heart or visualization of bowel or stomach beside the heart.

*Prognosis:* Factors affecting prognosis are enlisted in **Box 3**.

*Fetal surgery* is offered on experimental basis in the form of plugging of trachea which will prevent egress of lung fluid required for stimulating lung growth.[21]

*Labor and delivery:* Vaginal delivery is not contraindicated. Immediate intubation after delivery is required.

## Esophageal Atresia with or without Tracheoesophageal Fistula

*Incidence:* 3 in 10,000 live births.[22]

*Diagnosis:* The most common antenatal presentation is polyhydramnios and failure to visualize the fetal stomach more so if noted after 20 weeks. A repeat examination within a few days should be done. Careful search for other anomalies is done, fetal karyotyping should be offered as abnormality is seen in 10% of the cases. It is also associated with syndromes such as VATER or VACTERL association and DiGeorge sequence.

*Prognosis:* Termination of pregnancy can be offered if diagnosis is done before viability especially if associated abnormalities are present. Continuing pregnancies are managed by providing normal obstetric care. Therapeutic amniocentesis can be done.

Labor and delivery are not influenced by malformation. Immediate postdelivery care is given. Surgery is done after the condition of the infant is stable. The outcome of surgery is generally good.

*Recurrence risk:* Generally, sporadic but may be familial.

## Duodenal Atresia

*Incidence:* 1 in 6,000 live births.

*Diagnosis:* Sonographic diagnosis is made by appearance of "double bubble" and presence of hydramnios **(Fig. 23)**.

*Prognosis:* Associated anomalies are present in 50% cases; chromosomal abnormality is seen in 30% cases. Detailed ultrasonographic assessment is required. As there is high-risk of heart abnormality, fetal echocardiography is also advised. Prognosis for the condition if isolated is good. Operative mortality rate is 4% with long-term survival as 86%.

*Recurrence risk:* It is low.

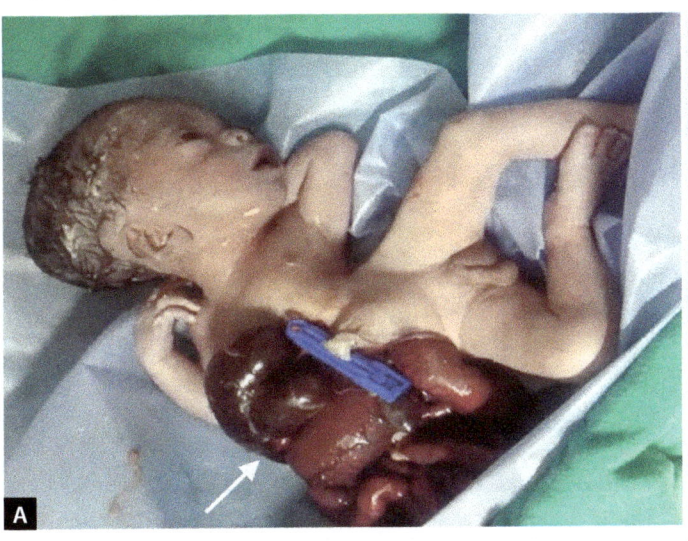
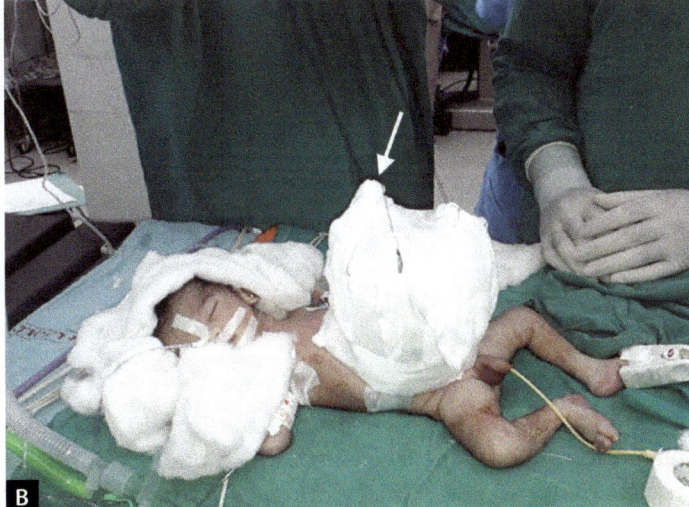

**Figs. 22A and B:** (A) Abdominal wall defect in the baby was seen on the right of cord insertion, there was no membrane covering, the cord is inserted at its normal position indicating gastroschisis; (B) Live baby with gastroschisis, being managed conservatively till stabilization.

**BOX 3:** Factors that affect prognosis of diaphragmatic hernia.
- Additional associated anomalies
- Early diagnosis (<25 weeks' gestation)
- Liver in the chest
- Lower lung to head ratio (LHR) or lung volume
- Right-sided diaphragmatic hernia
- Bilateral diaphragmatic hernia

## SKELETAL SYSTEM

*Incidence:* Prevalence of skeletal dysplasia is 1 in 5,000 stillbirths.

### Bone Length Abnormalities

If the length of any of the long bones is found to be smaller than the gestational age, it must be confirmed. Measurements of all long bones must be compared with nomograms available for limb biometry. Values less than 4 SD below the mean definitely indicate skeletal dysplasia. The values between −2 and −4 SD can be due to syndromic causes, chromosomal cause, or due to intrauterine growth restriction.

Short limbs can be micromelic (shortening of whole limb), rhizomelic (shortening of proximal part), mesomelic (shortening of middle part) or acromelic (shortening of distal part of limb). The various conditions associated with different types of shortening of limbs are described in **Table 4**.

After detection of abnormal length of bone, evaluation of density, bending, presence or absence of fractures is done **(Fig. 24)**. Density of long bones is adjudged by presence or absence of acoustic shadow behind the bone, intracranial visibility and whether the skull is compressed by the transducer.

Detailed examination of the skull, its shape and size, face for clefting, thorax for length and breadth, spine for kyphosis

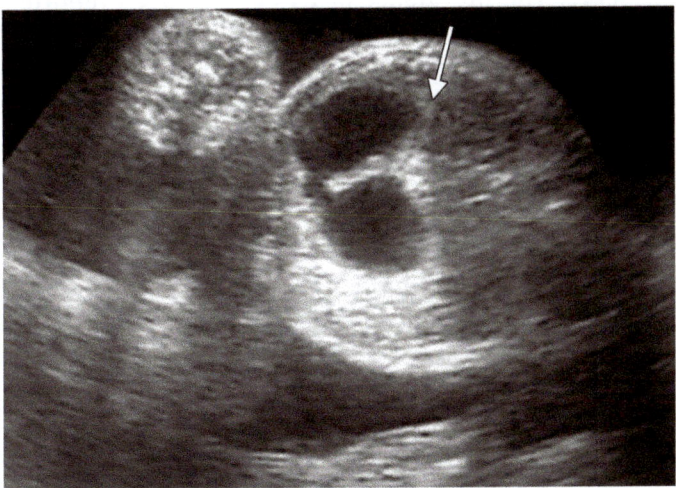

**Fig. 23:** Transverse scan of upper abdomen of fetus with duodenal atresia. A typical double bubble is seen.

**TABLE 4:** Types of shortening of limbs.

| Rhizomelia | Mesomelia | Micromelia |
|---|---|---|
| Thanatophoric dysplasia | Ellis van Creveld (chondroectodermal dysplasia) | Achondrogenesis |
| Chondrodysplasia punctata | Robert syndrome | Short rib polydactyly |
| Congenital short femur | | Osteogenesis imperfecta |
| Achondroplasia | | |

and scoliosis, digits for its number, and foot for clubbing is noted to aid in diagnosis. Systemic examination especially cardiac and renal should be done.

*Postnatal examination:* Infantogram is done which should include anteroposterior and lateral view—thoracic and lumbar spine, lateral view—cervical spine and skull, anteroposterior view of pelvis, chest, long bones and hands.

Other studies like chromosomal analysis are advised in all cases. DNA testing may be done for some cases.

*Counseling:* It is to be provided after gathering all information. Counseling is to be provided by obstetrician and the geneticist both. The parents are informed about the recurrence risk in future pregnancies. Management plans for antenatal diagnosis in future pregnancy should also be explained.

## Hydrops Fetalis

### Definition

It is the presence of excessive extracellular fluid in the interstitial compartment secondary to disruption of normal intravascular and interstitial homeostatic mechanisms. Sonographic diagnosis of hydrops requires accumulation of fluid in two or more cavities **(Figs. 25 and 26)**.

*Incidence:* The prevalence of 1:1,000 has been reported. Fetal hydrops has been classified into immune (IH) and nonimmune hydrops (NIH). The ratio of NIH to IH has been reported to be 9:1. The etiology of nonimmune hydrops according to a recent meta-analysis is given in **Table 5**.

### Prognosis

Although, few cases of spontaneous remission of nonimmune hydrops have been reported the prognosis in majority of the infants is universally poor with perinatal mortality rate ranging from 70 to 90%.

### Management and Treatment

Identification of the hydropic infant is easy but the real difficulty lies in identifying the underlying cause, determining the appropriate therapy, and optimal time of delivery. After identification of a hydropic infant, the first step is to rule out isoimmunization as the possible cause. Whether due to rhesus or any other antibody, this can be done by performing

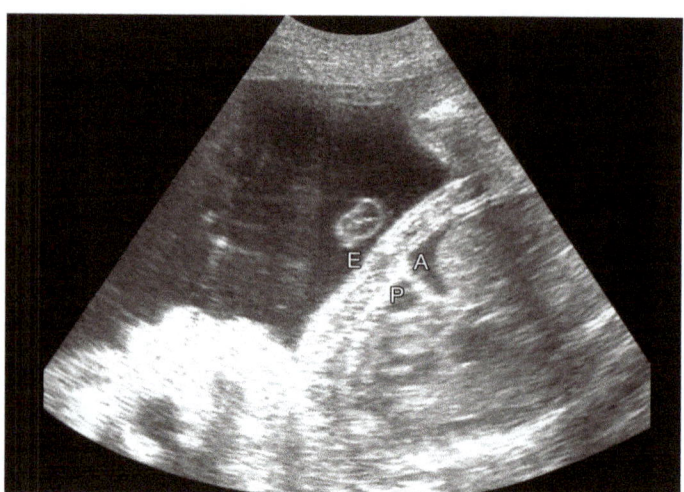

**Fig. 25:** Longitudinal scan of the fetus showing pleural effusion (P), ascitis (A), and skin edema (E).

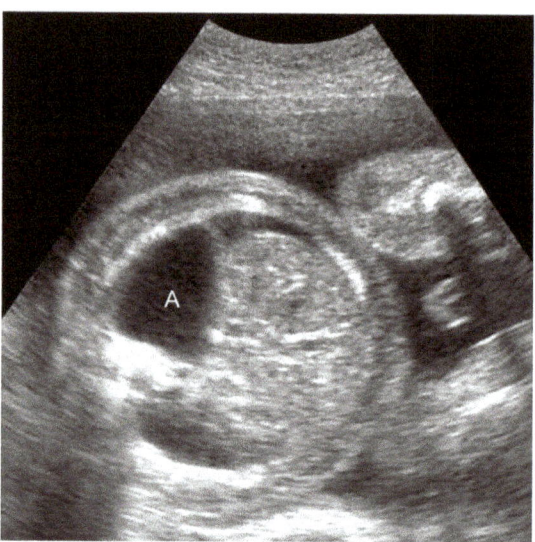

**Fig. 26:** Transverse scan of the fetal abdomen showing ascitis (A).

**TABLE 5:** Etiology of nonimmune hydrops.

| Causes | Incidence (%) |
| --- | --- |
| Cardiovascular | 21.7 |
| Hematologic | 10.4 |
| Chromosomal | 13.4 |
| Syndrome | 4.4 |
| Lymphatic dysplasia | 5.7 |
| Inborn errors of metabolism | 1.1 |
| Infections | 6.7 |
| Thoracic | 6.0 |
| Urinary tract malformations | 2.3 |
| Extra thoracic tumors | 0.7 |
| Twin–twin transfusion syndrome | 5.6 |
| Gastrointestinal | 0.5 |
| Miscellaneous | 3.7 |
| Idiopathic | 17.8 |

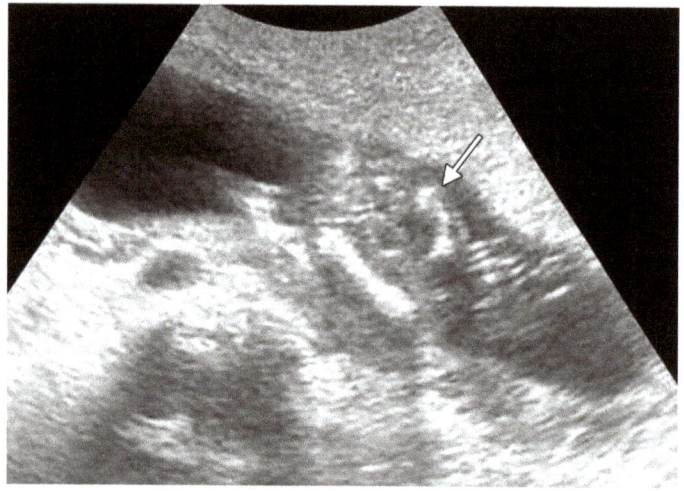

**Fig. 24:** Scan showing normal right femur but short and bent left femur.

> **BOX 4:** Laboratory investigations in hydrops fetalis.
>
> *Blood tests:*
> - Complete blood count
> - ABO type and rhesus antigen status
> - Indirect Coombs' test
> - Kleihauer Betke stain test
> - Acute phase titers
> - Toxoplasmosis
> - Cytomegalovirus
> - Serological test of syphilis (VDRL)
> - G6PD deficiency screen
>
> *Amniotic fluid tests:*
> - Karyotyping
> - L:S ratio after viability

an indirect Coombs' test. A detailed ultrasound examination along with fetal echocardiography is the next step to exclude congenital anomalies in fetus and placenta. Maternal blood tests and amniotic fluid test, as given in the **Box 4**, are also done to reach at a diagnosis. In most of the cases this diagnostic workup fails to give a definitive diagnosis. Management decision at this point depends upon gestational age. Before viability, the option of pregnancy termination should be given. The prognosis before viability is poor. If decision for continuation is taken, the dilemma is when to deliver. The risk of an intrauterine death has to be weighed against the risk of premature delivery with increased total lung water in the baby which would compound the problem of treating respiratory distress.

The approach for expectant management is to follow the fetus with frequent ultrasound examinations and biophysical profile until the clinical picture deteriorates or lung maturity is determined by L:S ratio of amniotic fluid. If preeclampsia is associated, delivery is indicated. A chance of cesarean section is increased due to soft tissue dystocia and associated polyhydramnios. Patients are to be explained that chances of survival of fetus postdelivery are minimal.

The prognosis of nonimmune hydrops is good in selected groups such as cardiac dysrhythmias amenable to transplacental medical therapy. In fetomaternal hemorrhage, intrauterine transfusion can be done. In rare cause such as G6PD deficiency, removal of offending agent followed by intrauterine transfusion or delivery depending upon the gestational age can be done successfully.

## ROLE OF FETAL SURGERIES AND EXIT PROCEDURE

Sala et al. after reviewing the fetal surgical procedures stated that in utero fetal surgery interventions are currently considered in selected cases of congenital diaphragmatic hernia, cystic pulmonary abnormalities, amniotic band sequence, selected congenital heart abnormalities, myelomeningocele, sacrococcygeal teratoma, obstructive uropathy, and complications of twin pregnancy. Randomized controlled trials (RCTs) have demonstrated an advantage for open fetal surgery of myelomeningocele and for fetoscopic selective laser coagulation of placental vessels in twin-to-twin transfusion syndrome. The evidence for other fetal surgery interventions, such as tracheal occlusion in congenital diaphragmatic hernia, excision of lung lesions, fetal balloon cardiac valvuloplasty, and vesicoamniotic shunting for obstructive uropathy, is more limited.[23] Conditions amenable to intrauterine surgical treatment are rare; the mother may consider termination of pregnancy as an option for many of them; treatment can be lifesaving but in itself carries risks to both the infant (preterm premature rupture of the membranes, preterm delivery) and the mother. Moreover, there is scanty information on long-term outcomes. It is recommended that fetal surgery procedures be performed in centers with extensive facilities and expertise.

The ex utero intrapartum treatment (EXIT) procedure was initially developed to secure the airway in fetuses at delivery after they had undergone in utero tracheal occlusion for congenital diaphragmatic hernia. Indications for the EXIT procedure have been expanded to include any delivery in which prenatal diagnosis indicates neonatal airway compromise, such as large neck masses and congenital high airway obstruction syndrome, or when a difficult resuscitation is anticipated such as with large lung lesions. Uteroplacental blood flow and gas exchange are maintained through the use of inhalational anesthetics to allow optimal uterine relaxation with partial delivery of the fetus and amnioinfusion to sustain uterine distension. Using the EXIT procedure, sufficient time is provided on placental bypass to perform life-saving procedures, such as bronchoscopy, laryngoscopy, endotracheal intubation, tracheostomy, cannulation for extracorporeal membrane oxygenation, and resection of lung masses or resection of neck masses in a controlled setting, thus avoiding a potential catastrophe.[24]

## NEED FOR EXAMINING FETUS, STILLBIRTH OR NEONATE

If a malformation is severe enough to require termination of pregnancy or if it is not treatable then generally no further investigations are carried out. However, the information sufficient to take decision for termination of pregnancy may be totally inadequate to provide genetic counseling for the next pregnancy. The grieving family members may not be interested in knowing the cause of such mishap at that moment, but soon they may be concerned whether it can happen again in next pregnancy. To be prepared to answer this question appropriate investigations and autopsy must be carried out when a malformed baby is born.

Every fetus terminated due to prenatal ultrasonographic diagnosis of malformations needs to be examined after termination. It is essential not only for audit of ultrasonographer's skill but also for providing correct genetic counseling to the family. This is because even with best ultrasonographic setup, autopsy shows additional findings in about 44–49% of cases.[25] These findings may be missed or may not be detectable by USG and may change in about 25–30% of the cases. Thus, genetic counseling based on ultrasonographic diagnosis may be erroneous.

In a recent study by Kumar et al. out of 403 cases of stillbirth and abortion, consent for autopsy was given in 312. Most common defect was craniovertebral defect followed by genitourinary anomaly. The autopsy finding correlated with USG findings fully in 63.5% cases, there were additional findings altering diagnosis in 24.7% cases and the diagnosis completely changed in 11.8% cases. Additional findings on autopsy helped in reaching at a diagnosis and counseling accordingly.[26]

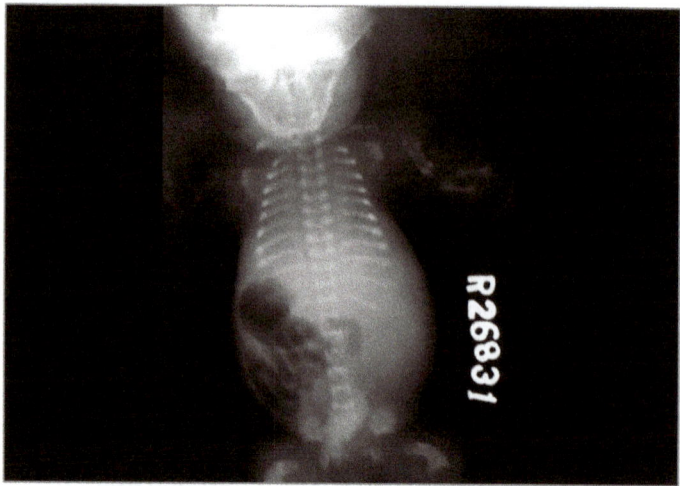

**Fig. 27:** Radiograph of the infant with thanatophoric dysplasia.

## Clinical Examination

The clinical examination includes careful observation and measurements. A photograph is much better than lengthy description and also provides opportunity to get second opinion especially from clinical geneticist.

## Chromosomal Study

Chromosomal study is indicated in presence of malformations, fetal hydrops, intrauterine growth restriction, and oligohydramnios or previous fetal loss. The sample can be aseptically collected from cord or fetal heart in a heparinized syringe.

## Radiographic Study

Anterior and lateral radiographs are mandatory especially if skeletal dysplasia is suspected **(Fig. 27)**.

## Fetal Autopsy

Gross autopsy is extremely useful for separating subjects into normal and abnormal. If autopsy is not possible immediately, fetus can be stored in 10% formalin for transportation **(Figs. 28 and 29)**.

## Histopathology

Directed histopathological examination is required if gross abnormality is detected. For example, it is useful in the diagnosis of polycystic kidney disease **(Fig. 28)**.

## Examination of Placenta and Cord

Fetal death can be attributable to placenta or cord abnormality in 15% cases. In cases of intrauterine infection, placental histology may provide important information.

The uptake of perinatal autopsy services totally depends upon awareness among obstetricians regarding its use and utility.

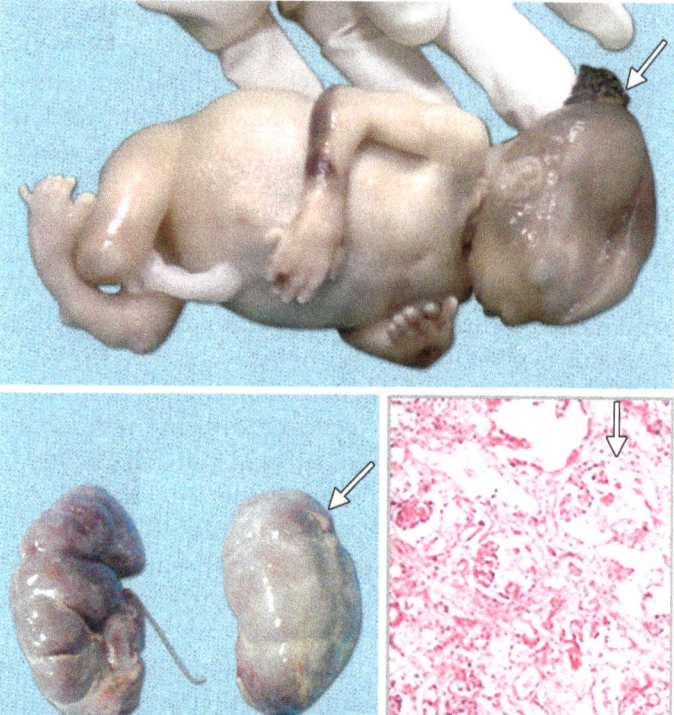

**Fig. 28:** Autopsy showing encephalocele, polydactyly, bilateral polycystic kidney with histopathological confirmation features suggestive of Meckel–Gruber syndrome.

## EXPERIENCE AT OUR CENTER

A prospective study of all women with prenatally detected major congenital malformations was carried out at our center. Postnatal follow-up of live born babies was carried out for 1 year there was no live birth in cases such as anencephaly, iniencephaly, bilateral renal agenesis, gastroschisis, and cystic hygroma. Survival at 1 year was less than 25% in spina bifida, bilateral cystic kidneys, complex cardiac disease, and nonimmune hydrops fetalis. In cases

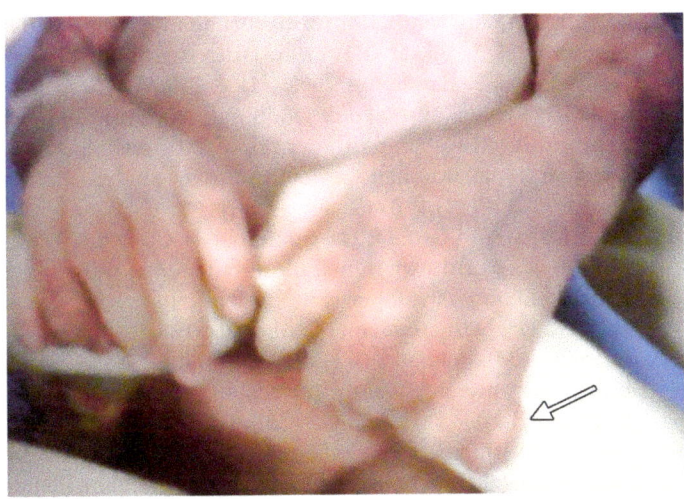

**Fig. 29:** Polydactyly in the same fetus suggesting the diagnosis of Meckel–Gruber syndrome, which has 25% recurrence risk in next pregnancy

with mild hydrocephalus or unilateral and mild renal disease, the survival was over 75%.[27]

In India, the majority of cases with congenital anomalies present late in gestation. As per the recent Medical Termination of Pregnancy (Amendment) Act, 2021, pregnancy beyond 20 weeks and up to 24 weeks can be terminated if two medical practioners are of the opinion that if the child were born, it would suffer from serious physical or mental abnormality. In cases where pregnancy is continued, full support along with quality antenatal and neonatal case should be given.

## KEY POINTS

- Approximately 3% of neonates have a major congenital malformation.
- Majority of birth defects occur in families with no prior history of birth defect.
- Most fetal structures can be visualized at 12–13 weeks.
- For measurement of NT, the optimal gestational age is 11–13 weeks 6 days.
- Biochemical screening for NTD is done by maternal serum alpha fetoprotein estimation.
- In anencephaly, pregnancy can be terminated at any period of gestation as it is lethal.
- In spina bifida, about 75% will have mild-to-severe paralysis and only 17% have normal continence on late follow-up.
- The risk in the next pregnancy is 4% if NTD is due to a multifactorial cause.
- After birth of one affected child, periconceptional administration of folic acid can reduce recurrence risk of NTD in the next baby in up to 70% cases.
- Genetic sonography has a sensitivity of 50–93% for detecting fetal aneuploidy.
- Cardiac malformations are the most common birth defects.
- Associated malformations with cardiac malformations are seen in 10% of cases of congenital malformation. Chromosomal abnormality is seen in 10–40%, hence, a detailed ultrasound evaluation and karyotyping is advised.
- After diagnosis of cardiac anomaly, multidisciplinary approach involving pediatric cardiologist, cardiac surgeon, obstetrician, and geneticist is required.
- Counseling of the patient after diagnosis should involve the description of malformation, possibility of surgical correction, chances of short- and long-term survival, quality of life expected after correction and hazards of surgery.
- Follow-up with echocardiography is done every 2–4 weeks.
- The delivery of fetuses with heart defect is to be done at a tertiary care center: most fetuses tolerate labor well and can be allowed vaginal delivery.
- Baby is to be assessed by pediatric cardiologist at birth and managed accordingly.
- If one child is affected the risk of recurrence in second child is 2–5%. The chance of heart disease in child, if father is affected, is 2% and, if mother is affected it is 6%.
- In hydrocephalus amniocentesis for karyotyping is done as abnormal karyotype may be associated in up to 10% of the affected fetus.
- Parents are to be counseled that the overall mortality rate ranges from 15 to 70% in severe hydrocephalus. Cognitive impairment may be seen in up to 70%.
- The prognosis of unilateral hydronephrosis is good but is uniformly bad in case of bilateral affection and when associated oligohydramnios is present.
- Infantile polycystic kidney disease (IPKD) appears as bilaterally enlarged, homogeneously hyperechoic kidneys that retain their shape. It is autosomal recessive and the risk of recurrence is 25%.
- The fetal prognosis depends on presence of pulmonary hypoplasia. If the mean vertical pocket of amniotic fluid on ultrasound is 10 mm, pulmonary hypoplasia is unlikely to occur.[18]
- For prediction of postnatal renal function, fetal urinalysis can be done with invasive testing.
- There is lack of high-quality evidence to guide clinical practice regarding prenatal bladder drainage. In utero drainage may improve survival in severely affected fetuses by improving renal function but in the long-term chronic renal failure is a rule. Many may require renal transplant.
- Fetal intervention is not done in unilateral cases, or when there is isolated uropathy with normal renal parenchyma or normal renal function.
- In case of fetal death, examination after delivery must be done. Renal tissue is to be sent for histopathological examination.
- Fetal DNA must be tested if the termination is done for suspected genetic renal abnormality such as polycystic kidney disease.

- In omphalocele, karyotypic abnormality is seen in up to 50% cases.
- In gastroschisis, the probability of associated chromosomal abnormality is <1%.
- The measurement of long bone less than 4 SD below mean definitely indicates skeletal dysplasia.
- Although, few cases of spontaneous remission of nonimmune hydrops have been reported, the prognosis in majority of the infants is universally poor with perinatal mortality rate ranging from 70 to 90%.
- Although fetal surgeries have been tried in certain problems such as congenital diaphragmatic hernia, excision of lung lesions, spinabifida, etc., these should be performed in centers with extensive facilities and expertise.
- There is need for examining the affected fetus, stillborn or neonate to arrive at etiological diagnosis for counseling regarding risk in next pregnancy.
- A photograph, infantogram, and chromosomal study are indicated in presence of malformations. Tissue directed histopathological examination is also required.

## REFERENCES

1. Toufaily MH, Westgate MN, Lin AE, Holmes LB. Causes of congenital malformations. Birth Defects Res. 2018;110(2):87-91.
2. Sepulveda W, Sebire NJ, Hughes K, Odibo A, Nicolaides KH. The lambda sign at 10–14 weeks of gestation as a predictor of chorionicity in twin pregnancies. Ultrasound Obstet Gynecol. 1996;7:421-3.
3. Goldstein SR. Embryonic death in early pregnancy: a new look at first trimester. Obstet Gynecol. 1994;83:738-40.
4. Maruotti GM, Saccone G, Morlando M, Martinelli P. First-trimester ultrasound determination of chorionicity in twin gestations using the lambda sign: a systematic review and meta-analysis. Eur J Obstet Gynecol Reprod Biol. 2016;202:66-70.
5. Carvalho JS, Senat MV, Schwarzler P, Ville Y. Increased nuchal translucency and ventricular septal defect in the fetus. Circulation. 1999;99:E10.
6. Snijders RJ, Noble P, Sebire N, Souka A, Nicolaides KH. UK multicentre project on assessment of risk of trisomy 21 by maternal age and nuchal translucency thickness at 10–14 weeks of gestation. Lancet. 1998;351:343-6.
7. Circero S, Curcio P, Papageorghiou A, Sonek J, Nicolaides K. Absence of nasal bone in fetuses with trisomy 21 at 11–14 weeks of gestation: an observational study. Lancet. 2001;358:1665-7.
8. Cameron A, Nimrod C, Nicholson S, Harder J, Davies D, Fritzler M. Evaluation of fetal cardiac dysarrhythmias with two dimensional, M mode, and pulsed Doppler ultrasonography. Am J Obstet Gynacol. 1998;158:286.
9. Oudijk MA, Ruskamp JM, Ambachsheer BE, Ververs TF, Stoutenbeek P, Visser GH, et al. Drug treatment of fetal tachycardias. Pediatr Drugs. 2002;4(1):49-63.
10. Hill GD, Kovach JR, Saudek DE, Singh AK, Wehrheim K, Frommelt MA. Transplacental treatment of fetal tachycardia: a systematic review and meta-analysis. Prenat Diagn. 2017;37(11):1076-83.
11. Khol T, Sharland G, Allan LD, Gembruch U, Chaoui R, Lopes LM,, et al. World experience of percutaneous ultrasound guided balloon valvuloplasty in human fetuses with severe aortic valve obstruction. Am J Cardiol. 2000;85:1230-3.
12. Bowman RM, McLone DG, Grant JA, Tomita T, Ito JA. Spina bifida outcome: a 25-year prospective. Pediatr Neurosurg. 2001;34:114-20.
13. Brunner JP, Tulipan N, Paschall RL, Boehm FH, Walsh WF, Silva SR, et al. Fetal surgery for myelomeningocele and incidence of shunt dependent hydrocephalus. JAMA. 1999;282:1819-25.
14. Holzgreve W, Evans MI. Non-vascular needle and shunt placement for fetal therapy. West J Med. 1993;159(3):333-40.
15. Cavalheiro S, Moron AF, Zymberg ST, Dastoli P. Fetal hydrocephalus: prenatal treatment. Childs Nerv Syst. 2003;19:561-73.
16. Cohen MM Jr, Shoita K. Teratogenesis of holoprosencephaly. Am J Med Genet. 2002;109:1-15.
17. Ouzounian JG, Castro MA, Fresquez M, al-Sulyman OM, Kovacs BW. Prognostic significance of antenatally detected fetal pylectasis. Ultrasound Obstet Gynacol. 1995;7(6):424-8.
18. Salihu HM, Boos R, Schmidt W. Omphalocele and gastroschisis. J Obstet Gynecol. 2002;22:489-83, 738-40.
19. Babcook C, Hedrick MH, Goldstein RB, Callen PW, Harrison MR, Adzick NS, et al. Gastroschisis: can sonography of fetal bowel accurately predict postnatal outcome? J Ultrasound Med. 1994;13:701-6.
20. Blakelock R, Upadhyay V, Kimble R, Pease P, Kolbe A, Harding J. Is a normally functioning gastrointestinal tract necessary for normal growth in late gestation? Pediatr Surg Int. 1998;13:17-20.
21. Quinn TM, Adzick NS. Fetal surgery. Obstet Gynecol Clin North Am. 1997;24:143-57.
22. Shulman A, Mazkareth R, Zalel Y, Kuint J, Lipitz S, Avigad I, et al. Prenatal identification of esophageal atresia: the role of ultrasonography for evaluation of functional anatomy. Prenat Diagn. 2002;22:669-74.
23. Sala P, Prefumo F, Pastorino D, Buffi D, Gaggero CR, Foppiano M, et al. Fetal surgery: an overview. Obstet Gynecol Surv. 2014;69(4):218-28.
24. Moldenhauer JS. Ex utero intrapartum therapy. Semin Pediatr Surg. 2013;22(1):44-9.
25. Snowdon C, Elbourne DR, Garcia J. Perinatal pathology in the context of a clinical trial: a review of the literature. Arch Dis Child Fetal Neonatal Edn. 2004;89(3):F200-3.
26. Kumar M, Singh A, Gupta U, Anand R, Thakur S. Relevance of labor room fetal autopsy in increasing its acceptance. J Matern Fetal Neonatal Med. 2014;27:1-6.
27. Kumar M, Sharma S, Bhagat M, Gupta U, Anand R, Puri A, et al. Postnatal outcome of congenital anomalies in low resource setting. Prenat Diagn. 2013;33(10):983-9.

# Recurrent Pregnancy Loss

*Sangeeta Gupta, Shivangini Rana*

## INTRODUCTION

Recurrent pregnancy loss (RPL) is a source of mental trauma and distress to both, the couples and the clinicians. It is a daunting task for the obstetrician to strike a balance between the required and the unnecessary workup, as the latter usually stems from desperation to achieve a successful pregnancy. Despite extensive workup of couples, in about 50% of cases, no etiology is delineated. The greatest challenge lies in the diverse causes of RPL, majority of which are still unexplained. In this chapter, the pathophysiology and the management of RPL will be reviewed.

## DEFINITION

There is a lack of consensus regarding the number of miscarriages used to define RPL and regarding inclusion of biochemical pregnancies in RPL.

Recurrent pregnancy loss is defined as three or more consecutive pregnancy losses before 24 weeks of gestation by the Royal College of Obstetricians and Gynaecologists (RCOG).[1] The German, Austrian, and Swiss Societies of Gynecology and Obstetrics (DGGG/OEGGG/SGGG) also consider RPL as ≥3 consecutive losses.[2]

As per the Federation of Obstetric and Gynaecological Societies of India (FOGSI), RPL is defined as three or more consecutive spontaneous losses before 20 weeks of pregnancy.[3]

The American Society for Reproductive Medicine (ASRM) defines RPL as two or more failed clinical pregnancies after ultrasound or histopathological confirmation.[4]

The European Society of Human Reproduction and Embryology (ESHRE) defines RPL as two or more pregnancy losses till 24 weeks of gestation. This includes nonvisualized pregnancies confirmed by serum or urine beta human chorionic gonadotropin (hCG) including biochemical pregnancies and pregnancies of unknown location. In the nonvisualized pregnancy loss group, pregnancy losses after 6 weeks are included, where an ultrasound examination was only done following complete expulsion or no ultrasound was done after heavy bleeding: it includes pregnancies that would have been diagnosed as clinical abortions in case an earlier ultrasound scan had been done.[5] It excludes molar and ectopic pregnancies and it also excludes implantation failures.[5]

Incidence of RPL is about 1–3% if the criteria used is three or more losses whereas this figure rises to 5% where definition is revised to two or more losses.[6,7]

There is still a debate on whether couple should be investigated after two or three miscarriages. This should be a part of shared decision making with the couple, taking into account the available resources. Certain scenarios may warrant an early investigation:
- History of infertility
- Female partner is more than 35 years
- Cardiac activity documented in previous loss
- Previous products of conception having a normal karyotype.[8]

It has been suggested that a threshold of three or more losses should be used for epidemiological studies while clinical evaluation may be done after two first-trimester pregnancy losses.[4]

Recurrent pregnancy loss can also be categorized as primary or secondary. Primary RPL refers to RPL without a prior viable pregnancy and in secondary RPL at least one viable pregnancy has occurred previously. It has been studied that there is no difference between the two in terms of live births, but primary RPL is associated with adverse obstetric outcomes.[8,9]

## RISK FACTORS AND ETIOLOGIES

Many etiologies have been implicated in RPL, however, in more than 50% of the cases the cause remains unexplained.[4] In the following section, we overview the likely role of various risk factors and etiologies in RPL, evaluate evidence for workup and management options that can be offered.

### Age

The risk of miscarriages increases with age of the woman. A fall in the number and quality of oocytes is seen with advancing maternal age. Least risk from RPL is between the ages of 20 and 35 years of the female partner according to many studies and the risk of such losses rises sharply after 40 years of maternal age.[5,8]

Though increase in paternal age is associated with miscarriages, but no specific mention has been made with regards to RPL.[5]

## Obstetric History

History of *previous pregnancy losses is an important prognostic factor* along with maternal age; number of previous losses increase the future miscarriage risk.[8]

## Genetic Factors

Chromosomal abnormalities account for most of the spontaneous miscarriages; out of which about 90% are numerical (aneuploidy, polyploidy)—the most common being trisomy—and others are structural abnormalities (translocation, inversion) and mosaicism. The risk of oocyte aneuploidy increases with maternal age. Advancing maternal age is associated with poor ovarian reserve and increased segregation errors.[8]

The balanced translocations have an incidence of 2–5% in couples with RPL compared with 0.7% of the general population. A carrier of a balanced reciprocal or a balanced Robertsonian translocation has a normal phenotype. However, their gametes might be balanced or unbalanced genetically. The unbalanced gametes on combining with the gametes of partners who are not affected by these chromosomal abnormalities, result in pregnancy losses in majority of the cases and in the few cases that do not abort, they cause malformations.[4,8] There is lack of consensus among various guidelines regarding testing the karyotype of the parents and the evaluation of the abortus or pregnancy tissue.

### Evaluation of the Products of Conception

The analysis of the abortus tells us about genetic abnormalities like aneuploidies and translocations as well as morphologically abnormal products of conception. In some cases, the abortus is chromosomally and phenotypically normal and the couple needs to be evaluated for other causes of RPL. Genetic analysis of the pregnancy tissue can be done by many methods like conventional karyotyping, fluorescence in situ hybridization (FISH) or array-based comparative genomic hybridization (array-CGH). Out of these, array-CGH is the recommended technique as it has reduced contamination by the maternal tissues and being a molecular technique it overcomes the limitations of conventional karyotyping, i.e., failure of culture in the products of conception.[10,11] The evaluation of pregnancy tissue is recommended at the third loss or if the loss follows after initiation of therapy for a remedial cause of RPL.[4,5]

### Parental Karyotyping

The RCOG and ESHRE proposed selective parental karyotyping after individual risk assessment. It can be recommended on the basis of genetic history like translocations in the products of conception, history of congenital abnormalities in the previous births as well as family history of unbalanced chromosomal translocations in an offspring. For other couples, the benefit of karyotyping is limited. In cases where abortus is not evaluated or there is a culture failure, karyotyping may be offered to parents.[1,5]

### Treatment

Genetic counseling is important when a structural genetic factor is identified. The likelihood of a subsequent healthy live birth depends on the chromosome(s) involved and the type of rearrangement. When one of the partners has a structural genetic abnormality, preimplantation genetic testing (PGT), amniocentesis, or chorionic villus sampling are options to detect the genetic abnormality in the fetus. Treatment options include PGT, with transfer of unaffected embryos or the use of donor gametes. However, use of PGT and in vitro fertilization (IVF) is not routinely advised as it has lower live birth rates than natural conception.[12]

## Anatomic Causes

Anatomic distortions such as congenital uterine anomalies, uterine adhesions, submucous myomas, and endometrial polyps have been associated with RPL. These causes can be divided into congenital and acquired.

### Congenital Causes

Congenital uterine anomalies usually cause losses due to decreased volume of the uterus and hampered blood supply. The anomalies associated are unicornuate uterus, uterus didelphys, bicornuate uterus, arcuate uterus, and uterine septum. It has been studied that women with septate and bicornuate uteri have increased second trimester losses as compared to women with unexplained RPL.[13]

In the light of these findings, all women with RPL should have evaluation of uterine anatomy as a part of their workup.

The gold standard in this case is laparoscopy with hysteroscopy, which allows for the direct visualization of the uterus. The only problem lies in the invasiveness and cost of the procedure.

The conventional two-dimensional (2D) ultrasound and hysterosalpingography (HSG) are popular methods for screening of uterine anomalies. But the low sensitivity of the 2D ultrasound and the inability of HSG to distinguish different types of anomalies, limit their use.[5,14]

Uterine imaging is enhanced by saline infusion sonohysterography (SIS), which uses fluid to show the uterus and its cavity. It can diagnose and classify uterine anomalies and allows simultaneous evaluation of tubal patency. It has higher sensitivity and specificity than HSG and hysteroscopy. It may be uncomfortable for some women due to the use of fluid.[5,15]

On the other hand, a three-dimensional (3D) ultrasound has the advantage of delineating the external and internal contours of the uterus, having high sensitivity and specificity and is noninvasive. It can distinguish between the various congenital malformations. Therefore, it is the preferred technique when it comes to the diagnosis of uterine malformations.[5,14]

*Magnetic resonance imaging (MRI)* is excellent when it comes to looking at the cavity, fundus, external structure of the uterus and also the associated renal abnormalities, but it is still not considered a first-line investigation because of its cost and no other added diagnostic benefit over 3D ultrasound. It can be used where 3D ultrasound is not available. It also cannot replace the gold standard-laparoscopy and hysteroscopy.[5]

## Acquired Causes

Submucous myomas, endometrial polyps, and uterine adhesions can be possible causes of RPL and can also have associated bleeding disorders, amenorrhea and dysmenorrhea. But their clear cut role in RPL is still not established. Though various imaging modalities are used in their diagnosis, hysteroscopy is the gold standard.[5,16]

## Treatment

The treatment options vary depending on the type of malformations. Hysteroscopic septal resection is the treatment of choice for septate uterus using hysteroscopic scissors and electrodes. Many studies show a decrease in miscarriage rates in RPL after septal resection. But the impact of septal resection on future fertility is still not clear. Hence, further randomized controlled trials (RCTs) are needed to compare hysteroscopic resection of septum with expectant management in cases of RPL in terms of risks and benefits.[5] However, ASRM proposes that it may be reasonable to opt for septal resection in cases with prior pregnancy loss or poor obstetrical outcome.[4,17]

Metroplasty or uterine reconstruction for other uterine anomalies is not recommended by ESHRE. Another treatment option to be kept in mind for couples with RPL and congenital uterine anomalies, which cannot be repaired is IVF with surrogacy.[5]

In case of uterine adhesions, the treatment is *hysteroscopic adhesiolysis*. Some studies have shown the benefit of surgical removal of adhesions in cases of RPL but a weighed choice has to be made due to the lack of conclusive evidence. Stem cell therapy as a nonsurgical treatment option for uterine adhesions is under study.[5,18]

Until better quality evidence emerges, the ASRM and DGGG/OEGGG/SGGG propose that it is reasonable to undertake surgical correction in cases of significant uterine cavity defects associated with fibroids and polyps.[2,4]

The hysteroscopic procedures cited above are not risk free, but in trained hands, are low risks.

## Cervical Weakness

Cervical incompetency is a known cause of second trimester losses. The diagnosis is clinical with a suggestive history of painless cervical dilatation or a history of spontaneous rupture of membranes followed by expulsion of fetus.[1]

## Treatment

In women with a history of second trimester losses and suspected cervical insufficiency, it is strongly recommended to monitor the cervical length with ultrasound in a serial manner. In these women cervical stitch should be applied before 24 weeks of gestation if the ultrasound shows a cervical length of <25 mm. If the history is clearly indicative of cervical weakness, cervical stitch may be applied between 12 and 14 weeks, electively.[1,19,20] Due to inconclusive evidence with regards to benefits of cerclage and possible harm associated with it, ESHRE is cautious in recommending cerclage for RPL but strongly recommends ultrasound surveillance.[5]

## Thrombophilia

Thrombophilias can be hereditary or acquired and are often studied in relation to RPL. The acquired thrombophilia is an important cause of RPL whereas there is very little evidence to support association of hereditary thrombophilia with RPL.

## Hereditary Thrombophilia

Hereditary thrombophilia, like factor V Leiden mutation, prothrombin mutation and protein C, protein S, and antithrombin deficiency have been evaluated in cases of pregnancy loss and their association is debated and not confirmed. Both ESHRE and ASRM do not recommend the routine screening for hereditary thrombophilia in RPL.[4,5]

## Acquired Thrombophilia

Antiphospholipid syndrome (APS) is found in 5-20% of women with recurrent miscarriage and is considered the most important treatable cause.[4,21] APS is an acquired thrombophilia and also an autoimmune disorder in which the antibodies are directed toward self. The antibodies cause thrombosis, further leading to pregnancy complications. Its diagnosis requires at least one clinical and one laboratory criteria. The laboratory test results must be obtained twice, at least 12 weeks apart. The testing for APS antibodies (ACA, LA, and β2 glycoprotein) is generally done 6 weeks after the pregnancy loss.[7] It is recommended to investigate women for APS even after two pregnancy losses as a part of the evaluation of RPL.[5,22]

## Treatment

The treatment of thrombophilia in RPL is aimed at preventing the thrombotic events and improving implantation and suppressing the immune response (immunological treatments).

*Treatment of RPL with hereditary thrombophilia:* In these cases no beneficial effect of anticoagulants was seen for prevention of pregnancy loss. These agents can be given for the prevention of venous thromboembolism and for research. Studies on steroids and intravenous immunoglobulins in hereditary thrombophilia and RPL are still awaited.[5]

*Treatment of RPL with APS:* Studies show benefits of combined treatment with aspirin and heparin rather than aspirin alone. ESHRE also recommends treatment with aspirin (75–100 mg) and heparin in those patients who have three or more pregnancy losses and who fulfill the laboratory criteria of APS. Low dose aspirin should be started before conception and heparin [unfractionated heparin (UFH) or low molecular weight heparin (LMWH)] should be added to the treatment after the pregnancy test comes positive. This treatment should be continued till delivery. RCOG also considers treatment with aspirin and heparin in patients of RPL with APS. They do not recommend the use of steroids and IV immunoglobulins in treatment of women with APS and RPL as no improvement in live births is seen. UFH is prescribed in the dose of 5,000–10,000 units subcutaneous twice daily and LMWH 40 mg SC once daily. LMWH has lower chances of causing osteoporosis and heparin-induced thrombocytopenia than UFH, a higher antithrombotic ratio and a longer half-life, thus requiring less monitoring and can be prescribed as once daily. Pregnancies with APS receiving aspirin and heparin should be monitored closely as they are still at risk when it comes to pre-eclampsia, fetal growth restriction and preterm births.[1,5,8]

## Immunological Causes

Theoretically, any disturbance in the normal maternal alloimmune response to paternal antigens can lead to pregnancy loss. Various immunological mechanisms have been studied in RPL like the production of cytotoxic antibodies in the mother, cytokine dysregulation, antigenic similarity of the mother and father which leads to failure in the production of maternal blocking antibody and also dysregulation of the immune response at the fetomaternal junction. Let us understand the various plausible factors one by one.

Human leukocyte antigen (HLA) complex is a group of proteins involved in the immune response. It is located on chromosome 6 and consists of polymorphic genes. In theory, increased HLA compatibility between couples was said to decrease the production of maternal blocking antibodies, which leads to pregnancy loss. However, the evidence to support such claims is inconsistent. ESHRE and RCOG do not recommend HLA testing of couples routinely in recurrent miscarriages. In pregnancy, there is generally a production of anti-inflammatory cytokines by T-helper-2 cells. The predominance of T-helper-1 cells and production of proinflammatory cytokines like interleukin 2 and tumor necrosis factor alpha (TNF-alpha) has been suggested as a possible mechanism in RPL. But further research is required before routinely prescribing testing for cytokines in all patients of recurrent miscarriages.[1,5]

Antinuclear antibodies (ANAs), as the name suggests, are the antibodies against the cell nucleus. Association between ANA and RPL has been established by majority of case-controlled studies, hence testing for ANA could be considered in such couples.

Natural killer (NK) cells are found in the peripheral blood and in the endometrium. The routine testing for NK cells is not recommended in patients with repeated miscarriages as per the current evidence.

Testing for anti-HLA antibodies and anti-HY antibodies is also not recommended.[5,8]

### Treatment

*Immunotherapy:* Currently, the use of immunotherapeutic options for RPL lack evidence. The treatment options available for women with these immune biomarkers including paternal leukocyte immunization, third party donor leukocytes, trophoblast membranes, and intravenous immunoglobulins have been studied widely in recurrent miscarriages. The Cochrane review, 2014, on immunotherapy in RPL does not show any benefit of these treatment modalities in terms of live births and miscarriage rates as compared to placebo. Intralipid infusion which acts by decreasing the NK cells and proinflammatory cytokines has also been studied in one RCT. In this intralipid infusion has shown to increase chemical pregnancy rates in IVF patients with RPL with high peripheral NK cells. Other treatment options like TNF-alpha inhibiting factor and granulocyte colony-stimulating factor require further research in RPL.[1,5]

## Hormonal and Metabolic Factors

### Thyroid Disorders

Abnormalities of the thyroid have been implicated in adverse pregnancy outcomes including pregnancy loss. Hypothyroidism has many manifestations and can be overt or subclinical. A higher than normal serum thyroid-stimulating hormone (TSH) level with a normal free thyroxine (T4) is called subclinical hypothyroidism (SCH). Overt hypothyroidism is characterized by high serum TSH levels (usually >10 mIU/L) and free T4 levels, which are subnormal.

Thyroid peroxidase autoantibodies (TPO Ab) are also studied in relation to RPL. Women with TPO Ab can be euthyroid or hypothyroid.

As a result of various studies, it has been found that there is a link between SCH as well as presence of TPO Ab and recurrent miscarriages. Due to the high prevalence of these disorders in women with RPL, ESHRE recommends routine testing of the TSH and TPO Ab levels in women with RPL. Also in cases of abnormality in the TSH and TPO Ab levels, it is recommended to screen for free T4.[5,23]

## Treatment

Ideally, a female with thyroid disorder should be referred to a physician or an endocrinologist.

- *Overt hypothyroid:* Chronic overt hypothyroidism should always be corrected with levothyroxine as it has many effects on pregnancy and is very essential for the neurological maturation and development of the fetus as the fetal thyroid does not produce thyroid hormone before 10-13 weeks of gestation. Federation of Obstetric and Gynaecological Societies of India (FOGSI) suggests increasing dose of thyroxine by 30–50% when pregnancy is diagnosed.
- *Euthyroid with TPO Ab:* The evidence for treatment of euthyroid females with levothyroxine in RPL having thyroid autoantibodies is also inadequate.[24] Available data does not show increase in live births with treatment. *The thyroid antibodies and levothyroxine trial (TABLET)* is a large multicenter RCT in UK, which compares euthyroid TPO Ab positive females treated with levothyroxine versus placebo. It led to the conclusion that there was no difference in the outcomes of the two groups. Further the results of this trial also lead one to think that an unfavorable immune environment could be a cause of RPL in these females, rather than a relative deficiency of thyroid hormone.[5,25]
- *Subclinical hypothyroid:* In patients with SCH with the presence of thyroid autoantibodies, levothyroxine should be given in case TSH is above trimester specific cut offs. Treatment should be given in cases of SCH if TSH is > 10 mIU/L irrespective of the antibody status. Evidence suggests that the treatment of subclinical hypothyroidism in RPL should be considered after weighing the benefits and risks. Larger RCTs are needed on this topic as the evidence is still insufficient. Also lower IQ of the child has been reported with levothyroxine treatment in pregnancy in a prospective cohort study by Korevaar et al., so a cautious decision needs to be made.[5,26,27]

## Polycystic Ovarian Syndrome and Insulin Metabolism

The most common endocrinopathy affecting reproductive age group females is polycystic ovarian syndrome (PCOS) with a prevalence of 8–13% depending on the population studied. It has metabolic, reproductive, and psychological impact on the patients, thereby making it a complex entity. PCOS as a probable cause of RPL is still uncertain as many other factors are common to both PCOS and RPL like obesity, hyperandrogenism, luteinizing hormone (LH) hypersecretion, hyperinsulinemia, and thrombophilia. Considering the current evidence, evaluation of PCOS, fasting insulin and fasting glucose is not recommended in couples with RPL to improve the outcome of next pregnancy according to ESHRE. In RPL, well-controlled diabetes mellitus is not considered as a risk factor.[4,5,28,29]

*Treatment:* ESHRE does not recommend the routine use of metformin, an insulin sensitizing drug, in pregnancy in females with recurrent pregnancy loss and PCOS due to lack of proper evidence. Meta-analysis of 17 RCTs has also shown no effect of metformin on sporadic miscarriage risk when administered preconceptionally in women with PCOS and infertility. Trials for use of metformin prepregnancy in RPL are still needed.[1,5]

## Luteal Phase Defect

Luteal phase defect (LPD) can be broadly defined as a short luteal phase interval (<12 days) with normal progesterone level, normal luteal phase length with decreased production of progesterone, or an insufficient response of the endometrium to otherwise normal progesterone levels. These mechanisms are further thought to influence implantation and pregnancy outcome. The various tests employed to diagnose LPD are midluteal phase single serum progesterone levels, timed endometrial biopsy, preovulatory follicular diameter, basal body temperature, and salivary progesterone levels. Further evidence is needed to attribute LPD as a cause of RPL. Thus, it is not recommended to screen for LPD in recurrent miscarriages.

*Treatment:* There is not enough evidence to support the use of progesterone or hCG in LPD with RPL.[5,30]

## Prolactin Disorder

Hyperprolactinemia impacts the hypothalamic-pituitary-ovarian axis and causes disruption of folliculogenesis, oocyte maturation, and luteal phase. More clinical studies are needed justifying the role of prolactin in RPL and as of now routine testing for prolactin disorders is not recommended in RPL, in the absence of features like oligomenorrhea and amenorrhea. Prolactin disorders are also associated with other problems like luteal phase defects, PCOS and stress thereby the link may not be direct with RPL.

*Treatment:* Both ASRM/ESHRE are of the common consensus that in patients with hyperprolactinemia, treatment with dopamine agonists has been seen to improve pregnancy outcomes in RPL.[4,5,31]

## Other Factors

According to ESHRE, testing for androgens, LH levels, plasma homocysteine levels and vitamin D are not recommended in patients suffering from RPL.[5]

## Infections

Recurrent pregnancy loss has no association with toxoplasmosis, rubella, cytomegalovirus, and herpes infections, hence, screening for TORCH infections is not recommended in RPL.[1]

## Endometritis

Chronic endometritis is mostly an asymptomatic state, in which the endometrial stroma has infiltration of plasma cells with edema. It is detected by biopsy or immunohistochemistry with antibodies to CD138. It has been viewed as a cause of RPL in which antibiotics as a treatment modality improve live births, but further research and trials are required.[5,19]

## Male Factors

There is moderate evidence correlating poor sperm quality with RPL especially increased sperm DNA fragmentation. Further research is needed in this area, so sperm selection is not recommended in RPL. Also sperm damage by unhealthy habits (smoking, excessive exercise, and obesity) has been reported. Therefore, partner is advised against excessive alcohol consumption, and excessive exercise; cessation of smoking and attainment of normal body weight is advised.[5]

## Unexplained

In majority of the cases the cause of RPL remains unexplained.

In such cases, certain immunological factors and inflammatory mediators are considered to contribute.

In these cases, immense psychological support with counseling in a dedicated early pregnancy unit goes a long way without pharmacological treatment. Tender loving care (TLC), which includes mental support with weekly check-ups and advice to avoid heavy work, travel, and intercourse, is very important. In such cases, one should resist unnecessary treatments.

The treatment of unexplained RPL with lymphocyte immunization therapy, intravenous immunoglobulins and glucocorticoids is not recommended; these may be associated with many adverse effects which may be life-threatening. The evidence to support treatment with intralipid therapy and G-CSF is also lacking. In unexplained RPL, heparin and aspirin use is also not recommended. There is also insufficient evidence to support endometrial scratching and multivitamins in these couples. Hence, one should be judicious with the treatment prescribed for unexplained RPL.[4,5]

## Behavioral Modifications

- *Smoking:* Smoking has an adverse impact on pregnancy. Therefore, it is recommended for couples with RPL to quit smoking.
- *Alcohol consumption:* ESHRE recommends limiting alcohol intake in RPL as it is a possible cause.
- *Abnormal body mass index (BMI):* Couples with RPL should be informed that maternal obesity or being significantly underweight is associated with obstetric complications and could have a negative impact on their chances of a live birth and on their general health. Striving for a healthy normal range BMI is recommended.[32]
- *Stress:* There is an association between stress and pregnancy loss but whether it is the cause or effect is still unclear.
- *Caffeine intake:* Few studies show a link between caffeine intake and pregnancy loss depending on quantity taken. In one study there was a linear association between mild (<150 mg/day), moderate (150–300 mg/day), and high (>300 mg/day) caffeine intake and pregnancy loss. But evidence is still inconsistent.[5,33]

## ROLE OF PROGESTERONES

In theory, progesterone has a number of benefits in pregnancy; it helps in implantation, affects cytokine balance between Th1 and Th2 cells, inhibits NK cells, inhibits release of arachidonic acid, and prevents the contractility of myometrium and cervical dilatation. It is necessary for the establishment and maintenance of pregnancy.

The Progesterone in Recurrent Miscarriage (PROMISE) trial is a large, high quality, double-blinded trial which included 836 women with idiopathic recurrent miscarriages. The women were given 400 mg of vaginal micronized progesterone twice daily after confirmation of pregnancy or placebo. It was observed that the live birth and the miscarriage rates in both the groups were the same.

The effects of natural and synthetic progesterone in the first trimester were further evaluated in a meta-analysis of 10 RCTs (including the PROMISE trial) in 1,586 women with idiopathic RPL. In eight studies involving synthetic progesterone, higher live births, and decreased miscarriages were seen. However, the drawback of this meta-analysis was that various dosages, routes, and formulations of progesterone were used and the studies that were taken into account were done over a span of 60 years.

Current evidence suggests that there is no role of vaginal progesterone in unexplained RPL on the live births. However, there is some evidence to suggest that supplementation with oral dydrogesterone is effective in RPL. More trials are needed to validate this and also that progesterone supplementation from the luteal phase is more beneficial than after a positive pregnancy test.[5,17,34,35]

FOGSI recommends the following dosage of progesterone for use in RPL:

- *Oral dydrogesterone:* 10 mg BD till 20 weeks of pregnancy
- *Micronized progesterone:* 400 mg/day vaginally till 20 weeks of pregnancy.[3]

## INDIAN PERSPECTIVE

Many Indian studies also have tried to determine the various factors linked with RPL. In the study by Rao V et al. the frequency of hypothyroidism in women with recurrent pregnancy loss in first trimester was assessed. A statistically significant relationship of hypothyroidism with recurrent pregnancy loss in the first trimester was demonstrated and it was concluded that the diagnosis and treatment of hypothyroidism could result in a successful outcome in subsequent pregnancies.[36] Another study by Suryanarayana et al. suggested that the occurrence of the CYP1A1*2A allele was a probable risk factor in idiopathic recurrent miscarriages. There was no association with the other polymorphisms and combinations.[37] Vettriselvi et al. also studied the association between polymorphisms in angiotensin converting enzyme (ACE) and methylene tetrahydrofolate reductase (MTHFR) genes and recurrent pregnancy loss by a case-control study in South Indian women. No association was found between MTHFR C677T and ACE insertion deletion polymorphisms in RPL in South Indian women.[38] The role of MTHFR C677T in recurrent pregnancy losses in North Indian women because of hyperhomocysteinemia was studied by Puri et al. It was found that low vitamin $B_{12}$ increases homocysteine, specifically among mothers carrying T allele. The role of vitamin $B_{12}$ in the prevention of RPL in North Indian women is highlighted by this study.[39] Agrawal et al. studied IL-1 gene cluster variants among the couples with RPL and compared them with healthy controls. IL-1 gene cluster polymorphisms were found among RPL patients and controls invariably.[40] However, these sporadic data need further evaluation.

## CONCLUSION

The multiplicity of recommendations in the literature poses a dilemma for the caregivers. However, individualizing the patients on the basis of background risk and clinical profile will assist in taking a pragmatic and realistic approach to such cases. The cornerstone is supportive care along with directing therapy towards treatable causes, if any. The couples should be reassured that the cumulative chances of a successful pregnancy within 5 years are 60–75% with supportive care alone.[41] A variety of potential therapeutic interventions have been explored, but for most the evidence base remains equivocal, warranting further research into the pathophysiology of recurrent miscarriage and the evolving treatment options.

## KEY POINTS

- The negative prognostic factors for having further miscarriages due to any etiology are increasing maternal age and number of previous miscarriages. The presence of concurrent subfertility also increases the likelihood of another pregnancy loss.
- Parental karyotyping may be offered to couples with RPL especially those with suggestive genetic history.
- Imaging of the uterus should be done in all cases of RPL. 3D USG is the preferred technique. ASRM concluded that it is reasonable to consider surgical correction for septate and cavity-distorting lesions.
- Both ESHRE and ASRM do not recommend screening for hereditary thrombophilia.
- APS is the most important treatable cause for RPL. Hence, all cases of RPL should be screened for APS. It is recommended to treat such cases with aspirin and heparin.
- Various immunological factors have been linked with RPL, but their clear cut role is still controversial. Immunotherapy is expensive and can have serious side effects.
- It is recommended to test the TSH and TPO Ab levels in all females with RPL. There is inadequate evidence to support the treatment of euthyroid females with TPO Ab, but the presence of TPO Ab influence the treatment of subclinical hypothyroidism.
- Majority of the cases of RPL have an unexplained cause. Psychological support and tender loving care in such cases play a very important role.

## REFERENCES

1. Royal College of Obstetricians and Gynaecologists. The Investigation and Treatment of Couples with Recurrent First-Trimester and Second Trimester Miscarriage. London (UK): Royal College of Obstetricians and Gynaecologists (RCOG); 2011. p. 18.
2. Toth B, Würfel W, Bohlmann M, Zschocke J, Rudnik-Schöneborn S, Nawroth F, et al. Recurrent miscarriage: diagnostic and therapeutic procedures. Guideline of the DGGG, OEGGG and SGGG (S2k-Level, AWMF Registry Number 015/050). Geburtshilfe Frauenheilkd. 2018;78(4):364-81.
3. FOGSI Position Statement on the Use of Progestogens. Federation of Obstetric and Gynecological Societies of India; 2015.
4. American Society for Reproductive Medicine. Evaluation and treatment of recurrent pregnancy loss: a committee opinion. Fertil Steril. 2012;98:1103-11.
5. European Society of Human Reproduction and Embryology (2017). The Guideline Development Group on Recurrent Pregnancy Loss [online]. Available from: https://www.eshre.eu/Guidelines-and-Legal/Guidelines/Recurrent-pregnancy-loss. [Last accessed July, 2021].
6. Stephenson M. Cytogenetic analysis of miscarriages from couples with recurrent miscarriage: a case-control study. Human Reprod. 2002;17(2):446-51.
7. Choi TY Lee HM, Park WK, Jeong SY, Moon HS. Spontaneous abortion and recurrent miscarriage: a comparison of cytogenetic diagnosis in 250 cases. Obstet Gynecol Sci. 2014;57:518-25.
8. Fritz M, Speroff L. Recurrent Early Pregnancy Loss. In: Clinical Gynecologic Endocrinology and Infertility, 8th edition. Philadelphia, US: Lippincott Williams & Wilkins; 2015. pp.1191-220.
9. Shapira E, Ratzon R, Shoham-Vardi I, Serjienko R, Mazor M, Bashiri A. Primary vs. secondary recurrent pregnancy loss – epidemiological characteristics, etiology, and next pregnancy outcome. J Perinat Med. 2012;40(4):389-96.
10. Kudesia R, Li M, Smith J, Patel A, Williams Z. Rescue karyotyping: a case series of array-based comparative genomic hybridization evaluation of archival conceptual tissue. Reprod Biol Endocrinol. 2014;12:19.

11. Mathur N, Triplett L, Stephenson MD. Miscarriage chromosome testing: utility of comparative genomic hybridization with reflex microsatellite analysis in preserved miscarriage tissue. Fertil Steril. 2014;101:1349-52.
12. Ikuma S, Sato T, Sugiura-Ogasawara M, Nagayoshi M, Tanaka A, Takeda S. Preimplantation genetic diagnosis and natural conception: a comparison of live birth rates in patients with recurrent pregnancy loss associated with translocation. Plos One. 2015;10(6):e0129958.
13. Saravelos S, Cocksedge K, Li T. The pattern of pregnancy loss in women with congenital uterine anomalies and recurrent miscarriage. Reprod BioMed Online. 2010;20(3):416-22.
14. Saravelos S, Cocksedge K, Li T. Prevalence and diagnosis of congenital uterine anomalies in women with reproductive failure: a critical appraisal. Hum Reprod Update. 2008;14:415-29.
15. Tur-Kaspa I, Gal M, Hartman M, Hartman J, Hartman A. A prospective evaluation of uterine abnormalities by saline infusion sonohysterography in 1,009 women with infertility or abnormal uterine bleeding. Fertil Steril. 2006;86:1731-35.
16. Makris N, Kalmantis K, Skartados N, Papadimitriou A, Mantzaris G, Antsaklis A. Three-dimensional hysterosonography versus hysteroscopy for the detection of intracavitary uterine abnormalities. Int J Gynaecol Obstet. 2007;97:6-9.
17. Homer H. Modern management of recurrent miscarriage. Aust N Z J Obstet Gynaecol. 2019;59:36-44.
18. Santamaria X, Cabanillas S, Cervello I, Arbona C, Raga F, Ferro J, et al. Autologous cell therapy with CD133+ bone marrow-derived stem cells for refractory Asherman's syndrome and endometrial atrophy: a pilot cohort study. Hum Reprod. 2016;31:1087-96.
19. Pandey D, Gupta S. Current update on recurrent pregnancy loss. J Basic Clin Reprod Sci. 2019;8(1).
20. Ressel GW. ACOG Releases Bulletin on Managing Cervical Insufficiency. Am Fam Physician. 2004;69:436-9
21. El Hachem H, Crepaux V, May-Panloup P, Descamps P, Legendre G, Bouet PE. Recurrent pregnancy loss: current perspectives. Int J Womens Health. 2017;9:331-345.
22. van den Boogaard E, Cohn DM, Korevaar JC, Dawood F, Vissenberg R, Middeldorp S, et al. Number and sequence of preceding miscarriages and maternal age for the prediction of antiphospholipid syndrome in women with recurrent miscarriage. Fertil Steril. 2013;99:188-92.
23. FIGO Working Group on Good Clinical Practice in Maternal-Fetal Medicine. Good clinical practice advice: Thyroid and pregnancy. Int J Gynecol Obstet. 2019;144:347-51.
24. Practice Committee of the American Society for Reproductive Medicine. Subclinical hypothyroidism in the infertile female population: a guideline. Fertil Steril. 2015;104(3):545-53.
25. Dosiou C, Stagnaro-Green A. The TABLET trial: limitations and implications. BMC Med. 2019;17(1).
26. Alexander EK, Pearce EN, Brent GA, Brown RS, Chen H, Dosiou C, et al. 2017 Guidelines of the American Thyroid Association for the Diagnosis and Management of Thyroid Disease During Pregnancy and the Postpartum. Thyroid. 2017;27:315-89.
27. Korevaar TI, Muetzel R, Medici M, Chaker L, Jaddoe VW, de Rijke YB, et al. Association of maternal thyroid function during early pregnancy with offspring IQ and brain morphology in childhood: a population-based prospective cohort study. Lancet Diabetes Endocrinol. 2016;4:35-43.
28. Teede H, Misso M, Costello M, Dokras A, Laven J, Moran L, et al. Recommendations from the international evidence-based guideline for the assessment and management of polycystic ovary syndrome. Fertil Steril. 2018;110(3):364-79.
29. Ke RW. Endocrine basis for recurrent pregnancy loss. Obstet Gynecol Clin North Am. 2014;41:103-12
30. Miller P, Soules M. Luteal Phase Deficiency: Pathophysiology, Diagnosis, and Treatment. London: Global Library of Women's Medicine; 2009.
31. Hirahara F, Andoh N, Sawai K, Hirabuki T, Uemura T, Minaguchi H. Hyperprolactinemic recurrent miscarriage and results of randomized bromocriptine treatment trials. Fertil Steril. 1998;70:246-52.
32. Boots CE, Bernardi LA, Stephenson MD. Frequency of euploid miscarriage is increased in obese women with recurrent early pregnancy loss. Fertil Steril. 2014;102:455-9.
33. Stefanidou EM, Caramellino L, Patriarca A, Menato G. Maternal caffeine consumption and sine causa recurrent miscarriage. Eur J Obstet Gynecol Reprod Biol. 2011;158:220-4.
34. Coomarasamy A, Devall A, Brosens J, Quenby S, Stephenson M, Sierra S, et al. Micronized vaginal progesterone to prevent miscarriage: a critical evaluation of randomized evidence. Am J Obstet Gynecol. 2020;223(2):167-76.
35. Saccone G, Schoen C, Franasiak JM, Scott RT Jr, Berghella V. Supplementation with progestogens in the first trimester of pregnancy to prevent miscarriage in women with unexplained recurrent miscarriage: a systematic review and meta-analysis of randomized, controlled trials. Fertil Steril. 2017;107:430-438e3.
36. Rao V, Lakshmi A, Sadhnani M. Prevalence of hypothyroidism in recurrent pregnancy loss in first trimester. Indian J Med Sci. 2008;62(9):357.
37. Suryanarayana V, Deenadayal M, Singh L. Association of *CYP1A1* gene polymorphism with recurrent pregnancy loss in the South Indian population. Human Reprod. 2004;19(11):2648-52.
38. Vettriselvi V, Vijayalakshmi K, Paul S, Venkatachalam P. *ACE* and *MTHFR* gene polymorphisms in unexplained recurrent pregnancy loss. J Obstet Gynaecol Res. 2008;34(3):301-6.
39. Puri M, Kaur L, Walia G, Mukhopadhhyay R, Sachdeva M, Trivedi S, et al. MTHFR C677T polymorphism, folate, vitamin B12 and homocysteine in recurrent pregnancy losses: a case control study among north Indian women. J Perinat Med. 2013;41(5):1-6.
40. Agrawal S, Parveen F, Faridi R, Prakash S. Interleukin-1 gene cluster variants and recurrent pregnancy loss among North Indian women: retrospective study and meta-analysis. Reprod BioMed Online. 2012;24(3):342-51.
41. Lund M, Kamper-Jørgensen M, Nielsen HS, Lidegaard Ø, Andersen AM, Christiansen OB. Prognosis for live birth in women with recurrent miscarriage: what is the best measure of success? Obstet Gynecol. 2012;119:37-43.

# CHAPTER 5

# Antepartum Hemorrhage

*Madhu Goel, Monika Bhatia, Shubha Sagar Trivedi*

## INTRODUCTION

Antepartum hemorrhage (APH) continues to be one of the most serious complications of pregnancy and is an important cause of maternal and perinatal morbidity and mortality. APH is defined as bleeding from or into the genital tract after the period of viability but before the delivery of baby. As per the Royal College of Obstetricians and Gynaecologists (RCOG), bleeding from $24^{+0}$ weeks of pregnancy and before the birth of baby is considered APH.[1] APH occurs in about 3–5% of all pregnancies.[2]

Complete assessment and management of APH in a well-equipped hospital with facilities for resuscitation, replacement of blood and blood products, and expertise in operative delivery improve the maternal and fetal outcome. Massive and uncontrollable hemorrhage can occur in this condition; prompt and aggressive management by an experienced team can save lives.

## CAUSES OF ANTEPARTUM HEMORRHAGE

Antepartum hemorrhage can occur due to a variety of causes. These could be placental, extraplacental, vasa previa or indeterminate **(Flowchart 1)**. Most common are placental causes and include placenta previa and abruptio placentae. Abruptio placentae also called accidental hemorrhage, refers to premature separation of a normally situated placenta in the upper segment of the uterus, whereas placenta previa is conventionally defined as the presence of placenta in lower uterine segment. However, the term placenta previa should be used when the placenta lies directly over the internal os. For pregnancies at more than 16 weeks of gestation, the term low-lying placenta should be used when the placental edge is less than 20 mm from the internal os on transabdominal or transvaginal scanning (TVS).[3] Extraplacental causes of APH are uncommon and include cervical or vaginal lesions such as cervical polyp, varicose veins, cervicitis, and neoplasms, especially carcinoma of the cervix. Rarely, APH is due to vasa previa where fetal vessels lie below the presenting part and blood loss in this situation is fetal. It is a rare but important cause of fetal loss in APH. In about one-third cases of APH, no definite cause is found, and these are classified as indeterminate, unexplained, or unclassified APH. Excessive show may also present as APH but can be diagnosed by the associated mucoid discharge.

Rarely bleeding from hemorrhoids or urinary tract may be confused with vaginal bleeding.

## PLACENTA PREVIA

Placenta previa and low-lying placenta are important causes of APH. The incidence of placenta previa has increased because of the increasing rates of cesarean sections, increasing maternal age at conception, and increase in IVF pregnancies.

### Incidence of Placenta Previa

Placenta previa occurs in about 0.3% of pregnancies.[4]

The frequency with which the zygote implants in the lower part of the uterus is much higher but many of these pregnancies end in early pregnancy losses. In many others, the placenta migrates consequent to differential growth of lower uterine segment as compared to upper and comes to lie in the upper uterine segment. The incidence of placenta previa diagnosed by TVS at 15–20 weeks was reported to

**Flowchart 1:** Causes of antepartum hemorrhage.

be 1.1%; but only 14% of these persisted until delivery.[5] A recent study also reported that the majority of the placenta previa detected in second trimester no longer overlie the internal os in the third trimester. The overlying distance of the placenta, a previous cesarean delivery, and assisted reproductive technology (ART) were found to increase the risk of persistence of a placenta previa.[6]

## Etiology

Various factors predisposing to placenta previa are described here.

*Uterine scars and pathology:* Placenta previa is found more commonly in women with previous history of cesarean section, myomectomy, endometritis, manual removal of placenta, and dilatation and curettage. Incidence of placenta previa rises with number of previous cesarean sections with resultant increase in the risk of life-threatening placenta accreta spectrum (PAS); hence the need to reduce the incidence of cesarean section and to promote vaginal delivery wherever possible. Previous cesarean delivery increases the risk of occurrence of placenta previa from 0.65% after one cesarean to 10% after four or more cesarean sections.

*Multiparity:* The incidence of placenta previa is much higher in parous women. An incidence of 2.2% in women with parity 5 or more has been reported.[7]

*Advanced maternal age:* Advanced maternal age is associated with an increased risk of placenta previa. Older nulliparous as well as older multiparous women were found to be at high odds of placenta previa (adjOR, 2.02; 95% CI, 1.68–2.44 and adjOR, 2.11; 95% CI, 1.83–2.44, respectively).[8]

*Placental size:* Incidence of placenta previa is higher in twin pregnancy, presumably because of large placental size.

*Assisted conception:* Possibly due to increase in multiple pregnancies with assisted conception.

*Placental pathology:* Marginal or velamentous cord insertion, succenturiate lobe, bipartite placenta, and fenestrated placenta are more commonly associated with placenta previa.

*Smoking:* It increases the risk of placenta previa, may be due to compensatory placental enlargement.

*Previous history of placenta previa:* Incidence of placenta previa is higher in a woman with previous history of placenta previa. It is 4–6% which is almost 8–12 times higher. A 4.8% recurrence rate of placenta previa has been reported in the second birth.[9]

## Associated Conditions

*Abnormal placentation:* PAS disorders may be associated with placenta previa, especially if there is a previous cesarean scar. A recent meta-analysis concluded that cesarean delivery appeared as a consistent risk factor for placenta previa, placenta accreta, and placental abruption in subsequent pregnancy.[10]

*Malpresentations:* Placenta previa and low-lying placenta prevent engagement of fetal head and may predispose to malpresentation. It is often associated with high-floating head, breech presentation, oblique, or transverse lie.

*Congenital anomalies:* Incidence of fetal congenital anomalies is almost twice as high in women with placenta previa. The reason is not known.

## Classification

Originally, placenta lying in lower uterine segment was labeled as placenta previa and was graded from 1 to 4, depending upon the distance of placental edge from internal os. More recently, a multidisciplinary workshop of American Institute of Ultrasound in Medicine has recommended that the term placenta previa should be used when the placenta lies directly over the internal os and the term low-lying placenta should be used when placental edge is less than 20 mm from the internal os on transabdominal or transvaginal sonography after 16 weeks of gestation.[11]

The term complete previa has been used in the past to describe a placenta that covers the cervical os and marginal previa when it is less than 2 cm from internal os.

## Clinical Features

Placenta previa may be asymptomatic. A high head, oblique lie or transverse lie should arouse the suspicion of placenta previa. Many a times, placenta previa presents as APH. Painless, causeless, and recurrent bleeding in late pregnancy is strongly suggestive of placenta previa.

The onset of bleeding is usually sudden, it may follow intercourse, although in most cases, it is causeless. The bleeding may vary from being slight to profuse; usually the first bout of bleeding is threatening but not alarming and stops spontaneously, only to recur later. The subsequent bouts of bleeding can be heavier and massive.

Bleeding in some cases may not occur till the onset of labor. PAS should be suspected in such cases.

The absence of abdominal pain and uterine contractions has classically been considered an important distinguishing feature between placenta previa and accidental hemorrhage. However, placental separation in placenta previa may incite mild uterine contractions sometimes, which usually cease subsequently. Hence, sonography must be done in all cases of bleeding during second half of pregnancy to exclude placenta previa.

The general condition of the woman corresponds to the amount of blood loss. If the bleeding has been profuse, the signs of hypovolemic shock will be present. There may be restlessness, agitation, syncope, anxiety, or confusion. Pallor, cold and clammy skin, tachycardia, hypotension, and dyspnea denote significant bleeding. Oliguria and anuria are signs of persistent hypovolemic shock.

On abdominal examination, the size of the uterus corresponds to the period of gestation. The uterus is relaxed, soft without any area of tenderness. The fetal parts are easily palpable in contrast to placental abruption where fetal parts are difficult to palpate because of the tense and tender uterus. The presenting part is usually high, and fetus may be in oblique or transverse lie. Fetal heart sounds are present unless there is a major degree of placental separation or hypovolemic shock.

## Diagnosis

Most of the cases of placenta previa are diagnosed on a routine transabdominal anomaly scan at 18–20 weeks and confirmed on subsequent ultrasound, abdominal and/or transvaginal, at 32 and 36 weeks.

However, placenta previa should be suspected in any woman who presents with causeless, painless vaginal bleeding after 20 weeks of pregnancy with no previous ultrasound report. Clinical features must always be kept in mind in such patients.

Diagnosis is confirmed on ultrasonography. Transvaginal sonography is an accurate and safe diagnostic procedure for confirming placenta previa. In women with placenta previa, placental cord insertion should be evaluated to rule out the possibility of vasa previa in case insertion is velamentous.

An evaluation for presence of placenta accreta, increta, or percreta (PAS) is indicated, especially in cases of placenta previa with previous cesarean section and in cases with other high-risk factors for placenta accreta.

## Management of Placenta Previa

Management of placenta previa and low-lying placenta diagnosed at 18-20 weeks scan (fetal anomaly scan) depends on the clinical course and subsequent scans and is summarized in **Flowchart 2**.

Placenta previa may be asymptomatic or may present with recurrent bleeding episodes, sometimes profuse, and it may be associated with placenta accreta. Management is thus, described accordingly.

### Management of Asymptomatic Women Diagnosed at Second Trimester Ultrasound Scan

The patient is usually diagnosed with placenta previa or low-lying placenta in the second trimester scan where the

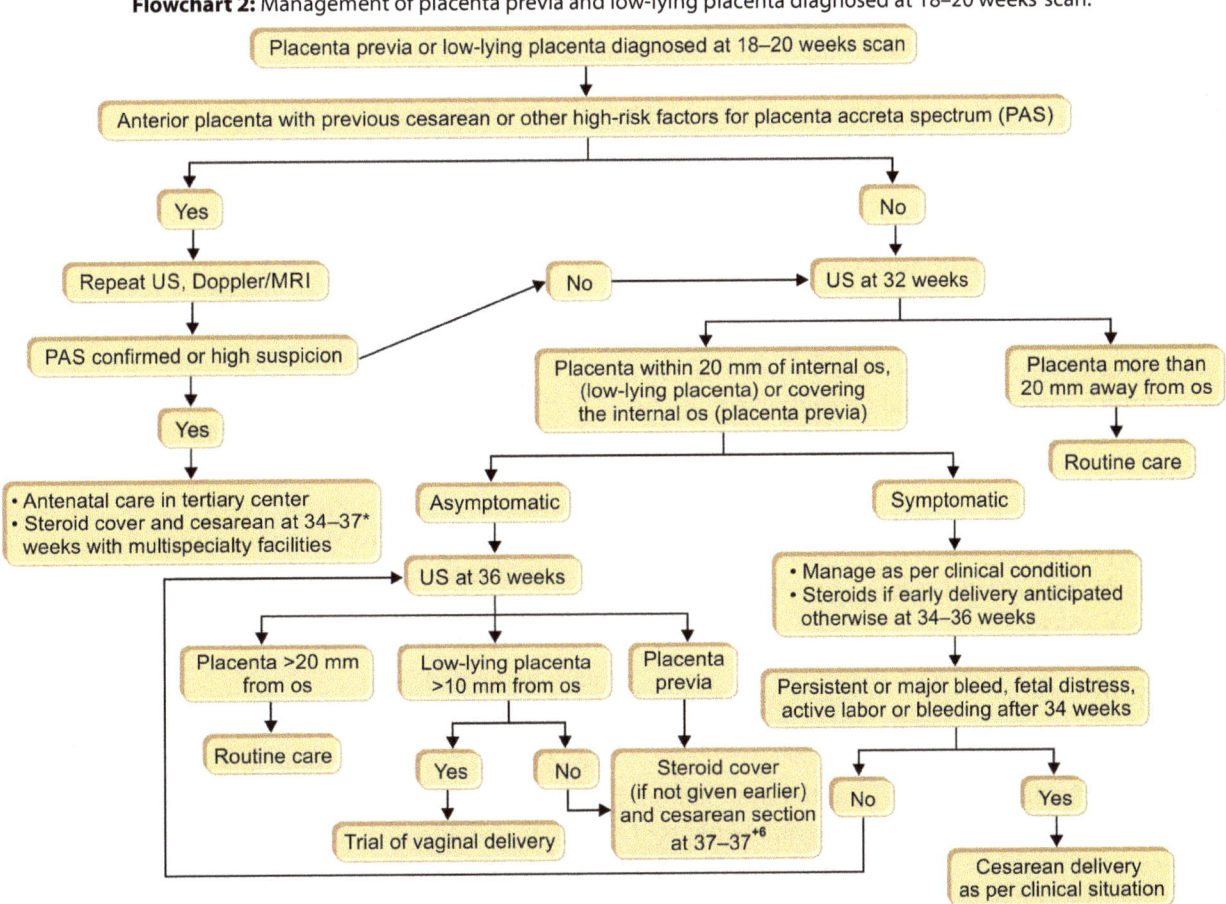

**Flowchart 2:** Management of placenta previa and low-lying placenta diagnosed at 18–20 weeks' scan.

*Society for Maternal and Fetal Medicine Recommendations, 2017.[12]

placental edge is either covering the internal os or is within 20 mm from the internal os. These patients should have routine antenatal care. In addition, they should be advised to avoid intercourse, avoid lifting heavy weights, and should be made aware of the chances of spotting or bleeding and to report in the hospital in case they have bleeding per vaginum.

*Repeat ultrasound:* A transvaginal ultrasound is repeated at 32 weeks in these patients. If the placental edge is more than 2 cm away from the internal os, the patient continues with routine antenatal care. In those with persistent placenta previa or low-lying placenta, TVS is repeated at 36 weeks.

Vasa previa should be ruled out on ultrasound in these cases as it can occur in patients with resolution of placenta previa.

As per RCOG guidelines, cervical length should also be measured at the time of scan as this may help in decision making in management of asymptomatic women with placenta previa. A short cervical length on TVS before 34 weeks has been shown to be associated with increased risk of preterm delivery and excessive bleeding at cesarean section.[11]

*Antenatal corticosteroids:* A single course of antenatal corticosteroids between 34 and 35$^{+6}$ weeks is recommended in women with placenta previa and low-lying placenta, which may be given prior to 34 weeks of gestation in women at higher risk of preterm birth.[11] Society for Maternal-Fetal Medicine (SMFM) recommends administration of antenatal corticosteroids to women who are eligible and are managed expectantly, the gestational age is between 34 and 36$^{+6}$ weeks, and antenatal corticosteroids have not been given earlier (Grade 1A).[12]

*Hospital or home management:* A decision is taken regarding hospital or home management after considering all the factors. An asymptomatic placenta previa can be managed at home provided the woman can reach hospital immediately in case bleeding occurs. Studies have not shown any difference regarding maternal or fetal morbidity with home management versus hospitalization prior to the first bleed in these women.[11]

*Route and time of delivery:* According to RCOG guidelines, in cases of placenta previa, i.e., where the placental edge covers the internal os at 36 weeks scan, cesarean delivery is planned between 36 and 37 weeks.[11]

Society for Maternal-Fetal Medicine, however, recommends delivery at 36 to 37$^{+6}$ weeks of gestation for stable women with placenta previa without bleeding or other obstetric complications.[12]

If the placental edge does not cover the os but is <2 cm from the internal os (low-lying placenta), the risks and benefits of a trial of labor should be discussed with the patient. The risk of bleeding increases as the distance between the placental edge and internal os decreases.

In a recent systematic review and meta-analysis, it was found that vaginal delivery was successful in 43% cases when placental distance from internal os (IOD) was 0–10 mm, 85% when the distance was 11–20 mm, and 82% when IOD was >20 mm. A shorter IOD had a higher chance of APH. They concluded that low-lying placenta is not a contraindication for trial of labor.[13]

Vasa previa is sometimes associated with low-lying placenta and should be looked for, which, if present, is an indication for elective cesarean.

## Management of Women Who Present with Active Bleeding

Many women with placenta previa, diagnosed or undiagnosed, present with bleeding per vaginum. All women with APH should be admitted to the hospital. One should be prepared to manage massive hemorrhage and preterm delivery in a woman with placenta previa.

*Management in hospital:* All women admitted with APH should have an immediate overall assessment to establish if any urgent intervention is required as in women with continued or profuse bleeding. Resuscitation is initiated, if indicated.

If there is no maternal or fetal compromise, a detailed assessment is done.

- A comprehensive history is taken. Gestational age is calculated by last menstrual period or previous ultrasonography (USG) done in early pregnancy. Information about placental localization on previous ultrasounds and its relationship to previous scars, if any, is reviewed.
- Assessment of general condition of patient is done. Maternal pulse, blood pressure, respiratory rate, and oxygen saturation are recorded. Pallor is assessed for its presence and severity. Presence of pallor, tachycardia, tachypnea, and hypotension are signs of excessive blood loss, and patient may be in hemorrhagic shock.

Estimate of the amount of blood loss is done. Exact assessment may be difficult. Vulva is inspected to assess the amount of blood loss, its color, and to determine whether bleeding has stopped or is continuing. A pregnant woman with APH presenting in hemorrhagic shock has already lost 15–20% of her circulating blood volume (1–1.5 L, approximately).

*Abdominal examination:* It is important to exclude uterine tenderness, increased tone, and contractions and to note whether uterine fundal height is corresponding with gestational age or is more as in placental abruption. Lie and presentation should be noted. In placenta previa, the uterus is usually soft, relaxed, nontender with fundal height corresponding to the period of gestation.

Fetal heart is auscultated for any evidence of fetal distress. No per speculum or per vaginal examination is done in patients with active bleeding as it can incite hemorrhage.

An intravenous line is established with wide bore cannula no. 16 or 18. Ringers lactate or normal saline is infused to achieve or maintain hemodynamic stability and adequate urine output (at least 30 mL/h).

A blood sample is taken for full blood count, blood group and type, cross-matching, and for coagulation studies. Transfusion of blood products in a woman with an actively bleeding placenta previa should be guided by the volume of blood loss and changes in hemodynamic parameters, e.g., blood pressure, maternal and fetal heart rates, peripheral perfusion, and urine output, as well as the hemoglobin level. The volume replacement is done at the rate of 3 mL of crystalloid or 2 mL of colloid for every mL of blood loss till packed cell volume is arranged.

If possible, an USG should be performed for placental localization, confirmation of lie, to rule out associated abruption, and for fetal well-being.

No tocolytic drugs should be administered in an actively bleeding patient with threatened preterm labor. If the patient is not actively bleeding, the tocolytics may be administered in preterm placenta previa for 48 hours to provide corticosteroid cover to the fetus.[14]

A course of corticosteroids should be given to women with preterm pregnancy. However, if she must be taken for emergency cesarean section, one should administer the first dose of corticosteroids and not wait for 48 hours. In Rh-negative patient, anti-D should be given in women presenting with APH. Readministration is not necessary, if the bleeding/delivery occur within 3 weeks of the last injection.

Magnesium sulfate therapy for neuroprotection in pregnancies between 24 and 32 weeks is indicated in cases where a decision to deliver within 24 hours but not emergently is taken. Emergency delivery should not be delayed for administration of magnesium sulfate.

Depending on the maturity of fetus, amount of bleeding, maternal and fetal condition, and whether the woman is in labor or not, further management can be expectant or active.

*Expectant management:* Aim of the expectant management is to prolong the pregnancy till the fetus matures. It is indicated when the following conditions are present:
- Preterm pregnancy
- Live fetus
- No serious fetal malformations
- Bleeding is not excessive
- Patient is hemodynamically stable
- Patient is not in labor.

Absolute bed rest is advised till at least 48 hours after the bleeding stops. Careful monitoring of pulse, blood pressure, fundal height, fetal heart rate, and vaginal bleeding is done. Antenatal steroids for fetal lung maturity should be administered in women with gestation between 24 and $36^{+6}$ weeks. Rh-negative woman should be given anti-D immunoglobulin. Ultrasound examination, if not done earlier, is done to localize placenta and to exclude any fetal malformation. Anti-anemic treatment in form of hematinics is given and woman is kept in hospital under observation. Use of cervical cerclage to prevent bleeding and prolong pregnancy is not recommended. Tocolytics have been tried with a view to prolong the pregnancy but are not advocated for lack of evidence. Very cautiously tocolysis is sometimes given for antenatal corticosteroid cover in women with APH and uterine activity. Expectant management is continued till fetal maturity is attained or if bleeding continues or becomes excessive.

Most women who initially present with symptomatic placenta previa respond to conservative treatment and do not require immediate delivery but they are at high risk of recurrent bleeds and 25–40% requiring emergency delivery because of bleeding.

Prolonged hospitalization may be required and is a safer option. Decision to discharge the woman depends on her condition, the number of episodes of bleeding, proximity to the hospital, as well as likely compliance. Carefully selected women with placenta previa whose bleeding has stopped for a minimum of 48 hours and who have no other pregnancy complications can be discharged after explaining the risks and proper counseling. They should understand that there is a risk of profuse bleeding and they should be able to reach the hospital immediately.

*Active management:* Active management of placenta previa involves delivering the woman by cesarean section. It is indicated, if there is severe and persistent vaginal bleeding or if maternal hemodynamic stability cannot be achieved or maintained. In cases where there is significant vaginal bleeding after 34 weeks of gestation, neonatal benefits from avoiding preterm birth decrease with advancing gestational age and the maternal risks from persistent or recurrent bleeding increase, hence delivery is indicated. Delivery is also indicated in symptomatic women with placenta previa, if she is in labor, there is fetal distress or pregnancy is 36 weeks or more **(Box 1)**.

---

**BOX 1:** Indications of active management of placenta previa.

- The woman is in labor
- There is fetal distress
- If there is severe and persistent vaginal bleeding or if maternal hemodynamic stability cannot be achieved or maintained
- Significant vaginal bleeding after 34 weeks of gestation—the neonatal benefits from avoiding preterm birth decrease with advancing gestational age and the maternal risks from persistent or recurrent bleeding probably increase
- Intrauterine fetal death or congenitally malformed baby
- In women who have been asymptomatic or on expectant treatment and reach 37 weeks of pregnancy

*Cesarean section in placenta previa:* Cesarean section is required in all cases of placenta previa where placenta lies over the internal os and it is the recommended treatment.

Cesarean section should be performed by a senior obstetrician along with a senior anesthesiologist. Blood should be available in all cases. Antenatal evaluation for PAS is recommended especially in anterior placenta previa in women with previous cesarean section.

The choice of anesthetic technique for cesarean section for placenta previa must be made by the anesthetist in consultation with obstetrician and the patient. General anesthesia had been advocated in the past but there is increasing evidence to support the safety of regional block with decreased blood loss.

Lower segment cesarean section is preferred, and it must be performed by an experienced obstetrician. An ultrasound done prior to cesarean section may help in planning the incision on the uterus and access the membranes avoiding the placenta. Care should be taken while giving an incision on the lower segment as it is highly vascular in such cases. In cases where placenta is implanted anteriorly, the placenta is either separated manually to reach the margin of the placenta or cut through; membranes are ruptured and baby delivered. In both these conditions, the cord must be clamped promptly to prevent further fetal blood loss. Complete hemostasis should be achieved in all cases.

Diffuse and profuse bleeding may occur from the placental bed because placental site is in the lower uterine segment which does not contract and retract as efficiently as the upper segment. Medical and surgical interventions to stop the bleeding are required simultaneously. Uterotonics, including oxytocin, methylergonovine maleate (Methergine), 15 methyl prostaglandin F2 alpha (Carboprost), or misoprostol should be used systematically to manage uterine atony. Tranexamic acid one gram (10 mL of a 100 mg/mL solution) is infused over 10-20 minutes. It can be given along with uterotonic drugs. It can also be given prophylactically to decrease blood loss.

For hemostasis at placental site, packing or pressure with gauze may stop or decrease the bleeding. Hemostatic sutures are applied, over sewing the placental site or interrupted sutures can be placed. Intrauterine balloon tamponade and uterine compression sutures have been described for controlling bleeding.

In cases of focal placenta accreta with persistent bleeding, excision may be done if the area is small and easily accessible.

If bleeding persists, bilateral uterine artery ligation or internal iliac artery ligation may be required and is often effective.

Rapid replacement of blood and blood products should be carried out for stabilization of patient's hemodynamic status.

If all the measures fail to control the bleeding, timely hysterectomy may be lifesaving and should not be delayed.

Newborn must be monitored carefully and may require blood transfusion.

*Delivery in a woman with low-lying placenta:* The optimal route for delivery of pregnancies where the distance between the placental edge and internal os is 0-20 mm is debatable.

Although a variety of factors influence the decision to perform cesarean delivery, a trial of labor can be given in patients in whom the placenta is more than 10 mm away from the internal os.[6,8,14] In these cases, the fetal head may tamponade the adjacent placenta, thus preventing hemorrhage.

If this distance is ≤ 10 mm, there is high risk of intrapartum hemorrhage necessitating emergency cesarean delivery.

If a trial of vaginal delivery with a low-lying placenta is attempted, the facilities to perform an emergency cesarean delivery should be there. Early artificial rupture of membranes (ARM) may be considered in these cases.

## ■ PLACENTA ACCRETA SPECTRUM

Placenta accreta spectrum, formerly known as morbidly adherent placenta, refers to the range of pathologic adherence of the placenta, including placenta increta, percreta, and placenta accreta.[15]

Placenta accreta is when the villi simply adhere to the myometrium; placenta increta, when the villi invade the myometrium **(Fig. 1)**; and placenta percreta, when villi invade the full thickness of the myometrium including the uterine serosa and sometimes bladder, ureter and other adjacent pelvic structures. Variations in the lateral extension of myometrial invasion also divide PAS disorders into the focal, partial, or total categories, depending on the number of placental cotyledons involved.[16]

Placenta accreta spectrum carries high risk of maternal mortality and morbidity and its incidence is increasing globally.

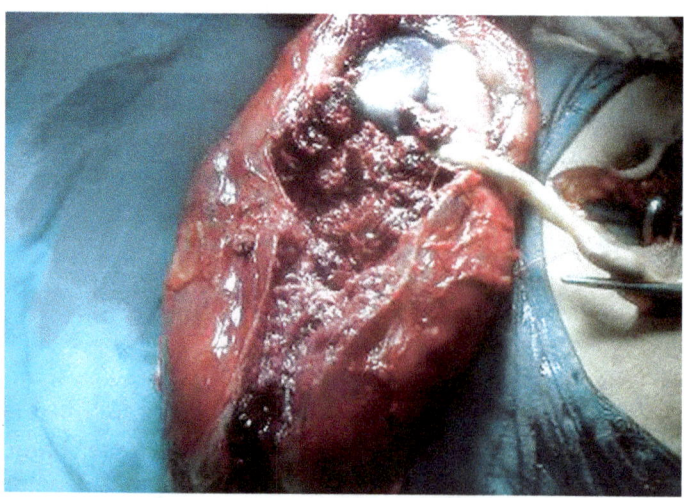

**Fig. 1:** Placenta increta.

It is essential to identify this condition before or during delivery, particularly the invasive forms.

Variable incidence has been reported across the world ranging from 1 in 300 to 1 in 2,000 pregnancies. The incidence of PAS is increasing because of the increasing rates of cesarean section. In a large multicentric US cohort study, it was found that in women with placenta previa and previous cesarean delivery, the risk of placenta accreta was 3%, 11%, 40%, 61%, and 67% for first, second, third, fourth, and fifth or more cesarean deliveries, respectively.[17]

## Risk Factors for Placenta Accreta Spectrum

The most common risk factor for PAS is previous cesarean, more the number of previous cesarean sections, higher is the risk for PAS. Placenta previa is another significant risk factor. Other risk factors include advanced maternal age, multiparity, prior uterine surgeries, previous history of dilatation and curettage, and Asherman's syndrome. Previous cesarean with anterior placenta previa should alert the obstetrician to the presence of placenta accreta.

## Diagnosis

Diagnosing PAS in antenatal period is crucial.

Placenta accreta spectrum must be looked for in all pregnancies with high-risk factors listed above especially in women with previous cesarean section diagnosed with placenta previa on second and third trimester ultrasound. Features of PAS include multiple vascular lacunae within the placenta, loss of the normal hypoechoic zone between the placenta and myometrium, decreased retroplacental myometrial thickness (less than 1 mm), abnormalities of the uterine serosa–bladder interface, and extension of placenta into myometrium, serosa, or bladder. However, ultrasound does not rule out PAS and hence index of clinical suspicion should remain high in the presence of high-risk factors. Color Doppler can further help in the diagnosis of PAS. MRI complements ultrasound and helps to assess the depth of penetration of placenta and is especially useful in posterior placenta.

## Management

Placenta accreta spectrum disorders are emerging as one of the most serious obstetric complications, and causing significant maternal mortality and morbidity worldwide. As per ACOG Obstetric Care Consensus 2018, outcomes in PAS are optimized when delivery occurs at a level III (subspecialty care), or level IV (regional perinatal healthcare centers) before the onset of labor or bleeding.[15]

### Timing of Delivery in PAS

In the absence of risk factors for preterm delivery in women with PAS, planned delivery at $35^{+0}$ to $36^{+6}$ weeks of gestation is said to provide the best balance between fetal maturity and the risk of unscheduled delivery.[11] FIGO consensus guidelines suggest that women who are stable with no prepartum hemorrhage, preterm premature rupture of membranes, or uterine contractions may be considered for planned delivery at 36–37 weeks.

However, contingency plan for emergency cesarean/hysterectomy, massive blood transfusion, and multidisciplinary management of the patient should be in place.

### Preoperative Management

- Optimization of hemoglobin of the patient antenatally.
- Risk of postpartum hemorrhage (PPH), need for hysterectomy, ICU care, and elective ventilation are to be explained and informed consent taken.
- Arrange requisite amount of blood. Massive blood transfusion may be required in some cases.
- Senior obstetrician and anesthetist should be present.
- Multidisciplinary involvement in preoperative planning.
- Schedule cesarean section at 34 to $36^{+6}$ weeks in a facility equipped to manage PAS.
- Antenatal corticosteroids.

### Intraoperative Management

The best approach to PAS is cesarean hysterectomy with placenta left in situ. Attempt to separate the placenta should not be made.

Depending upon the individual case and imaging results, surgical planning is done. Vertical abdominal incision may be preferable in women with morbidly adherent placenta or where difficulties are anticipated in approaching the lower segment.

Evaluation is carried out to plan the uterine incision. In placenta previa accreta, incision in the uterus is given above the site of placental edge and upper segment cesarean is preferable.

It is important that after delivery of the baby, injection oxytocin is withheld, no attempt is made to separate the placenta otherwise there can be torrential hemorrhage.

In case the diagnosis of placenta accreta is not certain, spontaneous separation of placenta should be awaited. In absence of spontaneous separation, a decision for expectant management or hysterectomy is taken depending upon the preplanned management or the clinical situation.

In women with major degree of placenta accreta, hysterectomy is a safer option. Although successful conservative management has been described, there is limited evidence to support it in placenta percreta.[3]

Expectant management may, however, be required in unsuspected, emergency cases where expertise or facilities for emergency hysterectomy are not available and patient is not bleeding. Expectant management may also be done if the patient is not bleeding and fertility is an issue. In expectant management, cord is cut close to placenta and uterus is closed. Careful monitoring and observation are continued for any vaginal bleeding in postoperative period.

The woman and her relative must be informed that hysterectomy may be required later because of complications such as hemorrhage and sepsis. Placenta is expelled or resorbed in some; but about 20–40% need hysterectomy. Uterine artery embolization and postoperative methotrexate have been tried with variable results.

In case hysterectomy is planned, all measures should be taken to minimize the blood loss. In cases of adherent bladder, separation may be done after bilateral uterine artery ligation. Internal iliac artery ligation or uterine artery embolization may be required in cases with excessive bleeding. Placing of balloon-tipped intra-arterial catheters in internal iliac arteries preoperatively has been described. These are inflated after delivery to occlude the vessels and reduce the blood loss. These catheters can also be used to embolize the vessels.

### Planned Delayed Hysterectomy

Planned delayed or secondary hysterectomy is an alternative "definitive" surgical management for PAS disorders where extensive invasion of surrounding structures renders immediate hysterectomy extremely difficult.[16] Decreased vascularity, involution of uterus, and placental resorption make delayed hysterectomy easier and can be performed 3–12 weeks postpartum. The risk of coagulopathy, sepsis, and hemorrhage must be kept in mind with full preparedness for a difficult emergency hysterectomy at any time. Conventionally, these hysterectomies are performed by laparotomy, but laparoscopic approach including robotic surgery has been described in selected cases with an aim to reduce morbidity.[18,19]

## ABRUPTIO PLACENTA

Abruptio placenta, also known as ablatio placenta or accidental hemorrhage, is a serious condition that despite the modern medical advances cannot be predicted or prevented and can lead to high fetal loss and maternal complications. Abruptio placentae, the premature separation of a normally situated placenta accounts for 30% of cases of APH. It occurs in about 0.5–1% of deliveries,[20] the severe form occurring in about 1 in 500 deliveries.

### Etiology

The exact cause of separation of normally situated placenta is not always known.

Following are some of the conditions which lead to abruptio placentae:
- *External trauma*: Fall or blow on abdomen or rarely external cephalic version.
- Acute decompression of polyhydramnios. Sudden diminution of surface area of uterus where placenta is attached leads to placental detachment.
- Preterm rupture of membranes predisposes to placental abruption.
- Hypertension is the most commonly associated condition with placental abruption. In severe abruption, gestational hypertension or chronic hypertension was found in 50% of the cases. In milder form of abruption, the incidence of hypertension is not high.
- Other predisposing factors include advanced maternal age, multiparity, uterine leiomyoma, smoking, and previous history of abruption (10% risk of recurrence), ART pregnancy, and cocaine abuse.
- Folic acid deficiency though implicated has not been proved to be the cause of abruption.
- First trimester bleeding predisposes to abruption.
- In many cases, no cause is found. Although not proven, congenital or acquired thrombophilia may be responsible in some cases.

### Pathophysiology

Placental abruption is initiated by hemorrhage into the decidua basalis. As the decidual hematoma expands, it separates and compresses the placenta. The blood may separate the membranes and escape vaginally giving rise to revealed type of abruptio placentae **(Figs. 2A and B)**. The placental detachment is usually incomplete with this and complications are fewer and less severe. The revealed form of abruptio placentae is more common and is found in approximately 80% of the cases. In early stages, there may not be any clinical features suggestive of abruption. On inspection of the placenta after delivery, a circumscribed depression with dark clotted blood is found. Abruption, if recent, however may not show any evidence of separation on placental examination following delivery.

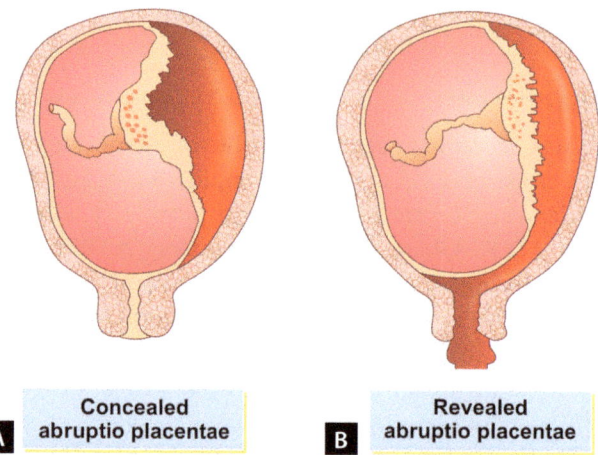

**Figs. 2A and B:** Types of abruptio placentae. (A) Concealed abruptio placentae; (B) Revealed abruptio placentae.

In concealed variety, the placental margins or the membranes remain adherent to the uterine wall and blood keeps collecting behind the placenta. This is a severe form of abruptio placentae and is seen in about 20% of the cases. Following the separation of the placenta, the blood does not escape out but is retained behind the placenta within the uterine cavity. Fetal death, coagulation disorders, and other maternal complications are more common with concealed variety of abruption. Blood may enter the amniotic cavity after breaking through the membranes. In some cases, the fetal head which is closely applied to the cervix may prevent the blood to escape.

In more severe form of concealed placental abruption, widespread extravasation of blood occurs into the uterine musculature and beneath the serosa giving rise to Couvelaire uterus which appears ecchymotic and purple on laparotomy. These myometrial hematomas do not interfere with uterine contractility and do not warrant hysterectomy.

## Clinical Features

Clinical presentation may vary depending upon the severity and type of abruption whether concealed or revealed. In mild cases, there may not be any symptoms or signs.

In majority of the cases, vaginal bleeding is the predominant feature and is found in about 70–80% of the cases. Bleeding is most often associated with abdominal pain. Back pain and uterine contractions may be observed in some cases. Uterine tenderness and rigidity are present in most of these cases and are important signs of placental abruption. Depending on the severity of abruption, fetal heart sounds may or may not be present. Fetal distress is found in about 50% of the cases and fetal death occurs in about 15% of the cases.

In mild cases of abruption, vaginal bleeding may not be associated with abdominal pain and may not produce any signs of abruption. Uterus may feel nontense and nontender. Diagnosis is made on examination of placenta after delivery, which reveals a retroplacental clot.

Typical signs of placental separation may be absent initially in a case of abruptio placentae. As the blood collects behind the placenta, the uterus becomes tender and tense and the uterine height may rise. Hence, every woman who presents with vaginal bleeding must be monitored carefully to detect this condition. Uterine tenderness and rigidity may be absent in abruption of a posteriorly situated placenta.

In severe forms of concealed hemorrhage, no vaginal bleeding may be observed but the uterus is found to be tense and tender and fetal heart sounds are usually absent. The woman may develop a hemorrhagic diathesis due to disseminated intravascular coagulation (DIC) with depletion of fibrinogen as well as other clotting factors. This may lead to active bleeding from all the sites. Hypovolemic shock and renal failure may develop.

## Diagnosis

Diagnosis of abruptio placentae is clinical and high index of suspicion is required to diagnose mild and atypical cases. All cases of vaginal bleeding or pain in latter half of pregnancy and those with history of trauma must be evaluated and observed carefully to diagnose or exclude abruption. Ultrasound is not always helpful in diagnosing abruptio placentae, it may be normal in these cases, but it helps to exclude placenta previa. There may be no findings on ultrasound in revealed abruption as there is no retroplacental clot. Retroplacental clot, if present, may take a variety of appearances from hypoechoic to isoechoic to hyperechoic and the diagnosis of abruption may be confused by the retroplacental complex which appears hyperechoic on ultrasound. The hyperechoic retroplacental complex which is usually no more than 2 cm in thickness demonstrates very high blood flow by color Doppler. When the retroplacental clot is large, ultrasound identifies it as hyperechoic or isoechoic compared with the placenta. This echogenicity may also be misinterpreted as a thick placenta. In women on expectant management with small retroplacental clot, resolution of the clot appears hyperechoic within 1 week and sonolucent within 2 weeks.

Depending upon the degree of abruption and its clinical effects, the cases are graded as follows:

*Grade 0:* Clinical features suggestive of placental separation are absent; the diagnosis is made retrospectively when retroplacental clots are detected incidentally following delivery.

*Grade I:* There is hemorrhage with uterine irritability and pain, but there is no maternal or fetal compromise.

*Grade II:* In this grade, APH is accompanied by classic features of abruptio placentae and the fetus is alive. The uterus is tense and tender and fetal heart abnormalities are present.

*Grade III:* Along with the features of grade II, there is fetal death. It has associated maternal shock, coagulation failure, or renal failure.

## Management of Abruptio Placentae

Management of abruptio placentae depends on the severity of the case and on the condition of the mother and the fetus. All cases require intensive monitoring and individualized management **(Flowchart 3)**.

In cases of mild abruption, where the uterus is soft and nontender, the pregnancy should be terminated by induction of labor with low rupture of membranes and oxytocin. Many cases of abruption are already in established labor and only ARM is done. They may not require oxytocin.

Careful watch on progress of labor, condition of woman and fetus is important. Signs of hemorrhage, revealed or concealed, should be looked for. Vital signs, uterine height,

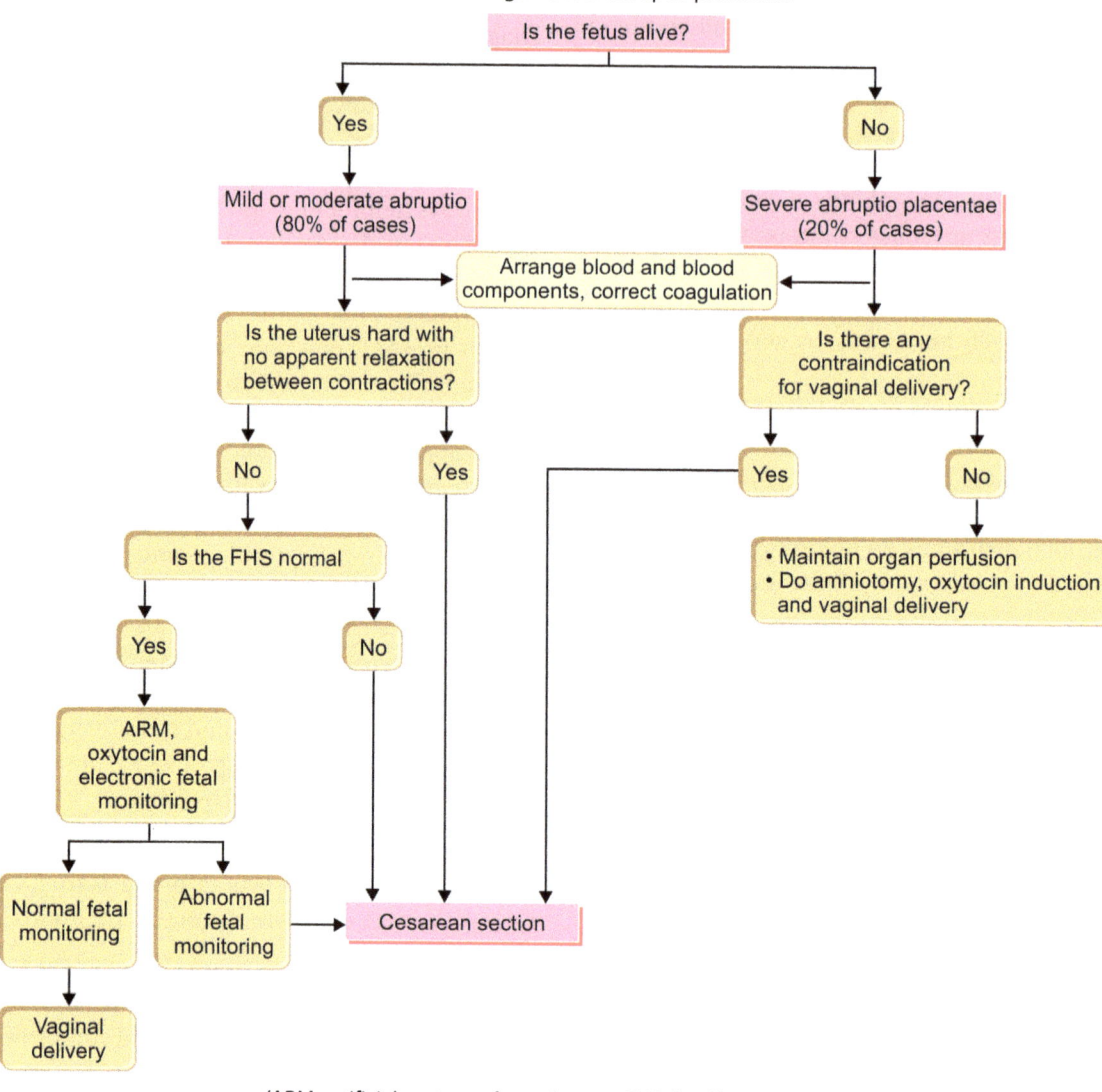

Flowchart 3: Management of abruptio placentae.

(ARM: artificial rupture of membranes; FHS: fetal heart sound)

vaginal bleeding, urinary output, and coagulation profile should be carefully monitored. Blood and fresh frozen plasma (FFP) should be arranged. An early delivery of fetus with adequate replacement of fluid or blood and careful monitoring results in good outcome. Cesarean section is indicated, if patient deteriorates or fetal distress develops. Coagulation profile, if found to be abnormal, should be promptly treated.

If the fetus is alive and the uterus is rigid, it implies that the abruption is large but is less than 50%, chances of fetal distress are high and therefore, patient should be prepared for immediate cesarean section with blood and fluid replacement. Coagulation profile should be checked, and if deranged must be corrected promptly prior to cesarean section.

Women with fetal death should preferably be delivered vaginally. Amniotomy should be done as soon as possible and if required, oxytocin drip is started. Strict watch on uterine contractions is maintained as the uterus is hypertonic. Careful monitoring of vital signs, coagulation profile, and urinary output is important.

Women with severe pre-eclampsia with abruption may appear to be normotensive despite excessive blood loss. The blood loss with severe abruptio placentae associated with fetal death was often found to be about half the total blood volume.[21]

These patients, therefore, require prompt and adequate transfusion of fluids and blood. Two wide bore intravenous access lines should be established to allow rapid administration of fluids and blood. Hematocrit and coagulation studies should be done 4–8 hourly depending on the grade of placental abruption. Indwelling urinary catheter should be inserted and urine output is monitored. Hematocrit should be maintained at 30% or more, to sustain the oxygen carrying capacity of the blood. Urinary output of at least 30 mL/h signifies effective intravascular volume and prevents acute tubular or cortical necrosis, an important cause of maternal mortality in abruptio placentae.

Central venous pressure may be monitored by putting a catheter in internal jugular vein and maintaining it at 10 cm of water. This helps in preventing fluid overload. Lung bases must be auscultated for any crepts suggestive of fluid overload.

Third stage of labor should be managed actively. Oxytocin infusion and uterine massage is usually sufficient to prevent PPH. Total blood loss should be estimated, retroplacental clots must be measured and recorded. Very often the blood loss is underestimated, and woman may go into hypovolemic shock. Close monitoring must be continued after delivery with special watch for PPH and urinary output.

Only in very mild cases of placental abruption with slight bleeding where fetus is preterm and maternal, and fetal condition is stable, expectant treatment can be given in the hospital under very close supervision. Periodic ultrasound examinations are done to monitor fetal growth and the size of the clot. Tocolysis to prolong pregnancy is not advocated in case the woman goes into preterm labor.

In cases with incidental finding of a small retroplacental clot on ultrasound, conservative management with careful monitoring is advisable. Predisposing factors such as smoking or hypertension should be looked for and managed.

### Management of Coagulopathy

In severe abruption, acute DIC may occur leading to fall in fibrinogen levels, other coagulation factors and elevation of fibrin degradation products and D-dimers. Fibrinogen levels may fall below 140 mg/dL and there may be fall in platelet count along with prolongation of partial thromboplastin time (PTT) and prothrombin time (PT). In absence of facilities for coagulation studies, a simple bedside clot observation test is invaluable in managing these cases. Venous blood sample is drawn and is placed in a clean dry test tube. It is observed for clot formation and clot lysis. Failure of clot formation within 10 minutes or dissolution of a firm clot when the tube is gently shaken at the end of an hour suggests clotting deficiency due to lack of fibrinogen, platelets, and other coagulation factors.

Aggressive blood and coagulation factors replacement should be carried out. As per RCOG guidelines, up to 4 units of FFP and 10 units of cryoprecipitates may be given while awaiting the results of coagulation studies.[1]

Platelet transfusion in a bleeding patient is indicated if count is below 50,000/mm$^3$ and in all patients with a platelet count less than 20,000/mm$^3$ even if there is no bleeding. Coagulation defect must be corrected if cesarean section is to be carried out. Platelet count of at least 50,000/mm$^3$ and 80,000/mm$^3$, respectively for vaginal delivery and cesarean section is desirable.

### Acute Kidney Injury

Acute kidney injury (AKI) or renal dysfunction is rare with lesser degrees of placental abruption but is seen in cases when there is delayed or incomplete treatment of hypovolemia. AKI is usually reversible and long-term prognosis is good. Renal dysfunction is more likely in cases of preeclampsia. The possibility of renal cortical or tubular necrosis must be considered if oliguria persists after an adequate intravascular volume has been restored. An attempt should be made to improve renal circulation and promote diuresis by increasing fluid volume under close monitoring. If renal failure persists, dialysis is indicated.

### Prognosis

*Maternal:* Maternal mortality in abruptio placentae ranges from 0.5 to 5%. Hemorrhage, coagulation failure, hypovolemic shock, and renal failure are responsible for high mortality. Early diagnosis and prompt and definitive therapy result in lowered maternal mortality and morbidity. In a large, population-based study, women with placental abruption in the first or a later pregnancy were found to have a 1.8-fold increased risk of CVD mortality later in life.[22] The recurrence risk of abruption is 6–17% after previous one abruption and 25% after previous two abruptions.

*Fetal:* Perinatal mortality rates of 4–68% have been reported and depend upon the severity of the abruption and the neonatal facilities available. Live-born infants have a high morbidity due to hypoxia, birth trauma, and prematurity. Neonatal anemia may be marked in these cases.

## OTHER CAUSES OF ANTEPARTUM HEMORRHAGE

Besides placenta previa and abruptio placentae, APH is caused by incidental causes, marginal placenta, and vasa previa.

### Local Lesions of Cervix

These include cervicitis, cervical erosion, polyps, varicose veins in vagina or cervix, and cancer cervix. Per speculum examination will reveal these lesions but they may coexist with other causes of APH-like placenta previa, which should therefore, be excluded.

### Vasa Previa

This is a rare condition occurring in 1 in 2,000–3,000 deliveries.[23] Clinically, it presents as fetal distress and is confirmed by testing vaginal blood for presence of fetal hemoglobin in cases of APH. Cesarean section is indicated, if fetal blood is detected. Fetal mortality is high, if the condition is not diagnosed. Antenatal diagnosis with Doppler ultrasound has been advocated in high-risk cases, that is, those with low-lying placenta, velamentous insertion of cord, multifetal pregnancies, and those following IVF.[24] Ultrasound done at the time of anomaly scan has high accuracy and low-false positive rate in diagnosing vasa previa, although about 20% of these may resolve by third trimester.

Routine screening for presence of vasa previa at the time of anomaly scan, however, is not recommended but it is useful to look for it in high-risk cases such as those with low-lying placenta. In the presence of confirmed vasa previa in the third trimester, elective cesarean section should be done prior to the onset of labor.[25]

Society for Maternal-Fetal Medicine recommends delivery between 34 and 37 weeks of gestation for stable women with vasa previa (Grade 1B).[12]

### Indeterminate or Unexplained Bleeding

Many cases of APH have no evidence of placenta previa, abruption, or any local cause. The cause of bleeding in these cases is not known. It can be due to marginal separation of placenta in some cases. The bleeding is usually slight. Increased risk of preterm births, NICU admission, and a lower birthweight have been observed in these cases.[26] Perinatal mortality is high in this group. The management of these patients is individualized, and is usually expectant till 38 weeks. Close maternal and fetal monitoring is required.

### KEY POINTS

- Antepartum hemorrhage is defined as bleeding from or into the genital tract after the period of viability of pregnancy but before delivery of the baby and occurs in 3–5% of all pregnancies.
- Antepartum hemorrhage can be due to placental, extraplacental, and indeterminate causes or rarely, it can be due to vasa previa.
- When the placenta lies directly on the internal os, it is called placenta previa, and when it is within 2 cm of internal os, it is labeled as low-lying placenta and these occur in about 1 in 200 deliveries.
- Placenta accreta spectrum (morbidly adherent placenta) must be suspected in cases of anterior placenta previa in women with previous cesarean section and these cases should be managed as a case of placenta accreta, unless proved otherwise.
- Placenta accreta spectrum disorders carry a high risk of massive hemorrhage, high morbidity and mortality and should be managed in specialist centers with multidisciplinary facilities.
- Bleeding in placenta previa is painless, causeless, and recurrent, the uterus is soft and nontender, usually the presenting part is high or there may be malpresentation. Diagnosis is confirmed by ultrasound.
- Expectant treatment is given, if pregnancy is less than 36 weeks, fetus is live with no serious congenital malformation, bleeding is not excessive, patient is not in labor and is hemodynamically stable.
- Delivery is indicated, if pregnancy is more than 36 weeks or if the patient is in labor, bleeding is excessive, or fetus is dead or malformed.
- Antenatal corticosteroids should be administered to women who are eligible and are managed expectantly, the gestational age is between 34 and $36^{+6}$ weeks, and antenatal corticosteroids have not previously been given.
- Cesarean section is the treatment of choice in placenta previa; trial of vaginal delivery can be given in selected cases of low-lying placenta.
- Abruptio placentae is the premature separation of normally situated placenta and occurs in about 1% of deliveries.
- Bleeding in abruptio placentae is usually associated with pain. Uterus is tense and tender, fetal parts are not easily made out and fetal heart may be absent. In concealed variety of abruptio placentae, there is no external bleeding, but patient may be in shock with all the other signs of abruptio placentae.
- Severe hemorrhage, shock, coagulation failure, and renal failure may be present in severe cases of abruptio placentae.
- Prompt and adequate administration of fluid, blood, and FFP; early delivery with careful monitoring of vital signs, coagulation profile, and urine output are included in the management of abruption.
- Vaginal delivery is preferred with careful fetal monitoring in mild cases of abruptio with relaxed uterus and also in cases with dead fetus.
- Cesarean section is indicated in severe cases of abruptio with a live fetus and in cases with associated conditions requiring cesarean section.
- Coagulation disorder, if present, must be corrected before surgical procedure.
- All women with APH are at high risk for PPH and should be managed appropriately.

### REFERENCES

1. RCOG. (2011). Antepartum hemorrhage. RCOG Green top guidelines No. 63. 1st edition. [online] Available from: https://www.rcog.org.uk/en/guidelines-research-services/guidelines/gtg63/. [Last Accessed December, 2020].
2. Calleja-Agius J, Custo R, Brincat MP, Calleja N. Placental abruption and placenta praevia. Eur Clin Obstet Gynaecol. 2006;2:121-7.
3. Reddy UM, Abuhamad AZ, Levine D, Saade GR; Fetal Imaging Workshop Invited Participants. Fetal imaging: executive summary of a joint NICHD, SMFM, AIUM, ACOG, American College of Radiology, Society for Pediatric Radiology, and Society of Radiologists in Ultrasound Fetal Imaging Workshop. J Ultrasound Med. 2014;33:745-57.
4. Cunningham FG, Leveno KJ, Bloom SL, Dashe JS, Hoffman BL, Casey BM, Spong CY (Eds). William's Obstetrics, 25th edition. New York: McGraw Hill Education; 2014.
5. Lauria MR, Smith RS, Treadwell MC, Comstock CH, Kirk JS, Lee W, et al. The use of second-trimester transvaginal sonography to predict placenta previa. Ultrasound Obstet Gynecol. 1996;8(5):337-40.

6. Jansen CHJR, Kleinrouweler CE, van Leeuwen L, Ruiter L, Mol BW, Pajkrt E. Which second trimester placenta previa remains a placenta previa in the third trimester: a prospective cohort study. Eur J Obstet Gynecol Reprod Biol. 2020;254:119-23.
7. Babinski A, Kerenyi T, Torok O, Grazi V, Lapinski RH, Bertwitz RL. Perinatal outcome in grand and greatgrand multipara: the effects of the parity on obstetric factors. Am J Obstet Gynecol. 1999;181(3):669-74.
8. Biro MA, Davey MA, Carolan M, Kealy M. Advanced maternal age and obstetric morbidity for women giving birth in Victoria, Australia: a population-based study. Aust NZJ Obstet Gynaecol. 2012;52(3):229-34.
9. Roberts CL, Algert CS, Warrendorf J, Olive EC, Morris JM, Ford JB. Trends and recurrence of placenta previa: a population-based study. Aust N Z J Obstet Gynaecol. 2012;52(5):483-6.
10. Klar M, Michels KB. Cesarean section and placental disorders in subsequent pregnancies: a meta-analysis. J Perinat Med. 2014;42(5):571-83.
11. Jauniaux E, Alfirevic Z, Bhide AG, Belfort MA, Burton GJ, Collins SL, et al. Placenta praevia and placenta accreta: diagnosis and management. Green-top Guideline No. 27a. BJOG. 2019;126(1):e1-48.
12. Society for Maternal-Fetal Medicine (SMFM). Consult Series #44: Management of bleeding in the late preterm period. Am J Obstet Gynecol. 2018;218(1):B2-8.
13. Jansen C, de Mooij YM, Blomaard CM, Derks JB, van Leeuwen E, Limpens J, et al. Vaginal delivery in women with a low-lying placenta: a systematic review and meta-analysis. BJOG. 2019;126(9):1118-26.
14. Bose DA, Assel BG, Hill JB, Chauhan SP. Maintenance tocolytics for preterm symptomatic placenta previa: a review. Am J Perinatol. 2011;28(1):45-50.
15. Cahill AG, Beigi R, Heine RP, Silver RM, Wax JR. Placenta accreta spectrum. Am J Obstet Gynecol. 2018;219(6):B2-16.
16. Allen L, Jauniaux E, Hobson S, Papillon-Smith J. FIGO Consensus Guidelines on Placenta Accreta Spectrum Disorders: nonconservative surgical management. Int J Gynecol Obstet. 2018;140(3):281-90.
17. Silver RM, Landon MB, Rouse DJ, Leveno KJ, Spong CY, Thom EA, et al; National Institute of Child Health and Human Development Maternal-Fetal Medicine Units Network. Maternal morbidity associated with multiple repeat cesarean deliveries. Obstet Gynecol. 2006;107(6):1226-32.
18. Arendas K, Lortie KJ, Singh SS. Delayed laparoscopic management of placenta increta. J Obstet Gynaecol Can. 2012;34(2):186-9.
19. Rupley DM, Tergas AI, Palmerola KL, Burke WM. Robotically assisted delayed total laparoscopic hysterectomy for placenta percreta. Gynecol Oncol Rep. 2016;17:53-5.
20. Giordano R, Cacciatore A, Cignini P, Vigna R, Romano M. Antepartum hemorrhage. J Perinat Med. 2010;4(1):12-6.
21. Pritchard JA, Brekken AL. Clinical and laboratory studies on severe abruptio placentae. Am J Obstet Gynecol. 1967;97(5):681-700.
22. DeRoo L, Skjærven R, Wilcox A, Klungsøyr K, Wikström AK, Morken NH, et al. Placental abruption and long-term maternal cardiovascular disease mortality: a population-based registry study in Norway and Sweden. Eur J Epidemiol. 2016;31(5):501-11.
23. Smorgick N, Tovbin Y, Ushakov F, Vaknin Z, Barzilay B, Herman A, et al. Is neonatal risk from vasa previa preventable? The 20 year experience from a single medical centre. J Clin Ultrasound. 2010;38(3):118-22.
24. Sinha P, Kaushik S, Kuruba N, Beweley S. Vasa previa: a missed diagnosis. J Obstet Gynecol. 2008;28(6):600.
25. Jauniaux ERM, Alfirevic Z, Bhide AG, Burton GJ, Collins SL, Silver R; on behalf of the Royal College of Obstetricians and Gynaecologists. Vasa praevia: diagnosis and management. Green-top Guideline No. 27b. BJOG. 2018.
26. McCormack RA, Doherty DA, Magann EF, Hutchinson M, Newnham JP. Antepartum bleeding of unknown origin in the second half of pregnancy and pregnancy outcome. BJOG. 2008;115(11):1451-7.

# CHAPTER 6

# Multifetal Pregnancy

*Reena Yadav*

## INTRODUCTION

Multifetal gestation is a high-risk pregnancy. The frequency of multifetal pregnancy varies worldwide. The rate of twins and other higher order multiple births have increased remarkably in the last three decades.[1] The increase is basically iatrogenic because of treatment of infertility using ovulation induction drugs and assisted-reproductive techniques (ART). The increase is also because of the shift toward an older maternal age at conception, when multifetal gestations are more likely to occur naturally. These changes translate into significantly greater proportion of multiples among premature and low-birth weight infants. Preterm birth and growth aberrations are indeed the most important adverse consequences of so-called epidemic of multiple gestations. The main complication with multifetal gestations is spontaneous preterm birth and resultant infant morbidity and mortality. Multiple interventions have been evaluated so as to prolong these gestations and improve outcome, none has been found to be effective.[2] The perinatal mortality rate associated with multiple pregnancy increases as the number of fetuses increase and relates to higher incidence of preterm delivery, fetal growth restriction (FGR), fetal anomaly, antepartum hemorrhage, and preeclampsia. Apart from major complications of pregnancy, the mother is more likely to suffer from minor ailments of pregnancy.

## PREVALENCE

The incidence of monozygotic twins is relatively constant worldwide at 1 in 250 pregnancies and is not influenced by factors like maternal age, heredity, etc., except use of ART, which are associated with an increased incidence.[3] The incidence of dizygotic twinning and higher order birth rates vary widely and are affected by maternal age, parity, family or personal history, racial background, and use of ART.

### Monozygotic Pregnancy

Delayed transfer of fertilized ovum through the fallopian tube increases the risk of its splitting into two. ART increases the risk of monozygotic twinning to 1 in 50 as compared to 1 in 250 following natural conceptions. Several mechanisms have been proposed to explain the increased risk associated with ART. Extended culture and blastocyst transfer with in vitro fertilization (IVF), micromanipulation of zona pellucida with intracytoplasmic sperm injection (ICSI), and minor trauma to the blastocyst during ART may lead to increased incidence of monozygotic twins.[4]

The type of monozygotic pregnancy is decided by timing of division (**Fig. 1**). In 30% of monozygotic twins, the division occurs before the formation of inner cell mass, i.e., in less than 72 hours of fertilization, resulting in diamniotic, dichorionic multifetal pregnancy with two embryos, two amnions, two chorions, and a separate placenta for each fetus. In 70% cases, division occurs when inner cell mass has already formed and cells destined to form chorion are differentiated, i.e., between 4 and 8 days, resulting in two embryos of diamniotic, monochorionic type with a single placenta (**Fig. 2**). Rarely division occurs after 8 days when the chorion and amnion have already differentiated; two embryos of monoamniotic, monochorionic type develop. If division is delayed even further, when embryonic disk is formed, it will lead to incomplete cleavage resulting in conjoined twins.

### Dizygotic Twins

Dizygotic twins result from fertilization of two different ova and each twin has its own placenta and amniotic sac. They are always diamniotic-dichorionic type. The frequency of dizygotic twins is influenced by a number of factors like race, heredity, maternal age parity, nutritional factors, ovulation induction drugs, ART, etc. Recent research confirmed that taller women and women with a body mass index > 30 kg/m$^2$ are at greater risk of dizygotic twinning.[5]

### Race

Frequency of multifetal pregnancy is more in blacks as compared to whites. In some areas of Africa, it is found to be 1 in every 20 births. In white women, it is 1 in 100 pregnancies as compared to nonwhite where it is 1 in 80. These differences may be because of the racial variations in the levels of follicular stimulating hormones.[3]

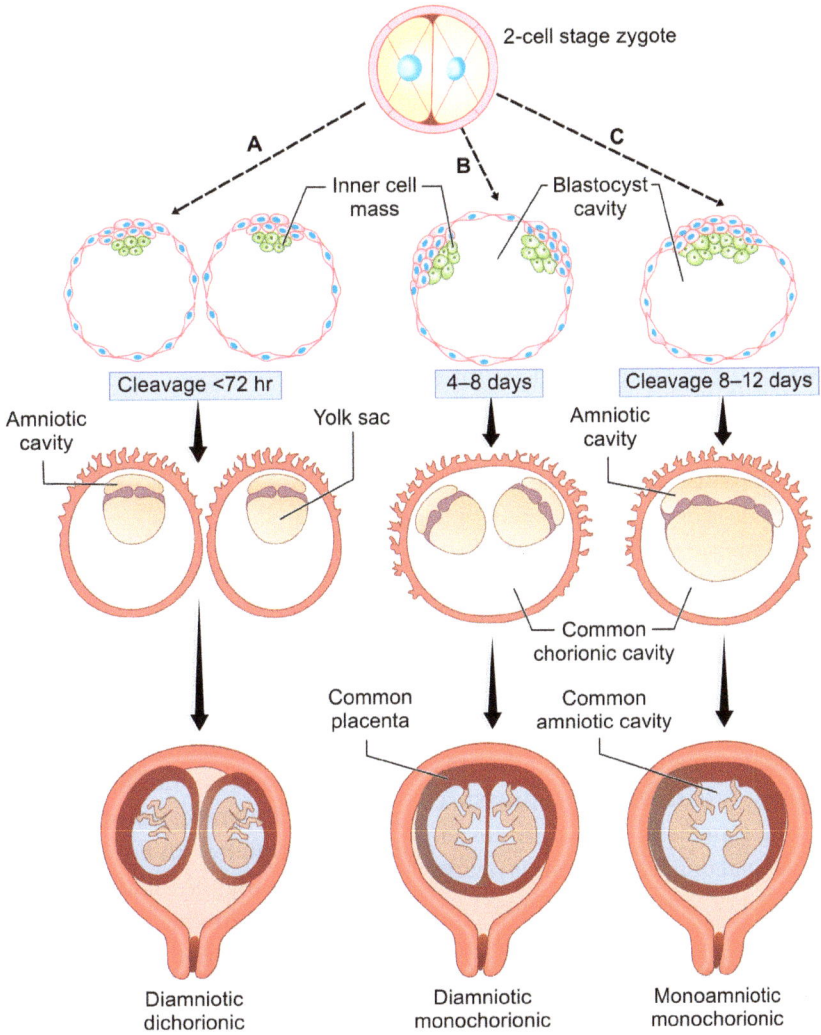

**Fig. 1:** Monozygotic twins.

## Maternal Age and Parity

Increasing maternal age and parity have been shown to increase the incidence of multifetal pregnancy. As the age advances, hormonal stimulation increases the rate of multiple ovulations especially around 35 years of age. The reported incidence at 35 years of age is 2%. Similarly, in grandmultipara with parity four or more, the frequency of multifetal pregnancy is almost doubled (2% after four pregnancies) as compared to first pregnancy.[6]

## Heredity

Family history of multifetal pregnancy in mother or sister is much more important as compared to that in father and his family. One explanation given is that tendency to release multiple ova is inherited and dizygotic twinning may be influenced by an autosomal dominant gene.[7]

## Ovulation Induction Drugs

Induction of ovulation by clomiphene citrate or by gonadotropins with hCG markedly enhances the likelihood of multiple ovulations. With clomiphene, the frequency of multifetal pregnancy varies from 6 to 12%, while with gonadotropins it is 16–40%.[3]

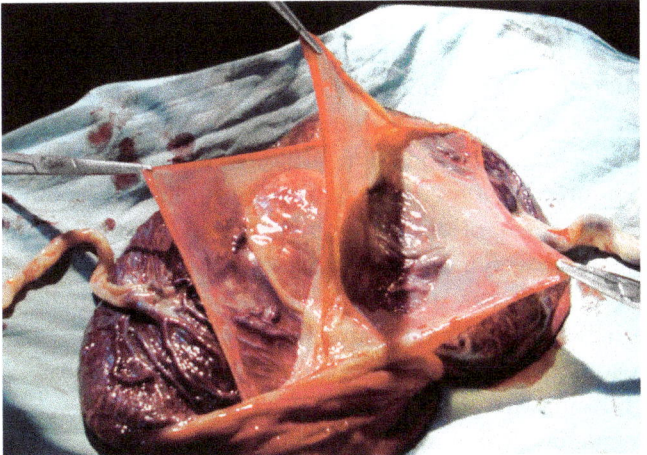

**Fig. 2:** Monochorionic diamniotic placenta.

## Assisted Reproductive Technique

Assisted reproductive technique procedures use superovulation, retrieval of multiple ova, and subsequent transfer of two or more embryos into the uterine cavity after fertilization results in multifetal pregnancy.

## PHYSIOLOGICAL CHANGES

The degree of maternal physiological changes is greater with multifetal pregnancy compared to singleton pregnancy. Women with multifetal pregnancy have excessive nausea and vomiting. The maternal blood volume expansion is greater in multifetal pregnancy. It is about 50–60% in twin pregnancy. The increase in requirements of both iron and folic acid along with marked increase in blood volume predispose the woman to increased incidence of anemia.[8] Cardiac output is also increased by 20% as compared to that in singleton pregnancy predominantly because of increased stroke volume.[9] As far as arterial blood pressure change is concerned, the diastolic blood pressure is lower at 20 weeks of gestation as compared to singleton but increase is more toward term. The increase is at least 15 mm Hg in 95% of women with multifetal pregnancy as compared to 54% of singleton pregnancies.[10] Uterus with its contents may achieve a volume of 10 L or more. This extra weight carried with multiple gestations exaggerates the minor ailments of pregnancy like backache, breathlessness, pressure symptoms, difficulty in walking especially in third trimester. The average blood loss with vaginal delivery of twins is nearly 500 mL more than with the delivery of a singleton fetus.

## MATERNAL AND FETAL RISKS

Higher order pregnancies confer significant risk to both mother and fetuses and reduce the chance of both a live birth or birth of a child without significant handicap. Medical complications are more common in women with multifetal gestation than singleton gestations. These include hyperemesis gravidarum, gestational diabetes mellitus, hypertension, anemia, hemorrhage, cesarean delivery, and postpartum depression. Although these complications are more common in women with multifetal pregnancy, the management of these complications follows the same strategy as with a singleton gestation, maternal morbidity is seven-fold greater in multiple gestations than in singletons. Perinatal mortality rates are four-fold higher for twins and six-fold higher for triplets, and cerebral palsy rates are 1–1.5% in twins and 7.8% in triplets.[11] Mackay et al., reported pregnancy-related mortality among women with multifetal pregnancy. In their study, the risk of maternal death in twins and higher order pregnancies was 3.6 times that of women with singleton pregnancies. The leading causes of death were embolism, hypertensive disorders of pregnancy, hemorrhage, and infection. They concluded that women with multifetal pregnancies have a significantly higher risk of pregnancy-related death than their counterparts with singleton pregnancies and that holds true for all women regardless of their age, race, marital status, and level of education.[12]

## Maternal Risks

### Hydramnios

Hydramnios may occur in one or both amniotic sacs. It is one of the important causes of preterm delivery. Acute hydramnios is more in monochorionic pregnancy. It may be caused by fetal anomalies. In some cases, there may not be any apparent cause. The reported incidence is 12%.[13]

### Hypertension

The incidence of hypertensive disorders of pregnancy is higher in multiple pregnancies. The occurrence of hypertensive disorders is proportional to the total fetal number, with twins it is 12.7% and with triplets at 20%.[14] Multifetal gestations have significantly higher rates of preeclampsia associated complications such as preterm delivery and abruptio placentae.[15] Primigravidae with multifetal pregnancy are at almost 5 times more risk of developing preeclampsia as compared to one with singleton pregnancy and for multigravida risk is 10 times greater.[16] The rate of severe preeclampsia is significantly higher in women carrying triplets.[17] In a recent study, Bdolah et al. reported a 2–3 times higher incidence of preeclampsia in multifetal pregnancy than singleton pregnancy. They demonstrated that excess placental secretion of a circulating antiangiogenic molecule, soluble fms-like tyrosine kinase1 (sFlt1) may have pivotal role in the pathogenesis of preeclampsia. This molecule acts by antagonizing placental growth factor (PlGF). The ratio of sFlt1/PlGF, was found to be a more reliable index of the circulating angiogenic state rather than either marker alone, and hence was a better predictor for risk of preeclampsia. Circulating sFlt1 concentrations were 2.2 times higher in maternal serum samples from twin pregnancy compared to singleton pregnancy. PlGF concentrations did not differ significantly between twin and singleton pregnancy. But the mean sFlt1/PlGF ratio was 2.2 times higher in twin pregnancy than in singleton pregnancy. These findings suggest that increased placental mass with accompanying increase in circulating sFlt1 may contribute to increased susceptibility to preeclampsia in women with multifetal pregnancy.[15] As per one study, ART pregnancies were at increased relative risk of 2.1 of developing mild and severe preeclampsia even after controlling for maternal age and parity.[18]

### Antepartum Hemorrhage

Risk of placental abruption is more with twins especially after the delivery of first fetus. Increased size of placenta or multiple placentae may encroach upon lower uterine segment, thereby increasing the chances of placenta previa.[19]

## Malpresentations

Most common presentation is both vertex. Other combinations are first vertex-second breech, first breech-second vertex, first transverse-second vertex, and so on. Nonvertex presentations increase chances of operative intervention including both, operative vaginal delivery and cesarean section.

## Preterm Labor

Preterm birth is one of the major causes of neonatal morbidity and mortality. Spontaneous preterm labor accounts for a large proportion of preterm births associated with multifetal pregnancy. The rate of preterm birth varies from 30 to 50%. The mean duration of pregnancy decreases as the number of fetuses increase in utero. The mean gestational age in twins is 35 weeks.[1]

The mean gestational age for triplets at delivery is reported as 32.2 ± 3.2 weeks.[20] Strauss et al.[21] reported the mean gestational age of 31.5, 29.5, and 28.4 weeks for triplets, quadruplets and quintuplets, respectively. The risk of preterm birth to the mother is associated with need for the hospitalization and use of tocolysis with its harmful side effects. Preterm premature rupture of membranes occurs more frequently in multifetal pregnancy.

## Postpartum Hemorrhage (PPH)

In multifetal pregnancies, over distention of uterus may weaken the contraction and retraction of uterine muscles and cause increase risk for PPH following delivery. A study by Shunj et al.[22] reported the risk of PPH in twin pregnancy as 24% and reported it to be more, if gestational age is more than 39 weeks or when the labor was induced.[22] Large surface area of placenta is also responsible for increased risk for PPH.[23]

# Fetal Risks

## Abortion

The rate of abortion is more in multifetal gestation than in singleton. Monochorionic abortuses greatly outnumber dichorionic abortuses implicating monozygosity as a risk factor for spontaneous abortion. The rate of missed abortion is approximately twice as compared to singleton at 10–14 weeks of gestation.[24] Sometimes during the first trimester, one or more of the multifetal gestation sacs fail to develop and get absorbed. This is known as vanishing twin syndrome where pregnancy has been diagnosed initially by ultrasonography (USG) as multifetal but later on, one or more gestation sac disappears. Women with vanishing twin may present with slight vaginal bleeding in first trimester. The reported incidence ranges from 10 to 20% with most cases occurring prior to 12 weeks.[25] The prognosis of the remaining fetus at that early gestation is good.[26] Sometimes one of the twin fetus dies and gets compressed between uterine wall and later presents as fetus papyraceus (**Fig. 3**).

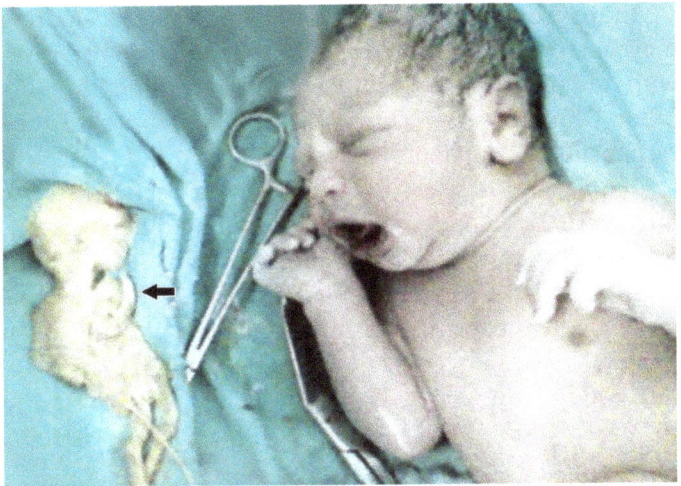

**Fig. 3:** Fetus papyraceus.

## Low-birth Weight

Chances of babies being born with low-birth weight are more in multifetal gestations as compared to singletons. This is both because of increased incidence of prematurity as well as intrauterine growth restriction. Larger the number of fetuses, greater the degree of growth restriction and increased are chances of small for gestational age babies, which is about 27% in twins and 46% in triplets.[21,27]

Growth abnormalities, which include FGR and weight discordancy between twins are common in multifetal pregnancy.[28] Accurate dating of pregnancy and knowledge of the chorionicity are essential and both can reliably be determined by first trimester USG.[29] The risk of growth restriction is much more in monochorionic twins.[30] A fetus is considered small for gestational age, if both abdominal circumference and estimated fetal weight is below tenth percentile. The chance of both fetuses being low-birth weight is twice as high in monochorionic gestations (17%) as compared to dichorionic twins (8%).[6] There can be growth discordancy between two fetuses. The parameters to detect growth discordancy are the abdominal circumference and birth weight. A difference of 20 mm in abdominal circumference after 24 weeks and birth weight difference of 20% are suggestive of discordant growth. The incidence of discordancy is 12% in twins and 34% in triplets.[31] Growth discordancy complicates both monochorionic as well as dichorionic multifetal gestations, however the growth pattern and underlying pathophysiology is different. The onset of discordancy is unpredictable in monochorionic twins, it is usually apparent late in pregnancy.[32] The possible reasons for discordancy in monozygotic twins could be either unequal allocation of blastomeres between monochorionic embryos or vascular anastomoses within the placenta causing unequal distribution of nutrients and oxygen.

In dizygotic multiple gestations, unequal placentation may be responsible for size difference between fetuses with one placenta receiving better blood supply than the other. Difference in genetic growth potential may also be responsible for different sizes.

Fetal risks associated with growth restriction are intrauterine death, neurological morbidity due to chronic oxygen and nutrient deprivation. Growth discordancy and restriction together increase risk of adverse perinatal outcome. Growth discordant monochorionic twins are at a higher risk of adverse outcome than growth discordant dichorionic twins.[33]

### Congenital Malformations

The prevalence of malformations is much more in multifetal pregnancy compared to singleton with a reported rate of 4% as compared to 2% in singletons.[34] In twins with known chorionicity, the prevalence of congenital anomalies in monochorionic twins is reported as 6% compared to 3% in dichorionic twins.[34] The rate is increased for all major anomalies except chromosomal abnormalities. The increase is almost entirely due to high incidence of structural defects. Structural anomalies are 1.2–2 times more common in twins than in singletons. Most studies do not subgroup incidence of congenital anomalies by either zygosity or placentation. It seems rate of anomalies per fetus in dizygotic twin is same as singleton whereas for monozygotic twins, rate is 2–3 times higher. Abnormalities associated with twins are neural tube defects, brain defects, facial clefts, gastrointestinal defects, anterior abdominal wall defects, and cardiac defects.[6] Exact mechanisms of structural anomalies in monozygotic twins are unknown. It is possible that the twinning process itself is teratogenic owing to unequal distribution of inner cell mass. Vascular events in early embryogenesis and later fetal life might account for part of the discordant brain and heart anomalies. The presence of cardiac anomalies in monozygotic twins is reported to be 2.3% as compared to 0.6% in general population.[6]

There are some problems specific to monochorionic multifetal pregnancy like conjoined twins; twin reversed arterial perfusion (TRAP) and twin-to-twin transfusion syndrome (TTTS).

### Monoamniotic Twins

The incidence is 1 in 10,000 pregnancies and constitutes 1% of monozygotic twins.[35] The umbilical cords insert close to each other with multiple deep and superficial anastomoses connecting placental stem vessels of the twins.[36] The diagnosis can reliably be made in first trimester by the presence of single yolk sac, one amniotic cavity containing two fetal poles and a single placenta. High fetal mortality is associated with this type of twins. The reported chance of fetal demise is 10%.[10] Monoamniotic twins are at increased risk of congenital anomalies and sudden intrauterine death.[37] Intertwining of their umbilical cords, a common cause of death, is estimated to complicate at least half of the cases. Umbilical cords of twins frequently entangle, but the factors which lead to pathological umbilical vessel constriction during entanglement are unknown. Increased fetal surveillance and delivery by cesarean section as soon as fetal lung maturity is achieved (usually between 32 and 33 weeks) can decrease the mortality rate.

### Conjoined Twins (Fig. 4)

Conjoined twins should be excluded whenever there is monoamniotic twin pregnancy. Incidence of conjoined twin is 1 in 50,000 pregnancies. The diagnosis is possible as early as in first trimester by the close and fixed apposition of the fetal bodies with fusion of the skin lines at some point.[38] Depending upon the part of the body involved in fusion, there are various types of conjoined twins, e.g., thoracopagus, pyopagus, ischiopagus, craniopagus. Diagnosis can be easily made later in pregnancy on USG when two heads or two breeches are always at same level. Once diagnosis is made, it is imperative that a complete workup be undertaken to determine shared anatomy, which guides management and determines prognosis. Intrauterine death occurs in 60% of conjoined twins and those who are live born, majority of them die because of severe anomalies or as a consequence of surgery to separate them.[39] There is only 18% survival rate of one twin from ultrasonographic diagnosis to successful separation. Unless the conjoined twins are very small or macerated, delivery needs to be done by cesarean section.

### Twin Reversed Arterial Perfusion Sequence/Acardiac Twin (Fig. 5)

It is one of the rare but serious complications of monochorionic monozygotic twins. The syndrome occurs in 1%

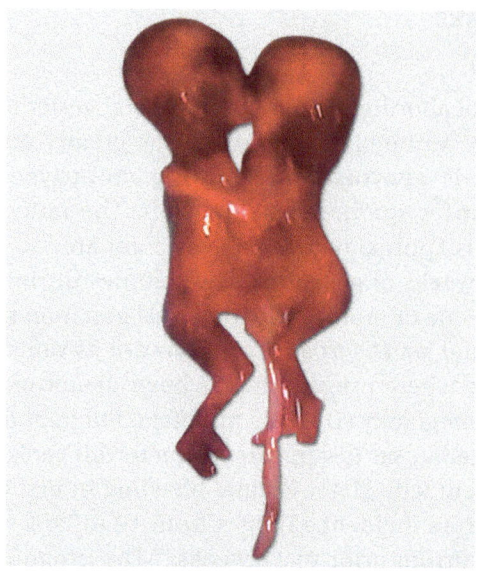

**Fig. 4:** Conjoined twins.

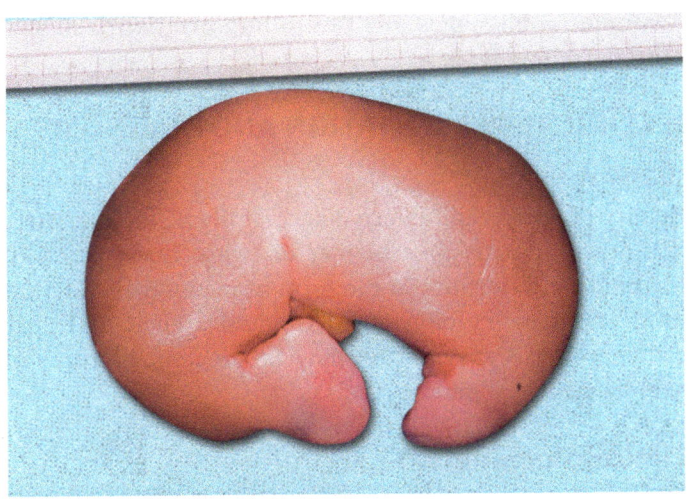

**Fig. 5:** Acardiac twin.

of monochorionic multiple gestations. There is one normal donor twin and the other with absent heart and other structures. It is hypothesized that there is large artery-to-artery shunt in placenta and perfusion pressure is more in the donor twin, so the recipient receives reverse blood flow from its sibling, this blood flow preferentially goes in the iliac vessels thus perfuse only the lower part of the body leading to disruption and deterioration of growth and development of upper part of body. This is also known as TRAP sequence. TRAP sequence in the recipient twin causes hypoxia particularly to the cephalic pole leading to acardia, acephaly, and abnormalities of upper part of body. The pump twin is at high risk, due to hazards of congestive heart failure from a prolonged high output state and also the risk of prematurity. The mortality rate is reported to be between 50 and 70% for the pump twin.[40] At least 20% of monozygotic pump twin can be expected to have congenital anomalies and 55% of these die in neonatal period. Early ultrasound prenatal diagnosis is difficult because this condition only becomes pronounced in later pregnancy. Classically, the Doppler ultrasound finding in acardiac twin demonstrate the absence of cardiac movement, a reverse or abnormal blood flow through the umbilical cord, a poorly defined head and trunk and abnormal upperlimb.[6]

The optimal management of acardiac twin is controversial because of the rarity of this condition and widely varied presentation but the objective is to achieve survival of pump twin. Since, the mortality of pump twin is very high, therefore invasive procedures to occlude blood flow to acardiac twin have been practiced by most authors. Interruption of vascular communication between donor and recipient at around 20 weeks of gestation can improve the survival of the normal twin. Such procedures include endoscopic umbilical cord ligation, ultrasound-guided thermocoagulation of the umbilical cord, endoscopic laser coagulation of umbilical artery, and radiofrequency ablation.[41-43] These vessels can be ligated or ablated in utero. A systematic review of minimally invasive techniques, i.e., radiofrequency ablation and monopolar coagulation aiming to occlude vascular supply to acardiac twin has shown an overall pump twin survival rate of 76%.[44] A conservative approach has been described by Sullivan et al. from 10 cases of acardiac twin in which the neonatal mortality of the pump twin was reported to be lower than that from invasive management. Nine of ten women delivered healthy pump twin from noninvasive management. Their management included two weekly serial USG, fetal echocardiography, Doppler flow study, along with performing a nonstress test, and a biophysical profile. It appears from their study that expectant management with close surveillance in an antenatally diagnosed TRAP sequence deserves consideration.[45]

*Twin-to-Twin Transfusion Syndrome*

Vascular anastomoses are present mostly in monochorionic twins. Most of these communications are hemodynamically balanced. In 10–15% of monochorionic twins, a chronic imbalance develops resulting in TTTS.[6] When significant shunts are present between fetuses, they can cause TTTS, exact incidence of which is not known. In this syndrome, blood is transfused from donor to the recipient such that donor become anemic and growth restricted and the recipient becomes polycythemic and may develop circulatory overload and features of hydrops. Neurological damage like cerebral palsy, microcephaly, and porencephaly are serious complications associated with vascular anastomoses in twin pregnancy. Damage is most likely by ischemic necrosis leading to cavitary brain damage.

In the donor twin, ischemia results from hypotension and anemia. In the recipient twin, ischemia is because of unstable blood pressure and episodes of severe hypotension.[46] Spontaneous abortion, preterm delivery, and fetal death may occur from cardiac failure in recipient and from poor perfusion in donor. TTTS usually occurs between 15 and 26 weeks. Monitoring for feto-fetal transfusion syndrome is not carried out in the first trimester but should be started using ultrasound (including identifying membrane folding) from 16 weeks and repeated fortnightly until 24 weeks. Fetal weight discordance should be estimated using two or more biometric parameters at each ultrasound scan from 20 weeks, with a difference of 25% or more considered a clinically important indicator of intrauterine growth restriction (IUGR).[47]

The diagnosis of twin-to-twin transfusion is difficult. Antenatal criteria recommended for defining TTTS include the following: same sex fetuses, monochorionicity with placental vascular anastomoses, weight difference of more than 20%, hydramnios in the larger twin, oligoamnios in the smaller twin, and the hemoglobin difference greater than 5 g/dL.[48] Staging for TTTS is defined by Quintero et al.[2,41]

- *Stage 1:* Monochorionic-diamniotic gestation with oligohydramnios [maximum vertical pocket (MVP) less than 2 cm] and polyhydramnios (MVP >8 cm)
- *Stage 2:* Absent (empty) bladder in donor
- *Stage 3:* Abnormal Doppler USG findings, absent or reversed diastolic flow in umbilical artery, absent or reversed diastolic flow in ductus venosus or umbilical vein pulsatile flow
- *Stage 4:* Hydrops
- *Stage 5:* Death of one or both twins.

The postnatal diagnosis is based on discordancy in weight of 15–20% and a hemoglobin difference of 5 g% or more. But there can be a number of reasons like anomalies and infection for discordancy.

Pathophysiology of TTTS is explained on angio-architectural basis. There are two types of vascular anastomoses, superficial and deep. Superficial anastomoses are arterio-arterial or veno-venous. They are bidirectional anastomoses. Arteriovenous (AV) anastomoses are usually referred as deep anastomoses. They occur at capillary level, deep in a shared cotyledon receiving arterial supply from one twin and providing venous drainage to the other twin. The AV anastomoses allow flow in one direction only, thus create imbalance in the inter-fetal transfusion leading to TTTS.[49]

Discordant nuchal translucency of at least 20% can be used to screen early loss and TTTS.[48] Recent Doppler-based longitudinal study through AV anastomoses shows that it is their size rather than their number and direction that determine transfusional complications in monochorionic twins. In monochorionic diamniotic twin with transmitted pattern in umbilical artery there is increased risk of sudden death and abnormal cranial lesions in the larger cotwin.[50]

Once diagnosis has been made, the prognosis depends on gestational age and severity of the syndrome.

Several therapies are currently used for twin-to-twin transfusion including amnioreduction, septostomy, laser ablation of vascular anastomoses, and selective feticides by cord occlusion. Selective reduction has generally been considered when severe amniotic fluid and growth disturbances develop early. Selection of the twin to be terminated is based on the evidence of damage to either fetus. Various techniques include injection of an occlusive substance into the umbilical vein, fetoscopic ligation, monopolar coagulation, or bipolar cautery of umbilical cord.[50,51]

Cochrane review[52] of various interventions for TTTS reported that laser coagulation resulted in less overall death as compared to amnioreduction (48% vs. 59%), less perinatal death (26% vs. 44%), and neonatal death (8% vs. 24%). There is no difference in perinatal outcome between amnioreduction and septostomy. Their results suggest that endoscopic laser coagulation should be considered in the treatment of all stages of TTTS to improve perinatal and neonatal outcome.

# CLINICAL PRESENTATION AND DIAGNOSIS

## History

History of advanced maternal age, family history of twins, grand-multiparity, past history of twins, and history of treatment of infertility in the form of ovulation induction drugs or pregnancy following ART should be elicited. History of hyperemesis gravidarum may be present. Features of anemia may be apparent.

## Clinical Examination

The height of uterus is more than the period of amenorrhea, evident especially in second trimester around 20 weeks. Between 20 and 30 weeks fundal height, on an average is about 5 cm greater than expected for singleton of same age.[53] On palpation of the abdomen, multiple fetal parts are palpable, two fetal heads may be appreciated in different maternal quadrants. The palpation is difficult, if hydramnios is present or the woman is obese. In twin pregnancy, two distinct fetal hearts can be heard with an area of silence in between the two, with a difference of minimum 10 beats per minute.

## Ultrasonography

With the use of USG, multiple gestation sacs can be seen as early as 5 weeks. Chorionicity should be determined by ultrasound as it is important for prognosis. If the scan is performed at 10–14 weeks of gestation, twin peak sign can be seen, which is an echogenic chorionic projection of tissue between the dividing membranes, which is present in dichorionic twins[54] **(Fig. 6)** and a T-sign when there is only a thin line (two amnions) with no echogenic tissue in between, suggestive of monochorionic twins **(Fig. 7)**. A retrospective observational study to determine the accuracy of USG in

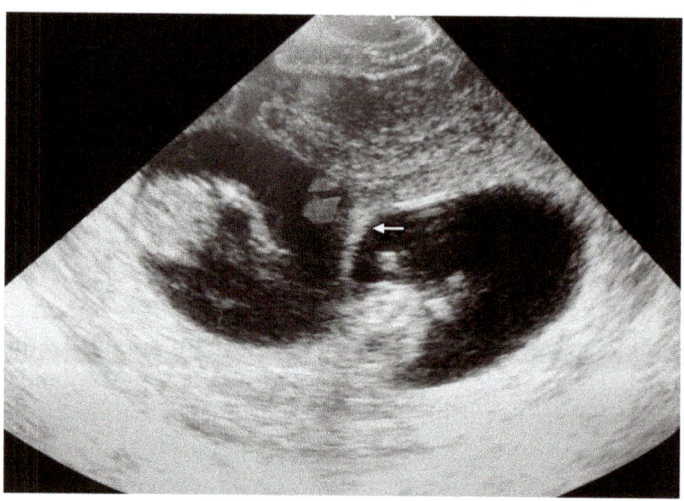

**Fig. 6:** Twin peak sign.

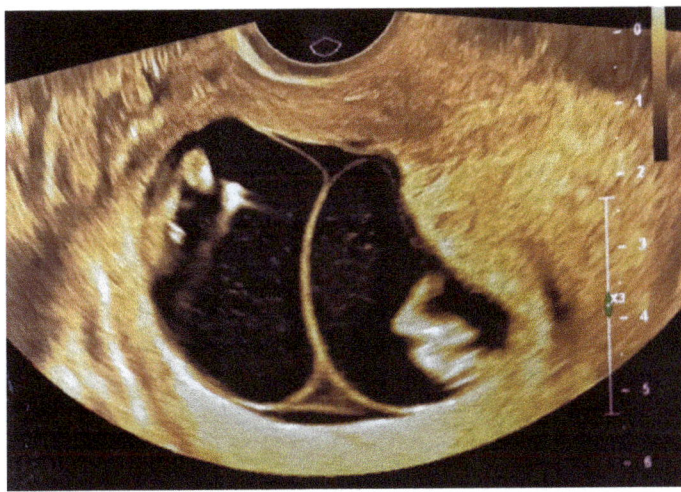

**Fig. 7:** Monochorionic diamniotic at 12 weeks of gestation.

establishing chorionicity at 11–14 weeks of gestation was conducted by Dias et al. They concluded that the pregnancies can be considered monochorionic in the presence of T-sign and dichorionic in the presence of Lambda sign.[55]

As gestation age increases this sign disappears. The dividing membrane is thicker in dichorionic twins, the cut off of 2 mm is mentioned in literature.[56] A standard method of nomenclature, for use in the first trimester of twin pregnancies, in predicting the presenting twin in subsequent scans and at delivery was analyzed by Dias et al.[57] At 11–14 weeks ultrasound assessment, the fetus in the gestational sac closer to the maternal cervix was designated as Twin-1 and relative orientation of the fetuses to each other defined as either lateral (left or right) or vertical (top or bottom). The analysis included 416 twin pregnancies, with 378 (90.9%) judged to have a lateral and 38 (9.1%) a vertical orientation. Although none of the vertically orientated twin pairs changed their presenting order between first scan and the last scan prior to delivery, 32 (8.5%, 95% CI 5.9–11.8%) of the laterally orientated twin pairs changed presenting order. There were 108 discordant sex twin pregnancies with ultrasound data available in the third trimester. Of these, 17 (15.7%) changed presentation between final scan and delivery, with the change significantly higher ($p = 0.0319$) for twins delivered by cesarean section (15 of 74, 20.3%) than by vaginal delivery (2 of 34, –5.9%).

It was noted that the orientation of the gestational sac remains unchanged throughout pregnancy because the base of the inter twin membrane is fixed, although the fetuses in a lateral orientation may move up or down within the sac, thereby changing which fetus is closest to the cervix. Consequently, the authors concluded that the antenatal labeling of twins according to lateral (left or right) or vertical (top or bottom) orientation is more reliable and reproducible than labeling according to proximity to the cervix, although they noted that the method cannot be used for monoamniotic twin pregnancies because there is no intertwin membrane.

Confusion arising from inconsistent identification of fetuses may result in lack of continuity in biometric assessment and has potentially serious implications where invasive prenatal diagnosis is needed.[57]

For confirming diagnosis of twins, ideally two heads or two abdomens should be seen in same plane to avoid scanning the same fetus twice and interpreting it as twins. Routine mid trimester USG examination can detect almost all multifetal gestation (99%) before 26th week.[58] Higher order multiple gestations are difficult to evaluate. With detail mid trimester scan, structural congenital abnormalities can be identified.

## Prenatal Screening and Diagnosis

All women with multifetal gestations, regardless of age, are candidates for routine aneuploidy screening. In the presence of multiple fetuses, the probability that one or more fetuses will be affected with a trisomy increases and thus results in higher overall risk to the pregnancy than attributed to the maternal age alone. However, several limitations must be considered when screening for aneuploidy in multifetal gestation. Serum screening tests are not as sensitive in women with twin or triplet gestation as compared to singleton in part because analyte levels must be estimated mathematical modeling. In addition, analytes from normal and the affected fetuses enter the maternal serum and in effect average together, thus potentially masking the abnormal levels of the affected fetus. Nuchal translucency screening in the first trimester with the option of chorionic villus sampling (CVS) and earlier selective reduction may be desirable in some cases. In twin pregnancy, the first trimester screening that combines maternal age, nuchal translucency, and biochemistry identifies approximately 75–85% of pregnancies with Down syndrome and 66.7% with trisomy 18.[59] As far as triplet is concerned, the experience is limited but nuchal translucency measurement is feasible and screening using maternal age and nuchal translucency has been validated for detection of Down syndrome and trisomy 18.[59]

Amniocentesis and CVS can be performed in women with multiple gestations who desire definitive testing for genetic anomalies. The procedure associated loss rate is slightly increased compared to loss rate with singleton pregnancy. There can be technical difficulties when performing CVS and amniocentesis in multiple gestations. There is risk of sampling error. Sampling error can be avoided while doing amniocentesis. After performing it in first sac, indigo carmine may be injected in to that sac before removing the needle. A second needle is used to sample the second sac and if a clear sample is obtained, it ensures that two different sacs have been sampled. When aneuploidy is diagnosed, women should be counseled regarding the options for pregnancy management, if only one fetus is affected. These include continuing the pregnancy without intervention, terminating the entire pregnancy, or selective reduction of affected fetus.

## MANAGEMENT

### Antenatal Management

Following the diagnosis of multifetal pregnancy, it is important to explain the need for regular antenatal care to the pregnant woman. This allows the mother to make appropriate changes in her lifestyle. For multifetal pregnancies, there is a growing body of evidence linking good maternal nutrition and weight gain to positive perinatal outcome including decrease in incidence of low-birth weight and very low-birth weight infants. Nutritional intervention appears to have important clinical implications for infant morbidity and mortality. Nutritional counseling can help women improve and maximize their intake of nutrients such as iron, folate, essential fatty acids, and calcium. Calorie consumption should be increased by about 300 kcal/day.[60]

Frequent antenatal visits at every 2 weeks from second trimester onward can lead to early detection of hypertension. Clinical assessment of fetal growth has poor correlation with fetal size in twin pregnancy. It is difficult to detect early discordant growth clinically. An overall clinical assessment should, however, include maternal weight gain, symphysio-fundal height, and abdominal girth.

Having established the correct gestational age of twin pregnancy by first and second trimester scan, ultrasound examination between 18 and 22 weeks of gestation for fetal anatomy, amniotic fluid, placentation, and growth is recommended. Fetal growth in uncomplicated twin pregnancies occurs at a similar rate as singletons until approximately 28–32 weeks of gestation when growth rate of twins slows. It is helpful to commence serial USG measurements for fetal growth especially in third trimester every 4 weeks in dichorionic and every 2 weeks in monochorionic pregnancies. Assessment of amniotic fluid volume is also important.

### Discordant Fetal Growth

Discordant fetal growth in multifetal pregnancies is most commonly defined as a 20% difference in estimated fetal weight between larger and smaller fetus. Whether growth discordant multiple gestations without a structural anomaly, aneuploidy, oligohydramnios or FGR are at risk for adverse outcome is debatable. Though discordant but appropriate for gestational age growth are not at increased risk of fetal or neonatal morbidity and mortality.

When discordant growth is identified, Doppler evaluation of vascular resistance may provide a measurement of fetal well-being. Increased resistance and diminished diastolic flow often accompanies growth restriction. Nonstress test or biophysical profile is commonly used in the management of multifetal pregnancy. Care must be taken to evaluate each fetus separately.

### Prediction of Preterm Labor

Lim et al.[61] conducted a systematic review of the literature on cervical length as a predictor of preterm birth in women with multiple pregnancies. Meta-analysis using a bivariate model showed a strong association between short cervical length in the second trimester and preterm birth in multiple pregnancies. Sensitivity and specificity for preterm birth before 34 weeks were determined from receiver operating characteristic (ROC) curves for cervical length 35 mm (78% and 66%, respectively), 30 mm (41% and 87%), 25 mm (36% and 94%), and 20 mm (30% and 94%). The authors concluded that women with a short cervix are at increased risk of preterm birth, but sensitivity associated with this measure is low, indicating that many women with a multiple pregnancy will deliver prematurely despite a long cervix in the second trimester. Furthermore, as there are no effective preventative strategies, the authors concluded that there is currently no place in routine clinical practice for cervical length measurement in this population. However, this evidence suggests that studies to evaluate interventions to prevent preterm birth in multiple pregnancies should focus on women with short cervix, who may be at increased risk.[61]

Preterm labor and subsequent birth present greatest risk to the fetus. It is difficult to predict which patient will go in preterm labor. Cervical assessment and fetal fibronectin levels predict preterm labor. Cervical assessment by digital examination or by USG has been suggested as a useful way to evaluate the risk of preterm labor. At 24 weeks, a cervical length of 25 mm or less is the best predictor of birth before 32 weeks.[62] In multifetal gestations, a positive fibronectin test at 28–30 weeks is associated with preterm birth before 32 weeks.[63] Women with multifetal gestations at 24 weeks who had a closed internal os on digital cervical examination, a normal cervical length on USG, and a normal fetal fibronectin test are at a low risk to deliver before 32 weeks.[64] The use of various screening methods for preterm labor in asymptomatic women with multifetal pregnancies is not recommended. In symptomatic women, fetal fibronectin test result or short cervical length alone is poor predictor and they should not be used exclusively to direct management in the setting of acute symptoms.[2]

### Management of Preterm Labor in Multifetal Gestation

Several antenatal interventions have been tried to reduce the risk of preterm birth in multifetal gestations. These include bed rest in hospital, use of tocolysis, and prophylactic cerclage. It has been shown by various studies that bed rest in hospital in an uncomplicated multifetal pregnancy neither reduces the risk of preterm birth nor does it lead to reduction in perinatal mortality.[65] The Cochrane review of randomized trial of routine hospitalization for bed rest shows an increased likelihood of preterm birth.[66] The value of admission for rest in higher order multifetal gestations is uncertain. One study in triplets showed reduction in preterm birth after hospitalization.[67] Limited physical activities, early work leave, more frequent antenatal checkups and USG examination and maternal education on the risks of preterm delivery have been advocated to be effective in reducing preterm births in multifetal gestations.[3]

Tocolytic therapy may provide short-term prolongation of pregnancy, which enables the administration of antenatal corticosteroids as well as transport to tertiary care facility, if indicated. Calcium channel blockers like nifedipine or nonsteroidal anti-inflammatory drugs should be first line treatment. Although there is dearth of large-scale randomized trials of multifetal gestations alone, this conclusion came from trials that included both singleton and multifetal gestation. So, a brief course of tocolysis may be considered for up to 48 hours in setting of acute preterm labor in order to allow corticosteroids to be administered. There is no evidence that tocolytic therapy improves neonatal outcome in multiple gestation. Tocolysis with betamimetics is not recommended in multifetal gestations. It can have harmful effect in multifetal pregnancy. This is in part because of increased plasma volume and cardiovascular demands in the pregnant woman. Women with multiple gestations have significantly more cardiovascular complications with the use of betamimetic tocolytic agents.[3]

Prophylactic cervical cerclage has not shown any benefit in various studies as regard improvement in neonatal outcome.[67,68] Elective cerclage contributes little in prolongation of gestational age at the time of delivery in women with twin pregnancy.[69] It seems prudent to reserve cervical cerclage for cases with evidence of cervical incompetence. Interventions to prevent spontaneous preterm birth in twin or triplet pregnancies including bed rest at home or in hospital, intramuscular or vaginal progesterone, cervical cerclage, or oral tocolytics are not found to be effective in various studies. Nevertheless, the evidence suggests that, although progesterone has a place in preventing preterm births in singleton pregnancies, there appears to be no such benefit in multiple pregnancies, even in women with short cervix. The conclusion drawn from the study is not to use intramuscular or vaginal progesterone to prevent preterm birth in multiple pregnancies.[70] As per ACOG Practice bulletin (2016), progesterone treatment does not reduce the incidence of spontaneous preterm birth in unselected women with twin or triplet pregnancy and therefore, is not recommended.[2]

A meta-analysis published by Romero et al. in 2017 showed that administration of vaginal progesterone to asymptomatic women with a twin gestation and a sonographic short cervix in the mid-trimester reduces the risk of preterm birth occurring at <30 to <35 gestational weeks, neonatal mortality and some measures of neonatal morbidity, without any demonstrable deleterious effects on childhood neurodevelopment.[71]

NICE guidelines-2019, did not make any recommendation on vaginal progesterone for preventing preterm birth in twin pregnancies because of emerging evidence in this area.[72]

Corticosteroids should be given in women with multifetal pregnancy who are at risk for preterm birth before 34 weeks or when there is a chance of preterm termination because of maternal indication.[73] Guidelines for use of corticosteroids are same as for singleton pregnancy, i.e., two doses of 12 mg of betamethasone intramuscularly 24 hours apart or dexamethasone 6 mg 12 hours apart total four doses intramuscularly.

Magnesium sulfate for fetal neuroprotection has been advocated. Meta-analysis of several randomized trials have shown that prenatal administration of magnesium sulfate reduces the severity and risk of cerebral palsy in infants if administered when birth is anticipated before 32 weeks of gestation, regardless of fetal number.[2]

### Timing of Delivery in Women with Multiple Gestations

On an average, women with twin pregnancies give birth at approximately 36 weeks of gestation. The risk of perinatal mortality begins to increase again in twin pregnancies at approximately 38 weeks of gestation. There are no large randomized control trials demonstrating clearly the optimal time of delivery. ACOG 2016 and NICE 2019 have made the following recommendations for timing of delivery for uncomplicated twin gestation.

- Women with uncomplicated dichorionic diamniotic twin gestations can undergo delivery at 38 weeks of gestation.
- Women with uncomplicated monochorionic diamniotic twin gestation can undergo delivery between 34 and 37 weeks of gestation.
- Women with uncomplicated monochorionic monoamniotic twin gestations can undergo delivery at 32–34 weeks of gestation.
- Women with uncomplicated trichorionic triamniotic or dichorionic triamniotic pregnancy should undergo delivery at 35 weeks of gestation.
- Women with monochorionic triamniotic triplet pregnancy, the timing of birth should be decided and discussed with each woman individually.
- Women who decline planned birth at the recommended gestation age, should be seen weekly and USG scan should be offered at each visit to assess amniotic fluid volume and Doppler of the umbilical artery flow of each baby in addition to fetal growth scan.

## Route of Delivery

The optimal route of delivery in women with twin pregnancy depends on type of twins, fetal presentation, and gestational age.

- Women with monoamniotic twin gestation should undergo cesarean section to avoid an umbilical cord complication of nonpresenting twin at the time of delivery of first twin.
- Diamniotic twins whose presenting fetus is vertex are candidates for vaginal delivery regardless of the presentation of the second twin provided that an obstetrician with experience in vaginal breech delivery and internal podalic version is available.
- When the first twin is not cephalic, cesarean section should be offered.
- Women with previous low transverse cesarean section and uncomplicated twin pregnancy with presenting fetus vertex may be considered for trial of labor. Delivery may be complicated by the need for internal fetal manipulation or emergent cesarean section.
- The optimal route of delivery for women with higher order multiple gestation remains unknown. As per NICE 2019 guidelines,[72] cesarean section should be offered to women with triplet pregnancy at the time of planned birth, i.e., 35 weeks or earlier if any complication is diagnosed in her pregnancy requiring early delivery or when the women is in established labor and gestational age suggests that there is reasonable chance of survival of the babies.

## Intrapartum Management

*Recommendations for intrapartum management of twins include:*[3]

- Delivery preferably at a tertiary level unit.
- An expert obstetrician should be there throughout labor and preferably two obstetricians during delivery.
- An intravenous line should be established early in labor.
- Blood should be sent for cross matching. All blood transfusion products should be available.
- An ultrasound scan should be performed once the woman is in established labor to confirm which twin is which and to locate fetal hearts.[40]
- Continuous electronic monitoring of both the fetuses should be done. Use of dual channel cardiotocography monitors to allow simultaneous monitoring of both fetal hearts is advocated. Documentation on the cardiograph and on the clinical records depicting which cardiography trace belongs to which baby and systematic assessments of both cardiographs should be done at least hourly and more frequently, if there are concerns.
- Maternal pulse should be monitored electronically and displayed simultaneously on the same cardiography trace.
- As per recent NICE guidelines, if abdominal monitoring is unsuccessful or there is concern about synchronicity of the fetal hearts, once the membrane rupture and cervix is dilated, internal electronic monitoring of the presenting fetus can be carried out. Fetal scalp electrode is applied to the first baby (only after 34 weeks and if there are no contraindications) while continuing abdominal monitoring of the second baby.[40,72]
- An experienced anesthesiologist should be available.
- Two pediatricians, one of whom is skilled in neonatal resuscitation should be present at the time of birth.
- Sonography should be available to evaluate the lie and presentation of the second fetus after the delivery of the first twin.

## Vaginal Delivery

When first twin is presenting as cephalic, with no other associated complications, mother is allowed to go in spontaneous labor. Continuous monitoring of labor and of both the fetuses is done. When the cervix is fully dilated, delivery of first twin is conducted as in singleton fetus. Following the delivery of first twin, cord is doubly clamped and cut, placental end of the cord remains clamped. The lie, presentation, and size of the second twin are assessed by abdominal and vaginal examination. Continue to monitor the second baby using cardiotocography. If lie is longitudinal and uterine contractions are good, let the presenting part enter the pelvis then rupture of membrane and conduct the delivery of second twin.

If uterine contractions subside after the delivery of first twin, start oxytocin drip for stimulation of uterine activity. Once contractions set in, do amniotomy and delivery proceeds with maternal efforts during contractions. Continuous monitoring of second twin is recommended as there are more chances of intrapartum asphyxia.

If the second twin is cephalic, deliver it in the same way as the first. If second twin is an average sized breech, with a flexed head and no fetopelvic disproportion, conduct assisted breech delivery.

If the second twin is in transverse lie, one can do external cephalic version (ECV). Usually, it is easy to do ECV for second twin because of laxity of abdominal wall and a short distance that the head has to traverse in transverse lie. If it fails, then internal podalic version with breech extraction can be carried out under anesthesia.

Controversial discussions have taken place on the importance of time interval between the birth of first and second twin. Stein et al. analyzed 4,110 twin pregnancies and studied the impact of twin-to-twin interval on neonatal outcome. Complications after the delivery of the first twin such as fetal distress, placental abruption, and cord prolapse were related to increased time interval. Vaginal operative delivery and cesarean section rates were associated with increased time interval and a decline in mean umbilical arterial pH, base excess and fetal acidosis consequent to it. They concluded that twin-to-twin time interval seems to be an independent factor for adverse short-term outcome of the second twin.[74] The risk of fetal distress and acidosis is increased if twin-twin interval exceeds 30 minutes.[75]

At times there is need to hasten the delivery of second twin in conditions like cord prolapse or nonreassuring fetal heart pattern or when signs of abruptio placentae appear. In such cases if second twin is in cephalic presentation at brim, high vacuum can be used for its delivery. In case of breech presentation, breech extraction or cesarean section is advocated. In case it is transverse lie, internal podalic version with breech extraction under anesthesia or cesarean section is indicated.

As far as induction of labor is concerned, if an uncomplicated twin pregnancy does not go in labor by expected date of delivery, then labor should be induced if there is no contraindication to it. Multifetal pregnancy should not be allowed to go beyond expected date of delivery because of increased chances of fetal distress and perinatal mortality. Other indications for induction are associated complications like preeclampsia and FGR.[13]

As far as labor analgesia is concerned, epidural analgesia is recommended.[76] It provides excellent pain relief, but one should be cautious in multifetal pregnancy because of increased risk of supine hypotension during labor and delivery.

Active management of third stage should be done after the birth of last baby, as over distention of uterus leads to increased risk of PPH. In vaginal birth, 10 IU of oxytocin is given by intramuscular injection immediately after birth of last baby and before the cord is clamped and cut. In a cesarean section, 5 IU of oxytocin is given by intravenous injection immediately after the birth of last baby and before the cord is clamped and cut.[72]

### Indications of Cesarean in Multifetal Pregnancy

*The various indications of cesarean section in multiple pregnancies are listed here:*

- Monoamniotic twins
- Triplet and higher order births
- Viable conjoined twins
- When the first twin is non-cephalic, cesarean section is often preferred[77]
- *Cesarean delivery of second twin, if:*
  - Second twin is larger and cephalopelvic disproportion anticipated.
  - Second twin is in transverse lie and obstetrician is not skilled in the performing internal podalic version.
  - When cervix contracts and thickens after delivery of first twin and does not dilate subsequently.
- Nonreassuring fetal heart rate develops. If there is suspicious cardiotocography, and vaginal birth cannot be achieved within 20 minutes, consider performing cesarean section.[72]
- Placental abruption following delivery of first twin.

## Postpartum Management

During postnatal period, taking care of two or more babies may be stressful for the mother. Breastfeeding should be encouraged, though at times it may be insufficient for two or more babies. There is an increased risk of infection and subinvolution of uterus. Maternal nutrition should be given special attention. Supplementation of iron and calcium should continue for a minimum of 3 months. A high percentage of depression is reported in mothers of twins, so additional support should be provided. Women should be provided information regarding postpartum contraception and helped to decide the most appropriate method for her.

## SPECIAL SITUATIONS

### Single Fetal Demise

Sometimes one fetus dies in utero and pregnancy continues with one living fetus. In the first trimester, a substantial number of women undergo spontaneous reduction of one or more fetuses, commonly referred as vanishing twin. The probability of this reduction increases with the number of gestational sacs, 36% for twins, 53% for triplets, and 65% for quadruplets. In the second trimester and third trimester, up to 5% of twins and 17% of triplets undergo death of one or more fetuses. Risk of single fetal death in twin pregnancy as reported by Saito et al.[78] is 6.2%. In general population scanned between 10 and 14 weeks of gestation, the prevalence of single fetal demise is reported as 4% in dichorionic twins and 1% in monochorionic twins, double intrauterine fetal death as 1.6% in dichorionic and 2% in monochorionic twins.[24]

Chorionicity influences the rate of loss, predicts outcome in the survivor. Gross unequal placental sharing and hemodynamic imbalance in monochorionic twins may cause single fetal demise. Whereas in dichorionic twins it may be because of discordant chromosomal or structural anomalies or suboptimal placentation. After 14 weeks onward, single fetal death occurs in 2% of dichorionic and 4% of monochorionic twin pregnancies.[6] In a metanalysis by Danon et al. it was found that consequent to the demise of one twin after 14 weeks of gestation, the risk of death in the cotwin was 15% in monochorionic gestations and 3% for dichorionic gestations.[79] The prognosis of surviving twin depends on the period of gestation at the time of death, chorionicity, length of time between the death and the delivery of the surviving twin. Early demise such as in first trimester does not appear to increase the risk of death in surviving twin. Later in gestation, demise of one of the fetuses could trigger coagulation abnormalities in the mother. Very few cases of maternal coagulopathy have been reported after single fetal demise. The surviving twin has an extremely high risk of cerebral palsy and cerebral impairment.[80] The risk of neurologic abnormality in the surviving twin is greater in monochorionic gestations (18%) versus dichorionic gestations (1%).[81] The management decision should be based on the cause of death and the risk to the surviving twin. Majority of the cases of fetal death in multifetal pregnancy involve monochorionic placentation. Evidence indicates that morbidity in the survivor is almost always due to vascular anastomoses. Although death of cotwin in a monochorionic pregnancy in the late second trimester or early third trimester is associated with significant morbidity and mortality in the other fetus, immediate delivery of the surviving twin has not been demonstrated to be of benefit. Therefore, if such a situation arises before 34 weeks, management should be based on the condition of the mother or the surviving fetus. If there is no such indication, then delivery before 34 weeks of gestation is not recommended. When death of one dichorionic twin is due to congenital anomaly, it should not affect the other fetus. Santema et al. studied 29 cases with single fetal demise. The cause of death was not clear in all. They recommended conservative management of the living fetus.[82]

## Locked Twins (Fig. 8)

This is one of the very rare complications of twin pregnancy during labor. Incidence reported is 1 in 90,000 cases. The types of locking described are vertex-vertex, breech-vertex, vertex-transverse. There is a chance of locking when two fetal sacs appear together in the pelvis and the twins are less than average in size. As for locking of two forecoming heads, this seldom results in serious consequences, as the second head can nearly always be pushed out of the way. Much more serious variety is locking of after coming head of first child by the forecoming head of the second child. The risk of death of first twin is very high, as is the risk of fetal hypoxia for second twin. An attempt should be made to push up and hold up the head of second while delivering the first twin by breech extraction under anesthesia. If it is unsuccessful and baby is still alive, immediate cesarean section is indicated. But, if because of prolonged asphyxia first twin is already dead, the usual course is to decapitate the first and deliver the second twin and finally remove the severed head. Cesarean section is indicated if obstetrician is not an expert in doing decapitation. During cesarean section, the head of the first twin is maneuvered upward, enabling birth of the second twin's head and body. The first twin may then be delivered.

## SELECTIVE REDUCTION AND TERMINATION

Although most professional societies have issued guidelines to reduce the number of embryos to be transferred during ART, the incidence of multifetal pregnancies remains unacceptably high. The negative psychological, social, and medical consequences for the patients and their offspring outweigh the benefits in term of increased success rate. Multifetal reduction is an ethically acceptable solution if and only if the physician has taken all reasonable steps to prevent the occurrence of multiple pregnancies.[83] Reduction of higher order multiple gestation to twin is associated with lower rate of maternal complications, preterm birth, and neonatal death. When there is higher order multiple gestation, reduction to two or three fetuses may improve the chances of survival of the remaining fetuses. Fetal reduction to twins was associated with lower rates of preterm birth, very preterm birth, low birth weight, very low birth weight, and fetal reduction to singletons was associated with lower rates of preterm birth and low birth weight. Women should be counseled on the potential risks and benefits of fetal reduction.[84]

Reduction is done early in pregnancy. It can be done transcervically, transvaginally, or transabdominally. The easiest route is transabdominal. Reduction is performed between 10 and 13 weeks because at this gestation whatever chances of spontaneous abortion are there, it is already over and remaining fetuses can be evaluated sonographically. The dead fetus is too small and will be absorbed and its chances of affecting remaining fetuses are very less. The risk of aborting the entire pregnancy because of the procedure is minimal. The smallest or anomalous fetus is chosen for reduction. Potassium chloride is injected under USG guidance into the heart of selected fetus. Pregnancy loss rate reported maximum up to 4.5% in cases of triplet who were reduced to twins.

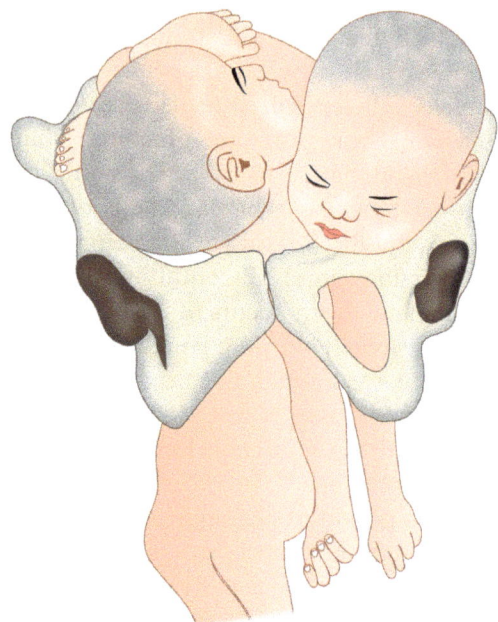

**Fig. 8:** Locking of twins.

When the fetuses are discordant for structural or genetic abnormalities, in that case selective termination can be done. Since anomalies are discovered mostly in second trimester, selective termination is performed later in gestation than selective reduction and risk involved is more than the selective reduction which is done early in gestation. Selective termination is usually performed only when the anomaly is severe but not lethal. For selective termination, precise diagnosis for the anomalous fetus and absolute certainty of fetal location should be known. Women should be counseled and discussion should include the morbidity and mortality rates expected if the pregnancy is continued and morbidity and mortality rates expected with surviving twins or triplets and the risk of procedure itself.[85] Decision for continuation of pregnancy without intervention or of selective termination is exclusively of the women. Risks involved are abortion of the remaining fetuses, abortion or retention of wrong fetus, damage without death to the fetus, preterm labor, discordant or growth restricted fetuses and maternal complication which include potential infection, hemorrhage or disseminated intravascular coagulopathy because of retained product of conception.[86,87]

## KEY POINTS

- Determination of chorionicity should be done at 10–14 weeks in multifetal pregnancy.
- Because of increased rate of complications associated with monochorionicity, increased surveillance to be maintained.
- All women with multiple gestation, regardless of age, should be subjected to routine aneuploidy screening.
- Women with higher order pregnancy should be counseled regarding the risk of prematurity and be offered the option of fetal reduction.
- Interventions like prophylactic cerclage, prophylactic tocolysis, routine hospitalization and bed rest have not been found to decrease neonatal morbidity or mortality. So not recommended routinely.
- Regular ultrasound assessment of growth and umbilical artery Doppler should be done.
- Magnesium sulfate is recommended if birth is anticipated before 32 weeks of gestation regardless of number of fetuses.
- One course of antenatal corticosteroids should be administered between 24 and 34 weeks of gestation in case there is risk of delivery within 7 days.
- Women with one previous lower segment cesarean section, who are otherwise for vaginal delivery, may be considered for trial of labor.
- Women with uncomplicated monochorionic monoamniotic twin gestation can undergo cesarean section at 32–34 weeks of gestation.
- Women with diamniotic twin pregnancy at 32 completed weeks or later; with presenting fetus as vertex, regardless of presentation of second twin, can undergo vaginal delivery provided the obstetrician experienced in internal podalic version and vaginal breech delivery, is available.
- Continuous monitoring of each fetus should be done during labor.
- Epidural analgesia, if available, should be offered.
- Experienced obstetrician, pediatrician, neonatal nurse, and anesthetist should be available at delivery.

## REFERENCES

1. Martin JA, Hamilton BE, Ventura SJ, Menacker F, Park MM, Sutton PD. Births: final data for 2001. Natl Vital Stat Rep. 2002;51(2):1-102.
2. Committee on Practice Bulletins—Obstetrics, Society for Maternal-Fetal Medicine. Practice Bulletin No. 169. Multifetal gestations: twin, triplet, and higher-order multifetal pregnancies. Obstet Gynecol. 2016;128(4):e131-46.
3. Cunninham FG, Leveno KJ, Bloom SL, Hauth JC, Gilstrap L, Wenstrom KD. Mutiple gestation. In: Cunninham FG, Leveno KJ, Bloom SL, Hauth JC, Gilstrap L, Wenstrom KD (Eds). Williams Obstetrics, 22nd edition. New York: McGraw Hill; 2006. pp. 911-43.
4. Alikani M, Ceckleniak NA, Walters E, Cohen J. Monozygotic twining following assisted conception: an analysis of 81 consecutive cases. Hum Reprod. 2003;18(9):1937-43.
5. Hoekstra C, Zhao ZZ, Lambalk CB, Willemsen G, Martin NG, Boomsma DI, et al. Dizygotic twinning. Hum Reprod Update. 2008;14(1):27-47.
6. Liesbeth L, Deprest J. Fetal problems in multifetal pregnancy. In: James DK, Steer PJ, Weiner CP, Gonk B (Eds). High Risk Pregnancy, Management Options, 3rd edition, Philadelphia: Elsevier (Saunders); 2006. pp. 524-60.
7. Meulemans WJ, Lewis CM, Boomsma DL. Genetic modelling of dizygotic twinning in pedigrees of spontaneous dizygotic twins. Am J Med Genetics. 1996;61:258.
8. Kametas SJ, McAuliffe F, Krampl E. Maternal cardiac function in twin pregnancy. Obstet Gynecol. 2003;102:806.
9. Campbell DM. Maternal adaptation in twin pregnancy. Semin Perinatol. 1986;10:14.
10. Krafft A, Breymann C, Streich J. Haemoglobin concentration in multiple versus singleton pregnancies. Retrospective evidence for physiology not pathology. Eur J Obstet Reprod Biol. 2001;99:184-7.
11. Wimalasundera RC, Trew G, Fisk NM. Reducing the incidence of twin and triplets. Best Pract Res Clin Obstet Gynaecol. 2003;17(2):309-29.
12. Mackay AP, Berg J, King JC, Duran C, Chang J. Pregnancy related mortality among women with multifetal pregnancies. Obstet Gynecol. 2006;107(3):563-8.
13. Crowther CA, Dodd JM. Multiple pregnancy. In: James DK, Steer PJ, Weiner CP, Gonik B (Eds). High Risk Pregnancy, Management Options, 3rd edition. Philadelphia: Elsevier (Saunders); 2006. pp. 1276-92.
14. Day MC, Barton JR, O'Brien JM, Istwan NB, Sibai BM. The effect of fetal number on the development of hypertensive condition of pregnancy. Obstet Gynaecol. 2005;106:927-31.

15. Bdolah Y, Lam C, Raja Kumar A, Shivalingappa V, Mutter W, Sachs BP, et al. Twin pregnancy and risk of preeclampsia: bigger placenta or relative ischaemia. Am J Obstet Gynecol. 2008;198(4):428-36.
16. Campbel D, MacGillivray L. Preeclampsia in twin pregnancies: Incidence and outcome. Hypertens Pregnancy. 1999;18:197-207.
17. Mastrobattista JM, Skupski DW, Monga M. The rate of severe preeclampsia is increased in triplet as compared to twin pregnancy. Am J Pernatol. 1997;14:263.
18. Lynch A, McDuffie R Jr, Murphy J, Faber K, Orleans M. Preeclampsia in multiple gestation: the role of assisted reproductive technologies. Obstet Gynecol. 2002;99(3):445-51.
19. Ananth C, Demissie K, Smulian J, Vintzileos A. Placenta previa in singleton and twin births in United States, 1989 through 1998. A comparison of risk factor profiles and associated conditions. Am J Obstet Gynecol. 2003;188:275-81.
20. Hruby E, Sass L, Gorbe E, Hupuczi P, Papp Z. The maternal and fetal outcome of 122 triplet pregnancies. Orv Hetil. 2007;148(49):2315-28.
21. Strauss A, Peak B, Genzl-Boroviezeny, Schulze A, Janssen U, Hepp H. Multifetal gestations—maternal and perinatal outcome of 112 pregnancies. Fetal Diagn Ther. 2002;17(4):209-17.
22. Shunj S, Fumi K, Nozomi O, Nagayama C, Nakagawa M, Inde Y, et al. Risk of postpartum haemorrhage after vaginal delivery of twins. J Nippon Med Sch. 2007;74:414-7.
23. Conde-Agudelo A, Belizán JM, Lindmark G. Maternal morbidity and mortality associated with multiple gestations. Obstet Gynecol. 2000;95:899-904.
24. Sebire N, Thorton S, Hughes K. The prevalence and consequence of missed abortion in twin pregnancies at 10-14 weeks of gestation. BJOG. 1997;104:847-8.
25. Tummers P, De Sutter P, Dhont M. Risk of spontaneous abortion in singleton and twin pregnancies after IVF/ICSI. Hum Reprod. 2003;18(8):1720-3.
26. Stein Kampf MP, Whitten SJ, Hammond KR. Effect of spontaneous pregnancy reduction on obstetric outcome. J Reprod Med. 2005;50(8):603-6.
27. Ananth CV, Vintzieos AM, Shen-Schwarz S, Smulian JC, Lai YL. Standards of birth weight in twin gestations stratified by placental chorionicity. Obstet Gynecol. 1998;91:917-24.
28. Cleary-Goldman J, D'Alton ME. Growth abnormalities and multiple gestations. Semin Perinatol. 2008;32(3):2006-12.
29. Caroll SGM, Soothill PW, Abdel-Fattah SA, Porter H, Montague I, Kyle PM. Prediction of chorionicity in twin pregnancies at 10-14 weeks of gestations. BJOG. 2002;109:182-6.
30. Lynch A, McDuffie RC, Murphy J. The contribution of assisted conception, chorionicity and other risk factors to very low birth weight in twin cohort. BJOG. 2003;110(4):405-10.
31. Fountain SA, Morrison JJ, Smith SK, Winston RM. Ultrasonography growth measurements in triplet pregnancies. J Perinat Med. 1995;23:257-63.
32. Senoo M, Okamuro K, Murotsuki J, Yaegashi N, Uehara S, Yajima A. Growth pattern of different chorionicity evaluated by sonography biometry. Obstet Gynecol. 2000;95:656-61.
33. Victoria A, Mora G, Arias F. Perinatal outcome, placental pathology and severity of discordance in monochorionic and dichorionic twins. Obstet Gynecol. 2001;97(2):310-5.
34. Glinianaia SV, RanKin J, Wright C. Congenital anomalies in twins: a register based study. Hum Reprod. 2008;23(6):1306-11.
35. Hall JG. Twinning. Lancet. 2003;362:735.
36. Bajoria R. Abundant vascular anastomses in monoamniotic versus diamniotic placentas. Am J Obstet Gynecol. 1998;179:788-93.
37. Allen VM, Windrim R, Barret J. Management of monoamniotic twin pregnancies: a case series and systemic review of literature. BJOG. 2001;108:931.
38. Lam YH, Sin SY, Lam C, Lee CP, Tang MH, Tse HY. Prenatal sonographic diagnosis of conjoined twins in the first trimester: two case reports. Ultrasound Obstet Gynecol. 1998;11(4):289-91.
39. Spitz L, Kiely FM. Experience and management of conjoined twins. Br J Surg. 2002;89:1188-92.
40. Nik Lah NA, Che Yaakob CA, Othman MS, Nik Mahmood NM. Twin reverse arterial perfusion sequence. Singapore Med J. 2007;48(12):335-7.
41. Quintero RA, Chmait RH, Murakoshi T, Pankrac Z, Swiatkowska M, Bornick PW, et al. Surgical management of twin reversed arterial perfusion. Am J Obstet Gynecol. 2006;194:982-91.
42. Hecher K, Lewi L, Gratacos E, Huber A, Ville Y, Deprest J. Twin reversed arterial perfused fetoscopic laser coagulation of placental anastomosis or the umbilical cord. Ultrasound Obstet Gynecol. 2006;28:688-91.
43. Hirose M, Murata A, Kita N, Aotani H, Takebayashi K, Noda Y. Successful intrauterine treatment with radiofrequency ablation in a case of acardiac twin pregnancy complicated with hydropic pump twin. Ultrasound Obstet Gynecol. 2004;23:509-12.
44. Tan TY, Sepal Veda N. Acardiac twin: a systemic review of minimally invasive treatment modalities. Ultrasound Obstet Gynecol. 2003;22:409-19.
45. Sullivan AE, Varner MW, Ball RG. The management of acardiac twins: a conservative approach. Am J Obstet Gynecol. 2003;189:1310.
46. Larroche JC, Droulle P, Delezoide AL. Brain damage in monozygous twins. Biol Neonate. 1990;57:261.
47. Memmo A, Dias T, Mahsud-Dornan S. Prediction of selective fetal growth restriction and twin-to-twin transfusion syndrome in monochorionic twins. BJOG. 2012;119:417-21.
48. Bruner JP, Rosemond RL. Twin-to-twin transfusion syndrome. A subset of twin oligohydoamnios-polyhydroamnios sequence. Am J Obstet Gynecol. 1993;169:925.
49. Wee LY, Muslim I. Perinatal complications of monochorionic placentation. Curr Opin Obstet Gynecol. 2007;19(6):554-60.
50. Challis D, Gratcos E, Deprest JA. Cord occlusion techniques for selective termination in monochorionic twins. J Perinat Med. 1999;27:327.
51. Donner C, Shahabi S, Thomas D. Selective feticide by embolisation in twin-twin transfusion syndrome: a report of two cases. J Reprod Med. 1997;42:747.
52. Roberts D, Gates S, Kilby M, Neilson JP. Interventions for twin-twin transfusion syndrome: a Cochrane review. Ultrasound Obstet Gynecol. 2008;31(6):701-11.
53. Rouse DJ, Skopee GS, Zlanik FJ. Fundal height as predictor of preterm twin delivery. Obstet Gynecol. 1993;81:211.
54. Sepulveda W, Sebire N, Hughes K. The Lambda sign at 10-14 weeks of pregnancy as a predictor of chorionicity in twin pregnancies. Ultrasound Obstet Gynecol. 1996;7:421-3.
55. Dias T, Arcangeli T, Bhinde A, Napolitano R, Mahsud-Dornan S, Thilaganathan B. First trimester ultrasound determination

56. Sepulveda W. Chorionicity determination in twin pregnancy; double trouble? Ultrasound Obstet Gynecol. 1997;10:79-81.
57. Dias T, Ladd S, Mahsud-Dornan S, Bhide A, Papageorghiou AT, Thilaganathan B. Systematic labeling of twin pregnancies on ultrasound. Ultrasound Obstet Gynecol. 2011; 38:130-3.
58. LeFevre ML, Bain RP, Ewigman BG. A randomized trial of prenatal ultrasonographic screening: impact on maternal management and outcome. RADIUS study group. Am J Obstet. 1993;169(3):483-9.
59. Sepulveda W, Wong AE, Casasbuenas A. Nuchal translucency and nasal bone in first trimester ultrasound screening for aneuploidy in multiple pregnancies. Ultrasound Obstet Gynaecol. 2009;33:152-6.
60. Roem K. Nutritional management of multiple pregnancies. Twin Res. 2003;6(6):514-9.
61. Lim AC, Hegeman MA, Huis In 't Veld MA, Opmeer BC, Bruinse HW, Mol BW. Cervical length measurement for the prediction of preterm birth in multiple pregnancies: asystematic review and bivariate meta-analysis. Ultrasound Obstet Gynecol. 2011;38:10-17.
62. Souka AP, Heath V, Flint S. Cervical length at 23 weeks in twins in predicting spontaneous preterm delivery. Obstet Gynecol. 1999;94:450.
63. Wennerholm U, Holm BN, Mattsby-Baltzer I, Nielsen T, Platz-Christensen J, Sundell G, et al. Fetal fibronectin, endotoxin, bacterial vaginosis and cervical length as predictors of preterm birth and neonatal morbidity in twin pregnancies. BJOG. 1997;104:1398-404.
64. McMahon KS, Neerhof MG, Haney EL, Thomas HA, Silver RK, Peaceman AM. Prematurity in multiple gestations: identification of patients who are at low risk. Am J Obstet Gynecol. 2002;186:1137.
65. Dodd JM, Crowther CA. Hospitalisation for bed rest for women with a triplet pregnancy: an abandoned randomized controlled trial and meta-analysis. BMC Pregnancy Childbirth. 2005;5:8.
66. Crowther CA, Verkuyl DA, Ashworth MF, Bannerman C, Ashurst HM. The effects of hospitalization for bed rest on duration of gestatation, fetal growth and neonatal morbidity in triplet pregnancy. Acta Genet Med Gemellol. 1991;40:63-8.
67. Elimian A, Figueroa R, Nigam S, Verma U, Tejani N, Kirshenbaum N. Perinatal outcome of triplet gestation: does pro-phylactic encerclage make a difference? J Matern Fetal Med. 1999;8:119.
68. Newman RB, Krombach S, Myers MC, McGee DL. Effect of cerclage on obstetrical outcome in twin gestations with shortened cervical length. Am J Obstet Gynecol. 2002;186:634.
69. EsKander M, Shafiq H, Almushail MA, Sobande A, Bahar AM. Cervical cerclage for prevention of preterm birth in women with twin pregnancy. Int J Gynecol Obstet. 2007;99(2):110-12.
70. Lim AC, Schuit E, Bloemenkamp K, Bernardus RE, Duvekot JJ, Erwich JJHM, et al. 17α-hydroxyprogesterone caproate for the prevention of adverse neonatal outcome in multiple pregnancies. Obstet Gynecol. 2011;118:513-20.
71. Romero R, Conde-Agudelo A, El-Refaie W, Rode L, Brizot ML, Cetingoz E, et al. Vaginal progesterone decreases preterm birth and neonatal morbidity and mortality in women with a twin gestation and a short cervix: an updated meta-analysis of individual patient data. Ultrasound Obstet Gynecol. 2017;49(3):303-14.
72. NICE (2019). Twin and triplet pregnancy. NICE guideline [NG137] [online]. Available from: https://www.nice.org.uk/guidance/ng137. [Last accessed July, 2021].
73. Crowley P. Prophylactic corticosteroids for preterm birth. Cochrane Database Syst Rev. 2000;(2):CD000065.
74. Stein W, Misselwitz B, Schmidt S. Twin-to-twin delivery time interval: Influencing factor and effect on short-term outcome of the second twin. Acta Obstet Gynecol Scan. 2008;87(3):346-53.
75. Leung T, Tam W. Effects of twin-to-twin delivery interval on umbilical cord blood gas in the second twin. BJOG. 2002;109:1424-5.
76. Koffel B. Abnormal presentation and multiple gestation. In: Chestnut DH (Ed). Obstetrical Anesthesia, 2nd edition. St Louis, Mosby: Elsevier;1999. pp. 694.
77. Hutton E, Hannah M, Barret J. Use of external cephalic version for breech pregnancy and mode of delivery for breech and twin pregnancy: a survey of Canadian practitioners. J Obstet Gynecol Can. 2002;24:804-10.
78. Saito K, Ohtsu Y, Amano K. Perinatal outcome and management of single fetal death in twin pregnancy: a case series and review. J Perinat Med. 1999;27:473.
79. Danon D, Sekar R, Hack KE, Fisk NM. Increased still birth in uncomplicated monochorionic twin pregnancies: a systematic review and meta-analysis. Obstet Gynecol. 2013;121:1318-26.
80. Pharoah PO, Adi Y. Consequences of in-utero death in a twin pregnancy. Lancet. 2000;355:1597.
81. Hillman SC, Morris RK, Kilby MD. Co-twin prognosis after single fetal death: a systematic review and meta-analysis. Obstet Gynecol. 2011;118:928-40.
82. Santema JG, Swaak AM, Wallenburg HCS. Expectant management of twin pregnancy with single fetal death. BJOG. 1995;102:26.
83. Pennings G. Avoiding multiple pregnancies in ART. Multiple pregnancies: a test case of moral quality of medically assisted reproduction. Hum Reprod. 2000;15(12):2466-9.
84. Neda R, Tehila A, Joseph T, Tracy P. Perinatal outcomes in multifetal pregnancy following fetal reduction. CMAJ. 2017;189(18):652-8.
85. Committee Opinion No. 719: Multifetal Pregnancy Reduction. Obstet Gynecol. 2017;130(3):e158-63.
86. Evans MI, Berkowitz RL, Wapner RJ, Carpenter RJ, Goldberg JD, Ayoub MA, et al. Improvement in outcome of multifetal pregnancy reduction with increased experience. Am J Obstet Gynecol. 2001;184:97.
87. Dodd J, Crowther C. Reduction of the number of fetuses for women with triplet and higher order multiple pregnancies. Cochrane Database Syst Rev. 2003;(2):CD003932.

# CHAPTER 7

# Fetal Growth Restriction

*Kanwal Gujral, Sakshi Nayar*

## INTRODUCTION

Fetal growth restriction (FGR) is a common complication associated with pregnancy. It is defined as the failure of a fetus to grow to its biologically determined growth potential. It accounts for a perinatal mortality rate of 80–120/1,000 total births, which is 6–10 times higher than that of appropriate for gestational age (AGA) fetuses. It also contributes to 50% of all still births.[1]

## DEFINITION

There is a lack of consensus as regards to the definition of FGR. Different societies use different criteria to diagnose FGR. American College of Obstetricians and Gynecologists (ACOG) and Society of Obstetricians and Gynaecologists of Canada (SOGC) define FGR as estimated fetal weight (EFW) below the 10th centile for gestational age (GA), whereas Royal College of Obstetricians and Gynaecologists (RCOG) additionally considers abdominal circumference (AC) <10th centile also as FGR.[2-4] Terms small for gestation age (SGA) and FGR are often used interchangeably whereas not all SGA fetuses are growth restricted. Some SGA fetuses are constitutionally small and are at low risk of adverse perinatal outcomes. On the contrary, some appropriate for GA fetuses may have aberrant growth (FGR) and may be at risk of still birth. However, all fetuses with a weight < 3rd centile are diagnosed as FGR.

Some authorities classify FGR as early onset (GA < 32 weeks) or late onset (GA ≥ 32 weeks) depending upon the timing of the presentation.[5,6] These were earlier referred to as symmetrical and asymmetrical respectively.

To rest this dilemma a panel of experts reached a consensus on the definition of FGR by Delphi procedure in 2016.[7] The defining parameters were solitary (single parameter sufficient to diagnose FGR) or contributory (parameter that required other abnormal parameters for diagnosis). The group also defined the percentile cut-off value for individual parameter. The criteria are applicable only in the absence of congenital anomalies. **Table 1** describes the criteria.

In nutshell, Delphi consensus has standardized the definition of early and late onset FGR (LOFGR) using biometry along with functional parameters, as against conventional definition based on biometry alone.

**TABLE 1:** Delphi consensus definition of FGR in the absence of congenital anomalies.

| Early FGR: | Late FGR: |
|---|---|
| • GA < 32 weeks | • GA ≥ 32 weeks |
| • AC/EFW <3rd centile or UA-AEDF | • AC/EFW <3rd centile |
| Or | Or |
| • AC/EFW <10th centile combined with: | • At least two out of three of the following: |
| – Ut-A-PI >95th centile and/or | – AC/EFW <10th centile |
| – UA-PI >95th centile | – AC/EFW crossing centiles >2 quartiles on growth centiles |
| | – CPR <5th centile or UA-PI >95th centile |

(AC: abdominal circumference; AEDF: absent end diastolic flow; CPR: cerebroplacental ratio; EFW: estimated fetal weight; FGR: fetal growth restriction; GA: gestational age; PI: pulsatility index; UA: umbilical artery; UtA: uterine artery)

**TABLE 2:** Etiology of fetal growth restriction.

| Maternal conditions | Fetal conditions | Placental conditions |
|---|---|---|
| • Chronic hypertension | • Infection | • Chorioangioma |
| • Pre-eclampsia | • Congenital malformation | • Infarction |
| • Pregestational diabetes | • Aneuploidy | • Circumvallate placenta |
| • Cardiovascular disease | • Multiple Pregnancies | • Confined placental mosaicism |
| • Substance abuse | | • Obliterative vasculopathy of placental bed |
| • Autoimmune conditions | | |
| • Poor nutritional state | | |
| • Medications | | |
| • High altitude | | |

## ETIOLOGY

It revolves around maternal, fetal, and placental disorders as depicted in **Table 2**.

## PATHOPHYSIOLOGY

### Early Onset Fetal Growth Restriction

Early onset FGR (EOFGR) differs from LOFGR in its response to hypoxia besides timing of the onset. It starts early in gestation (<32 weeks), responds to hypoxia or chronic

> **BOX 1:** Compensation to decompensation.
>
> - Decrease in umbilical venous volume and liver size
> - Abdominal circumference lag—1st biometric sign
> - Increased umbilical artery Doppler resistance
> - Flow redistribution—middle cerebral artery (MCA) compensatory vasodilatation
> - Decreased amniotic fluid
> - Absent end-diastolic velocity (AEDV) in umbilical artery
> - Loss of fetal movements, variability
> - Reversed end-diastolic flow in umbilical artery
> - Ductus venosus (DV) a-wave absent or reversal
> - Biophysical profile (BPP) or score (BPS) decline—nonreactive nonstress test (NST) and late decelerations
> - Fetal circulatory collapse and death

**TABLE 3:** Differential features between the clinical phenotypes of FGR.

| | Early onset FGR | Late onset FGR |
|---|---|---|
| Prevalence | 0.5–1% | 5–10% |
| Challenge | Management | Detection and diagnosis |
| Evidence of placental disease | • High<br>• 70% abnormal umbilical Doppler<br>• 60% association with pre-eclampsia<br>• Severe angiogenic disbalance | • Low<br>• <10% abnormal umbilical Doppler<br>• 15% association with pre-eclampsia<br>• Mild angiogenic disbalance |
| Pathophysiology and oxygen delivered to the brain | • Hypoxia +/+<br>• Systemic cardiovascular adaptation | • Hypoxia +/-<br>• Central cardiovascular adaptation |
| Clinical impact | High mortality and morbidity | Low mortality/morbidity + high prevalence = large etiological fraction of adverse outcomes |

(FGR: fetal growth restriction)

deprivation in a hierarchical manner from compensation to decompensation phase, which is as given in **Box 1**.[5]

Fetuses with EOFGR usually show these changes from arterial to venous circulation, but at times cardiovascular (Doppler) and behavioral response of fetus (BPP) can occur independent of each other resulting in discordant Doppler and BPP changes. Therefore, an integrated surveillance approach using multivessel Doppler and BPP is the recommended management approach.

## Late Onset Fetal Growth Restriction

Late onset FGR does not depict these changes in a sequential manner. Fetal metabolic needs are greater than placental capacity, even in the absence of placental insufficiency. Umbilical artery Doppler (UAD) can be normal in up to 20% of cases. Even with a normal UAD, cerebral redistribution can occur resulting in dilated MCA and low pulsatility index (PI), and decreased cerebroplacental ratio (CPR) (PI of MCA/PI of UAD) precedes MCA dilatation. This indicates that brain sparing is imminent. LOFGR is a significant clinical problem, which can frequently go undetected and contribute to over 50% of unanticipated still births. Therefore, more frequent monitoring is required.[8,9]

In a recent review, Figueras et al. have summarized main differential features between the clinical phenotypes of FGR[10] (**Table 3**).

## ■ DIAGNOSIS

*Dating of pregnancy*: Correct dating early in pregnancy helps to identify FGR later. Clinical information of last menstrual period (LMP), regular cycles, and no hormonal contraception in preceding 3 months establishes dates by Naegele's rule. In case of uncertain dates or inadequate information, ultrasound measurement of crown rump length in first trimester and fetal biometry in 2nd trimester are accurate in establishing dates ± 5–7 days and 7–10 days respectively. If the clinical dates and ultrasound dates are within 1 week of each other then clinical dates are taken as correct dates. On the other hand, if there is disparity of >7 days between the two, ultrasound date is presumed to be the correct one. A repeat ultrasound after 2–3 weeks showing adequate interval growth further establishes the correctness of ultrasound date. If growth lag is seen, it is the setting of early FGR.

## Maternal Medical History and Characteristics

Medical conditions such as hypertension, autoimmune disease, thrombophilia, and chronic kidney disease increase the risk of FGR. Maternal characteristics such as abnormal body mass index (BMI) (<20 kg/m$^2$ or >30 kg/m$^2$), anemia, poor nutrition, and addictions are also associated with FGR. A detailed list of associated major and minor risk factors depicted in **Table 6** should be assessed at first prenatal visit.

## Obstetric History

Obstetric risk factors associated with increased risk in FGR include previous SGA (2 fold increase), previous still birth (6 fold increase), and previous pre-eclampsia (10 fold increase).

## Clinical Examination

After a complete history, a detailed general physical examination including height, weight, BMI, assessment of anemia, and nutritional status should be carried out.

### Symphysis Fundal Height and Abdominal Girth

Carefully performed serial symphysis fundal height (SFH) is a simple, safe, inexpensive, and a reasonably accurate screening method to detect FGR. If measurement is < 2–3 cm from the expected height (normally, it is 20 cm at 20 weeks, with a linear rise of 1 cm/week), inappropriate fetal growth is suspected. Ideally, measurement should be plotted on a customized centile chart. A single measurement below the 10th centile or serial measurements showing a static or a slow growth needs further evaluation.

Abdominal girth in inches corresponds to weeks of pregnancy. Maternal obesity, presence of fibroids, abnormal lie, and deeply engaged head limit the predictive accuracy of clinical examination.

## INVESTIGATIONS

### Ultrasonography: Biometry

This is the mainstay in diagnosis of FGR. AC or EFW < 10th centile for GA is the recommended cut-off for diagnosis based on the population or customized growth charts. AC is the first parameter to depict a decelerated growth. Combining head, abdomen, and femur dimensions has shown to optimize the accuracy whereas little increment or improvement is gained by adding other biometric measurements. Sensitivity of AC is 96–100%, of femur length (FL) is 20–45%, of head circumference (HC)/AC is 70%, of FL/AC is 63%, and of EFW it is 87% for detecting FGR.[11]

One recent meta-analysis has highlighted that AC is comparable to EFW in predicting SGA, on the other hand, the largest prospective study favors EFW over other biometric parameters.[12,13]

Customized growth charts are computer generated, customized for each individual taking into account maternal characteristics—height, weight, parity, and ethnicity. Gestational network, GROW (gestation-related optimal weight) growth chart taking account of SFH, and expected fetal weight is one such example.[14]

Recently, "intergrowth 21st project" studied fetal growth of 4,607 low-risk healthy pregnancies with adequate nutritional status across eight countries. All pregnancies were assessed for ultrasound measurement of fetal HC, bi-parietal diameter (BPD), occipital frontal diameter (OFD), AC, and FL every 4–5 weeks from 14 weeks till 42 weeks of gestation. The best fitting curves at 3rd, 5th, 10th, 90th, 95th, and 97th centile were generated according to the GA.[15] Intergrowth-21st truly represents international fetal growth standards although at present, there is no consensus on its superiority over population customized growth charts. RCOG recommends use of GROW chart.

## DOPPLER ASSESSMENT

### Uterine Artery Doppler (UtAD)

Trophoblast invasion into uterine vessels occurs early in 2nd trimester. This results into dilated spiral arterioles, formation of low pressure, high flow shunts and a 10–12 folds increase in perfusion. The uterine velocity waveform shows a continuous forward flow through diastole till 26 weeks of pregnancy with little increase beyond that. A systolic/diastolic (S/D) ratio of <2.6, resistance index (RI) < 0.7, and PI < 1.0 from 26 weeks onward are normal values. Mean PI > 95th centile (UtAD) and presence of notch at 12 weeks of pregnancy may be the first change to arouse suspicion of impending FGR and persistence into second and third trimester further substantiates it **(Figs. 1 and 2)**.

### Umbilical Artery Doppler

As GA advances, UAD waveforms show progressive increase in end-diastolic velocity from 2nd trimester onward till 40 weeks of gestation and this reflects in progressive decrease in S/D ratio, PI, and RI indices. A S/D ratio of 3, RI of 0.5, and PI of 1 at 30 weeks are taken as normal values **(Fig. 3)**.

PI >95th centile with end-diastolic flow, absent end-diastolic flow (AEDF), and reverse end-diastolic flow (REDF) corresponds to placental insufficiency of ≥50%, ≥70%, and

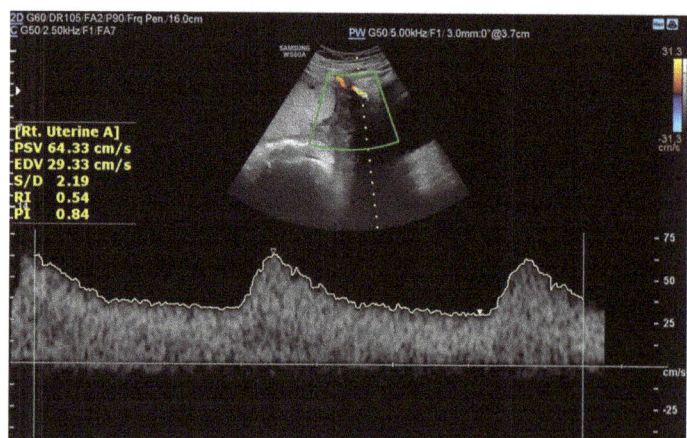

**Fig. 1:** Normal uterine artery Doppler. (PSV: peak systolic velocity; EDV: end-diastolic velocity; S/D: systolic/diastolic; RI: resistance index; PI: pulsatility index)

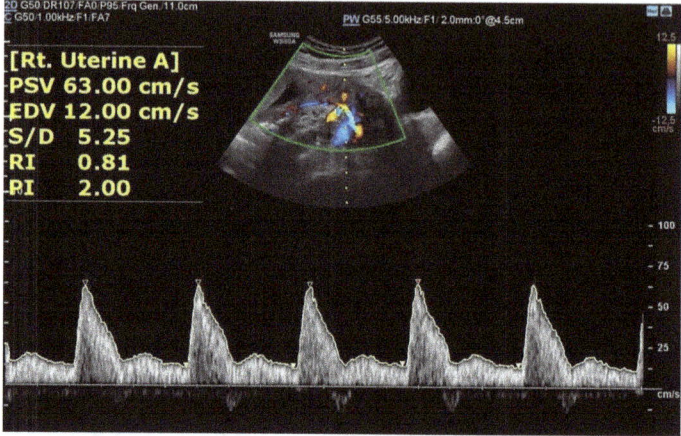

**Fig. 2:** Uterine artery increased impedance and notch. (PSV: peak systolic velocity; EDV: end-diastolic velocity; S/D: systolic/diastolic; RI: resistance index; PI: pulsatility index)

# Fetal Growth Restriction

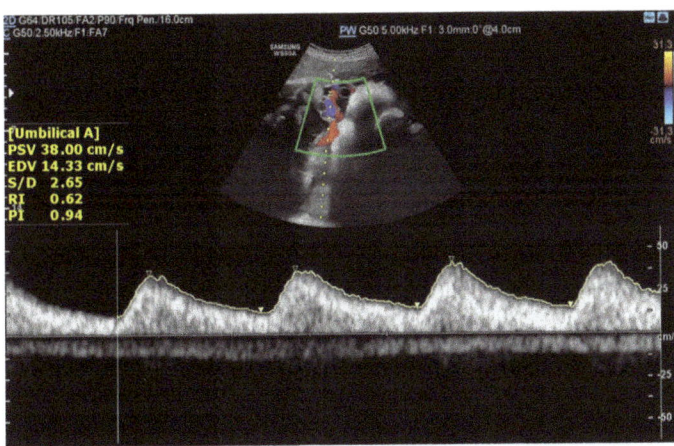

**Fig. 3:** Normal umbilical artery Doppler. (PSV: peak systolic velocity; EDV: end-diastolic velocity; S/D: systolic/diastolic; RI: resistance index; PI: pulsatility index)

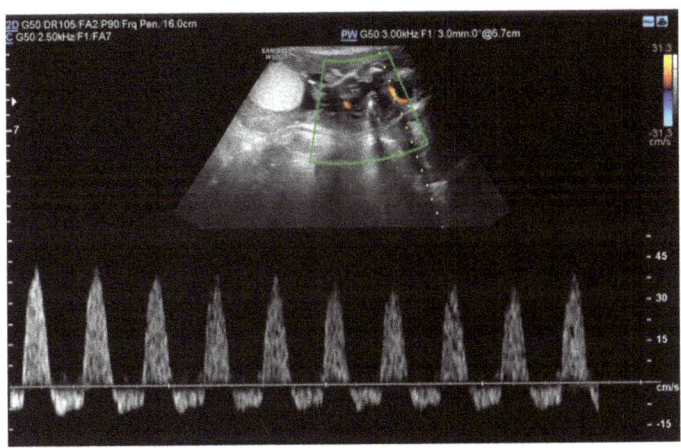

**Fig. 6:** Umbilical artery Doppler-reverse end-diastolic velocity.

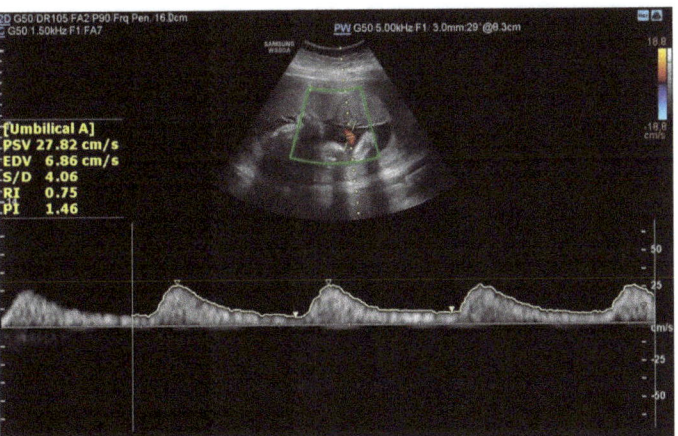

**Fig. 4:** Umbilical artery Doppler > 95th centile. (PSV: peak systolic velocity; EDV: end-diastolic velocity; S/D: systolic/diastolic; RI: resistance index; PI: pulsatility index)

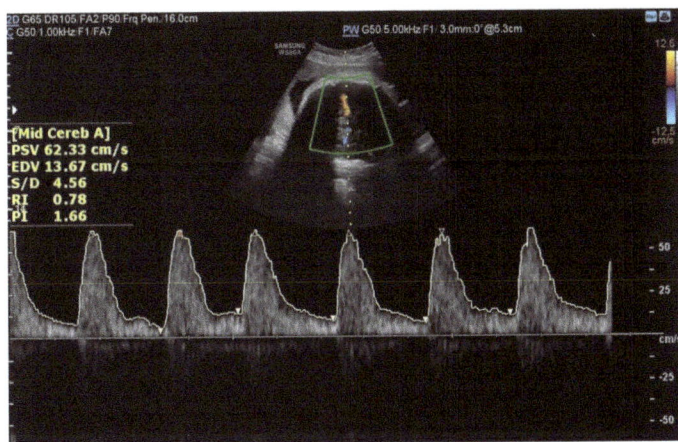

**Fig. 7:** Normal middle cerebral artery. (PSV: peak systolic velocity; EDV: end-diastolic velocity; S/D: systolic/diastolic; RI: resistance index; PI: pulsatility index)

## Middle Cerebral Artery and Cerebroplacental Ratio

In a normally grown fetus low vascular impedance shunts are seen in MCA throughout the gestation. Values of MCA S/D, PI, and RI are always higher than umbilical artery indices across weeks of gestation. Therefore at any given time CPR (MCA PI/UAD PI) is >1. In a growth restricted fetus because of increased impedance in umbilical arteries, redistribution of blood flow, an increase of blood flow in diastole in MCA resulting into dilated MCA. This is also called brain sparing effect. MCA indices thus become lower than UAD indices and CPR falls. Ratio of <1 indicates hypoxia (**Fig. 7**).

## Venous Doppler: Ductus Venosus and Umbilical Vein

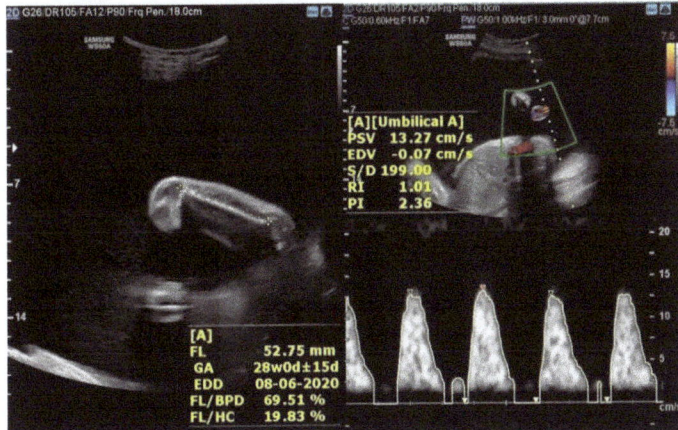

**Fig. 5:** Umbilical artery Doppler-absent end-diastolic velocity. (PSV: peak systolic velocity; EDV: end-diastolic velocity; S/D: systolic/diastolic; RI: resistance index; PI: pulsatility index; FL: femur length; GA: gestational age; EDD: expected date of delivery; BPD: bi-parietal diameter; HC: head circumference)

≥90% respectively (**Figs. 4 to 6**).[16] Most of the ultrasound machines have built in charts of Doppler parameters at 5th, 10th, 50th, and 95th centile for a quick reference.

Among the venous Dopplers, DV is the most commonly interrogated vessel. DV originates from umbilical vein before it turns to right to join the portal vein. It carries highly oxygenated blood from umbilical vein to right atrium and then via patent foramen ovale to left atrium. Oxygenated blood finally reaches cerebral circulation. DV normally exhibits a pulsatile triphasic waveform pattern—systole (S), diastole (D), and atrial systole (A). When hypoxia supervenes as in a growth restricted fetus, DV dilates to accommodate a major portion of oxygenated blood in right atrium. This results in increased PI. With further worsening of hypoxia and resulting acidemia, the phase of DV corresponding to atrial contraction becomes reversed (a wave reversal). Due to this backward flow of venous circulation, the normally *nonpulsatile* umbilical vein becomes pulsatile indicating right heart failure. Umbilical vein pulsations indicate impending fetal death **(Figs. 8 to 10)**.

## Cardiotocography: Nonstress Test

Conventional NST is the most commonly used fetal surveillance test, but it has high inter- and intraobserver variability. False nonreactive tests are up to 50%. For preterm fetus < 32 weeks an acceleration of 10 beats/minute (bpm) for 10 seconds suffices instead of 15 beats/minute for 15 second.

Computerized cardiotocography (cCTG) is more objective and consistent. Short-term variation (STV) ≤3 ms indicates metabolic acidemia in fetus. It is preferred over conventional CTG for surveillance of FGR fetus.

## Biophysical Profile

It is a marker for acute as well as chronic hypoxia. Acute variables are NST, fetal tone, breathing, and gross body movements. Chronic variable is measurement of amniotic fluid by amniotic fluid index (AFI) or single deepest pocket (SDP). Normal value for AFI is (9–19 cm) and for SDP it is ≥2 cm, and AFI < 5 cm or SDP < 1 cm are defined as oligoamnios. Acute hypoxemia will result in loss of any acute variable but AF remains normal. Repeated episodes of hypoxemia with recovery in between causes decrease in AF, but acute variable may be normal. Profound and severe hypoxia will produce both oligoamnios and loss of acute variables. A score of 2 is given to each variable if present, 0 if variable is absent or inadequate. Score of 8/10 or 10/10 is considered as normal, 6/10 needs repeat testing. Score of ≤4/10 is ominous.

It is important to remember that both abnormal BPP and CTG reflect an advanced stage of fetal distress. CTG and BPP get affected in later stages of hypoxia, much after arterial Doppler and venous Doppler changes (see pathophysiology). For preterm FGR, BPP, and CTG are poor predicates of fetal acidemia. Ductus vein Doppler is the preferred testing modality.

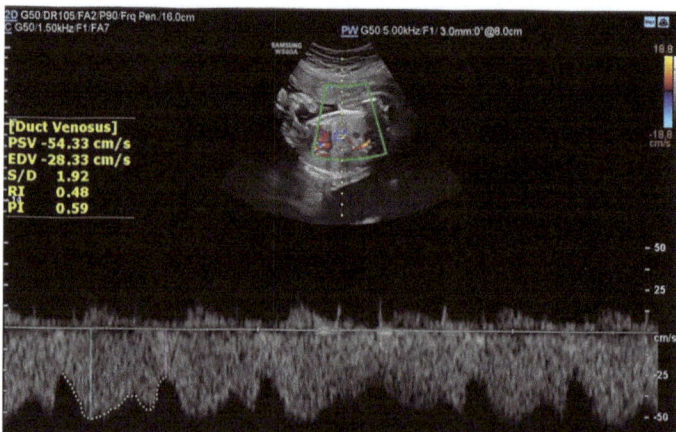

**Fig. 8:** Normal ductus venosus. (PSV: peak systolic velocity; EDV: end-diastolic velocity; S/D: systolic/diastolic; RI: resistance index; PI: pulsatility index)

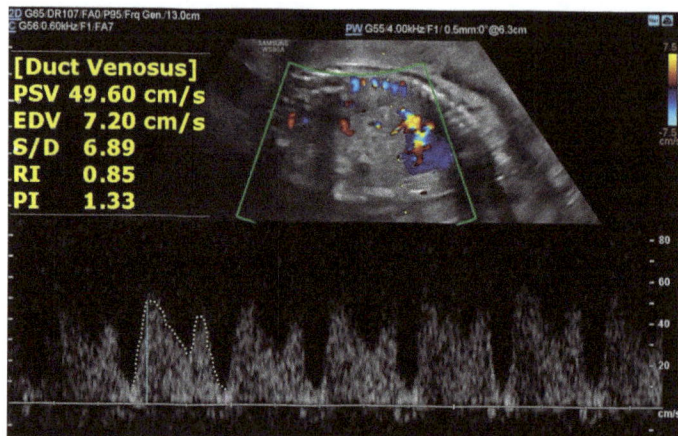

**Fig. 9:** Ductus venosus increased resistance. (PSV: peak systolic velocity; EDV: end-diastolic velocity; S/D: systolic/diastolic; RI: resistance index; PI: pulsatility index)

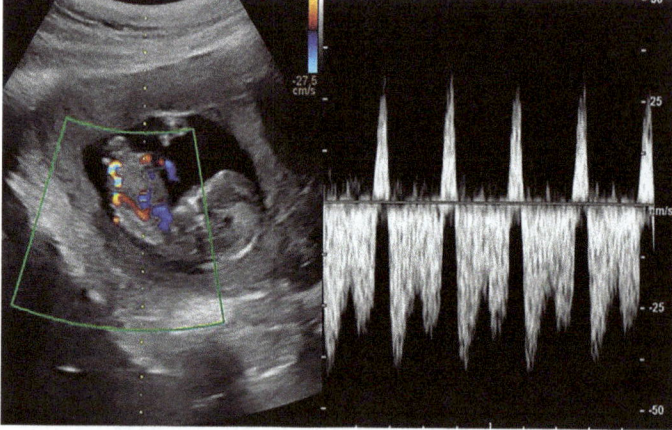

**Fig. 10:** Ductus venosus—a wave reversal.

## Detection of Fetal Anomalies

Ten percent of FGR fetuses have structural anomalies. Careful assessment of fetal anatomy and soft markers for chromosomal anomalies is a mandatory investigation for FGR. Gastroschisis, omphalocele, and congenital heart defects are some of the associated anomalies. Fetal echo is recommended.

## Chromosomal Analysis

Incidence of chromosomal abnormalities is 10–40% in a structurally malformed growth restricted fetus as against 2% of a normally formed growth restricted fetus. Therefore, karyotyping analysis, preferably AF microarray is recommended in all EOFGR, FGR <3rd centile, presence of structural malformations or soft markers on ultrasound.

## Tests for Maternal and Fetal Infections

Fetal infections account for <5% of all FGRs. So, workup of fetal infection should be undertaken if clinically suspected, as in case of positive maternal serology or ultrasound features suggestive of fetal infection. Common infections associated with FGR are cytomegalovirus (CMV), toxoplasmosis, malaria or occasionally syphilis.

## MANAGEMENT OF EARLY ONSET OF FETAL GROWTH RESTRICTION

Step by step management of EOFGR is depicted in **Flowchart 1**.

## Monitoring for Hypoxia

Once FGR is established and necessary workup is done, crux of management lies in monitoring for hypoxia.

Although UAD is the primary monitoring tool, and integrated surveillance approach utilizing uterine artery Doppler, UAD, MCA Doppler, CTG, and BPP is the usual practice. DV is mapped once UAD shows absent end-diastolic velocity (AEDV) and reverse end-diastolic velocity (REDV). Frequency of monitoring is determined by results of previous findings. Generally monitoring is recommended fortnightly, if initial UAD is normal, weekly if it is >95th centile, biweekly with AEDV, and daily with REDV. RCOG also agrees with this surveillance pattern, and also cautions that CTG and amniotic fluid volume (AFV) should not be used for preterm SGA fetuses. Check of interval growth of fetus is recommended in 2-3 weeks.

Stage-based management of EOFGR has been described by Figueras and Gratacos[17] **(Table 4)**.

## Timing of Delivery

Broadly, delivery should be considered when chances of outside survival are greater than that in utero, after carefully evaluating the institutional data on quality survivals as per the GA and birth weight. The Growth Restriction Intervention Trial (GRIT) has indicated that early delivery was associated with fewer still births but more neonatal deaths as against late delivery. Long-term follow-up showed no difference.[18,19]

Randomized Umbilical and Fetal Flow in Europe (TRUFFLE) trial has reported no significant difference in survivors without handicap, if intervened at early ductus changes, late ductus changes or STV at CTG. Delayed delivery till late ductus changes, improved survival without handicap but increased still birth rates.[20] Timings and indications of delivery are depicted in **Table 5**.

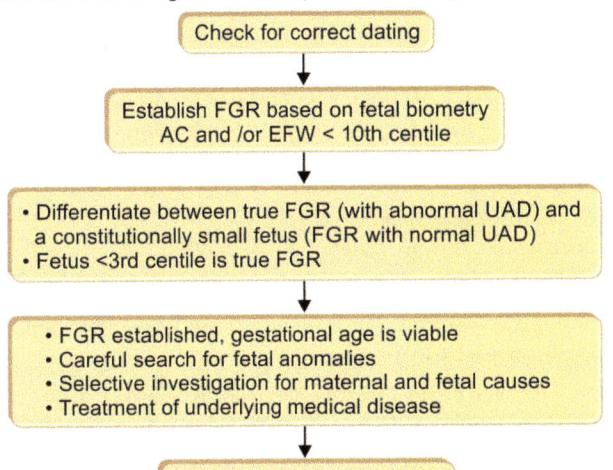

**Flowchart 1:** Management of early onset of fetal growth restriction.

(AC: abdominal circumference; EFW: estimated fetal weight; FGR: fetal growth restriction; UAD: umbilical artery Doppler)

**TABLE 4:** Stage based monitoring and timing of delivery of FGR fetuses.

| Stage | Criteria | Management |
|---|---|---|
| Stage 1 FGR: Severe smallness or mild placental insufficiency | Abnormal uterine artery/umbilical artery (UA)/MCA Doppler/CPR | • Weekly monitoring<br>• Delivery beyond 37 weeks |
| Stage 2 FGR: Severe placental insufficiency | UA–AEDV | • Biweekly monitoring<br>• Delivery ≥ 34 weeks |
| Stage 3 FGR: Advanced fetal deterioration Low-risk of fetal acidosis | UA–REDV DV > 95th centile | • Daily/alternate day monitoring<br>• Delivery at 30–32 weeks |
| Stage 4 FGR: High suspicion of fetal acidosis or death | Spontaneous fetal heart rate decelerations Reduced short-term variability on computerized cardiotocography Reverse atrial flow in DV | • Monitoring every 12–24 hours<br>• Delivery ≥ 26 weeks |

(AEDV: absent end-diastolic velocity; CPR: cerebroplacental ratio; DV: ductus venosus; FGR: fetal growth restriction; MCA: middle cerebral artery; REDV: reverse end-diastolic velocity)

## Mode of Delivery

Early onset FGR fetuses are generally hypoxic, oligoamniotic, and they withstand labor stress poorly. Cesarean section is the preferred mode of delivery. Normal delivery can be tried, if cervix is ripe and facilities for continuous CTG are available.

It is advisable to send umbilical cord blood analysis to establish neonatal baseline acid-base status.

| TABLE 5: Timings and indications of delivery. | |
| --- | --- |
| Monitoring | Timings/Indications of delivery |
| UAD end diastolic flow present | ≥ 37–38 weeks GA |
| AEDV | 32–34 weeks GA |
| REDV | 30–32 weeks GA |

Deliver any time during course of monitoring if:
- BPP ≤ 4/10, oligoamnios
- Ductus venosus a-wave absent or reversal
- Large decelerations on CTG
- STV changes on cCTG
- No interval growth in 3 weeks

(AEDV: absent end-diastolic velocity; BPP: biophysical profile; cCTG: computerized cardiotocography; GA: gestational age; REDV: reverse end-diastolic velocity; STV: short-term variation; UAD: umbilical artery Doppler)

> **BOX 2:** Indications for delivery.
>
> *Indications for delivery:*
> - GA ≥ 38 weeks
> - MCA < 5th centile
> - CPR < 1
> - BPP ≤ 4/10
> - Abnormal CTG
>
> (BPP: biophysical profile; CPR: cerebroplacental ratio; CTG: cardiotocography; GA: gestational age; MCA: middle cerebral artery)

## *Corticosteroids*

One course of corticosteroids between 24 and 34 weeks has proven its benefit in improving fetal lung maturity as in preterm babies. Antenatal corticosteroids are recommended for women where delivery is anticipated between $34^{+0}$ and $36^{+6}$ weeks and who have not received a course earlier.[2] Studies have shown that fetuses with AEDV who depicted transient improvement in blood flow after glucocorticoid administration had better outcomes than fetuses who did not show improvement.[21-23]

## *Magnesium Sulfate*

Magnesium sulfate use 12–24 hours prior to delivery has shown to reduce death, cerebral palsy, and gross motor dysfunction in neonates.[24] Dose is 4–6 g I/V loading dose followed by 1–2 g/hour for a maximum period of 24 hours prior to delivery in GA < 32 weeks.

## OTHER THERAPIES

Therapies for treatment of FGR are largely ineffective. Bed rest, maternal nutrient supplementation, calcium channel blockers, betamimetics, maternal oxygenation, plasma volume expansion, and transcutaneous electrostimulation have not shown any benefit for improving FGR as indicated by Cochrane reviews.[25-31]

*Sildenafil:* A systematic review and meta-analysis on 22 animal studies and two human randomized controlled trials (RCTs) had reported that sildenafil improved fetal growth in FGR and pre-eclampsia pregnancies as compared to healthy pregnancies with no pre-eclampsia and there was a positive correlation between dosage and fetal growth.[32] Recommended dose is 25 mg orally three times a day.

Sildenafil therapy in dismal prognosis early-onset intrauterine growth restriction (STRIDER) trial was launched in 2014 in five countries to evaluate the role of sildenafil in pregnancies between 20 weeks and $29^{+6}$ weeks with severe FGR, likely placental in origin. The primary outcome was live baby at term and no serious adverse neonatal morbidities. Trial was stopped prematurely in Netherlands because of a higher incidence of persistent pulmonary artery hypertension and overall neonatal death in sildenafil arm. Strider consortium has firmly concluded that clinicians should stop prescribing sildenafil for FGR.[33]

Role of newer therapies such as vascular endothelial growth factor, gene therapy, lipid lowering drug–Pravastatin are under research.

## Termination of Pregnancy

Mid-trimester severe FGR with AEDV or REDV carry extremely poor prognosis, termination of pregnancy is an option.

## LATE ONSET FETAL GROWTH RESTRICTION: MANAGEMENT

Gestational age here is not of concern. Weekly monitoring by UAD, MCA, and CPR is recommended. Indications for delivery are set in **Box 2**.

Normal vaginal delivery with continuous CTG is the preferred mode. Cesarean section is advised only for obstetric indications.

A recent review has outlined fetal surveillance methods, frequency, use of corticosteroids and $MgSO_4$, timing, and mode of delivery as per existing guidelines across various countries.[34]

## PREVENTION AND SCREENING OF FETAL GROWTH RESTRICTION

Prepregnancy optimization of medical conditions, substance abuse cessation, achievement of normal BMI, and adequate nutritional care are some of the strategies to prevent FGR.

During pregnancy—identification of risk factors at first prenatal visit is recommended **(Table 6)**.

Once a woman is identified at risk, mean uterine artery PI at 12 weeks is measured at the time of aneuploidy screen involving nuchal translucency scan, pregnancy-associated plasma protein-A (PAPP-A), and human chorionic gonadotropin (hCG). Mean uterine PI >95th centile or PAPP-A < 0.4 puts the patient at risk of pre-eclampsia and subsequent FGR. Initiation of aspirin prophylaxis from 14 weeks onward is recommended.

The ASPREE trial has firmly established that aspirin at a dose of 150 mg at bedtime achieves maximum benefit to reduce preterm pre-eclampsia and hence growth restriction.[35]

Further assessment of uterine artery Doppler at 22–24 weeks pregnancy is recommended since an abnormal Doppler at this stage again puts the patient at risk of FGR.

Monitoring for fetal growth is further assessed at 28–30 weeks along with uterine artery Doppler and UAD. FGR detection at this stage or earlier requires intensified surveillance as discussed earlier.

**TABLE 6:** During pregnancy—identification of risk factors at first antenatal visit.

| Minor risk factors | Major risk factors |
|---|---|
| • Maternal age ≥ 35 years | • Maternal age > 40 years |
| • IVF singleton pregnancy | • Smoker > 11 cigarettes/day |
| • Nulliparity | • Paternal SGA |
| • BMI < 20 kg/m² | • Cocaine |
| • BMI 25–34.9 kg/m² | • Daily vigorous exercise |
| • Smoker 1–10 cigarettes/day | • Previous SGA baby |
| • Low fruit intake prepregnancy | • Previous still birth |
| • Previous pre-eclampsia | • Maternal SGA |
| • Pregnancy interval < 6 months | • Chronic hypertension |
| • Pregnancy interval ≥ 60 months | • Diabetes with vascular disease |
| | • Renal impairment |
| | • Antiphospholipid syndrome |
| | • Heavy bleeding similar to menses |
| | • PAPP-A < 0.4 MoM |

(BMI: body mass index; IVF: in vitro fertilization; MoM: multiples of the median; PAPP-A: pregnancy associated plasma protein-A; SGA: small for gestational age)

## NEONATAL MORBIDITIES

Neonatal morbidities are as depicted in **Table 7**.[36]

## KEY POINTS

- Fetal growth restriction complicates 10% of all pregnancies and is associated with high perinatal mortality, morbidity besides long-term neurological handicap in neonates.
- Delphi consensus has standardized the definition of both EOFGR and LOFGR using biometry along with functional parameters, as against conventional definition based on biometry.
- Etiology revolves around maternal, fetal, and placental disorders.
- Early onset FGR (<32 weeks) responds to hypoxia in a sequential manner from compensation to decompensation phase depicting changes from arterial to venous circulation to behavioral state of fetus.
- Late onset FGR (≥32 weeks) does not depict these changes in a sequential manner. UAD is abnormal only in 10% of cases. Cerebral redistribution can occur even with a normal UAD.
- Diagnosis is based on SFH and ultrasonic fetal biometry along with Doppler assessment.
- It is mandatory to rule out structural anomalies in all cases of EOFGR.
- Karyotyping analysis is indicated in EOFGR, FGR <3rd centile, presence of structural malformations or soft markers on ultrasound.

**TABLE 7:** Neonatal morbidities in fetal growth restriction.

| | Cardiovascular morbidity | Respiratory morbidity | Neurological morbidity | Others |
|---|---|---|---|---|
| Neonatal period | • Early hypotension<br>• Persistent fetal circulation/PPHTN<br>• Structural heart changes<br>• Vessel wall rigidity<br>• Cardiac function issues<br>• Late systemic hypertension<br>• Secondary pulmonary hypertension | • Increased need for respiratory/ventilator support<br>• Meconium aspiration syndrome<br>• Pulmonary hemorrhage<br>• Bronchopulmonary dysplasia | • Perinatal asphyxia<br>• Microcephaly<br>• Cranial ultrasound abnormalities (IVH and PVL)<br>• White matter and gray matter changes on MRI<br>• Functional and DTI MRI changes<br>• General movement assessment abnormalities<br>• EEG abnormalities | • Hypoglycemia<br>• Hypocalcemia<br>• Hypothermia<br>• Sepsis<br>• Jaundice<br>• Polycythemia<br>• Prolonged NICU stay<br>• Feed intolerance<br>• Delay in establishment of feeds<br>• Necrotizing enterocolitis<br>• Renal tubular injury<br>• Retinopathy of prematurity |
| Long-term impact | • Hypertension and ischemic heart disease<br>• Stroke<br>• Atherosclerosis | • Chronic respiratory insufficiency<br>• Reactive airway disease | *Neurodevelopmental issues:*<br>• Behavioral problems<br>• Learning difficulties<br>• Cerebral palsy<br>• Dementia<br>• Mental health issues | • Failure to thrive<br>• Obesity immune dysfunction<br>• Osteoporosis<br>• Metabolic syndrome<br>• Renal issues<br>• Hormonal issues<br>• Cancer<br>• Shortened life span |

(PPHTN: portopulmonary hypertension; IVH: intraventricular hemorrhage; PVL: periventricular leukomalacia; DTI: diffusion tensor imaging; MRI: magnetic resonance imaging; NICU: neonatal intensive care unit; EEG: electroencephalography)

- Workup of fetal infections is indicated on clinical suspicion, positive maternal serology or ultrasound features suggestive of fetal infections.
- Stage-based management and timing of delivery are widely practiced.
- Generally, weekly monitoring if umbilical artery end-diastolic flow is present, biweekly with AEDV, and daily with REDV is recommended. Ductus vein Doppler and cCTG are added once REDV is present.
- Delivery is recommended at ≥37–38 weeks if UAD end-diastolic flow is present, at 32–34 weeks with AEDV, and at 30–32 weeks with REDV. Delivery is also indicated if during the course of monitoring BPP of 4/10 or less, presence of severe oligoamnios, ductus vein changes, large decelerations on CTG, STV changes on cCTG, and no interval growth in 3 weeks.
- Magnesium sulfate for fetal and neonatal neuroprotection should be considered for deliveries before 32 weeks.
- Antenatal corticosteroids are recommended for women where delivery is anticipated before $36^{+6}$ weeks and who have not received a course of antenatal steroids earlier.
- For LOFGR weekly monitoring by UAD, MCA, and CPR, and delivery at ≥38 weeks is recommended.
- Therapies for treatment of FGR are largely ineffective.
- Screening for FGR involves identification of risk factors at first prenatal visit, uterine artery Doppler, and biomarkers at 12 weeks. If identified "at risk", initiation of aspirin prophylaxis from 14 weeks onward is the key preventive intervention.

## REFERENCES

1. Bashat AA, Galan LH. Intrauterine growth restriction. In: Gabbe MD, Neibyl JR, Simpson JL (Eds). Normal and Problem Pregnancies, 6th edition. Philadelphia: Elsevier Publication; 2017. pp. 737-69.
2. American College of Obstetrician and Gynaecologists Committee on Practice Bulletins—Obstetrics and the Society for maternal-fetal medicine. ACOG Practice bulletin no. 204: fetal growth restriction. Obstet Gynecol. 2019; 133(2):e97-e109.
3. Lausman A, Kingdom J; Maternal Fetal Medicine Committee. Intrauterine growth restriction: screening, diagnosis, and management. J Obstet Gynaecol Can. 2013;35(8):741-8.
4. RCOG. Green Top Guidelines No. 31. The Investigation and Management of the Small-for-Gestational Age. Fetus. 2014;1-34.
5. Baschat AA. Fetal growth restriction–from observation to intervention. J Perinat Med. 2010;38(3):239-46.
6. Savchev S, Figueras F, Sanz-Cortes M, Cruz-Lemini M, Triunfo S, Botet F, et al. Evaluation of an optimal gestational age cut-off for the definition of early and late onset fetal growth restriction. Fetal Diagn Ther. 2014;36(2):99-105.
7. Gordijn SJ, Beune IM, Thilaganathan B, Papageorghiou A, Baschat AA, Bakers PN, et al. Consensus definition of fetal growth restriction: a Delphi procedure. Ultrasound Obstet Gynecol. 2016;48(3):333-9.
8. Vladareanu R, Burnei A, Constantinescu S. Timing and mode of delivery of the infant with IUGR. In: Studd J, Tan SL, Chernevak FA (Eds). Current Progress in Obstetrics and Gynecology, 2nd edition. New Delhi: Tree Life Media; 2014. pp. 135-50.
9. Oros D, Figueras F, Cruz-Martinez R, Meler E, Munmany M, Gratacos E. Longitudinal changes in uterine, umbilical and fetal cerebral Doppler indices in late-onset small-for-gestational age fetuses. Ultrasound Obstet Gynecol. 2011;37(2):191-5.
10. Figueras F, Caradeux J, Crispi F, Eixarch E, Peguero A, Gratacos E. Diagnosis and surveillance of late-onset fetal growth restriction. Am J Obstet Gynecol. 2018;218(2S):S790-802.
11. Coyaji KA, Otiv S. Fetal growth restriction. In: Krishna U, Tank DK, Daftary SN (Eds). Pregnancy at Risk, 4th edition. New Delhi: FOGSI Publication, Jaypee Brothers Medical Publisher (P) Ltd.; 2001. p. 268.
12. Blue NR, Yordan JMP, Holbrook BD, Nirgudkar PA, Mozurkewich EL. Abdominal circumference alone versus estimated fetal weight after 24 weeks to predict small or large for gestational age at birth: a meta-analysis. Am J Perinatol. 2017;34(11):1115-24.
13. Fadigas C, Saiid Y, Gonzalez R, Poon LC, Nicolaides KH. Prediction of small-for-gestational-age neonates: screening by fetal biometry at 35-37 weeks. Ultrasound Obstet Gynecol. 2015;45(5):559-65.
14. Gestation network. Growth Charts. [online] Available from: https://www.gestation.net/growthcharts.htm [Last accessed July, 2021].
15. Papageorghiou AT, Ohuma EO, Altman DG, Todros T, Ismail LC, Lambert A, et al. International standards for fetal growth based on serial ultrasound measurements: the Fetal Growth Longitudinal Study of the INTERGROWTH-21st Project. Lancet. 2014;384(9946):869-79.
16. Alfirevic Z, Stampalija T, Gyte GM. Fetal and umbilical Doppler ultrasound in high-risk pregnancies. Cochrane Database Syst Rev. 2010;(1):CD007529.
17. Figueras F, Gratacos E. An integrated approach to fetal growth restriction. Best Pract Res Clin Obstet Gynaecol. 2017;38:48-58.
18. When do obstetricians recommend delivery for a high-risk preterm growth-retarded fetus? The GRIT Study Group. Growth Restriction Intervention Trial. Eur J Obstet Gynecol Reprod Biol. 1996;67(2):121-6.
19. Thornton JG, Hornbuckle J, Vail A, Spiegelhalter DJ, Levene M. Infant wellbeing at 2 years of age in the Growth Restriction Intervention Trial (GRIT): multicentred randomised controlled trial. Lancet. 2004;364(9433):513-20.
20. Lees CC, Marlow N, van Wassenaer-Leemhuis A, Arabin B, Bilardo CM, Brezinka C, et al. 2 year neurodevelopmental and intermediate perinatal outcomes in infants with very preterm fetal growth restriction (TRUFFLE): a randomized trial. Lancet. 2015;385(9983):2162-72.
21. Robertson MC, Murila F, Tong S, Baker LS, Yu VY, Wallace EM. Predicting perinatal outcome through changes in umbilical artery Doppler studies after antenatal corticosteroids in the growth-restricted fetus. Obstet Gynecol. 2009;113(3):636-40.
22. Simchen MJ, Alkazaleh F, Adamson SL, Windrim R, Telford J, Beyene J, et al. The fetal cardiovascular response to antenatal steroids in severe early-onset intrauterine growth restriction. Am J Obstet Gynecol. 2004;190(2):296-304.
23. Nozaki AM, Francisco RP, Fonseca ES, Miyadahira S, Zugaib M. Fetal hemodynamic changes following maternal

betamethasone administration in pregnancies with fetal growth restriction and absent end-diastolic flow in the umbilical artery. Acta Obstet Gynecol Scand. 2009;88(3):350-4.
24. Doyle LW, Crowther CA, Middleton R, Marret S, Rouse D. Magnessium sulphate for women at risk of preterm births for neuroprotection of the fetus. Cochrane Database Syst Rev. 2009;(1):CD004661.
25. Gülmezoglu AM, Hofmeyr GJ. Bed rest in hospital for suspected impaired fetal growth. Cochrane Database Syst Rev. 2000;1996(2):CD000034.
26. Say L, Gülmezoglu AM, Hofmeyr GJ. Maternal nutrient supplementation for suspected impaired fetal growth. Cochrane Database Syst Rev. 2003;(1):CD000148.
27. Gülmezoglu AM, Hofmeyr GJ. Calcium channel blockers for potential impaired fetal growth. Cochrane Database Syst Rev. 2000;1996(2):CD000049.
28. Gülmezoglu AM, Hofmeyr GJ. Betamimetics for suspected impaired fetal growth. Cochrane Database Syst Rev. 2001;(4):CD000036.
29. Say L, Gülmezoglu AM, Hofmeyr GJ. Maternal oxygen administration for suspected impaired fetal growth. Cochrane Database Syst Rev. 2003;(1):CD000137.
30. Gülmezoglu AM, Hofmeyr GJ. Plasma volume expansion for suspected impaired fetal growth. Cochrane Database Syst Rev. 2000;1996(2):CD000167.
31. Gülmezoglu AM, Hofmeyr GJ. Transcutaneous electrostimulation for suspected placental insufficiency (diagnosed by Doppler studies). Cochrane Database Syst Rev. 1996(2):CD000079.
32. Paauw ND, Terstappen F, Ganzevoort W, Joles JA, Gremmels H, Lely AT. Sildenafil during pregnancy: a preclinical meta-analysis on fetal growth and maternal blood pressure. Hypertension. 2017;70(5):998-1006.
33. Groom KM, Ganzevoort W, Alfirevic Z, Lim K, Papageorghiou AT. Clinical should stop prescribing sildenafil for fetal growth restriction (FGR) comment from the STRIDER Consortium. Ultrasound Obstet Gynecol. 2018;52(3):295-6.
34. McCowan LM, Figueras F, Anderson NH. Evidence-based national guidelines for the management of suspected fetal growth restriction: comparison, consensus, and controversy. Am J Obstet Gynecol. 2018;218(2S):S855-68.
35. Rolnik DL, Wright D, Poon LC, O'Gorman N, Syngelaki A, de Paco Matallana C, et al. Aspirin versus placebo in Pregnancies at high risk for preterm preeclampsia. N Engl J Med. 2017;377(7):613-22.
36. Malhotra A, Allison BJ, Castillo-Melendez M, Jenkin G, Polglase GR, Miller SL. Neonatal morbidities of fetal growth restriction: pathophysiology and impact. Front. Endocrinol (Lausanne). 2019;10:55.

# Antepartum Fetal Surveillance

*Anubhuti Rana, Seema Singhal*

## INTRODUCTION

The assessment of the fetus in the uterus remains a challenge to the obstetrician because of the inability to perform a direct examination. With the evolution of technology, more specific assessment of the fetus is possible now. As fetal compromise has varied etiology, tests which are developed for fetal surveillance should be able to assess both acute fetal asphyxia and chronic disease states. The main aim of antepartum fetal surveillance is to prevent adverse perinatal outcomes as most of the damage sustained by the fetus is during the antenatal period rather than arising during labor.

## OBJECTIVES OF ANTEPARTUM FETAL SURVEILLANCE

The objectives of fetal surveillance are to assess fetal well-being to:
- Identify fetuses at risk of intrauterine death or neonatal morbidity or mortality.
- Identify potential risks early to allow timely interventions, thereby improving neonatal outcomes.

## INDICATIONS OF FETAL SURVEILLANCE

Antepartum fetal surveillance is recommended for pregnancies with high risk of antepartum fetal demise. Currently, there are multiple maternal and fetal indications to perform antepartum fetal surveillance, however, none of the tests have shown definitive improvement in fetal outcomes. The conditions which typically require antepartum fetal surveillance are listed in **Box 1**.

### Physiological Basis of Antepartum Fetal Surveillance

It is a known fact that level of activity, muscular tone, and fetal heart rate (FHR) pattern of human fetus are sensitive to hypoxemia and acidemia.[1] Chronic hypoxia as in cases of fetal growth restriction (FGR) leads to redistribution of blood flow, reduced renal perfusion and subsequent oligohydramnios.[2] Hypoxia when severe may result in detectable sequence of biophysical changes from physiological adaptation to decompensation leading to metabolic acidosis and resultant fetal compromise.

Various antepartum fetal surveillance techniques that are available are useful to identify the fetus that may be undergoing such changes and provides an opportunity to intervene. However, these tests can neither reflect the duration and severity of hypoxemia nor can they predict or prevent the fetal compromise that occurs due to acute events such as cord prolapse and abruption. The correlation between degree of hypoxemia and acidemia and fetal well-being indices is not precisely known. However, studies have shown that fetal umbilical vein blood pH of $7.28 \pm 0.11$ is associated with abnormal fetal surveillance test results and values of $7.16 \pm 0.08$ are associated with abnormal fetal movements.[3]

Therefore, the tests used for antepartum fetal surveillance aim to improve perinatal outcomes by decreasing the incidence of still births and long-term neurologic impairments, minimize perinatal morbidity by optimizing the timing of delivery, and identifying the fetuses at highest risk of hypoxia during labor and to prevent avoidable interventions in low-risk pregnancies.

The timing of initiation and frequency of testing should be individualized and should mirror the risk factors associated with the index pregnancy.

**BOX 1:** Indications for antepartum fetal surveillance.
- Fetal growth restriction
- Amniotic fluid abnormalities (oligohydramnios/polyhydramnios)
- Prolonged pregnancy > 42 weeks
- Diabetes mellitus
- Hypertensive disorders of pregnancy (chronic hypertension and pre-eclampsia)
- Renal disease
- Collagen vascular disorders
- Alloimmunization
- Maternal thyrotoxicosis
- Severe anemia or maternal hemoglobin disorder
- Prior unexplained fetal death
- Third-trimester vaginal bleeding
- Decreased fetal movements
- Abnormal or irregular fetal heart rate (FHR) on auscultation
- Multiple gestation
- Intrahepatic cholestasis of pregnancy

## Timing of Initiation

It is usually recommended between 30 and 32 weeks; however, it may be done earlier depending on the severity of disease and at a gestational age when the fetus is considered viable. Timing of fetal surveillance depends on the prognosis for neonatal survival and severity of maternal disease.

There is no optimal regimen and usually the tests are recommended once a week, but more frequent testing can be done depending on clinical situation. In case the indication is not persisting, the test need not be repeated.[1] Since a mode of surveillance which is appropriate for one condition may not be appropriate for another, a condition-specific antenatal testing is recommended.

## Frequency of Testing

The tests are usually performed weekly or twice weekly. More frequent testing may be warranted (daily or even more often) to assist in deciding the timing of delivery with an aim to maximize the period of gestation while avoiding intrauterine fetal morbidity.

## ANTEPARTUM FETAL SURVEILLANCE TECHNIQUES

Various techniques are used for antepartum fetal surveillance, which include:
- Fetal movement assessment
- Contraction stress test/oxytocin challenge test (CST/OCT)
- Nonstress test (NST)
- Biophysical profile (BPP) and modified biophysical profile (MBPP)
- Doppler velocimetry.

## Fetal Movement Assessment (Fetal Kick Count)

Most women are aware of fetal movements around 16–18 weeks of gestation as a sensation of a discrete kick, flutter or roll but perception of fetal movements is maximum at around 28–32 weeks. The assessment of fetal kick count is based upon a well-known fact that fetal movements decrease in response to hypoxemia. The advantage of this method is that it has no contraindications and is simple, inexpensive, noninvasive, and understandable to patients. Thus, daily fetal movement counting is a method which can be used by all pregnant women routinely. Presence of good fetal movements reflects fetal well-being and is an indirect measure of normal fetal acid-base status. Women perceive about 80% of fetal movements that can be visualized by ultrasound.[4] A decrease in fetal movements is often associated with adverse perinatal outcomes including intrapartum fetal compromise, fetal mortality, and stillbirth.[5,6]

However, there are many factors which influence maternally perceived fetal movements, some of which are as follows:
- *Maternal factors* such as activity, obesity, ingestion of medications or drugs that depress or increase fetal movements. Methadone depresses fetal movements whereas cocaine increases fetal movements.
- *Fetal factors* such as behavioral states, gestational age, and congenital anomalies (e.g., neuromuscular disorders and fetal akinesia syndrome).
- *Uterine factors* such as placental location, amniotic fluid volume (AFV), etc.

The ideal duration for counting movements is unclear. While numerous approaches have been formulated, the most popular one is to have the patient count distinct fetal movements while lying on her left side.[7] Cardiff method of counting ten movements in a timespan of up to 12 hours is also reassuring. Another reliable method involves counting fetal movements for 1 hour after each of three main meals in left lateral position, and total movements perceived should be more than or equal to ten. If the count is not reassuring further evaluation is recommended.

## Contraction Stress Test/Oxytocin Challenge Test

This test is of historical interest and is rarely performed nowadays due to easy availability of other tests for fetal surveillance, which are easier to perform and are noninvasive.

The CST evaluates the changes in FHR in response to uterine contractions. It operates upon the assumption that a marginally adequate fetal oxygenation, with the uterus at rest, will worsen in the presence of uterine contractions. Intermittent fetal hypoxemia occurring during uterine contractions results in late decelerations of the FHR in the suboptimal oxygenated fetus.[8] Uterine contractions may also result in variable decelerations, in the setting of oligohydramnios, secondary to cord compression.

### Technique of CST

Lying in lateral recumbent position, the patient has an external fetal monitor to record both the FHR and uterine contractions simultaneously for a 20–30 minutes interval. The FHR and uterine contractions are monitored, and a baseline trace is recorded. The contractions are considered satisfactory if there are at least 3 contractions of ≥40-second duration in a 10-minute interval. If fewer in number, contractions are induced with nipple stimulation or administration of intravenous oxytocin. Nipple stimulation is usually sufficient to induce a satisfactory contraction pattern. Patient is instructed to rub one nipple gently, through her clothing for 2 minutes or until a contraction begins. Patient is advised to restart after 5 minutes if the first stimulation does not induce satisfactory contractions (3 contractions in 10 minutes). Oxytocin infusion (0.5–1.0 mU/min) may also be used to stimulate contractions; rate is doubled every 15–20 minutes till a satisfactory contraction pattern is observed.

### Interpretation of Results

The CST is interpreted based on presence/absence of late FHR decelerations (decelerations reaching their lowest point following the contraction peak and persisting beyond the end of contraction). The results may be as follows:[9]

- *Negative:* When no late FHR decelerations or no significant variable FHR decelerations are seen.
- *Positive:* When late FHR decelerations are seen following ≥50% of contractions (even in presence of <3 contractions in 10 minutes).
- *Equivocal-suspicious:* When intermittent late FHR decelerations or significant variable FHR decelerations are seen.
- *Equivocal-hyperstimulation:* When FHR decelerations are seen in the setting of contractions that are more frequent than every 2 minutes or lasting >90 seconds.
- *Unsatisfactory:* <3 contractions in 10 minutes or an uninterpretable tracing.

Relative contraindications to CST include conditions at high risk for preterm labor, in presence of preterm rupture of membranes, placenta previa, and history of previous uterine surgery, myomectomy or classical cesarean section scar, among others.

The most common result is a negative CST, which indicates adequate fetal oxygenation during contractions and reflects good fetal outcomes (that is less than 1% antepartum fetal death within a week of a negative test). However, this test will not predict acute fetal compromise unrelated to placental insufficiency, such as in cord prolapse.[10,11] Fetal deaths after a negative CST are often due to abruption, congenital malformations, and poor glucose control in diabetics. A positive CST reflects uteroplacental insufficiency and is associated with adverse perinatal outcomes and increased chances of intrauterine deaths.[9] The most important limitation of CST in predicting fetal outcome is its high false positivity, which has been reported to be as high as 50% with a very poor positive predictive value of 9–15%; although, the negative predictive value is very high (99.8%).

## Nonstress Test

Fetal heart rate acceleration in relation to fetal movements is a reliable indicator of a fetus with a normal autonomic function. Absent FHR reactivity may be commonly seen with the fetal sleep cycle but can also reflect central nervous system (CNS) depression and fetal acidosis. FHR is monitored using a transducer, while a tocodynamometer may be used to record uterine contractions, if any **(Figs. 1 and 2)**. Fetal activity is also recorded with the results displayed on the strip; however, the patient need not document fetal movement for the test to be interpreted. The purpose of NST is to identify both a normal fetus and those with asphyxia or hypoxia. The NST as compared with CST has the advantage of lesser time, easier interpretability, no requirement of oxytocin, and lack of any contraindications.[12]

The tracing is categorized as reactive (normal) or nonreactive. The most widely accepted definition of reactivity is presence of ≥2 FHR accelerations reaching at least 15 bpm above the baseline, each lasting >15 seconds within a 20-minute period **(Fig. 3)**.[13]

Routine NST interpretation does not take gestational age into account, however, it is an important consideration.[14] Preterm fetuses are less likely to have FHR accelerations with fetal movements. At <32 weeks period of gestation, ≥2 accelerations peaking at ≥10 bpm above baseline, each lasting ≥10 seconds occurring within a 20-minute period is considered normal. The frequency and amplitude of accelerations increase as gestation advances. Preterm fetuses may also normally exhibit FHR decelerations between 20 and 30 weeks. NST in a neurologically healthy preterm fetus may frequently be nonreactive; between 24 and 28 weeks,

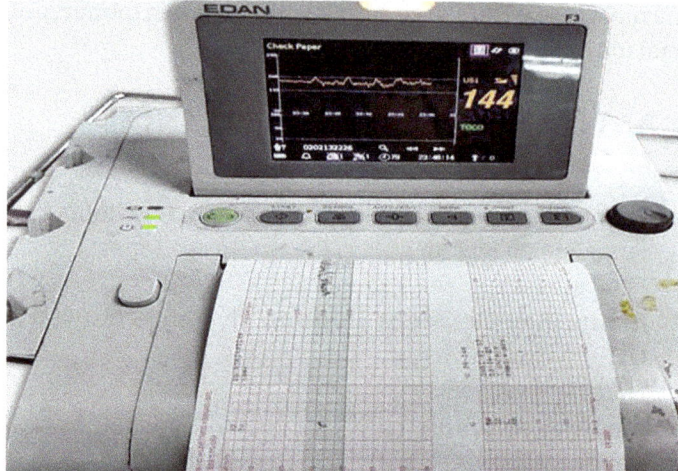

**Fig. 1:** Equipment used for recording the fetal heart rate with the result being displayed on the monitor as well as paper strip.

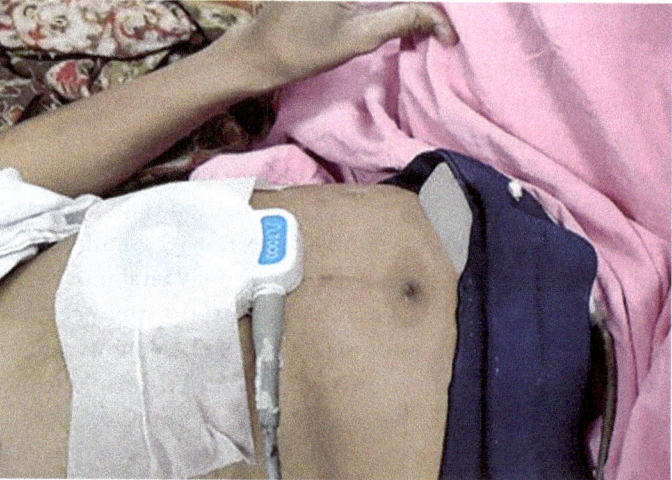

**Fig. 2:** Fetal heart rate (FHR) is monitored using a transducer (below with blue belt), while a tocodynamometer may be used to record uterine contractions (above), if any.

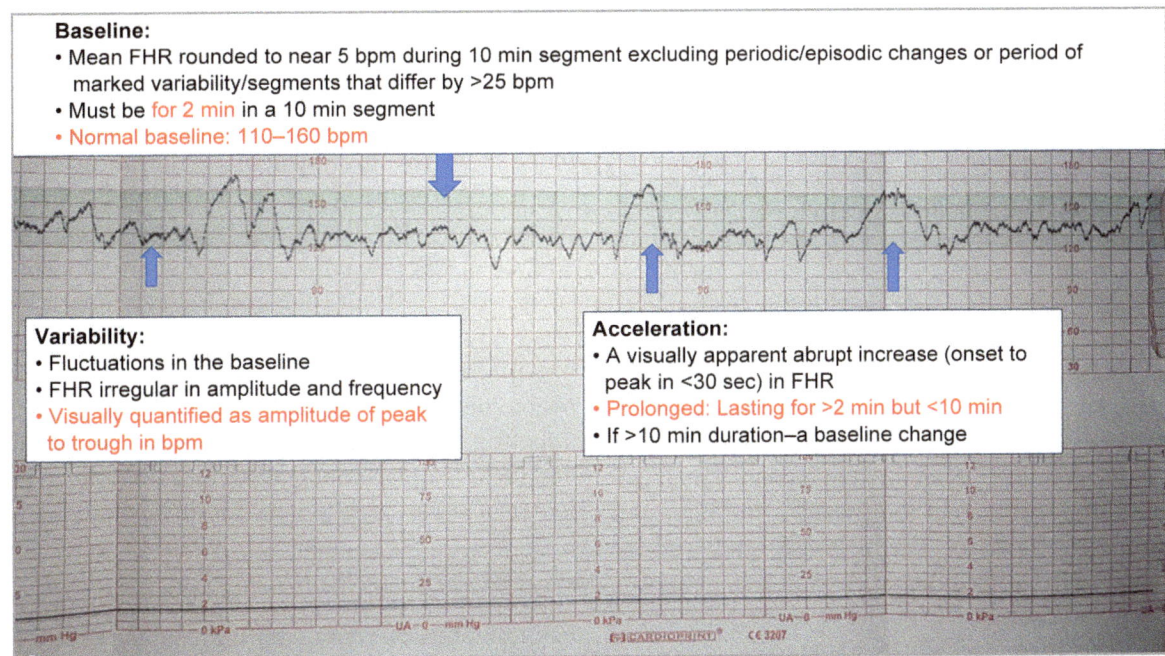

**Fig. 3:** Trace of a reactive nonstress test (NST) depicting the baseline heart rate, variability, and accelerations in a patient with term pregnancy.

up to half of the NSTs may be nonreactive, while from 28 to 32 weeks, up to 15% of NSTs may be nonreactive. It may be prudent to extend the tracing for 40 minutes to take the fetal sleep-wake cycle into account, because it may take this long for a healthy term fetus to display two FHR accelerations. If, after 40 minutes (from the start of testing), the criteria are still not met, the test is considered nonreactive. At preliminary testing, almost 85% of high-risk patients have a reactive NST, while the remaining 15% have a nonreactive NST.[15] Factors which result in a nonreactive NST are fetal hypoxia, asphyxia, behavioral states, gestational age, depressants (narcotics, phenobarbital) beta-blockers, and smoking.[16] There is no effect on reactivity by maternal glucose administration, transabdominal fetal manipulation, and changing maternal position (if not causing supine hypotension syndrome).

It is important to note that whenever NST is performed during antenatal period, there is no exposure of stress to the fetus and the uterus is relaxed. However, if any uterine activity is present, this could be called as a spontaneous contraction test.[17] This differs from CST as contractions are spontaneous and frequency of contractions may not be as required in CST. However, decelerations of the fetal heart in association with such spontaneous uterine activity should be evaluated. Society of Obstetricians and Gynaecologists of Canada (SOGC) clinical practice guidelines[17] classify NST as normal, atypical or abnormal. A normal NST has a baseline FHR of 110–160 bpm, variability of 6–25 bpm or ≤5 (absent or minimal) for <40 minutes, no decelerations and accelerations as described above for term and preterm fetus respectively. An atypical NST has a baseline FHR of 100–110 bpm or >160 bpm for <30 minutes, variability of ≤5 for 40–80 minutes, variable decelerations of 30–60 seconds, and ≤2 accelerations with respective amplitude and duration in term and preterm fetus in 40–80 minutes. An abnormal NST has a baseline FHR showing bradycardia (<100 bpm) or tachycardia (>160 bpm for >30 minutes), variability of ≤5 bpm for ≥80 minutes or ≥25 bpm for >10 minutes or sinusoidal pattern, variable decelerations > 60 seconds, or late decelerations and ≤2 accelerations with respective amplitude and duration in term and preterm fetus in >80 minutes. Based upon this classification, further assessment is required in case of an atypical NST and an urgent action with complete appraisal of the scenario and even immediate delivery may be required in case of abnormal NST.

### Frequency of Performing NST

American College of Obstetricians and Gynecologists (ACOG) recommends that NST is typically repeated at weekly intervals, although certain high-risk conditions may warrant twice weekly testing.[8] NST is not ideal for primary fetal surveillance as it fails to recognize early stages of fetal distress. While the false-negative rate of the test is extremely low (3.2/1,000), the false-positive rate is very high, indicating the low probability of serious fetal problems even when the NST is positive (nonreactive).[18] Therefore, in the setting of a nonreactive NST, the time of NST should be extended or the test should be repeated in 30 minutes or other forms of testing like BPP should be proceeded with and if possible, the factors potentially causing nonreactive results (e.g., smoking) should be modified. A reactive FHR after extended NST is also found to be associated with good fetal outcome; persistent absence of reactivity, however, may be associated fetal compromise in most cases.[19]

### Vibroacoustic Stimulation

Vibroacoustic stimulation (VAS) is a test of fetal well-being in which the fetus is stimulated in utero by using an artificial larynx which elicits a startle response and the effect of this response on FHR is studied. It has an advantage of differentiating normal fetal sleep from asphyxia.

### Method

Artificial larynx can be placed on the mother's abdomen over the fetal vertex and a stimulus of 1–2-second duration is applied. It can be repeated up to 3 times at 1-minute intervals for progressively extended durations up to 3 seconds to provoke FHR accelerations. Normal fetal response includes FHR accelerations, increase in long-term variability, and gross fetal body movements. This test can safely reduce testing time without compromising detection of acidemic fetus.[20] It is safe and harmless to the fetus. A combination of VAS and NST has a higher sensitivity in detecting abnormal outcomes (66% vs. 39%) compared to NST alone.[21]

## Biophysical Profile

It was first described by Manning et al. and provides a fair assessment of risk of intrauterine fetal mortality in near future.[22] The BPP is performed using real time ultrasonography to assess fetal biophysical activities including fetal breathing movements, fetal body movements, fetal tone, and AFV over a 30-minute period. The BPP assesses both acute markers (FHR reactivity, fetal breathing movements, and tone) and chronic markers (AFV) of fetal well-being. The first step in BPP is performing a NST following which a real-time sonography is performed to assess other parameters. The observation is continued till normal activity is observed or 30 minutes of continuous scanning have elapsed. The presence of normal BPP implies that CNS of fetus is intact, and that fetus is not significantly hypoxic. However, it has limited value in predicting longitudinal deterioration, which is better evaluated using Doppler velocimetry.

A scoring system assigns a numeric value (usually 0 or 2) to each of the biophysical components **(Table 1)**. In the original score given by Manning,[22] each of the five parameters (FHR, breathing, tone, gross body movements, and AFV) were assigned either a score of 2 (normal) or 0 (abnormal) with no scores in between. As a result, there was no intermediate score here some movements or tone was present but did not fit into criteria for a score of 2. To overcome this limitation, Vintzileos et al. in 1983 proposed a scoring system which had provision of intermediate scores and included placental grading as a variable. A normal score (score of >8) predicts a nonacidotic fetus.[23]

### Physiologic Basis for the Biophysical Profile

Each biophysical parameter represents normal functioning of a particular area of the CNS, which develops at an expected gestational age. Vintzileos et al. proposed the gradual hypoxia concept, which states that the biophysical activity which develops last becomes abnormal earliest, in fetal academia/infection.[23]

- The CNS center controlling fetal tone, located in subcortical area develops earliest at around 7.5 weeks.
- The CNS center controlling body movements develop at 8.5–9.5 weeks in cortex nuclei.
- The CNS center controlling breathing movements develop after 20–21 weeks in the ventral surface of 4th ventricle.
- The CNS center controlling FHR reactivity is functional by the end of the 2nd or start of third trimester.

Therefore, in early stages of fetal compromise, there are FHR reactivity and breathing abnormalities, the tone is abolished last of all.

**TABLE 1:** Biophysical profile scoring.

| Variable | Normal (score = 2) | Abnormal (score = 0) |
| --- | --- | --- |
| Fetal breathing movements | More than one episode lasting >30 seconds, in 30 minutes | • Absent fetal breathing movements<br>• No episode lasting >30 seconds, in 30 minutes |
| Gross body movements | Three or more discrete body or limb movements, in 30 minutes (Simultaneous movement of the limb and trunk should be counted as a single movement) An episode of active continuous movement is considered as one movement | • Less than three episodes of gross body movements, in 30 minutes<br>• Absent fetal movements |
| Fetal tone | At least one episode of active extension with return to flexion of fetal limb(s) or trunk. Opening and closing of hand is considered normal tone | Slow extension with return to partial flexion or movement of limb in full extension |
| Reactive FHR | Two or more episodes of FHR acceleration of >15 bpm lasting for at least 15 seconds associated with fetal movement, in 30 minutes | Less than two episodes of FHR acceleration of >15 bpm or FHR acceleration of <15 bpm, in 30 minutes |
| Amniotic fluid volume (AFV) | At least one pocket of fluid measuring 2 cm in vertical axis and horizontal dimension should be at least 1 cm | Either no pocket or largest pocket measuring <2 cm in vertical axis |

## Interpretation of Biophysical Profile and Pregnancy Management

- A score of 10 is interpreted as normal, nonasphyxiated fetus, and no intervention is indicated. It is recommended to repeat the test weekly, except in diabetics and in postterm pregnancy, where it must be done twice weekly.
- A score of 8 with normal fluid also indicates a normal nonasphyxiated fetus and no intervention is indicated and repeat testing is recommended as per protocol.
- Score of 8 with oligohydramnios is suspicious of chronic fetal hypoxia and delivery is recommended if >37 weeks, otherwise repeat testing is recommended.
- Score of 6 indicates possible fetal asphyxia and the recommended management is:
  - If abnormal AFV: Delivery
  - If normal AFV and period of gestation >36 weeks with favorable cervix: Delivery
  - If normal AFV and period of gestation <36 weeks, then test should be repeated
  - If repeat test <6: Delivery
  - If repeat test > 6: Observe and repeat as per protocol.
- Score of 4 is considered probable fetal asphyxia and the recommended management is:
  - *>32 weeks:* Delivery
  - *<32 weeks:* Test should be repeated same day; if repeat BPP score is <6, deliver.
- A score of 0-2 is almost certain of fetal asphyxia and immediate delivery is recommended.

Application of BPP to high-risk population results in a remarkable improvement in perinatal mortality rates.[24] While absence of fetal breathing movement is best predictive of fetal distress in labor (even better than a nonreactive NST), lack of fetal movement is best predictive of fetal death.[25] A normal BPP indicates a low-risk of still birth. The false-negative rate of the BPP (that is fetal demise within a week of a normal test) is reported to be 0.645/1,000.[25,26]

The frequency of BPP testing (1–2/week) is arbitrary, but more frequent testing can be done depending on individual judgment, training, preferences, and experience. A variety of medications especially magnesium sulfate and corticosteroids, commonly used in obstetric practice have significant effects on the BPP. If one is not aware of the effects of medications on the BPP, inappropriate interpretation of the results may occur resulting in the possibility of iatrogenic and unnecessary premature delivery. Corticosteroids and magnesium sulfate decrease the FHR variability and fetal breathing movements but have no effects on fetal tone or AFV.[27,28]

## Modified Biophysical Profile

The MBPP includes NST which is an acute marker of fetal acid-base status and AFV which indicates chronic uteroplacental function. It was proposed to reduce the time taken for assessment of BPP and is used by many centers as a primary means of antepartum fetal surveillance. The amniotic fluid index (AFI) is the total of the deepest cord-free pocket of amniotic fluid (in cm) in each of the four maternal uterine quadrants. AFI > 5 cm is considered adequate.[29] The MBPP score is considered normal in the presence of a reactive NST and AFI > 5 cm. A management protocol is suggested based on the interpretation of MBPP:[30]

- If NST is reactive and AFV is normal—twice weekly testing is recommended or may be more intensive monitoring as per indication of testing.
- If NST is reactive with oligohydramnios—delivery is recommended if gestation is >36 weeks. But if gestation is <36 weeks then Doppler with increased frequency of testing should be done.
- If NST is nonreactive, complete BPP is done and management is according to its results.

It was observed that the still birth rate within a week of normal MBPP was 0.8/1,000 women which was similar as the full BPP with the advantage of reduced time for assessment.

## Doppler Ultrasonography

Doppler ultrasonography is used to measure the blood flow in maternal and fetal blood vessels to assess the hemodynamic components of vascular resistance **(Table 2)**.

Doppler ultrasound is useful in predicting complications, especially FGR and pre-eclampsia and helps to differentiate between FGR and small-for-gestational age (SGA) fetus. Apart from above, Dopplers have now added a new dimension to the definition of FGR as per the Delphi consensus. Thus, performing a Doppler has become increasingly useful in day-to-day clinical practice.

The commonly calculated flow indices include the following:
- Systolic to diastolic ratio (S/D)
- Resistance index (S-D/S)
- Pulsatility index (S-D/A).

### Fetal Arterial Doppler

*Umbilical artery:* The normal Doppler flow pattern of umbilical artery is a low resistance waveform, with increasing end-diastolic flow with advancing gestation **(Fig. 4)**.[31,32] Thus, the S/D ratio gradually reduces from about 4.0 at 20

**TABLE 2:** Doppler velocimetry of various vessels and clinical information.

| Vessel | Clinical information |
| --- | --- |
| Uterine artery | Maternal (resistance to uterus) |
| Umbilical artery | Placental (resistance to placenta) |
| Middle cerebral artery | Fetal (fetal adaptation to flow resistance change) |
| Ductus venosus | Fetal (fetal cardiac function) |

weeks of gestation to 2.0 at term; S/D ratio is usually <3 after 30 weeks.[33] It should be preferably measured in a pocket free of umbilical cord loops and optimally done in the absence of fetal breathing movements.

Umbilical arterial waveforms indicate the placental circulation status. The increase in end-diastolic flow with advancing gestation is consequent to the increase in number of tertiary stem villi. In a normal pregnancy, this results in progressive decrease in pulsatility index (PI) as gestation advances. However, conditions affecting the small muscular arteries in these villi cause a progressive decrease in end-diastolic flow consequently increasing the PI as gestation advances, until it becomes absent and with subsequent flow reversal during diastole **(Figs. 5 to 7)**.[34] In addition, it must be always remembered that rather than an absolute value, it is the centile value at a particular gestation which may be clinically more relevant.

Abnormal Doppler parameters in the umbilical artery are associated with high rates of still birth and neurological impairment. Absent or reversed end-diastolic flow (AREDF) indicates damage to about 60–70% of the villous vascular tree (advanced placental compromise).[35] REDF is associated with adverse perinatal outcomes (sensitivity and specificity of 60%), independent of prematurity. A systematic review including 16 randomized trials (over 10,000 high-risk patients) observed that using Doppler ultrasound velocimetry was associated with decreased perinatal mortality (OR: 0.71, 95% CI 0.52–0.98).[36] It is important to note the fetuses with early-onset FGR follow a stepwise sequence of changes in umbilical artery Doppler over a period of time. However, the umbilical artery Doppler cannot be used as a stand-alone measurement in fetuses with late-onset IUGR as the placental disease is mild in these cases and might not be reflected appropriately in Doppler of umbilical artery.

*Middle cerebral artery:* The normal Doppler flow pattern of middle cerebral artery (MCA) is a high-resistance circulation with a continuous forward flow. The ideal location to measure it as the proximal part of the vessel **(Fig. 8)**.

In fetal hypoxemia, brain sparing reflex occurs whereby redistribution of blood flow occurs as a fetal adaptation to hypoxemia which results in increased blood flow to brain, heart, and adrenals with reduced flow to peripheral and placental circulation.[37] Increased MCA diastolic flow indicates fetal compromise which is reflected by a low PI **(Fig. 9)**. Moreover, like umbilical artery Doppler values, there are specific PI values for each gestation. Abnormality in this vessel correlates with neonatal acidosis and neurological impairment. The measurements of this vessel are particularly valuable in identification and prediction of adverse outcomes among fetuses with late-onset IUGR, independent of umbilical artery Doppler which may be normal as placental disease is mild in these fetuses. Thus, it is very important to remember that umbilical artery Doppler is no longer used as a stand-alone standard criterion for detection of FGR as it will lead to missing out of high number of late-onset FGR cases. Also, the changes in this vessel correlate with an increased cesarean rates which may be clinically relevant as labor induction at term is the current

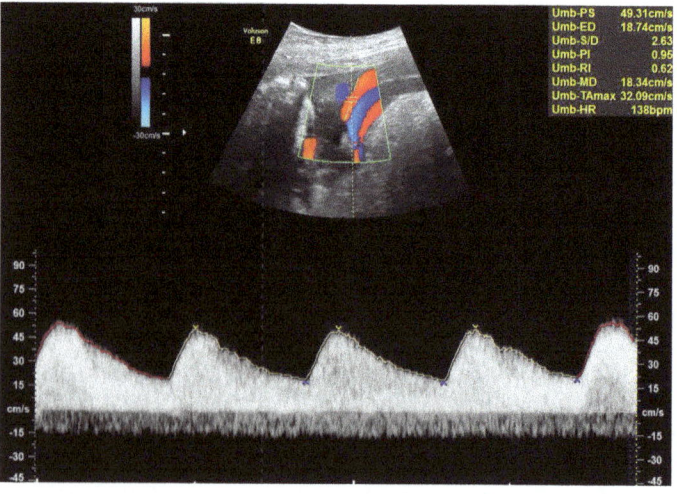

**Fig. 4:** Normal Doppler flow pattern in umbilical artery with good diastolic flow.

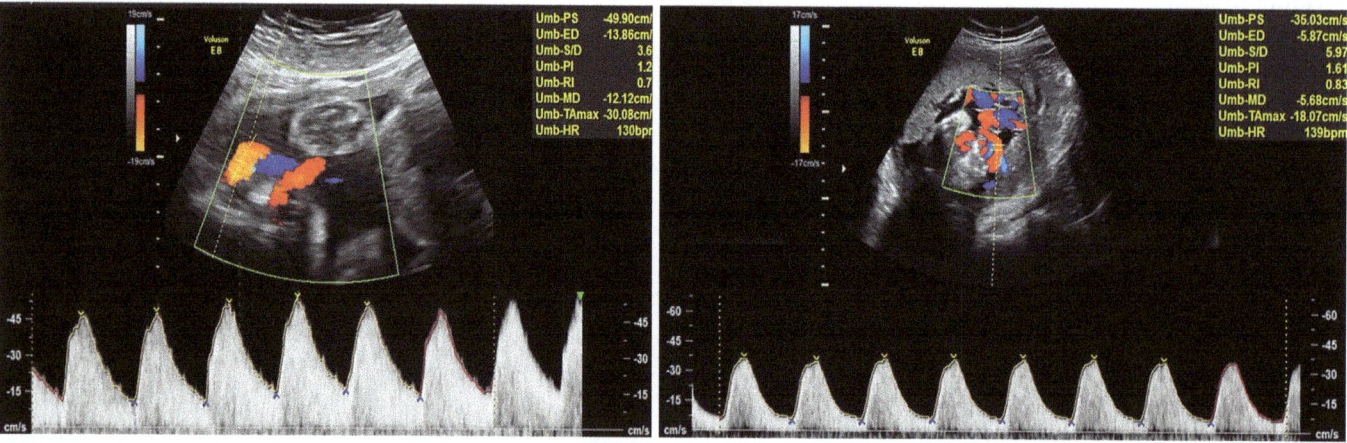

**Fig. 5:** Doppler of the umbilical artery depicting progressive decrease in end-diastolic flow consequently increasing the pulsatility index (PI) as gestation advances. It is seen in conditions such as fetal growth restriction or pre-eclampsia in which the small muscular arteries in villi are affected.

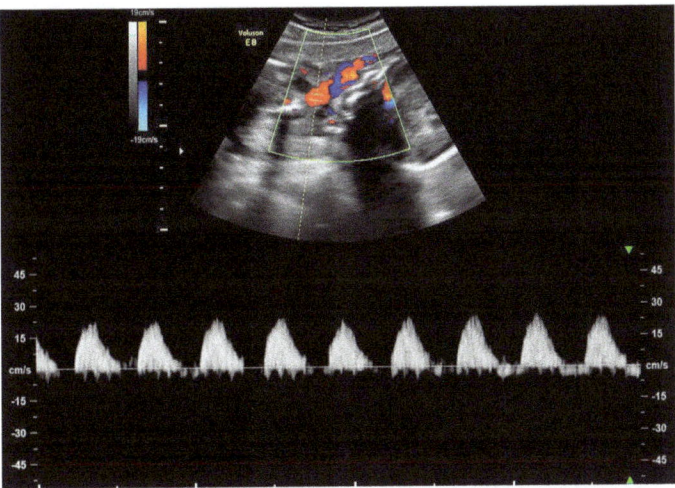

**Fig. 6:** Doppler of the umbilical artery depicting absent end-diastolic flow suggestive of advanced placental compromise.

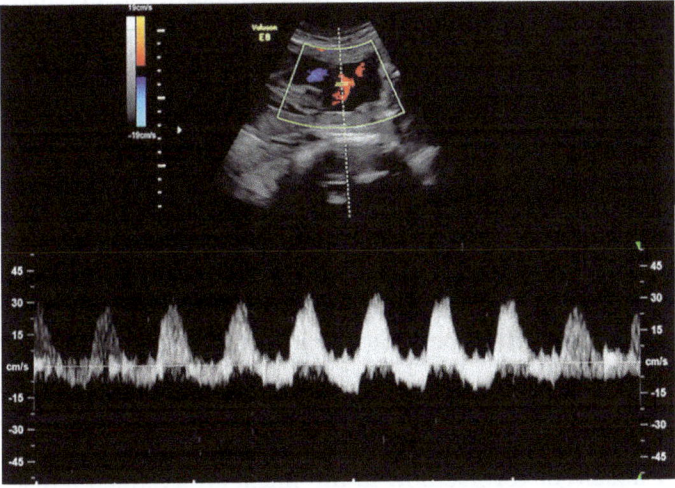

**Fig. 7:** Doppler of the umbilical artery depicting reversed end-diastolic flow suggestive of damage to 60–70% of villi in the placenta.

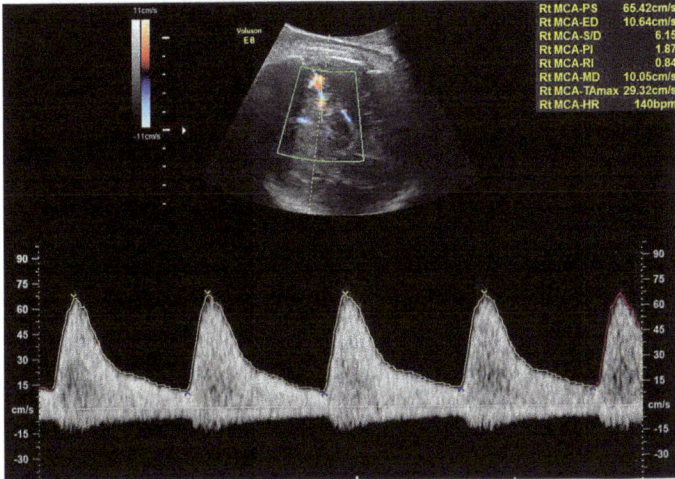

**Fig. 8:** Doppler of the middle cerebral artery depicting a high resistance, continuous forward flow with minimal diastolic flow.

standard of care in late-onset fetuses. In addition, it is noted that cerebroplacental ratio (CPR) which is defined as MCA PI value divided by umbilical artery PI value is used to identify

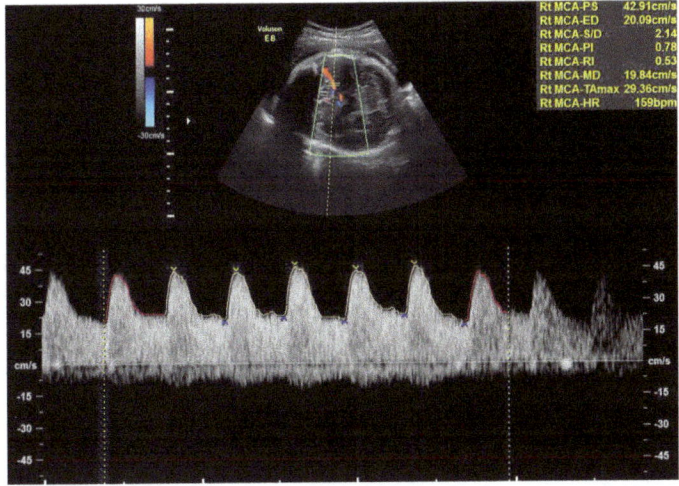

**Fig. 9:** Doppler of the middle cerebral artery depicting increased diastolic flow reflecting brain sparing as shown by increasing diastolic flow and a low pulsatility index.

the fetuses in whom the placental insufficiency is associated with altered cerebral blood flow.[38] Ratio of <1.0 indicates severe neonatal morbidity and CPR <5th centile for gestation is very good predictor of adverse outcome. Use of CPR for monitoring improves the sensitivity of umbilical artery and MCA Doppler, as increased placental resistance (reflected in umbilical artery) can be associated with reduced cerebral resistance (reflected in MCA). In addition, CPR can be decreased even while its individual components are within normal limits.

### Fetal Venous Doppler

*Basis of fetal venous Doppler:* The flow velocity waveforms in great veins such as ductus venosus (DV), inferior vena cava (IVC), and umbilical vein have been studied. The Doppler waveform in the central fetal veins are influenced by the central venous pressure which reflects cardiac function. In cases of fetal growth restriction (FGR), the changes in arterial circulation have a major effect on afterload, preload, and cardiac contractility. High resistance in umbilical circulation leads to increased right ventricular afterload. In the most compromised fetuses, low resistance in cerebral circulation reduces the left ventricular afterload. With further hypoxemia myocardial contractility and cardiac output fall.[39]

### Fetal Ductus Venosus and Inferior Vena Cava

Doppler evaluation of fetal veins combined with umbilical artery assessment may be useful for predicting outcomes in FGR.[40,41] The fetal precordial veins (DV and IVC) and the umbilical vein are the vessels most evaluated in clinical practice. Umbilical venous blood flow is continuous in normal pregnancies >15 weeks of gestation. In pathological states, such as FGR, flow may be pulsatile, reflecting the cardiac dysfunction due to increased afterload. The DV is resistant to alterations in flow, except in severe FGR.[42]

The measurement of DV is done where it branches from umbilical vein, at the site of aliasing **(Fig. 10)**. The abnormality in the DV blood flow is the single best parameter to predict the short-term risk of fetal demise, especially in early-onset FGR fetuses. Also, monitoring of flow in the DV can help in surveillance of early-onset FGR cases with AREDF with progressively increasing PI, subsequently absent a wave and finally reversal of a wave **(Figs. 11 and 12)**. The timing of delivery in these cases can also be based on the changes in the blood flow in DV giving the fetus the possible benefit gained from each day in-utero.

### Maternal Uterine Circulation

It is measured at a site where the uterine artery crosses the hypogastric vessels. With advancing gestation, a progressive decrease in impedance is noted in uterine circulation. Abnormal uterine artery waveforms in late second and third trimester have an increased risk of complications such as FGR, pre-eclampsia, and preterm delivery.[43] Uterine artery PI > 95th centile for a particular gestation is also used as a criterion to diagnose fetus with FGR. However, the major role of this vessel is in first and second trimester for prediction of pre-eclampsia.

### Clinical Implications of Doppler in Fetal Compromise

Doppler studies can be used in the evaluation of fetal compromise in high-risk pregnancy.[44] They are used to identify high-risk pregnancy, diagnose FGR, and confirm the potential for fetal compromise. Use of umbilical artery Doppler assumes that placental vascular lesions underlie all fetal compromise except in cases of acute fetal deterioration, e.g., placental abruption. Meta-analysis has established that women with high-risk pregnancies with a compromised fetus should have access to Doppler studies of the umbilical artery.[45] Cerebral Doppler defines the redistribution of cardiac output and assumes a very significant role in fetuses with late-onset FGR. Venous Doppler defines changes in cardiac load and contractility. Timing of delivery can be based on DV Doppler in early-onset FGR cases and it showed improvement in developmental outcomes at 2 years of age as per the TRUFFLE (Trial of Randomized Umbilical and Fetal Flow in Europe).[46]

The value and the use of Doppler parameters to make decisions for fetuses with growth restriction have been described by the Barcelona group who have proposed the stage based management of FGR based on the Doppler parameters. In early-onset FGR, the fetus follows a long sequence of Doppler changes in the various vessels including umbilical artery and DV. It starts with raised PI followed by absent or reverse flow in umbilical artery. Such fetuses can be monitored by changes in DV Doppler till absent or reversal in DV giving them the potential benefit gained by each day in-utero. However, in late-onset IUGR, there is limited role of umbilical artery as a stand-alone criterion and it is the changes in the MCA and the CPR which aids in

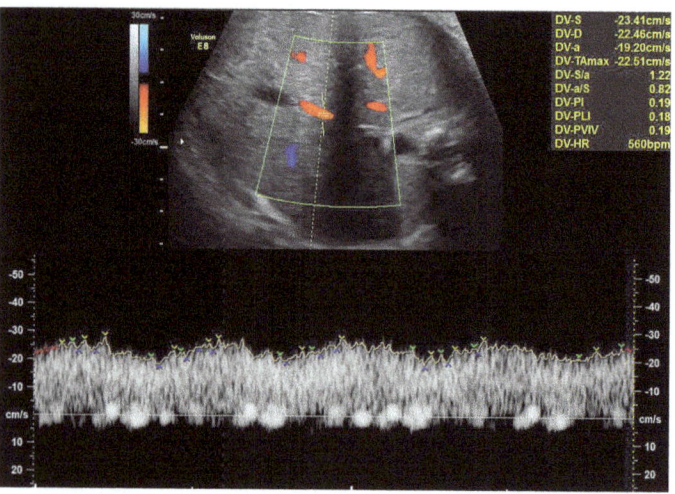

**Fig. 10:** Doppler of the ductus venosus depicting normal triphasic waveform.

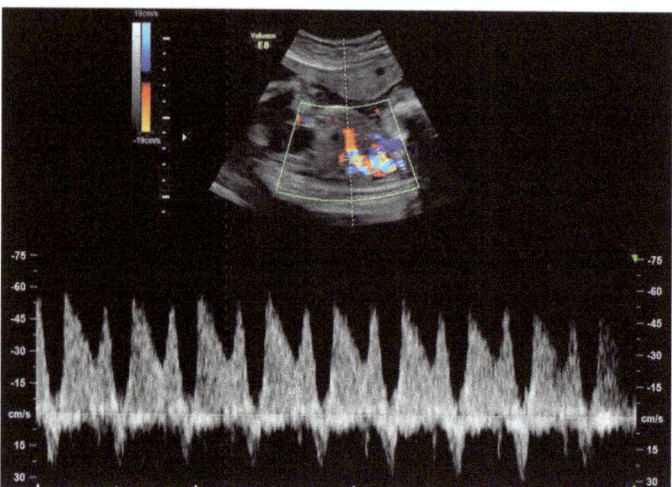

**Fig. 11:** Doppler of the ductus venosus showing increased pulsatility index (PI).

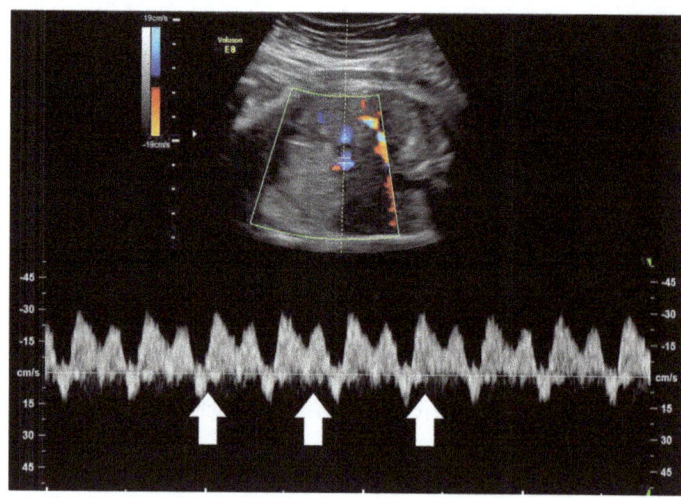

**Fig. 12:** Doppler of the ductus venosus depicting reversal of a wave which is an ominous sign of fetal compromise.

diagnosis as well as timing of delivery too. In fetuses with late-onset IUGR, with brain sparing, there is gradual increase in diastolic flow in MCA leading to decreasing PI values of the MCA and decreasing centile values of the CPR.

## Management of Abnormal Test Results

The results of an abnormal antepartum surveillance test are usually followed by an additional test due to high false-positive rates, e.g., if NST is abnormal then, it is advisable to do a BPP and get more information about fetus rather than considering termination of pregnancy. Another important factor that needs to be considered is clinical situation, e.g., in a temporary maternal condition, such as diabetic ketoacidosis, prompt treatment of the maternal condition may improve fetal oxygenation and subsequent normal test result.[1] In chronic conditions, overall clinical assessment that includes gestational age, severity of disease, and pattern of abnormal result (decelerations, absent variability, or bradycardia; BPP score 10 vs. 4) may guide further management. Hence, any abnormal result should be considered keeping the overall clinical scenario in mind. If delivery cannot be planned (e.g., extreme prematurity) then test should not be conducted as no further management will be done based on the test result.[1]

## Implications in Clinical Practice

Pregnancies are categorized as high risk or low risk, based on the presence or absence of complicating factors. In low-risk pregnancies, usual assessment tools include maternal monitoring of fetal movements, measurement of symphysis-fundal height (SFH), and fetal heart auscultation.[47] SFH is measured from 24 weeks onward at 2–3 weekly intervals. Abdominal palpation alone has a sensitivity and specificity of 21% and 96%, respectively for detection of SGA fetuses. SFH measurement results in small improvement in prediction of growth abnormalities, with a sensitivity and specificity of 27% and 88%, respectively.[47] While customized growth charts developed on the basis of SFH do not improve perinatal outcomes, their use reduces the number of ultrasonograms requested for assessment of fetal growth and it can be used as a simple, inexpensive tool in out-patient department (OPD) in case of nonavailability of ultrasound machine.[48] For monitoring low-risk pregnancies, only daily fetal movement count has a proven value.[47] No evidence-based guideline recommends the routine use of ultrasound (excluding a dating and anomaly scan) and Doppler velocimetry in low-risk pregnancies.[1]

In all high-risk pregnancies, appropriate surveillance should be performed in accordance with the clinical situation.[47] Although studies have described the use of NST and BPP for monitoring high-risk pregnancies, the superiority of one method over the other is unclear. The choice depends on multiple factors, including gestational age, availability, presence of a congenital anomaly, ability to monitor the FHR (e.g., a fetus with cardiac arrhythmia cannot be monitored with NST), and cost.[49] The pregnancies that are complicated by placental insufficiency, fetal assessment should be done at appropriate intervals with fetal biometry and growth velocity scans, Doppler of various vessels based on stage-based management protocol for FGR, and AFV. In cases with early-onset FGR, fetus with AEDF should be delivered by 32–34 weeks and fetuses with REDF by 30–32 weeks with cesarean section as mode of delivery for both, however, each case needs to individualize based on the overall clinical picture. The fetuses with early-onset FGR with AREDF can be strictly monitored with DV Doppler. The indication for delivery in early-onset FGR is abnormal NST, abnormal DV Doppler, and/or abnormal BPP. In cases with late-onset FGR, CPR or MCA-PI along with NST and BPP should be used for surveillance and umbilical artery Doppler is not valid anymore as a stand-alone test as it only identifies severe placental insufficiency, failing to pick mild disease characterized in late-onset FGR. The timing of birth in late-onset FGR is around 37 weeks and routine cesarean is not indicated for isolated FGR with normal or even abnormal Doppler examination. It is also important to differentiate a small fetus from an FGR fetus with increased risk of perinatal morbidity and it can be done based on only Doppler findings.[50]

## CONCLUSION

The principal aim of antepartum fetal surveillance is to detect fetuses at risk and plan an appropriate intervention to increase the likelihood of favorable perinatal outcome. Different pathophysiological processes can place the fetus at risk with the efficacy of the various fetal tests depending on the underlying condition. The best approach is a longitudinal surveillance beginning with integrated fetal testing (including Doppler velocimetry, FHR analysis, and assessment of BPP) as a combination of tests improves the prediction of acidemia and still birth compared with single tests and no one test is ideal for all high-risk fetuses. The monitoring frequency depends on gestational age, clinical speed of deterioration, and associated risk of impending fetal acidemia. Therefore, multiple parameter assessment or combinations of different tests may often be the optimal surveillance strategy.[51]

## KEY POINTS

- Antepartum surveillance of the fetus helps in detecting fetal compromise (acidemia), so that timely intervention can be done. It can detect both acute and chronic disease states.
- Fetal movement monitoring is a simple, inexpensive, and noninvasive method of antepartum surveillance.

- The relationship between decreased fetal activity and poor perinatal outcome has been well-established.
- FHR reactivity reflects normal fetal autonomic function and well-being.
- Preterm fetuses are less likely to have FHR accelerations in association with fetal movements.
- The negative predictive value of an NST is very high with a reactive NST predicting good perinatal outcome in about 95% of cases; however, the false-positive rate of a nonreactive NST is very high.
- The normal fetal response to VAS includes FHR reactivity along with increase in long-term FHR variability and gross body movements. VAS can safely reduce testing time without compromising detection of the acidemic fetus.
- The BPP is unique in that it assesses both acute and chronic markers of fetal condition.
- The "gradual hypoxia concept" implies that the biophysical activity which develops last becomes abnormal earliest, in fetal acidemia/infection. Accordingly, early stages of fetal compromise show abnormalities in FHR reactivity and breathing, while movement and tone are generally not affected until later stages.
- The interpretation of FHR patterns should incorporate knowledge of gestational age, maternal condition, medication, and other factors that could influence FHR components.
- The use of umbilical artery Doppler flow velocity waveforms to study high-risk pregnancy is associated with a 32% reduction in perinatal mortality.
- Throughout pregnancy, there is a progressive decrease in resistance to blood flow to the placenta in the umbilical arteries as the placenta grows and this is reflected by changing pattern of the umbilical artery flow velocity waveforms.
- The presence of a high-resistance pattern in the umbilical artery is manifested as increased S/D ratio, absent or REDF and is associated with an increased risk of FGR, fetal distress in utero, fetal distress in labor, and need for early delivery.
- In the MCA, a pattern of low resistance predicts fetal hypoxia.
- The central fetal veins like DV and IVC show changes in flow velocity waveforms in condition of fetal compromise. Retardation of flow velocity in the DV waveform at the time of atrial systole indicates developing fetal hypoxemia.
- A high-resistance pattern in the uterine artery flow waveform is signaled by low-diastolic flow velocities and the non-disappearance of diastolic notch by late second trimester. This predicts pregnancy at risk of pre-eclampsia and FGR.
- Abnormality in the umbilical artery flow velocity waveform signals developing placental vascular pathology, which may lead to fetal hypoxemia and acidosis. Changes in the fetal MCA, and DV waveform correlate with the degree of hypoxemia and fetal condition.

## REFERENCES

1. Practice Bulletin no. 145: antepartum fetal surveillance. Obstet Gynecol. 2014;124(1):182-92.
2. Seeds AE. Current concepts of amniotic fluid dynamics. Am J Obstet Gynecol. 1980;138(5):575-86.
3. Manning FA, Snijders R, Harman CR, Nicolaides K, Menticoglou S, Morrison I. Fetal biophysical profile score. VI. Correlation with antepartum umbilical venous fetal pH. Am J Obstet Gynecol. 1993;169(4):755-63.
4. Rayburn WF. Clinical significance of perceptible fetal motion. Am J Obstet Gynecol. 1980;138(2):210-2.
5. Pearson JF, Weaver JB. Fetal activity and fetal wellbeing: an evaluation. Br Med J. 1976;1(6021):1305-7.
6. Rayburn WF. Antepartum fetal assessment: monitoring fetal activity. Clin Perinatol. 1982;(9):231-52.
7. Moore TR, Piacquadio K. A prospective evaluation of fetal movement screening to reduce the incidence of antepartum fetal death. Am J Obstet Gynecol. 1989;160(5 Pt 1):1075-80.
8. American College of Obstetricians and Gynecologists. Antepartum fetal surveillance. Washington: ACOG Practice Bulletin no. 9; 1999. p. 911.
9. Freeman RK, Anderson G, Dorchester W. A prospective multi-institutional study of antepartum fetal heart rate monitoring. I. Risk of perinatal mortality according to antepartum fetal heart rate test results. Am J Obstet Gynecol. 1982;143(7):771-7.
10. Evertson LR, Gauthier RJ, Collea JV. Fetal demise following negative contraction stress tests. Obstet Gynecol. 1978;51(6):671-3.
11. Lagrew DC Jr. The contraction stress test. Clin Obstet Gynecol. 1995;38(1):11-25.
12. Keegan KA Jr, Paul RH, Broussard PM, McCart D, Smith MA. Antepartum fetal heart testing. V. The nonstress test—an outpatient approach. Am J Obstet Gynecol. 1980;136(1):81-3.
13. Evertson LR, Gauthier RJ, Schifrin BS, Paul RH. Antepartum fetal heart rate testing. I. Evolution of the nonstress test. Am J Obstet Gynecol. 1979;133(1):29-33.
14. Navot D, Yaffe H, Sadovsky E. The ratio of fetal heart rate accelerations to fetal movements according to gestational age. Am J Obstet Gynecol. 1984;149(1):92-4.
15. Phelan JP. The nonstress test: a review of 3,000 tests. Am J Obstet Gynecol. 1981;139(1):7-10.
16. Margulis E, Binder D, Cohen AW. The effect of propranolol on the nonstress test. Am J Obstet Gynecol. 1984;148(3):340-1.
17. Liston R, Sawchuck D, Young D. No. 197a-Fetal Health Surveillance: Antepartum Consensus Guideline. J Obstet Gynaecol Can. 2018;40(4):e251-71.
18. Devoe LD, Castillo RA, Sherline DM. The nonstress test as a diagnostic test: a critical reappraisal. Am J Obstet Gynecol. 1985;152(8):1047-53.
19. Devoe LD, McKenzie J, Searle NS, Sherline DM. Clinical sequelae of the extended nonstress test. Am J Obstet Gynecol. 1985;151(8):1074-8.
20. Smith CV, Phelan JP, Platt LD, Broussard P, Paul RH. Fetal acoustic stimulation testing. II. A randomized clinical comparison with the nonstress test. Am J Obstet Gynecol. 1986;155(1):131-4.

21. Trudinger BJ, Boylan P. Antepartum fetal heart rate monitoring: value of sound stimulation. Obstet Gynecol. 1980;55(2):265-8.
22. Manning FA, Platt LD, Sipos L. Antepartum fetal evaluation: development of a fetal biophysical profile. Am J Obstet Gynecol. 1980;136(6):787-95.
23. Vintzileos AM, Campbell WA Ingardia CJ, Nochimson DJ. The fetal biophysical profile and its predictive value. Obstet Gynecol. 1983;62(3):271-8.
24. Manning FA, Harman CR, Morrison I, Menticoglou SM, Lange IR, Johnson JM. Fetal assessment based on fetal biophysical profile scoring. IV. An analysis of perinatal morbidity and mortality. Am J Obstet Gynecol. 1990;162(3):703-9.
25. Manning FA, Morrison I, Lange IR, Harman CR, Chamberlain PF. Fetal assessment based on fetal biophysical profile scoring: Experience in 12620 referred high risk pregnancies. Perinatal mortality by frequency and etiology. Am J Obstet Gynecol. 1985;151(3):343-50.
26. Platt LD, Eglinton GS, Sipos L, Broussard PM, Paul RH. Further experience with the fetal biophysical profile. Obstet Gynecol. 1983;61(4):480-5.
27. Deren O, Karaer C, Onderoglu L, Yigit N, Durukan T, Bahado-Singh RO. The effects of steroids on the biophyisical profile and Doppler indices of umbilical and middle cerebral arteries in healthy preterm fetuses. Eur J Obstet Gynecol Reprod Biol. 2001;99(1):72-6.
28. Carlan SJ, O'Brien WF. The effect of magnesium sulfate on the biophysical profile of normal term fetus. Obstet Gynecol. 1991;77(5):681-4.
29. Rutherford SE, Phelan JP, Smith CV, Jacobs N. The four quadrant assessment of amniotic fluid volume: an adjunct to antepartum fetal heart rate testing. Obstet Gynecol. 1987;70(3 Pt 1):353-6.
30. Vintzileos AM, Knuppel RA. Multiple parameter biophysical testing in the prediction of fetal acid base status. Clin Perinatol. 1994;21(4):823-48.
31. Fleischer A, Schulman H, Farmakides G, Bracero L, Blattner P, Randolph G. Umbilical artery waveforms and intrauterine growth retardation. Am J Obstet Gynecol. 1985;151(4):502-5.
32. Ott WJ. The diagnosis of altered fetal growth. Obstet Gynecol Clin North Am. 1988;15(2):237-63.
33. Fleischer A, Schulman H, Farmakides G, Bracero L, Grunfeld L, Rochelson B, et al. Uterine artery Doppler velocimetry in pregnant women with hypertension. Am J Obstet Gynecol. 1986;154(4):806-13.
34. Trudinger BJ, Stevens D, Connelly A, Hales JR, Alexander G, Bradley L, et al. Umbilical artery flow velocity waveforms and placental resistance: the effects of embolization of the umbilical circulation. Am J Obstet Gynecol. 1987;157(6):1443-8.
35. Kingdom JC, Burrell SJ, Kaufmann P. Pathology and clinical implications of abnormal umbilical artery Doppler waveforms. Ultrasound Obstet Gynecol. 1997;9(4):271-86.
36. Alfirevic Z, Stampalija T, Gyte GM. Fetal and umbilical Doppler ultrasound in high-risk pregnancies. Cochrane Database Syst Rev. 2017;6(6):CD007529.
37. Mari G, Deter RL. Middle cerebral artery flow velocity waveforms in normal and small for gestational age fetuses. Am J Obstet Gynecol. 1992;166(4):1262-70.
38. Arias F. Accuracy of the middle cerebral to umbilical artery resistance index ratio in the production of neonatal outcome in patients at high risk for fetal and neonatal complications. Am J Obstet Gynecol. 1994;171(6):1541-5.
39. Reece EA, Hobbins JC, Norman F, et al., (Eds). Doppler ultrasonography and fetal well-being. In: Handbook of Clinical Obstetrics: Fetus and Mother, 3rd edition. US: Blackwell Publishing Ltd; 2008. pp. 575-6.
40. Baschat AA, Gembruch U, Reiss I, Gortner L, Weiner CP, Harman CR. Relationship between arterial and venous Doppler and perinatal outcome in fetal growth restriction. Ultrasound Obstet Gynecol. 2000;16(5):407-13.
41. Kiserud T, Kessler J, Ebbing C, Rasmussen S. Ductus venosus shunting in growth-restricted fetuses and the effect of umbilical circulatory compromise. Ultrasound Obstet Gynecol. 2006;28(2):143-9.
42. Kiserud T, Eik-Nes SH, Blaas HG, Hellevik LR, Simensen B. Ductus venosus blood velocity and the umbilical circulation in the seriously growth-retarded fetus. Ultrasound Obstet Gynecol. 1994;4(2):109-14.
43. Hernandez-Andrade E, Brodszki J, Lingman G, Gudmundsson S, Molin J, Marsál K. Uterine artery score and perinatal outcome. Ultrasound Obstet Gynecol. 2002;19(5):438-42.
44. Reece EA, Hobbins JC, Norman F, et al., (Eds). Doppler ultrasonography and fetal well-being. In: The Handbook of Clinical Obstetrics: Fetus and Mother, 3rd edition. US: Blackwell Publishing Ltd; 2008. p. 577.
45. Laudy JA, Gaillard JL, van der Anker JN, Tibboel D, Wladimiroff JW. Doppler ultrasound imaging: a new technique detect lung hypoplasia before birth? Ultrasound Obstet Gynecol. 1996;7(3):189-92.
46. Thornton JG, Hornbuckle J, Vail A, Spiegelhalter DJ, Levene M; The GRIT study group. Infant wellbeing at 2 years of age in the growth restricted intervention trial (GRIT): multicentered randomized controlled trial. Lancet. 2004;364(9433):513-20.
47. Jones NW. Assessing antepartum fetal health. Obstetrics, Gynaecology and Reproductive Medicine. 2011;21(6):164-8.
48. Gelbaya TA, Nardo LG. Customised fetal growth chart: a systematic review. J Obstet Gynaecol. 2005;25(5):445-50.
49. Bishop EH. Fetal acceleration test. Am J Obstet Gynecol. 1981;141(8):905-9.
50. Royal College of Obstetricians and Gynaecologists. The Investigation and Management of the Small-for-Gestational-Age Fetus (Green-top guideline no. 31). UK: RCOG; 2013.
51. Kontopoulos EV, Vintzileos AM. Condition-specific antepartum fetal testing. Am J Obstet Gynecol. 2004;191(5):1546-51.

# CHAPTER 9

# Polyhydramnios Oligohydramnios

*Prabha Lal*

## INTRODUCTION

Amniotic fluid is a faintly alkaline (pH 7.2) watery content of amniotic sac where fetus grows. It is the sum of inflow and outflow of fluid into amniotic sac and reflects fetal fluid balance. It is primarily of fetal origin with a small maternal contribution via extraplacental membranes. Exact site of origin differs according to the gestational age. In the first trimester, it is mainly a transudate of plasma with transudation occurring across the maternal surface of uterine decidua-placental surface and directly through the non-keratinized skin of fetus acting as a membrane up to 24 weeks. Later in gestation, it is the fetal urine and fetal lung secretions which contribute to its formation so that the components of amniotic fluid at term include urea and creatinine. Fetal urine is the most fundamental source of amniotic fluid as evidenced by the complete absence of liquor in fetal renal agenesis. Compositionally, 98–99% is water and rest are solids such as proteins (0.25%), uric acid and creatinine (2%). Levels of electrolytes such as sodium and potassium are low at term.

Amniotic fluid is not a static collection of fluid but is rather dynamic whose volume is maintained by a circulatory process of fetal lung and urine production balanced by swallowing and absorption directly across the amnion into the fetal circulation. Earliest detection of amniotic fluid occurs at 8 weeks of gestation and its volume progressively increases with increasing age of gestation. Amniotic fluid is 30 mL at 10 weeks, 190 mL at 16 weeks and 800–1,000 mL at 32–35 weeks gestation. Thereafter, it declines to 550 mL by 42 weeks.[1]

Amniotic fluid provides the fetus a protective, low resistance environment suitable for growth and development. It also reflects the maternal hydration because the fluid shifts freely across the placenta predominantly in response to osmotic gradient.

## ASSESSMENT OF AMNIOTIC FLUID VOLUME

- Clinical assessment is done by careful manual palpation of the uterus and it gives a fairly good idea of amount of liquor; whether it appears to be normal, reduced or is excessive. It is subjective but initial clinical assessment is useful as it prompts further evaluation and confirmation in case liquor volume appears abnormal.

  Symphysio-fundal height (SFH) estimation also raises suspicion of abnormal quantity of liquor and needs confirmation.
- Ultrasonography (USG) is the method of choice for assessing the liquor volume. This is done by estimation of deepest vertical pocket (DVP) or measuring amniotic fluid index (AFI) and is reliable for diagnosis of both oligo- and polyhydramnios.
  - *AFI:* It is calculated by dividing uterus into 4 quadrants by the midline and transverse axis at the level of umbilicus and measuring the deepest vertical pool free of fetal parts and umbilical cord. Measurements of all 4 quadrants are added to give AFI.[2] The normal AFI is 5–24 cm.
  - *DVP:* Measuring the single deepest vertical pocket gives the most accurate assessment of amniotic fluid volume (AFV). AFI has been reported to overestimate clinically insignificant oligohydramnios with the concern that it may lead to unnecessary interventions with no significant difference in outcome.[3] It is also useful in cases of multiple pregnancy, measuring DVP in each sac.
- *Dye dilution method:* It is an invasive method for determining the AFV and is usually used in research settings. A predetermined amount of dye is injected into the amniotic sac and after allowing time for its mixing and distribution, amniotic fluid is sampled for estimating dye concentration and volume of amniotic fluid is calculated.

## DISORDERS OF AMNIOTIC FLUID

### Incidence

Amniotic fluid derangements are classified as hydramnios (polyhydramnios) and oligohydramnios. Hydramnios occurs in 1–3.5% of all pregnancies. However, it is severe in only 5% of these disorders. The prevalence of oligohydramnios, defined as AFI < 5, is 8%; but it is only 1%, if criteria of DVP < 2 cm is considered.

# POLYHYDRAMNIOS

Polyhydramnios is defined as excess of liquor amnii in the amniotic cavity of a gravid uterus. It is suspected clinically and confirmed sonographically. It is defined as DVP of 8 cm or more, or an AFI of 24 cm or more or AFI greater than the 95th centile for a given gestational age.

Hydramnios is generally classified as mild, moderate and severe depending on the amount of liquor **(Table 1)** and is found in 65–70%, 20% and less than 15% of cases, respectively.[4]

Polyhydramnios may be acute or chronic in onset or a combination of both.

*Acute polyhydramnios:* Patients are usually symptomatic. It develops rapidly within a few days in mid-pregnancy (16–20 weeks) and is most commonly associated with monozygotic twin pregnancy with recipient twin-to-twin transfusion syndrome (RTTTS) and usually ends in preterm labor (PTL) at around 28 weeks.[5] Any other chromosomal or structural anomaly in the fetus should be ruled out in the second trimester itself.

*Chronic polyhydramnios:* It is more common than the acute form, develops in late pregnancy and is mostly idiopathic in origin. Accumulation of fluid occurs gradually, patient tolerates the excessive abdominal distention with relatively less discomfort and it usually does not require intervention.

## Etiology

Polyhydramnios, also called hydramnios, could be because of maternal, fetal or placental causes **(Flowchart 1)** but majority of cases of hydramnios are idiopathic. The likelihood of a fetal abnormality varies with degree of polyhydramnios, being 1%, 2% and 11%, in cases of mild, moderate and severe hydramnios, respectively.[6] Hydramnios may be because of impaired fetal swallowing, overproduction of fetal urine due to a high-output cardiac state, renal abnormality, or osmotic fetal diuresis.

Inability of fetus to swallow amniotic fluid may be due to various reasons such as tracheoesophageal fistula, duodenal atresia, pyloric stenosis and neuromuscular disorders like myotonic dystrophy etc.

Polyhydramnios presenting in late pregnancy is frequently associated with maternal uncontrolled diabetes and alloimmunization. Alloimmunization can cause fetal anemia leading to hydrops fetalis and polyhydramnios.

Congenital infections, such as parvovirus, cytomegalovirus or syphilis can cause polyhydramnios by a variety of mechanisms, including anemia or cardiac dysfunction.

It has also been postulated that polyhydramnios could be physiologic in cases where the fetus is large, as larger fetuses have higher urine output[4] and studies have reported that many cases of idiopathic polyhydramnios are associated with fetal weight of more than 4,000 g.[7]

## Complications Associated with Polyhydramnios

### Maternal Complications

*During pregnancy:* Maternal complications in polyhydramnios during pregnancy are usually due to over distention of uterus. Patients usually complain of discomfort and in severe cases, she may complain of dyspnea for which she has to adopt an upright posture to get relief. Pressure effects on major venous system give rise to edema of lower extremities, vulva and lower abdominal wall. Very rarely pressure on ureters can give rise to oliguria. Intra-amniotic pressure is markedly raised in women with severe polyhydramnios causing increased risk of preterm prelabor rupture of membranes and preterm labor. Other maternal complications include malpresentations and unstable lie leading to increased risk of cesarean section.

*During labor:* There is increased risk of malpresentations and rupture of membranes leading to cord prolapse. Rupture of membranes in polyhydramnios is associated with sudden decompression of uterine cavity which can cause severe abruptio placentae.[10]

There can be uterine inertia leading to dysfunctional labor. All these can result in increased incidence of cesarean section, atonic postpartum hemorrhage, retained placenta and shock.

### Fetal Complications

Increased perinatal morbidity and mortality associated with polyhydramnios is due to presence of congenital anomalies, preterm premature rupture of membranes or preterm delivery. Perinatal morbidity is directly related to the severity of polyhydramnios. Increased rates of newborn intensive care unit (NICU) admissions[11] and lower 5 minutes Apgar scores have been reported.[12]

Increased intra-amniotic pressure due to polyhydramnios adversely affects uteroplacental perfusion resulting in hypoxia and acidemia. This hypothesis is supported by the observation of increased blood flow after amnioreduction.

Fetal hypoxia may be secondary to cord prolapse and abruptio placentae.

**TABLE 1:** Types of hydramnios.[4]

| | Deepest vertical pocket | Amniotic fluid index |
|---|---|---|
| Mild hydramnios | 8–11 cm | 24–29.9 cm |
| Moderate hydramnios | 12–15 cm | 30–34.9 cm |
| Severe hydramnios | >15 cm | ≥35 cm |

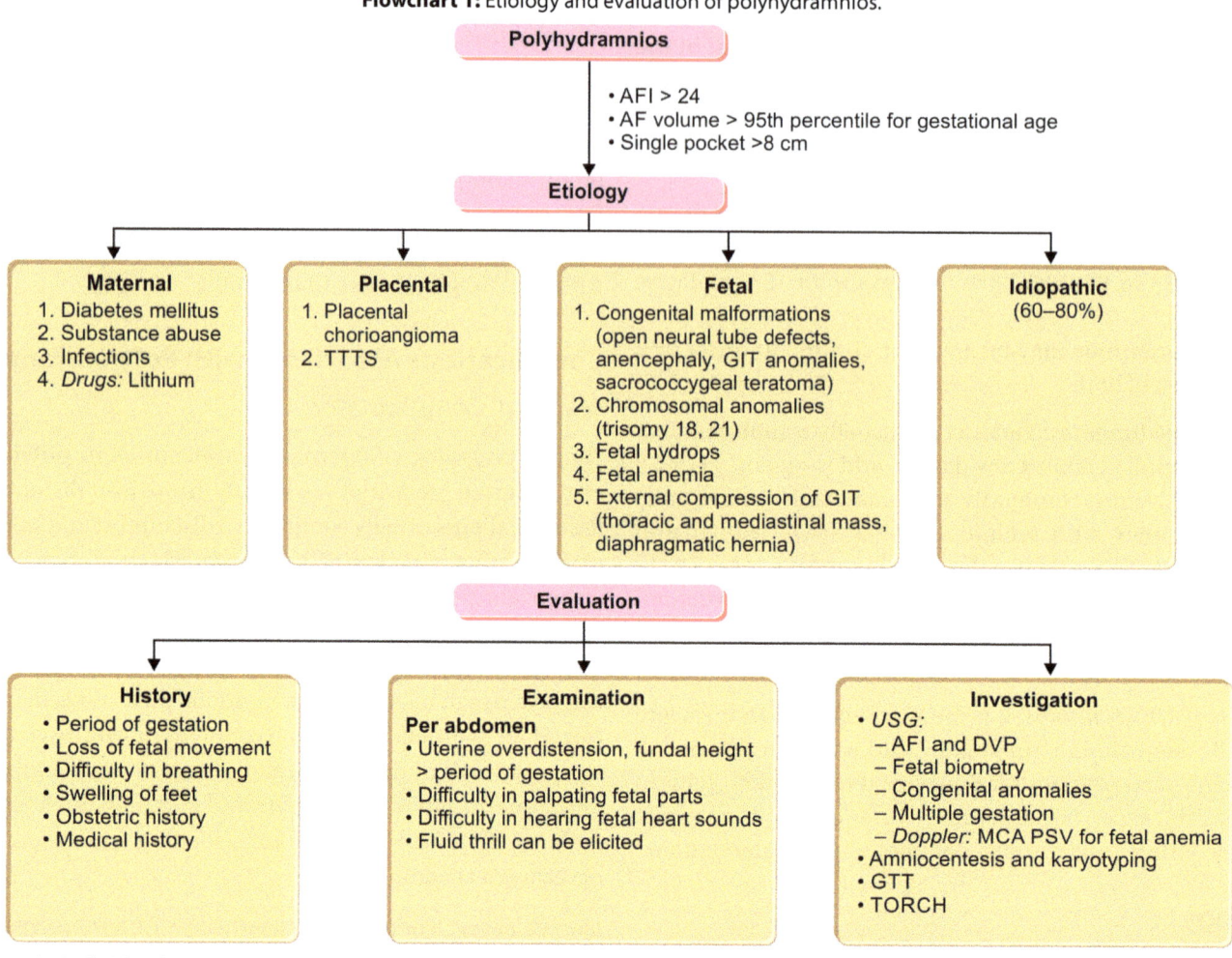

Flowchart 1: Etiology and evaluation of polyhydramnios.

(AFI: amniotic fluid index; DVP: deepest vertical pocket; GIT: gastrointestinal tract; GTT: glucose tolerance test; MCA: middle cerebral artery; PSV: peak systolic velocity; TORCH: toxoplasma, rubella, cytomegalovirus, herpes infection; TTTS: twin-to-twin transfusion syndrome; USG: ultrasonography)

## Diagnosis

The clinician must have a high index of suspicion in women with risk factors. Diagnosis is suspected on clinical findings of fundal height more than period of gestation (POG), difficulty in palpating fetal parts due to overdistended uterus and inability to hear fetal heart sounds. The diagnosis is confirmed on USG.

Differential diagnosis includes multiple pregnancy, macrosomia, etc.

## Investigations

*Ultrasound:*
- To confirm the diagnosis
- To assess degree of polyhydramnios
- Look for presence of multiple gestation
- Estimate the fetal weight
- Diagnose congenital fetal anomalies
- Study fetal bladder dynamics
- Do a guided amniocentesis for karyotyping and viral infections, if indicated.
- To see recipient bladder fullness in monochorionic twins in twin-to-twin transfusion syndrome (TTTS)

*Blood sugar estimation or glucose tolerance test (GTT):* It is indicated to rule out maternal diabetes.

*Serological studies:* For alloimmunization and for evidence of TORCH infection.

*Doppler study:*
- For middle cerebral artery peak systolic velocity (MCA-PSV) estimation in cases of suspected fetal anemia.
- For diagnosis and management of chorioangioma.
- For diagnosis of utero placental insufficiency.

Etiology and evaluation of polyhydramnios is depicted in **Flowchart 1**.

## Management

### Principles of Treatment of Polyhydramnios

- Relieve symptoms
- Prolong the pregnancy till fetal maturity

- To give appropriate treatment in cases of known etiologies.

*Mild polyhydramnios*
Expectant line of management with bed rest and monitoring is advocated. Resolution rate of approximately 37% has been reported in cases of idiopathic hydramnios diagnosed earlier in pregnancy and with lower mean AFV.[7]

*Moderate-to-severe polyhydramnios*
For progressive hydramnios re-evaluation should be done. Rescreening for diabetes may be done. Repeat sonography may reveal underlying fetal anomaly.

## Treating the Cause

Cases where the etiology is obvious, treatment is given to correct the condition responsible for polyhydramnios, e.g., polyhydramnios in cases of diabetes needs tight glycemic control.

Twin-to-twin transfusion syndrome may be treated by therapeutic amniocentesis or fetoscopic laser ablation of the communicating vessels.

For polyhydramnios associated with fetal hydrops secondary to fetal anemia, the direct intravascular transfusion of erythrocytes (or infusion into the fetal abdomen) may improve the fetal hematocrit and fetal congestive heart failure, thereby allowing prolongation of the pregnancy and improving survival. Many other intrauterine interventions for various congenital anomalies are under study.

Genetic counseling should be provided in cases of congenital fetal anomalies.

## Ultrasonography

Serial USG to monitor the AFV and document fetal growth may be required in cases of idiopathic polyhydramnios.

## Steroid Cover

Steroids to enhance fetal lung maturity are given if preterm delivery is anticipated. There is higher incidence of preterm labor secondary to overdistention of the uterus.

## Amnioreduction

Treatment is usually required during mid or early third trimester in these patients. Criteria for treatment are: AFI > 40 cm or DVP > 12 cm. It may be in the form of amnioreduction, either by drugs or invasive intervention.

*Medical Amnioreduction*

*Indomethacin:* It is a prostaglandin synthetase inhibitor, given in a dose of 50–200 mg per day. It antagonizes the antidiuretic effect of vasopressin on the collecting tubules of kidney and enhances proximal tubular reabsorption of water and sodium. This leads to decrease in urine output in fetus. It is usually discontinued by 32 weeks because of the associated neonatal morbidity in later gestation. Morbidity includes premature closure of ductus arteriosus, cerebral vasoconstriction in the fetus and impaired renal function.[13] As per SMFM (Society for Maternal-Fetal Medicine) guidelines it is not recommended for the sole purpose of decreasing amniotic fluid in polyhydramnios because of its side effects.[4]

*Invasive Amnioreduction*

It is done in moderate to severe polyhydramnios where patient is symptomatic. Informed consent is taken after counseling the patient about the procedure and its merits and demerits. A risk of 0.3% fetal loss due to chorioamnionitis and preterm labor is explained.

*Procedure:* After due aseptic precautions, an 18 gauge needle is inserted through the locally anesthetized abdominal wall under USG guidance avoiding placenta and lateral wall. Mid anterior uterine wall is selected for entering the uterine cavity. Confirmation of intra-amniotic needle tip location and membrane tenting is done by aspiration of an aliquot of amniotic fluid. Diagnostic sample is collected and sent for karyotyping. Next a three-way cannula is attached to the needle hub and slow aspiration or drainage of fluid is started at the rate of 500 mL per hour with the help of a 50 mL syringe or slow continuous drainage till the DVP or AFI is at the upper limit of normal. The continuous drainage of amniotic fluid is controlled with screw clamp. Anti-D is given to pregnant women who are Rh-negative. Nonstress test (NST) is done after the procedure if gestation is more than 26–28 weeks especially if it was complicated or the fetus was compromised. Serial amnioreduction is done if AFI is >40–45 cm or DVP goes >12 cm.

## Intrapartum Management

Tertiary level care with maternal-fetal medicine unit is preferable, not only in cases with fetal anomalies but also in those with idiopathic hydramnios because fetal anomaly may be detected after birth in some of these cases.

- Polyhydramnios may be associated with abnormal presentation.[14] Ultrasonography is indicated if clinically malpresentation is suspected. External version, if not contraindicated, may be performed for transverse lie or breech presentation.
- Careful monitoring is required during labor as dysfunctional labor is common in polyhydramnios.[15]
- Sudden rupture of membranes may cause abruptio placenta. "Controlled" amniotomy is performed especially in moderate to severe hydramnios using a spinal or pudendal block needle and allowing liquor amnii to flow out slowly.[4] Fixing the head at pelvic brim

by an assistant, abdominally, helps to prevent cord prolapse.

- Non-reassuring fetal heart rate tracings have been reported to be more frequent with polyhydramnios, hence careful fetal monitoring is to be done. An increased risk of operative vaginal delivery in the presence of polyhydramnios has also been reported.[15]
- Even in the absence of diabetes, idiopathic polyhydramnios is reported to be associated with macrosomia in approximately 15-30% of cases leading to higher risk of cesarean.[4]

## Postpartum Management

There is increased risk for postpartum hemorrhage even in the presence of mild polyhydramnios. Active management of third stage of labor, careful watch for uterine atony and postpartum hemorrhage should be maintained. Blood and blood products should be available.

## Neonatal Care

Specialized neonatal care may be required even in cases labeled as "idiopathic" polyhydramnios as structural abnormalities or genetic syndromes may be detected in the neonate. Transient tachypnea of the newborn is also common in polyhydramnios. Admission to NICU may be required.

## ■ OLIGOHYDRAMNIOS

### Definition

Oligohydramnios is defined as AFV below the 5th percentile for gestational age. More commonly in clinical practice, sonographic assessment of AFI, which is an integral part of biophysical profile, of less than 5 cm is used as a criteria to label patients as having oligohydramnios. A DVP of less than 2 cm also constitutes oligohydramnios

### Etiology

Oligohydramnios can be due to maternal or fetal causes, which are shown in **Flowchart 2**. Basic mechanism of amniotic fluid production in early gestation differs from that in the later period. In early gestation before the establishment of fetal urine production and fetal swallowing, the most important mechanism of amniotic fluid maintenance in the amniotic sac is passive movement of water down the solute gradient. After 17-18 weeks, fetal urine production and later respiratory secretion of fluids are major sources of amniotic fluid. Therefore, even in congenital absence of fetal kidneys, AFV may appear normal before 17 weeks.

A study by Manning et al. demonstrated decreased AFV in fetal growth restriction.[16]

Earlier studies were suggestive of chronic fetal hypoxia due to placental insufficiency to be the cause of oligohydramnios, consequent to reduced urine output and reduced renal perfusion with brain sparing effect. Studies by Brace show that placental insufficiency may be a cause of increased intramembranous absorption of water into fetal and maternal vascular compartment, rather than reduced fetal urinary output.[1]

Oligohydramnios can be early onset or late onset. Early onset oligohydramnios occurs in early mid-trimester and congenital anomalies are mainly responsible. Congenital renal anomalies account for 33-51% cases and include bilateral renal agenesis, bilateral multicystic kidneys, infantile polycystic kidney disease and lower urinary tract obstruction like posterior urethral valves. Chromosomal anomalies such as aneuploidy (4%) cause symmetrical early onset fetal growth restriction (FGR) with severe oligohydramnios. Congenital toxoplasma, rubella and CMV infection also cause severe FGR.

Late onset oligohydramnios is due to term prelabor rupture of membranes and complicates 3-17% of term pregnancies. Other causes include late onset fetal growth restriction (FGR), post-maturity and prolonged use of maternal medications such as indomethacin, sulindac, ACE inhibitors and angiotensin-receptor blockers.

The etiology and evaluation of oligohydramnios is depicted in **Flowchart 2**.

### Complications

#### Maternal

Oligohydramnios per se is asymptomatic in the mother. Underlying causes of oligohydramnios such as preeclampsia, PPROM and increased rate of cesarean deliveries and intrauterine deaths may adversely affect maternal health.

#### Fetal

Pulmonary hypoplasia and skeletal deformities are two important complications of oligohydramnios and are known as oligohydramnios deformation syndrome or oligohydramnios sequence.

Renal malformation, with oligohydramnios, was found in 25%, of autopsies.[17]

Severe oligohydramnios for more than 14 days after premature rupture of membranes at less than 25 weeks' gestation was found to have a high neonatal mortality.[18]

The crucial canalicular phase of lung development occurs around 16-25 weeks of pregnancy. Therefore, the severity of development of pulmonary hypoplasia is related to the gestational age. Patients with earlier onset of oligohydramnios have more severe hypoplasia. Further, hypoplasia also depends upon severity and duration of oligohydramnios.[19]

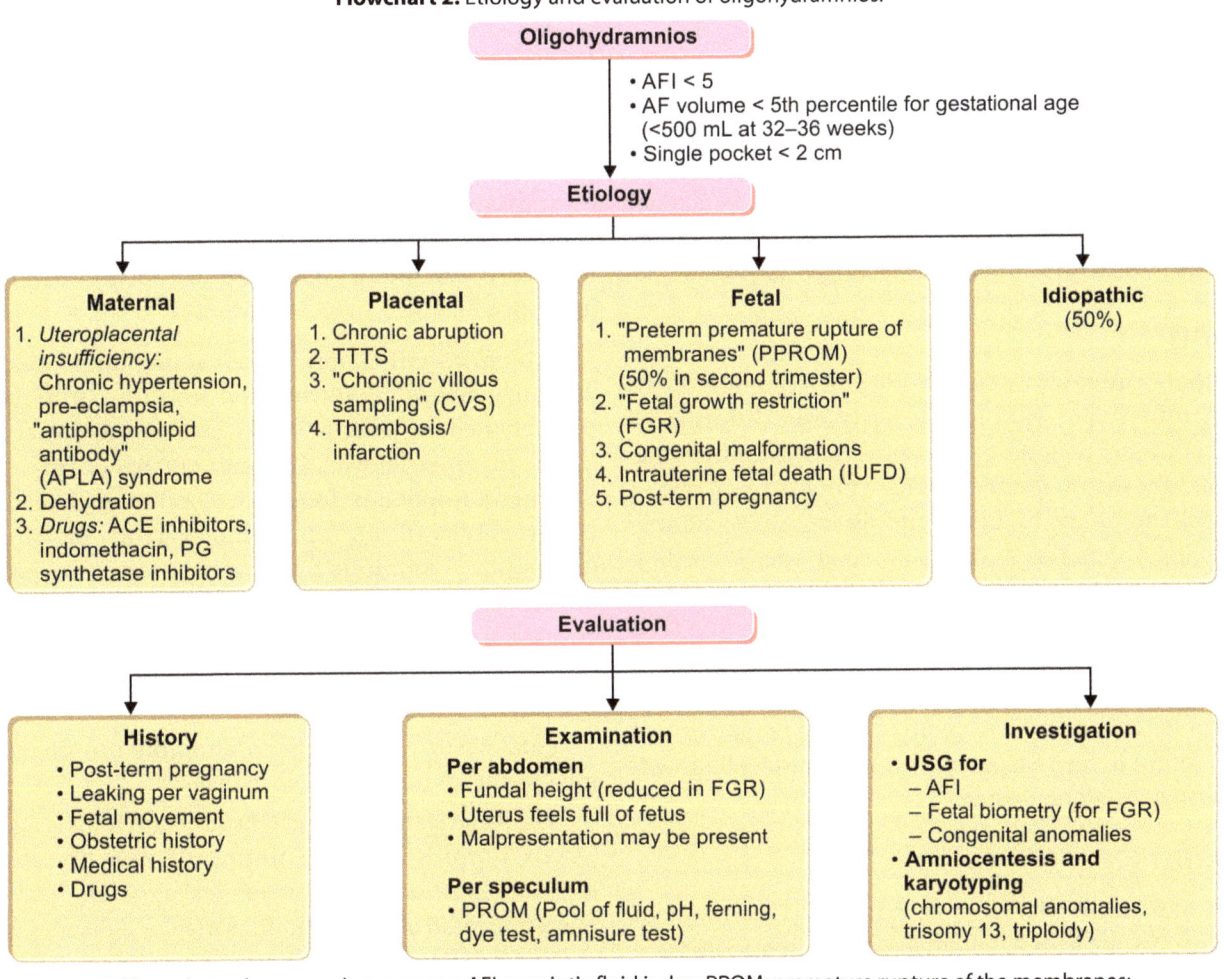

Flowchart 2: Etiology and evaluation of oligohydramnios.

(ACE: angiotensin-converting-enzyme; AFI: amniotic fluid index; PROM: premature rupture of the membranes; TTTS: twin-to-twin transfusion syndrome; USG: ultrasonogrphy)

It results from thoracic compression which may prevent chest wall excursion and lung expansion, loss of fetal breathing, reduced lung inflow, failure to retain amniotic fluid outflow by impaired lung growth.

Various skeletal deformities are seen secondary to oligohydramnios, e.g., talipes equinovarus, curved lower limbs, spinal deformity, etc. The severity depends upon the duration of oligohydramnios. It occurs as a result of adhesion of fetal surface with amniotic membrane following uterine pressure, less intrauterine space and lack of cushioning effect of amniotic fluid. Risk of low birth weight babies is up to 13%. Perinatal mortality is increased specially in cases of PPROM with gestational age less than 29 weeks. Newborn survival rate can be improved with better obstetric and neonatal care.

## Diagnosis

### History

Correct diagnosis of oligohydramnios is essential for optimal outcome.

History of passage of gush of clear fluid per vaginum followed by persistent leak is suggestive of PROM. Any history of infections (TORCH) in early pregnancy, drug intake, smoking, alcoholism, heart disease, type I diabetes with history of vascular involvement, lupus erythematosus, any past history of stillbirth, recurrent abortions or mid-trimester loss should be elicited.

### Symptoms and Signs

There may be no specific symptoms except those due to complicating features. On abdominal palpation uterine height may appear less than period of gestation. Uterus may feel full of fetus. Malpresentation is more common in these cases.

### Investigations

Ultrasound is indicated to confirm the diagnosis and its severity, further investigations are done to find out the possible etiology. USG level II is indicated to diagnose various congenital anomalies such as bilateral renal agenesis, lower urinary tract obstruction (LUTO) and infantile polycystic kidneys.[16]

Demonstration of early symmetrical IUGR indicates possibility of chromosomal abnormalities such as trisomy 18 and aneuploidy. Hourly filling and emptying of bladder excludes presence of renal agenesis.

The various tests done are maternal serology for toxoplasma, rubella, CMV and herpes simplex (TORCH) infections, antiphospholipid antibody (APA), lupus-anticoagulant antibody (LAC). Doppler study is done to diagnose placental insufficiency and visualize the fetal renal arteries. Karyotyping and diagnostic amniocentesis is done to rule out chromosomal anomalies and congenital infections.

## Prognosis

The ultimate prognosis depends on the gestational age at onset, underlying etiology, severity and duration of oligohydramnios. Second trimester oligohydramnios has 50% chances of major anomalies with a poor survival rate of 10%. Oligohydramnios in third trimester have 22% chances of congenital anomalies and 85% survival rate. According to Chamberlain et al., in absence of anomalies, perinatal mortality rate is 10.9% when DVP < 1 cm and 3.8% when DVP is <2 cm. Isolated oligohydramnios in the absence of PROM, congenital abnormalities and maternal comorbidities such as diabetes and hypertension has an excellent prognosis and not been found to be associated with impaired fetal growth and adverse perinatal outcome.[20]

## Treatment

Bed rest and limited activity is advised. Treatment of underlying etiology with a definitive treatment option, such as in pregnancy-induced hypertension (PIH), is initiated. Patients with suspected FGR are monitored with enhanced fetal surveillance in form of daily fetal movement count, biophysical profile and umbilical artery Doppler flow studies. Glucocorticoids are administered where premature termination is anticipated as in severe FGR. Either 2 doses of 12 mg betamethasone 24 hours apart or 4 doses of injection dexamethasone, 6 mg each every 12 hourly for 48 hours is given. Elective induction at 36 weeks is recommended; earlier intervention is indicated if NST is not reassuring and when there is absent or reversal of end diastolic flow in umbilical artery.

In PPROM, a close watch is kept for early detection of signs and symptoms of chorioamnionitis. Prophylactic antibiotics are started in PPROM. Maternal hydration is suggested to improve AFV. Drinking of 2 liters of fluid before USG in patients with normal pregnancy and oligohydramnios, increases the AFI by 2.01 cm. This short-term improvement in AFI can continue long-term if maternal hydration is continued at the rate of 2 liters per day for a week.[21]

A recent systematic-literature-review and meta-analysis to evaluate efficacy of maternal hydration in cases of isolated oligohydramnios concluded that maternal oral hydration was effective in improving AFV but its effect on perinatal outcome was not found to be very clear.[22]

Serial amnioinfusion have been used to prevent pulmonary hypoplasia in selected euploid fetuses with functioning renal tissue to improve outcome. However, most patients with mid-trimester PPROM are unsuitable as fluid leaks out immediately.[23] A systematic review and meta-analysis of randomized and observational studies on transabdominal amnioinfusion for premature preterm rupture of membranes found that serial amnioinfusion increased the latency period and reduced the perinatal mortality.[24]

*Amnioinfusion:* It is done under sonographic guidance. A 20 gauge needle is introduced into the amniotic cavity through the mid-anterior uterine wall avoiding placenta and lateral myometrial wall. Infusion of 0.9% normal saline or Hartman's solution is done with 50 mL syringe till the AFI is 20 cm or DVP of 6 cm. Concomitant karyotyping can be done on the initial amniotic fluid aspirate. After the procedure, umbilical artery flow is checked by Doppler and pads are checked for leaking. Repeat amnioinfusion is done at weekly intervals. NST is performed if the fetus is beyond period of viability.

Fetal cystoscopy has been attempted to diagnose and treat posterior urethral valve with laser.

The American College of Obstetricians and Gynecologists (ACOG) states that the timing of delivery should be individualized based on the clinical situation. Isolated and uncomplicated oligohydramnios may be delivered at 36–37$^{+6}$ or later, if diagnosed later.[25]

## ■ KEY POINTS

- Earliest detection of amniotic fluid occurs by 8 weeks.
- AFV is 30 mL at 10 weeks, 190 mL at 16 weeks and level gradually increases to peak volume of 800–1,000 mL at 32–35 weeks. Thereafter, it declines to 550 mL by 42 weeks.
- Transudation from maternal plasma is the source during early gestation but beyond 17 weeks fetal urination and lung secretions are the main sources.
- Polyhydramnios is sonographically defined as AFI of >25 cm or DVP of > 8 cm.
- Hydramnios occurs in 1–3.5% of pregnancies and is severe in 5% of cases. Majority of cases are idiopathic. In severe cases 80% have a known underlying etiology such as congenital fetal anomalies, diabetes mellitus, lithium therapy and substance abuse.
- Fetal abnormalities are associated in 1%, 2% and 11% of cases of mild, moderate and severe polyhydramnios, respectively.
- Maternal complications are due to uterine overdistention and major venous system compression.
- Fetal complications include spontaneous preterm birth in 22% of cases.

- Direct method of assessment like dye dilution methods are cumbersome and not routinely used. Ultrasonography is the main modality of assessment.
- In moderate to severe cases, amnioreduction by either drugs or invasive intervention is required.
- Oligohydramnios is sonographically defined as AFI of < 5 cm or DVP of < 2 cm.
- Early onset oligohydramnios is usually due to PPROM and congenital anomalies. Late onset is due to term PROM, late onset FGR and postmaturity.
- Investigations include ultrasonography and serological studies for alloimmunization and congenital infections.
- Ultrasonography helps to assess degree of oligohydramnios, presence of FGR, fetal and uterine blood flow studies and presence of fetal anomalies.
- Pulmonary hypoplasia and skeletal deformities are two important complications of oligohydramnios.
- Management involves treating the cause, increased surveillance, maternal hydration, amnioinfusion and delivery, if fetal or maternal condition indicates.

## REFERENCES

1. Brace RA. Amniotic fluid dynamics. In: Creasy RK, Resnik R (Eds). Maternal Fetal Medicine: Principles and Practice. Philadelphia: Elsevier; 2004. pp. 45-54.
2. Moor TR. Superiority of the four quadrant sum over the single deepest pocket technique in ultrasonographic identification of abnormal amniotic fluid volume. Am J Obstet Gynaecol. 1990;163(3):762-7.
3. Magann EF, Chauhan SP, Doherty DA, Magann MI, Morrison JC. The evidence for abandoning the amniotic fluid index in favor of the single deepest pocket. Am J Perinatal. 2007;24(09):549-55.
4. Dashe JS, Pressman EK, Hibbard JU. Evaluation and management of polyhydramnios. Society for Maternal-Fetal Medicine Consult series #46. Am J Obstet Gynecol. 2018;219(4):B2-B8.
5. Duncan KR, Denbow M, Fisk NM. The etiology and management of twin to twin transfusion syndrome: prenatal diagnosis. 1997;17:1227-36.
6. Dashe JS, McIntiro DD Ramus RM. Hydramnios: anomaly prevalence and sonographic detection. Obstet Gynecol. 2002;100:134-9.
7. Odibo IN, Newville TM, Ounpraseuth ST, Dixon M, Lutgendorf MA, Foglia LM, et al. Idiopathic polyhydramnios: persistence across gestation and impact on pregnancy outcomes. Eur J Obstet Gynecol Reprod Biol. 2016;199:175-8.
8. Vink JY, Poggi SH, Ghidini A, Spong CY. Amniotic fluid index and birth weight: is there a relationship in diabetic with poor glycemic control? Am J Obstet Gynaecol. 2006;195:848-50.
9. Ang MS, Thorp JA, Parisi VM. Maternal lithium therapy and polyhydramnios. Obstet Gynaecol. 1990;76:517-9.
10. Khazaei S, Jenabi E. The association between polyhydramnios and the risk of placenta abruption: a meta-analysis. J Matern Fetal Neonatal Med. 2020;33(17):3035-40.
11. Khan S, Donnelly J. Outcome of pregnancy in women diagnosed with idiopathic polyhydramnios. Aust N Z J Obstet Gynaecol. 2017;57(1):57-62.
12. Luo QQ, Zou L, Gao H, Zheng YF, Zhao Y, Zhang WY. Idiopathic polyhydramnios at term and pregnancy outcomes: a multicenter observational study. J Matern Fetal Neonatal Med. 2017;30(14):1755-9.
13. Mamopoulos M, Assimakopoulos E, Reece EA, Andreou A, Zheng XZ, Mantalenakis S. Maternal indomethacin therapy in the treatment of polyhydramnios. Am J Obstet Gynecol. 1990;162(5):1225-9.
14. Panting-Kemp A, Nguyen T, Chang E, Quillen E, Castro L. Idiopathic polyhydramnios and perinatal outcome. Am J Obstet Gynecol. 1999;181(5 Pt 1):1079-82.
15. Aviram A, Salzer L, Hiersch L, Ashwal E, Golan G, Pardo J, et al. Association of isolated polyhydramnios at or beyond 34 weeks of gestation and pregnancy outcome. Obstet Gynecol. 2015;125:825-32.
16. Manning FA, Hill LM, Platt LD. Qualitative amniotic fluid volume determination by ultrasound: antepartum detection of intrauterine growth retardation. Am J Obstet Gynaecol. 1981;139(3):254-8.
18. Kilbride HW, Yeast J, Thibeault DW. Defining limits of survival: lethal pulmonary hypoplasia after midtrimester rupture of membrane. Am J Obstet Gynaecol. 1996;175(3Pt 1):675-81.
19. Chauhan SP, Sanderson M, Hendrix NW, Magann EF, Devoe LD, et al. Perinatal outcome and AFI in antepartum and intrapartum periods: a meta-analysis. Am J Obstet Gynaecol. 1999;181(6):1473-8.
20. Zhang J, Troendle J, Meikle S, Klebanoff MA, Rayburn WF. Isolated oligohydramnios is not associated with adverse perinatal outcomes. BJOG. 2004;111(3):220-5.
21. Kilpatick SJ, Safford KL, Pomeroy T, Hoedt L, Scheerer L, Laros RK. Maternal hydration increases amniotic fluid index. Obstet Gynaecol. 1991;78(6):1098-102.
22. Gizzo S, Noventa M, Vitagliano A, Dall'Asta A, D'Antona D, Aldrich CJ, et al. An update on maternal hydration strategies for amniotic fluid improvement in isolated oligohydramnios and normohydramnios: evidence from a systematic review of literature and meta-analysis. PLoS One. 2015;10(12): e0144334.
23. Fisk NM, Ronderos-Dumit D, Soliani A, Vaughan J, Rodeck CH. Diagnostic and therapeutic transabdominal amnioinfusion in oligohydramnios. Obstet Gynaecol. 1991;78(2):270-8.
24. Porat S, Amsalem H, Shah PS, Murphy KE. Transabdominal amnioinfusion for premature preterm rupture of membranes: a systematic review and meta-analysis of randomized and observational studies. Am J Obstet Gynecol. 2012;207:393.
25. ACOG. ACOG Committee Opinion No. 764: Medically indicated late-preterm and early-term deliveries. Obstet Gynecol. 2019;133(2):e151.

# CHAPTER 10

# Preterm Labor

*Kanika Chopra, Monika Bhatia, Shubha Sagar Trivedi*

## ■ INTRODUCTION

Preterm birth complicates 10–15% of all pregnancies and is a leading cause of neonatal morbidity and mortality.[1] More than 60% burden worldwide is from South East Asian and sub-Saharan African countries.[1] Idiopathic preterm labor accounts for about 40% of all preterm births, 35% of preterm births follow preterm prelabor rupture of membranes (PPROM), and around 25% are iatrogenic because of obstetric or medical complications of pregnancy. Preterm delivery can be associated with immediate and long-term neonatal complications such as respiratory distress syndrome, intraventricular hemorrhage, apnea, necrotizing enterocolitis, retinopathy of prematurity as well as long-term disabilities including mental retardation, cerebral palsy, chronic lung disease, gastrointestinal problems, vision and hearing loss, and poor neurodevelopment outcomes. The neonatal outcome is dependent on the gestational age at delivery and associated complications such as infection. The lower the gestational age, higher the risk of mortality and morbidity. The management of preterm labor involves identification of high-risk women, prevention, and treatment.

Preterm labor is defined as onset of regular uterine contractions after the period of viability but prior to completed 37 weeks of pregnancy which leads to progressive cervical change. Usually <10% of women with a clinical diagnosis of preterm labor deliver within a week of presentation.[2]

Onset of preterm labor is usually determined by clinical criteria which include uterine contractions occurring at a frequency of 4 in 20 minutes or 8 in 60 minutes accompanied by progressive change in cervical dilatation and/or effacement; or at the initial presentation, there are regular contractions and cervical dilation of at least 2 cm.[2,3]

Threatened preterm labor may be diagnosed when there are documented uterine contractions but no evidence of cervical change.

Though, the survival rates for preterm babies have improved over the last decade because of better neonatal facilities, every effort should be made to inhibit preterm labor after careful patient selection, which may allow time for in utero transfer of a pregnancy at risk to an appropriate tertiary referral center, administration of glucocorticosteroids and antibiotic prophylaxis to reduce the risk of neonatal sepsis where required.

## ■ ETIOPATHOGENESIS

The etiopathogenesis of preterm labor is not well-understood, it is often not clear whether preterm labor represents early idiopathic activation of the normal labor process or results from a pathologic mechanism. The underlying biochemical and hormonal mechanisms of parturition are quite complex and intricate. The process is heralded by an increase in myometrial gap junctions, oxytocin receptors, enhanced myometrial contractile efficiency, and changes in cervical collagens and matrix. This complex cascade results in contractions, effacement of the cervix, and ultimately expulsion of the fetus. Several theories are proposed regarding the initiation of labor.[3]

### Activation of Hypothalamic Pituitary Axis

As parturition nears, the fetal-adrenal axis becomes more sensitive to adrenocorticotropic hormone, increasing the secretion of cortisol. Both fetal and maternal stress can lead to early activation of the axis. Maternal stress could be due to environmental factors and medical conditions such as hypertension, renal disease, heart disease, etc. Fetal stress may be associated with growth restriction and abnormal placentation. Cortisol stimulates corticotropin-releasing hormone (CRH) release in the decidua, trophoblast, and membranes which in turn activates the maternal and fetal hypothalamic-pituitary axis (HPA). Cortisol then stimulates trophoblast 17α-hydroxylase activity, which decreases progesterone secretion and leads to a subsequent increase in estrogen production. This reversal in the estrogen/progesterone ratio results in increased prostaglandin formation, initiating a cascade of events that culminate in labor and subsequent delivery. Although, this mechanism is well-documented in sheep, its role in humans has not been confirmed.

## Pathologic Uterine Overdistention

The stretching of myometrium as in multiple gestation and polyhydramnios causes formation of gap junctions leading to upregulation of oxytocin receptors and production of prostaglandins, which leads to cervical ripening and uterine contractions.[4]

## Decidual Hemorrhage

Vaginal bleeding in placenta previa and abruptio placentae can predispose to preterm birth. Following decidual hemorrhage, tissue factor is released which interacts with various hemostatic factors to generate thrombin which in turn binds to the decidual membrane receptors upregulating the expression of proteases and metalloproteinases leading to cervical ripening and uterine contractions.

## Inflammation/Infection

Microbiological studies suggest that intrauterine infection might account for 25–40% of preterm births.[5] Clinical and subclinical chorioamnionitis have been found to be more common in preterm than in term pregnancies. It has been shown that there is overgrowth of potential pathogens in the vagina or cervix associated with bacterial vaginosis and the most commonly isolated organisms include *Ureaplasma urealyticum, Fusobacterium,* and *Mycoplasma hominis.* Following amnio-chorionic decidual infection, activated macrophages and granulocytes release proinflammatory substances such as cytokines and matrix metalloproteinases. These in turn stimulate prostaglandin production and ripen the cervix triggering preterm labor. In addition, some organisms directly produce proteases, collagenases, elastases, and phospholipase A2 which can degrade the fetal membranes and stimulate uterine contractions.

## Abnormal Cervical Function

The function of cervix is to retain the pregnancy within the uterus and to prevent ascent of potential bacterial pathogens from vagina. It has been shown that cervical length,[6] strength, and quality of cervical mucus contribute toward this function. Conditions such as diethylstilbestrol (DES) exposure in utero, congenital anomalies in the genital tract (bicornuate, subseptate or unicornuate uterus), previous cervical surgery (conization of cervix), and cervical incompetence lead to cervical weakness hampering normal functioning.

## ▮ PREDICTION

Prediction is the first step toward prevention. Hence, prediction of preterm labor is important. The aim of prediction is firstly to identify those asymptomatic women who are at high-risk of preterm labor. Secondly, to determine the risk of delivery within the next 7 days in symptomatic women who present with threatened preterm labor so that appropriate and timely intervention can be done. Any method used to predict labor should be safe, sensitive, specific, and preferably inexpensive. While such an ideal method still eludes the medical community, the various methods that are being used presently are discussed here.

## Risk Scoring

To identify the women who are at high-risk of preterm labor "risk score" is calculated. The demographic profile of preterm labor has been used as a basis for the evolution of various scoring systems. Various parameters such as maternal age, race, educational status, social status, marital status, smoking, cocaine use, prepregnancy weight, and weight gain during pregnancy are taken into account for predicting preterm labor. While the clinical validity of risk scoring systems is still debatable, it is important to recognize that some of these factors such as smoking are preventable and alerts the obstetrician to the possibility of preterm labor. Some of the important risk factors associated with preterm delivery are highlighted in **Box 1**. History of one preterm birth is associated with a recurrence risk of 20%, ranging from 15.8 to 30%.[7] The risk of preterm labor is also increased in women who have experienced one or more second trimester abortions.

## Home Uterine Activity Monitoring

It has been shown that women destined to develop preterm labor show an increase in the frequency of uterine contractions at least a week in advance.

This increased frequency, however, is not perceived by the women. Ambulatory home uterine activity monitoring was introduced with the intention of recording this increased frequency and initiating therapeutic intervention before the actual onset of preterm labor.

> **BOX 1:** Risk factors associated with preterm delivery.
>
> - Maternal age (<20 years or >40 years)
> - History of preterm delivery (increased risk of 1.5–2 times)
> - Multiple pregnancy
> - Polyhydramnios/oligohydramnios
> - Previous cervical conization or loop electrosurgical excision procedure
> - Shortened length of cervix of <25 mm before 28 weeks of gestation
> - Vaginal bleeding specially after first trimester
> - Premature rupture of membranes
> - Bacterial vaginosis
> - Intrauterine infection
> - Urinary/genital tract infection
> - Periodontal disease
> - Cocaine/heroin use/smoking
> - Short interpregnancy interval
> - In vitro fertilization (IVF)
> - Intra-abdominal surgery
> - Low prepregnancy weight (<19.8 kg/m$^2$)
> - Overweight/obesity

This system provides for the recording of uterine activity. It consists of a patient unit and a practitioner unit. The patient unit consists of light weight external pressure device or sensor based on the guard ring principle, a transmission device, and a recorder. The recorder can store uterine activity data up to 3 hours. Transmission occurs through a telephone to the obstetrician's unit.

The baseline tone is 0 mm Hg and the peak deviation from the baseline tone is considered proportional to intensity. Contractions with duration of 35 seconds or longer and with an amplitude of >5 mm Hg are considered significant.

Until the 30th week of pregnancy, 1 contraction/hour in primi and 2 contractions/hour in multigravida are accepted as normal. Beyond 30th week usually 2 contractions/hour are normal. More than 3 contractions/hour between 26 and 28 weeks and >5 contractions/hour between 30 and 32 weeks are considered to be predictive of preterm labor and an indication for therapeutic intervention.

As with all other predictors of preterm labor, the clinical validity of this method is also open to debate. While some authorities strongly advocate it and show improved neonatal outcomes when therapeutic interventions are initiated on the basis of home uterine monitoring, others argue that there has been no significant decrease in the incidence of preterm births and the benefit is mainly due to close nursing supervision and remarkable patient education and there is no real need for such an expensive form of screening.

## Biochemical Markers

Various biochemical markers have been advocated to predict preterm labor. These are currently under study:
- Salivary estriol to progesterone ratio
- Salivary estriol
- Serum collagenase
- Neutrophil collagenase
- Tissue inhibitor of metalloproteinase (TIMP)
- Serum relaxin
- Corticotropin releasing hormone.

## Mediators of Inflammation and Infection

It has been postulated that infection predisposes to preterm labor. Hence, an attempt has been made to detect the mediators of inflammation and infection and their association with preterm labor. Cervical interleukin-6 (IL-6) and tumor necrosis factor (TNF) levels have been correlated with the risk of preterm delivery. However, most of these mediators have been shown to be of no practical help in predicting preterm labor.

## Cervical Assessment

Cervical length in the general obstetrical population is relatively stable over the first two trimesters. The natural history of cervical length change may be useful in identifying women at increased risk of spontaneous preterm birth. Serial assessment of cervical length is useful to detct the changes in cervix.

It is proposed that full bladder may falsely elongate the cervix and precise anatomic landmarks of internal and external os are difficult to visualize, so some authorities recommend scanning the woman with both full and empty bladder. Endovaginal ultrasound is the preferred option as compared to transabdominal examination. Shortening of the cervix (< 25 mm), widening of endocervical canal, thinning of lower uterine segment, and bulging of membranes in the endocervical canal are predictive of preterm labor. Transperineal cervical sonography has recently been advocated and has the advantage of avoiding vaginal instrumentation.

Thus, cervical length measurement can be used to identify increased risk of preterm birth in high-risk asymptomatic women at <24 weeks. However, because of poor positive predictive value and sensitivity and lack of proven effective interventions, routine transvaginal cervical length assessment is not recommended in asymptomatic high-risk women beyond 24 weeks and in asymptomatic women at low-risk.

In women presenting with suspected preterm labor, transvaginal sonographic assessment of cervical length may be useful in determining who is at high-risk of preterm delivery and may be helpful in preventing unnecessary intervention. It is unclear whether this information results in a reduced risk of preterm birth.[8]

## Cervicovaginal Fibronectin

A relatively new method proposed for the screening of preterm labor is the assessment of fetal fibronectin (FFN) in the cervicovaginal secretions in symptomatic women with preterm labor between 24- and 36-weeks' gestation with intact membranes and cervical dilatation <3 cm to assess the risk of preterm delivery within the next 7 days. Fibronectin is a glycoprotein produced by fetal amnion, hepatocytes, malignant cells, fibroblasts, and endothelial cells. It is present in high concentration in maternal blood and amniotic fluid. FFN can be detected in vaginal secretions just prior to onset of labor and appears to reflect stromal remodeling of cervix prior to labor. It is detected by enzyme-linked immunosorbent assay (ELISA) and a value of >50 ng/mL is considered to be a positive result. False positive result may occur due to bleeding, digital examination, vaginal ultrasound or intercourse. Lubricant on speculum may give false negative result.

Increased levels are associated with increased risk of preterm labor in both low- and high-risk women and is considered to be the most effective predictors of preterm labor.[9] A negative test suggests low-risk of delivery within 7 days.

A recent Cochrane review concluded that management based on knowledge of FFN results may reduce preterm birth before 37 weeks (20.7%) versus controls without such knowledge (29.2%) but may make little or no difference to preterm birth before 34 weeks or maternal hospitalization.[10]

## PREVENTION

The identification of women at high-risk of preterm delivery remains a major challenge. Most of the methods discussed have shown a suboptimal correlation with subsequent preterm birth. This is primarily because the single greatest risk factor is a history of preterm labor, so delivery cannot be reliably predicted in the first pregnancy. Thus, in clinical practice, the determination of risk, therefore, tends to be based on obstetric history and management restricted to avoidance of certain factors, identification and treatment of bacterial vaginosis, using progesterone or cervical cerclage for asymptomatic high-risk women.

For symptomatic women who present with threatened preterm labor, FFN and cervical length are indicators of the risk of preterm delivery, and provide guidance to subsequent change in management such as use of steroids and tocolysis.

### Prepregnancy Initiative

Ideally, prepregnancy counseling should be done in all women. Not only preterm labor but a variety of other obstetrical problems can be markedly reduced by prepregnancy counseling. Childbearing at right age, adequate spacing between pregnancies, avoidance of multiple medical termination of pregnancy (MTP), and avoidance of smoking are some of the measures that can be initiated. Optimization of weight in cases of overweight and obese women prior to pregnancy by structured diet plan and exercise can also help by preventing preterm birth.[11]

As association has been found between in vitro fertilization (IVF) and preterm labor as well, it is considered that IVF should be performed carefully in patients with other high-risks for preterm labor. Also, single embryo transfer is considered better than multiple embryo transfer.[12]

### Patient Education

Education of patient is of utmost importance. All women should be adequately counseled regarding the risk of preterm labor and to seek early medical care if warning signs and symptoms of preterm labor in the form of low dull backache, menstrual like cramps, increase in vaginal discharge or uterine contractions develop.

### Behavioral Alteration

In patients who are at high-risk for preterm labor some of the further given measures would be beneficial.

- Limitation of physical activity
- Coital abstinence
- Cessation of smoking.

### Treatment of Infection

Bacterial vaginosis is a polymicrobial condition associated with preterm delivery. It is not yet clear whether low-risk women should be screened and treated as various studies have shown conflicting results. In a meta-analysis of 2011, it was found that treatment of symptomatic bacterial vaginosis with clindamycin was shown to decrease the risk of preterm labor.[13] In contrast, a Cochrane review of 2013, showed no effect of treatment of asymptomatic bacterial vaginosis in decreasing preterm birth before 37 weeks.[14]

Given the evidence available, it seems reasonable to screen women for bacterial vaginosis if they are at high-risk of preterm delivery. Treatment should be given to those in whom a diagnosis is made. Systemic metronidazole or topical clindamycin are the mainstay of treatment.

Asymptomatic bacteriuria is associated with preterm birth, so screening and its treatment is of value in preventing preterm birth.

### Cervical Cerclage

This form of treatment is mainly helpful for patients with cervical incompetence. It has also been used by some authorities for prevention of preterm birth. A recent Royal College of Obstetricians and Gynaecologists (RCOG) guideline recommends cervical cerclage for women with singleton pregnancy who have a previous history of preterm birth and a cervical length of 25 mm or less before 24 weeks of pregnancy. It is recommended between 16 and 24 weeks of pregnancy.[15]

### Progesterone Therapy

It is well-known that progesterone promotes and maintains pregnancy in women. Administration of progesterone for the prevention of preterm labor has therefore been investigated in recent clinical trials especially for women at high-risk of preterm labor. Both 17α-hydroxyprogesterone caproate (17-OHP) and natural vaginal progesterone have been reported to considerably reduce the risk of early delivery in high-risk women. The group of women who benefit most from 17-OHP supplementation are those who have experienced a prior spontaneous preterm birth <34 weeks. Progesterone supplementation should generally be initiated between 16 and 24 weeks of gestation and treatment should be continued through 34 weeks of gestation. Progesterone supplementation has also been recommended for the prevention of preterm labor in women with cervical length shortening (≤2.5 cm) on transvaginal ultrasound in the mid-trimester before 24 weeks. To prevent spontaneous preterm birth, vaginal progesterone is also recommended in women with twin pregnancy and a cervical length of ≤ 2.5 cm on transvaginal ultrasound between 16 to 24 weeks and by extrapolating the data of twins, it has been recommended in higher order multifetal pregnancy.[16]

## DIAGNOSIS

The diagnosis is based on clinical criteria of regular uterine contractions associated with cervical change. Although, the diagnosis is straightforward in advanced preterm labor, it is difficult to make the diagnosis accurately with lesser degrees of dilatation and effacement. The pregnant women may initially present with nonspecific features such as sense of pelvic pressure, backache, menstrual like cramps, and periodic painless or painful tightening of the abdomen with mucoid discharge per vaginum which may or may not be mixed with blood. Digital examination done to assess cervical dilatation and effacement may or may not be able to identify cases which will progress to preterm birth. Digital examination should be done only after ruling out preterm premature rupture of membranes and placenta previa. If FFN testing is available, it should be done on vaginal sample from posterior fornix which should be collected before digital examination. Preterm labor is unlikely if FFN is <50 ng/mL.[17] Cervical length, 15 mm or less on ultrasonography suggests preterm labor.

## MANAGEMENT

All women with symptoms of preterm labor need to be thoroughly evaluated for any underlying predisposing factors. A complete history including accurate estimation of period of gestation is recorded. Additionally, any associated medical or obstetric conditions should be evaluated which might contraindicate tocolytic therapy. This is followed by a complete clinical examination particularly the fundal height, presentation, estimated fetal weight, and per-speculum examination to rule out any evidence of infection, leaking, bleeding, and to collect vaginal and cervical swabs for cultures as required. Sample may also be collected for FFN. If cervix is found to be closed on speculum examination, a digital examination can be avoided unless there is a strong possibility of cord presentation or prolapse.

The laboratory evaluation of these women is aimed at etiological workup, differentiating between threatened and established preterm labor, and establishing fetal well-being. It also predicts the risk of delivery in next 7 days in those with threatened preterm labor. The workup includes the following:

- Complete blood count with differential count—to look for evidence of infection.
- Urine routine, microscopy and culture—to exclude urinary tract infection.
- Vaginal wet mount preparation for bacterial vaginosis and trichomoniasis.
- Cervical cultures for *Neisseria* and *Chlamydia*.
- *Fetal fibronectin assay*: It has been shown to be a better predictor than clinical indices as it has high negative predictive value. FFN assay should not be done within 48 hours of sexual intercourse or in presence of bleeding, as it can be falsely elevated.
- Ultrasound is done for gestational age, number of fetuses, fetal size and biometry, gross congenital anomaly, placental localization, any subchorionic hemorrhage and grading, amniotic fluid index, and cervical length.
- Cardiotocography is useful for confirming fetal well-being.

The goals of treatment in women admitted with preterm labor include the following:

- Delay the delivery with the help of tocolysis where beneficial, so that:
  - Corticosteroids can be administered
  - In utero transfer to a tertiary care center can be arranged, if required, thereby reducing the neonatal morbidity.
- Treat the infection, if present.
- In women with threatened preterm labor, decisions regarding further management are based on gestational age, estimated fetal weight, contraindications to labor suppression, if any, and results of screening tests.
- The woman is admitted for observation, offered analgesia and is monitored for preterm labor.
- If uterine contractions are not observed or are very infrequent and the pain resolves; cervix is long, and undilated she may be discharged home with instruction to return if pains or uterine contractions restart. She is asked to follow-up as an outpatient within 7 days or earlier, if required.
- If FFN has been done and is negative and there is no evidence of cervical change, cervical length is >3 cm on transvaginal ultrasound, in that case there is <1% chance of delivery within the next 7 days.[3]
- If FFN is positive and or there is evidence of cervical change and or the cervical length is <20 mm, there is an increased risk of delivery within next 7 days.
- As per National Institute for Healthcare and Excellence (NICE) guidelines, in suspected preterm labor and in absence of transvaginal ultrasound measurement of cervical length or FFN testing to exclude preterm labor, treatment consistent with that of diagnosed preterm labor should be offered.[17]
- The American College of Obstetricians and Gynecologists (ACOG) also states that the positive predictive value of a positive FFN test result or a short cervix alone is poor and should not be used exclusively to direct management in the setting of acute symptoms.[2]
- Hence, during clinical observation if contractions are regular and painful, the woman should be admitted,

administered analgesics, steroids, and tocolysis, and monitored carefully. Tocolysis is given after ruling out contraindications to suppression of labor (*see* **Table 1**). Continuous fetal monitoring with cardiotocography is started. Management based on screening with FFN is shown in **Flowchart 1**.[18]

The interventions for the management of pregnancies with preterm labor include the following:

### Restriction of Physical Activity

Bed rest is one of the most commonly prescribed interventions used for the prevention and/or treatment of threatened preterm labor. However, there are no prospective randomized studies that have independently evaluated the effectiveness of bed rest for the prevention of preterm labor. Although, a reduction of physical activity may seem appropriate for some women at risk of preterm birth, a Cochrane review has confirmed that there is insufficient evidence to support or refute the usefulness of this intervention, especially when extended to full bed rest. The risk of venous thromboembolism associated with prolonged bed rest also has to be kept in mind.

### Hydration/Sedation

Another common practice used for the initial treatment of preterm labor is oral or intravenous hydration. This is based on physiologic evidence that hypovolemia may be associated with increased uterine activity and women in preterm labor may have plasma volumes below normal. Intravenous hydration is not without risk, especially because administration of tocolytics with intravenous hydration may place the patient at increased risk for pulmonary edema.

Sedation is also a commonly used intervention in women with premature contractions. There is limited data documenting the efficacy of sedation in preterm labor and current literature does not support the use of hydration and or sedation as the initial treatment of preterm labor.

### Corticosteroids

Antenatal glucocorticoid therapy results in a significant decrease in the incidence of respiratory distress syndrome associated with a decrease in perinatal mortality in newborns born between 24 and 34 weeks and has become the standard of care. Recent data supports the use of steroids for cases in late preterm labor within 34 weeks and $36^{+6/7}$ weeks, who are at risk of delivering within 7 days. It helps in decreasing neonatal respiratory morbidity. The incidence of intraventricular hemorrhage and necrotizing enterocolitis is also lower. The optimal benefits appeared >24 hours after the start of treatment, peak at 48 hours, and last for 7 days. According to recent NICE guidelines, repeat courses of maternal corticosteroids should not be offered routinely but should be taken into account the interval since the end of last course, gestational age, and the likelihood of delivery within 48 hours.

A single repeat course of antenatal corticosteroids should, therefore, be considered in women who are <34 weeks of gestation, who are at risk of preterm delivery within the next 7 days, and whose prior course of antenatal corticosteroids was administered >14 days previously. Rescue course corticosteroids could be provided as early as 7 days from the prior dose, if indicated by the clinical scenario.

Long-term follow-up of infants exposed in utero to a single course of antenatal corticosteroid therapy has not demonstrated any adverse effect on growth, physical development, motor or cognitive skills, or school progress at 3 and 6 years.[19] The commonly utilized steroids for the enhancement of fetal maturity are betamethasone (12 mg intramuscularly every 24 hours, two doses) or dexamethasone (6 mg intramuscularly every 12 hours, four doses). These two glucocorticoids have been identified as most appropriate for antenatal use as they readily cross the placenta and have long half-lives and limited mineralocorticoid activity. There is no significant difference in efficacy between the two.

If mother has diabetes mellitus (gestational or overt), monitor blood glucose of the mother and plan management of blood sugar levels accordingly.

### Magnesium Sulfate for Neuroprotection

Magnesium sulfate is used in cases of expected preterm deliveries in <32 weeks of gestation owing to its effect of decreasing neurological morbidities in the neonates

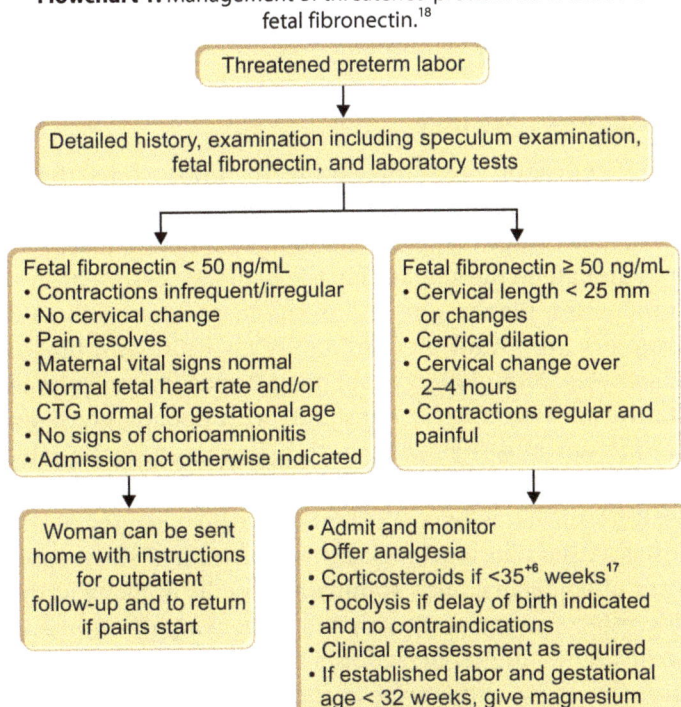

**Flowchart 1:** Management of threatened preterm labor based on fetal fibronectin.[18]

(CTG: cardiotocography)

born preterm. Various meta-analysis confirm this benefit. The standard protocol of using magnesium sulfate for this purpose has to be individualized by the institutions taking into consideration the larger trials undertaken. The dose recommended is 4–6 g IV loading dose followed by 1 g/hour for 24 hours or till delivery whichever is sooner. If delivery is imminent within next 4 hours, start magnesium sulfate immediately.[18] The maternal monitoring is done in the same way as when used for anti-seizure prophylaxis or tocolysis.[20]

## Antibiotics

Preterm labor, especially at <30 weeks of gestation, has been associated with occult upper genital tract infection. Many, if not all, of the bacterial species involved in this occult infection are capable of inciting an inflammatory response, which ultimately may culminate in preterm labor and delivery. Antibiotics therefore have the potential to prevent and/or treat spontaneous preterm labor. This use has been extensively studied with mixed results. A recent Cochrane meta-analysis compared antibiotic therapy with a placebo for the treatment of documented preterm labor. Overall, the use of antibiotics was not associated with reduction in perinatal and infant mortality or preterm birth. The only positive health benefit was significantly decreased risk for maternal infection in women who had received antibiotics. Thus, antibiotic therapy for women in preterm labor should be limited to group B *Streptococcus* (GBS) prophylaxis, women with PPROM or treatment of a specific infection and not for the sole purpose of preventing preterm delivery.

## Tocolysis

Tocolytic agents aimed at inhibiting contractions of the uterus have been used to prolong pregnancy. This may improve perinatal outcomes by allowing the fetus to mature before being born, allow time for antenatal corticosteroid administration for lung maturation, magnesium sulfate administration for neuroprotection, and allow time for in utero transfer to a tertiary care center with neonatal intensive care facilities, if needed. Ideally, tocolytics should not be used beyond 48 hours.

Tocolysis is contraindicated when the maternal and fetal risks of prolonging pregnancy or the risks associated with tocolytic drugs are greater than the risks associated with preterm birth. It should not be used before the period of viability and generally after 34 weeks. Contraindications to tocolytic therapy for suppression of labor are given in **Table 1**.

The ideal tocolytic agent is one which is effective in prolonging pregnancy but has no side effects for the mother or the infant. Several tocolytic agents have been used including betamimetics, calcium channel blockers (CCBs), prostaglandin synthetase inhibitors, magnesium sulfate, nitric oxide donor, and oxytocin receptor antagonists (ORAs). Mechanism of action, their dose and administration have been described in detail here. **Table 2** illustrates the contraindications to the use of each drug along with their maternal and fetal side effects.

**TABLE 1:** Contraindications to tocolytic therapy.

| Maternal | Fetal |
|---|---|
| • Severe pre-eclampsia and eclampsia<br>• Chorioamnionitis<br>• Antepartum hemorrhage<br>• Cervical dilatation > 4 cm<br>• Maternal conditions such as cardiac arrhythmias/valvular heart disease, acute respiratory distress syndrome (ARDS)/pulmonary edema, and hyperthyroidism | • Nonreassuring fetal status<br>• Intrauterine fetal death<br>• Congenital anomalies incompatible with life<br>• Period of gestation ≥ 34 weeks<br>• Before the age of viability* |

*Sometimes used before viability in cases requiring intra-abdominal surgery.

## Betamimetics

Like the endogenous catecholamines epinephrine and norepinephrine, this class of drugs stimulate all beta-adrenergic receptors present throughout the body. Betamimetics include ritodrine, terbutaline, albuterol, fenoterol, hexoprenaline, isoxsuprine, metaproterenol, nylidrin, orciprenaline, and salbutamol. They have been used extensively as tocolytic agents but are no longer recommended. Ritodrine, isoxsuprine and terbutaline are the beta-2 receptor agonists and were most commonly used.

### Mechanism of Action

Three types of beta-adrenergic receptors have been described in humans: beta-1 receptors are prevalent in the heart, small intestine, and adipose tissue; beta-2 receptors predominate in the smooth muscle of blood vessels, uterus, bronchioles, diaphragm, and in the liver; whereas beta-3 receptors are found predominantly on white and brown adipocytes. Stimulation of the beta-2 receptors results in uterine smooth muscle relaxation with hepatic glycogen production and insulin secretion from pancreatic islet cells. Although, some beta-sympathomimetic agents have been proposed as beta-2 receptor selective agents, at the dosages used pharmacologically, stimulation of all receptor types often occurs. Such stimulation results in many of the side effects associated with the beta-sympathomimetic agents. Beta-adrenergic agonists activate adenyl cyclase to form Cyclic 3',5'-adenosine monophosphate (cAMP). The increased cellular levels of cAMP decrease myosin light-chain kinase (MLCK) activity, both by phosphorylation of the

**TABLE 2:** Contraindications and side effects associated with tocolytic agents.[45]

| Tocolytic agent | Contraindications | Maternal side effects | Fetal side effects |
|---|---|---|---|
| Betamimetic | • Tachycardia sensitive cardiac disease<br>• Uncontrolled diabetes mellitus | • Tachycardia<br>• Hypotension<br>• Tremors (10–15%), palpitation (33%) pulmonary edema (3–5%)<br>• Hypoglycemia and hyperkalemia | • Fetal tachycardia<br>• Neonatal hypoglycemia<br>• Neonatal hyperbilirubinemia |
| Calcium channel blocker | • Hypotension<br>• Aortic insufficiency | • Dizziness and flushing<br>• Hypotension<br>• Deranged hepatic transaminases | Nil |
| Magnesium sulfate | • Myasthenia gravis | • Flushing, diaphoresis, and nausea<br>• Loss of deep tendon reflexes<br>• Respiratory depression<br>• Cardiac arrest | Neonatal depression |
| Prostaglandin synthetase inhibitor | • Hepatic dysfunction<br>• Renal dysfunction<br>• Platelet dysfunction and bleeding disorder<br>• Peptic ulcer disease<br>• Asthma<br>• Hypersensitivity to drug | • Nausea and vomiting<br>• Gastritis | • Constriction of ductus arteriosus<br>• Oligohydramnios<br>• Necrotizing enterocolitis |
| Oxytocin antagonist | Not known | Nausea, vomiting, headache, chest pain, and dysgeusia | Nil |
| Nitric oxide donor | • Hypotension | Nausea, vomiting, headache, and lightheadedness | Nil |

MLCK itself and by reducing intracellular calcium through increasing calcium uptake by sarcoplasmic reticulum and results in decreased myocyte contractility.

## Ritodrine

Ritodrine is the only medication among betamimetics approved by the United States Food and Drug Administration (US FDA) for the treatment of preterm labor, but it was withdrawn from US market voluntarily in 1983.[21] Ritodrine is a rapid acting drug, it is metabolized in the liver and excreted in the urine. It can be administered intravenously, intramuscularly, or orally.

Treatment usually begins with intravenous infusion to allow maximal bioavailability. Serum levels reach 75% of maximum within 20 minutes of infusion. There is an initial half-life of 6–9 minutes followed by a second half-life of 2–3 hours and elimination time of 2.5 hours. For intravenous administration, the infusion is begun at 50–100 µg/min and increased every 20 minutes till either uterine quiescence is achieved or unacceptable side effects occur, or a maximum infusion rate of 350 µg/min is reached. Once labor is inhibited, the labor inhibiting infusion rate is maintained for 60 minutes and then decreased by 50 µg/min every 30 minutes until the lowest effective rate is achieved (but not <50 µg/min). The lowest effective infusion rate is then arbitrarily maintained for 12 hours. If labor recurs within this 12-hour period, the process is repeated.[22] Tachyphylaxis may occur after prolonged exposure, therefore, the myometrium may remain quiescent longer with pulsatile administration of lower doses. The patient should be closely monitored for pulse, blood pressure, fluid balance, cardiac status, and electrolytes, including potassium and glucose. Oral ritodrine is used for maintenance of tocolysis with approximately 30% of an oral dose absorbed.[23]

## Terbutaline

Terbutaline is used as off-label betamimetic as it is not approved by the US FDA for tocolysis. It is not recommended because life-threatening adverse effects has been reported. It has been administered by intravenous, subcutaneous, and oral routes. The intravenous infusion rate of terbutaline is generally started at 2.5–5 µg/min and increased every 20 minutes by increments of 5 µg/min to a maximum of 25 µg/min. Once labor is inhibited, the labor inhibiting rate is sustained for 60 minutes and thereafter reduced by 2.5 µg/min every 30 minutes until the lowest effective dose is established. This rate is maintained for 12 hours. Subcutaneous administration is also used for acute tocolysis with a typical dose of 0.25 mg subcutaneously every 1–6 hours with repeated dosing titrated to uterine activity and maternal side effects, stopping the dose at a pulse rate >120 bpm. A rapid onset of action is seen in 3–5 minutes after subcutaneous administration. Orally administered terbutaline has mostly been used to prevent recurrence of already inhibited contractions. Generally, a dose of 2.5–5 mg every 4–6 hours, titrated by patient response and maternal pulse is used, it has been shown to be superior to oral ritodrine in preventing recurrent preterm labor and prolonging pregnancy.[24]

### Efficacy

According to a recently published Cochrane review betamimetics help to delay birth, which may give time to allow women to be transferred to tertiary care or to complete a course of antenatal corticosteroids, the data was not enough to support the use of any particular betamimetic.[25] However, frequent unpleasant and sometimes potential life-threatening adverse effects are a concern and NICE guidelines advise against their use for preterm labor.

## Calcium Channel Blockers (CCBs)

Nifedipine is the most common CCB used for tocolysis. CCBs have the advantage of oral formulation and when tocolysis is indicated for women in preterm labor, CCBs are often preferred over other tocolytic agents, mainly betamimetics.

### Mechanism of Action

These agents inhibit the influx of calcium ions through the voltage-dependent calcium channels in the muscle cell membrane and reduce uterine vascular resistance. They may also inhibit release of intracellular calcium from sarcolemma stores and increase calcium efflux from the cell. The resultant decrease in intracellular free calcium leads to inhibition of calcium-dependent MLCK phosphorylation and results in decreased myometrial activity.

### Dosage and Administration

Nifedipine is administered orally and is nearly completely absorbed from the gastrointestinal tract after ingestion. Onset of action after oral nifedipine is <20 minutes and maximum plasma concentrations occur within 15–90 minutes after oral administration.[26,27] Nifedipine is almost completely metabolized in the liver and 70–80% is excreted by the kidneys and 30% through bowel. An appropriate dosing regimen of nifedipine for the treatment of preterm labor has not been demonstrated and different dosing regimens were used in various study protocols. One recommended regimen is to administer 10 mg orally every 20 minutes for up to four doses followed by 20 mg orally every 4–8 hours.[28] Others have administered an initial loading dose of 30 mg, followed-up by 10–20 mg doses every 4–6 hours. RCOG recommends an initial dose of 20 mg followed by 10–20 mg three to four times daily, adjusted according to uterine activity for up to 48 hours. A total dose above 60 mg has shown to be associated with 3- to 4-fold increase in adverse events.[29]

Concomitant use with magnesium sulfate should be avoided because of reports of neuromuscular blockade and profound hypotension.

### Contraindications

Contraindications to the use of nifedipine or any of the CCBs include hypotension, congestive heart failure, and aortic stenosis.

### Efficacy

According to a systematic review comparing the effects of CCBs (mainly nifedipine) with other tocolytic agents (mainly betamimetics), CCBs were reported to be more effective tocolytic agents (less births within 7 days of initiation of treatment and before 34 weeks gestation) with improvement in some clinically important neonatal outcomes (less respiratory distress syndrome, intraventricular hemorrhage, necrotizing enterocolitis, and jaundice) and a marked reduction in adverse maternal side effects. Also, there is the advantage of oral formulation. They concluded that when tocolysis is indicated for women in preterm labor, CCBs are preferable to other tocolytic agents, mainly betamimetics.[30]

Calcium channel blockers, mainly nifedipine, for women in preterm labor have benefits over placebo or no treatment in terms of postponement of birth thus, allowing time for administration of antenatal corticosteroids and transfer to higher level care. CCBs were shown to have benefits over betamimetics with respect to prolongation of pregnancy, serious neonatal morbidity, and maternal adverse effects. CCBs may also have some benefits over oxytocin receptor antagonists (ORAs) and magnesium sulfate, although ORAs result in fewer maternal adverse effects.[31]

## Magnesium Sulfate

### Mechanism of Action

The exact mechanism by which magnesium sulfate acts is not well-known. The mechanism appears to be via the competitive inhibition of calcium at the voltage-operated calcium channels at the plasma membrane of the myocytes leading to hyperpolarization of the membrane. Magnesium may directly compete with intracellular calcium by decreasing the calcium-calmodulin binding affinity to MLCK, thereby inhibiting myometrial contractility.[32-34]

### Dosage and Administration

Magnesium sulfate must be administered intravenously to achieve therapeutic levels, it is excreted primarily by the kidneys. The recommended dosing consists of an initial loading dose of 4–6 g intravenously over 20 minutes in 100 mL fluid followed by continuous maintenance infusion of 1–3 g/h. Individual titration to uterine quiescence and maternal side effects is recommended. Maternal toxicity can be assessed clinically by monitoring the respiratory rate, deep tendon reflexes, and urine output or by evaluation of serum magnesium concentrations which should be maintained in the range of 5–8 mg/dL which is considered therapeutic for inhibiting myometrial activity. Once uterine quiescence is achieved, the patient is generally maintained at the lowest effective infusion rate for 12-24 hours which is then tapered and stopped.

## *Efficacy*

Though magnesium sulfate has been widely used as a tocolytic for many years, systematic review by Cochrane revealed the surprising fact that the evidence to support its use was sparse and generally of poor quality. The currently available evidence shows magnesium sulfate to be ineffective in delaying preterm birth and thus, it cannot be recommended as a tocolytic agent for women in preterm labor. However, it was less likely than betamimetics to cause maternal side effects, although compared with other tocolytics it was more likely to cause maternal side effects. Administration of magnesium sulfate to women considered at risk of preterm birth reduces the risk of cerebral palsy.[35]

## Prostaglandin Synthetase Inhibitors

Prostaglandins have been shown to have a significant role in the labor process. Prostaglandins stimulate myometrial gap junction formation and raise intracellular calcium levels by increasing calcium influx across the cell membrane and stimulating calcium release from the sarcoplasmic reticulum. Prostaglandin synthetase inhibitors are reversible competitive inhibitors of cyclooxygenase (COX), blocking the conversion of free arachidonic acid to prostaglandin. Because prostaglandin E and F series are mediators of uterine contractions, a decrease in production results in decreased contractile activity therefore, this pathway represents a key target for pharmacological intervention. Indomethacin is the most commonly used agent in this class, but other agents such as sulindac and ketorolac have also been used. Indomethacin should not be used in gestation >32 weeks owing to its effect on ductus arteriosus causing its constriction.

Because of the potential adverse fetal and neonatal effects, indomethacin should be considered only if gestational age is $<28^{+0}$ weeks and other tocolytics have failed to achieve tocolysis or are contraindicated.[18]

Indomethacin is usually administered orally or rectally. A loading dose of 50-100 mg is followed by 25 mg orally every 4-6 hours for 48 hours, a total 24-hour dose not > 200 mg.[36,37]

According to a recent Cochrane database systematic review, COX inhibitors inhibit uterine contractions, are easily administered and appear to have fewer maternal side-effects. However, adverse effects have been reported in the fetus and newborn as a result of exposure to COX inhibitors. The authors concluded that there is insufficient evidence on which to base decisions about the role of COX inhibition for women in preterm labor.[38]

## Oxytocin Receptor Antagonists (ORAs)
### *Mechanism of Action*

Atosiban is a selective oxytocin-vasopressin receptor antagonist capable of inhibiting oxytocin induced myometrial contractions. The mechanism appears to be competitive inhibition of oxytocin receptors in the myometrium and decidua. Oxytocin stimulates contractions by stimulating the conversion of phosphatidylinositol to inositol triphosphate. This binds to a protein in the sarcoplasmic reticulum leading to calcium release into the cytoplasm. Thus, oxytocin antagonists result in a decrease in intracellular free calcium that results in decreased myometrial contractility.

### *Dosage and Administration*

Atosiban is a nonapeptide. Atosiban has not been approved by the FDA, but is licensed in the United Kingdom (UK) for treatment of threatened preterm labor. Atosiban is typically administered intravenously, beginning with a single bolus of 6.75 mg over 1 minute, followed immediately by a 300 μg/min intravenous infusion for 3 hours and then 100 μg/min for up to 45 hours.[39] Atosiban is not active orally.

## Nitric Oxide Donors

Nitric oxide is a potent endogenous hormone that facilitates smooth muscle relaxation in the vasculature, the gut, and the uterus. Nitric oxide donors which have been used for tocolysis include nitroglycerin and glyceryl trinitrate. Clinical use of these agents for the treatment of preterm labor remains experimental.

### *Mechanism of Action*

Nitric oxide donors, activate the cyclic guanosine monophosphate pathway involved in smooth muscle relaxation. The activation of cyclic guanosine monophosphate results in decreased intracellular free calcium that leads to decreased activation of MLCK and decreased myometrial contractility.

### *Dosage and Administration*

Nitric oxide donors have been administered intravenously and by transdermal patch. The dosing and administration have varied in studies but are primarily titrated to cessation of contractions while maintaining adequate blood pressure. The transdermal regimen used is an initial 10 mg transdermal glyceryl trinitrate patch applied to the skin of the abdomen. If after 1 hour, there was no reduction in contraction frequency or strength, an additional patch was applied. No more than two patches were administered simultaneously, and these were left in place for 24 hours after which they were removed and patient reassessed.

## Combination Tocolytic Therapy

Few studies have assessed the concomitant use of two labor inhibiting agents. While there was a suggestion of improved efficacy in one trial this has not been supported by other trials.[40,41] Side effects with combined regimen were found to be significantly increased. Given, the limited and conflicting data on efficacy and safety, it is not recommended to use combined therapy for labor inhibition.

## Maintenance Tocolytic Therapy

Patients who are successfully treated for an acute episode of preterm labor remain at risk for having recurrent episodes of preterm labor. Maintenance tocolytic therapy has been used in these patients with the hope that the risk of recurrence will decrease. But a meta-analysis has shown that maintenance tocolytic therapy was not associated with a significant reduction in the rates of recurrent preterm labor or preterm delivery and thus is not recommended.[42]

## Role of Tocolytics in Multiple Gestation

The indication for using tocolytics is similar to singleton gestation, with a higher associated risk of pulmonary edema. There is no role of giving prophylactic tocolytics in these cases.

## Summary of Tocolytics

Thus, to summarize, although treatment with tocolytics can significantly reduce the rate of delivery within 48 hours and 7 days, they have not been shown to improve perinatal outcomes, but do have adverse health effects on women.[43] In a systematic review of 49 clinical guidelines for prevention and management of preterm birth, however, it was found that there is a consensus on the use of short-term tocolysis among the various clinical guidelines.[44]

However, they do appear to delay delivery long enough for successful administration of corticosteroids. Therefore, as a general rule, if tocolytics are given, they should be given concomitantly with corticosteroids. Candidates for labor inhibition must be evaluated and chosen carefully with the goals of labor inhibition clearly defined in each situation. Though the ideal tocolytic agent has not yet been discovered, the choice of pharmacologic agent must be tailored to the individual patient with particular attention to side effects of and contraindications to these potent medications so as to choose the tocolytic most suitable to the individual patient. Maternal and fetal status should be closely monitored with frequent reassessment during therapy to identify the evolution of contraindications to labor inhibition, such as infection and specific side effects and toxicities. Labor inhibition therapy should be stopped if the risks outweigh the benefits of continuing therapy.

There is the advantage of oral formulations. NICE guidelines suggest nifedipine for tocolysis, atosiban if nifedipine is contraindicated and betamimetics are not advocated for tocolysis.

Once a pregnancy has continued beyond 34 weeks, fetal survival rate is within 1% of the term survival and long-term sequelae are also rare. Hence, tocolysis is not given as it may not provide additional benefit.

## Rescue Cervical Cerclage

As per NICE guidelines, "rescue" cervical cerclage should be considered for women with 16 to $27^{+6}$ weeks of pregnancy and a dilated cervix and exposed, intact fetal membranes.[17]

## Conduct of Labor and Delivery

Women in preterm labor should deliver in a tertiary care setting equipped with neonatal intensive care unit. For singleton vertex presentation vaginal birth is recommended unless there are contraindications to vaginal birth or there is maternal indication of cesarean section.[46]

Preterm babies, however, are at an increased risk of intrapartum asphyxia and there should be relatively low threshold for delivery by cesarean in presence of fetal heart rate (FHR) abnormalities. Apgar scores are often low in these babies due to physiologically immature nervous system. This needs to be differentiated from asphyxia by routine cord blood pH. Vaginal birth is preferred unless there are other indications of cesarean delivery. The route of delivery of very low birth weight infants is debatable. A recent Cochrane review inferred that there is not enough evidence to evaluate the use of a policy of planned immediate cesarean delivery for preterm babies.[46]

As per NICE guidelines there are no known benefits or harms for the baby from cesarean section, but cesarean section should be considered for women with preterm labor between $26^{+0}$ and $36^{+6}$ weeks of pregnancy with breech presentation.[17]

The World Health Organization (WHO), however, does not recommend routine delivery by cesarean section for the purpose of improving preterm newborn outcomes, regardless of cephalic or breech presentation.[47] Increased short- and long-term maternal morbidity with cesarean section needs to be considered.

During cesarean section it is important to ascertain that the uterine incision is adequate for extracting the fetus without delay to avoid unnecessary trauma. This often requires a vertical incision especially when the lower uterine segment is incompletely developed. During vaginal delivery a generous episiotomy should be considered, especially if the perineum is rigid to reduce the risk of injury. There is no evidence supporting elective forceps delivery for protecting the fetal head.

**BOX 2:** Management of preterm labor.
- Reduction of physical activity
- Analgesia
- Steroids
- Magnesium sulfate (If gestational age <32 weeks)
- Antibiotics (in presence of premature rupture of membranes or signs of chorioamnionitis)
- *Tocolytics:* Nifedipine preferred, oxytocin receptor antagonists if nifedipine contraindicated[17]
- Informed consent
- In-utero transfer to higher facility if necessary, after informing referral center
- Delivery in a tertiary care setting equipped with neonatal intensive care unit

**TABLE 3:** Survival of neonates as per gestational age.

| Gestational age (weeks) | Birth weight (g) | Survivors (%) | Intact survivors* (%) |
|---|---|---|---|
| 24–25 | 500–750 | 60 | 35 |
| 25–27 | 751–1,000 | 75 | 60 |
| 28–29 | 1,001–1,250 | 90 | 80 |
| 30–31 | 1,251–1,500 | 96 | 90 |
| 32–33 | 1,501–1,750 | 99 | 98 |
| 34–35 | 1,751–2,000 | 100 | 99 |

*Intact defined as not blind, deaf, retarded, or with cerebral palsy.

**TABLE 4:** Problems in premature newborn.

| System | Problems |
|---|---|
| Neurological | Perinatal depression and intracranial hemorrhage |
| Temperature regulation | Hypothermia and hyperthermia |
| Ophthalmologic | Retinopathy of prematurity |
| Respiratory | Apnea, hyaline membrane disease, and bronchopulmonary dysplasia |
| Cardiovascular | Hypotension, patent ductus arteriosus, and congestive heart failure |
| Gastrointestinal | Necrotizing enterocolitis |
| Renal | Acid base and electrolyte imbalance due to low glomerular filtration rate |
| Hematological | Anemia and hyperbilirubinemia |
| Metabolic | Hypoglycemia and hypocalcemia |
| Immunological | Increased risk of infection |

Delayed cord clamping is preferred. A wait of at least 30 seconds, but no longer than 3 minutes, before clamping the cord is advocated, if the mother and baby are stable. It is also recommended to hold the baby at or below the level of the placenta before clamping the cord.

Management of preterm labor is summarized in **Box 2**.

## NEONATAL OUTCOME

The prognosis for the preterm infant depends on the level of neonatal care in the delivery room and nursery. The gestational age is a more important predictor of neonatal outcome as compared to the weight. The babies require to be monitored for side effects due to tocolytic agents. Even in babies who survive, there is a risk of short- and long-term morbidity. Some associated conditions are acute and amenable to treatment but others such as cerebral palsy, neurodevelopmental delay, and pulmonary disorders can result in long-term severe disability.

Neonatal morbidity and survival vary widely across centers depending on facilities making generalization difficult. However, a rough guide is presented in **Table 3** to facilitate decision-making and counseling.

The problems of prematurity which are related to difficulty in extrauterine adaptation due to immaturity of organ systems are given in **Table 4**.

## KEY POINTS

- Preterm birth is defined as delivery of the baby after the period of viability and before 37 weeks of pregnancy.
- Preterm birth complicates 10–15% of all pregnancies and is a leading cause of neonatal morbidity and mortality.
- Idiopathic preterm labor accounts for about 40% of all preterm births.
- Assessment of risk of preterm delivery should be done at each antenatal visit concentrating on identification of modifiable risk factors.
- In women with a single fetal pregnancy and a history of spontaneous preterm delivery, progesterone supplementation is beneficial starting at 16–24 weeks' gestation and continuing through 34 weeks' gestation.
- Diagnostic goals are to identify etiology and to differentiate true from false preterm labor.
- Cervical length estimation by ultrasound along with FFN testing have been used to differentiate true from false preterm labor. A negative fibronectin and a long cervix are strong negative predictors of imminent preterm birth.
- Therapeutic goal is to identify and treat the subgroup of women who will benefit from antibiotics, tocolysis, and corticosteroids.
- Pregnancies between 24 and 34 weeks of gestation or estimated fetal weight between 600 and 2,500 g with no evidence of infection, benefit from tocolysis.
- Acute tocolysis is used to allow enough time for the effect of steroids, and to allow in-utero transfer to a tertiary care center, if required.
- Maintenance therapy with tocolytics is ineffective and is not recommended.
- Contraindications to use of tocolysis such as severe pre-eclampsia, eclampsia, chorioamnionitis, etc. must be ruled out.
- Calcium channel blocker, nifedipine is the preferred tocolytic. Beta-adrenergic receptor agonists, terbutaline, and ritodrine are effective but can have serious side effects and are usually used for uterine tachysystole.

- There is limited role of bed rest, hydration, and sedation in these women.
- Antibiotics are indicated only for those with documented infection, for GBS prophylaxis and in women with preterm PROM.
- Routine delivery by cesarean section for the purpose of improving preterm newborn outcomes is not recommended.
- These women should deliver in a tertiary care setting equipped with neonatal intensive care unit.

## REFERENCES

1. Blencowe H, Cousens S, Chou D, Oestergaard M, Say L, Moller AB, et al. Born too soon: the global epidemiology of 15 million preterm birth. Reprod Health. 2013;10(Suppl 1):52.
2. ACOG. Practice Bulletin No 171: management of preterm labour. Obstet Gynecol. 2016;128(4):e155-64.
3. Berghella V. Management of preterm labor. In: Queenan JT, Spong CY, Lockwood CJ Management of high-risk pregnancy/edited by, 5th edition. US: Blackwell Publishing Ltd; 2007. pp. 354-61.
4. Ou CW, Chen ZQ, Qi S, Lye SJ. Increased expression of the rat myometrial oxytocin receptor messenger ribonucleic acid during labor requires both mechanical and hormonal signals. Biol Reprod. 1998;59(5):1055-61.
5. Goldenberg RL, Hauth JC, Andrews WW. Intrauterine infection and preterm delivery. N Engl J Med. 2000;342(20):1500-7.
6. Andersen HF, Nugent CE, Wanty SD, Hayashi RH. Prediction of risk for preterm delivery by ultrasonographic measurement of cervical length. Am J Obstet Gynecol. 1990;163(3):859-67.
7. Kazemier BM, Buijs PE, Mignini L, Limpens J, de Groot CJ, Mol BW. Impact of obstetrics history on the risk of spontaneous preterm birth in singleton and multiple pregnancies: a systematic review. BJOG. 2014;121(10):1197-205, discussion 1209.
8. Butt K, Lim K, Crane JM. No. 257-Ultrasonographic cervical length assessment in predicting preterm birth in singleton pregnancies. J Obstet Gynaecol Can. 2018;40(2):e151-64.
9. Peaceman AM, Andrews WW, Thorp JM, Cliver SP, Lukes A, Iams JD, et al. Fetal fibronectin as a predictor of preterm birth in a patient with symptoms: a multicenter trial. Am J Obstet Gynecol. 1997;177(1):13-8.
10. Berghella V, Saccone G. Fetal fibronectin testing for reducing the risk of preterm birth. Cochrane Database Syst Rev. 2019;7(7):CD006843.
11. Cnattingius S, Villamor E, Johansson S, Edstedt Bonamy AK, Persson M, Wikström AK, et al. Maternal obesity and risk of preterm delivery. JAMA. 2013;309(22):2362-70.
12. Grady R, Alavi N, Vale R, Khandwala M, McDonald SD. Elective single embryo transfer and perinatal outcome: a systematic review and meta-analysis. Fertil Steril. 2012;97(2):324-31.
13. Lamont RF, Nhan Chang CL, Sobel JD, Workowski K, Conde-Agudelo A, Romero R. Treatment of abnormal vaginal flora in early pregnancy with clindamycin for the prevention of spontaneous preterm birth: a systematic review and meta-analysis. Am J Obstet Gynecol. 2011;205(3):177-90.
14. Brocklehurst P, Gordon A, Heatley E, Milan SJ. Antibiotic for treatment of bacterial vaginosis in pregnancy. Cochrane Database Sys Rev. 2013;(1):CD000262.
15. Szychowski JM, Owen J, Hankins G, Iams JD, Sheffield JS, Perez-Delboy A, et al. Can the optimal cervical length for placing ultrasound indicated cerclage be identified? Ultrasound Obstet Gynecol. 2016;48(1):43-7.
16. Jain V, McDonald SD, Mundle WR, Farine D. Guideline No. 398: Progesterone for Prevention of Spontaneous Preterm Birth. J Obstet Gynaecol Can. 2020;42(6):806-12.
17. NICE guideline (2015). Preterm labour and birth. [online] Available from: https://www.nice.org.uk/guidance/ng25/resources/preterm-labour-and-birth-pdf-1837333576645 [Last accessed July, 2021].
18. Queensland Clinical Guidelines (2020). Queensland Maternity and Neonatal Clinical Guideline: Preterm labour and birth. [online] Available from: https://www.health.qld.gov.au/__data/assets/pdf_file/0019/140149/g-ptl.pdf [Last accessed July, 2021].
19. Royal College of Obstetricians and Gynaecologists (2010). Antenatal corticosteroids to reduce neonatal morbidity and mortality. Green top guideline No. 7. [online] Available from: https://www.glowm.com/pdf/Antenatal%20Corticosteroids%20to%20Reduce%20Neonatal%20Morbidity.pdf [Last accessed July, 2021].
20. Rouse DJ, Hirtz DG, Thom E, Varner MW, Spong CY, Mercer BM, et al. A randomized controlled trial of magnesium sulfate for prevention of cerebral palsy. N Engl J Med. 2008;359(9):895-905.
21. Cunningham FG, Leveno KJ, Bloom SL, Dashe JS, Hoffman BL, Casey BM, et al. Preterm birth. Williams Obstetrics, 25th edition. New York: McGraw Hill; 2018. pp. 1240-90.
22. Caritis SN, Venkataramanan R, Darby MJ, Chiao JP, Krew M. Pharmacokinetics of ritodrine administered intravenously. Recommendations for changes in the current regimen. Am J Obstet Gynecol. 1990;162(2):429-37.
23. The Canadian Preterm Labor Investigators Group. The treatment of preterm labor with beta-adrenergic agonist ritodrine. N Engl J Med. 1992;327(5):308-12.
24. Caritis SN, Toig G, Heddinger L, Ashmead G. A double-blind study comparing ritodrine and terbutaline in the treatment of preterm labor. Am J Obstet Gynecol. 1984;150(1):7-14.
25. Neilson JP, West HM, Dowswell T. Betamimetics for inhibiting preterm labour. Cochrane Database Syst Rev. 2014;(2):CD004352.
26. Garcia-Velasco JA, Gonzalez GA. A prospective randomized trial of nifedipine vs. ritodrine in threatened preterm labor. Int J Gynaecol Obstet. 1998;61(3):239-44.
27. Ferguson JE 2nd, Schutz T, Pershe R, Stevenson DK, Blaschke T. Nifedipine pharmacokinetics in preterm labor tocolysis. Am J Obstet Gynecol. 1989;161(6 Pt 1):1485-90.
28. Papatsonis DN, Van Geijn HP, Ader HJ, Lange FM, Bleker OP, Dekker GA. Nifedipine and ritodrine in the management of preterm labor: a randomized multicenter trial. Obstet Gynecol. 1997;90(2):230-4.
29. Royal College of Obstetricians and Gynaecologists (2011). Tocolysis for women in preterm labour. Green top guideline No. 1b. [online] Available from: https://www.rcog.org.uk/en/guidelines-research-services/guidelines/gtg1b/ [Last accessed July, 2021].
30. King JF, Flenady VJ, Papatsonis DN, Dekker GA, Carbonne B. Calcium channel blockers for inhibiting preterm labour. Cochrane Database Syst Rev. 2003;(1):CD002255.

31. Flenady V, Wojcieszek AM, Papatsonis DN, Stock OM, Murray L, Jardine LA, et al. Calcium channel blockers for inhibiting preterm labour and birth. Cochrane Database Syst Rev. 2014;2014(6):CD002255.
32. Monga M, Creasy RK. Pharmacologic management of preterm labor. Semin Perinatol. 1995;19(1):84-96.
33. Sanborn BM. Ion channels and the control of myometrial electrical activity. Semin Perinatol. 1995;19(1):31-40.
34. Ohki S, Ikura M, Zhang M. Identification of magnesium binding sites and the role of magnesium on target recognition by calmodulin. Biochemistry. 1997;36(14):4309-16.
35. Doyle LW, Crowther CA, Middleton P, Marret S, Rouse D. Magnesium sulphate for women at risk of preterm birth for neuroprotection of the fetus. Cochrane Database Syst Rev. 2009;(1):CD004661.
36. Niebyl JR, Blake DA, White RD, Kumor KM, Dubin NH, Robinson JC, et al. The inhibition of premature labor with indomethacin. Am J Obstet Gynecol. 1980;136(8):1014-9.
37. Zuckerman H, Shalev E, Gilad G, Katzuni E. Further study of the inhibition of premature labor by indomethacin. Part II double-blind study. J Perinat Med. 1984;12(1):25-9.
38. Reinebrant HE, Pileggi-Castro C, Romero CL, Dos Santos RA, Kumar S, Souza JP, et al. Cyclo-oxygenase (COX) inhibitors for treating preterm labour. Cochrane Database Syst Rev. 2015;2015(6):CD001992.
39. Romero R, Sibai BM, Sanchez-Ramos L, Valenzuela GJ, Veille JC, Tabor B, et al. An oxytocin receptor antagonist (atosiban) in the treatment of preterm labor: a randomized, double-blind, placebo-controlled trial with tocolytic rescue. Am J Obstet Gynecol. 2000;182(5):1173-83.
40. Hatjis C, Swain M, Nelson LH, Meis PJ, Ernest JM. Efficacy of combined administration of magnesium sulfate and ritodrine in the treatment of preterm labor. Obstet Gynecol. 1987;69(3 Pt 1):317-22.
41. Ferguson JE 2nd, Hensleigh PA, Kredenster D. Adjunctive use of magnesium sulfate with ritodrine for preterm labor tocolysis. Am J Obstet Gynecol. 1984;148(2):166-71.
42. Sanchez-Ramos L, Kaunitz AM, Gaudier FL, Delke I. Efficacy of maintenance therapy after acute tocolysis: a meta-analysis. Am J Obstet Gynecol. 1999;181(2):484-90.
43. Gyetvai K, Hannah ME, Hodnett ED, Ohlsson A. Tocolytics for preterm labor: a systematic review. Obstet Gynecol. 1999;94(5 Pt 2):869-77.
44. Medley N, Poljak B, Mammarella S, Alfirevic Z. Clinical guidelines for prevention and management of preterm birth: a systematic review. BJOG. 2018;125(11):1361-9.
45. Rundell K, Panchal B. Preterm labor: prevention and management. Am Fam Physician. 2017;95(6):366-72.
46. Alfirevic Z, Milan SJ, Livio S. Caesarean section versus vaginal delivery for preterm birth in singletons. Cochrane Database Syst Rev. 2013;2013(9):CD000078.
47. World Health Organization. WHO recommendation on the optimal mode of birth for women in refractory preterm labour; 2015.

# Premature Rupture of Membranes

*Sharda Patra*

## DEFINITION AND INCIDENCE

Premature rupture of membranes or prelabor rupture of membrane (PROM) is rupture of fetal membranes in the absence of uterine contractions regardless of gestational age.[1,2] Rupture of membranes occurring after 37 completed weeks of gestation is known as term PROM and that occurring before 37 weeks is preterm PROM (PPROM). The overall incidence of premature rupture of the fetal membranes (PROM) is 5–10% of all pregnancies[2] that of term PROM 8% and preterm PROM 2–4%. PPROM is the leading cause of premature birth and accounts for approximately 18–20% of perinatal deaths.[2] Despite significant advances in perinatal care, PPROM continues to be an important obstetrical complication due to its poorly understood etiopathogenesis, diagnostic dilemmas, and controversial management strategies.

## ETIOPATHOGENESIS

A number of mechanisms have been proposed for PROM. These are intrinsic membrane weakness due to defect in collagen synthesis, increased collagen degradation, ascending overt or subclinical infection, and mechanical stress due to distention **(Flowchart 1)**.[3-5]

## FACTORS PREDISPOSING TO PREMATURE RUPTURE OF MEMBRANE

The various factors which can predispose a woman to PROM are listed in **Table 1**.[2,6] However, most often PPROM occurs in otherwise healthy women without an identifiable risk factor.[2] Of the various predisposing factors, women with previous history of PPROM have a 14-fold increased risk of developing PPROM and three-fold increased risk of preterm birth in subsequent pregnancy. There is a three-to-seven fold risk of PROM in women with history of second or third-trimester bleeding in index pregnancy.[2] Moreover, antepartum bleeding in more than one trimester also increases the risk of PPROM three-to-seven-fold.[7]

A short cervix (<25 mm) on transvaginal ultrasonography with a positive fetal fibronectin is also associated with PPROM in both nulliparous and multiparous women.[8] There is a strong link between hypertension, diabetes mellitus,

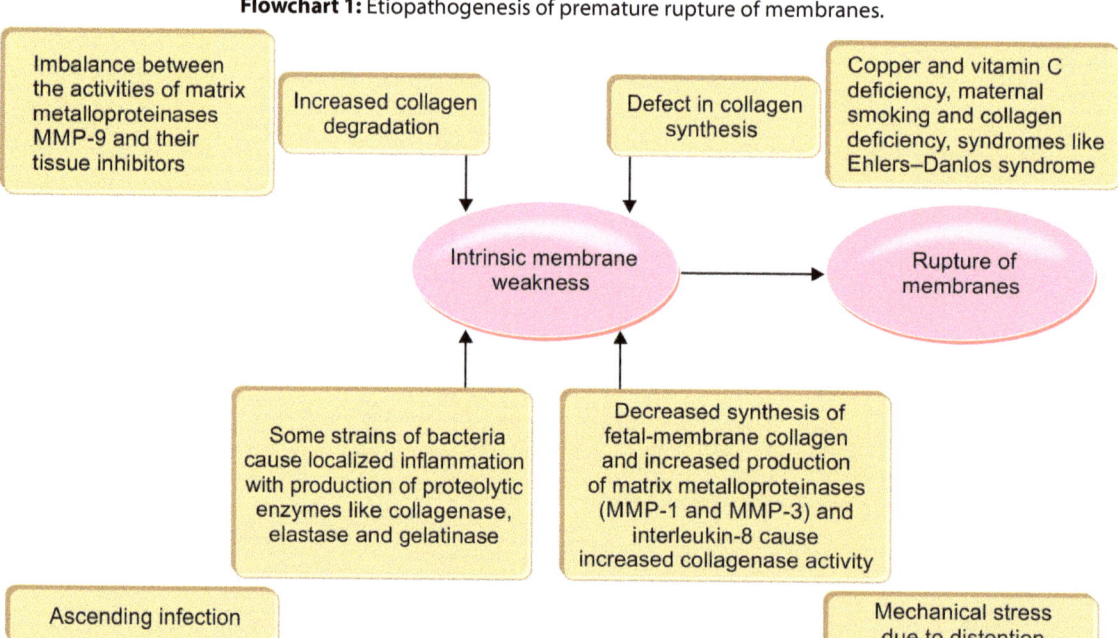

**Flowchart 1:** Etiopathogenesis of premature rupture of membranes.

| TABLE 1: Predisposing factors for premature rupture of membranes.[2,6] |||
|---|---|---|
| Obstetric history |||
| Past pregnancy | Present pregnancy | Medical factors |
| • Preterm premature rupture of membranes (PPROM) | • Antepartum vaginal bleeding—1st, 2nd, and 3rd trimester | • Collagen vascular disorders (such as Ehlers–Danlos syndrome and systemic lupus erythematosus) |
| • Preterm labor | • Placental abruption | • Cigarette smoking |
| • Prior cervical conization | • Advanced cervical dilatation (cervical insufficiency)<br>• Cervical shortening in the 2nd trimester (< 2.5 cm)<br>• Uterine overdistention (polyhydramnios and multiple pregnancy)<br>• Intra-amniotic infection (chorioamnionitis)<br>• Procedures—amniocentesis and chorionic villus sampling | • Nutritional deficiencies of copper and ascorbic acid |

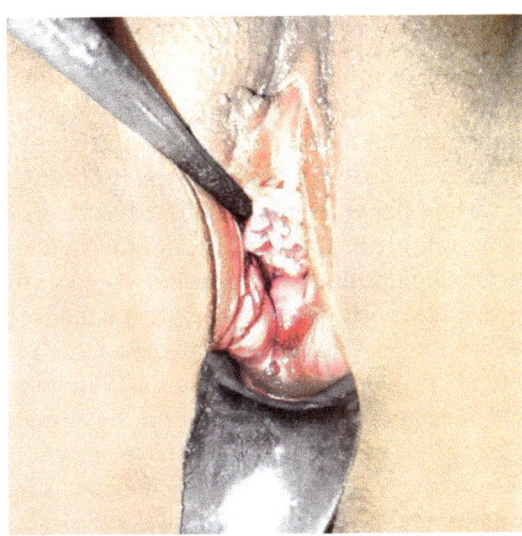

**Fig. 1:** Pooling of liquor seen on per speculum examination of patients with PROM. (PROM: premature rupture of membranes)

amnionitis, and abruption in current pregnancy and PROM.[9] Women with Ehlers-Danlos syndrome are highly susceptible to PROM, but interestingly there is no correlation between Marfan syndrome and PROM despite the fact that both are collagen deficiency syndromes.[2,9] Presence of trichomoniasis and group B streptococcal infection strongly predisposes to PROM. However, a weaker link between PROM and bacterial vaginosis has been reported.[9-11] The risk of PROM increases two to four-fold among smokers compared to nonsmokers. Certain procedures such as amniocentesis and chorionic villus sampling also cause PROM in 1.2% and 0.7% of pregnant women respectively.[12] Factors such as sexual intercourse, speculum examination, maternal exercise, and parity are not known to be associated with preterm PROM.[13]

## CLINICAL PRESENTATION AND DIAGNOSIS

### History

Women with PROM often present with a typical history of sudden gush of clear or pale yellow fluid from the vagina. However, many women may present with history of intermittent or constant leaking of small amounts of fluid or just a sensation of wetness within the vagina or on the perineum. In the initial evaluation, it is essential to note the duration, amount, and persistence of fluid leakage. Conditions such as urinary incontinence, recent vaginal or cervical infection, recent sexual activity, and douching should be ruled out for a correct diagnosis. Timely and accurate diagnosis of PROM allows for gestational age-specific obstetric intervention and is critical to optimize pregnancy outcome. A false positive diagnosis of PROM especially PPROM may lead to unnecessary obstetric interventions, including hospitalization, administration of antibiotics, corticosteroids, and even induction of labor.

### Per Speculum Examination

The next step in the diagnosis of PROM includes a sterile per speculum examination to demonstrate leaking. Pooling of fluid in the posterior fornix or leakage of fluid from the cervical os confirms the diagnosis of PROM (**Fig. 1**). If no amniotic fluid is immediately visible, the woman is asked to push or do Valsalva maneuver or cough to express amniotic fluid from the cervical os. A sterile speculum examination not only helps in the diagnosis of PROM but also allows for inspection of the cervix for any local cervical lesion such as cervicitis; cord prolapse, cervical dilatation, and effacement and also allows to take high vaginal swab for culture. A per vaginum examination should be avoided for risk of intrauterine infection and preterm labor.[14] Moreover, per vaginum examination adds little to the information obtained by the speculum examination unless the patient is in active labor or immediate delivery is planned. At times the findings at speculum examination are doubtful or equivocal. However, per speculum examination carries a 12% false negative rate in cases where there is slow fluid leak or any associated bleeding, or in absence of the classic "gush of fluid".[15] In these women two simple and practical bedside tests—nitrazine test and fern test can help to diagnose PROM.

### Nitrazine Test

This is based on the principle of differentiating amniotic fluid from the vaginal secretions by the pH. Amniotic fluid has a pH ranging from 7.0 to 7.7 compared to the acidic vaginal pH in pregnancy of 3.8–4.2. Nitrazine test is positive when a yellow nitrazine paper (impregnated with sodium-dinitro-phenylozonapthol-disulfonate) turns blue by coming in contact with amniotic fluid. However, in 5% of cases the result can be either false positive or false negative. It is false positive in the presence of alkaline fluids in the vagina, such as blood, seminal fluid, soap or bacterial vaginosis. With intermittent prolonged leakage, small high leaks or if the amniotic fluid is diluted by other vaginal fluids, it is false negative. Hence, the sensitivity and specificity of this test in diagnosing PROM ranges from 90 to 97% and 16 to 70%, respectively.[16]

### Fern Test (Fig. 2)

This is another test to confirm presence of amniotic fluid in the vagina. Fluid from the posterior vaginal fornix is swabbed onto a glass slide and allowed to dry for at least 10 minutes. Amniotic fluid produces a delicate ferning pattern in contrast to the thick and wide arborization pattern of dried cervical mucus under low power microscope. This method, however, is not sufficiently accurate. It may produce false results in as many as 30% of the cases. False-positive fern test may result from well estrogenized cervical mucus or a fingerprint on the microscope slide. False negative result can be due to inadequate amniotic fluid on the swab or heavy contamination with vaginal discharge or blood.

Though, these two tests are very simple and easy to perform, the main drawback with these two tests is their high rate of inaccuracy which increase progressively when >1 hour has elapsed since membranes rupture and the tests become inconclusive after 24 hours.[17] None of the traditional procedures have proven to be entirely satisfactory in isolation, but combination of any two of the following produces a diagnostic accuracy of 93.1%.[18]

- A positive history
- A positive nitrazine test
- A positive fern test.

Due to nonavailability of nitrazine paper it is no more recommended.[19] In cases where PROM is prolonged and associated with oligohydramnios, examination by ultrasound may be of value in supporting the diagnosis of PROM.

### Ultrasonography

Evidence of diminished amniotic fluid volume either by clinical examination or ultrasound alone cannot confirm the diagnosis, but may help to suggest PROM in an appropriate clinical setting. Approximately 50–70% of women with PROM have low amniotic fluid volume on initial ultrasonography. The presence of anhydramnios or severe oligohydramnios combined with a characteristic history of leaking per vaginum is highly suggestive of rupture of membranes. Sometimes, oligohydramnios may not be detected even in women with confirmed PROM, possibly because the drainage slowly becomes intermittent or even stops once the presenting part descends and acts as a plug, preventing further drainage. Hence, the accuracy of ultrasound quantification of amniotic fluid in confirmation of PROM remains inconclusive.[19,20] Conditions causing anhydramnios/oligohydramnios such as fetal renal agenesis, obstructive uropathy, or severe uteroplacental insufficiency should be excluded before the diagnosis of PROM is made on the basis of ultrasonography.[21]

### Indigo Carmine Test

Another method of confirming PROM is instillation of 1 mL indigo carmine diluted in 9 mL of sterile saline into the amniotic cavity transabdominally under ultrasound guidance. Blue staining of a tampon kept vaginally after 1.5 hours indicates leakage of amniotic fluid. Inherent risks of intra-amniotic dye injection include trauma, bleeding, infection, and preterm labor.[22] However, a "negative dye test" may occur if the membranes seal after previous amniotic fluid leakage.

### Newer Tests

Owing to the limitations of the conventional tests for diagnosis of PROM, newer and more objective tests are emerging. These tests are based primarily on the identification of one or more biochemical markers in the cervicovaginal discharge. Several such markers such as alpha-fetoprotein, fetal fibronectin, prolactin, subunit of human chorionic gonadotropin, creatinine, urea, lactate, insulin-like growth factor binding protein-1 (IGFBP-1), and placental alpha microglobulin-1 (PAMG-1) can be identified. As a general rule, these tests are either too invasive or too cumbersome

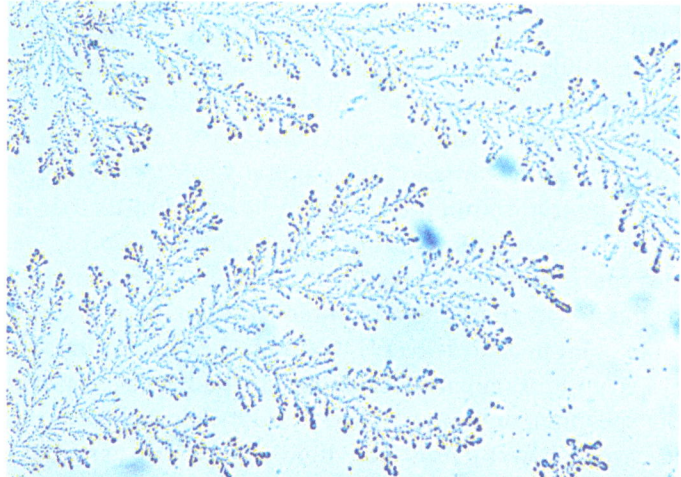

**Fig. 2:** Ferning pattern seen on microscopic examination of cervicovaginal discharge in patients with PPROM. (PPROM: preterm premature rupture of membranes)

or too expensive to have a routine application in clinical practice. However, the tests based on detection of proteomic markers like IGFBP-1 and PAMG-1 have come up with very convincing results.

## AmniSure

AmniSure test is a Food and Drug Administration (FDA) approved, immunoassay, slide test for PAMG-1. This test is simple, easy to perform, rapid (5–10 minutes), noninvasive, and does not require a speculum examination. In this test sterile swab is inserted into the vagina for 1 minute and placed into a vial containing a solvent for 1 minute. An AmniSure test strip is dipped into the vial and the test result is revealed by the presence of one or two lines within the next 10 minutes. One visible line indicates a negative result for amniotic fluid, two visible lines a positive result, and no visible lines indicate an invalid result. False results appear after 15 minutes. PAMG-1 is a placental protein that is abundant in amniotic fluid (2,000–25,000 ng/mL) but is present in far lower concentrations in maternal blood (5–25 ng/mL). The protein is present in even lower concentrations in cervicovaginal secretions (0.05–0.2 ng/mL). This 10,000-fold difference in concentration between amniotic fluid and cervicovaginal secretions makes PAMG-1 a very attractive marker for PROM. The minimum detection threshold of AmniSure immunoassay is 5 ng/mL, which is sufficiently sensitive to detect PROM with an accuracy of approximately 99%. The test has a very high sensitivity of 96.5%, specificity of 98.2%, positive predictive value of 98.2%, and a negative predictive value of 96.5%.[6,23-25]

### Actim® Premature Rupture of Membranes Test

It is a new FDA approved, immunoassay, slide test for IGFBP-1. In this test sterile swab is inserted into the vagina for 1 minute and placed into a vial containing a solvent for 1 minute. An Actim® PROM test strip is dipped into the vial and the test result is revealed by the presence of one or two lines within the next 5 minutes. One visible line indicates a negative result for amniotic fluid, two visible lines a positive result, and no visible lines indicate an invalid result. A test read after 5 minutes gives a negative result. IGFBP-1 is an excreted protein synthesized in the decidual cells and fetal liver and detected in amniotic fluid throughout pregnancy. It is abundant in amniotic fluid (10,500–350,000 µg/L) but is present in far lower concentrations in maternal blood (29–300 µg/L). The minimum detection threshold of actim PROM immunoassay is >25 µg/L unlike that of PAMG-1. The test has a very high sensitivity of 98.2%, specificity of 95.8%, positive predictive value of 96.0%, and a negative predictive value of 98.0%.[25]

A very recent review on the accuracy of these two tests suggested that the overall accuracy of Actim® PROM and AmniSure® for the detection of PROM are comparable if used in the same clinical population.[26]

## AmnioSense

It is an absorbent pad, 12 × 4 cm with a central strip that changes color from yellow to blue or green when it comes in contact with a fluid of pH > 5.2. Once dried this strip when meets urine reverts to its original color. The ammonium in the urine detaches the conjugate-based nitrazine molecules, hence the color reverts. Each pad can be worn for up to 12 hours and can detect as little as 2 drops of amniotic fluid. The reported AmnioSense pad test sensitivity is 100% and a specificity between 65 and 90%. Thus, a negative AmnioSense result indicates intact membranes in term and preterm gestations in 99% of cases. A positive result, however, suggests only a 70% chance of ruptured membranes, and thereby warrants confirmation or further investigations to identify infections.[27,28] It is indicated in pregnant women with unexplained vaginal wetness and those with small leaks at frequent intervals difficult to be detected clinically. The available evidence regarding the use of rapid immunoassay test kit devices to detect PROM is inadequate to form firm conclusions regarding its safety, efficacy, and how this testing will impact clinical outcomes for the pregnant woman and the neonates, in comparison to established methods of PROM detection. There is a need for larger randomized controlled trials before the clinical utility of these protein markers tests in suspected PROM can be established.[29,30]

These commercially available kits, at the most, should be considered selectively relative to standard methods of diagnosis (**Flowchart 2**).[19,31]

## CLINICAL COURSE IN PREMATURE RUPTURE OF MEMBRANES

The optimum clinical course of PROM is of short latency followed by labor and delivery. The interval from ruptured membranes to delivery is the latent period. The risk of infection to both mother and fetus increases with prolongation of latent period. Factors affecting latency are gestational age, degree of oligohydramnios, etc. An inverse relation exists between the gestational age at the time of PROM and latent period. At term, in the absence of any obstetric intervention, 50% of women with PROM will go into labor spontaneously within 12 hours, 70% within 24 hours, 85% within 48 hours, and 95% within 72 hours.[6] In women with PPROM remote from term, 50% will go into labor within 24–48 hours and 70–90% within 7 days.[6] Furthermore, women with PPROM at 24–28 weeks of gestation are likely to have a longer latent period than those with PPROM closer to term. This was observed in a study that the latency at 20–26 weeks' gestation, was 12 days and at 32–34 weeks' gestation, it was only 4 days.[3] The latent period is shorter in women who have severe

**Flowchart 2:** Diagnostic algorithmic work-up of a pregnant woman with leaking per vaginum.

```
Woman complaints of watery discharge P/v
                │
                ▼
    Clinical and obstetric examination
                │
                ▼
Fundal height less than or same as period of gestation
              Clinically less liquor
                │
                ▼
         Per speculum examination
                │
                ▼
Direct observation of amniotic fluid leaking from the cervical os and pooling in the Posterior fornix
         │                          │
        Yes                         No
         │                          │
         ▼                          ▼
Gold standard for diagnosis    Woman asked to cough
    Confirms PROM                   │
                                    ▼
                          Leakage through os observed
                            │                │
                           Yes               No
                                              │
                                              ▼
                                            USG
                                       Liquor and AFI
                                        │         │
                                     AFI low    Normal
                                        │         │
                                        ▼         ▼
                        Bedside test—fern test    PROM ruled out
                         or commercial tests
```

(AFI: amniotic fluid index; PROM: premature rupture of membranes; P/v: per vaginum; USG: ultrasonography)

oligohydramnios.[32] Evidence of excessive thinning of the myometrium at the fundal region of the uterus in a patient who is not in labor with PPROM (<12 mm) as measured by transabdominal ultrasound has been associated with a shorter latency interval. A fundal myometrial thickness <12.1 mm was 93.7% sensitive and 63.6% specific for the identification of women whose latent period was <120 hours.[33] Twin pregnancies complicated by PPROM have a shorter latent period than singleton pregnancies.

## MATERNAL AND PERINATAL COMPLICATIONS

Premature rupture of membrane is associated with a high-risk of maternal and perinatal complications **(Table 2)**. Maternal complications include clinically evident intra-amniotic infection and postpartum endometritis. Chorioamnionitis occurs in 13–60% of women with PPROM as compared to 1% at term PROM.[1,2] The risk of chorioamnionitis is higher in women with PPROM remote from term, with prolonged leaking, presence of severe oligohydramnios, and multiple per vaginal examinations.[6] The incidence of postpartum endometritis with PPROM is 2–13%. There is an increased risk of cord prolapse, especially in pregnancies with a nonvertex presentation.[1,2] The risk of cesarean delivery with its attendant surgical risks increase in PPROM as compared to term PROM. Severe oligohydramnios leading to cord compression and nonreassuring fetal testing (fetal distress) in labor further adds to the increased risk of cesarean delivery.[1,2] PPROM may lead to abruptio placentae in 4–12% of cases.[6]

**TABLE 2:** Maternal and perinatal risks of preterm premature rupture of membranes (PROM).

| Maternal risks | Neonatal risks |
|---|---|
| • Chorioamnionitis | • Prematurity |
| • Placental abruption | • Infection |
| • Malpresentation | • Cord prolapse |
| • Dysfunctional labor | • Cord compression |
| • Cesarean section | • Pulmonary hypoplasia |
| • Postpartum endometritis | • Skeletal compression deformities |

The perinatal complications are more common with PPROM as compared to term PROM. There is a 4-fold increase in perinatal mortality and a 3-fold increase in neonatal morbidity with PPROM. Respiratory distress syndrome (RDS) which occurs in 10–40% of women with PPROM is responsible for 40–70% of neonatal deaths. Polymicrobial intra-amniotic infection, which occurs in 15–30% of women with PPROM accounts for 3–20% of neonatal deaths and intraventricular hemorrhage (IVH).[2,34] Other neonatal complications related to severity and duration of PPROM include pulmonary hypoplasia, which develop in 26% of babies born following PPROM prior to 22 weeks, skeletal deformities which complicate 12% of PPROM, and neurodevelopmental impairment.[6] Infection, cord accident, and other factors contribute to 1–2% of intrauterine fetal demise (still birth) after PPROM.

Neonatal sepsis occurs in 7–25% of babies born to women with chorioamnionitis.[30] Sepsis is almost twice as likely to be fatal in premature neonates as in term neonates. In majority of the cases of PPROM, premature delivery occurs. The overall perinatal survival is rare prior to 24 weeks of gestation. The survival rate increases from 36% at 24 weeks of gestation to 90% at 29 weeks. Significant morbidity also decreases with increasing birth weight and gestational age. Prolongation of gestation by as little as 1 week in PPROM prior to 28 weeks of gestation has profound effects on neonatal morbidity and mortality.[35]

## MANAGEMENT OF PREMATURE RUPTURE OF MEMBRANES

Management of PROM for each patient has to be individualized according to factors such as gestational age, duration of leaking, whether patient is in labor or not, fetal presentation, fetal heart rate (FHR) tracing pattern, and presence or absence of chorioamnionitis. In addition, the level of available neonatal care also plays an important role in deciding the course of management.

### Initial Evaluation

All pregnant women presenting with a history of watery discharge per vaginum should be hospitalized and subjected to a detailed clinical examination and laboratory tests to confirm the diagnosis of PROM. This is followed by an assessment of various factors important in planning the line of management.

### Management Options

The management can be broadly classified into:
- Management of term PROM
- Management of PPROM

### Management of Term Premature Rupture of Membranes

*Active versus expectant management:* Most patients go in spontaneous labor within 24 hours of rupture of membranes at term. The major question regarding management of these patients is whether to allow them to enter labor spontaneously or to induce labor. The major risk at this gestational age is of intrauterine infection which increases with the duration of rupture of membrane. The risk of chorioamnionitis with term PROM has been reported to be <10% and increases to 24% after 24 hours of PROM. Evidence supports that induction of labor as opposed to expectant management decreases the risk of chorioamnionitis without increasing the cesarean delivery rate.[2,36]

Proper counseling should be followed by an informed consent regarding the risks and benefits of termination of pregnancy from the woman and her relatives. The next step in clinical management is to determine whether the cervix is favorable for induction of labor or not. If the cervix is favorable, induction of labor with oxytocin infusion is recommended.[2] During induction of labor with oxytocin, a sufficient period of adequate contractions (at least 12–18 hours) should be allowed for the latent phase of labor to progress before diagnosing failed induction and moving to cesarean delivery.[36] However, if the cervix is unfavorable, labor may be induced with prostaglandins (PE) either intracervical PGE2 gel 0.5 mg every 6 hours for two doses or intravaginal, oral or sub-lingual misoprostol 25 µg every 6 hours for a maximum of 5 doses.[2]

*Fetomaternal monitoring:* Maternal pulse, temperature, and auscultation of fetal heart should be done every 4–8 hourly.[37] A complete blood count (CBC) should be sent for a baseline total leukocyte count (TLC) and differential leukocyte count (DLC). A high count may indicate the beginning of ascending genital tract infection. High vaginal swab should be sent on admission for any vaginal infection. Intrapartum fetal monitoring in the form of intermittent FHR auscultation should be done.[19]

*Prophylactic antibiotics:* The routine use of prophylactic antibiotics in women with term PROM has not been proved to reduce the incidence of infectious morbidity. Although, therapeutic antibiotics should be started preferably in women with prolonged leaking (>18 hours) or with any evidence of chorioamnionitis such as persistent elevation of the maternal or FHR, maternal pyrexia, marked leukocytosis, or uterine tenderness. Prophylactic antibiotics should also be utilized in properly selected patients for the prevention of group B streptococcal infections and women requiring prophylaxis for bacterial endocarditis.[2,38,39]

### Management of Preterm Premature Rupture of Membranes

The management issues relating to PPROM occurring between 24 and 37 weeks gestation are far more complex than PROM at term. Several areas of controversies exist regarding the best medical approach to the management of PROM remote from term. The most important factors that need to be balanced in formulating a management plan is the risk of prematurity and risk of infection to the neonate with its associated morbidity and mortality depending upon the gestational age and availability of neonatal intensive care. Taking the above facts into consideration women with PPROM can be further subdivided into those between 34 and 37 weeks and those below 34 weeks. In absence of intensive neonatal care unit, women with PPROM (<34 weeks) should be transferred to a tertiary care facility with sufficient support from neonatology unit. The management options in patients with PPROM include expectant management and immediate delivery, and each has its own advantages and disadvantages. However, if managed judiciously the benefits of expectant management outweigh its risks before 34 weeks of gestation. Hence, a proper selection of patients should be done for each type of management.[40]

*Immediate delivery:* Immediate termination of pregnancy irrespective of the gestational age is indicated in women with:
- Signs and/or symptoms suggestive of chorioamnionitis
- Signs of fetal distress as evidenced by meconium-stained liquor with or without abnormal FHR patterns
- Abruptio placentae
- Severe oligohydramnios.

*Expectant management:* In the absence of an indication for immediate delivery and a period of gestation < $34^{0/7}$ weeks, an expectant approach should be opted. The risks and potential benefits of expectant management should be discussed with the patient and her family and an informed consent should be obtained. The major aim of the expectant management of PPROM is to prolong pregnancy so as to achieve fetal lung maturity and to identify when clinically significant chorioamnionitis is evolving and deliver the fetus at the right time. A delay in identification of this can lead to septicemia in the mother and neonate with its adverse sequelae. The maternal and fetal status should be evaluated daily and the safety and potential benefits of expectant management should be reassessed. If the condition remains stable, the immature fetus may benefit from expectant management, even if for a short period, as it allows administration of steroids and antibiotics. The decision to continue pregnancy with expectant management in PPROM should only be made following a detailed maternal and fetal evaluation on admission including a per speculum examination to collect discharge or swabs either from the cervix or posterior fornix for bacteriological culture to diagnose any subclinical infection. Electronic FHR monitoring and uterine activity monitoring is carried out to identify occult umbilical cord compression and presence of any uterine contractions.

It is important to remember that nonstress test (NST) at <32 weeks of gestation may be false nonreactive in an immature but otherwise healthy fetus. However, after a reactive baseline test, a subsequent nonreactive test should be considered abnormal or suspicious.[2,36]

Once pregnancy reaches 34 weeks, the benefit from expectant management of PPROM is unclear and the risks of infection may outweigh any potential benefits. Traditionally, delivery has been recommended in cases of PPROM after 34 weeks of gestation but a recent large randomized study has suggested benefits of expectant management in cases with gestational age between 34 weeks and $36^{+6/7}$ weeks; hospital admission and careful monitoring however, is necessary.[41] In women with late PPROM, that is between 34 and $36^{+6/7}$ weeks, immediate delivery resulted in higher rates of RDS, intensive care unit (ICU) admissions, and cesarean deliveries as compared to those with expectant management.[42] Decision regarding expectant management should be taken on individual basis after assessing the benefit and risk, from both maternal and neonatal perspectives, and in consultation with the woman. Expectant management, however, should not extend beyond 37 weeks of gestation.

## COMPONENTS OF EXPECTANT MANAGEMENT

The basic components of expectant management are:
- Maternal monitoring
- Fetal monitoring
- Drug treatment

### Maternal Monitoring (Table 3)

The woman is advised adequate bed rest and subjected to close monitoring of vital parameters every 4-8 hourly especially pulse and temperature. Though, tachycardia and fever are crude and late indicators of evolving chorioamnionitis, but these are easy to perform and are noninvasive. The woman is daily observed for leaking as regards its amount, color, and odor. Daily per abdomen examination is done to assess amount of liquor, any uterine tenderness, uterine contractions, and FHR.

**TABLE 3:** Routine maternal–fetal surveillance.

| Maternal parameters | Fetal parameters |
|---|---|
| Maternal pulse—4 times a day | Ultrasonography—2 weekly to assess fetal growth |
| Maternal temperature—4 times a day | USG for AFI for estimation of liquor—weekly |
| Observe amount, consistency, color, and odor of discharge daily | Biophysical score (BPS) according to CTG |
| TLC/DLC—Three times a week | |
| C-reactive protein measurement | |

(AFI: amniotic fluid index; CTG: cardiotocography; DLC: differential leukocyte count; TLC: total leukocyte count; USG: ultrasonography)

> **BOX 1:** Investigations in preterm premature rupture of membranes.
>
> - Urine for microscopy and culture
> - Amniotic fluid collected on per speculum, for microbiological culture
> - Microscopic examination of the cervicovaginal discharge for evidence of "ferning"
> - High vaginal swab for Gram's staining and culture
> - Endocervical swab for *Neisseria gonorrhoeae* and *Chlamydia*
> - Urethral and anorectal swab culture in women suspicious of genital infection

> **BOX 2:** Signs and symptoms of chorioamnionitis.
>
> - Maternal fever > 38°C with any two of the following:
>   - Increased white cell count (>15,000/cm$^2$)
>   - Maternal tachycardia (>100 bpm)
>   - Fetal tachycardia (>160 bpm)
>   - Uterine tenderness
>   - Offensive smelling vaginal discharge
>   - C-reactive protein raised

## *Investigations (Box 1)*

All baseline investigations including CBC with peripheral smear examination, urine routine and microscopy examination, high vaginal swab for culture and sensitivity, and estimation of C-reactive protein (CRP) should be done. This is to be followed by daily total and differential white blood cell count (TLC/DLC) if leaking persists or every 72 hours if leaking stops. White blood cell count and level of CRP are possibly better predictors of evolving chorioamnionitis. The patient should be closely observed for signs and symptoms of chorioamnionitis as detailed in **Box 2**. In the absence of other pre-existing infections, the presence of fever exceeding 38°C or 100.4°F with or without uterine tenderness and/or maternal or fetal tachycardia is suggestive of chorioamnionitis. It is important to remember that a rising maternal blood leukocyte count may be consequent to administration of antenatal corticosteroids and may persist for 5–7 days.[2,13]

However, in the absence of clinical evidence of infection, serial monitoring of leukocyte counts and other markers of inflammation such as CRP and weekly high vaginal swab cultures have not proved useful.[19,36]

## Fetal Monitoring

There is no consensus on the optimal frequency of assessment, but an acceptable strategy would include periodic ultrasonographic monitoring of fetal growth and periodic FHR monitoring.[36] Fetal monitoring should be performed at least once a day. Daily fetal movement count (DFMC) and intermittent FHR auscultation should be done.

Cardiotocography, biophysical profile score, and Doppler velocimetry are useful but have limitation in predicting intrauterine fetal infection.[19]

Ultrasonography is usually performed once or twice a week to assess fetal growth and liquor volume. Ultrasonographic examination for fetal growth, fetal well-being, and amniotic fluid index should be used liberally to ensure appropriateness of continued expectant management. A scan will provide information on gestational age, presentation, placental position, and fetal weight to assist in planning for delivery and counseling on neonatal outcomes. While oligohydramnios has been associated with shorter latency and chorioamnionitis, it alone is not an indication for delivery when other tests of surveillance are reassuring. Digital cervical examination is to be avoided as far as possible throughout expectant management. It should only be done to decide the mode of delivery not the timing of delivery.

## Drug Treatment

This includes administration of antibiotics to prevent chorioamnionitis and steroids to enhance fetal lung maturity **(Table 4)**.

### *Prophylactic Antibiotic Therapy*

Once a decision to manage a patient expectantly has been made, institution of prophylactic antibiotics should be considered. A number of antibiotic regimens have been advocated for use in patients with PPROM.

Based on various recommendation either a combination of ampicillin 2 g and erythromycin 250 mg intravenously every 6 hours for 48 hours, followed by oral amoxicillin 250 mg and erythromycin 333 mg every 8 hours for 5 days[2,36,43] or oral erythromycin 250 mg four times a day for 10 days or until the woman is in established labor can be instituted.[19] Women receiving prophylactic antibiotics showed increased latency of up to 3 weeks despite discontinuation of the antibiotics after 7 days. Substitution with a single oral dose of azithromycin in situations where erythromycin is not available or not tolerated could be an alternative.[36]

It is advisable to administer appropriate antibiotics for intrapartum group B *Streptococcus* prophylaxis to women who are carriers or whose status is unknown and PROM is for >18 hours even if these patients have previously received a course of antibiotics after PPROM. Intravenous penicillin is the treatment of choice. Benzylpenicillin 3 g IV loading dose is given as soon as possible, followed by 1.2 g IV every 4 hours until delivery and a minimum of 4 hours of antibiotics is recommended prior to delivery.[39,38,44]

### *Antenatal Corticosteroid Treatment*

A single course of corticosteroids should be administered to pregnant women between $24^{0/7}$ weeks and $34^{0/7}$ weeks of gestation with PPROM to reduce the risk of neonatal RDS, IVH, and necrotizing enterocolitis (NEC).[19,36] Corticosteroids decrease perinatal morbidity and mortality after PPROM.[2,36]

**TABLE 4:** Drug treatment during expectant management.

| Drug | Recommended dose | Remark |
| --- | --- | --- |
| Antenatal steroids | *Betamethasone*: 12 mg IM every 24 hours × 2 doses. OR *Dexamethasone*: 6 mg IM every 12 hours × 4 doses. | Should be given to women with PPROM from 24 to 34 weeks of gestation Can be considered up to 35$^{+6}$ weeks' gestation. (Grade A) (RCOG) |
| Prophylactic antibiotic | *Ampicillin*: 2 g IV every 6 hours Plus *Erythromycin*: 250 mg IV every 6 hours × 48 hours followed by amoxicillin 250 mg PO every 8 hours for 5 days Plus erythromycin 333 mg PO every 8 hours for 5 days. Or Oral erythromycin 250 mg four times a day for 10 days Or a single dose of Azithromycin 1g in situations where erythromycin is not available or is not tolerable | If penicillin allergy, low-risk: Cefazolin 1 g IV every 8 hours × 48 hours and erythromycin 250 mg IV every 6 hours × 48 hours followed by: Cephalexin 500 mg PO every 6 hours × 5 days |
| Magnesium sulfate | Magnesium sulfate, IV: Bolus 4 g over 40 minutes, then infuse 2 g/hour maintenance dose from premixed 20 g/500 mL bag until delivery or until 12 hours of therapy. (If preterm delivery seems unlikely after 12 hours of therapy, discontinue therapy) | Intravenous magnesium sulfate should be offered between 24$^{+0}$ and 29$^{+6}$ weeks of gestation. (Grade A) (RCOG, 2019) Can be considered to <32 weeks when delivery is expected within 24 hours in established labor or having a planned preterm birth within 24 hours |

(IM; intramuscular; PPROM: preterm premature rupture of membranes; RCOG: Royal College of Obstetricians and Gynecologists)

The recommended schedule of antenatal corticosteroid is two doses of 12 mg of betamethasone given intramuscularly (IM) at 24-hour intervals or four doses of dexamethasone 6 mg given IM at 12-hour intervals.[45] A course of corticosteroids should also be considered for patients who present with PPROM at 34$^{+0}$–36$^{+6/7}$ weeks of gestation who are going to be managed expectantly, have not received a previous course of steroids, and who are scheduled for delivery in >24 hours and <7 days.[36]

Administration of antenatal steroids for pregnancies that present with PPROM in the 22nd week of gestation is also reasonable if delivery in the next 7 days is anticipated and the family desires aggressive neonatal intervention after thorough consultation with maternal-fetal medicine and neonatology specialists.[46]

A single rescue course of betamethasone can be given in pregnancies up to 34 weeks of gestation who are at high risk of delivery within 7 days and prior exposure > 14 days earlier.[47]

### Tocolytics

The use of tocolytic drugs in patients of PPROM is controversial. Tocolytic therapy may prolong the latent period for a short time but does not appear to improve neonatal outcome.[48]

In the absence of adequate data, a short course of tocolysis after PPROM to allow initiation of antibiotics, administration of corticosteroid, and maternal transport may be considered, however, long-term therapy in patients with PPROM is not recommended.[2,19,36]

In the setting of ruptured membranes with active labor, therapeutic tocolysis has not been shown to prolong latency or improve neonatal outcomes. Therefore, therapeutic tocolysis is not recommended.[19,36]

### Magnesium Sulfate for Fetal Neuroprotection

Recently, several randomized trials have shown the beneficial effect of magnesium sulfate on fetal neuroprotection when administered to women with PPROM < 32 weeks with risk of imminent delivery. Though, there are many regimens but an optimal treatment regimen for fetal neuroprotection still remains unclear. However, a single dose of 40 mL infusion of 0.1 g/mL of MgSO$_4$ (4 g) solution given over 30 minutes has shown to reduce the risk of cerebral palsy in surviving infants (RR, 0.71; 95% CI, 0.55–0.91).[49-51] As per the recent recommendations, women with PPROM before 32 weeks of gestation, who are thought to be at risk of imminent delivery, should be considered candidates for fetal neuroprotective treatment with intravenous magnesium sulfate regardless of the treatment regimen.[19,36]

### Timing of Delivery

The timing of delivery should be individualized taking into consideration the clinical condition, gestational age, and woman's preference. As per the recent Royal College of Obstetricians and Gynecologists (RCOG) guidelines, if there are no contraindications to continuation of pregnancy, expectant management with careful monitoring can be offered in cases of PPROM till 37$^{+0}$ weeks of pregnancy.[19] Continuation of expectant management until 37 weeks in a well dated pregnancy with no indication of termination such as chorioamnionitis, fetal distress, and vaginal bleeding and where leaking stops with adequate liquor is considered a reasonable approach.[36] Expectant management, however, should not be extended beyond 37 weeks.

### Mode of Delivery

In the absence of any fetal or maternal compromise and cephalic presentation, vaginal delivery is usually indicated.

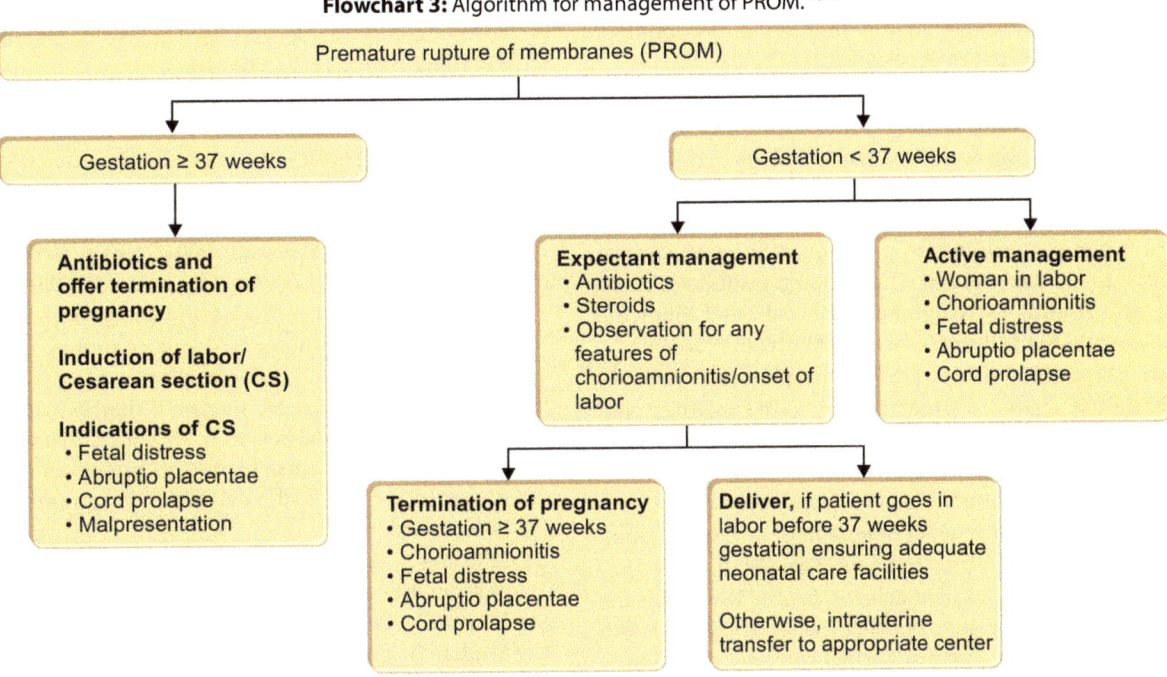

Flowchart 3: Algorithm for management of PROM.[41,42]

Where the presentation is breech, decision need to be individualized as there is no evidence to suggest that cesarean section improves neonatal outcome. The management of PROM is summarized in **Flowchart 3**.

## KEY POINTS

- Premature rupture of membranes complicates 5–10% of all pregnancies. PPROM occurs in 2–4% of all pregnancies and is associated with 18–20% of all perinatal deaths.
- The etiopathogenesis of PROM is still unknown however; infection remains the major contributor in its genesis.
- The fetal membranes serve as a barrier to ascending infection. Once the membranes rupture, both the mother and fetus are at risk for infection and other complications.
- Premature rupture of membrane is largely a clinical diagnosis. Three clinical signs of PROM documented on sterile speculum examination are visual pooling of fluid in the vagina or leakage of fluid from the cervical os, an alkaline pH of cervicovaginal discharge, and/or microscopic ferning of the cervicovaginal discharge on drying.
- The initial management of a woman presenting with suspected PROM should focus on confirming the diagnosis, documenting correct gestational age, assessing fetal well-being, and deciding on the plan of management.
- The management of term PROM includes admission to hospital and induction of labor.
- Immediate termination of pregnancy irrespective of the gestational age should be done in women with signs and symptoms suggestive of chorioamnionitis, severe oligohydramnios, and signs of fetal distress evidenced by meconium stained liquor with or without abnormal FHR patterns and abruptio placentae.
- Management options in PPROM include admission to hospital, careful fetomaternal monitoring, administration of antenatal corticosteroids, and broad-spectrum antibiotics.
- Women with PPROM before $32^{0/7}$ weeks of gestation who are thought to be at risk of imminent delivery should be considered candidates for fetal neuroprotective treatment with intravenous magnesium sulfate.
- In the absence of fetal or maternal compromise, expectant management can be continued in hospital with careful monitoring till 37 weeks of pregnancy but should not be extended beyond 37 weeks.

## REFERENCES

1. ACOG practice bulletin. Premature rupture of membranes. Clinical management guidelines for obstetrician-gynecologists. Number 1, June 1998. American College of Obstetricians and Gynecologists. Int J Gynaecol Obstet. 1998;63(1):75-84.
2. ACOG Committee on Practice Bulletins-Obstetrics. ACOG Practice Bulletin No. 80: premature rupture of membranes. Clinical management guidelines for obstetrician-gynecologists. Obstet Gynecol. 2007;109(4):1007-19.
3. Bryant-Greenwood GD, Millar LK. Human fetal membranes: their preterm premature rupture Biol Reprod. 2000;63(6):1575-9.
4. Parry S, Strauss JF 3rd. Premature rupture of the fetal membranes. N Engl J Med. 1998;338(10):663-70.
5. Kumar D, Moore RM, Mercer BM, Mansour JM, Redline RW, Moore JJ. The physiology of fetal membrane weakening and rupture: insights gained from the determination of physical properties revisited. Placenta. 2016;42:59-73.

6. Caughey AB, Robinson JN, Norwitz ER. Contemporary diagnosis and management of preterm premature rupture of membranes. Rev Obstet Gynecol. 2008;1(1):11-22.
7. Lykke JA, Dideriksen KL, Lidegaard O, Langhoff-Roos J. First-trimester vaginal bleeding and complications later in pregnancy. Obstet Gynecol. 2010;115(5):935-44.
8. Mercer BM, Goldenberg RL, Meis PJ, Moawad AH, Shellhaas C, Das A, et al. The Preterm Prediction Study: prediction of preterm premature rupture of membranes through clinical findings and ancillary testing. The National Institute of Child Health and Human Development Maternal-Fetal Medicine Units Network. Am J Obstet Gynecol. 2000;183(3):738-45.
9. Medina TM, Ashley Hill D. Preterm premature rupture of membranes: diagnosis and management. Am Fam Physician. 2006;73(4):659-64.
10. Romero R, Chaiworapongsa T, Kuivaniemi H, Tromp G. Bacterial vaginosis, the inflammatory response and the risk of preterm birth: a role for genetic epidemiology in the prevention of preterm birth. Am J Obstet Gynecol. 2004;190(6):1509-19.
11. Hillier SL, Nugent RP, Eschenbach DA, Krohn MA, Gibbs RS, Martin DH, et al. Association between bacterial vaginosis and preterm delivery of a low-birth-weight infant. The vaginal infections and prematurity Study Group. N Engl J Med. 1995;333(26):1737-42.
12. Allen SR. Epidemiology of premature rupture of the fetal membranes. Clin Obstet Gynecol. 1991;34(4):685-93.
13. Royal College of Obstetricians and Gynaecologists (RCOG). Preterm prelabour rupture of membranes (Green-top Guideline no. 44). London (UK): Royal College of Obstetricians and Gynaecologists (RCOG); 2006. p. 11.
14. Lewis DF, Major CA, Towers CV, Asrat T, Harding JA, Garite TJ. Effects of digital vaginal examinations on latency period in preterm premature rupture of membranes. Obstet Gynecol. 1992;80(4):630-4.
15. Ladfors L, Mattsson LA, Eriksson M, Fall O. Is a speculum examination sufficient for excluding the diagnosis of ruptured fetal membranes? Acta Obstet Gynecol Scand. 1997;76(8):739-42.
16. Gorodeski IG, Haimovitz L, Bahari CM. Reevaluation of the pH, ferning and Nile blue sulphate staining methods in pregnant women with premature rupture of the fetal membranes. J Perinat Med. 1982;10(6):286-92.
17. de Haan HH, Offermans PM, Smits F, Schouten HJ, Peeters LL. Value of the fern test to confirm or reject the diagnosis of ruptured membranes in modest in nonlaboring women presenting with nonspecific vaginal fluid loss. Am J Perinatol. 1994;11(1):46-50.
18. Friedman ML, McElin TW. Diagnosis of ruptured fetal membranes. Clinical study and review of the literature. Am J Obstet Gynecol. 1969;104(4):544-50
19. Thomson AJ, Royal College of Obstetricians and Gynaecologists. Care of Women Presenting with Suspected Preterm Prelabour Rupture of Membranes from 24+0 Weeks of Gestation. Green-top Guideline No. 73. BJOJ. 2019;126(9):e152-66.
20. Robson MS, Turner MJ, Stronge JM, O'Herlihy CO. Is amniotic fluid quantitation of value in the diagnosis and conservative management of prelabour membrane rupture at term? Br J Obstet Gynaecol. 1990;97(4):324-8.
21. Naylor CS, Gregory K, Hobel C. Premature rupture of the membranes: an evidence-based approach to clinical care. Am J Perinatol. 2001;18(7):397-413.
22. Gibbs RS, Blanco JD. Premature rupture of the membranes. Obstet Gynecol. 1982;60(6):671-9.
23. Cousins LM, Smok DP, Lovett SM, Poeltler DM. Amnisure placental alpha macroglobulin-1 rapid immunoassay versus standard diagnostic methods for detection of rupture of membranes. Am J Perinatol. 2005;22(6):317-20.
24. Lee SE, Park JS, Norwitz ER, Kim KW, Park HS, Jun JK. Measurement of placental alpha-microglobulin-1 in cervicovaginal discharge to diagnose rupture of membranes. Obstet Gynecol. 2007;109(3):634-40.
25. Palacio M, Kühnert M, Berger R, Larios CL, Marcellin L. Meta-analysis of studies on biochemical marker tests for the diagnosis of premature rupture of membranes: comparison of performance indexes. BMC Pregnancy Childbirth. 2014,14:183.
26. Igbinosa I, Moore FA 3rd, Johnson C, Block JE. Comparison of rapid immunoassays for rupture of fetal membranes. BMC Pregnancy Childbirth. 2017;17(1):128.
27. Mulhair L, Carter J, Poston L, Seed P, Briley A. Prospective cohort study investigating the reliability of the AmnioSens method for detection of spontaneous rupture of membranes. BJOG. 2009;116(2):313-8.
28. Bornstein J, Geva A, Solt I, Fait V, Schoenfeld A, Shoham HK, et al. Nonintrusive diagnosis of premature ruptured amniotic membranes using a novel polymer. Am J Perinatol. 2006;23(6):351-4.
29. van der Ham DP, van der Ham DP, van Teeffelen AS, Mol BW. Prelabour rupture of membranes: overview of diagnostic methods. Curr Opin Obstet Gynecol. 2012;24(6):408-12.
30. Canadian Agency for drugs and technologies in Health (CADTH). (2012). AmniSure versus fern testing to assess the rupture of fetal membranes in pregnant women: a review of the comparative accuracy, cost-effectiveness, and guidelines. Rapid Response Report: summary with critical appraisal. [online] Available from: http:// www.cadth.ca/media/pdf/htis/mar-2012/RC0341%20 Amnisure%20Final.pdf [Last accessed July, 2021].
31. US Food and Drug Administration. (2018). Risks associated with use of rupture of membranes tests—letter to health care providers. Silver Spring, MD: FDA. [online] Available from: https://www.fda.gov/medical-devices/letters-health-care-providers/risks-associated-use-rupture-membranes-tests-letter-health-care-providers (Level III) [Last accessed July, 2021].
32. Pergialiotis V, Bellos I, Fanaki M, Antsaklis A, Loutradis D, Daskalakis G. The impact of residual oligohydramnios following preterm premature rupture of membranes on adverse pregnancy outcomes: a meta-analysis. Am J Obstet Gynecol. 2020;222(6):628-30.
33. Buhimschi CS, Buhimschi IA, Norwitz ER, Sfakianaki AK, Hamar B, Copel JA, et al. Sonographic myometrial thickness predicts the latency interval of women with preterm premature rupture of the membranes and oligohydramnios. Am J Obstet Gynecol. 2005;193(3 Pt 1):762-70.
34. Greenwald JL. Premature rupture of the membranes: diagnostic and management strategies. Am Fam Physician. 1993;48(2):293-306.

35. Mercer B, Milluzzi C, Collin M. Periviable birth at 20 to 26 weeks of gestation: proximate causes, previous obstetric history and recurrence risk. Am J Obstet Gynecol. 2005;193(3 Pt 2):1175-80.
36. Prelabor rupture of membranes: ACOG Practice Bulletin, No. 217. Obstet Gynecol. 2020;135(3):e80-97.
37. Royal College of Obstetricians and Gynaecologists (RCOG). Preterm prelabour rupture of membranes (Green-top Guideline no. 44). London (UK): Royal College of Obstetricians and Gynaecologists (RCOG); 2010.
38. Schrag S, Gorwitz R, Fultz-Butts K, Schuchat A. Prevention of perinatal group B streptococcal disease. Revised guidelines from CDC. MMWR Recomm Rep. 2002;51(RR-11):1-22.
39. American College of Obstetricians and Gynecologists. ACOG Committee Opinion: number 279, December 2002. Prevention of early-onset group B streptococcal disease in newborns. Obstet Gynecol. 2002;100(6):1405-12.
40. Lorthe E, Ancel PY, Torchin H, Kaminski M, Langer B, Subtil D, et al. Impact of Latency Duration on the Prognosis of Preterm Infants after Preterm Premature Rupture of Membranes at 24 to 32 Weeks' Gestation: A National Population-Based Cohort Study. J Pediatr. 2017; 182:47-52.e2.
41. Morris JM, Roberts CL, Bowen JR, Patterson JA, Bond DM, Algert CS, et al. Immediate delivery compared with expectant management after preterm pre-labour rupture of the membranes close to term (PPROMT trial): a randomised controlled trial. Lancet. 2016;387(10017):444-52.
42. Quist-Nelson J, de Ruigh AA, Seidler AL, van der Ham DP, Willekes C, Berghella V, et al. Immediate delivery compared with expectant management in late preterm prelabor rupture of membranes: an individual participant data meta-analysis. Obstet Gynecol. 2018;131(2):269-79.
43. Committee on Practice Bulletins-Obstetrics. ACOG Practice Bulletin No. 199: Use of Prophylactic Antibiotics in Labor and Delivery. Obstet Gynecol. 2018;132(3):e103-19.
44. Chatzakis C, Papatheodorou S, Sarafidis K, Dinas K, Makrydimas G, Sotiriadis A. Effect on perinatal outcome of prophylactic antibiotics in preterm prelabor rupture of membranes: network meta-analysis of randomized controlled trials. Ultrasound Obstet Gynecol. 2020;55(1):20-31.
45. Roberts D, Brown J, Medley N, Dalziel SR. Antenatal corticosteroids for accelerating fetal lung maturation for women at risk of preterm birth. Cochrane Database Syst Rev. 2017;3(3):CD004454.
46. Park CK, Isayama T, McDonald SD. Antenatal Corticosteroid Therapy Before 24 Weeks of Gestation: a systematic review and meta-analysis. Obstet Gynecol. 2016;127(4):715-25.
47. Committee on Obstetric Practice. Committee Opinion No. 713: Antenatal Corticosteroid Therapy for Fetal Maturation. Obstet Gynecol 2017;130(2):e102-9.
48. Mackeen AD, Seibel-Seamon J, Muhammad J, Baxter JK, Berghella V. Tocolytics for preterm premature rupture of membranes. Cochrane Database Syst Rev. 2014;(2):CD007062.
49. Rouse DJ, Hirtz DG, Thom E, Varner MW, Spong CY, Mercer BM, et al. A randomized, controlled trial of magnesium sulfate for the prevention of cerebral palsy. N Engl J Med. 2008;359(9):895-905.
50. Marret S, Marpeau L, Zupan-Simunek V, Eurin D, Leveque C, Hellot MF, et al. Magnesium sulphate given before very-preterm birth to protect infant brain: the randomized controlled PREMAG trial. BJOG. 2007;114(3):310-8.
51. Crowther CA, Hiller JE, Doyle LW, Haslam RR. Effect of magnesium sulfate given for neuroprotection before preterm birth: a randomized controlled trial. JAMA. 2003;290(20):2669-76.

# CHAPTER 12

# Prolonged Pregnancy

*Amita Suneja, Sandhya Jain, Raksha Soni*

## ■ INTRODUCTION

Prolonged pregnancy is a common clinical situation and causes considerable anxiety to women and the treating obstetrician. Because of the associated perinatal morbidity and mortality as well as increased maternal morbidity, it demands accurate diagnosis, antenatal fetal surveillance and timely intervention.

The terms post-term, prolonged, postdates and postmature are often used interchangeably to signify pregnancies that have exceeded a duration considered to be the upper limit of normal. However, postmature, postmaturity syndrome and dysmaturity are not synonyms to post-term pregnancy, rather are used to describe an infant of pathologically prolonged pregnancy with recognizable clinical features.[1] Post-term or prolonged pregnancy is the preferred expression for an extended pregnancy.

## ■ DEFINITION

Latest definition of prolonged pregnancy, endorsed by the American College of Obstetricians and Gynecologists (ACOG)[2] and WHO[3] is 42 completed weeks (294 days) or more from the first day of last menstrual period (LMP) in women with a regular 28 days menstrual cycle. Pregnancies between 41 weeks 1 day and 41 weeks 6 days, although in the 42nd week, do not complete 42 weeks until the 7th day has elapsed.

The ACOG defines early term ($37^{0/7}$ weeks of gestation through $38^{6/7}$ weeks of gestation), full term ($39^{0/7}$ weeks of gestation through $40^{6/7}$ weeks of gestation), late term ($41^{0/7}$ weeks of gestation through $41^{6/7}$ weeks of gestation), and post-term ($42^{0/7}$ weeks of gestation and beyond) to more accurately describe deliveries occurring at or beyond $37^{0/7}$ weeks of gestation.[4]

## ■ EPIDEMIOLOGY

The estimated date of confinement or delivery (EDD) is calculated as 40 weeks after the first day of LMP, assuming normal 28 days cycle (Naegele's formula). About 1% of women deliver on the day of EDD. The incidence of post-term pregnancy is about 7% of all pregnancies.[1] As per an Indian study, incidence of pregnancy beyond 42 weeks was 1.25%.[5] The prevalence of prolonged pregnancy across the world varies from 3 to 12% and is affected by accuracy of gestational age estimation, complications in pregnancy demanding early termination and adoption of elective induction of labor (IOL) before 41 weeks gestation.[6-8]

## ■ PREDISPOSING FACTORS

### Demographic Factors

Certain maternal demographic factors have been related to prolonged pregnancy such as primiparity, higher socioeconomic class, overweight, obesity (BMI >35 kg/m$^2$), sedentary lifestyle, elderly multipara and increased fish consumption in first two trimesters.[1,9] Smoking is associated with preterm birth rather than post-term, however mechanisms are poorly understood.[10]

### Ethnic Factors

Babies of different ethnic origin most likely mature at different rates. Studies have shown that the median gestational length is 39 completed weeks in Black and Asian women in comparison to 40 completed weeks in White European women. This explains an almost threefold increased risk of cesarean section delivery in nulliparous black females when induced for postdated pregnancy.[11,12]

### Biological and Genetic Factors

A woman with single previous prolonged pregnancy has a 30% chance of recurrence which suggests that prolonged pregnancies are biologically determined. Few studies have observed this tendency of recurrence of prolonged pregnancy across generations especially in Swedish women.[13,14]

The genetic influence on the initiation of parturition may differ for preterm, term, and post-term births. Paternal genes contributing to fetal genome, when expressed preferentially through genomic imprinting tend to optimize the fetal outcome by maintaining the pregnancy and fetal growth. As pregnancy progresses influence of fetal genetic factors increases indicating an important role of paternal genes in post-term birth.[13]

## Fetoplacental Factors

Fetoplacental factors have been seen to predispose to post-term pregnancy. These include anencephaly, adrenal hypoplasia, and X-linked placental sulfatase deficiency. These cause a lack of the usually high estrogen levels of normal pregnancy which is essential for labor initiation. Estrogen helps in initiation of labor by increasing the release of oxytocin from posterior pituitary, stimulates oxytocin receptor synthesis in myometrium and decidua, accelerates prostaglandin, myometrial contractile protein synthesis and also increases excitability of myometrial cell membranes. A relative fetal adrenocortical deficiency may contribute to delay in onset of labor and an increased risk of intrapartum hypoxia and even death in post-term pregnancy. Infants born post-term may have an inherent biological defect, since it has been found that there is increased risk of demise up to 2 years of age; sudden infant death syndrome is also more common in them.

## Other Factors

In term laboring women cervical nitric acid release helps in cervical ripening and therefore its reduced levels may be a factor for prolonged pregnancy.[15]

## PATHOPHYSIOLOGY

### Postmaturity Syndrome

The postmature infant has wrinkled, patchy, peeling skin and body wasting; nails are long and neonate looks old and worrisome. These changes are due to loss of vernix caseosa, subcutaneous fat and lanugo. Most of them are not growth restricted. The incidence of the postmaturity syndrome increases with the length of pregnancy and at 42 weeks, postmaturity affects about 20% of fetuses.[16]

### Placental Dysfunction

The concept that postmaturity is due to placental insufficiency has persisted despite an absence of morphological or significant qualitative findings. It has been reported that placental apoptosis (i.e., programmed cell death), significantly increases at 41 to 42 completed weeks. The post-term placenta shows a decrease in length and diameter of chorionic villi, fibrinoid necrosis, and accelerated atherosis of vessels. There are foci of hemorrhagic infarcts and calcium deposition.[16] The post-term fetus may continue to gain weight, though at a slower rate between 38 and 42 weeks. This at least suggests that placental function is not compromised.

### Amniotic Fluid Changes

There are quantitative and qualitative changes with prolongation of pregnancy. The amniotic fluid volume reaches a peak of 1,000 mL at 38 weeks and decreases to 800 mL at 40 weeks. It further decreases with prolonged gestation; the mechanism seems to be diminished production of urine by the fetus. Oligohydramnios has been associated with cord compression, fetal heart rate abnormalities, meconium-stained amniotic fluid, and fetal acidosis.[2] Fetal heart tracing shows variable decelerations and saltatory baseline pattern consistent with cord occlusion due to oligohydramnios. At term, the fluid becomes milky and cloudy due to abundant flakes of vernix caseosa. It becomes greenish-yellow with passage of meconium. Meconium also makes it thick and viscous increasing the chances of 'meconium aspiration syndrome'.

### Fetal Macrosomia

Gestational age influences birth weight and the risk of macrosomia. Post-term pregnancy is associated with macrosomia and related complications with an OR of 1.9.[17] Among all women in the United States in 2014, the risk of birth weight more than 4,500 g increases from 1.3% at 39 weeks of gestation to 2.9% when gestational age exceeds 41 weeks.[18] However, the ACOG guidelines do not support a policy of early labor induction in women at term who have suspected macrosomia.[19] Moreover, vaginal delivery is not contraindicated for women with estimated fetal weight up to 5,000 g. Cesarean delivery is recommended for estimated fetal weight greater than 4,500 g in the presence of prolonged second stage of labor or arrest of descent.

## DIAGNOSIS

The management of pregnancy beyond 40 weeks gestation relies on an accurate assessment of the gestational age. Dating gestational age with LMP alone assumes both accurate recall by the patient and ovulation on 14th day of the menstrual cycle. The duration of follicular phase may vary from 7 to 21 days; also, delayed ovulation is an important cause of perceived prolonged pregnancy. First trimester ultrasound should be offered, ideally between 11 and 14 weeks, to all women, as it is a more accurate assessment of gestational age than LMP with fewer pregnancies prolonged past $41^{+0}$ weeks (I-A).[19] In case of a difference of more than 5 days between gestational age dated using the last menstrual period and first trimester ultrasound, the estimated date of delivery should be adjusted as per the first trimester ultrasound. If there is a difference of greater than 10 days between gestational ages dated using the LMP and second trimester ultrasound, the estimated date of delivery should be adjusted as per the second trimester ultrasound. When there has been both a first and second trimester ultrasound, gestational age should be determined by the earliest ultrasound.[20]

## FETOMATERNAL OUTCOME

### Fetal Outcome

In postdated pregnancy, especially after 41 weeks' fetal complications increase mainly due to increasing fetal weight, decline in placental function, oligohydramnios which increases chances of cord compression, and meconium aspiration. Therefore, there is increased risk of fetal hypoxia, asphyxia, intracranial damage, meconium aspiration syndrome (MAS), macrosomia, bone fracture, peripheral nerve paralysis, atelectasis, hypoglycemia, intrauterine death and stillbirths.

Perinatal mortality after 42 weeks is twice as compared to the perinatal mortality at 40 weeks and by 44 weeks the rate is increased up to threefold.[21] The risk of unexplained intrauterine fetal demise is 1 in 926 at 40 weeks; 1 in 826 at 41 weeks; 1 in 769 at 42 weeks and 1 in 633 at 43 weeks.[22] In the Indian study incidence of still birth in post-term pregnancies beyond 42 weeks, was found to be 5.9%.[5] Intrauterine infections, placental insufficiency, cord compression and meconium aspiration are main contributors to the excess perinatal deaths.

## Neonatal Outcome

Neonates born at ≥41 weeks of gestation experience a one-third greater risk of neonatal mortality than term neonates born at 38–40 weeks of gestation. Neonates are at risk for hypoglycemia, polycythemia, respiratory distress syndrome, pneumonia, persistent pulmonary hypertension, birth fractures and Erb's palsy. They are at increased risk for intellectual disabilities, hypoxic ischemic encephalopathy, brain damage, seizure disorders and cerebral palsy. In a study, risk for CP was found to be higher in earlier or later delivery as compared to term delivery, with relative risk reaching 1.9 at 37 weeks (95% CI, 1.6–2.3) and 1.4 at 42 weeks (95% CI, 1.2–1.6).[23]

## Maternal Outcome

Maternal morbidity increases due to increase in endomyometritis, labor dystocia, perineal injuries, operative vaginal deliveries, cesarean section and postpartum hemorrhage.[23] There is considerable maternal anxiety once they go beyond the estimated date of confinement; moreover, many women find the physical burden of pregnancy at or near term to be intolerable.

## MANAGEMENT OF PREGNANCY BEYOND 40 WEEKS GESTATION

Pregnancies complicated by gestational diabetes, hypertension, or other high-risk conditions should be managed according to guidelines for those conditions and should not be allowed to go postdated. Low-risk patients should be offered induction of labor at 41 weeks. The risks and benefits of labor induction versus expectant management should be discussed with the patient at 41 weeks gestation. With appropriate obstetric and neonatal care, the absolute mortality rate is low with either management option.

## Recommendations for Induction of Labor

Worldwide, different countries have their own guidelines for induction of labor in uncomplicated singleton term pregnancies. In a recent Cochrane review of 30 RCTs (2018), policy of labor induction as compared to expectant management at or beyond term, is found to be associated with fewer perinatal deaths, fewer cesarean sections and more operative vaginal births.[24] NICU admissions were lower and fewer babies had low Apgar scores with induction. World Health Organization (2018) has recommended induction of labor for women, who are known with certainty to have reached 41 weeks (>40 weeks + 7 days) of gestation and are not at gestational age less than 41 weeks.[3]

NICE guidelines (2019) and The Society of Obstetricians and Gynecologists of Canada (SOGC, 2017) recommend that women with uncomplicated pregnancies should usually be offered induction of labor between $41^{+0}$ and $42^{+0}$ weeks to avoid the risks of prolonged pregnancy.[20,25] However, ACOG states that induction of labor is recommended after $42^{+0}$ weeks and by $42^{6/7}$ weeks of gestation (level A); IOL can be considered, between $41^{0/7}$ weeks and $42^{0/7}$ weeks of gestation (level B).[2]

South Australian Perinatal Practice Guideline (SAPPG 2020) also states that the risk of fetal death in singleton pregnancies increases with gestational age and is 0.44 per 1,000 live births at $40^{+0}$ weeks' gestation, 0.76 per 1,000 live births at $41^{+0}$ weeks' gestation and 1.38 per 1,000 live births at $42^{+0}$ weeks' gestation. As per this guideline, women with uncomplicated pregnancies should be offered induction of labor between $41^{+0}$ and $41^{+3}$ weeks to avoid the risks of prolonged pregnancy and waiting until $42^{+0}$ is not recommended.[26]

The exact timing should take into account the woman's preferences and local circumstances. Women who decline induction of labor should be offered increased antenatal monitoring consisting of at least twice weekly cardiotocography and ultrasound estimation of maximum amniotic pool. During labor, it is recommended to do early rupture of membranes to detect meconium stained liquor. Fetal heart rate monitoring should preferably be continuous where facilities are available. **Flowchart 1** summarizes management of post-term pregnancy.

## FETAL MONITORING

When the physician and patient chooses expectant management of a low-risk prolonged pregnancy, fetal monitoring should be performed which often includes daily fetal movement count, twice-weekly nonstress test (NST), biophysical profile (BPP), modified BPP (a combination of NST and AFI), and Doppler velocimetry of umbilical artery. Antenatal testing in the post-term pregnancy should include at least a NST and an assessment of amniotic fluid volume.[20]

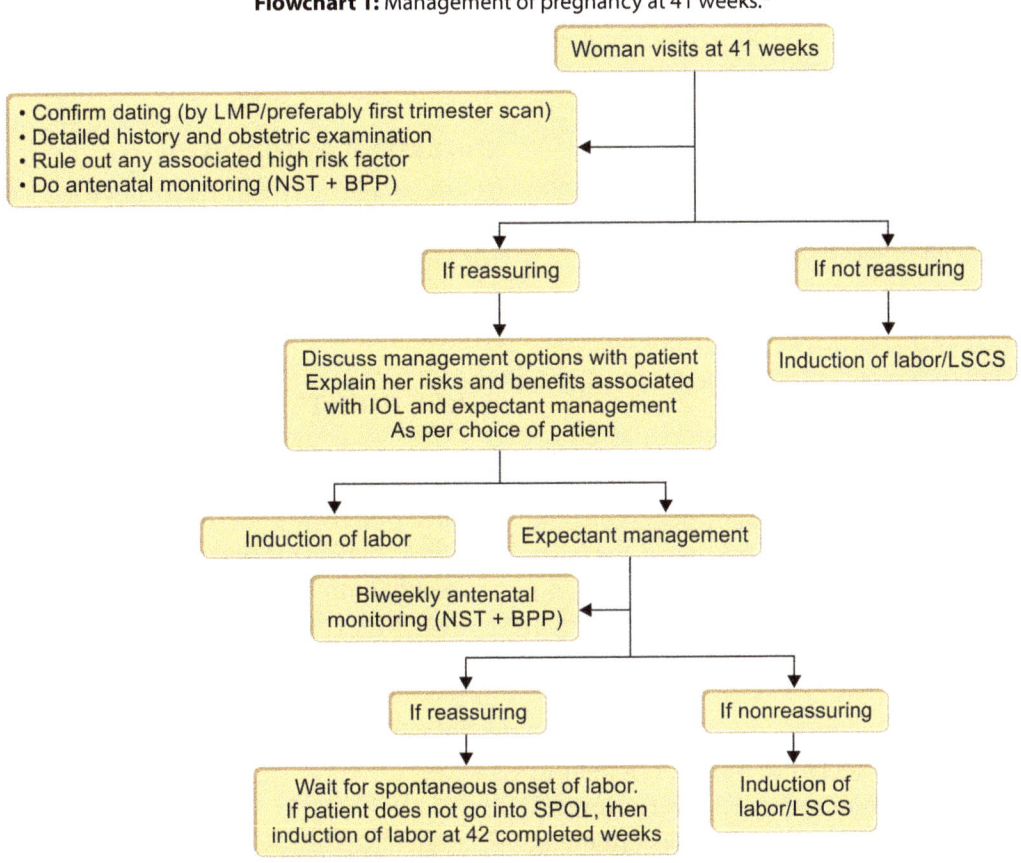

**Flowchart 1:** Management of pregnancy at 41 weeks.*

*WHO recommends induction of labor at 41 weeks.[3]
(BPP: biophysical profile; IOL: induction of labor; LMP: last menstrual period; LSCS: lower segment cesarean section; NST: nonstress test; SPOL: spontaneous onset of labor)

There is insufficient data to define optimal type or frequency of testing.[2] The American College of Obstetricians and Gynecologists has given a Level C recommendation (consensus and expert opinion) for initiation of fetal surveillance between 41 and 42 weeks because of evidence that perinatal morbidity and mortality increase as gestational age advances and that a twice weekly assessment of amniotic fluid and an NST should be adequate.[2]

For the outcome of stillbirth, a reactive NST has a negative predictive value of 99.8%, and a modified BPP or full BPP has a negative predictive value greater than 99.9%.[27] The efficacies of the tests do not relate to acute compromising events such as abruption or prolapsed umbilical cord. The positive predictive values of abnormal antenatal monitoring are more difficult to estimate but generally are lower. Using surrogate markers of fetal distress as an outcome, a nonreactive NST has a positive predictive value of approximately 10%, and an abnormal modified BPP has a positive predictive value of 40%.

Several studies have evaluated importance of detecting oligohydramnios in post-term pregnancies. For amniotic fluid assessment, measurement of the single deepest vertical pocket (at least 2 cm) seems a better choice since the use of the amniotic fluid index is associated with over diagnosis of oligohydramnios, with resultant increase in the rate of induction of labor without improvement in peripartum outcomes.[28]

Umbilical artery Doppler velocimetry may be of benefit only in pregnancies complicated by intrauterine growth restriction; middle cerebral artery Doppler velocimetry is still investigational.

# PREVENTION OF POST-TERM PREGNANCY

## Sweeping (or Stripping) of Membranes

Sweeping (or stripping) of membranes of the lower uterine segment has been reported to stimulate the onset of labor. Women should be offered the option of membrane sweeping commencing at 38 to 41 weeks, following a discussion of risks and benefits (I-A).[20] During a vaginal examination, the fetal membranes are separated from the cervix and lower uterine segment as far as possible, sweeping a finger inserted through the cervical os to 360° if possible. This procedure necessitates a sufficiently dilated cervix, usually representing a favorable Bishop score. When the cervix is closed, some clinicians attempt to stretch the cervix open or perform cervical massage. Sweeping results in the release of endogenous prostaglandins, softening the cervix and augmenting oxytocin-induced uterine contractions. Membrane sweeping is generally most efficacious in nulliparous women with unfavorable Bishop score. A Cochrane review in 2005 assessed 22 trials involving sweeping of membranes and recommended that routine use of sweeping of membranes from 38 weeks of pregnancy onward does not seem to produce clinically important benefits. When used as a means for induction of labor, the reduction in the use of more formal methods of induction needs to be balanced against women's discomfort and other adverse effects.[29]

According to a recent study sweeping of the membranes appears an effective and safe procedure in reducing the incidence of elective induction of labor and duration of pregnancy at term in low-risk population.[30]

Another recent large meta-analysis and review involving seven studies consisting of 2,252 participants concluded that membrane sweeping improves the likelihood of spontaneous labor when performed from 38 weeks of gestation onwards and therefore reduces the need for induction of labor for postmaturity without any undue side effects to the mother or baby.[31]

## Nipple Stimulation

Nipple stimulation has been shown to be of no benefit in reducing the incidence of post-term pregnancy. However, a Cochrane review on breast stimulation for cervical ripening and induction of labor concluded that breast stimulation appears beneficial in reducing the number of women not in labor after 72 hours, and reducing postpartum hemorrhage rates. It should not be used in high-risk women and further studies are required before recommending its adoption in practice.[32]

## Unprotected Sexual Intercourse

Human semen is the biological source that is presumed to contain the highest prostaglandin concentration. Unprotected sexual intercourse may stimulate labor due to the physical stimulation of the lower uterine segment, or endogenous release of oxytocin or from the direct action of prostaglandins in semen. Some studies show that unprotected sexual intercourse results in earlier onset of labor, reduction in post-term pregnancy rates and fewer interventions with labor induction. However, a Cochrane review concluded that the role of sexual intercourse as a method of induction of labor is uncertain and that further studies of sufficient power are needed to assess its value.[33,34]

## Acupuncture

The Shanghai College of Traditional Medicine recommends acupuncture for labor induction and is used routinely for this purpose in some societies without posing any significant maternal or fetal risks.[35,36] A Cochrane review on this issue concluded that although acupuncture improved cervical maturity to a certain extent, there was no reduction in cesarean section rate.[37] However, because of paucity of trial data, role of acupuncture in labor induction needs further evaluation.[38]

## Outpatient Misoprostol

In the recent past various studies have been carried out to explore the use of outpatient misoprostol to prevent prolonged pregnancy and all have consistently revealed favorable results.[39,40] However, larger studies are needed to get it into clinical practice.[40]

## ■ KEY POINTS

- Prolonged pregnancy is defined as pregnancy beyond 42 completed weeks (294 days) calculating from the first day of last menstrual period.
- The perinatal mortality rate (i.e., stillbirths plus neonatal deaths) approximately doubles by 42 weeks gestation and is four to six times greater at 44 weeks.
- First trimester ultrasound should be offered, ideally between 11 and 14 weeks to all women, as it is a more accurate assessment of gestational age than last menstrual period with fewer pregnancies prolonged past $41^{+0}$ weeks (I-A).
- Low-risk women should be offered induction of labor at 41 weeks.
- Antenatal testing used in the monitoring of the 41 to 42 weeks pregnancy should include biweekly NST and an assessment of amniotic fluid volume (I-A).
- Elective induction of labor at or beyond 41 weeks is effective in reducing perinatal morbidity and mortality associated with post-term pregnancies compared with expectant management, and should be offered to women with post-term pregnancies.
- Effective communication between obstetrician and patient, along with a discussion of the risks and benefits involved, is critical in ensuring that informed decisions are made.

## ■ REFERENCES

1. Galal M, Symonds I, Murray H, Petraglia F, Smith R. Postterm pregnancy. Facts Views Vis Obgyn. 2012,4(3):175-87.
2. American College of Obstetricians and Gynecologists. Practice Bulletin No 146: Management of Late Term and Post Term Pregnancies. Obstet Gynaecol. 2014;124(2 Pt 1):390-6.
3. WHO. WHO recommendations on induction of labor. Geneva: World Health Organization; 2018.
4. ACOG Committee Opinion No 579: Definition of term pregnancy. Obstet. Gynecol. 2013;122:1139.
5. Priya Shankar, Hemalatha KR. Study of maternal and foetal outcome in post-term pregnancies. Int J Reprod Contracept Obstet Gynaecol. 2017;6(7):3147-50.
6. MedScape. (2013). Post-term pregnancy. [online] Available from: http://emedicinemedscape.com/article/261369-overview. [Last Accessed July, 2021].

7. Mandruzzato G, Alfirevic Z, Chervenak F, Gruenebaum A, Heimstad R, Heinonen S, et al. Guidelines for the management of post term pregnancy. J Perinat Med. 2010;38(2)111-9.
8. Mya KS, Laopaiboon M, Vogel JP, Cecatti JG, Souza JP, Gulmezoglu AM, et al. Management of pregnancy at and beyond 41 completed weeks of gestation in low-risk women: a secondary analysis of two WHO multi-country surveys on maternal and newborn health. Reprod Health. 2017;14:141
9. Slen SF, Osterdal ML, Salvig JD. Duration of pregnancy in relation to seafood intake during early and mid-pregnancy: prospective cohort. Eur J Epidemiol. 2006;21(10):749-58.
10. Roos N, Sahlin L, Ekman-Ordeberg G, Kieler H, Stephansson O. Maternal risk factors for postterm pregnancy and cesarean delivery following labor induction. Actaobstetrician et Gynaecologica. 2010;89:1003-10.
11. Patel R, Steer P, Doyle P, Little MO, Elliott P. Does gestation vary by ethnic group? A London-based study of over 122,000 pregnancies with spontaneous onset of labor. Int J Epidemiol. 2004;33(1):107-13.
12. Papoutsis D, Antonakou A, Tzavara C. The effect of ethnic variation on the success of induced labour in nulliparous women with postdates pregnancies. Scientifica. 2016:9569725.
13. Oberg AS, Frisell T, Svenssonet AC. Maternal and fetal genetic contributions to postterm birth: familial clustering in a population-based sample of 475,429 Swedish births. Am J Epidemiol. 2013;177(6);531-7.
14. Mogren I, Stenlund H, Hogberg U. Recurrence of prolonged pregnancy. Int. J Epidemiology. 1999;28:253.
15. Vaisanen-Tommiska M, Nuutila M, Ylikorkala O. Cervical nitric oxide release in women post-term. Obstet Gynecol. 2004;103:657.
16. GLOWN. (2008). Postdatism. [online] Available from: https://www.glowm.com/section-view/heading/Postdatism/item/123#.YPU-QpgzbIU. [Last Accessed July, 2021].
17. Nkwabong E, Tangho GR. Risk factors for macrosomia. J Obstet Gynaecol India. 2015;65(4):226-9.
18. Hamilton BE, Martin JA, Osterman MJ, Curtin SC, Matthews TJ. Births: final data for 2014. Natl Vital Stat Rep. 2015;64(12):1-64.
19. American College of Obstetrics and Gynecology. Macrosomia. 2020;135(1):e18-e35
20. The Society of Obstetricians and Gynaecologists of Canada. Clinical practice guideline No. 214. Guidelines for the Management of pregnancy at 41+0 to 42+0 weeks. J Obstet Gynaecol Canada. 2017;39(8):E164-E174.
21. Prakash V, Kandalgaonkar S, Kose V. Fetomaternal outcome in postdated pregnancy. Int J Reprod Contracept Obstet Gynecol. 2019;8(5):1899-906.
22. Edlow AG, Norwitz ER. Endocrine diseases of pregnancy. Yen Jaffe Reprod Endocrinol. 2019,662-708.e17.
23. Markestad T. Cerebral palsy among term and postterm births. J Am Med Assoc. 2010;304(9):976-82.
24. Middleton P, Shepherd E, Crowther CA. Induction of labour for improving birth outcomes for women at or beyond term. Cochrane Database Syst Rev. 2018;5(5):CD004945.
25. NICE. Induction of labour overview. Manchester: NICE; 2019.
26. South Australian Perinatal Practice Guidelines (SAPPG). Clinical Guideline Prolonged Pregnancy. 2017.
27. ACOG Practice Bulletin Number 145: Antepartum Fetal Surveillance. Obstet Gynecol. 2014;124:182-92.
28. Nabhan AF, Abdelmoula YA. Amniotic fluid index versus single deepest vertical pocket as a screening test for preventing adverse pregnancy outcome. Cochrane Database Syst Rev. 2008;3:CD006593.
29. Boulvain M, Stan C, Irion O. Membrane sweeping for induction of labour. Cochrane Database Syst Rev. 2005;25;(1):CD000451.
30. MG Nyamzi, Isah DA, Offiong RA, Isah AY. Effectiveness of sweeping of membranes in reducing the incidence of elective induction of labor for postdate pregnancies. Arch Med Surg. 2019;15-21.
31. Avdiyovski H, Haith-Cooper M, Scally A. Membrane sweeping at term to promote spontaneous labour and reduce the likelihood of a formal induction of labour for postmaturity: a systematic review and meta-analysis. J Obstet Gynaecol. 2019;39(1):54-62.
32. Kavanagh J, Kelly AJ, Thomas J. Sexual intercourse for cervical ripening and induction of labour. Cochrane Database Syst Rev. 2001;(2):CD003093.
33. Tan PC, Yow CM, Omar SZ. Coitus and orgasm at term: effect on spontaneous labour and pregnancy outcome. Singapore Med J. 2009;50:1062-8.
34. Tan PC, Andi A, Azmi N, Noraihan MN. Effect of coitus at term on length of gestation, induction of labor, and mode of delivery. Obstet Gynecol. 2006;108:134-40.
35. West Z. Acupuncture within the National Health Service: a personal perspective. Complement Ther Nurs Midwifery. 1997;3:83-6.
36. Neri I, Fazzio M, Menghini S. Non-stress test changes during acupuncture plus moxibustion on BL67 point in breech presentation. J Soc Gynecol Investig. 2002;9:158-62.
37. Smith CA, Armour M, Dahlen HG. Acupuncture or acupressure for induction of labour. Cochrane Database Syst Rev. 2017:10:CD002962.
38. Rabl M, Ahner R, Bitschnau M. Acupuncture for cervical ripening and induction of labor at term—a randomized controlled trial. Wien KlinWochenschr. 2001;113:942-6.
39. Mostaghel N, Nakhaee F, Amiri Z. Outpatient vaginal misoprostol and its effect on post term pregnancy. Middle East J Fam Med. 2009;7(4):14-7.
40. Jindal N, Vaid NB. Outpatient-based misoprostol to prevent prolonged pregnancy. Int J Res Med Sci. 2017;5(5):2085.

# CHAPTER 13

# Rh Negative Pregnancy

*Aruna Nigam, Sumedha Sharma*

## INTRODUCTION

Rhesus (Rh) alloimmunization occurs when an Rh-negative woman's immune system is sensitized to Rh antigen present on the surface of the Rh-positive fetal erythrocytes resulting in production of anti-D antibodies. These antibodies (IgG) can cross the placenta in subsequent pregnancies and cause hemolysis of fetal erythrocytes in Rh positive fetus. This antibody mediated hemolysis of fetal erythrocytes is known as hemolytic disease of the fetus and newborn (HDFN) and can have varied manifestations due to the resultant anemia and hyperbilirubinemia. Advances in the invasive fetal therapy have greatly improved the survival rates of even severely affected fetuses. Intensive monitoring, intrauterine transfusions (IUT), timely delivery, intensive neonatal care, and exchange transfusions are required during the management of these cases to decrease the fetal and neonatal morbidity and mortality.

The common causes of maternal sensitization during pregnancy include fetomaternal hemorrhage (FMH) associated with delivery, trauma, spontaneous or induced abortion, ectopic pregnancy, and invasive obstetric procedures such as chorionic villous biopsy and amniocentesis.

## PREVALENCE

In India, rate of Rh negative pregnancy varies between 3 and 5.7%.[1] The incidence of alloimmunization also called isoimmunization varies greatly among the populations. In a hospital based study from Delhi, the overall prevalence of alloantibodies was 1.25%, alloimmunization rates in the D antigen-negative and D antigen-positive groups were 10.7% and 0.12%, respectively.[2] In this study anti-D was found to be most common and other alloantibodies found included anti-C, anti-M, anti-S and anti-c. Widespread use of anti-D immune globulin to prevent red cell alloimmunization has resulted in a relative increase in the number of cases of non-Rh-D alloimmunization causing fetal anemia and hemolytic disease of the newborn. Hundreds of other distinct antigens, known as "minor" antigens, are present on the red blood cell surface. Many cases of alloimmunization due to these minor antigens are caused by incompatible blood transfusion. Overall, antibodies to minor antigens occur in 1.5–2.5% of obstetric patients.[3] However, antibodies to D antigen remain most common. In India, the incidence of Rh sensitization during pregnancy has been reported to be 1.9% with a perinatal loss between 1 and 2.5%.[4] The main causes of Rh sensitization appear to be lack of awareness and omission of routine testing of pregnant women for ABO and Rh group especially in rural setups, scarcity of laboratory facility for testing and ignorance about use of anti-D for the prevention of isoimmunization in certain situations or administration of inadequate dose of anti-D.

## PATHOPHYSIOLOGY OF RHESUS ALLOIMMUNIZATION

There are several classes of antigens which can cause fetal or neonatal hemolytic disease and others which do not cause HDFN (**Table 1**). There are three major rhesus antigen groups; D, c/C, e/E. The rhesus locus is present on the short arm of chromosome one. The D antigen is the most immunogenic of all the Rh antigens. Rh antigens are present in varying gene frequencies and combinations. The capital and small letters are used for referring to the different alleles of these antigens.

Unlike C and E antigens which have c and e alleles, D antigen does not have d allele and d refers to the absence of the D allele.

The primary immune response to the D antigen is weak and develops over 6 weeks to 12 months. The initial antibodies are of IgM types that do not cross the placenta hence the first pregnancy is not typically at risk of isoimmunization. IgG antibodies become detectable within 6 months of exposure. A second antigen challenge generates anamnestic response

**TABLE 1:** Antigens and hemolytic disease of the fetus and newborn (HDFN).[3,5,6]

| Antigens that cause HDFN | Antigens that do not cause HDFN |
|---|---|
| • Rh: D, E, c, C, $C_w$, e | • Lewis: $Le_a$, $Le_b$ |
| • Kell: $K_1$, $Kp_a$, k, $Js_a$, $Js_b$ | • Lutheran: $Lu_a$, $Lu_b$ |
| • Duffy: $Fy^a$ | • Duffy: $Fy_b$ |
| • MNS: M, S, s, N | • $Jk_b$ |
| • Kidd: $Jk_a$ | |

that is both rapid and almost exclusive for IgG antibodies which cross the placenta, thus posing the risk of severe fetal disease.

There are three phases of fetal hematopoiesis: (1) mesoblastic, (2) hepatic, and (3) myeloid related to three major organs. Erythropoiesis commences in the yolk sac on day 21 (mesoblastic phase), then moves to the liver (hepatic phase) and finally to the bone marrow at the 16th week of gestation (myeloid phase). The decreasing contribution of the liver is characterized by the exponential decrease in the number of erythroblasts. The Rh antigens are well-developed by day 30 of gestation, in contrast to ABO antigens which are poorly expressed on the fetal RBC. Anti-D antibody triggered hemolysis is not complement mediated, rather anti-D coated RBC are destroyed extravascularly by the reticuloendothelial system at a faster than normal rate. The response of the affected fetus varies depending on the quantity and subclass of IgG antibody, the efficiency of placental passage, the avidity with which the antibody binds to the antigen site, the maternal human leukocyte antigen (HLA) make up, the maturity and efficiency of reticuloendothelial system.[7]

Hemolytic anemia may occur whenever the erythrocyte lifespan declines below 70-90 days and hematopoietic system can no longer meet the demands. Erythropoiesis may occur anywhere in the fetoplacental unit. Both the liver and the spleen are enlarged secondary to extramedullary erythropoiesis and congestion. Erythroblasts are released into peripheral circulation, hence the term erythroblastosis fetalis. The greater the number of erythroblasts in the circulation, the greater the likelihood that an antenatal transfusion therapy may be necessary. All fetal sequelae of hemolytic disease relate to the development of anemia. In general, fetus tolerates mild-to-moderate anemia well. However, metabolic alterations develop as the anemia worsens. As the fetal RBCs are principal fetal buffer, metabolic acidemia with hyperlactatemia develops in fetuses with severe anemia. Most important causative factor in the development of fetal hydrops is cardiac dysfunction, possibly secondary to insufficient oxygen carrying capacity. This dysfunction is detectable immediately prior to development of hydrops and resolves rapidly after transfusion with consequent increase in the fetal oxygen carrying capacity.

Hyperbilirubinemia secondary to hemolysis is an important component of alloimmune hemolytic disease. Heme pigment is first converted to biliverdin by heme oxygenase and then to water-insoluble and lipid-soluble bilirubin (the indirect fraction) by biliverdin reductase. Both the fetus and the neonates have reduced levels of glucuronyl transferase, the enzyme necessary to produce water-soluble diglucuronide. Indirect bilirubin unbound to albumin penetrates the lipid neuronal membrane and produces cell death. Thus, the neonates with severe hyperbilirubinemia are at risk of developing encephalopathy (kernicterus).

Kernicterus and jaundice due to erythroblastosis fetalis are not manifested during intrauterine life, since accumulation of the pigment is prevented by its removal through the placental circulation and metabolism in the maternal liver. However, after birth, the newborn liver cannot effectively handle the large amount of pigment released during the brisk hemolytic process and this leads to rapid increase in serum bilirubin and eventual tissue deposition. The concentration of bilirubin necessary to cause kernicterus rises with the gestational age. A term neonate can tolerate a total bilirubin of 25 mg/dL, but an extremely preterm neonate is at risk of developing kernicterus at 12 mg/dL. Affected neonates are initially lethargic and then become hypertonic, with hyperextended neck arched back and flexed knees, elbows, and wrist. Newborn has poor sucking, loss of Moro reflex, bulging fontanelle, seizures and ultimately develop apneic episodes. Neural tissue in the auditory center is particularly sensitive to indirect bilirubin. Ten percent of survivors often have profound neurosensory deafness and choreoathetoid spastic cerebral palsy.

## FETOMATERNAL HEMORRHAGE

Fetomaternal hemorrhage refers to the entry of fetal blood into the maternal circulation before or during delivery.[8] Some degree of FMH occurs in most of the pregnancies without any adverse consequences to the mother or fetus. The incidence of massive FMH, defined as entry of 30 mL of fetal blood in maternal circulation, is 0.3% whereas it is 80 mL in 0.1% of pregnancies.[9] Massive FMH is associated with adverse outcomes such as stillbirth, hypoxic ischemic encephalopathy (HIE), prematurity and severe anemia in neonate. It can be diagnosed with tests such as Kleihauer-Betke test, flow cytometry and liquid chromatography.

In Rh negative pregnant women carrying Rh positive fetus, FMH can act as a sensitizing event leading to antibody response. Depending on whether the exposure is occurring for the first time or is a recurring event, IgM or IgG antibodies are produced.

Conditions under which FMH can occur and cause maternal alloimmunization in Rh negative woman with Rh positive fetus are listed in **Box 1**. These are indications for administration of anti-D immunoglobulin.

## MANAGEMENT OF RHESUS NEGATIVE PREGNANCY

The blood group and Rh type should be done in all pregnant women at their first prenatal visit and an antibody screening is also recommended. If the mother is Rh negative, the Rh phenotype status of husband should be determined, the paternity needs to be certain. If the husband or partner is Rh negative, the baby will be Rh negative and pregnancy should be managed like any other normal pregnancy.

In case the baby's father is Rh positive, the probability that the fetus will be Rh positive is substantial and therefore, Rh alloimmunization may occur during pregnancy. In such cases it is important to know whether the Rh negative woman is alloimmunized or not, hence she should be tested for presence of RhD antibodies by indirect anti globulin test (indirect Coombs' test). Further management will depend on whether she is positive for the antibodies or not (nonimmunized), and if she has the antibodies then whether it is her first affected pregnancy, or she already has history of previously affected pregnancy.

There could be another group of Rh positive women, alloimmunized against non-D Rh antigens or against other blood group systems.

## Management of Rh Negative Nonalloimmunized Woman (Flowchart 1)

The fetus of an Rh negative mother with Rh positive father will either be Rh positive or Rh negative depending on the father's zygosity. If the father is homozygous with DD antigen, the baby will inherit D and will be Rh positive but in case father is heterozygous with Dd antigen, baby can inherit D or d and thus has a 50% chance of being Rh negative. If the fetal blood group can be determined in early pregnancy, then the pregnancy carrying Rh positive fetus only needs to be monitored for alloimmunization. Pregnant mothers with Rh negative fetus do not carry any risks of alloimmunization are monitored as any other pregnancy.

### Methods of Determining the Rh Status of the Fetus

The fetal Rh genotype can be determined by using cells collected by invasive methods such as chorionic villus sampling (CVS) biopsy or amniocentesis or by noninvasive test involving assessment of cell free fetal DNA in maternal blood.

Although, CVS has the advantage of being done early in pregnancy, it increases the risk of alloimmunization, if the fetus is Rh positive. Amniocentesis can be done to obtain fetal cells for Rh factor determination. Polymerase chain reaction (PCR) test can also be used to determine the fetal genotype in the amniocytes. But, performing these tests early in pregnancy has its own risks and complications, so these are routinely not performed for determining fetal phenotype.

Noninvasive prenatal test (NIPT) offers the possibility to determine the fetal Rh status in early pregnancy using maternal blood and assessing cell free fetal DNA. It is a highly accurate and reliable method.[11,12] Noninvasive fetal genotyping using maternal blood is now possible for D, C, c, E, e and K antigens. The Royal College of Obstetricians and Gynaecologists (RCOG) recommends this test for the relevant antigen when maternal red cell antibodies are present.[13] NIPT, however, is not freely available at present but routine availability soon may allow consideration of routine immunoprophylaxis only in pregnant women carrying Rh positive fetuses.

### Monitoring of Nonalloimmunized Pregnancy

Possibility of Rh sensitization during antenatal period is small, thus antibody screening is performed only at 28 weeks

> **BOX 1:** Conditions associated with fetomaternal hemorrhage.
> - Spontaneous abortion (first* and second trimester)
> - Induced abortion (medical and surgical)
> - Ectopic pregnancy
> - Evacuation for molar pregnancy (partial mole)
> - Intrauterine death
> - APH (abruption and placenta previa)
> - Normal pregnancy (during antenatal period and delivery)
> - During cesarean section
> - During invasive procedures—amniocentesis, chorionic villus sampling, cordocentesis, fetoscopy
> - External cephalic version
> - Manual removal of placenta
> - Maternal blunt abdominal trauma
>
> *ACOG recommends anti-D prophylaxis in cases of spontaneous first-trimester miscarriage, especially those that are later in the first trimester. Although the risk of alloimmunization is low (1.5–2%) but consequences can be significant, hence RhD immunoglobulin should be considered. If instrumentation is done then immunoglobulin should be given as the risk of alloimmunization is 4–5%.[10]

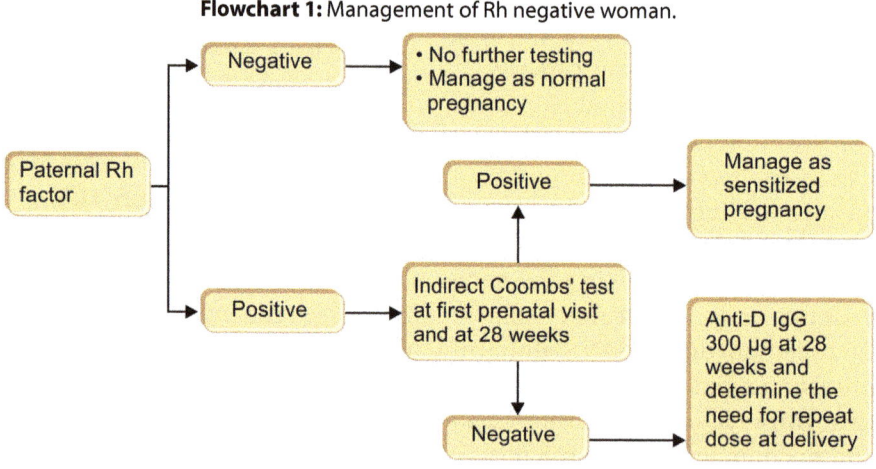

Flowchart 1: Management of Rh negative woman.

before the administration of anti-D immunoglobulin. Current guidelines for the management of Rh negative women are that if antibody screen by indirect Coombs' test (ICT) is negative at first prenatal visit, the screen is repeated at 28 weeks and 300 µg anti-D is administered if test remains negative. If at any time, the antibody screening test is positive, which means the woman is Rh alloimmunized, she is managed as described under management of alloimmunized woman.

The Rh negative gravida who remains unsensitized during pregnancy and receives anti-D immunoglobulin antenatally should be administered anti-D immunoglobulin in the postpartum period if the baby is Rh positive.

After the antepartum administration of anti-D immunoglobulin, the antibody screening will detect anti-D antibodies in the mother's serum, but the titer should not be greater than 1:4 at term. An antibody titer greater than 1:4 at term most probably results from alloimmunization rather than anti-D immunoglobulin administration. Therefore, once 300 µg of anti-D has been given to pregnant woman, repeat ICT is not required. If such a woman experiences some sensitizing event that can result in the FMH, then Kleihauer–Betke test should be done to assess the fetomaternal hemorrhage to decide whether any further dose of anti-D is required.

It is recommended that Kleihauer–Betke screening should be performed in all the RhD negative nonsensitized women at the time of delivery to identify additional requirement of anti-D immunoglobulin injection. This is especially indicated in the following conditions:
- Traumatic deliveries
- Cesarean section
- Stillbirths
- Twin delivery
- Unexplained fetal death
- History of abdominal trauma during third trimester.

The usual dosage of 300 µg anti-D immunoglobulin can neutralize the antigenic potential of up to 30 mL of fetal blood (15 mL of fetal red cells) and it prevents Rh alloimmunization in 90% of cases. In less than 1% of cases in which the volume of FMH exceeds 30 mL, Kleihauer–Betke test is used to quantitate the volume of FMH and administration of the appropriate dose of anti-D IgG (i.e., 10 µg/mL fetal blood). The basic principle behind this test is that acid denatures the adult hemoglobin present in RBCs and not the fetal hemoglobin which is resistant to it. The maternal blood is examined on a counting chamber after fixation with 80% of ethanol and hematoxylin staining. The amount of fetal blood in the maternal circulation can be approximated from the number of fetal red cells.

Flow cytometry offers an alternative technique for quantifying the size of FMH.[14] It has a number of advantages in that the results are more accurate and more reproducible than those from the Kleihauer–Betke test and that it detects RhD positive cells, making it particularly helpful in patients with high HbF levels. Not all hospitals will have ready access to a flow cytometer. Flow cytometry is most effectively employed in those cases where a Kleihauer screening test indicates a large FMH which requires accurate quantitation and follow-up.

Initially, qualitative screening test, rosette assay can be done which detects FMH greater than 4 mL and, if it is positive quantitative testing such as the Kleihauer–Betke test can be done.

Anti-D immunoglobulin administration in postpartum period may be withheld if the last administration was given less than 21 days before delivery and passively acquired antibodies are still demonstrable on the antibody screen.[7] The rosette test may also be performed in maternal blood to assess the need for further administration of anti-D immunoglobulin.

## Prophylaxis Following Sensitizing Events before Delivery

Anti-D immunoglobulin should be given to all nonsensitized RhD negative women following potential sensitizing events during pregnancy.

A dose of 50 µg is recommended for prophylaxis following sensitizing events up to 12 weeks of pregnancy. As most hospitals and the pharmacy do not have 50 µg preparation available, 300 µg is often administered without any harm. For all events after 12 weeks, 300 µg (1,500 IU) of anti-D immunoglobulin should be given followed by a test to identify FMH greater than 4 mL red cells and additional anti-D IgG needs to be given as required.[15] Not more than 5 units (5 prefilled syringe) of anti-D can be given in a 24 hours period by intramuscular route and if more dose is required in the event of large FMH, intravenous route of anti-D preparation is used. Routine antenatal anti-D Ig prophylaxis (RAADP) should be regarded as a separate entity and administered regardless of, and in addition to, any anti-D Ig that may have been given for a potentially sensitizing event.[15] Anti-D immunoglobulin is best given intramuscularly into the deltoid muscle as injections into the gluteal region may only reach the subcutaneous tissues and absorption may be delayed. It should be given via subcutaneous or intravenous route (different preparations are available) if the women is suffering from some bleeding disorder. For successful immunoprophylaxis, anti-D immunoglobulin should be given as soon as possible after the sensitizing event but always within 72 hours. If it is not given within 72 hours, every effort should still be made to administer the anti-D immunoglobulin, as a dose given within 28 days may provide some protection.

## Management of Rh Negative, Alloimmunized Pregnant Woman

The management of Rh negative immunized pregnant woman is shown in **Flowchart 2**.

## Management of First Affected Pregnancy Diagnosed by Presence of Rh antibodies

Rh negative woman found to have Rh antibodies in early pregnancy with no previous affected pregnancy can be managed by monitoring RhD antibody titers. Only in first affected pregnancy, Rh antibody titers can be used to determine the risk of fetal anemia. The rationale being that the association between the antibody titers and fetal affection that exists in the first affected pregnancy is lost during subsequent gestations. In majority of first immunized pregnancies the anti-Rh antibody concentration is low and rarely exceeds the critical level of most laboratories. Critical titer is that titer at which there is significant risk of severe erythroblastosis fetalis and hydrops and in most centers this is between 1:8 and 1:32.[3]

- Serum antibody titers are done in these women every 4 weeks and if antibody titers remain below critical level up to 36 weeks, the woman should be delivered by elective induction between 38 and 40 weeks and the birth of unaffected or mildly affected fetus should be anticipated.
- If the titers are found to be at or above the critical level (1:16) or there is a significant rise in titer between two consequent samples (two tube dilution), even if the upper dilution does not reach the critical level, in both these conditions, further testing of antibody titers is not useful. The pregnancy should be monitored by middle cerebral artery-peak systolic velocity (MCA-PSV) determined by Doppler ultrasound.
- If MCA-PSV remains <1.5 MoM (multiples of the median) pregnancy may be continued till 37–38$^{+6}$ weeks.
- If MCA-PSV is >1.5, and pregnancy is more than 35 weeks woman may be delivered after giving steroid cover.
- Management of preterm woman with less than 35 weeks pregnancy and MSA-PSV > 1.5 MoM, is done in a specialized center with expertise in performing fetal

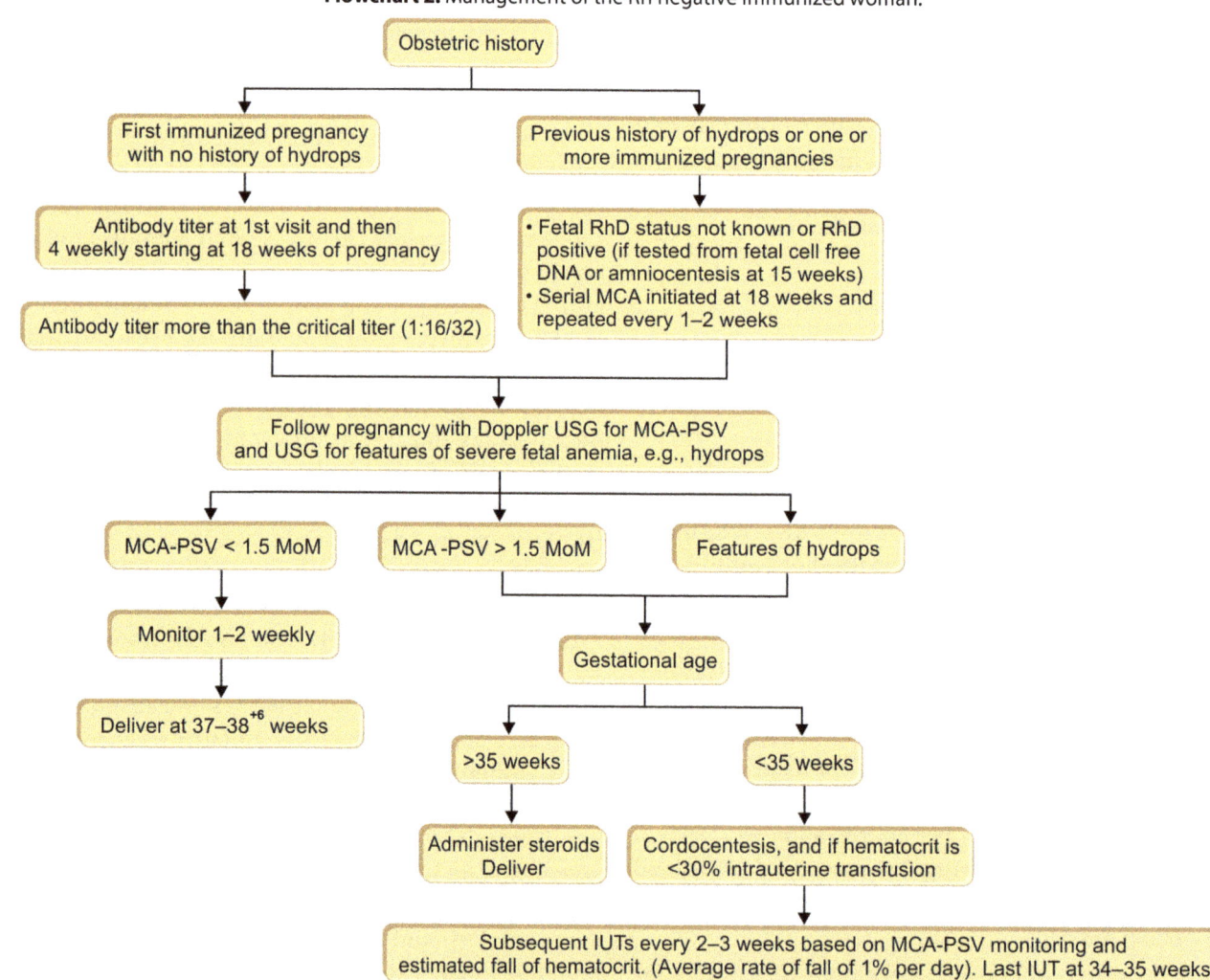

**Flowchart 2:** Management of the Rh negative immunized woman.

(IUT: intrauterine transfusion; MCA-PSV: middle cerebral artery-peak systolic velocity; MoM: multiples of the median; USG: ultrasonography)

blood sampling (FBS) by cordocentesis and if required, following it with IUT.

## Management of Women with Previous Affected Pregnancy

These pregnancies should be managed at a center where the expertise and facility for managing the isoimmunized pregnancies is available. If available, testing for fetal RhD status by NIPT in cases where paternal genotype is heterozygous is useful, because only the pregnancies with Rh positive fetus needs to be monitored. After the first affected pregnancy, the ability to predict fetal anemia from the maternal anti-D antibody titers is lost and these pregnancies should be monitored by MCA-PSV. Ultrasonography (USG) and MCA Doppler studies are done every 1–2 weeks depending on the trend.

### Ultrasonography

Ultrasonography is utilized in the management of Rh negative pregnancies to assess gestational age, fetal wellbeing, diagnose hydrops and guide amniocentesis, fetal blood sampling, and IUTs. In this capacity, USG has improved both the safety and success rate of noninvasive procedures and has helped to minimize invasive procedures. The sonographic findings consistent with hydrops include ascites, pleural and pericardial effusion and edema. Several other sonographic findings have been proposed as possible indicators of the future development of hydrops. These include polyhydramnios, increased placental thickness (>4 cm), dilation of the cardiac chambers, dilation of the umbilical vein, chronic enlargement of the spleen and liver and visualization of both sides of the fetal bowel wall. Serial ultrasounds 1–3 weekly can be used to document the progression of the disease and when used in combination with Doppler evaluation, it has been found to be more accurate than amniocentesis for detection of fetal anemia.[16]

### Middle Cerebral Artery Peak Systolic Velocity

It is a noninvasive tool for the diagnosis of fetal anemia. The principle behind this test is that there is an increased velocity of blood flow in the anemic fetuses due to increased cardiac output to enhance the oxygenation. In their studies of the MCA, Mari et al. demonstrated that increases in peak velocity of systolic blood flow in the MCA can be used to detect moderate and severe anemia in nonhydropic fetuses.[17,18] The MCA is utilized because it can be evaluated using a minimal angle of insonation.

Correct technique is a critical factor for determining PSV in the fetal MCA with Doppler USG.

*Technique:* The ultrasound probe is used to obtain a view adequate for the measurement of biparietal diameter and the vascular structures are identified with color Doppler. The MCA of the cerebral hemisphere closer to the ultrasound transducer is insonated few millimeters after its origin from the internal carotid artery but without including any part of this artery and taking care that angle of insonation is as close as possible to zero. The fetus should be resting, since activity will cause falsely elevated PSV values.[19] It is better to examine proximal one-third of MCA far from the ultrasound probe.[20] Typical waveforms are obtained and the PSV of at least three of them are measured and averaged.

The threshold for the diagnosis of fetal anemia is a value equal to or greater than 1.5 MoM for the gestational age. Abnormally elevated MCA-PSV has a sensitivity of 100% and a false-positive rate of 12% for the diagnosis of moderate-to-severe fetal anemia. Correct technique is a critical factor when determining PSV in the fetal MCA with Doppler USG.[3]

Cordocentesis and fetal blood sampling for detecting anemia is done if MCA-PSV is more than the cut-off value of 1.5 MoM. Intrauterine transfusion is indicated in the management of isoimmunized pregnancy if the fetus is anemic and not mature enough to be delivered. If fetal anemia is not treated, fetus is at the risk of developing hydrops and dying in utero. Reliable MCA-PSV values can be obtained as early as 18 weeks gestation. False positive rate of MCA-PSV increases after 35 weeks gestation.

### Amniotic Fluid Spectrophotometry

Amniotic fluid spectrophotometry (AFS) has been the mainstay of monitoring an alloimmunized pregnancy in the past but has been replaced by MCA-PSV. Society for Maternal-Fetal Medicine (SMFM) clinical guidelines suggest that amniotic fluid delta OD450 should not be used to diagnosis fetal anemia. Only in rare cases in which MCA Doppler studies cannot be performed, measuring the delta optical density 450 levels in amniotic fluid as a screening test for fetal anemia may be reasonable, although the accuracy may be limited in some cases, such as with anti-Kell alloimmunization.[21]

Amniotic fluid spectrophotometry is being described here for historical interest. AFS detects the presence and severity of fetal hemolysis. Amniotic fluid is obtained by ultrasound guided amniocentesis, transported to the laboratory in a light resistant container to prevent degradation of bilirubin, centrifuged and filtered. Fetal hemolysis is detected by using spectrophotometric measurements of bilirubin in amniotic fluid. It is an invasive procedure, needs to be done serially and is associated with the risks of intrauterine infection, rupture of membranes, preterm labor and fetomaternal hemorrhage leading to increased alloimmunization. Amniotic fluid containing high levels of bilirubin, such as that found in fetuses with severe hemolytic disease, is yellowish-brown. This observation by Liley in 1961 led to the development of this method to predict the severity of fetal hemolysis using spectrophotometric measurements of bilirubin in amniotic fluid (**Fig. 1**). Because the wavelength at which bilirubin absorbs light is 420–460 nm, the amount of shift in optical density from linearity at 450 nm (ΔOD450) in amniotic fluid samples can be used to estimate the degree of fetal hemolysis. The Queenan curve is a modification of the Liley curve to adjust for the relative inaccuracy of ΔOD450 readings in the early to middle second trimester (**Fig. 2**).

During normal pregnancy, ΔOD450 values change with gestational age and it is necessary to use adequate norms to correlate the laboratory values with fetal situation. In his original description, Liley recorded the ΔOD450 of 101 immunized patients on a semilogarithmic paper (gestational age in weeks on X-axis and ΔOD450 values on the Y-axis) and divided the graph in 3 zones. Mild or no hemolytic disease occurs in zone 1; intermediate disease in zone 2 (transitional between mild and severe hemolysis); and severe disease, including the development of hydrops within a week, in zone 3.

If the amniotic fluid values show an OD450 in zone 1, there is no immediate danger to the fetus and the procedure should be repeated in 4 weeks. If the OD450 remain in zone 1 amniocentesis is repeated every 4 weeks, the patient should be delivered at term gestation and the birth of unaffected or a mildly affected baby should be anticipated. If at any time the amniotic fluid shows an OD450 in zone 2, the procedure should be repeated in 1 week, since values in this zone may correspond to moderately or severely affected infants. If the following amniocentesis shows OD450 in zone 1, there is no need to repeat the amniocentesis before 4 weeks. If the following amniocentesis shows a decreasing trend but remains in zone 2, amniocentesis should be repeated in 2 weeks. If the following amniocentesis shows the same value as previous one and remain in zone 2 (horizontal trend), procedure should be repeated in another week and if the horizontal trend continues, cordocentesis and fetal hematocrit evaluation is indicated with exception of those patients who have achieved fetal lung maturity and better managed by immediate delivery.

If the initial amniotic fluid examination shows an OD450 in zone 3 or if any OD450 value previously in zone 1 or 2 moved to zone 3 (rising trend), the fetus may be in immediate danger of intrauterine death. Fetal blood sampling is indicated in these cases and IUT performed if the fetal hematocrit is less than 30%. Termination of the pregnancy is the treatment of choice where lung maturity has been achieved.

The main limitation of the Liley curve is that it starts at 26 weeks of gestation and extrapolation of the lines to earlier gestational ages is inaccurate. Queenan developed a curve for fetal assessment from 14 to 40 weeks, divided into 4 zones. The lower, first zone corresponds to non-affected fetus. Values in the second zone are indeterminate and do not permit a determination whether the fetus is affected or not.

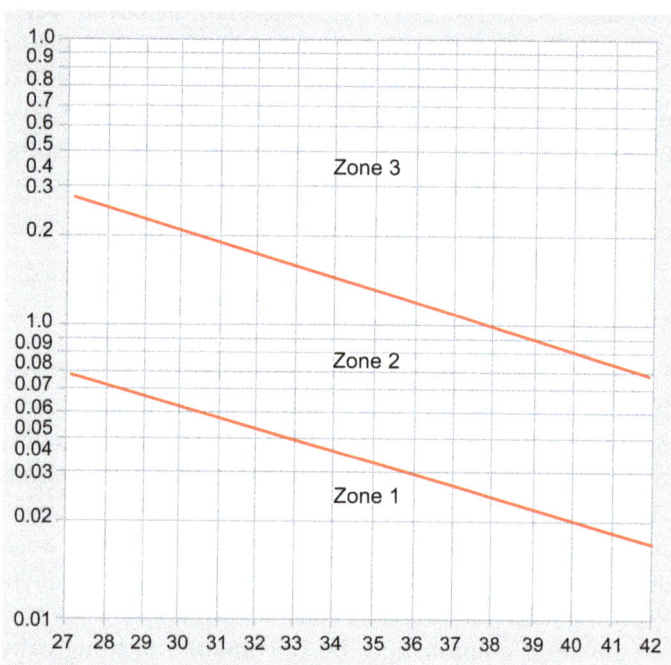

**Fig. 1:** Liley's graph to estimate severity of fetal anemia.

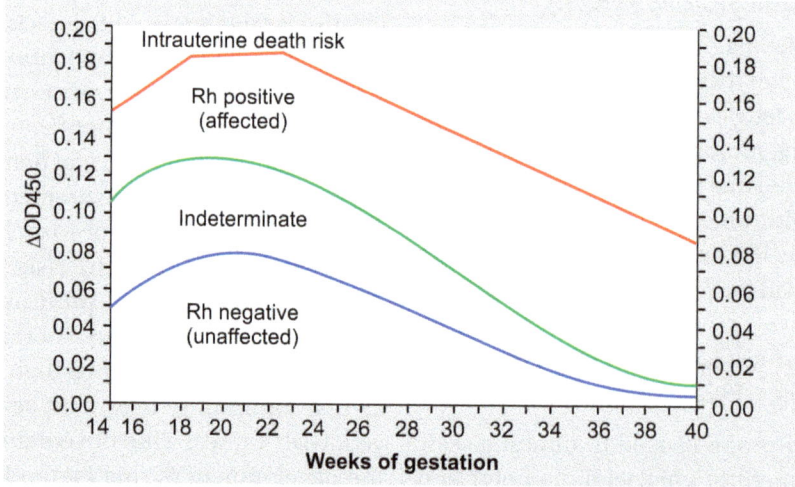

**Fig. 2:** Queenan curve (Curve for ΔOD450 values from 14 to 40 weeks of gestation).

The third zone corresponds to affected Rh positive fetus. The upper zone corresponds to the fetuses at risk of intrauterine death. In general, OD450 greater than 0.15 indicates severe immunization and the need for cordocentesis and early transfusion. Values below 0.09 indicate mild disease or no disease. Values between 0.09 and 0.15 will require repeat amniocentesis in 1 week. After 26 weeks the need for intervention can be determined by Liley's graph.

## FETAL BLOOD SAMPLING

The only definitive means of diagnosing fetal anemia and acidosis is via FBS, also known as cordocentesis or percutaneous umbilical blood sampling, which was first performed in the early 1980s. It allows direct access to the fetal circulation which can be used to analyze the fetal blood for hematocrit, fetal blood type, direct Coombs' test, reticulocyte count and fetal bilirubin. If fetal anemia, i.e., hematocrits <30%, is detected intrauterine transfusion is performed in the same sitting. Cordocentesis is not to be used only for purpose of diagnosis because of concerns regarding fetal and maternal complications which include fetomaternal hemorrhage, fetal loss (0.5–2% per procedure) placental abruption, fetal distress and amnionitis. Indications of FBS include raised MCA-PSV (>1.5 MoM), evidence of fetal hydrops on USG and elevation of OD450 values (80th percentile of zone 2 or zone 3 on Liley curve).

### Intrauterine Transfusion

Fetal transfusion therapy is done whenever the fetus is hydropic with significant anemia, i.e., hematocrit <30% as it is below the 2.5 percentile for all gestational ages greater than 20 weeks.

There are two types of IUT: (1) intraperitoneal and (2) intravascular. In both the methods, the procedure is carried out under visual control with real time ultrasound. In intraperitoneal transfusion, the blood is injected in the peritoneal cavity and transported by lymphatic system into the fetal bloodstream. In intravascular transfusion, the blood is injected directly in the umbilical circulation. They complement each other and either one or both may be used depending on the circumstances. Although, the direct intravascular transfusion is the procedure of choice, it is not without problems and it is preferable to perform an intraperitoneal transfusion if the approach to umbilical cord is difficult (posterior placenta, maternal obesity) or if a sample of blood cannot be obtained after several attempts. In the severely hydropic fetus, the intravascular approach offers the best possibility for successful fetal therapy. If access into the umbilical cord is difficult, it is possible to transfuse through intrahepatic portion of umbilical vein. When everything fails, access is done through the right ventricle of heart.

The blood to be transfused should be adult group O RhD negative, fresh when available and compatible with

**BOX 2:** Intravascular intrauterine transfusion.[21,22]

- Ultrasound is done to select site of fetal blood sampling and transfusion. Depending on fetal position and placental localization, it can be cord at placental or umbilicus insertion, free cord loop, or in intrahepatic vein.
- Fetal heart rate is checked.
- Maternal blood sample is drawn, and intravenous access is established, antibiotics may be given.
- Local anesthesia is given at the selected site of puncture on maternal abdomen.
- Paralytic agent vecuronium or atracurium may be given to stop the fetus from moving
- 20 or 22-gauge needle, depending on gestational age, is used to enter umbilical vein and 1 mL of fetal blood is drawn and tested for hemoglobin and hematocrit.
- Verification of correct placement of the needle is done by injecting a small amount of saline, followed by a fetal weight adjusted dose of muscle relaxant.
- Volume of blood to be transfused is calculated from fetal hematocrit.
- Slow transfusion is done under ultrasound control.
- Fetal heart is monitored.
- After the transfusion fetal blood is checked for final hematocrit.
- Puncture site is observed for any bleeding.
- Maternal and fetal monitoring is done

the mother. It should be negative for HIV, hepatitis B, C, and cytomegalovirus. It should also be irradiated to render it leukocyte poor to avoid "graft-versus-host" like complications in the fetus. The hematocrit of the prepared blood should be around 75–85%.

The amount of blood to be transfused can be calculated once the hematocrit or hemoglobin results are obtained. In general, 30–60 mL/kg of nonhydropic fetal weight is transfused because volumes higher than this may be difficult for the fetus to tolerate in intravascular transfusion.

Intravascular transfusion procedure is summarized in **Box 2**. Intraperitoneal transfusions require a greater volume of blood, roughly calculated as the following:

(Number of weeks' gestation – 20) × 10 mL

Blood in the peritoneal cavity is absorbed over a 7- to 10-day period.[21] After the transfusion, fetus should be monitored with continuous fetal monitoring for the ensuing 4 hours because decelerations of the fetal heart rate are common and must be managed cautiously.

Other complications following IUT include preterm prelabor rupture of membranes (PPROM), infection (chorioamnionitis) and preterm labor. As per SMFM clinical guidelines, timing of a second transfusion in fetuses with anemia, should be determined by MCA-PSV and, alternatively, a predicted decline in fetal hemoglobin may be used for timing the second procedure.[21]

The fall in hematocrits is about 1% per day. Timing of subsequent transfusions (third and beyond) should be individualized rather than based on MCA-PSV values.[21]

The goal of the procedure is to maintain the fetal hemoglobin value at greater than 9 g/dL. Serial IUTs are usually performed until 34 weeks gestation, beyond which time the risk of the procedure probably outweighs the benefits. This usually leads to delivery of the fetus by 34–37 weeks gestation.

## TIMING OF DELIVERY

Timing of delivery needs to be individualized. In cases with mild fetal hemolysis, the woman should be delivered by 37–38 weeks. In severe cases requiring repeated transfusions, risk of invasive procedures is to be balanced with risk of prematurity, last transfusion can be done at 30–32 weeks and delivery by 32–34 weeks after steroid administration. In cases where transfusion can be performed till 36 weeks, delivery can be accomplished by 37–38 weeks which results in overall improved neonatal outcome.[3]

### Intrapartum Care

The mode and place of delivery should be decided on standard obstetric grounds. Continuous electronic fetal heart monitoring is advisable during labor.[13] Cardiotocography (CTG) abnormalities such as sinusoidal pattern may be observed in anemic fetuses. Early cord clamping is advisable after delivery and milking of the cord should be avoided to reduce fetomaternal hemorrhage. Cord blood samples should be sent for blood group, direct antiglobulin test (DAT), hemoglobin and bilirubin levels. Care should be taken to leave some length of cord on the fetal side which may aid in neonatal exchange transfusions later.

## OTHER TREATMENT MODALITIES

Where there are high initial titers of antibody and history of fetal hydrops, plasmapheresis, promethazine, and IgG have been tried. The best evidence of benefit is for IgG administration. Voto et al. treated 69 women with extremely severe Rh alloimmunization. Thirty received IgG before 20 weeks, 400 mg/kg/day for 5 consecutive days every 2–3 weeks, followed by IUTs after 20 weeks and 39 received IUT only. They found significantly lower incidence of number of fetal deaths in women treated with the combination of IUT and IgG.[23]

A recent Cochrane data based systemic reviews concluded that randomized trials did not provide information to indicate whether the antenatal use of intravenous immunoglobulin is effective in the management of fetal red blood cell alloimmunization, although several case series have suggested a beneficial role in delaying the onset of fetal anemia requiring invasive intrauterine transfusion.[24]

## ABO INCOMPATIBILITY AND MINOR BLOOD GROUP ANTIGENS

The ABO incompatibility rarely causes fetal disease because the antibodies are often IgM which are not strongly expressed on the fetal erythrocyte. Lewis antibodies are most common of all the minor blood group antigens, but they are almost always IgM and do not pose a risk for fetal disease as the antigen is poorly expressed on erythrocytes. Therefore, risk for hemolysis is low.

Kidd, Kell, and Duffy are the most common minor antigens that cause perinatal hemolytic disease. Kell alloimmunization is of particular interest because of its different pathophysiology and particularly unpredictable clinical course as the anti-Kell antibodies damage or inhibit erythrocyte progenitors. Severe anemia and hydrops in this condition develops with low antibody titers and $\Delta OD450$ values. Management is as that of Rh isoimmunization with monitoring and intervention tailored to the individual circumstances.

## KEY POINTS

- Rh alloimmunization occurs when Rh negative woman's immune system is sensitized to Rh factor present on the surface of the Rh positive fetal erythrocytes stimulating the production of immunoglobulin G (IgG) antibodies. RhD alloimmunization remains the most important cause of HDFN.
- The blood group and Rh type should be checked in all pregnant women at their first prenatal visit and if possible, an antibody screening should be offered.
- Rh negative women are at risk of Rh alloimmunization if the fetus is Rh positive.
- Pregnant women with Rh negative fetus are not at risk of Rh alloimmunization; Rh negative fetus is not at risk of hemolytic disease even in Rh alloimmunized pregnancy.
- Fetus will be Rh negative if father is Rh negative.
- There is 50% chance of fetus being Rh negative if Rh positive father is heterozygous for RhD.
- Knowing fetal Rh status is useful in managing alloimmunized pregnancy because Rh negative fetus will not be affected. Fetal Rh status can be determined by CVS, amniocentesis or by testing cell free fetal DNA in maternal blood.
- All Rh negative women should be tested for presence of Rh antibodies. Fetus is not at risk of HDFN if antibodies are absent (nonalloimmunized pregnancy).
- Anti-D immunoglobulin effectively prevents maternal alloimmunization. It should be given to Rh negative, nonsensitized pregnant woman at 28 weeks of gestation and after any sensitizing event such as episodes of vaginal bleeding, amniocentesis, external cephalic version and after delivery of Rh positive child.
- The first alloimmunized pregnancy is managed by monitoring Rh antibody titers at monthly intervals after 18 weeks of gestation and if titers remain below the critical level, pregnancy can be continued till term.
- If anti-D titers exceed the critical level (>1:16), USG and Doppler for MCA-PSV is performed weekly for diagnosing fetal anemia.

- Pregnancy can be continued till 38$^{+6}$ weeks if MCA-PSV remains <1.5 MoM for gestational age.
- MCA-PSV > 1.5 MoM suggests the presence of fetal anemia.
- Alloimmunized woman with previous affected pregnancy is monitored with 1–2 weekly MCA-PSV (not by antibody titers) and USG. MCA-PSV > 1.5 suggests fetal anemia.
- Treatment of the significant fetal anemia prior to 34 weeks of gestation is cordocentesis, fetal blood sampling and if hematocrit is <30%, fetal blood transfusion. Intravascular transfusion is the procedure of choice.
- Successful transfusion eliminates the antenatal and largely the postnatal complications of fetal anemia.
- Delivery may be safely delayed until 37–38 weeks of gestation if intrauterine transfusion is done.
- By maintaining the hematocrit at high end, fetal erythropoiesis is minimized, reducing the risk of postnatal hyperbilirubinemia.

## REFERENCES

1. Salvi V. The clinician's approach to rhesus isoimmunization. In: Shah D, Salvi V (Eds). The Rh Factor. Mumbai: Perinatology Committee FOGSI; 1998. pp. 99.
2. Pahuja S, Gupta SK, Pujani M, Jain M. The prevalence of irregular erythrocyte antibodies among antenatal women in Delhi. Blood Transfus. 2011;9:388-93.
3. ACOG Practice Bulletin No. 192: management of alloimmunization during pregnancy. Obstet Gynecol. 2018;131(3):e82-e90.
4. Shah D, Shroff S. New approaches in the management of rhesus alloimmunization. In: Saraiya UB, Rao KA, Chatterjee A (Eds). Principles and Practice of Obstetrics and Gynaecology for Postgraduates. FOGSI Publication. New Delhi: Jaypee Brothers, Medical Publishers (P) Ltd. 2004. pp. 137.
5. Thompson DJ, Stults DZ, Daniel SJ. Anti-M antibody in pregnancy. Obstet Gynecol Surv. 1989;44(9):637-41.
6. Moise KJ. Hemolytic disease of the fetus and newborn. In: Creasy RK, Resnik R, Iams JD (Eds). Creasy and Resnik's Maternal-Fetal Medicine: Principles and Practice, 6th edition. Philadelphia: Saunders/Elsevier; 2009. pp. 477-503.
7. Weiner CP. Fetal hemolytic disease. In James D, Steer P, Weiner CP, Gonik B (Eds). High Risk Pregnancy, Management Options, 3rd edition. Philadelphia: Saunders/Elsevier; 2006. pp. 291-311.
8. Sebring ES, Polesky HF. Fetomaternal hemorrhage: incidence, risk factors, time of occurrence, and clinical effects. Transfusion. 1990;30(4):344-57.
9. Wylie BJ, D'Alton ME. Fetomaternal hemorrhage. Obstet Gynecol. 2010;115(5):1039-51.
10. Practice Bulletin No. 181: Prevention of RhD alloimmunization, Obstet Gynecol. 2017;130(2):e57-e70.
11. Manzanares S, Entrala C, Sanchez-Gila M, Fernandez-Rosado F, Cobo D, Martinez E, et al. Noninvasive fetal RhD status determination in early pregnancy. Fetal Diagn Ther. 2014;35:7-12.
12. Clausen FB, Dziegiel MB, Dziegiel MH. Noninvasive fetal RhD genotyping. Transfus Apher Sci. 2014;50:154-62.
13. RCOG Green Top Guideline No. 65. The Management of Women with Red Cell Antibodies during Pregnancy. London: RCOG; 2014.
14. Johnson PR, Tait RC, Austen EB, Shwe KH, Lee, D. Flow cytometry in diagnosis and management of large fetomaternal haemorrhage. J Clin Path. 1995;48:1005-8.
15. Qureshi H, Massey E, Kirwan D, Davies T, Robson S, White J, et al. British Society for Haematology. BCSH guideline for the use of anti-D immunoglobulin for the prevention of haemolytic disease of the fetus and newborn. Transfus Med. 2014;24(1):8-20.
16. Martinez-Portilla RJ, Lopez-Felix J, Hawkins-Villareal A, Villafan-Bernal JR, Paz y Miño F, Figueras F, et al. Performance of fetal middle cerebral artery peak systolic velocity for prediction of anemia in untransfused and transfused fetuses: systematic review and meta-analysis. Ultrasound Obstet Gynecol. 2019;54:722.
17. Mari G, Collaborative Group for diagnosis of fetal anemia with Doppler ultrasonography. Noninvasive diagnosis by Doppler ultrasonography of fetal anemia due maternal red-cell alloimmunization. N Eng J Med. 2000;342:9-14.
18. Mari G, Detti L, Oz U, Zimmerman R, Duerig P, Stefos T. Accurate prediction of fetal hemoglobin by Doppler ultrasonography. Obstet Gynecol. 2002;99:589-93.
19. Sallout BI, Fung KFK, Wen SW, Xia H. The effect of fetal behavioural status on middle cerebral artery peak systolic velocity. Am J Obstet Gynecol. 2004;191:1283-7.
20. Abel DE, Grambow SC, Brancazio LR, Hertzberg BS. Ultrasound assessment of fetal middle cerebral artery peak systolic velocity: a comparison of the near field versus far field. Am J Obstet Gynecol. 2003;189:986-9.
21. Mari G, Norton ME, Stone J, Berghella V, Sciscione AC, Tate D, et al. Society for Maternal-Fetal Medicine (SMFM) Clinical Guideline #8: the fetus at risk for anemia—diagnosis and management. Am J Obstet Gynecol. 2015;212:697.
22. Adama van Scheltema PN, Oepkes D. Intrauterine blood transfusion. ISBT Sci Series. 2010;5:1-6.
23. Voto LS, Mathet ER, Zapaterio JL, Orti J, Lede RL, Margulies M. High dose gammaglobulin (IVIG) followed by intrauterine transfusions (IUTs). A new alternative for the treatment of severe haemolytic disease. J Perinat Med. 1997;25:85-8.
24. Wong KS, Connan K, Rowlands S, Kornman LH, Savoia HF. Antenatal immunoglobulin for fetal red blood cell alloimmunization. Cochrane Database Syst Rev. 2013;(5):CD008267.

# Pregnancy in Previous Cesarean Section

*Shubham Bidhuri, Ritu Rana, Saritha Shamsunder*

## ■ INTRODUCTION

Pregnancy with previous cesarean section (CS) remains a topic of widespread public and professional concern. Globally, the increase in rates of CS over the last couple of decades, have led to an increase in proportion of women having pregnancies with previous cesarean, and thus increasing the pool of high-risk obstetric population. The CS rates have increased by 25–30% in the United States in the last decade, doubled to 22% in the United Kingdom, and reached up to 35% in Brazil and 25% in India. This increase is contributed to an increasing use of elective cesarean sections, and for indications like previous CS.[1] Nearly 60% of all elective cesarean sections have previous CS as an indication and up to 14% of emergency cesareans are in women with a previous cesarean. Vaginal birth-after-cesarean section (VBAC) has been advocated as a means of reducing the CS rate.[2] Multiple cesarean sections are a known cause of increased maternal and neonatal morbidity and mortality, and there is a systematic shift toward reducing CS rates not only based on evidence, but also to reduce costs. The current chapter explores the pool of evidence and current guidelines on management of pregnancy with the previous CS.

## ■ EFFECT ON FUTURE FERTILITY

One of the key concerns for all women, and to the obstetricians is the likely effect of any medical or surgical intervention, including CS on conception and future pregnancies. There is scanty evidence to suggest the relationship of previous cesarean delivery and future pregnancy rate and most of the studies are limited by several confounding factors, including the indications for the CS, and the choice of the women.[1,3-6] In a retrospective Cohort study in Scotland with a mean follow-up duration of 13 years, absence of conception was voluntary in 69% (CI, 66–73%) of the cases.[6] A systematic review of Cohort studies has shown that women with previous CS have got a 46% higher chance of not having or having fewer children after 5 years of first cesarean delivery (RR: 1.46; 95% CI: 1.07–1.99). The sterilization rates were also higher in these women.[3] It is also postulated that women who had their first child by CS may take longer to conceive because of pelvic adhesions, infections or placental bed disruption, which in turn may be influenced by the indication for CS.[7] As most of the evidences suggesting decrease in fertility are at the most level II,[1] it may be assumed that association between CS and subfertility is more likely to be caused by confounding rather than being causal.

## ■ ANTENATAL COMPLICATIONS

As an obstetrician, it is essential that we are aware of all the potential complications one can come across in post-CS pregnancies, not only to be able to look for and be prepared for all eventualities, but also to inform the couple and counsel them. Some of these complications are elaborated in the following sections.

As stated above, previous operative interventions can lead to postoperative infections, with resultant changes in the tubal lining. Also, healing can cause fibrosis and formation of scars and adhesions which are likely to affect implantation during early pregnancy, and subsequent development of the placenta.

### Ectopic Pregnancy

Cesarean section is a risk factor for subsequent ectopic pregnancies. Postoperative inflammation and infection seem to be the most likely cause. Although the risk is small, but due to the serious consequences of ectopic pregnancy, it is a clinically important factor.[8-10]

### Cesarean Scar Pregnancy

With increasing CS rate, this is getting more common than before. The pregnancy implants at the site of cesarean scar and usually presents as early as 5 weeks to as late as 16 weeks with symptoms of painless vaginal bleeding and abdominal pain. It can cause massive uncontrolled bleeding if uterine curettage is undertaken in the absence of diagnosis, which can occur in many cases.[10-12]

The CS scar has been reported to cause pathological changes like polyp formation, lymphocyte infiltration, capillary dilatation, and infiltration of the endometrial tissue.[13]

These in turn cause suboptimal implantation of the placenta, impaired decidualization, increased vascular malformations, which are known risk factors for placenta previa, placental abruption, and placenta accreta.[14] Placental location should be noted in patients with a history of prior uterine surgery. Placenta accreta should be ruled out in patients having placenta previa.

## Placenta Previa

The incidence of placenta previa is 0.4–0.8% for women with a previous CS as compared to 0.2–0.5% for women with a previous vaginal birth.[15-17] There is an exponential increase in the risk of placenta previa with increase in the number of cesarean sections and women with a combination of high parity and multiple repeat cesarean deliveries have the greatest likelihood of placenta previa **(Table 1)**. Shorter interdelivery time also increases the risk of placenta previa among such women.[15,18,19]

## Placental Abruption

Placental abruption complicates 1 in 100 pregnancies and is known to recur in subsequent pregnancies.[20-22] Abruption rates in pregnancy with a previous CS have been reported to be significantly higher than with previous vaginal birth (0.95% vs. 0.74%). Getahun et al. reported that the risk of abruption in third pregnancy increases by 30% after two consecutive cesarean deliveries (RR 1.3, 95% CI 1.0–1.8), and abruption rates increase if inter delivery period is less than a year. This increase is by 52% if previous delivery was vaginal and by 111% if previous delivery was by CS (RR 1.5, 95% CI 1.1–2.3).[23]

Relative risks are adjusted for maternal age, race, education, prenatal care, marital status, interpregnancy interval, and smoking and drinking during pregnancy.

## Placenta Accreta Spectrum

Placenta accreta spectrum, formerly known as morbidly adherent placenta, refers to the range of pathologic adherence of the placenta, including placenta increta, placenta percreta, and placenta accreta based on the depth of abnormal trophoblastic invasion of the myometrium. Overall incidence of placenta accreta is 1 in 2,500 pregnancies. Placenta accreta is usually associated with placenta previa and causes significant morbidity and mortality due to severe

**TABLE 1:** Association between cesarean delivery and placenta previa in subsequent pregnancies.

| No. of LSCS | Placenta previa incidence |
| --- | --- |
| 1 | 0.6% |
| 2 | 1.7% |
| 3 or more | 2.8% |

(LSCS: lower segment cesarean section)

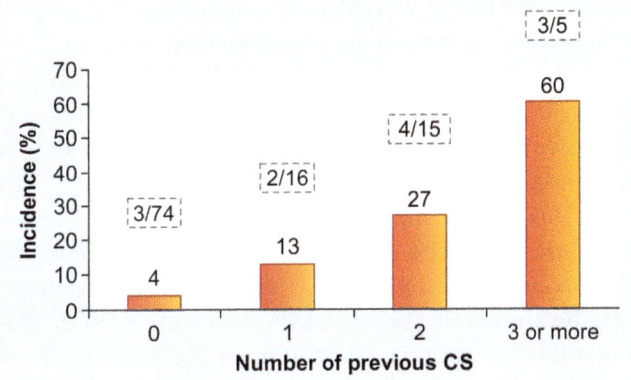

**Fig. 1:** Association between incidence of placenta previa accreta and number of previous cesarean sections.

**TABLE 2:** Association between cesarean delivery and placenta accreta in subsequent pregnancies.

| No. of LSCS | Placenta accreta without previa | Placenta accreta with previa |
| --- | --- | --- |
| 1 | 0.3–0.6% | 11–14% |
| 2 | 1.4% | 23–40% |
| 3 or more | 6.74% | Up to 67% |

(LSCS: lower segment cesarean section)

postpartum hemorrhage that can lead to hysterectomy.[24] There are case series reported on the incidence of placenta accreta in women with previous CS.[25,26] The risk of placenta accreta in placenta previa has been reported to increase from 4.1% in women with no previous CS to 60% in patients with three or more cesarean sections **(Fig. 1)**.[24] Risk of placenta accreta in previous CS is also related with presence of placenta previa, i.e., in presence of placenta previa, the risk of accreta was 3% as compared to 0.03% without placenta previa and this risk increases exponentially with number of cesarean sections **(Table 2)**.

## Stillbirth

Stillbirth rate in women who had no previous CS was 2 per 1,000 compared to 4 per 1,000 among women who had a previous CS. This risk depends on gestational age and increases especially after 34 weeks of gestation (hazard ratio 2.23, 95% CI 1.48–3.36).[27] It is important to remember that the absolute excess risk is still less than 1/1,000. One of the recent studies by Salihu et al. however, did not find any increase in stillbirth in women with previous CS.[28]

## MODE OF DELIVERY AFTER PREVIOUS CESAREAN SECTION: VBAC OR ELECTIVE REPEAT CS

In 1916, Cargin quoted "once a cesarean, always a cesarean". However, this was since almost all cesarean sections were performed by classical uterine incision. The turning point came in 1978 when Merrill and Gibbs safely attempted vaginal delivery in 83% of their patients with previous CS.[29] In 1980, the National Institute of Health (NIH) convened a conference called the National Consensus Development Conference on Cesarean Birth which released a report, recognizing VBAC as the safe mode of delivery.[30,31] The CS rate, however, continued to rise in spite of NIH report and American College of Obstetricians and Gynecologists (ACOG) consensus on VBAC. By 1996, the cesarean delivery rate in the United States was 20.7%, reached 29.1% in 2004 and is still increasing. The reason most likely is inability to make VBAC a norm in well-selected patients. This in turn is due to the lack of clear and robust evidence, which prevents establishment of a uniform protocol for VBAC and each case needs to be individualized. Physicians therefore find it difficult to give a confident explanation and women are afraid to take chances with this uncertainty about the grave outcomes of uterine rupture or failed VBAC. Medicolegal implications do not help either. It therefore becomes extremely important to have a full and evidence-based knowledge of factors that decide the safety and success of VBAC in order to enhance our counseling and decision making. Factors to anticipate before decision making include:

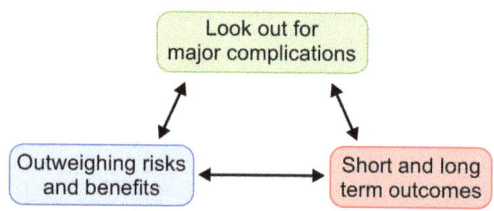

There are many studies pertaining to VBAC. However, the two landmark clinical studies which form most of the evidences for VBAC are from the research undertaken by Landon et al. and Macones et al.[32,33] In 2005, Macones did a large multicenter retrospective cohort study in North-East United States of over 25,000 patients with a history of at least one prior cesarean delivery and studied the maternal complications as well as factors determining success of VBAC.[32] The second study done by Landon et al. was a prospective cohort study of almost 46,000 women with a history of a prior cesarean delivery within the Maternal-Fetal-Medicine Units (MFMU) Network in US which looked not only at the maternal outcomes but also the neonatal outcomes and factors determining success rates of VBAC.[33] The latter is quoted as a stronger study as it was prospective and in addition to maternal outcomes it also assessed the neonatal outcomes.

Trial of labor after cesarean delivery (TOLAC) refers to a planned attempt to deliver vaginally by a woman who has had a previous cesarean delivery, regardless of the outcome. This method provides women who desire a vaginal delivery the possibility of achieving that goal—a VBAC. In addition to fulfilling a patient's preference for vaginal delivery, at an individual level, VBAC is associated with decreased maternal morbidity and a decreased risk of complications in future pregnancies as well as a decrease in the overall cesarean delivery rate at the population level.[34-36] However, although TOLAC is appropriate for many women, several factors increase the likelihood of a failed trial of labor, which in turn is associated with increased maternal and perinatal morbidity when compared with a successful trial of labor (i.e., VBAC) and elective repeat cesarean delivery.[32,33] Therefore, assessing the likelihood of a successful VBAC as well as the individual risks is important when determining who is an appropriate candidate for TOLAC.

## Factors Predicting Success Rates

The success rates of VBAC after one CS is approximately 72–76%. This has been shown by systematic reviews.[37-40] The knowledge of factors predicting success rates would enable us to apply them to an individual woman **(Table 3)**. However, the likelihood of achieving VBAC for an individual varies based on her demographic and obstetric characteristics. For example, women whose first cesarean delivery was performed because of an arrest of labor disorder are less likely to succeed in their attempt at VBAC than those whose first cesarean delivery was for a nonrecurring indication (e.g., breech presentation).[41] A good idea of the success rate of VBAC can be done at the first antenatal visit. The best available evidence remains to be Level 2 and 3 as discussed in **Table 3**.

### Antenatal Factors

Previous vaginal birth, particularly previous VBAC, is the single best predictor for successful VBAC and is associated with an approximately 87–90% planned VBAC success rate.[42-44] The success rate ranges from 63.3% with women having no previous VBAC to 91.6% for women with 4 or more prior

**TABLE 3:** Factors affecting success of VBAC.

| Favoring success | Reducing success |
|---|---|
| • Previous safe vaginal birth<br>• Previous successful VBAC<br>• Spontaneous onset of labor<br>• Uncomplicated pregnancy without other risk factors | • Previous cesarean section for dystocia<br>• Induction of labor<br>• Coexisting fetal, placental, or maternal conditions<br>• Maternal BMI greater than 30 kg/m<br>• Fetal macrosomia of 4 kg or more<br>• Advanced maternal age<br>• Short stature.<br>• More than one previous cesarean section<br>• Risk factors associated with an increased risk of uterine scar rupture |

(BMI: body mass index; VBAC: vaginal birth-after-cesarean section)

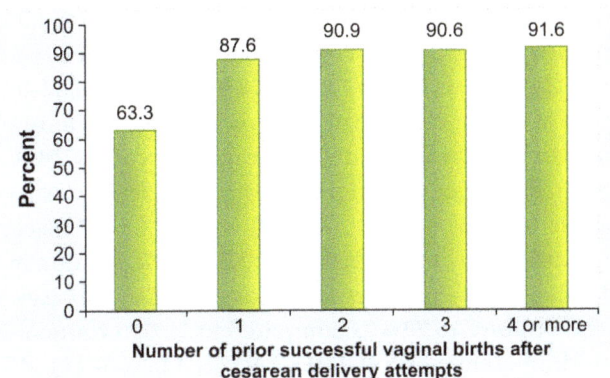

**Fig. 2:** Likelihood of successful vaginal birth after cesarean delivery (VBAC) according to the number of prior successful VBAC attempts.[45]

**TABLE 4:** Pregnancy and neonatal outcomes according to number of prior successful vaginal births after cesarean delivery.[33]

| Outcomes | Number of prior VBACs | | | |
| --- | --- | --- | --- | --- |
| | 0 (n = 9,012) | 1 (n = 2,900) | 2 or more (n = 1,620) | P value* |
| VBAC success | 63.3 | 87.6 | 90.9 | <0.001 |
| Uterine rupture | 0.87 | 0.45 | 0.43 | 0.01 |
| Uterine rupture if induced | 1.37 | 0.37 | 0.68 | 0.03 |
| Scar dehiscence | 0.94 | 0.24 | 0.25 | <0.001 |
| Hysterectomy | 0.23 | 0.17 | 0.06 | 0.15 |
| Surgical complications* | 0.45 | 0.17 | 0.12 | 0.008 |
| Thromboembolism† | 0.09 | 0 | 0 | 0.07 |
| Transfusion | 1.89 | 1.24 | 0.99 | 0.002 |
| Endometritis | 3.68 | 1.17 | 1.30 | <0.001 |
| Maternal death | 0.02 | 0 | 0 | 0.71 |
| 5 minute Apgar score ≤ 5 | 2.50 | 2.11 | 1.86 | 0.07 |
| Cord arterial pH ≤ 7.00 | 2.34 | 1.63 | 1.62 | 0.17 |
| Neonatal intensive care unit admission | 15.1 | 12.9 | 14.6 | 0.08 |
| Hypoxic ischemic encephalopathy | 0.17 | 0.07 | 0 | 0.05 |
| Infant death | 0.64 | 0.59 | 0.44 | 0.35 |

*Broad ligament hematoma, cystotomy, or bowel or ureteral injury.
†Deep vein thrombosis or pulmonary embolus.

VBAC **(Fig. 2)**.[45] The risk of scar rupture being 0.87% with no history of VBAC, and 0.45%, 0.38%, 0.54%, and 0.52% after one, two, three, and four or more successful VBAC, respectively **(Table 4)**. Second row of **Table 4** shows percentage risk of uterine rupture after number of successful VBACs respectively.

## Intrapartum

Favorable modified Bishops score is related to increase chance in VBAC being successful. First pelvic examination in labor can give some idea whether VBAC is likely to be successful or not. Bujold et al. in his study showed the success rates being 57.8%, 64.5%, 82.5%, and 97% for modified Bishops score being 0–2, 3–5, 6–8, and 9–11, respectively.[46] The success rate of VBAC is 81% versus 67% in women with spontaneous labor and induced labor, respectively. Further augmented labor with oxytocin has been shown to have a better success rate than induced labor but is less than that of spontaneous labor **(Table 5)**.[43]

To predict a successful TOLAC, there are various tools, which assess the multiple factors predicting VBAC. Flamm and Geiger Scoring System is among the popular ones. This scoring model provides reasonable predictability for VBAC and also consistent ability to identify women at risk for failed trial of labor. This scoring system includes following criteria- age of patient, history of previous vaginal delivery, indication of previous CS, cervical dilatation, and cervical effacement at time of admission.[47]

## Factors Related to Unsuccessful VBAC

### Antenatal

Many predictive nomograms have been suggested in the literature, which are simple and can calculate the VBAC success rate as soon as the first antenatal visit, based on simple variables. These models, however, have their own limitations and have not gained popularity.[44,48-51] They are applicable only to women at term with a previous uncomplicated CS. No previous vaginal birth as described earlier has got the VBAC success rate of only 63%.[45] Body mass index greater than 29 has been shown to decrease the success rate. These patients are almost 50% less likely to have VBAC success compared to their underweight counterparts (odds ratio 0.53, 95% CI 0.29–0.98, $p = 0.043$).[52]

Previous CS for dystocia decrease the success rates of VBAC.[43] Cervical dilatation achieved at the primary CS has also been found to play a role, and there has been controversy about the cervical dilatation in previous pregnancy before CS to the success rate of VBAC in current pregnancy. As a more generalization, the success rate of VBAC in women with previous CS for cervical dystocia in first and second stage is 75% and 65%, respectively, compared to 82% success rates when CS was done for other indication apart from cervical dystocia.[41] No correlation of the amount of cervical dilatation at previous CS and successful VBAC was found.[53] Previous preterm cesarean birth has comparable success rates but is associated with higher scar rupture rates.[54,55] Inter-delivery period of less than 24 months from previous cesarean birth is associated with lower VBAC success rate of 67%. Fetal weight of more than 4,000 g is also associated with decreased VBAC rates to as low as 62%.[43,56] Advanced maternal age, nonwhite ethnicity, short stature and fetus of male sex have all shown to reduce success rates.[57]

**TABLE 5:** Factors related to success rates of VBAC.[43]

| Characteristics | n (VBAC success %) | Odds ratio (95% CI) |
| --- | --- | --- |
| Previous cesarean delivery | | |
| Dystocia | 2,940 (63.5) | 0.34 (0.30–0.37) |
| Nonreassuring fetal well-being | 2,231 (72.6) | 0.51 (0.45–0.58) |
| Other | 1,718 (77.5) | 0.67 (0.58–0.76) |
| Malpresentation | 2,856 (83.8) | 1.0 |
| Prior uterine scar | | |
| Transverse | 8,688 (72.5) | 0.71 (0.64–0.79) |
| Unknown* | 2,002 (78.7) | 1.0 |
| Previous cesarean delivery | | |
| ≤2 years | 2,338 (67.8) | 0.70 (0.64–0.76) |
| >2 years* | 7,831 (75.2) | 1.0 |
| Previous vaginal delivery | | |
| Yes* | 6,121 (86.6) | 1.0 |
| No | 4,499 (60.9) | 0.24 (0.22–0.23) |
| Previous VBAC | | |
| Yes* | 4,166 (89.6) | 1.0 |
| No | 5,924 (64.4) | 0.21 (0.19–0.23) |
| Maternal disease† | | |
| Yes | 1,652 (70.1) | 0.81 (0.74–0.90) |
| No* | 9,038 (74.3) | 1.0 |
| Labor type | | |
| Induction | 2,569 (67.4) | 0.50 (0.45–0.55) |
| Augmented | 3,854 (73.9) | 0.68 (0.62–0.75) |
| Spontaneous* | 4,266 (80.6) | 1.0 |
| Admit cervical dilation (cm) | | |
| <4 | 5,384 (66.8) | 0.39 (0.36–0.48) |
| ≥4* | 4,980 (83.8) | 1.0 |
| Epidural anesthesia | | |
| Yes* | 7,850 (73.4) | 1.0 |
| No | 1,007 (50.4) | 0.37 (0.33–0.41) |
| Birth weight (g) | | |
| <2,500 | 267 (77.2) | 1.14 (0.89–1.47) |
| 2,500–3,999* | 9,486 (74.9) | 1.0 |
| ≥4,000 | 935 (62.0) | 0.55 (0.49–0.61) |
| Gestational age (wk/d) | | |
| 370/7–40 6/7* | 9,340 (75.0) | 1.0 |
| ≥41 | 1,350 (64.8) | 0.61 (0.55–0.68) |

*Reference group.
†Maternal diseases were defined as diabetes, asthma, thyroid disease, seizure disorder, pregestational chronic hypertension treated with medication, renal disease, connective tissue disease.

### Intrapartum

Apart from antenatal factors certain indicators during intrapartum period can affect the success rate of VBAC. Induction of labor decreases the rate of successful VBAC to 67% (OR 0.50, 95% CI 0.44–0.55) as compared to 80% in spontaneous labor. On the other hand augmented labor has got a VBAC success rate of 73.9% (OR 0.68, 95% CI 0.62–0.75). The MFMU Cesarean Registry also showed the following intrapartum factors related to decreased success of VBAC. In pregnancies 41 weeks or more of gestation, the VBAC success rates decrease to 65% as compared to 75% at 37 weeks to 40 weeks and 6 days (OR 0.61, 95% CI 0.55–0.68). Landon in his study also showed that epidural anesthesia increases the success of VBAC to 73% as compared to 50% in women with no epidural anesthesia (OR 0.37, 95% CI 0.33–0.41). When women present in labor with cervical dilatation of ≥4 cm, the chances of favorable outcome are increased. When all these unfavorable factors are present, successful VBAC is achieved in as few as only 30% of women.[43]

## Risks and Benefits of VBAC

The main evidence of VBAC on neonatal and pregnancy outcomes came from a study by Landon as shown in **Table 4**.[33]

### Maternal Risks

*Maternal morbidity and mortality:* This is usually associated with failure to achieve successful VBAC as morbidity otherwise is very low in cases of successful vaginal birth. The morbidity is mainly due to uterine rupture, emergency CS, blood transfusion, and endometritis. According to the best available evidence the rate of significant maternal complications for women undergoing VBAC are 5.5% compared with only 3.6% in women who had elective repeat CS (ERCS) **(Table 6)**. Maternal mortality does not increase significantly in women undergoing VBAC to those having planned ERCS.[33]

*Risk of uterine rupture:* Uterine rupture is the most dreaded complication of trial of scar. This results in severe maternal and neonatal morbidity. Risk of uterine rupture is 0.2–0.7% in planned VBAC after one previous CS and zero in women undergoing ERCS.[38,58-63] This is much higher than risk of rupture 1/10,000 to 1/20,000 in unscarred uterus. However, the more recent study by Macones et al. found the rate of uterine rupture in women attempting VBAC with one single prior cesarean as 0.98%.[32] Maternal complications are shown in **Table 6**.

*Risk associated with failed trial of VBAC:* The most important detrimental effect in cases of trial of VBAC is because of failed VBAC. Women who had successful VBAC had an overall morbidity of 2.4% whereas women who had failed attempted VBAC had a 14.1% incidence of morbidity.[43]

*Long-term complications of VBAC:* Vaginal birth may cause adverse effects on pelvic floor and bladder functions as with normal vaginal delivery. However, this in context to VBAC and ERCS still needs to be studied further.

**TABLE 6:** Maternal complications in women undergoing TOLAC.[43]

| Complications | Trial of labor (n = 17,898) n (%) | Elective repeat cesarean delivery (n = 15,801) n (%) | Odds ratio (95% CI) | P value |
|---|---|---|---|---|
| Uterine rupture | 124 (0.7) | 0 | - | <0.001 |
| Scar dehiscence* | 119 (0.7) | 76 (0.5) | 1.38 (1.04–1.85) | 0.03 |
| Hysterectomy | 41 (0.2) | 47 (0.3) | 0.77 (0.51–1.17) | 0.22 |
| Thromboembolism† | 7 (0.04) | 10 (0.1) | 0.62 (0.24–1.62) | 0.32 |
| Transfusion | 304 (1.7) | 158 (1.0) | 1.71 (1.41–2.08) | <0.001 |
| Endometritis | 517 (2.9) | 285 (1.8) | 1.62 (1.40–1.87) | <0.001 |
| Maternal death | 3 (0.02) | 7 (0.04) | 0.38 (0.10–1.46) | 0.21 |
| Other maternal adverse events‡ | 64 (0.4) | 52 (0.3) | 1.09 (0.75–1.57) | 0.66 |
| One or more of the above | 978 (5.5) | 563 (3.6) | 1.56 (1.41–1.74) | <0.001 |

*Not all women underwent examination of their scars after vaginal delivery
†Includes deep vein thrombosis or pulmonary embolism
‡Includes broad ligament hematoma, cystotomy, or bowel or ureteral injury

## Fetal Risks

*Antepartum stillbirth:* As explained earlier in the chapter, the risk of still birth (excluding malformations) is 2/1,000 in VBAC and 0.8/1,000 in ERCS (RR with VBAC 2.45; 95% CI 1.25-4.78; $p = 0.007$).[21,33] The risk is primarily due to increased chances of stillbirth after 34 weeks **(Table 7)**.

*Delivery-related perinatal death:* Though the risk of delivery-related perinatal death is increased by 12-fold in VBAC group than ERCS, the absolute risk is of the order of a nulliparous woman attempting vaginal delivery which is 1.3/1,000. Only 30% of these were due to uterine rupture. There is also a chance of 10% babies having severe asphyxia among the cases with uterine rupture which would lead to hypoxic ischemic encephalopathy or death.[27,63,64] It is important to note that although the fetal risks are more with VBAC but absolute risks are low. The pregnant woman and her partner should be counseled accordingly.

## Maternal and Fetal Benefits

The benefits are primarily shorter hospital stay and that women have more control on the labor. The respiratory morbidity in the newborn due to transient tachypnea of newborn is decreased in case of successful VBAC.

## Risks and Benefits of ERCS

### Maternal Risks

Women having ERCS have complication rate of 3.6% which is higher than women having successful VBAC.[33,59] This is attributed to routine complications of surgery like bleeding, thromboembolism, febrile morbidity, long-term bladder dysfunction, and prolonged recovery. In addition, there is an increased risk of future placental problems, subfertility, and ectopic pregnancies, as highlighted in the previous sections. Anesthetic complications are exceedingly rare, irrespective of planned VBAC or ERCS.

**TABLE 7:** Composite neonatal morbidity from elective repeat cesarean delivery and trial of labor after previous cesarean.[69]

| Neonatal risks | ERCD (%) | TOLAC (%) |
|---|---|---|
| Antepartum stillbirth | 0.21 | 0.10 |
| Intrapartum stillbirth | 0–0.004 | 0.01–0.04 |
| HIE | 0–0.32 | 0–0.89 |
| Perinatal mortality | 0.05 | 0.13 |
| Neonatal mortality | 0.06 | 0.11 |
| Respiratory morbidity | 5.4 | 5.4 |
| Transient tachypnea | 4.2 | 3.6 |

(ERCD: elective repeat cesarean delivery; HIE: hypoxic ischemic encephalopathy; TOLAC: trial of labor after cesarean delivery)

### Maternal Benefits

Elective repeat CS avoids the risks of failed VBAC and consequently all the complications associated with emergency CS. It also avoids pelvic floor and perineal trauma. Moreover, it is done under controlled circumstances with a full knowledge of time of delivery and woman can therefore plan relatively well.

### Fetal Risks

*Respiratory problems:* This is the main cause of morbidity in babies delivered by ERCS. ERCS is associated with 5-fold increase in transient tachypnea of the newborn (TTN) or respiratory distress syndrome (RDS).[65] Absolute risk of morbidity in ERCS group is 3.5-3.7% compared with 0.5-1.4% for VBAC.[64-66] Risk is more, if cesarean is performed before labor and in the earlier weeks of gestation after term. It is seen that the risk of asthma in neonates admitted with TTN is doubled as compared to those who are not.[66-68] The respiratory morbidity is 11.4%, 6.2%, and 1.5% at 37, 38, and 39 weeks of gestation, respectively **(Table 7)**.

### Fetal Benefits

They are from avoidance of any morbidity from scar rupture. The incidence of intrapartum hypoxic ischemic encephalopathy (HIE) at term is significantly greater in planned VBAC (7.8/10,000) compared with ERCS (zero rate).[59]

## Planned VBAC in Special Circumstances

In cases where previous CS was done by an uncomplicated low-transverse incision with an otherwise uncomplicated pregnancy, the success and complication rates have been studied by many published series.

### Preterm Birth

Preterm (24–36 weeks of gestation) planned VBAC has higher success rates when compared with women at term undergoing planned VBAC (82% vs. 74%). The risk of uterine rupture is also decreased though nonsignificantly.[70] Perinatal outcomes were similar with preterm VBAC and preterm ERCS. The Bishop's score of cervix should be taken into account as these women can have unfavorable cervix resistant to induction. Also, the risks of scar rupture associated with induction should be discussed well with the patient. However, women with preterm gestation who are in labor have a higher chance of successful VBAC and lesser rate of uterine rupture.

### Twin Gestation

It was initially thought that women with previous cesarean delivery and currently having twin pregnancy should be delivered by CS, but the evidence does not show any benefit of doing so. However, two recent studies by Cahil et al. and Varner et al. showed no increased maternal risk of VBAC associated with twins and comparable success rates of 75.7% in twins versus 75.4% in singletons.[71-73]

### Macrosomia

The concern for women with previous CS and macrosomic baby (>4,000 g) is primarily the decreased success rate of VBAC and secondly increased rate of rupture. In a study done by Landon et al., the success rate of trial of VBAC is 55–67% for pregnancies with infants weighing 4,000 g or more compared to 75–83% with smaller infants.[33] However, we do not have enough data to support the concern regarding increased rupture rates. It also should be acknowledged that antenatal estimation of fetal weight by ultrasound is not exactly accurate. It is important to be cautious in cases where the progress of labor is suboptimal as cephalopelvic disproportion could be one of the causes.

### Short Interdelivery Interval

Pregnancies in quick succession after previous cesarean delivery can cause suboptimal healing of the scar and increased chances of scar dehiscence and scar rupture. An interdelivery interval shorter than 18 months was reported to be associated with a significant increase of uterine rupture (odds ratio [OR], 3.0; 95% confidence interval [CI], 1.3-7.2)[74] while as per green top guidelines (2015) an interdelivery interval of less than 12 months is considered to potentially increase the risk of uterine rupture.[75]

### Gestation beyond 40 Weeks

Studies evaluating the association of gestational age with VBAC outcomes have consistently demonstrated decreased VBAC rates in women who undertake TOLAC beyond 40 weeks of gestation.[76-77] Although one study has shown an increased risk of uterine rupture beyond 40 weeks of gestation,[76] other studies, including the largest study evaluating this factor, have not found this association.[77]

## Contraindications to VBAC

There is limited evidence on safety of VBAC in more than one previous cesarean sections or type of previous uterine scar and therefore absolute risks are not known.[33,37,43,59,72,78] According to best possible evidence available, planned VBAC is contraindicated in:

- Previous uterine rupture (increases the risk of recurrent uterine rupture although the absolute rate is not known)
- Previous high-vertical classical CS (200–900/10,000 risk of uterine rupture)
- Three or more previous cesarean deliveries (reliable estimate of risk of rupture unknown)
- In certain extreme circumstances (such as miscarriage, intrauterine fetal death) for some women in the above groups, the vaginal route (although risky) may not necessarily be contraindicated
- Previous inverted T or J incision (190/10,000 risk of uterine rupture)
- Prior low-vertical incision (200/10,000 risk of uterine rupture).

The current practice in most units is to do an elective CS in women where uterine cavity was opened while myomectomy. However, the evidence is insufficient and conflicting on whether the risk of uterine rupture is increased in women with previous myomectomy or prior complex uterine surgery.[79]

## VBAC in Previous Two Cesarean Sections

There have been many published studies advocating vaginal delivery after multiple previous cesarean deliveries. These show an insignificant increased risk of scar rupture with VBAC after two previous cesarean sections as compared to VBAC after one CS (92/10,000 vs. 68/10,000) and slightly decreased success rates of VBAC (66% in previous two cesareans vs. 74% in previous one cesarean).[43]

A study by Macones et al., showed an insignificant increase in scar rupture between previous two cesarean sections and previous one CS, i.e., 1.8% versus 0.9%.[80] VBAC is therefore not a contraindication and can be offered in selected cases and should be consultant led. A recent systematic review showed a risk of scar rupture to be 1.36% in women with previous two CSs as compared to 0.71% after previous one CS.[81]

The Royal College of Obstetricians and Gynaecologists recommends that women with a prior history of even two previous uncomplicated low transverse CSs, in an otherwise uncomplicated pregnancy at term, with no contraindication for vaginal birth, may be considered suitable for planned VBAC. According to ACOG guidelines, having previous two cesarean sections may reduce the likelihood of VBAC success but should not preclude a trial of labor.[82]

## Uterine Rupture and Previous CS

Uterine rupture is defined as separation of the entire thickness of the uterine wall with extrusion of any portion of the fetal-placental unit often resulting in intraperitoneal or vaginal hemorrhage, need for hysterectomy, or bladder injury. As mentioned earlier, the uterine rupture rate in women undergoing trial of VBAC varies from 0.2 to 0.7%. It is an obstetric catastrophe that is associated with serious complications like need for blood transfusions, hysterectomy, damage to the genitourinary tract, severe neonatal morbidity, and even maternal and perinatal mortality. Chauhan et al. reviewed literature from 1989 to 2001 to study the morbidity related to uterine rupture and found that per thousand trial of VBAC, the morbidity related to uterine rupture was 1.8 for packed cell transfusion, 1.5 for pathologic fetal acidosis (cord pH < 7.00), 0.9 for hysterectomy, 0.8 for genitourinary injury, 0.4 for perinatal death, and 0.02 for maternal death **(Table 8)**.[38] Moreover, prompt delivery is needed to avoid permanent neonatal damage or death. It is by far the most common reason for women refusing trial of VBAC. There is lack of robust evidence in absence of randomized controlled trials and inadequately powered studies and most data is in the form of meta-analysis of retrospective studies.

There are certain predisposing factors which can increase this risk and we need to know them to counsel women accordingly. All the factors which contraindicate VBAC increase the chance of uterine rupture, if VBAC is still attempted. The type of previous uterine scar is an important factor determining the scar rupture rates. In study done by Landon et.al., the rates of rupture were 0.7% for women with one prior low-transverse incision, 2% for those with a prior low-vertical incision, 1.9% with a prior classical, inverted T or J incision who either presented in advanced labor or refused a repeated cesarean delivery, and 0.5% for those with an unknown type of prior incision **(Table 9)**. In women with previous classical CS, it would be advisable to do an ERCS earlier than 39 weeks as there is a chance of silent scar rupture and to minimize the risk of them going into labor before elective CS. A previous preterm cesarean delivery significantly increases the risk of subsequent uterine rupture as compared to women with previous CS at term (0.58% compared with 0.28%, $p < 0.001$).[55] The reason primarily is

**TABLE 8:** The complication rates related to scar rupture per 1,000 women attempting VBAC.[38]

| Complication | Risk/1,000 attempted VBAC |
| --- | --- |
| Uterine rupture | 5–7/1,000 |
| Perinatal death | 0.4–0.7/1,000 |
| Maternal death | 0.02/1,000 |
| Hysterectomy | 0.5–2/1,000 |
| Genitourinary injury | 0.8/1,000 |
| Blood transfusion | 1.8/1,000 |
| Fetal acidosis (cord pH < 7) | 1.5/1,000 |
| HIE | 0.4/1,000 |

(HIE: hypoxic ischemic encephalopathy; VBAC: vaginal birth-after-cesarean section)

**TABLE 9:** Estimated uterine rupture rates based on prior incision type.

| Prior incision type | Estimated rupture rate (%) |
| --- | --- |
| Classical | 1.9 |
| T-shaped | 1.9 |
| Low vertical | 2 |
| One low transverse | 0.2–0.9 |
| Prior preterm cesarean delivery | Increased (2 fold) |
| Prior uterine rupture | 2–6 |

due to suboptimal healing of a poorly formed lower segment in these women, as the risk of rupture was higher in women who had not gone into labor prior to CS. This together with a shorter inter-delivery period compounds the risk. Previous single layer closure has been found to increase the risk of uterine rupture by up to 6 times.[83] The risk of uterine rupture is also inversely related to interdelivery interval.[74] As discussed later in the chapter, induction of labor with prostaglandins increases scar rupture rates. A woman having successful vaginal birth, in any order, has got a protective factor from scar rupture and her chance of having it is five times less. Maternal age greater than 30 years is also associated with increased scar rupture. The risk is 3 times higher than for women younger than 30 years undergoing trial of VBAC. Maternal fever after a previous CS seems to be associated with increased risk of scar rupture but needs further studies.

## MANAGEMENT

### Antenatal Counseling

The antenatal counseling is based on the evidence given earlier in the chapter regarding success rates, complications, risk and benefits, and suitability of the patient for trial of VBAC or ERCS. It is vital to apply this evidence to the individual woman, according to her circumstances. Women with previous one uncomplicated lower-segment transverse CS, with an otherwise uncomplicated pregnancy, with no other contraindication for vaginal delivery can be given an option of planned VBAC or ERCS at term. An estimate of the likelihood of a successful trial of labor should be discussed.

This is important because the increased risk for morbidity in women attempting VBAC is primarily found in those who fail to achieve successful vaginal birth. The discussion should be well documented in the notes.

Previous operation notes should be seen to find the details of previous CS surgery. Any divergence from the routine low transverse incision should be discussed with a consultant.

Discussion should also be done regarding continuous intrapartum monitoring.[53] Future reproductive choices should be discussed as this can be important in decision making. In women planning future pregnancies, multiple cesarean sections increase the risk of severe maternal morbidity and mortality, e.g., placenta previa, placenta accreta, or percreta. Proper documentation is vital from medicolegal aspects. The decision should be made at least a few weeks before term. Informed consent is a must in these cases.

## Monitoring in Antenatal Period

### Role of USG

In women with placenta previa, possibility of placenta accreta should be ruled out by ultrasound or MRI. A consultant should be present during the CS with placenta previa/accreta with previous scar. Blood should be cross matched, senior anesthetist should be present and interventional radiologist should be kept available, if possible.

### Scar Thickness

There have been few observational studies showing the possible benefit of measuring scar thickness before trial of VBAC.[84-86] Even an arbitrary cut-off of 3.5 mm scar thickness has been used by some authors for selecting patients for trial of VBAC and showed good negative predictive value for scar rupture. However, the evidence is not robust enough for routine clinical practice.

### Timing of Elective Repeat CS or Planned VBAC

As up to 10% of women scheduled for ERCS go into labor before the 39th week, it is a good practice to have a plan for the event of labor starting prior to the scheduled date. For the same reason, 39 weeks seems to be a reasonable gestation to perform elective CS. The risk of respiratory morbidity in the neonate appears to be significantly low. However, in cases of planned VBAC, pregnancy should go till term and plan for induction of labor should be undertaken weighing the risks and benefits of postdated pregnancy. Apart from these factors, routine monitoring according to hospital protocol should be done.

## Management of Labor

### Intrapartum Support and Intervention during Planned VBAC

Knowing that there is a risk of 0.5–1.0% of scar rupture and consequent risk of fetal demise and morbidity, VBAC should be conducted in well-staffed and equipped units. About 6% of uterine ruptures will end in fetal demise and 0.5–19% can have hypoxic encephalopathy with long-term disability.[87] There should be adequate facilities for immediate CS and neonatal and maternal resuscitation. Intravenous access with grouping and saving of blood should be done in all these cases. Continuous cardiotocography (CTG) is recommended, as abnormality in the cardiotocograph is the most consistent finding in uterine rupture. CTG abnormalities are present in 55–87% of such cases.[58] Although abnormal cardiotocograph is usually the earliest warning sign, presence of any of the following should raise the suspicion of uterine scar rupture.

- Abnormal CTG
- Severe abdominal pain, especially if persisting between contractions
- Chest pain or shoulder tip pain
- Sudden onset of shortness of breath
- Acute onset scar tenderness
- Abnormal vaginal bleeding or hematuria
- Cessation of previously efficient uterine activity
- Maternal tachycardia, hypotension or shock
- Loss of station of the presenting part.

Epidural anesthesia is not contraindicated in planned VBAC. There is no evidence to show that masking of symptoms of uterine rupture due to epidural anesthesia increase the risk of maternal or perinatal morbidity. The routine use of intrauterine pressure catheters in the early detection of uterine scar rupture is not recommended.

### Induction and Augmentation

Induction of labor (regardless of the method of induction) and augmentation of labor with oxytocin are associated with a significantly greater risk of uterine rupture than with spontaneous labor without oxytocin augmentation ($p < 0.001$ for both).[21,33] Induction should be done after analyzing the risks and benefits of induction of labor. Women should be informed that there is a two- to three-fold increase in risk of uterine rupture and 1.5-fold increase in emergency CS due to induction and/or augmentation of labor compared with spontaneous labour.[88] However, some studies in literature do not suggest a significant increase in uterine rupture rates between women undergoing induction of labor with or without previous CS.[89] As the evidence is not strong enough, caution should be taken before induction of labor. The decision should be consultant led and induction should happen preferably in the labor ward.

### Prostaglandin Induction

The risk of uterine rupture is 0.4% in women with spontaneous labor. The best available evidence suggests a higher rupture rate in these cases. Prostaglandin induction with or without oxytocin augmentation compared with nonprostaglandin induction has a higher risk of uterine rupture of 1.4% versus 0.9%, respectively. In another study, the uterine rupture rate was found to be 0.87% versus 0.29%. Prostaglandin induction is also associated with a higher risk of perinatal death from uterine rupture. Prostaglandin E2 (dinoprostone) is associated with an increased risk of uterine rupture and should not be used except in rare circumstances.[63] Prostaglandin E1 (misoprostol) is found to have a high risk of uterine rupture and should not be used for induction of labor after CS.[90]

### Non-prostaglandin Induction

Induction of labor with oxytocin may be associated with an increased risk of uterine rupture. However, the exact rate of increase is not known.[69] Foley catheter may be safely used to ripen the cervix in a woman planning a VBAC.

### Augmentation of Labor

Oxytocin augmentation should be a consultant led decision. Oxytocin rate should be titrated such that it should not exceed the maximum rate of four contractions in 10 minutes. Early recognition and intervention for labor dystocia can prevent a proportion of uterine ruptures among women attempting VBAC and therefore progress of labor should be carefully assessed. Misoprostol (PGE1) should not be used for augmentation of labor as it increases the risk of uterine rupture.[90]

**Table 10** lists the rates of uterine rupture according to labor status. Majority of poor outcomes and litigations can be prevented, if labor is spontaneous, nonaugmented, and when appropriate actions are taken to detect fetal heart abnormalities.

## Management of Third Stage of Labor

Due to the presence of scar and its inability to contract, the possibility of postpartum hemorrhage is increased and therefore active management of third stage is recommended.

It is important not to attempt delivery of the placenta, if there are no signs of placental separation. Scan reports should be reviewed to see the site of placenta and possibility of placenta accreta should be kept in mind especially if the placenta is anterior. In case of such suspicion following should be done:

- Four units of blood should be cross matched.
- Explain to the patient about placenta accreta and the possible interventions that can be done and obtain consent from the patient.
- Consultant should be informed.
- Theater should be arranged for exploration and consent should be taken for manual removal of placenta and possible interventions in case of placenta accreta. Manual removal should only be done if a clear plane of cleavage is found between the uterus and placenta. If no such plane is found then it is extremely important not to attempt any separation, as this might lead to massive bleeding.

## Management Options in Cases of Placenta Accreta

- *Hysterectomy:* Evidence supports an aggressive surgical approach by means of hysterectomy in such cases unless preserving fertility is an issue. However, if the patient is not bleeding or fertility is an issue, expectant management can be done.
- *Expectant:* There have been many case reports and case series published where expectant management of placenta accreta has been used especially where conserving fertility is an issue.[91] This would involve leaving the whole placenta in and cutting the cord as close to the placenta as possible. However, close monitoring is required by means of weekly scans and monitoring for infection. The expectant management can be continued until placenta gets resorbed, which could take up to 6–10 months or until patient develops any signs or symptoms of infection or heavy bleeding. Role of methotrexate to help resorption is not known although some authors' have advocated its use in form of weekly injections. Beta hCG has been used by some authors to see the resorption of placenta but it does not predict the complications like heavy bleeding.
- *Conservative surgery:* Uterine artery embolization, internal artery ligation or embolization, and subendometrial

**TABLE 10:** Rates of uterine rupture according to labor status.[33]

| Type of labor | No. of patients | Uterine rupture no. (%) | Odds ratio (95% CI) | P value |
| --- | --- | --- | --- | --- |
| Spontaneous | 6,685 | 24 (0.4) | 1.00 | – |
| Augmented | 6,009 | 52 (0.9) | 2.42 (1.49–3.93) | <0.001 |
| Induced | 4,708 | 48 (1.0) | 2.86 (1.75–4.67) | <0.001 |
| With any prostaglandin, with or without oxytocin | 926 | 13 (1.4) | 3.95 (2.01–7.79) | <0.001 |
| With prostaglandins alone | 227 | 0 | – | – |
| With no prostaglandins* | 1,691 | 15 (0.9) | 2.48 (1.30–4.75) | 0.004 |
| With oxytocin alone | 1,864 | 20 (1.1) | 3.01 (1.66–5.46) | <0.001 |
| Not classified | 496 | 0 | – | – |

*Induction with no prostaglandins includes mechanical dilation with or without oxytocin.

vasopressin are other methods which have been reported in the literature. In many cases after conservative surgery a relaparotomy followed by hysterectomy is done under more controlled situation and with less bleeding and morbidity.

Triple P procedure is used in some regional centers in UK for conservative management of placenta percreta by means of perioperative placental localization and delivery of fetus by a transverse incision above the upper border of placenta, pelvic devascularization, placental nonseparation after delivery, and myometrial excision followed by uterine reconstruction.[92]

- In cases of late identification where removal of placenta has already been attempted, the placenta can be removed manually as much as possible. Oxytocics should be given in these cases to contract the uterus and intrauterine pressure balloon can be inserted for 24 hours. Antibiotic cover should be given and once the bleeding stops blunt curettage should be considered. Complications like uterine rupture while curettage and infection can occur and thus should be done with great care.

## Manual Exploration of Scar after VBAC

Although a lot of controversy exists on this issue, the current practice is not to routinely examine the lower uterine segment in a woman after a successful VBAC. The reasons are primarily no knowledge about the sensitivity and specificity of a manual assessment of the lower uterine segment for an occult rupture. Secondly, vigorous manual examination can damage or perforate the lower uterine segment.[72] However, in case of postpartum hemorrhage, it is important to ensure that bleeding is not coming from low-transverse scar.

## Postnatal Visit

All women undergoing emergency CS for failed VBAC should be debriefed about the events surrounding delivery and should be counseled about safe inter delivery time.

## Future Pregnancy after Uterine Rupture

If the site of the ruptured scar is confined to the lower segment of the uterus, the rate of repeat rupture or dehiscence in labor is 6%.[93] If the scar includes the upper segment of the uterus, the repeat rupture rate is reported to be as high as 32%[93,94] with the most recent report estimating the rate of recurrence to be 15%.[95] Given these rates, ACOG recommends that women who have had a previous uterine rupture give birth by repeat cesarean delivery before the onset of labor. In addition, because spontaneous labor is unpredictable and could occur before 39 weeks of gestation (the earliest recommended time for an elective delivery), like a history of a prior classical cesarean or myomectomy, the suggested timing of delivery between $36^{0/7}$ and $38^{6/7}$ weeks of gestation should be considered but can be individualized based on the clinical situation.

## Cost of VBAC Compared with Repeat CS

Although VBAC is known to be cost-effective as compared to ERCS, it is important to understand that VBAC is associated with high maternal and perinatal morbidity if there are no adequate facilities for close intrapartum monitoring in these women. This would in turn increase the costs incurred in further management of the mother and baby. It is therefore important for individual units to work out their own cost-effectiveness.

## Audit and Research

It is important to audit the practice around VBAC and ERCS. Further research needs to be done in form of randomized controlled trials to find more hard evidence.

## ■ KEY POINTS

- There is 46% higher chance of not having or having fewer children after 5 years of first CS delivery.
- The adjusted RR of placenta previa in subsequent pregnancy is 1.28 after one lower segment cesarean section (LSCS) in primiparous, 2.0 after two previous CS, and 4.0 after three previous CSs.
- Abruption rates in pregnancy with a previous CS are 0.95%, significantly higher than 0.74% with previous one vaginal birth.
- The risk of placenta previa accreta is 4% after vaginal delivery, 13% after one CS, 27% after two CS and 60% after three CS.
- Increase in stillbirth rate with previous CS is controversial.
- The success rates of VBAC after one CS is approximately 72–76%.
- Among many factors, previous vaginal birth, particularly previous VBAC, is the single best predictor for successful VBAC and is associated with an approximately 87–90% planned VBAC success rate.
- Cervical dilatation achieved at the primary cesarean for dystocia remains controversial in determining the VBAC success.
- Risk of uterine rupture is 0.2–0.7% in planned VBAC and zero in women undergoing ERCS.
- An interdelivery interval of less than 12 months increases the risk of uterine rupture.
- Successful VBAC had an overall morbidity of 2.4% whereas women who had failed attempted VBAC had a 14.1% incidence of morbidity.
- Maternal risk of repeat ERCS is primarily related to future reproductive problems. Fetal risks are primarily respiratory morbidity associated with 5-fold increase in TTN or RDS.
- Risk of delivery related perinatal death is increased by 12-fold in VBAC group than ERCS however the absolute risk is still small.

- VBAC between 26 and 37 weeks is associated with decreased scar rupture rates.
- Any previous uterine incision apart from lower segment transverse incision is a contraindication of planned VBAC.
- There is no clear evidence on safety of VBAC after myomectomy.
- VBAC in previous two cesarean sections is not contraindicated, however the evidence is very limited and the decision should be consultant led.
- An estimate of the likelihood of a successful trial of labor should be discussed with the patient and previous operation notes should be checked.
- Possibility of placenta accreta should be ruled out in cases of placenta previa.
- ERCS should be planned at around 39 weeks in usual circumstances.
- Trial of VBAC should be done in well-staffed unit with consultant support and adequate available resources for immediate CS and advanced neonatal and maternal resuscitation.
- About 6% of uterine ruptures will end in fetal demise and 0.5–19% can have hypoxic encephalopathy with long-term disability.
- There is a two- to three-fold increased risk of uterine rupture and around 1.5-fold increased risk of CS in induced and/or augmented labor compared with spontaneous labor.
- As far as the method of induction is concerned prostaglandins carry a higher rate of rupture than artificial rupture of membranes or oxytocin induction.
- Continuous monitoring by cardiotocograph should be done in women with trial of VBAC as its abnormality is the most consistent finding in uterine rupture and is present in 55–87% of these events.

## REFERENCES

1. Oral E, Elter K. The impact of cesarean birth on subsequent fertility. Curr Opin Obstet Gynecol. 2007;19:238-43.
2. Dodd J, Crowther C. Vaginal birth after caesarean versus elective repeat caesarean for women with a single prior caesarean birth: a systematic review of the literature. Aust NZ J Obstet Gynaecol. 2004;44:387-91.
3. Jolly J, Walker J, Bhabra K. Subsequent obstetric performance related to primary mode of delivery. Br J Obstet Gynaecol. 1999;106:227-32.
4. Hemminki E. Impact of caesarean section on future pregnancy—a review of cohort studies. Paediatr Perinat Epidemiol. 1996;10:366-79.
5. Collin SM, Marshall T, Filippi V. Caesarean section and subsequent fertility in sub-Saharan Africa. BJOG. 2006;113:276-83.
6. Bhattacharya S, Porter M, Harrild K, Naji A, Mollison J, van Teijlingen E, et al. Absence of conception after caesarean section: voluntary or involuntary? BJOG. 2006;113:268-75.
7. Murphy DJ, Stirrat GM, Heron J. The relationship between caesarean section and subfertility in a population-based sample of 14,541 pregnancies. Hum Reprod. 2002;17:1914-7.
8. Hemminki E, Merilainen J. Long-term effects of cesarean sections: Ectopic pregnancies and placental problems. Am J Obstet Gynecol. 1996;174:1569-74.
9. Kendrick JS, Tierney EF, Lawson HW, Strauss LT, Klein L, Atrash HK. Previous cesarean delivery and the risk of ectopic pregnancy. Obstet Gynecol. 1996;87:297-301.
10. Maymon R, Halperin R, Mendlovic S, Schneider D, Herman A. Ectopic pregnancies in a caesarean scar: review of the medical approach to an iatrogenic complication. Hum Reprod Update. 2004;10:515-23.
11. Halperin R, Schneider D, Mendlovic S, Pansky M, Herman A, Maymon R. Uterine-preserving emergency surgery for cesarean scar pregnancies: another medical solution to an iatrogenic problem. Fertil Steril. 2009;91(6):2623-7.
12. Ash A, Smith A, Maxwell D. Caesarean scar pregnancy. BJOG. 2007;114:253-63.
13. Morris H. Surgical pathology of the lower uterine segment caesarean section scar: is the scar a source of clinical symptoms? Int J Gynecol Pathol. 1995;14:16-20.
14. Jackson N. SP-B. Physical sequelae of caesarean section. Best Practice and research Clinical Obstet and Gynaecology. 2001;15:49-1.
15. Rasmussen S, Albrechtsen S, Dalaker K. Obstetric history and the risk of placenta previa. Acta Obstet Gynecol Scand. 2000;79:502-07.
16. Rageth JC, Juzi C, Grossenbacher H. Delivery after previous cesarean: a risk evaluation. Swiss Working Group of Obstetric and Gynecologic Institutions. Obstet Gynecol. 1999;93:332-7.
17. Lydon-Rochelle M, Holt VL, Easterling TR, Martin DP. First-birth cesarean and placental abruption or previa at second birth(1). Obstet Gynecol. 2001;97:765-9.
18. Gilliam M, Rosenberg D, Davis F. The likelihood of placenta previa with greater number of cesarean deliveries and higher parity. Obstet Gynecol. 2002;99:976-80.
19. Ananth CV, Smulian JC, Vintzileos AM. The association of placenta previa with history of cesarean delivery and abortion: a meta-analysis. Am J Obstet Gynecol. 1997;177:1071-8.
20. Ananth CV, Savitz DA, Williams MA. Placental abruption and its association with hypertension and prolonged rupture of membranes: a methodologic review and metaanalysis. Obstet Gynecol. 1996;88:309-18.
21. Ananth CV, Berkowitz GS, Savitz DA, Lapinski RH. Placental abruption and adverse perinatal outcomes. JAMA. 1999;282:1646-51.
22. Rasmussen S, Irgens LM, Dalaker K. The effect on the likelihood of further pregnancy of placental abruption and the rate of its recurrence. Br J Obstet Gynaecol. 1997;104:1292-5.
23. Getahun D, Oyelese Y, Salihu HM, Ananth CV. Previous cesarean delivery and risks of placenta previa and placental abruption. Obstet Gynecol. 2006;107:771-8.
24. Zaki ZM, Bahar AM, Ali ME, Albar HA, Gerais MA. Risk factors and morbidity in patients with placenta previa accreta compared to placenta previa non-accreta. Acta Obstet Gynecol Scand. 1998;77:391-4.
25. Clark SL, Koonings PP, Phelan JP. Placenta previa/accreta and prior cesarean section. Obstet Gynecol. 1985;66:89-92.

26. Miller DA, Chollet JA, Goodwin TM. Clinical risk factors for placenta previa-placenta accreta. Am J Obstet Gynecol. 1997;177:210-4.
27. Smith GC, Pell JP, Dobbie R. Caesarean section and risk of unexplained stillbirth in subsequent pregnancy. Lancet. 2003;362:1779-84.
28. Salihu HM, Sharma PP, Kristensen S, Blot C, Alio AP, Ananth CV, et al. Risk of stillbirth following a cesarean delivery: Black-white disparity. Obstet Gynecol. 2006;107:383-90.
29. Merrill BS, Gibbs CE. Planned vaginal delivery following cesarean section. Obstet Gynecol. 1978;52:50-2.
30. The National Institutes of Health Consensus Development statement on cesarean childbirth. A summary. J Reprod Med. 1981;26:103-12.
31. NIH consensus development statement on cesarean childbirth. The Cesarean Birth Task Force. Obstet Gynecol. 1981;57:537-45.
32. Macones GA, Peipert J, Nelson DB, Odibo A, Stevens EJ, Stamilio DM, et al. Maternal complications with vaginal birth after cesarean delivery: A multicenter study. Am J Obstet Gynecol. 2005;193:1656-62.
33. Landon MB, Hauth JC, Leveno KJ, Spong CY, Leindecker S, Varner MW, et al. Maternal and perinatal outcomes associated with a trial of labor after prior cesarean delivery. N Engl J Med. 2004;351:2581-9.
34. Little MO, Lyerly AD, Mitchell LM, Armstrong EM, Harris LH, Kukla R, et al. Mode of delivery: toward responsible inclusion of patient preferences. Obstet Gynecol. 2008;112:913-8.
35. Menacker F, Curtin SC. Trends in cesarean birth and vaginal birth after previous cesarean, 1991-99. Natl Vital Stat Rep. 2001;49:1-16.
36. Curtin SC, Gregory KD, Korst LM, Uddin SF. Maternal morbidity for vaginal and cesarean deliveries, according to previous cesarean history: new data from the birth certificate, 2013. Natl Vital Stat Rep. 2015;64(4):1-13.
37. Guise JM, Hashima J, Osterweil P. Evidence-based vaginal birth after caesarean section. Best Pract Res Clin Obstet Gynaecol. 2005;19:117-30.
38. Chauhan SP, Martin JN Jr, Henrichs CE, Morrison JC, Magann EF. Maternal and perinatal complications with uterine rupture in 142,075 patients who attempted vaginal birth after cesarean delivery: a review of the literature. Am J Obstet Gynecol. 2003;189:408-17.
39. Mozurkewich EL, Hutton EK. Elective repeat cesarean delivery versus trial of labor: a meta-analysis of the literature from 1989 to 1999. Am J Obstet Gynecol. 2000;183:1187-97.
40. Guise JM, Berlin M, McDonagh M, Osterweil P, Chan B, Helfand M. Safety of vaginal birth after cesarean: a systematic review. Obstet Gynecol. 2004;103:420-29.
41. Bujold E, Gauthier RJ. Should we allow a trial of labor after a previous cesarean for dystocia in the second stage of labor? Obstet Gynecol. 2001;98:652-5.
42. Gyamfi C, Juhasz G, Gyamfi P, Stone JL. Increased success of trial of labor after previous vaginal birth after cesarean. Obstet Gynecol. 2004;104:715-19.
43. Landon MB, Leindecker S, Spong CY, Hauth JC, Bloom S, Varner MW, et al. The MFMU Cesarean Registry: Factors affecting the success of trial of labor after previous cesarean delivery. Am J Obstet Gynecol. 2005;193:1016-23.
44. Smith GC, White IR, Pell JP, Dobbie R. Predicting cesarean section and uterine rupture among women attempting vaginal birth after prior cesarean section. PLoS Med. 2005;2:e252.
45. Mercer BM, Gilbert S, Landon MB, Spong CY, Leveno KJ, Rouse DJ, et al. Labor outcomes with increasing number of prior vaginal births after cesarean delivery. Obstet Gynecol. 2008;111:285-91.
46. Bujold E, Blackwell SC, Hendler I, Berman S, Sorokin Y, Gauthier RJ. Modified Bishop's score and induction of labor in patients with a previous cesarean delivery. Am J Obstet Gynecol. 2004;191:1644-8.
47. Patel RM, Kansara VM, Patel SK, Anand N. Impact of FLAMM scoring on cesarean section rate in previous one lower segment cesarean section patient. Int J Reprod Contracept Obstet Gynecol. 2016;5:3820-3.
48. Durnwald C, Mercer B. Vaginal birth after Cesarean delivery: Predicting success, risks of failure. J Matern Fetal Neonatal Med. 2004;15:388-93.
49. Hashima JN, Eden KB, Osterweil P, Nygren P, Guise JM. Predicting vaginal birth after cesarean delivery: a review of prognostic factors and screening tools. Am J Obstet Gynecol. 2004;190:547-55.
50. Dinsmoor MJ, Brock EL. Predicting failed trial of labor after primary cesarean delivery. Obstet Gynecol. 2004;103:282-6.
51. Macones GA, Cahill AG, Stamilio DM, Odibo A, Peipert J, Stevens EJ. Can uterine rupture in patients attempting vaginal birth after cesarean delivery be predicted? Am J Obstet Gynecol. 2006;195:1148-52.
52. Juhasz G, Gyamfi C, Gyamfi P, Tocce K, Stone JL. Effect of body mass index and excessive weight gain on success of vaginal birth after cesarean delivery. Obstet Gynecol. 2005;106:741-6.
53. Sachs BP, Kobelin C, Castro MA, Frigoletto F. The risks of lowering the cesarean-delivery rate. N Engl J Med. 1999;340:54-7.
54. Kwee A, Smink M, Van Der Laar R, Bruinse HW. Outcome of subsequent delivery after a previous early preterm cesarean section. J Matern Fetal Neonatal Med. 2007;20:33-57.
55. Sciscione AC, Landon MB, Leveno KJ, Spong CY, Macpherson C, Varner MW, et al. Previous preterm cesarean delivery and risk of subsequent uterine rupture. Obstet Gynecol. 2008;111:648-53.
56. Zelop CM, Shipp TD, Repke JT, Cohen A, Lieberman E. Outcomes of trial of labor following previous cesarean delivery among women with fetuses weighing >4000 g. Am J Obstet Gynecol. 2001;185:903-5.
57. Srinivas SK, Stamilio DM, Sammel MD, Stevens EJ, Peipert JF, Odibo AO, et al. Vaginal birth after caesarean delivery: does maternal age affect safety and success? Paediatr Perinat Epidemiol. 2007;21:114-20.
58. Guise JM, McDonagh MS, Osterweil P, Nygren P, Chan BK, Helfand M. Systematic review of the incidence and consequences of uterine rupture in women with previous caesarean section. BMJ. 2004;329:19-25.
59. McMahon MJ, Luther ER, Bowes WA Jr, Olshan AF. Comparison of a trial of labor with an elective second cesarean section. N Engl J Med. 1996;335:689-95.
60. Wen SW, Rusen ID, Walker M, Liston R, Kramer MS, Baskett T, et al. Comparison of maternal mortality and morbidity between trial of labor and elective cesarean section among

women with previous cesarean delivery. Am J Obstet Gynecol. 2004;191:1263-9.
61. Turner MJ, Agnew G, Langan H. Uterine rupture and labour after a previous low transverse caesarean section. BJOG. 2006;113:729-32.
62. Gardeil F, Daly S, Turner MJ. Uterine rupture in pregnancy reviewed. Eur J Obstet Gynecol Reprod Biol. 1994;56:107-10.
63. Smith GC, Pell JP, Pasupathy D, Dobbie R. Factors predisposing to perinatal death related to uterine rupture during attempted vaginal birth after caesarean section: retrospective cohort study. BMJ. 2004;329:375.
64. Smith GC, Pell JP, Cameron AD, Dobbie R. Risk of perinatal death associated with labor after previous cesarean delivery in uncomplicated term pregnancies. JAMA. 2002;287:2684-90.
65. Smith GC, Wood AM, White IR, Pell JP, Cameron AD, Dobbie R. Neonatal respiratory morbidity at term and the risk of childhood asthma. Arch Dis Child. 2004;89:956-60.
66. Morley GM. Mode of delivery and risk of respiratory diseases in newborns. Obstet Gynecol. 2001;97:1025-6.
67. Levine EM, Ghai V, Barton JJ, Strom CM. Mode of delivery and risk of respiratory diseases in newborns. Obstet Gynecol. 2001;97:439-42.
68. Richardson BS, Czikk MJ, daSilva O, Natale R. The impact of labor at term on measures of neonatal outcome. Am J Obstet Gynecol. 2005;192:219-26.
69. Guise JM, Eden K, Emeis C, Denman MA, Marshall N, Fu R, et al. Vaginal birth after cesarean: new insights. [Archived] Evidence Report/Technology Assessment No.191. AHRQ Publication No. 10–E003. Rockville (MD): Agency for Healthcare Research and Quality; 2010.
70. Quinones JN, Stamilio DM, Pare E, Peipert JF, Stevens E, Macones GA. The effect of prematurity on vaginal birth after cesarean delivery: Success and maternal morbidity. Obstet Gynecol. 2005;105:519-24.
71. Varner MW, Leindecker S, Spong CY, Moawad AH, Hauth JC, Landon MB, et al. The Maternal-Fetal Medicine Unit cesarean registry: Trial of labor with a twin gestation. Am J Obstet Gynecol. 2005;193:135-40.
72. Cahill AG, Macones GA. Vaginal birth after cesarean delivery: evidence-based practice. Clin Obstet Gynecol. 2007;50:518-25.
73. Cahill A, Stamilio DM, Pare E, Peipert JP, Stevens EJ, Nelson DB, et al. Vaginal birth after cesarean (VBAC) attempt in twin pregnancies: is it safe? Am J Obstet Gynecol. 2005;193:1050-5.
74. Bujold E, Gauthier RJ. Risk of uterine rupture associated with an interdelivery interval between 18 and 24 months. Obstet Gynecol. 2010;115(5):1003-6.
75. RCOG: Birth after previous cesarean birth. Green-top Guideline No. 45 October 2015.
76. Kiran TS, Chui YK, Bethel J, Bhal PS. Is gestational age an independent variable affecting uterine scar rupture rates? Eur J Obstet Gynecol Reprod Biol. 2006;126:68-71. (Level II-2)
77. Coassolo KM, Stamilio DM, Pare E, Peipert JF, Stevens E, Nelson DB, et al. Safety and efficacy of vaginal birth after cesarean attempts at or beyond 40 weeks of gestation. Obstet Gynecol. 2005;106:700-6.
78. Spaans WA, van der Vliet LM, Roell-Schorer EA, Bleker OP, van Roosmalen J. Trial of labour after two or three previous caesarean sections. Eur J Obstet Gynecol Reprod Biol. 2003;110:16-19.
79. Seracchioli R, Manuzzi L, Vianello F, Gualerzi B, Savelli L, Paradisi R, et al. Obstetric and delivery outcome of pregnancies achieved after laparoscopic myomectomy. Fertil Steril. 2006;86:159-65.
80. Macones GA, Cahill A, Pare E, Stamilio DM, Ratcliffe S, Stevens E, et al. Obstetric outcomes in women with two prior cesarean deliveries: is vaginal birth after cesarean delivery a viable option? Am J Obstet Gynecol. 2005;192:1223-8.
81. Tahseen S, Griffith M. Vaginal birth after two caesarean sections (VBAC-2)—a systematic review with meta-analysis of success rate and adverse outcomes of VBAC-2 versus VBAC-1 and repeat (third) caesarean sections. BJOG. 2010;117(1):5-19.
82. ACOG. ACOG Practice Bulletin Number 115: Vaginal birth after previous cesarean delivery. Obstet Gynecol. 2010;116(2 Pt 1):450-63.
83. Gyamfi C, Juhasz G, Gyamfi P, Blumenfeld Y, Stone JL. Single- versus double-layer uterine incision closure and uterine rupture. J Matern Fetal Neonatal Med. 2006;19:639-43.
84. Rozenberg P, Goffinet F, Phillippe HJ, Nisand I. Ultrasonographic measurement of lower uterine segment to assess risk of defects of scarred uterus. Lancet. 1996;347:281-4.
85. Rozenberg P, Goffinet F, Philippe HJ, Nisand I. Echographic measurement of the inferior uterine segment for assessing the risk of uterine rupture. J Gynecol Obstet Biol Reprod (Paris). 1997;26:513-19.
86. Rozenberg P, Goffinet F, Philippe HJ, Nisand I. Thickness of the lower uterine segment: Its influence in the management of patients with previous cesarean sections. Eur J Obstet Gynecol Reprod Biol. 1999;87:39-45.
87. Bonanno C, Clausing M. VBAC: a medicolegal perspective. Clin Perinatol. 2011;38:217-25.
88. Royal College of Obstetricians and Gynaecologists (2007). Birth after previous caesarean birth. Greentop Guideline No 45. Available from: https://www.rcog.org.uk/globalassets/documents/guidelines/gtg_45.pdf. [Last accessed July, 2021].
89. Locatelli A, Regalia AL, Ghidini A, Ciriello E, Biffi A, Pezzullo JC. Risks of induction of labour in women with a uterine scar from previous low transverse caesarean section. BJOG. 2004;111:1394-9.
90. SOGC clinical practice guidelines. Guidelines for vaginal birth after previous caesarean birth. Number 155 (Replaces guideline Number 147), February 2005. Int J Gynaecol Obstet. 2005;89:319-31.
91. Kayem G, Davy C, Goffinet F, Thomas C, Clément D, Cabrol D. Conservative versus extirpative management in cases of placenta accreta. Obstet Gynecol. 2004;104:531-6.
92. Chandraharan E, Rao S, Belli A, Arunkumaran S. The triple-P procedure as a conservative surgical alternative to peripartum hysterectomy for placenta percreta. Int J Gynaecol Obstet. 2012;117(2):191-4.
93. Ritchie EH. Pregnancy after rupture of the pregnant uterus. A report of 36 pregnancies and a study of cases reported since 1932. J Obstet Gynaecol Br Commonw. 1971;78:642-8.
94. Reyes-Ceja L, Cabrera R, Insfran E, Herrera-Lasso F. Pregnancy following previous uterine rupture. Study of 19 patients. Obstet Gynecol. 1969;34:387-9.
95. Eshkoli T, Weintraub AY, Baron J, Sheiner E. The significance of a uterine rupture in subsequent births. Arch Gynecol Obstet. 2015;292:799-803.

# CHAPTER 15

# Malpresentations

*Usha Gupta, Swati Agrawal*

## ■ INTRODUCTION

The fetus at term or at onset of labor normally assumes a longitudinal lie, flexed attitude with vertex presentation. When fetal part other than vertex presents at the pelvis, it is known as malpresentation. The various malpresentations include breech, shoulder, face, brow, and compound presentation. The most common malpresentation is the breech presentation in which, the lie is longitudinal and podalic pole of fetus occupies the lower uterine segment. Other malpresentations are due to a deviation from the normal flexed attitude of head in vertex presentation to full or partial extension of head resulting in face or brow presentations **(Fig. 1)**. Sometimes more than one fetal part presents in pelvis, e.g., a limb along with head, resulting in compound presentation.

## ■ PREVALENCE

The prevalence varies with the type of malpresentation. Breech presentation is seen in 3-4% of cases, shoulder presentation occurs in 0.3-0.5%, and face presentation occurs in 0.2-0.5%. Compound presentation and brow presentation are least common, being present in less than 0.2% of cases.

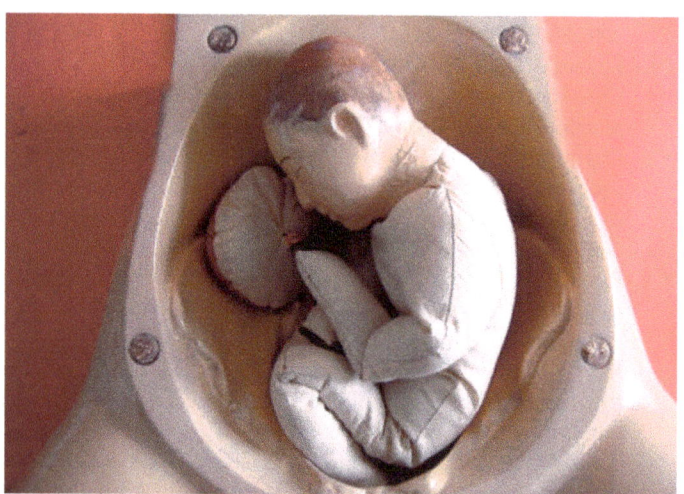

**Fig. 1:** Breech presentation—Flexed breech.

## ■ ETIOLOGY

In majority of cases, no cause of malpresentation is found.
However, following factors may be associated with various malpresentations.

- Increased mobility of fetus as occurs in prematurity or in hydramnios is associated with malpresentations. The prevalence of breech presentation at 28 weeks is 25% and at term it is about 3%.
- Contracted pelvic inlet, large fetus with resultant cephalopelvic disproportion, and pelvic tumors may prevent engagement of head at pelvic inlet leading to breech presentation.
- Diminished space in lower part of uterus due to low-lying placenta or uterine myomata, and fundal insertion of placenta are sometimes associated with breech presentation.
- Laxity of abdominal wall, as in multigravida, alters the vertical axis of uterus and consequently the vertical axis of fetus, which may result in transverse lie.
- Müllerian duct abnormalities of the uterus like subseptate uterus are often seen in cases of transverse lie. Septate uterus or uterus didelphys may be present in cases of breech presentation.
- Restricted mobility of fetus due to oligoamnios may prevent breech to turn into vertex presentation.
- Congenital malformations of the fetus like hydrocephaly and umbilical cord abnormalities like short cord are associated with breech presentation.
- Anencephaly and tumors of fetal neck and coils of cord round neck can cause face presentation.
- Autosomal trisomies, myotonic dystrophies, neurologic dysfunction of fetal muscles with imbalance between flexor and extensor muscles or joint contractures may lead to malpresentations like face and brow presentation.
- In multiple pregnancies, malpresentations are common.

## ■ CLINICAL PRESENTATION AND DIAGNOSIS

In the antenatal period, the woman usually has no complaints related to malpresentation. On routine palpation of abdomen, malpresentations can be detected. Whenever any malpresentation is observed, one must look for predisposing factors like uterine malformations, placenta previa, space occupying lesions like fibroid uterus, ovarian tumor, diminished or increased liquor volume, multiple pregnancy, and fetal malformations like anencephaly or hydrocephalus. However, in 50–75% of cases no predisposing or associated factor may be found.

It is important to diagnose malpresentation as it is likely to adversely impact labor. Eliciting a good history is important as it may give a clue to the possible cause of malpresentation. The woman may complain of bleeding per vaginum in case of placenta previa, pressure symptoms like dyspnea or difficulty in walking in case of excessive liquor or multiple pregnancies. Presence of head in fundus of uterus in cases of breech presentation at term may lead to discomfort in the hypochondrium or epigastric region.

A previous obstetric history of difficult labor, instrumental delivery, operative delivery, intrapartum still birth, asphyxiated baby, neonatal death may be elicited in case of contracted pelvis. Congenital malformations of the uterus may have been diagnosed prior to conception and there may be history of repeated malpresentations or bad obstetric history. In case of tumors of uterus, patient may have had menstrual disturbances or bladder pressure symptoms prior to getting pregnant or earlier ultrasound may have documented uterine or ovarian mass.

The woman may give history of premature rupture of membranes with or without prolapse of umbilical cord. There may be history suggestive of prolonged or obstructed labor in her previous pregnancy.

The management of the patient varies with the type of malpresentation.

The first step in management is correct diagnosis of the malpresentation and it can be made by careful palpation of abdomen.

## BREECH PRESENTATION

### Types of Breech

Breech presentation may be complete or incomplete **(Figs. 1 to 3)**. The relation between lower extremities and buttocks of breech presentation determines the type of breech.

### Complete or Flexed Breech (see Fig. 1)

In this the lower limbs of the fetus are flexed at both hip and knee joint. This is the least common variety of breech, being present in 4–12% of cases. Here, the presenting part comprises buttocks, feet and external genitalia. As the presenting part does not fit the pelvic brim well, the risk of cord prolapse is high (4–6%).

### Incomplete Breech

Incomplete breech may be extended or footling breech.

*Extended or frank breech* **(Fig. 2)**: Extended breech, also called frank breech, results when lower limbs of the fetus are flexed at hip joint but extended at knee joint. This is the most common type, being present in up to 60–70% of cases. Since the buttocks fit the pelvic brim well, chance of cord prolapse is only 0.5% in frank breech.

*Footling breech* **(Fig. 3)**: In this, the lower limb is extended at the hip joint and partially or fully flexed at knee joint resulting in foot or knee presentation. This is seen in 12–38% of the cases. Here, the presenting part fits poorly in the pelvis so the risk of cord prolapse is highest, being 15–18%.

## Clinical Examination

### Palpation of Abdomen

The height of uterus corresponds to the period of gestation unless the fetus has associated fetal growth restriction, congenital anomalies, hydramnios, or multiple pregnancies.

The fetal lie is longitudinal. Leopold's maneuvers reveal hard globular, smooth, round, and ballotable head of fetus

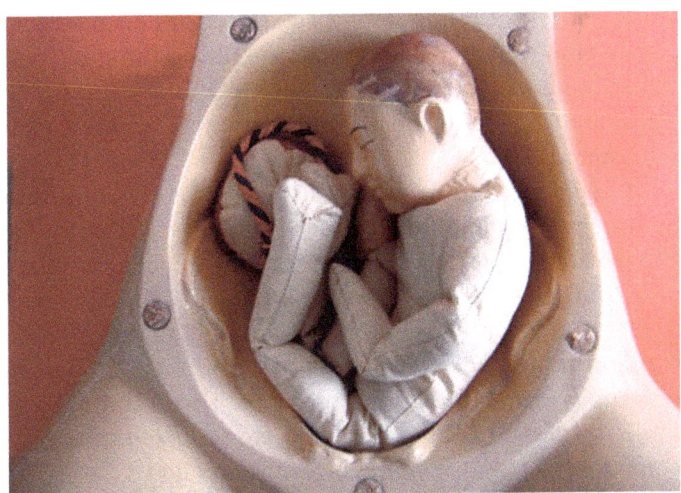

**Fig. 2:** Breech presentation—Extended breech.

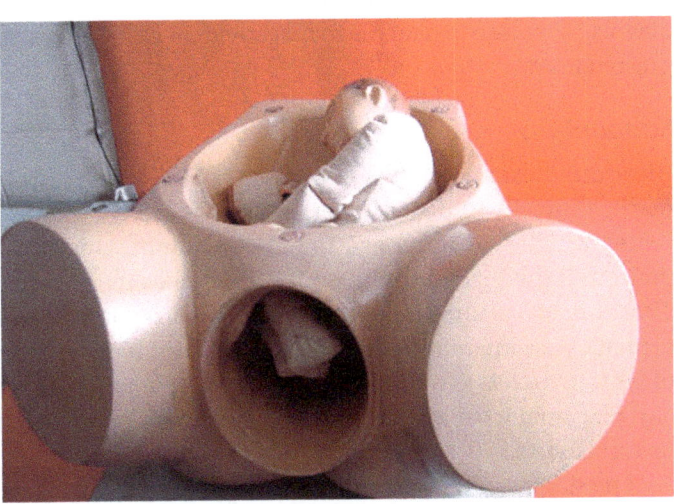

**Fig. 3:** Breech presentation—Footling breech.

in the fundal grip. The lateral grip is suggestive of back on one side and limbs on the other side. On superficial pelvic grip broad, soft, irregular podalic pole of the fetus, which is not ballotable is appreciated. Deep pelvic grip shows the relationship of the podalic pole to the pelvic brim. When breech is extended the head may not be well-appreciated as the limbs may be palpated alongside the head. The fetal heart is heard at the level of the umbilicus or above it.

*Per Vaginum Findings*

On vaginal examination, breech is felt as broad, soft, irregular part in contrast to hard globular head palpable in cephalic presentation. External genitalia and feet may be palpable confirming the diagnosis. The spinous processes of the fetal sacrum can be palpated easily and are diagnostic of breech presentation and its position. Breech has to be distinguished from the face. The anal opening may be mistaken for the mouth. In face presentation, the mouth is surrounded by the hard, alveolar ridges and forms the apex of a triangle with the malar prominences forming the base of the triangle. The examining finger may appreciate the sucking motion of the mouth, if the membranes are ruptured. In breech presentation, finger in the fetal anus feels the muscular resistance and it is in line of two ischial tuberosities. The examining finger in the fetal anus may be stained with meconium.

Breech presentation must also be differentiated from shoulder presentation and this can be done by feeling for the ribs which have a grid iron feel. Fetal hand can be identified by moving the thumb while foot in breech is distinguished by feeling the heel. One must also look for cord presentation if membranes are intact or for cord prolapse and cord pulsations if membranes are ruptured. The average risk of prolapse of cord is 3–5% in complete or flexed breech as compared to only 0.3% in cephalic presentation.

## Imaging Technique

Imaging techniques are required not only to confirm the diagnosis but also to plan the management in cases of breech presentation.

*Sonography*

Ultrasound examination is justified even if the diagnosis is made clinically in order to get additional information on issues which will influence the management. One must find out if there are any congenital anomalies in the fetus. These are two to three times higher in breech as compared to cephalic presentation. The type of breech, estimated weight of fetus, hyperextension of fetal head, multiple pregnancies and placental localization all can be accurately appreciated on ultrasound.

The degree of neck flexion or extension is an important parameter to decide whether vaginal delivery should be permitted or not. Full flexion of the cervical spine is the safest and most successful parameter for vaginal delivery. Hyperextension of fetal neck is when the angle of extension is more than 90 degrees. It occurs in less than 1% of cases, and is associated with arrest of delivery of head. It is an indication for cesarean section. As the degree of fetal neck extension can change, ultrasound should be repeated near delivery or in early labor. If sonography is uncertain, simple two-view radiography of abdomen will define head extension. Evaluation with more expensive techniques like computed tomography (CT) or magnetic resonance imaging (MRI) is rarely required.

More recently, obstetricians are using different radiological means for better assessment of maternal pelvis before delivery. The methods used are plain X-ray, one view computed tomography and magnetic resonance imaging. Data comparing these different modalities is lacking. Some workers have suggested specific measurements to permit vaginal delivery like inlet anteroposterior diameter ≥ 10.5 cm, inlet transverse diameter of ≥ 12.5 cm and mid-pelvic interspinous distance of ≥ 10.0 cm.[1,2] Others have suggested different values and different parameters.[3] Prediction of pelvic adequacy with MRI was associated with high success of vaginal delivery.[4] There are still other obstetricians who feel there is no need for pelvimetry by these techniques and RCOG does not include these in their guidelines.[5]

## Mechanism of Labor

The denominator in breech presentation is the sacrum and as in vertex there are eight positions, right and left sacroanterior position, sacroposterior, sacrolateral positions, direct sacroanterior and direct sacroposterior positions. The most common position is right sacroanterior (RSA).

During labor in RSA position, bitrochanteric diameter engages in the right oblique diameter of maternal pelvis. With increasing uterine contractions there is descent of buttocks till anterior buttock touches the pelvic floor at the level of ischial spines when it undergoes internal rotation by one eighth of a circle so that bi-trochanteric diameter comes to lie in anteroposterior diameter of outlet of maternal pelvis. Now, the anterior buttock hinges below the symphysis pubis and the posterior buttock is born by lateral flexion and anterior buttock slips out from beneath the symphysis pubis.

Delivery of the shoulders takes place next. The bisacromial diameter is 12 cm and engages in the right oblique diameter, undergoes descent and internal rotation similar to bitrochanteric diameter. The anterior shoulder hinges below the symphysis pubis and the posterior shoulder and the arm sweeps over perineum and are born.

The head now prepares to deliver. One of the two diameters, i.e., sub-occipito-frontal diameter which is 10 cm or sub-occipito-bregmatic diameter which is 9.5 cm engages in the left oblique diameter of the maternal pelvis, followed by descent and flexion. When the occiput touches the pelvic floor, it rotates by 45 degrees so that the sagittal suture lies in the anteroposterior diameter of maternal pelvis with the occiput anterior. Now, the sub-occiput hinges below the pubic symphysis and the head is born by flexion.

## Management of Breech Presentation

Women with breech presentation need closer follow up in antenatal period as there is higher risk of premature rupture of membranes and preterm labor. Besides standard antenatal care, detailed assessment is done, taking into consideration the woman's preference, to select the most appropriate management option. Various options available are external cephalic version (ECV), elective cesarean or breech vaginal delivery.

## External Cephalic Version

The risk of perinatal mortality is higher in vaginal breech delivery than vertex delivery, therefore, if breech presentation persists near term, the woman should be offered external cephalic version unless there is a contraindication. External cephalic version is the maneuver by which the fetus is rotated from breech presentation to cephalic presentation by manipulating it through maternal abdominal wall, externally.

The ECV is one of the most effective and safe procedures in modern obstetrics.[5] Its use is being recommended in guidelines of Royal College of Obstetricians and Gynaecologists (RCOG), American College of Obstetricians and Gynecologists (ACOG), and National Institute for Health and Care Excellence (NICE).[6-8]

Before attempting version, contraindications should be ruled out.[9,10]

### Contraindications to External Cephalic Version

- Hypertension or preeclampsia
- Scarred uterus like previous cesarean section, myomectomy, or uteroplasty
- Pelvic contraction or pelvic deformity
- Nonreassuring fetal status or any other evidence of antenatal fetal compromise[7]
- Fetal growth restriction
- History of antepartum hemorrhage
- Previous bad obstetric history
- Uterine malformations
- Prolonged leaking per-vaginum
- Multiple pregnancies
- Congenital anomaly of fetus
- Intrauterine death.

### Timing of External Cephalic Version

External cephalic version can be done anytime from 32 to 41 weeks of gestation, however, the best time is 37–38 weeks.

From 32 to 36 weeks, risk of reverting back to breech after successful version is high. Repeated attempts may be required and should any complication which requires termination of pregnancy occur, the fetus will be preterm with its attendant risks of prematurity.

At 37–38 weeks, the fetus is term and pregnancy can be terminated without any risk of prematurity, and the risk of reversion to breech is significantly reduced. However, the chances of failure of the procedure are higher as liquor is reduced.

### Procedure (Figs. 4A to C)

External cephalic version should be carried out in an area that has ready access to a facility equipped to perform an emergency cesarean section.

The woman should be counseled regarding the risks and benefit of ECV and consent taken.

To facilitate the procedure, sedatives like phenergan or opioids; tocolytics or even regional analgesia is sometimes used.

ACOG states that there is not enough consistent evidence to recommend conduction analgesia routinely for external version.[8]

Cochrane database of systematic reviews (2015) on the use of opioids, regional analgesia, amnioinfusion, moxibustion for facilitating ECV concluded that although parenteral beta stimulants were effective in facilitating successful ECV, data on adverse effects was insufficient.[9] Other tocolytics such as salbutamol, nitroglycerin, calcium channel blockers, hexaprenaline, and oxytocin receptor antagonist atosiban have also been used. The data on use of these agents, however, is limited and in some cases nonsupportive.[11-16]

To facilitate ECV, whether to use an intervention or not and which one to use, thus, depends on the choice and experience of health care provider.

The procedure is explained to the woman to allay anxiety. If an intervention is planned, it should be given at least 30 minutes prior to the procedure. The author prefers to use mild sedation in the form of 25 mg phenergan intramuscular and/or tocolytic, terbutaline 0.25 mg subcutaneously.

If version is done at 37 weeks or more, ultrasound to confirm the findings and monitor fetal heart, is useful.

The bladder should be empty and woman is asked to lie in dorsal supine position with legs flexed to 45 degrees at the hip joint. Abdomen is exposed and fetus palpated to ensure the exact position of the back. The fetal heart is heard or preferably a fetal cardiotocography should be carried out. It is preferable to rotate the fetus in the direction of its face called "the forward roll", to maintain an attitude of flexion. The head is held by one hand and the other hand supports the buttocks; the head is gently guided towards the pelvis and podalic pole is directed towards the fundus till fetal head

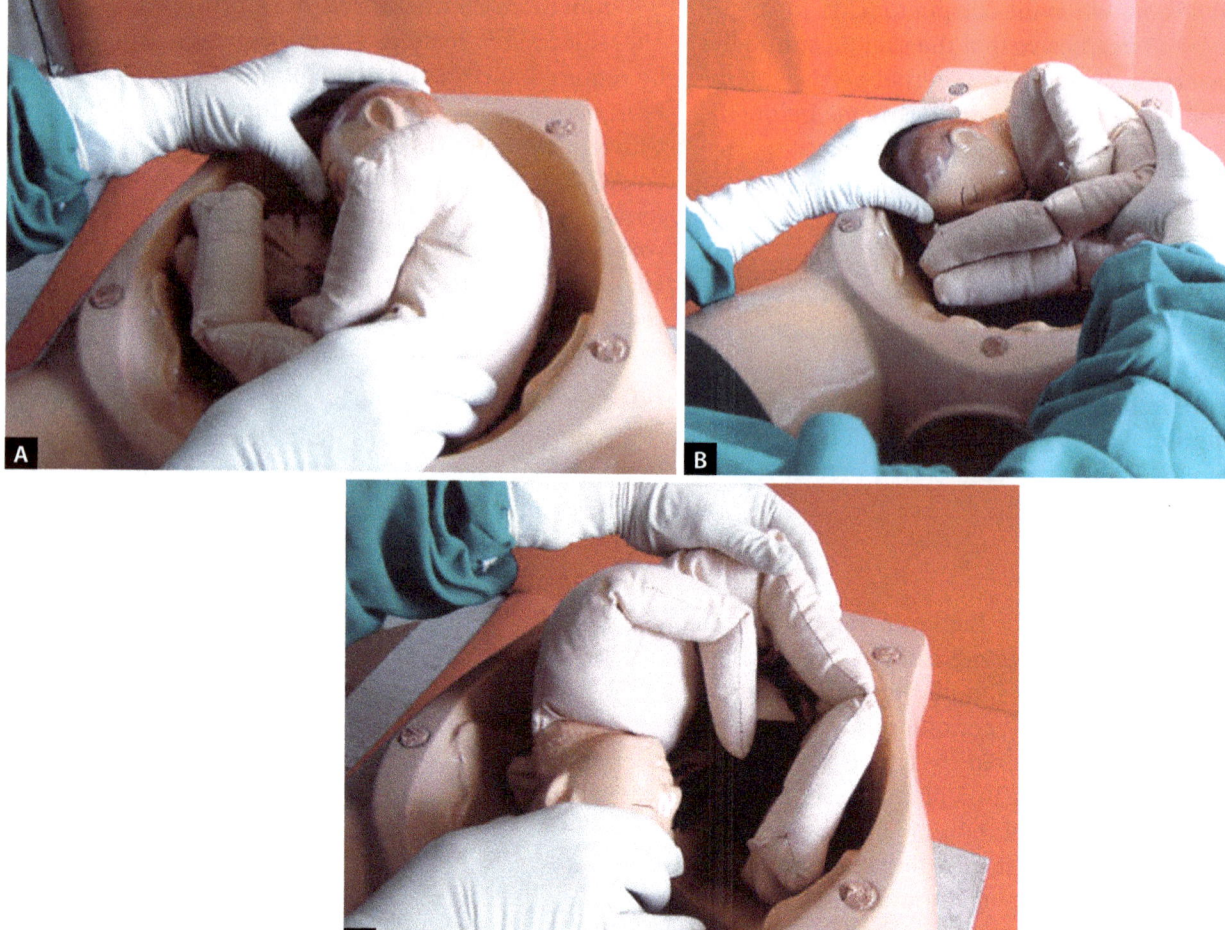

**Figs. 4A to C:** (A) External cephalic version—(A) Step I; (B) Step II; (C) Step III.

comes to occupy the lower uterine segment and the podalic pole occupies the fundus of uterus. An attempt is made to push the fetal head toward the pelvic inlet, so that chance of reversal is reduced. The fetal heart is checked as soon as version is completed and monitored. Vaginal bleeding or leaking should be looked for and abdomen observed for any evidence of tenderness. There should be no or minimal discomfort to the patient.

Success of version is reported to be 60–80%. Factors associated with successful version are lax abdomen as in multiparous women, adequate amniotic fluid, complete breech, unengaged presenting part, and posterior placenta.[10] Unsuccessful version may be due to decreased liquor, nulliparity, obesity, engaged presenting part, difficult palpation of fetal head as with frank breech, posterior position of the fetal back, extended legs, anterior placenta, or congenital malformations of the uterus like septate uterus.

### Complications of External Cephalic Version

External cephalic version is a safe procedure associated with a low complication rate of 0.5%.[17] The complications which can occur are:

- *Abruptio placentae:* Patient will complain of severe pain. One should look for bleeding per vaginum, evidence of fetal distress, signs of tenderness, and increased tone of the uterus. Patient will require an emergency cesarean section as she is not in labor and delivery per vaginum is likely to take a long time during which placental site bleeding can continue.
- *Fetal distress:* It may result from cord entanglement around the neck or other body parts of the fetus. If fetal distress persists and cord entanglement is suspected fetus should be reverted back to original position in an attempt to undo the cord entanglement. An emergency cesarean section may be required, if abnormal fetal heart tracing persists.
- Premature labor pains or premature rupture of membranes may occur.
- There is risk of fetomaternal hemorrhage and Rh isoimmunization. Fetomaternal hemorrhage occurs in about 6% of women; hence anti-D should be given to Rh negative women in a dose of 300 micrograms. Where possible, Kleihauer-Betke test should be done to determine the degree of hemorrhage as approximately 1% of patients require additional dose of anti-D.
- Very rarely serious complications such as uterine rupture and amniotic fluid embolization may occur.

If there are no complications, the woman may be sent home with advice to report if there are any complaints like decreased fetal movements, vaginal leaking or bleeding. She is advised to come back after 1 week for confirmation of fetal presentation.

In case the version is not successful due to increased tendency of uterus to contract, ECV may be done under cover of tocolytic agents as mentioned above. The commonly used tocolytic agents are ritodrine and terbutaline. The former can be given in a dose of 5–10 µg/min as intravenous infusion with frequent monitoring of pulse for tachycardia and blood pressure for hypotension. Terbutaline can also be given as subcutaneous injection of 250 µg prior to version. A placebo controlled randomized trial showed that terbutaline given before an attempted version in women at term with noncephalic presentations significantly increased the success rate of version and decreased the rate of cesarean delivery in labor.[18]

## Management of Breech at Term

The first decision to be made by the obstetrician is to determine the best route of delivery for the given mother and fetus. Several factors like gestational age, estimated weight of the fetus, tests of fetal well-being, maternal characteristics like height, pelvis adequacy, antenatal complications, hospital facilities, expertise of health care providers, and patient preference are taken into consideration to decide whether an abdominal route or vaginal route should be used for delivery. Risks versus benefit of the procedure are discussed with the patient preferably in antenatal period before onset of labor, consent taken and properly documented.

Elective cesarean section is offered as first line management in women who are expected to be at high risk for vaginal delivery

Indications for elective cesarean section are:
- *Footling breech presentation:* In this the progress of labor is slow as the presenting part acts as poor cervical dilator, chances of premature rupture of membranes and cord prolapse are high and delivery of fetal parts before full dilatation of cervix and entrapment of fetal head are high therefore cesarean is justified.
- *Breech with hyperextended head:* Arrest of aftercoming head of fetus and risk of fetal spinal injury is very high (21%) therefore cesarean section is done.
- *Low birth weight breech:* Breech fetus weighing 1,000–1,500 g has less risk of trauma if delivered by cesarean than if delivered vaginally. The cut off for doing cesarean section may vary from place to place, from <1,500 to <2,000 g estimated fetal weight (EFW).
- Severe growth restriction.
- Large fetus, more than 3.5 kg. In some countries 3.8 kg is taken as the cut off.
- Any degree of contracted pelvis or unfavorable shape of the pelvis. Cesarean section is indicated for minor degrees of contracted pelvis also and there is no place for trial of labor in breech presentation.
- Associated medical conditions like gestational hypertension, etc., are indications for cesarean section.
- Postdated pregnancy or biparietal diameter (BPD) more than 90 mm.
- Evidence of antenatal fetal compromise.
- Prior perinatal death or neonatal birth trauma.
- Lack of expertise in breech delivery.

### Planned Vaginal Delivery

Present thinking among obstetricians regarding vaginal delivery is influenced by several studies. Term Breech Trial Collaborative Group did a randomized multicentric study to compare planned cesarean section versus planned vaginal birth for breech presentation at term.[16] The group reported significantly lower perinatal mortality, neonatal mortality, and serious neonatal morbidity for the planned cesarean section group as compared to planned vaginal birth group but found no differences in terms of maternal mortality or serious maternal morbidity between groups. They therefore, concluded that planned cesarean section is better than planned vaginal birth for the term fetus in breech presentation.[19]

World Health Organization[20] evaluated one lakh deliveries from nine different Asian countries and reported better perinatal outcome with planned cesarean section as compared to planned vaginal delivery. Some other studies also reported lower neonatal mortality and morbidity rates with cesarean section.[21,22]

After this study, a number of countries included these recommendations in their hospital protocol for managing breech term deliveries with resultant increase in rate of lower segment cesarean section (LSCS) from 20 to 87%.

This high rate of cesarean in breech was a cause of concern and there was criticism of the Hannah trial as well. The various drawbacks that were pointed out were that 31% of women included in the trial did not have any ultrasound; growth restricted babies were also included; senior obstetrician was not present in 31.9% of births and no obstetrician was present in 13% of births. A number of large and multicentric studies were conducted in European countries, which observed that if strict selection criteria are applied, the perinatal deaths did not differ significantly between women who had planned cesarean section and planned vaginal breech delivery.[21-23] Most serious neonatal morbidities did not result in long-term disability or poor intellectual performance.[24-26] Fetal attitude and pelvic capacity were the most important parameters for successful outcome. It was also seen that women who had cesarean section had significantly higher rate of maternal complications than their counterparts who had vaginal breech delivery.

Subsequent studies[23] have also highlighted the fact that patients subjected to planned cesarean section for breech presentation had increased short-term maternal morbidity and long-term complications like uterine scar dehiscence or rupture, scar ectopic pregnancy, increased incidence of placenta previa or morbidly adherent placenta like placenta accrete, increta, or percreta in future pregnancies and these complications may pose considerable risk to the woman especially if she does not have access to proper health care.

The American College of Obstetricians and Gynecologists in 2012 modified its stance on breech presentation and delivery. Committee Opinion 340 states that, "decision regarding the mode of delivery should depend on the experience of the health care provider", and that "planned vaginal delivery of a term singleton breech fetus may be reasonable under hospital specific protocol guidelines". This was reaffirmed by ACOG in 2016.[27] RCOG also states that proper selection of pregnancies and skilled intrapartum care may allow planned vaginal birth to be nearly as safe as planned vaginal cephalic birth.[7] Therefore, there is need to revive the art of vaginal breech delivery and provide necessary skill to the concerned obstetricians for proper case selection and proper conduct of breech delivery where feasible.

## Management of Breech in Labor

Vaginal delivery should be considered in a set up where facilities for emergency cesarean section exist. Prior to undertaking a vaginal breech delivery, the woman should be informed about the risk of perinatal or neonatal mortality and that the short-term neonatal morbidity may be higher than that of planned cesarean delivery. Her informed consent should be documented. It is desirable to get an ultrasound done to estimate the fetal weight and position of fetal neck and legs whenever time and circumstances permit (RCOG).[7] Vaginal delivery is considered where:

- The estimated weight of breech is between 2.5 and 3.5 kg
- Gestational age from 37 to 41 weeks
- Frank breech or complete breech
- Fetal head is flexed
- Pelvis is adequate at all levels
- Absence of any associated obstetric complications like hypertension
- No evidence of antenatal fetal compromise.

As regards delivery from 32 to 37 weeks, i.e., the preterm breech, the fetal weight is more important than the gestational age for neonatal outcome.[28]

Planned cesarean section has been found to be associated with lower neonatal mortality rates for gestational age 24 to 31$^{+6}$ weeks in some studies.[29,30] While others observed conflicting results with no improved survival benefit to neonate with cesarean section for gestation less than 28 weeks.[28] Therefore, the decision for route of delivery in breech with gestational age less than 28 weeks should be based on individualized hospital protocol.

It is desirable to score the patient by Zatuchni-Andros score. If score is 4 or more, patient can be left for vaginal delivery. Bird and Mclein conducted a prospective study over 6 years employing the Zatuchni-Andros Breech Scoring Index and observed that when patients with a score of 4 or more were allowed to go in labor with meticulous supervision, a high rate of successful vaginal deliveries resulted and fetal mortality and morbidity rates were markedly reduced.[31,32]

On the other hand, when the score was 3 or less chances of success were poor. So, the authors recommended that patients whose breech score was 3 or less should have cesarean section. Further the authors were of the opinion that this breech assessment method was a valid method for selecting cases for vaginal delivery. They also observed that intravenous oxytocin could be safely used, when necessary, if the score was 4 or more.

The score is calculated as given in **Table 1**.

### Prerequisites for Conduct of Vaginal Delivery

Expert help should be available for conducting breech vaginal delivery and the following points should be kept in mind:

- An intravenous line with 16–18 G needle should be kept patent
- Cross-matched blood should be available
- Facilities for continuous electronic fetal monitoring or enough help for frequent auscultation of fetal heart should be available
- Anesthetist should be readily available. There is no contraindication to use of epidural analgesia once labor is established
- Pediatrician should be alerted
- Facilities for neonatal resuscitation should be available
- Instrument trolley should have all the instruments as for any normal vaginal delivery with an additional extra towel and a pair of long forceps preferably Piper's forceps.

**TABLE 1:** Zatuchni-Andros breech scoring index.

| Parameter | Score 0 | Score 1 | Score 2 |
| --- | --- | --- | --- |
| Parity | Nullipara | Multipara | |
| Gestational age | 39 weeks or more | 38 weeks | 37 weeks |
| Previous history of breech | None | One | Two |
| Estimated fetal weight | 8 lbs | 7–8 lbs | 7 lbs |
| Cervical dilatation at admission | 2 cm | 3 cm | 4 cm or more |
| Station of breech | –3 or more | –2 | –1 or less |

## Monitoring the Progress of Labor

Detailed examination of patient is done at admission and partogram maintained once labor starts. A careful watch is kept on the following:

- Vital parameters.
- Nutrition of the patient which should consist of small quantities of liquid diet that is rich in calories and electrolytes.
- The uterine contractions should be recorded. Their intensity and duration should increase progressively and interval decrease till about 3 contractions per 10 minutes are attained by late first stage of labor. If uterine contractions are inadequate, augmentation with oxytocin drip can be done.
- The fetal heart sounds (FHS) should be auscultated frequently or preferably continuous fetal electronic monitoring is done. If labor is progressing normally, the site of maximum intensity of fetal heart shifts to progressively lower level on the abdomen.
- Detailed pelvic examination with regard to cervical effacement, dilatation, type of breech, its station and state of membranes and cord should be assessed and recorded. Adequacy of pelvis should be noted. If all points are favorable for vaginal delivery subsequent progress is assessed from time to time.
- Patient should be encouraged to labor in left lateral position. When membranes rupture, a per vaginal examination is done to exclude cord prolapse and at the same time the cervical dilatation, effacement, and station of breech is noted.
- In general, labor progresses more slowly in breech presentation but if cervix is dilating progressively there is no need for any interference till patient enters second stage of labor.
- Epidural or other analgesia may be given as per patient need and hospital protocol.
- The patient is shifted to delivery table and placed in lithotomy position once the anterior buttock starts climbing the perineum.

## Conduct of Breech Delivery

### Spontaneous Breech Delivery

Spontaneous breech delivery is when the breech is expelled entirely spontaneously on its own without the need for any manipulation except for support to the neonate. This spontaneous expulsion occurs due to cardinal movements of different parts of the fetus within the maternal pelvis. This is possible if fetus is of average size, maternal pelvis is adequate and uterine contractions and maternal expulsive efforts are good. Usually however, some assistance is required mostly at the level of arms or head.

### Assisted Breech Delivery

Assisted breech delivery is when some manipulation is required to deliver different parts of the fetus.

Team members comprising anesthetist, pediatrician, and obstetrician well-versed with the art of breech delivery along with staff nurse and preferably another associate member should be present.

Cardinal rules of breech delivery:

- Watchful expectancy, with no unnecessary interference
- Never pull the breech from below
- Always encourage patient to push
- Keep the back of the baby anterior
- Ask the assistant to apply fundal or suprapubic pressure whenever required.

When breech starts climbing the perineum:

- Give liberal episiotomy after infiltration of the perineum with local anesthetic agent, pudendal block may be given unless epidural analgesia has already been given. Usually, mediolateral episiotomy is preferred due to its lower risk of complications like injury to anal sphincter.
- Allow the breech to deliver spontaneously till the umbilicus.
- Hold the baby by pelvi-femoral grip (**Fig. 5A**) and not by abdomen so as to avoid injury to fetal abdominal organs.
- Pull out a loop of cord to check for cord pulsations and for length of cord (**Fig. 5B**). If the cord is too short, it should be cut between two clamps. From now on, one should aim to deliver the fetus within 5 minutes. Too rapid delivery runs the risk of tearing of tentorium cerebelli and hence intracranial hemorrhage. Delay in delivery beyond 5 minutes can result in fetal asphyxia.
- Cover the baby with a towel so that it is easy to hold the baby and reduce the external stimuli to prevent premature attempts to breathe.
- The uterine contractions are monitored closely. If inadequate, oxytocin drip is started or if already on flow, the rate is increased to obtain good uterine contractions. During contractions encourage the patient to bear down during contractions.
- As the trunk starts emerging from below the symphysis pubis look for the inferior angle of scapula. If it is parallel to the spine it means the arms are flexed. If there is winging of the inferior angle of scapula, it means the arms are extended.
- As soon as the axilla is visible, feel for the arms across the chest of the fetus and gently hook them out. Now, the trunk and shoulders are disengaged.
- Suprapubic pressure is given by the assistant in backward and downward direction so that attitude of flexion of fetal head is maintained.
- Fetal head will often deliver spontaneously or delivered by Burn Marshall's technique as described in

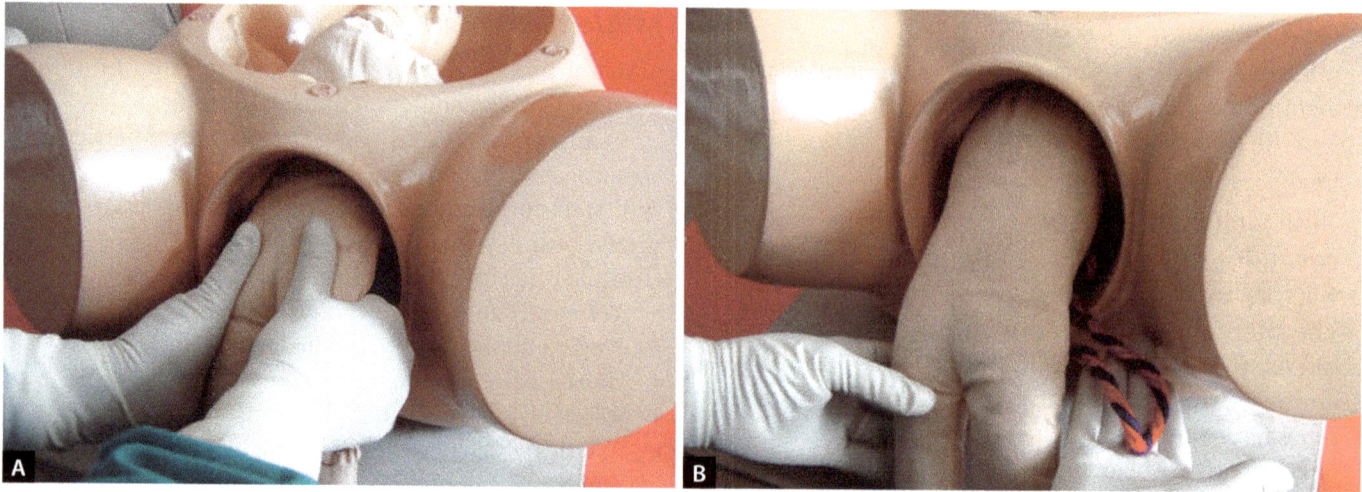

**Figs. 5A and B:** (A) Assisted breech delivery showing "pelvi-femoral" grip; (B) Umbilical cord—length and pulsations to be looked for.

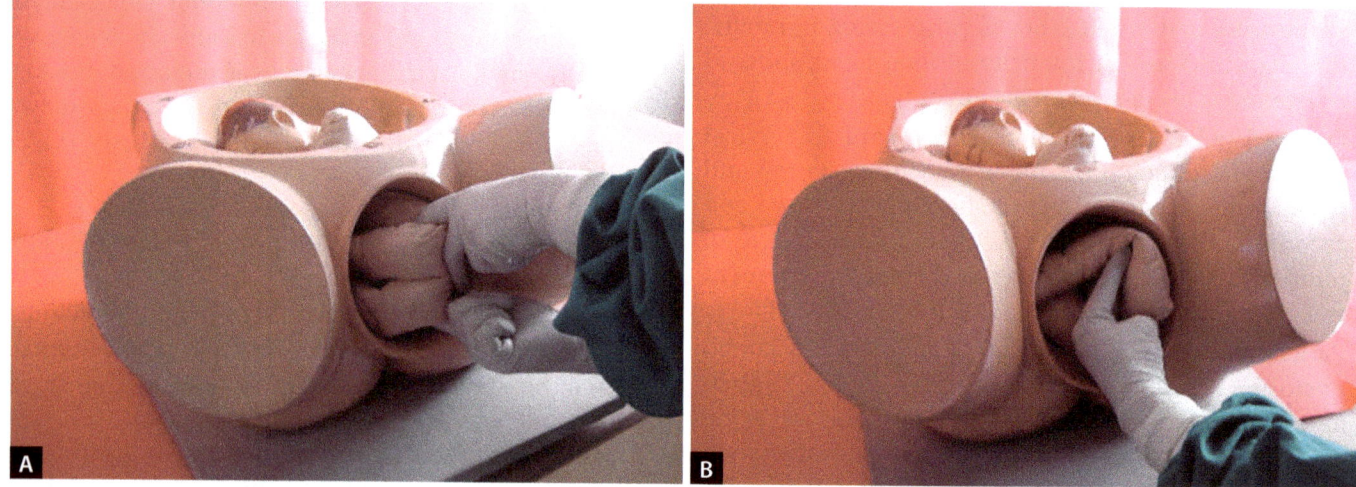

**Figs. 6A and B:** (A) Groin traction for extended legs impacted at outlet—note the pressure of the index fingers of the operator are toward pelvis to prevent injury to thighs; (B) Pinard's maneuver for delivery of extended legs impacted at midcavity or above. The index and middle finger of obstetrician press the popliteal fossa in a backward and outward direction. This causes the leg to fall across the abdomen of the baby and deliver.

**Figures 9A to C.** RCOG however recommends delivery of the head using Mauriceau-Smellie-Viet maneuver or with forceps as Burn Marshall technique may be associated with over-extension of the fetal neck.

- Baby is handed over to pediatrician. Oxytocic agents are given.
- Delivery of placenta, inspection of placenta, and perineum and stitching of episiotomy is completed.
- Patient is watched for postpartum hemorrhage (PPH).

## Overcoming Difficulties in Breech Delivery

### Difficulty in Delivery of Buttocks

The breech may be impacted low in the pelvis or the outlet. In this case, a liberal episiotomy may relieve the impaction. In some cases, groin traction (single or double) may be required. Index finger of one or both the hands of operator are placed in groins of the baby and steady gentle traction is made on the pelvis and not on the femur as its result can fracture femur **(Fig. 6A)**.

### Difficulty in Delivery of Legs

This is likely when the legs are extended. The legs get splinted alongside of the abdomen and chest. In this case two fingers of the right hand of the birth attendant should be passed up the thighs and the middle and index finger press on the popliteal fossa to flex the leg at the knee joint. This brings down the leg which can then be delivered easily. The second leg may deliver on its own or may require same maneuver as first leg. This is called Pinard's maneuver **(Fig. 6B)**.

### Extended Arms

One or both arms may be extended. This usually happens when traction is applied on the baby too early or the cervix is not fully dilated. There are two methods of delivery. The obstetrician must know which method to select.

*Lovset's maneuver* **(Figs. 7A to C):** This method is selected when there is mild extension or partial extension of the arms and the trunk is not too large to be impacted at the maternal outlet.

This is an extra pelvic maneuver. This works on the principle that the posterior arm is at lower level in the pelvis so when the fetus is rotated through 180 degrees the posterior arm will fall below the symphysis pubis and deliver as the anterior pelvis is deficient.

The fetus is grasped by the fetopelvic grip and drawn down till the inferior angle of the anterior scapula is visible below the symphysis pubis, the fetus is lifted and rotated by applying further traction to the trunk and carrying it away from the shoulder in question. Rotation is done in such a way that the back remains anterior and as it nears completion through 180 degrees the fetus is depressed so that the elbow, shoulder, and arm deliver in succession below the symphysis pubis. The other arm is hooked out from the sacral hollow. If any difficulty is encountered, fetus is again rotated in similar fashion to deliver the other arm.

*Classical method:* This method is justified when the fetus is large, impacted or with fully extended arms. This method is done under general anesthesia. In this the legs of the fetus are grasped by one hand of the obstetrician and body of the fetus is carried slightly upward and medially toward the abdomen of the mother. This depresses the posterior shoulder. It is important not to pull the trunk too low down in the pelvis as it will jam the shoulders along with the head making delivery of arms very difficult. The other hand is passed in the sacral hollow of the mother and the index and middle finger are passed along the dorsal aspect of the shoulder of the posterior arm of the fetus till it reaches beyond the elbow joint **(Fig. 8)**. Then the forearm is pressed so that the elbow joint flexes and the forearm drops across the face and chest of the fetus and is delivered. It is important not to catch the fingers or the humerus to pull on them for bringing down the arm as this will cause fracture of the arm. The anterior arm may now be delivered. The fetus is held and depressed in a downward and slightly lateral direction and two fingers of obstetrician are passed over anterior shoulder of fetus

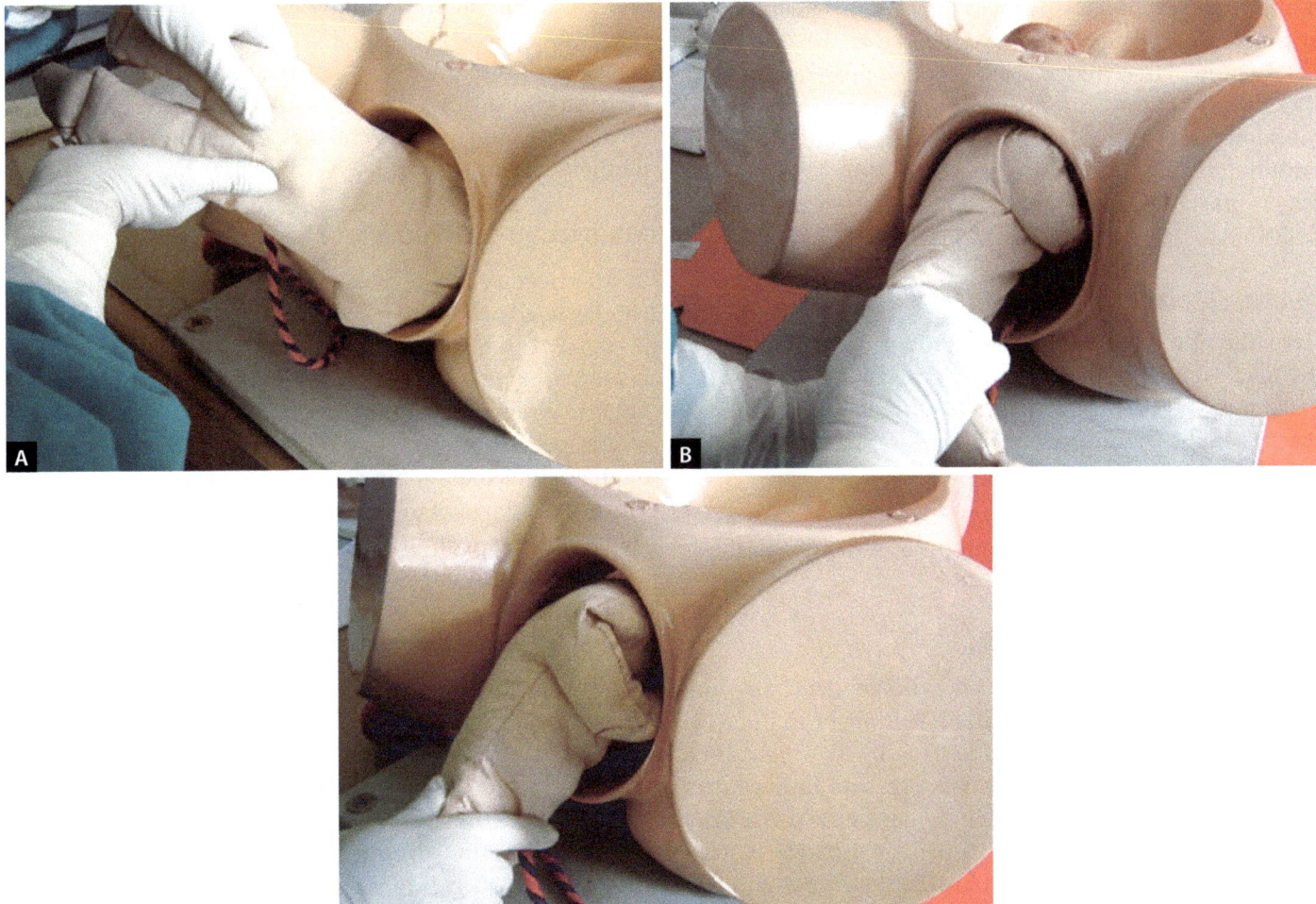

**Figs. 7A to C:** Lovset's maneuver for delivery of arms. (A) The baby is gently lifted up so that the posterior arm descends down in the sacral hollow; (B) The baby is rotated so that the posterior arm becomes anterior; (C) As the rotation is nearing completion gently depress the baby so that posterior arm which now becomes anterior descends below the symphysis pubis and can be delivered.

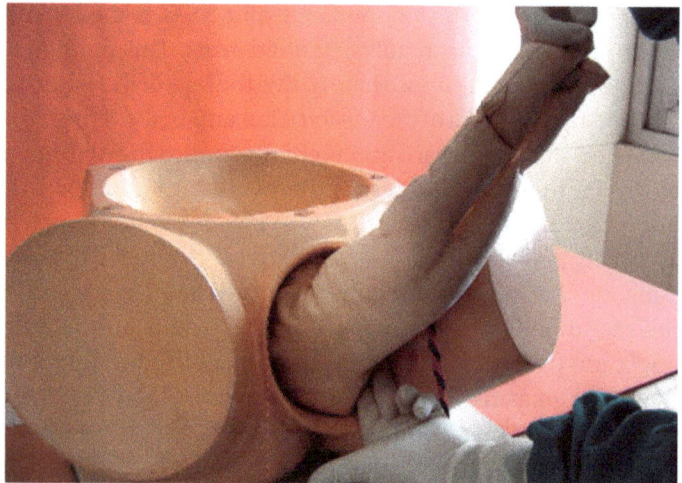

**Fig. 8:** Classical method of delivery of extended arms. The baby is gently lifted by its feet and its ventral aspect carried toward the abdomen of mother. This increases the space in sacral hollow. The index and middle finger of left hand of obstetrician are carried up the posterior arm of baby and passed above the elbow. The forearm is swept across the face of baby and delivered.

and is disengaged in the same manner as the posterior arm. If not possible, the fetus is rotated by 180° so that anterior arm becomes posterior and is delivered in the same way. For rotation of the child, it is important to push up the trunk slightly so that the chin does not enter the pelvic brim at the same time. The child should be held by the trunk with both hands, the thumbs are placed over the back and the fingers grasp the thorax and rotation is affected and the arm delivered as described for posterior arm.

### Nuchal Displacement of the Arm

Here, the arm is displaced behind the occiput. Rotation of the fetus is done in the direction of fingers, this causes the occiput to slip past the arm and the arm is brought in easy reach for delivery as in extended arms.

## Delivery of the Head

Delivery of head may be done by one of the methods described below.

### Burns and Marshall Technique

This method works well for an average size baby and uncomplicated breech. The patient is brought to the edge of the table and baby allowed to hang by its weight **(Fig. 9A)**. An assistant gives suprapubic pressure in backward and downward direction so that head enters the pelvic brim in well-flexed position. When the nape of the neck is seen, the feet of the baby are grasped between the index and ring finger with the middle finger between the two feet, a steady outward traction is maintained and the body of the baby carried in an arc shaped manner over the mother's abdomen **(Fig. 9B)**. It is important to ensure that the fulcrum is the nape of the neck and it rotates over the symphysis pubis. If traction is not maintained over the body once the nape of the neck is seen, it slips beneath the symphysis pubis and the rotation of the baby may occur over cervical vertebrae causing fracture of the neck and difficulty in delivery of the head **(Fig. 9C)**. If baby is large or nape of neck is not seen even when baby is suspended by its own weight for 1–2 minutes, delivery of the head should be done by alternative method. RCOG discourages the use of this method for delivery of the head due to concern of over extension of the fetal neck.[7]

### Delivery of the Aftercoming Head of Breech by Forceps

This method is superior to all other methods of delivery of the head as the pull is made directly to the head and flexion of the head is maintained with forceps. On the other hand, with all other methods the traction is through the spinal column which is more dangerous for the child.

For applying the forceps, it is very important that the head is in the pelvic cavity. The trunk and abdomen are wrapped in a towel and the assistant holds it upward so that it does not interfere with the application of the forceps **(Fig. 10A)**. The blades of the forceps are applied from ventral aspect of the fetus **(Fig. 10B)**. In this, the blades lie in the mentovertical plane. The pull is applied downward till the chin appears then the child is carried upward toward the mother's abdomen.

### Mauriceau-Smellie-Viet Maneuver

In Mauriceau-Smellie-Viet technique of delivering aftercoming head of breech, the assistant gives gentle suprapubic pressure. The obstetrician places the body of the child on his left arm with each leg of neonate on either side of his forearm and puts the index and middle fingers of this hand on the malar prominences of the baby and applies pressure on them, thus maintaining an attitude of flexion **(Fig. 11A)**. The middle finger of the right hand is placed on the cervical spine and the occiput whereas the ring and index finger are placed on either side of the shoulders of the baby. This splints the spine and provides protection to it. Traction is exerted in a backward and downward direction till the nape of the neck is seen below the symphysis pubis. Now, the baby is carried in upward direction toward the mother's abdomen, **(Fig. 11B)**.

### Delivery of Head with Occiput Posterior

On rare occasions, during delivery of the trunk the back rotates posteriorly, an event which can be prevented by facilitating anterior rotation of back once trunk is delivered till the umbilicus. The fetus is delivered using modified Prague maneuver. In this fingers are placed on either side of the shoulder and the feet grasped with other hand.

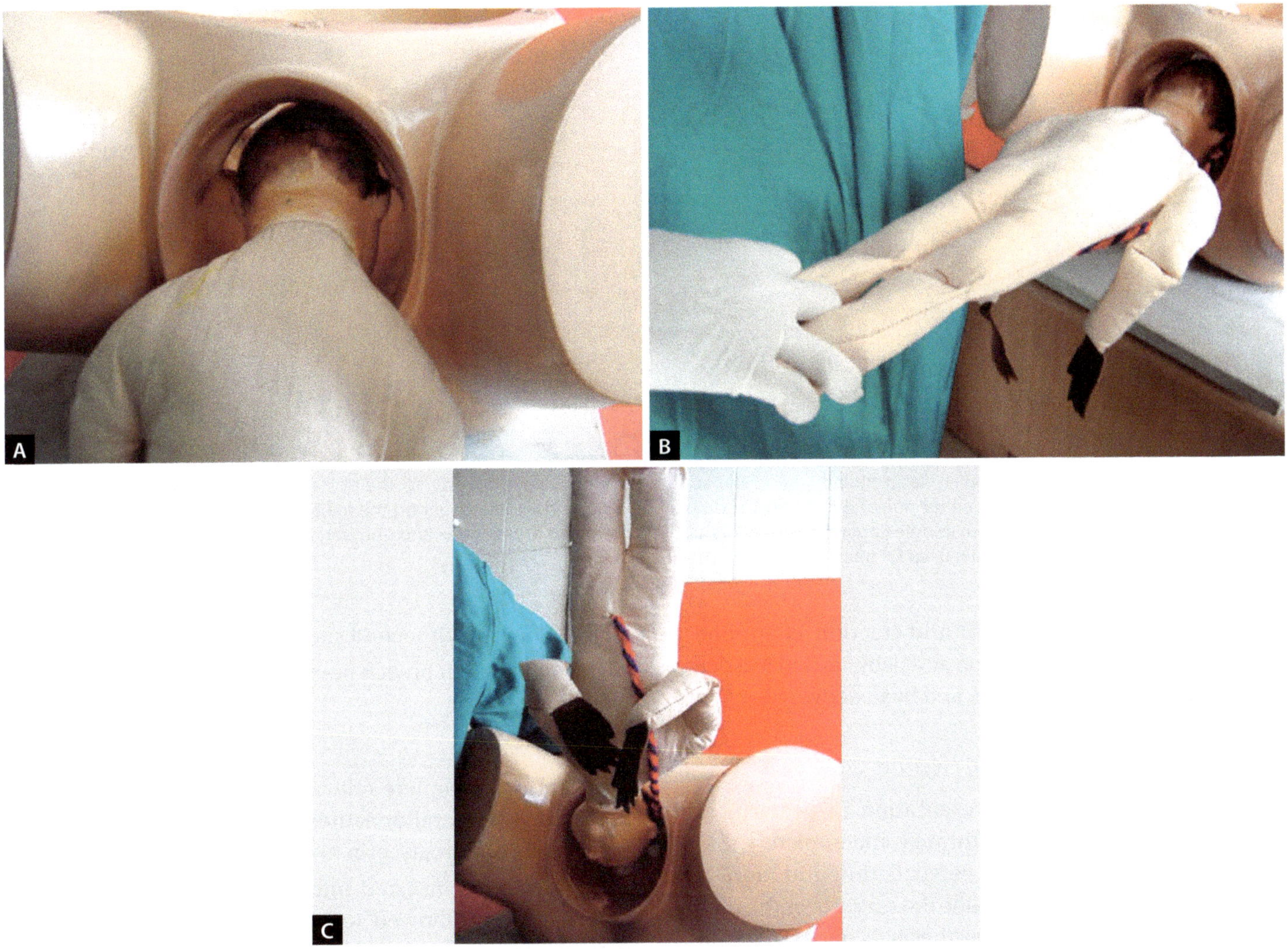

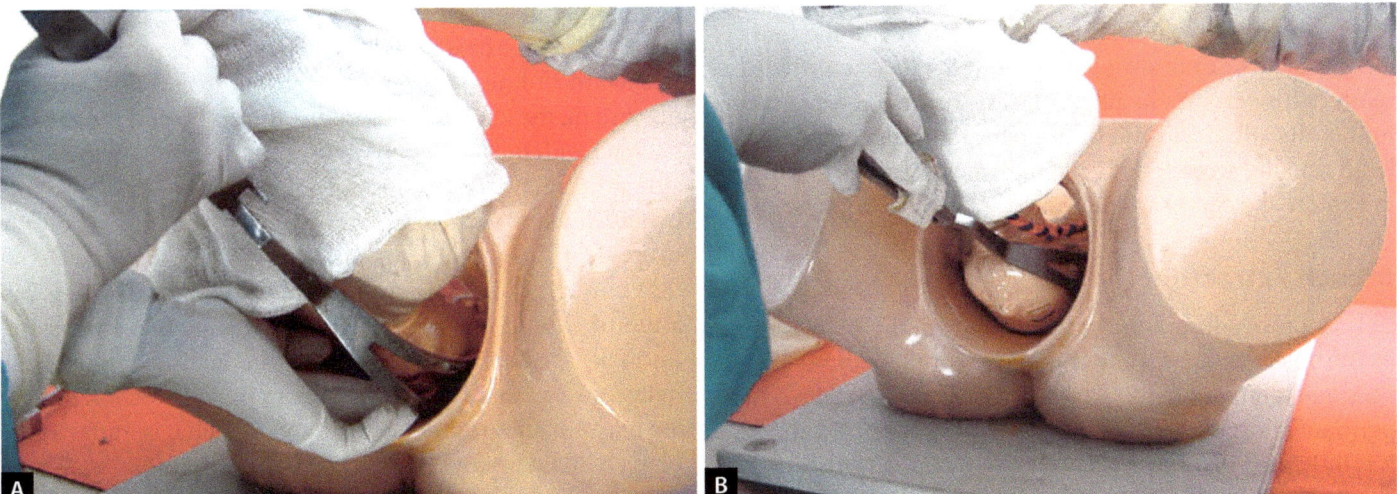

**Figs. 9A to C:** Burns and Marshall technique for delivery of aftercoming head of breech. (A) Patient is on edge of delivery table and baby is allowed to hang till nape of neck is seen; (B) Baby is held by the feet and traction applied in outward direction till the subocciput hinges below the symphysis pubis; (C) Maintaining outward traction the baby is carried across the abdomen of the mother in a wide arc with the fulcrum of rotation at subocciput. Note the fulcrum should be subocciput and not the cervical vertebrae to prevent injury to the cervical spine and spinal cord.

**Figs. 10A and B:** Forceps application for delivery of aftercoming head of breech. (A) The baby is wrapped in a sheet and gently lifted up to prevent it from interfering in the forceps application. The right blade of long midcavity or Piper forceps is introduced from the posterolateral aspect of maternal pelvis; (B) Cephalic application of both blades of forceps locked in position. Traction is first applied in downward and backward till chin appears and then in forward and upwards direction.

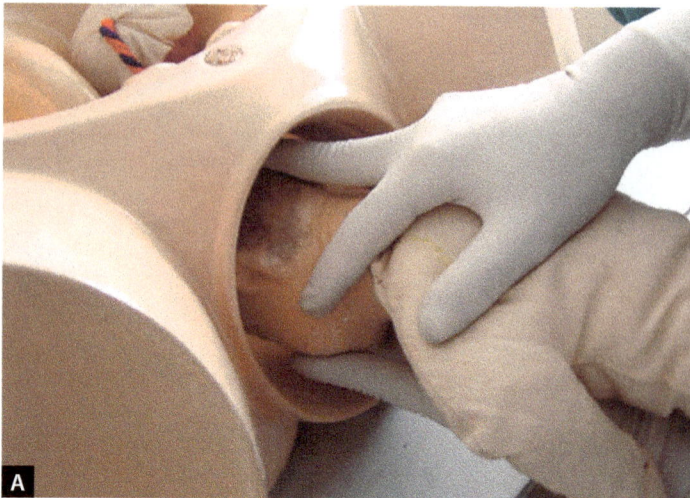 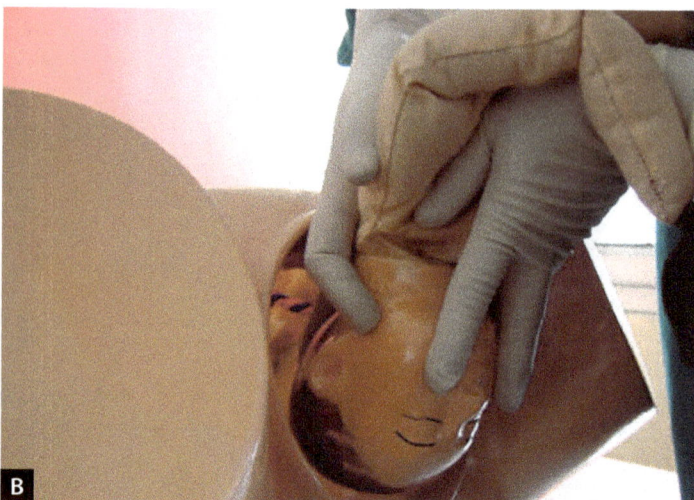

**Figs. 11A and B:** (A) Mauriceau-Smellie-Viet technique for delivery of aftercoming head of breech; (B) The obstetrician places the body of the baby astride the left arm with one leg on either side of the forearm and puts the index and middle finger on the malar prominences to flex the head. The right hand is placed on the head with middle finger on the occiput and neck to splint it. The index and ring finger rest astride the shoulders. The left hand flexes the head and right hand is used for traction to deliver the head.

Suprapubic pressure is given and traction is applied in upwards and forwards direction and baby carried 360 degree across the abdomen of mother and head delivered.

### Entrapment of Aftercoming Head

Occasionally, in footling presentation or preterm fetus the body of fetus is pushed through incompletely dilated cervix. In these cases, if the cervix is thin and more than 7 cm dilated, it is possible to slide the cervix over the occiput of the fetus under general anesthesia or under amylnitrate or nitroglycerin given by intravenous or sublingual route. If however, the cervix is thick or less than 7 cm dilated Duhrssen cervical incision at 2 and 10 o'clock or at 4 and/or 8 o'clock position will enlarge the cervical opening and help in safe delivery of fetus. It is important not to give cervical incision at 3 and 9 o'clock position as the branches of uterine artery can be involved resulting in profuse bleeding. If the fetus is already dead one option is craniotomy. In this a small incision made with scissors in nape of neck or through posterior fontanella will drain the brain matter and decompress the head causing an easy delivery of the head.[33,34] It is important to explore the cervix and uterus after delivery of placenta.

### Breech Extraction

This is a procedure done when delivery of the baby is done by the obstetrician without waiting for spontaneous delivery. This is seldom done nowadays as it is associated with a high perinatal mortality of 20%.

It is indicated in following conditions:
- Cord prolapse in second stage of labor and when delivery occurs in clinic/health center with no facilities for cesarean section or there is likely to be delay in performing cesarean section.
- Dead fetus with second stage arrest.
- Second twin in breech presentation with fetal distress.

### Technique

This requires complete relaxation of the uterus hence it is done under general anesthesia with use of halothane or amylnitrate or nitroglycerin to relax the uterine musculature.

One hand is inserted into the uterine cavity, and the anterior leg is followed to the foot. The heel of the foot is then grasped between the fingers and the thumb and traction is applied to it while the external hand steadies the uterus and applies counter pressure (**Figs. 12A and C**). It is important not to bring down the posterior leg as the anterior buttock will get caught at the symphysis pubis and hinder in extraction of the baby. Cord should be kept out of way by pushing it against the wall of the uterus if it is palpated during breech extraction. Steady gentle pressure is applied backward in line of curve of Carus and then forward and upward till the knee is visible at the introitus, now the thigh is grasped with the fingers on one side and thumb on the other side and traction is continued till the groin is visible. This brings down the other leg and when the posterior buttock distends the perineum, the anterior leg is pulled upward so that enough room is there to deliver the posterior leg. No attempt should be made to bring the leg down, rather the buttocks are delivered and then if the leg is extended, it is delivered by Pinard's maneuver. Sometimes, traction on one leg may not allow other leg to come down if it is impacted or being held up by any fetal part. In this case traction may have to be applied to the other heel and both legs brought down together.

Once both legs are born the baby is covered with towel and held with pelvi-femoral grip and delivery completed as

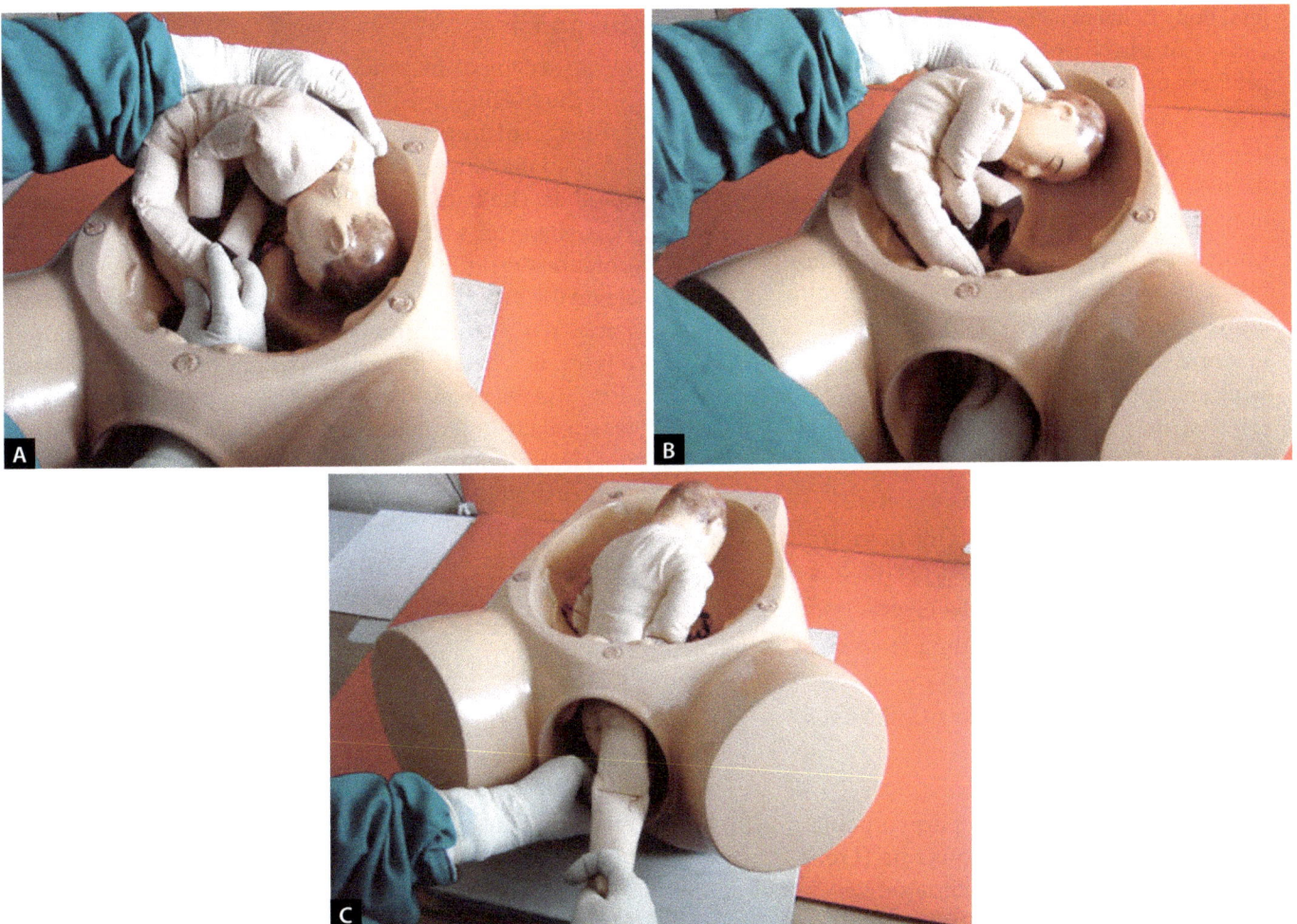

**Figs. 12A to C:** Internal podalic version. (A) The anterior leg of the baby is grasped by its foot. Note that posterior leg should not be brought down first as the anterior buttock will hinge against the symphysis pubis and prevent delivery of the baby; (B) The fundus of the uterus is steadied and leg brought down; (C) Maintain traction on the anterior leg till posterior leg comes within reach for delivery.

for assisted breech delivery, delivering trunk, arms and head by maneuvers described earlier.

Following delivery of baby, placenta is delivered and inspected, perineum explored for lacerations and episiotomy stitched as in normal delivery and usual precautions taken for preventing PPH.

## Cesarean Section for Breech

The breech should be delivered with care as injuries and difficulty can occur even when LSCS is done.

The difficulty may be encountered in extraction of a preterm breech baby when the lower segment is not formed. An adequate uterine incision is required to deliver the head otherwise the same injuries as in vaginal breech delivery will occur and benefit of cesarean section lost. A U-shaped incision is given after carefully reflecting the lower segment peritoneum. A low vertical incision has been suggested as alternative when lower uterine segment is not well-formed, care should be taken to prevent extension of incision into upper segment. When delivering breech through cesarean section incision it is important to deliver the baby slowly, making sure the baby is not pulled unduly which will cause extension of arms and head. The assistant should give fundal pressure and delivery conducted slowly. If legs are extended, Pinard's maneuver should be used. The head may require delivery by Mauriceau-Smellie-Viet technique. Forceps is avoided if baby is very preterm, below 32 weeks of gestation.

## Perinatal Outcome in Breech Delivery

The perinatal mortality associated with planned vaginal breech birth is approximately 2/1000. It is only marginally increased as compared to perinatal mortality in planned cephalic birth and cesarean section which is 1/1,000 and 0.5/1,000, respectively.[7] The lowest perinatal mortality is in frank breech, intermediate in flexed breech and is highest in footling breech.

### Causes of Perinatal Morbidity and Mortality

- Birth asphyxia: This can be due to arrest of the after-coming head in the pelvis or entrapment of the head due to incompletely dilated cervix, the latter being more common with preterm breech when the relatively small

fetal body delivers before cervix is dilated fully. The other causes of birth asphyxia are cord compression, cord prolapse or prolonged labor.
- Head injury: Intracranial hemorrhage can occur due to fracture of skull bones or due to sudden decompression on delivery of head or due to tentorial tears of the unmolded head.
- Congenital malformations: Lethal malformations like hydrocephaly, anencephaly and meningomyelocele are more common with breech presentation.
- Fracture of bones like femur, humerus, pelvis, clavicle, skull, spine, or any other bones can occur. In some cases, traction may separate scapular, humoral or femoral epiphyses.
- Spinal cord lacerations or transactions.
- Intraventricular hemorrhage or hemorrhage into the adrenals or hematomas of neck or shoulder muscles.
- Injury to viscera like liver, spleen, muscles, and genitalia.
- Injuries to nerve plexus leading to cervical or brachial nerve paralysis.
- Nonlethal malformations affecting the fetus.

## TRANSVERSE LIE

When long axis of the fetus is perpendicular to the long axis of uterus it is called transverse lie **(Fig. 13)**, whereas when it is at an angle it forms oblique lie. On abdominal examination, in transverse lie, the cephalic pole occupies one lumbar region and podalic pole occupies the opposite lumbar region. The denominator is the fetal acromion. The position of the fetus is determined by its back, being dorsoanterior when back is anterior, dorsoposterior when back is posterior, dorsosuperior when back is superior, and dorsoinferior when back is inferior.

### Incidence

It is 1 in 300 pregnancies at term.

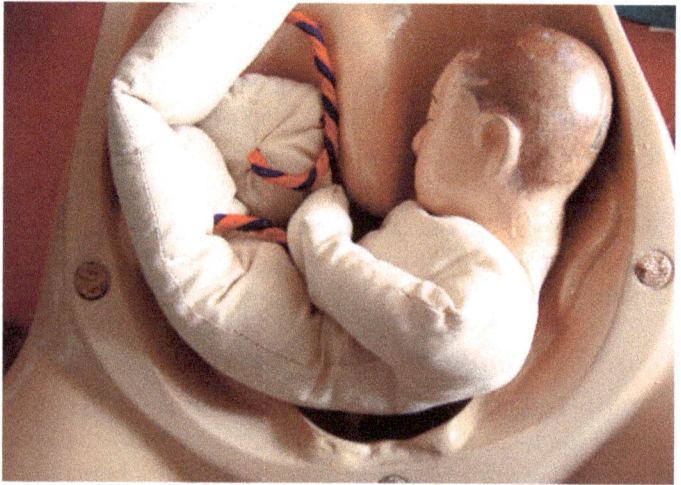

**Fig. 13:** Transverse lie—Dorsoinferior position.

### Diagnosis

On inspection of the abdomen the uterine ovoid appears wide and the height appears relatively shortened. On palpation the height of uterus appears less than period of gestation. On Leopold maneuvers the head is felt in one flank and breech in other. The back is readily palpable in dorsoanterior and dorsosuperior positions while it is less clearly palpable in dorsoposterior and dorsoinferior positions. Fetal heart is heard through the fetal shoulder and hence in dorsosuperior position it is along fundus of the uterus and in dorsoinferior it is low down near the pelvis. The position of fetal heart may first raise the suspicion of the presence of transverse lie. This is especially important if liquor is drained and fetal parts are not clearly defined.

Per vaginal examination may not be informative during pregnancy or early labor and should not be done without ruling out placenta previa. Diagnosis can be confirmed on ultrasound.

During labor, on per vaginal examination the bag of membranes may be conical in shape. The cervix is not well-applied to the presenting part and the soft parts are felt high up. The ribs of the thorax have a grid iron feel and this is a diagnostic feature of shoulder presentation. Sometimes vertebra is palpable or hand and cord may also be felt. With further dilatation of the cervix, axilla, and scapula may be palpated and in neglected cases the arm may be prolapsed.

### Management

#### Antenatal Period

An attempt should be made to correct the transverse lie after 36 weeks of gestation by external version, if there is no contraindication to it. If ECV fails or ECV is contraindicated, elective LSCS is done at 38–39 weeks of gestation.

#### Intrapartum Period

If patient comes in early labor and membranes are intact, ECV can be tried if there are no contraindications to vaginal delivery. If ECV fails or is contraindicated, cesarean section is performed.

If however, patient comes in late first stage of labor or in second stage or with rupture of membranes and liquor drained with fetal heart still present, it is safer to do cesarean section.

If the patient comes with an arm prolapsed and neglected shoulder presentation, the patient is carefully examined for any features of obstructed labor.

On general examination patient usually appears dehydrated, has tachycardia, fever, and acidotic breathing. The urine is high colored and may show presence of acetone. Abdominal examination may show Bandl's ring due to stretching of lower uterine segment. Abdominal palpation reveals the fetus to be in transverse lie. Often the liquor is completely drained hence it may be difficult to feel fetal parts. There may be tenderness in lower uterine segment if it is stretched. Occasionally, if uterus is ruptured, uterine contour may not be made out properly, fetal parts may be felt superficially, and retracted uterus may be felt separately. On auscultation, there may be fetal distress, or the fetal heart may be absent. The arm of the fetus prolapse out of the introitus and may get swollen and discolored. Per vaginal examination reveals the presence of fetal thorax or spine at brim or impacted in the pelvic inlet.

Management will depend on presence or absence of features of obstruction and FHS and includes correction of dehydration and other general measures.

If there are features of obstructed labor like presence of Bandl's ring, cesarean section is indicated even if FHS is absent as the risk of rupture uterus is very high with internal podalic version and breech extraction. If rupture of uterus has already occurred laparotomy with removal of fetus and placenta is done followed by repair of uterus or hysterectomy depending on the circumstances.

If fetal heart is absent but there are no features of obstructed labor, management will depend on the duration of rupture of membranes and the amount of liquor that has drained from the uterine cavity. If liquor is adequate and shoulder is not impacted in pelvis, the prolapsed arm is replaced and internal podalic version is done under general anesthesia and relaxation of the uterus. In most of the cases however, cesarean section is preferred and is considered a safer option.

If however liquor is drained, decapitation of the fetus can be tried if the fetal neck is within easy reach. For this, the prolapsed arm is pulled downwards and away from the neck by the assistant and the decapitation knife either Jardin's hook or the Gigley's saw is negotiated above the neck under cover of the left hand which is placed to protect the anterior vaginal wall. The hook is then rotated through 90 degrees and the left hand is shifted to the posterior vaginal wall. The neck is then severed off from the body by rotatory movements. Embryotomy scissors can also be used for cutting the neck. The body is then extracted by pulling on the prolapsed hand. The head is removed by putting finger in the mouth or crochet can be used for it. Before showing the neonate to the relatives it is important to suture the decapitated neck. **Flowchart 1** summarizes the management of a woman presenting with transverse lie.

After removal of the placenta the uterine cavity and genital tract should be explored to detect any genital tract injury. In all these cases, prophylactic oxytocic agents are used to prevent postpartum hemorrhage.

Destructive operations even on the dead fetus have been abandoned although the author is of the opinion that under exceptional circumstances these can be performed provided the operator is well versed with the technique as was the case with earlier obstetricians.[33]

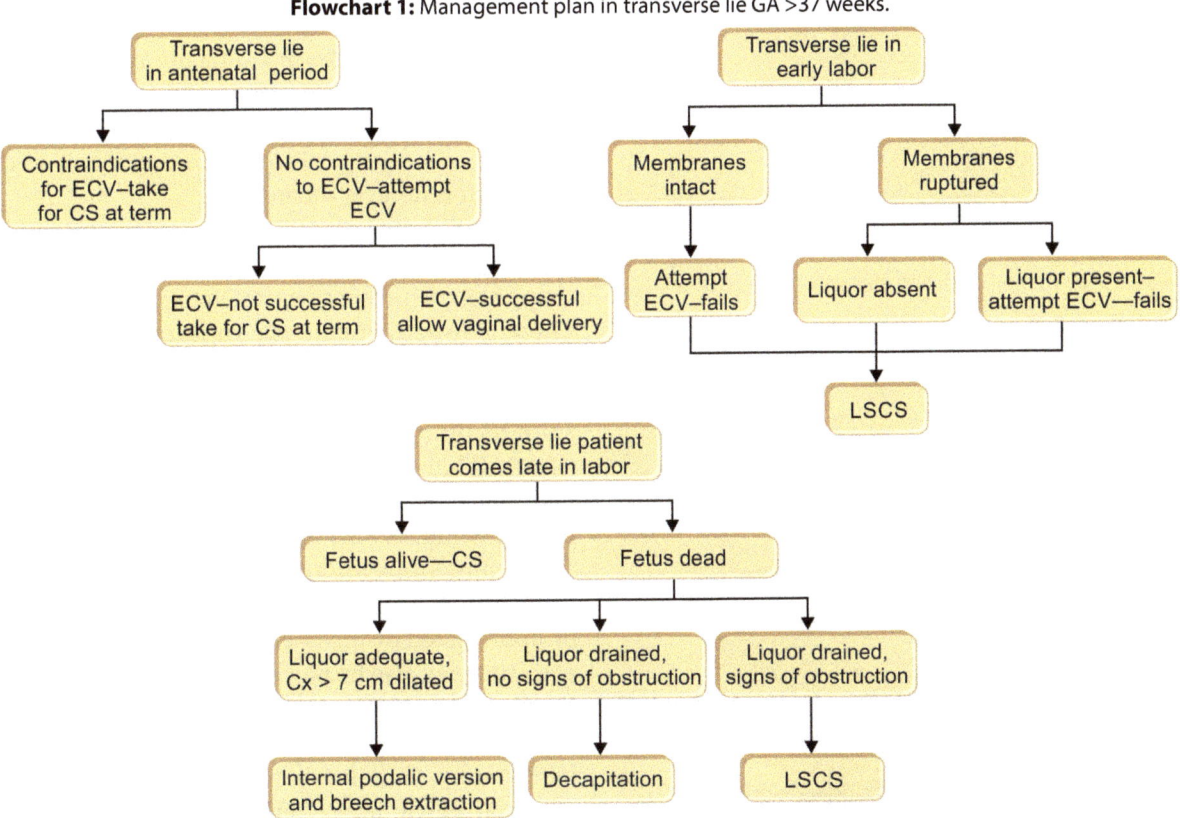

**Flowchart 1:** Management plan in transverse lie GA >37 weeks.

(Cx: cervix; LSCS: lower segment cesarean section; CS: cesarean section; ECV: external cephalic version; GA: gestational age)

# Malpresentations

## FACE PRESENTATION

Face presentation occurs when the lie of fetus is longitudinal and attitude of head is that of complete extension, mentum is the denominator and the engaging diameter is submento bregmatic (**Figs. 14 and 15**). The incidence of face presentation varies from 1 in 150 to 1 in 900 live births.

### Etiology

Exact cause is not known, some predisposing factors are:
- Contracted pelvis
- Multiparity with lax abdominal wall
- Congenital malformations of the fetus like anencephaly, congenital bronchocele
- Congenital tumors of the neck like goiter or multiple loops of cord or tight loop of cord round neck
- Certain shapes of the fetal head- like dolichocephaly
- Prematurity.

### Management

It is very important to diagnose this condition especially at onset of labor.

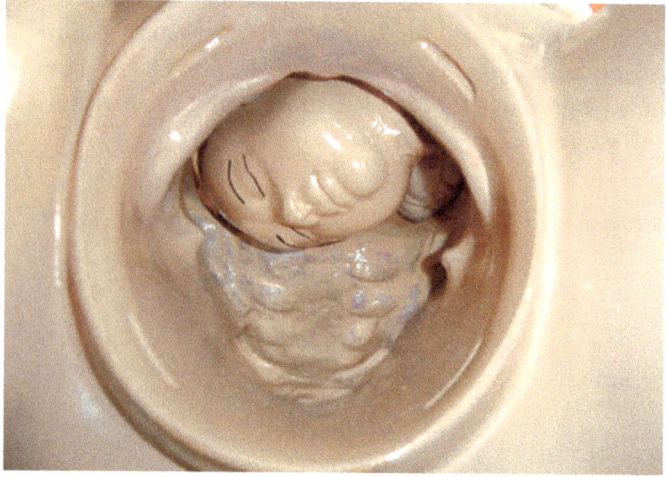

**Fig. 14:** Face presentation depicting mento-anterior position.

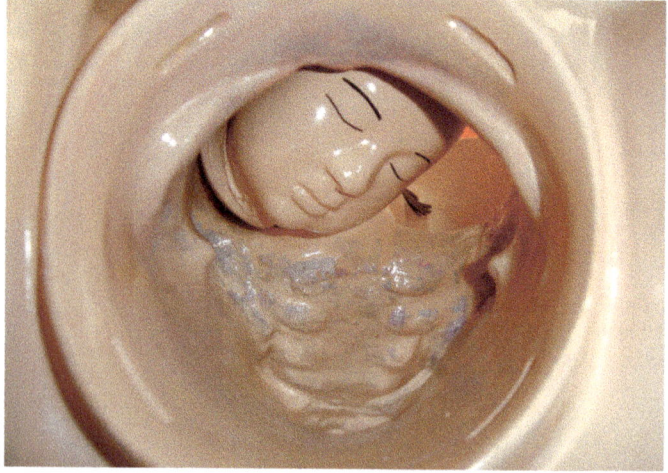

**Fig. 15:** Face presentation depicting mento-posterior position.

There are six positions in face presentation:
- Right and left mento anterior—most common accounts for 60–80% of the cases.
- Right and left mento posterior—20–25% are mento-posterior.
- Right or left mento lateral—10–12% are mento-transverse.

Vaginal delivery is not possible with persistent mento-posterior position unless the fetus is very small.

### Clinical Diagnosis

General physical examination of the patient will be normal except if she comes late in labor with unfavorable face position like mento-posterior position or with contracted pelvis, when there may be evidence of obstructed labor.

#### Abdominal Findings

It is often difficult to diagnose the condition as the extended head distends the lower uterine segment causing slight tenderness on palpation hence the muscles of lower abdomen may not relax to permit proper examination.

In face presentation, the occipital eminence is prominent and felt on a higher level than the sinciput. In the vertex presentation the occiput and back form one continuous curve with a slight depression at the neck whereas in face presentation, the continuity of the back is broken by a deep grove between the back and the occiput. This deep prominence can be mistaken for sinciput of a well-flexed head but a careful examination will reveal limbs of the baby to be on the opposite side of the prominence in face presentation whereas in vertex presentation the limbs will be on the same side as the sincipital prominence.

In mento-anterior positions the chest and limbs are felt anteriorly and back is not felt and fetal heart is easily heard. In mentoposterior position chest is difficult to define and fetal heart is not well-heard.

On per vaginal examination, if the membranes are intact the bag of membranes will appear conical instead of saucer shaped as the presenting part does not fit well in the pelvis. There is usually premature rupture of membranes or the membranes rupture early in the course of labor. The smooth rounded head is not palpated. Irregular parts are felt which are difficult to make out if the cervix is not dilated or only slightly dilated. When the cervix dilates and the presenting part lies within reach, one can palpate the opening of the mouth which is surrounded by the hard alveolar ridges. The mouth forms the apex of a triangle, the base of which is formed by the orbital ridges. The sucking movements may be appreciated by the finger in the mouth. The ridge of nose and chin may also be palpable and distinguishable if there is no edema of the face.

Diagnosis can be confirmed by ultrasound or by radiography. The later shows hyperextended head with facial bones at pelvic inlet. Early diagnosis improves perinatal outcome.

## Mechanism of Labor

The most common face presentation is left mento anterior. The lie is longitudinal, denominator is mentum and the engaging diameter is sub-mento bregmatic and it engages in right oblique diameter of maternal pelvis. With increasing uterine contractions, the face descends to the level of ischial spines and then undergoes internal rotation through one-eighth of a circle and further descent of head takes place till it reaches the pelvic floor when crowning takes place. The sub-mentum comes to lie below the symphysis pubis and the face is delivered by flexion. Rest of the delivery occurs as in the vertex presentation.

## Management in Labor

If any degree of contracted pelvis is associated with face presentation, LSCS should be considered as facial bones cannot undergo molding in labor, to overcome the mild pelvic contraction.

If the face is in mentoposterior, the likelihood of forward rotation to convert to anterior position late in labor in only 25%. Therefore, if baby is large and pelvis is borderline, cesarean section is justified.

In favorable face position and normal pelvis, vaginal delivery is permitted. The woman is allowed to go into spontaneous labor and is watched very carefully. Labor is often prolonged so a partogram is kept to watch for progress of labor and for evidence of fetal distress. If possible continuous electronic fetal heart rate monitoring should be done. No internal maneuvers should be done to convert face into vertex presentation. If progress of labor is arrested, an evaluation of its cause should be done and fetal heart auscultated. If progress is arrested with good uterine contractions LSCS should be done as the face cannot undergo molding and hence is less likely to deliver without risk to the fetus. If fetal distress is observed then too, LSCS is justified. If the progress of labor is tardy due to hypotonic uterine contractions, careful augmentation with oxytocin may be done.

Perinatal mortality for viable pregnancies varies from 0.6 to 5%.

## ■ BROW PRESENTATION

Brow is the part of the fetal head that is bounded anteriorly by the orbital ridges and posteriorly by the anterior fontanelle and coronal suture. When this part presents at the pelvic inlet, it is called brow presentation. It is the rarest presentation. The engaging diameter on fetal skull is mento-vertical which is 14 cm and since it is larger than any of the pelvic diameters, engagement cannot take place and fetus cannot deliver. It can only deliver by converting to either face or vertex presentation.

## Diagnosis

### Abdominal Palpation

On abdominal palpation the chin and occiput of the fetus can be palpated easily and are at same level on examination of pelvic grip.

### Vaginal Examination

The orbital ridges and root of the nose are easily palpable on one side and the anterior fontanel and coronal suture is palpable on the other side. The mouth and chin cannot be reached.

## Management

Cesarean section is done for persistent brow presentation.

## ■ COMPOUND PRESENTATION

When a limb of the fetus is present along the major presenting part, it is termed as compound presentation. The most common combination is an upper limb with the vertex.

## Diagnosis

It may be detected during routine pervaginal examination at the beginning of labor or more commonly it is suspected if there is arrest of progress of labor in the active phase or if there is failure of presenting part to engage despite good uterine contractions.

Diagnosis is made by vaginal examination when limb is palpated along with the other presenting part.

Compound presentation is most frequently associated with prematurity. It can also occur with ECV of breech presentation.

## Management

- Primary cesarean section is indicated, if there is associated cord presentation or nonreassuring fetal heart rate.
- In early labor, if no complications are present, one can wait and watch closely for the limb to retract on its own above the presenting part. During this stage, however, as the risk of cord compression or prolapse is high, continuous fetal monitoring is essential.
- In late first stage, the limb can be gently pushed up and reposited above the presenting part.
- If limb cannot be pushed up and/or signs of obstruction appear, cesarean section is to be done.
- Perinatal loss is increased as a result of cord prolapse, preterm delivery, and obstetric manipulation which may cause traumatic delivery.

## ■ KEY POINTS

- When the presenting part of the fetus is other than the vertex, it is called malpresentation and it occurs in 3–5% of cases.

- The most common malpresentation is breech presentation.
- Other malpresentations are face, brow, and compound presentation. Brow and compound presentations are the least common.
- Predisposing factors for malpresentations are uterine abnormalities or space occupying lesions, abnormal placental location, multigravida with lax abdominal wall, contracted pelvic inlet, congenital malformations of the fetus, amniotic fluid abnormalities, and multiple pregnancies.
- The first step in the management of malpresentation is its correct diagnosis as it is likely to impact labor.
- A good history, careful clinical examination and imaging techniques like ultrasound help in correct diagnosis of the type of malpresentation.
- Breech presentation in the antenatal period or early labor should be corrected by ECV if there are no contraindications.
- Contraindications for ECV are antepartum hemorrhage, PIH, scarred uterus, multiple pregnancy, bad obstetric history, uterine malformations, pelvic contraction, prolonged leaking and non-reassuring fetal status.
- ECV should be carried out in a place where facilities for emergency cesarean section are available.
- Complications of ECV include abruptio placentae, fetal distress, premature labor pains and premature rupture of membranes. Rarely uterine rupture and amniotic fluid embolism may occur.
- Rh negative women undergoing ECV should be given anti-D.
- Elective cesarean section for breech presentation is indicated for footling breech presentation, hyperextended head, low-birth weight breech, large fetus more than 3.5–3.8 kg, any degree of contracted pelvis or unfavorable shape of the pelvis, associated medical conditions, postdated pregnancy and nonreassuring fetal heart rate.
- As per ACOG guidelines 2012 and Committee Opinion with regard to breech delivery, "decision regarding the mode of delivery should depend on the experience of the health care provider", and that "planned vaginal delivery of a term singleton breech fetus may be reasonable under hospital specific protocol guidelines".
- RCOG also states that women with breech presentation should be informed that planned cesarean section leads to a small reduction in perinatal mortality compared with planned vaginal breech delivery. However, potential adverse consequences associated with cesarean section should also be discussed.
- Delivery by cesarean section is recommended in women with persistent breech presentation if risk factors for a poor outcome in planned vaginal breech birth are present.
- Transverse lie, after 34 weeks of gestation should be corrected by external cephalic version, if there is no contraindication to ECV
- If ECV fails or is contraindicated elective LSCS should be done at term.
- If patient comes with transverse lie in early labor and membranes are intact, ECV should be tried if there are no contraindications to it.
- If patient comes late in labor or with rupture of membranes and liquor drained out with fetal heart present, LSCS is the treatment of choice.
- If patient comes very late in labor or with neglected shoulder presentation and with features of obstruction, LSCS is justified even if FHS is absent due to risk of rupture of uterus.
- Face presentation should be differentiated from breech presentation by careful abdominal and vaginal examination.
- If any degree of contracted pelvis is associated with face presentation, LSCS should be done as facial bones cannot undergo molding in labor, to overcome the mild pelvic contraction.
- If the face is in mentoposterior position, the likelihood of forward rotation to convert to anterior position late in labor in only 25%, therefore, if baby is large and pelvis is borderline LSCS is justified.
- Cesarean section is indicated for persistent brow presentation.
- Cesarean section is indicated in compound presentation if there is associated cord presentation or non-reassuring fetal heart.
- In compound presentation, in early labor if no complications are present, wait and watch for the limb to retract on its own above the presenting part. During this stage, however, as the risk of cord compression or prolapse is high continuous fetal heart monitoring is essential.

# REFERENCES

1. Azria E, Le Meaux JP, Khoshnood B, Alexander S, Subtil D, Goffinet F, et al. Factors associated with adverse perinatal outcomes for term breech fetuses with planned vaginal delivery. Am J Obstet Gynecol. 2012;207(4):285.e.1.
2. Kotaska A, Monticoglou S, Gagnon R. SOGC clinical guidelines: vaginal delivery of breech presentation : No. 226, June 2009. Int J Gynaecol Obstet. 2009;107(2):169.
3. Michel S, Drain A, Closser E, Deruelle P, Ego A, Subtil D, et al. Evaluation of decision protocol for type of delivery of infants in breech presentation at term. Eur J Obstet Gynecol Reprod Biol. 2011;158(2):194-8.
4. Hoffmann J, Thomassen K, Stumpp P, Grothoff M, Engel C, Kahn T, et al. New MRI criteria for successful vaginal breech delivery in primiparae. PLoS One. 2016;11(8):e0161028.
5. Rosman AN, Guijt A, Viemmix F, Rijnders M, Mol BW, Kok M. Contraindications for external cephalic version in breech

position at term: a systematic review. Acta Obstet Gynecol Scand. 2013; 92(2): 137-42.
6. Royal College of Obstetricians and Gynaecologists Green –top Guideline No.20a, External Cephalic Version and Reducing incidence of Term Breech Presentation; 2017.
7. Royal College of Obstetricians and Gynaecologists Green–top Guideline No.20b, Management of Breech Presentation; 2017.
8. American College of Obstetricians and Gynecologists. External cephalic version. Practice Bulletin No 161; 2016a.
9. Cluver C, Gyte GML, Sinclair M, Dowswell T, Hofmeyr GJ. Interventions for helping to turn term breech babies to head first presentation when using external cephalic version Rev Cochrane Database Syst Rev. 2015;(2):CD000184.
10. Kok M, Cnossen J, Gravendeel L, van der Post J, Opmeer B, Mol BW. Clinical factors to predict the outcome of external cephalic version: a meta-analysis. Am J Obstet Gynecol. 2008;199(6):630.
11. Burgos j, Eguiguren N, Quintana E, Cobos P, Centeno Mdel M, Larrieta R, et al. Atosiban vs ritodine as a tocolytic in external cephalic version: a prospective cohort study. J Perinat Med. 2010;38(1):23.
12. Hilton J, Allan B, Swaby C, Wah R, Jarrell J, Wood S, et al. Intravenous nitroglycerin for external cephalic version, a randomized controlled trial. Obstet Gynecol. 2009;114(3):560.
13. Kok M, Bias JM, van Lith JM, Papatsonis DM, Kleiverda G, Hanny D, et al. Nifedipine as a uterine relaxant for external cephalic version: a randomized controlled trial. Obstet Gynecol. 2008;112:(2 Pt 1):271.
14. Vani S, Lau SY, Lim BK, Omar SZ, Tan PC. Intravenous salbutamol for external cephalic version. Int J Gynecol Obstet. 2009;104(1): 28.
15. Vetzel J, Vlemmix F, Opmeer BC, Molkenboer JF, Verhoeven CJ, van Pampus MG, et al. Atosiban versus fenoterol as a uterine relaxant for external cephalic version. BMJ. 2017;26:356.
16. Wilcox CB, Nassar N, Roberts CL. Effectiveness of nifedipine tocolysis to facilitate external cephalic version: a systematic review. BJOG. 2011;118 (4):423.
17. Collins S, Ellaway P, Harrington D, Pandit M, Impey LW. The complications of external cephalic version: results from 805 consecutive attempts. Br J Obstet Gynaecol. 2007;114(5):636-8.
18. Fernandez CO, Bloom S, Wendal G. A prospective, randomized blinded, comparison of terbutaline versus placebo for singleton term external cephalic version. Am J Obstet Gynecol. 1996;174:326.
19. Hannah ME, Hannah WJ, Hewson SA, Hodnett ED, Saigal S, Willan AR. Planned caesarean section versus planned vaginal birth for breech presentation at term: a randomized multicentre trial. Term Breech Trial Collaborative Group. Lancet.2000;356(9239):1375-83.
20. Lumbiganon P, Laopaiboon M, Gulmezoglu AM, Souza JP, Taneepanichskul S, Ruyan P, et al. Method of delivery and pregnancy outcome in Asia the WHO global survey on maternal and perinatal health 2007-08. Lancet. 2010; 375(9713):490.
21. Lyons J, Pressey T Bartholomew S, Liu S, Liston RM, Joseph KS et al. Delivery of breech presentation at term gestation in Canada, 2003-2011. Obstet Gynecol. 2015;125(5):1153.
22. Vistad I, Klungsoyr K, Albrechtsen S, Skjeldestad FE. Neonatal outcome of singleton term breech deliveries in Norway from 1991 to 2011. Acta Obstet Gynecol Scand. 2015;94(9):997.
23. Hofmeyr GJ, Hannah M, Lawrie TA. Planned caesarean section for term breech delivery. Cochrane Database Syst Rev. 2015;7: CD000166.
24. Glezerman M. Five years to the term breech trial: the rise and fall of a randomized controlled trial. Am J Obstet Gynecol. 2006;194(1):20.
25. Whyte H, Hannah ME, Saigal S, Hannah WJ, Hewson S, Amankwah K, et al. Outcomes of children at 2 years after planned cesarean birth versus planned vaginal birth for breech presentation at term. The International Randomised Term Breech Trial. Am J Obstet Gynecol. 2004;191(3):864.
26. Eide MG, Oyen N, Skjaerven R, Irgens LM, Bjerkedal T, Nilsen ST. Breech delivery and intelligence: a population-based study of 8,738 breech infants. Obstet Gynecol. 2005;105(1):4-11.
27. American College of Obstetricians and Gynecologists. Mode of term in singleton breech delivery. Committee Opinion No 340, July 2006, Reaffirmed 2016b.
28. Bergenhenegouwen LA, Meertens LJ, Schaaf J, Nijhuis JG, Mol BW, Kok M, et al. Vaginal breech delivery versus caesarean section in preterm breech delivery : a systematic review. Eur J Obstet Gynecol Reprod Biol. 2014;172:1.
29. Reddy UM, Zhang J, Sun L, Chen Z, Raju TN, Laughon SK. Neonatal mortality by attempted route of delivery in early preterm birth. Am J Obstet Gynecol. 2012;201(2):117.e.1.
30. Demirci O, Tugrul AS, Turgut A, Ceylan S, Eren S. Pregnancy outcome by mode of delivery among breech births. Arch Gynecol Obstet. 2012;285(2):297.
31. Bird CC, McElin TW. A six-year prospective study of term breech deliveries utilizing the Zatuchni-Andros prognostic scoring index. Am J Obstet Gynecol. 1975;121(4):551-8.
32. Bird CC, McElin TW. 500 consecutive term breech deliveries. Use of the Zatuchni-Androsprognostic scoring index. Obstet Gynecol. 1970;35(3):451-7.
33. Gupta U, Chitra R. Destructive operations still have a place in developing countries. Int J. Gynec Obstet. 1994;44:15.
34. Shrestha B, Gupta S, Chawnghlut L, Khaniya B. Fetal craniotomy. JNMA J Nepal Med Assoc. 2014;52(194):825-7.

# Anemia in Pregnancy

*Manju Puri, Nidhi Malhotra*

## INTRODUCTION

Anemia is a global public health problem with significant adverse impact on the health of individuals across all age groups, with preschool children and pregnant women being the most affected. According to World Health Organization (WHO), globally over 40% of pregnant women are anemic and the most affected regions are Southeast Asia and Africa. According to National Family Health Survey (NFHS)-4 (2015-16) in India 58.3% children and 50.3% pregnant women suffer from anemia. Majority suffer from nutritional deficiency anemia related to iron, folic acid, and vitamin $B_{12}$ deficiencies with iron deficiency anemia (IDA) as the most common. In India, anemia contributes to 20-40% maternal deaths directly or indirectly.[1] Of these 16% are direct deaths due to anemia.[2] Anemia is associated with an increase in incidence of preterm birth, fetal growth restriction (FGR) and low Apgar at birth with resultant increase in perinatal morbidity and mortality. Anemic mothers give birth to anemic infants who are more likely to suffer from cognitive and affective dysfunction and possibly long-term morbidities in the form of diabetes and cardiovascular (CVS) disease.[3] Prevalence of anemia has been described as a social imbalance worldwide. It is more prevalent in people with lower socioeconomic and educational status.[4]

## DEFINITION

Anemia is defined as a condition when the circulating levels of hemoglobin are qualitatively or quantitatively lower than normal. Anemia is diagnosed when the hemoglobin concentration is below the established cut-off levels in the blood. The criteria for diagnosing anemia are listed in **Table 1**.

The severity of anemia has been graded by Indian Council of Medical Research (ICMR) as given in **Table 2**.

## ETIOPATHOGENESIS OF ANEMIA IN PREGNANCY

Pregnancy is associated with a marked increase in blood volume, 40-45% above the prepregnant level. It is due to an increase in both plasma and red cell mass. The increase in plasma is more marked compared to red cell mass, hence, despite an increase in total hemoglobin content, there is a dilutional decrease in hemoglobin levels resulting in physiological anemia of pregnancy. It is characterized by hemoglobin level of <10.5 g/dL and no change in mean corpuscular volume (MCV) and mean corpuscular hemoglobin content (MCHC).

The increase in red cell mass is consequent to augmented erythropoiesis with associated increase in demand of various erythropoietic factors like iron, proteins, folic acid, vitamin $B_{12}$, vitamin C, vitamin A, pyridoxine, and trace elements like copper, zinc, cobalt. Inadequate dietary intake of these can result in nutritional deficiency anemia in pregnancy. Iron deficiency is most prevalent followed by folic acid and vitamin $B_{12}$ deficiency. Most often there is a combined deficiency manifesting as dimorphic anemia.

During pregnancy there is an additional requirement of about 1,000 mg of iron. Of this, approximately 300 mg is actively transported to the fetus and placenta, 500-600 mg is used for an increase in red cell mass and 100-250 mg is lost during delivery. About 150-300 mg of iron is conserved because of amenorrhea during pregnancy. Thus, an additional requirement of 4-6 mg/day of iron is there during pregnancy.

**TABLE 1:** Hemoglobin levels to diagnose anemia.

| | |
|---|---|
| Nonpregnant women | Hb < 12 g% |
| Pregnant women (WHO)[5] | Hb < 11 g%; hematocrit < 33% |
| Pregnant women (CDC 1999)[6] | • Hb < 11 g% (first and third trimester)<br>• Hb < 10.5 g% (second trimester); hematocrit < 31–32% |
| Postpartum women | Hb < 10 g%; hematocrit < 30% |

(WHO: World Health Organization; CDC: Centers for Disease Control and Prevention)

**TABLE 2:** Classification of anemia according to severity (ICMR).[7]

| Severity | Hemoglobin levels (g/dL) |
|---|---|
| Mild | 10.0–10.9 |
| Moderate | 7–9.9 |
| Severe | <7 |
| Very severe | <4 |

(ICMR: Indian Council of Medical Research)

This is lower in early pregnancy 2–3 mg/day but increases to 6–7 mg/day in late pregnancy.[8] A normal diet contains about 14 mg of iron. The average absorption of iron from normal diet is about 5–10% (1–2 mg) and is 3–4% if the diet is purely vegetarian. Iron absorption is increased in iron deficient state, but normal diet is inadequate in providing additional iron requirement during pregnancy and a daily supplement of 40–60 mg of elemental iron is needed by women during pregnancy.

The requirement of folic acid is also increased during pregnancy (400–800 µg/day). In developing countries, the diet is poor in folic acid due to low consumption of green leafy vegetables, fruits, nonvegetarian foods like liver, kidney, etc. Prolonged cooking further reduces the folic acid in diet. Pregnancy induced nausea and vomiting, malabsorption, worm infestation, use of goat's milk, and use of drugs like antiepileptics also contribute to decreased levels of folic acid during pregnancy.

During pregnancy vitamin $B_{12}$ is actively transported from the placenta to the fetus. Vitamin $B_{12}$ is found in foods of animal origin like meat, fish, eggs, and milk; and is not destroyed by heating. The daily requirement of vitamin $B_{12}$ (3 µg/day) is easily met by diet in nonvegetarians. However, in strict vegetarians, vitamin $B_{12}$ deficiency is common.

Other causes of anemia in pregnancy include chronic and acute blood loss. Chronic blood loss can result from parasitic infections like hookworm, trichuriasis, vesical, and intestinal schistosomiasis, etc. Acute blood loss is usually related to previous abortions or conditions like antepartum hemorrhage (APH) or postpartum hemorrhage (PPH) in previous pregnancies. Infections cause anemia by impairing erythropoiesis. Chronic or recurrent infections like urinary tract infection (UTI) and malaria are a common cause of anemia.

Genetic factors like thalassemia, sickle cell trait, and glucose-6-phosphate dehydrogenase deficiency can also cause anemia in pregnancy. These may be coexisting with nutritional deficiency anemia. Certain pregnancy-related conditions like HELLP in pregnancy-induced hypertension is associated with hemolytic anemia. Aplastic anemia is rarely seen in pregnancy.

The anemia in pregnancy can be classified as physiological or pathological. The pathological anemia can be classified based on etiology as shown in **Table 3**.

## CLINICAL FEATURES OF ANEMIA IN PREGNANCY

The spectrum of clinical presentation of anemia during pregnancy ranges from a completely asymptomatic woman with mild anemia to a very sick decompensated woman with severe anemia. It essentially depends upon the severity of anemia and other associated deficiencies. Although all pregnant women are at risk of developing anemia, those at higher risk are as shown in **Box 1**.

**TABLE 3:** Classification of anemia in pregnancy according to etiology.

*Acquired:*
- Nutritional deficiency anemia
- Iron deficiency
- Folic acid deficiency
- Vitamin $B_{12}$ deficiency
- Combined

*Hemorrhagic*
- *Acute blood loss:* Previous or current abortion, APH, PPH
- *Chronic blood loss:* Parasitic infections, piles

*Hemolytic*
- Autoimmune hemolytic

*Others*
- Infections
- Post bariatric surgery
- Hypothyroidism
- Chronic renal disease
- Aplastic

*Inherited:*
- Hemoglobinopathies
- Thalassemia
- Sickle cell disease
- Others

*Membrane defects*
- Spherocytosis
- Enzyme defects
- Elliptocytosis

*Enzyme defects*
- G6PD deficiency
- Pyruvate kinase deficiency

(APH: antepartum hemorrhage; PIH: pregnancy-induced hypertension; PPH: postpartum hemorrhage)

**BOX 1:** Pregnant women at high-risk of anemia.
- Young adolescent mothers
- Multiparous women especially those with short inter-pregnancy periods
- Women with multiple pregnancy
- Women from poor socioeconomic status

Women with mild-to-moderate anemia are usually asymptomatic. Those with severe anemia may complain of increasing pallor, weakness, easy fatigability, breathlessness, palpitation, swelling feet, or swelling all over the body. There may be no signs in mild anemia. However, in moderate to severe anemia there may be pallor, facial puffiness, raised jugular venous pressure (JVP), tachycardia, tachypnea, crepitations in lung bases, hepatosplenomegaly, pitting edema of abdominal wall and legs. Signs of various nutritional deficiencies like glossitis, stomatitis, cheilosis, etc., may be present.

## WORKUP OF PREGNANT WOMEN WITH ANEMIA

### History and Examination

A detailed history and thorough examination are important to assess the severity of problem and the probable cause of anemia. The onset of symptoms whether acute or insidious and the duration of symptoms should be inquired. The important points to be elicited in the history to arrive at a probable cause of anemia are as listed in **Table 4**.

A thorough head-to-toe general physical examination should be followed by a systemic examination. The various signs to be looked for are listed in **Table 5**.

**TABLE 4:** Important points to be elicited in history.

| Probable cause | Points elicited in history |
|---|---|
| Presence of infections (Malaria, UTI, TB) | Recurrent fever with chills and rigors, urinary complaints, prolonged cough with expectoration |
| Chronic loss of blood | Bleeding gums, piles, or worm infestation |
| Malabsorption | Bulky stools, chronic diarrhea |
| Bleeding or coagulation disorder | Petechiae, bruises, ecchymosis |
| Hemoglobinopathies | Repeated blood or blood component transfusion in self or family |
| Hemolysis | High-colored urine, discoloration of sclera, drug intake |
| Dietary deficiency | Detailed dietary history, cooking habits, etc. |
| Menstrual disorders | Cycle length, duration, amount of bleeding, passage of clots, etc. |
| Obstetric causes | Abortions, repeated childbirth, any complications like APH, PPH, blood transfusion, etc., in previous or current pregnancies |
| Contraceptives—IUCD | Use of IUCD with menorrhagia |

(APH: antepartum hemorrhage; PPH: postpartum hemorrhage; IUCD: intrauterine contraceptive device; TB: tuberculosis; UTI: urinary tract infection)

**TABLE 5:** Clinical examination in a pregnant woman with anemia.

| General physical examination | Systemic examination |
|---|---|
| Pulse rate (PR), BP, and respiratory rate (RR)<br>↑ PR, ↑ RR, suspect cardiac failure<br><br>Skin and mucosa<br>• Pallor<br>• Color of palmar creases<br>• Petechiae, ecchymosis (any bleeding tendency)<br><br>Eyes<br>• Pallor<br>• Icterus (hemolytic anemia)<br><br>Oral cavity<br>• Glossitis<br>• Stomatitis<br>• Cheilosis for any vitamin deficiency<br><br>Nails<br>• Pallor<br>• Platynychia or koilonychia<br>• Clubbing suggestive of chronic disease<br><br>Neck<br>• Lymphadenopathy in tuberculosis<br>• JVP raised in cardiac failure<br>• Thyroid enlargement suggestive of hypothyroidism<br><br>Legs<br>• Edema suggestive of hypoproteinemia<br>• Peripheral neuropathy present in vitamin $B_{12}$ deficiency | Chest examination<br>• Sternal tenderness for leukemia<br>• Any crepitations; fine basal for cardiac failure, coarse apical for tuberculosis<br><br>CVS examination<br>• Cardiac murmurs (Hemic murmurs)<br><br>Per abdomen<br>• Edema of abdominal wall suggestive of hypoproteinemia<br>• Hepatosplenomegaly for extra-medullary erythropoiesis, splenomegaly for hemolytic anemia<br>• Presence of free fluid suggestive of third space loss in hypoproteinemia<br><br>Obstetrical examination<br>• Abdominal examination<br>• Height of uterus<br>• Tone of uterus<br>• No. of fetuses<br>• Presentation<br>• Amount of liquor<br>• Fetal heart rate |

(BP: blood pressure; CVS: cardiovascular; JVP: jugular venous pressure)

## Investigations

The primary investigations in all pregnant women with anemia aim at assessing:
- Severity of anemia
- Type of anemia
- Cause of anemia.

### Severity of Anemia

Hemoglobin levels and hematocrit estimation are two simple investigations done to confirm the presence of anemia and assess the severity of anemia. It is recommended at booking visit and at 24–28 weeks by American College of Obstetricians and Gynecologists (ACOG) and 2019 UK guidelines.[9,10] However, as per Government of India (GoI) guidelines, hemoglobin estimation should be done thrice during antenatal period, at first visit, at 28–30 weeks and at 36 weeks.[7] Hemoglobin and hematocrit changes may reflect altered plasma volume and not a change in red cell mass. For example, in patients with severe dehydration due to protracted diarrhea or vomiting or third space loss as in preeclampsia there is a decrease in plasma volume relative to red cell mass resulting in hemoconcentration, and a falsely high hemoglobin levels.

### Type of Anemia

A complete blood count including blood indices and a peripheral smear help in the diagnosis of type of anemia. Peripheral smear provides information on the morphology of red blood cells (RBCs) like dimorphic picture where both microcytic and macrocytic cells are present but MCV may be normal. It also helps in detecting sickle cells, spherocytes, hemolysis, malarial parasite, etc. The differential diagnosis according to the type of anemia on peripheral smear is given in **Table 6**.

### Bone Marrow Activity

The gold standard for assessing bone marrow activity is by bone marrow aspiration but can be indirectly assessed by the reticulocyte count. A bone marrow sample stained for iron has been considered the gold standard for assessment of iron stores, but this is too invasive. Bone marrow aspiration is indicated rarely in the presence of abnormal cells on peripheral smear or for aplastic or refractory anemia in pregnancy.

The normal reticulocyte count is 0.5–1.5% of total RBCs. An increased reticulocyte count indicates increased bone

| TABLE 6: Differential diagnosis according to the types of anemia on peripheral smear. | |
|---|---|
| Types of anemia | Causes of anemia |
| Microcytic | Iron deficiency, thalassemia, chronic infections |
| Macrocytic | • *Megaloblastic (Impaired DNA synthesis, macro-ovalocytes seen):* Folic acid deficiency, vitamin $B_{12}$ deficiency<br>• *Non-megaloblastic (no macroovalocytes seen):* Liver disease, hypothyroidism, hemolytic anemia |
| Normocytic | • Post-hemorrhagic, renal, or hepatic disease, impaired marrow response, e.g., early iron deficiency, marrow hypoplasia, infiltrative disorder, myelodysplasia |
| Dimorphic | • Combined iron, folic acid and or vitamin $B_{12}$ deficiency |
| Hemolytic | • *Inherited:* Thalassemia, sickle cell disease, spherocytosis, G6PD deficiency, pyruvate kinase deficiency<br>• *Acquired:* Microangiopathic as in pregnancy-induced hypertension, cardiac hemolytic, autoimmune, pregnancy induced, infections, drugs |
| Pancytopenia | • *Megaloblastic:* Folic acid, vitamin $B_{12}$ deficiency<br>• *Aplastic:* Drugs, viral infections, exposure to toxic substances, etc. |

| TABLE 7: Investigations required for finding out the cause of anemia. | |
|---|---|
| Investigations | Causes of anemia |
| Peripheral smear | Morphology of red blood cell, malarial parasite, sickle cells, spherocytes, evidence of hemolysis, abnormal cells |
| Liver function tests | Liver disease, hemolysis |
| Renal function tests | Renal disease |
| Serum proteins | Hypoproteinemia |
| Electrophoresis/high performance liquid chromatography | Abnormal hemoglobin |
| Urine examination | Urinary tract infection, occult hematuria, schistosomiasis |
| Stool examination (three consecutive days) | Ova and cyst, occult blood |
| Bone marrow aspiration | Abnormal cells, iron stores, for aplastic or refractory anemia |
| X-ray chest (after shielding abdomen) | Pulmonary tuberculosis |

marrow activity as is seen in cases of hemolytic anemia, following acute blood loss and in women with IDA on treatment. In an anemic patient correction of reticulocyte count should be done as the RBC number is less and reticulocyte count may be spuriously high. Corrected reticulocyte count = % reticulocyte × hematocrit of patient/normal hematocrit for that age or:

Absolute reticulocyte count = % reticulocyte count × RBC count /L.

A corrected reticulocyte count of greater than 2% or an absolute count of more than $100 \times 10^6$/L indicate good marrow response.

## Cause of Anemia

The cause of anemia should be systematically found out and treated. The various investigations required for finding out the cause of anemia are listed in **Table 7**.

Further investigations are done depending on the type of anemia and the differential diagnosis thereof. The algorithm of an approach to anemia in pregnancy is summarized in the **Flowchart 1**.

## MATERNAL AND FETAL COMPLICATIONS

Anemia is an important cause of an increase in maternal and perinatal morbidity and mortality. It is associated with an increase in incidence of obstetric complications like preeclampsia, abruptio placentae, and preterm labor in antepartum period.[11] As these women are immunosuppressed they are predisposed to infections such as UTI and puerperal sepsis.[12] There is an increase in risk of PPH, subinvolution of uterus, puerperal sepsis, thromboembolism, lactation failure, and maternal mortality.[12,13]

The critical periods for women with severe anemia to decompensate are 3rd trimester at 28–30 weeks, in labor, immediately after delivery or in early puerperium. The congestive cardiac failure is due to inability of the hypoxic cardiac muscles to cope with the increase in pregnancy-induced cardiac load. The various causes of maternal mortality in anemic women during pregnancy and labor are congestive cardiac failure, cerebral anoxia, sepsis, and thromboembolism.

As regards the fetus, most of the nutrients are actively transported to the fetus across the placenta. There is placental hypertrophy associated with maternal anemia, which provides for an increase in oxygen transport to the fetus to compensate for decrease in circulating hemoglobin. An increased incidence of spontaneous abortions, prematurity, FGR, and intrauterine death have been reported with anemia. These children are more predisposed to have anemia and more susceptible to infections.[14] Infants born to anemic mothers are more likely to suffer from cognitive and affective dysfunction and possibly long-term morbidities in the form of diabetes and CVS disease.[3,15]

## BRIEF DESCRIPTION OF VARIOUS TYPES OF ANEMIA

### Iron Deficiency Anemia

This is the most common type of anemia in pregnancy. Pregnancy is associated with an increase in iron demand

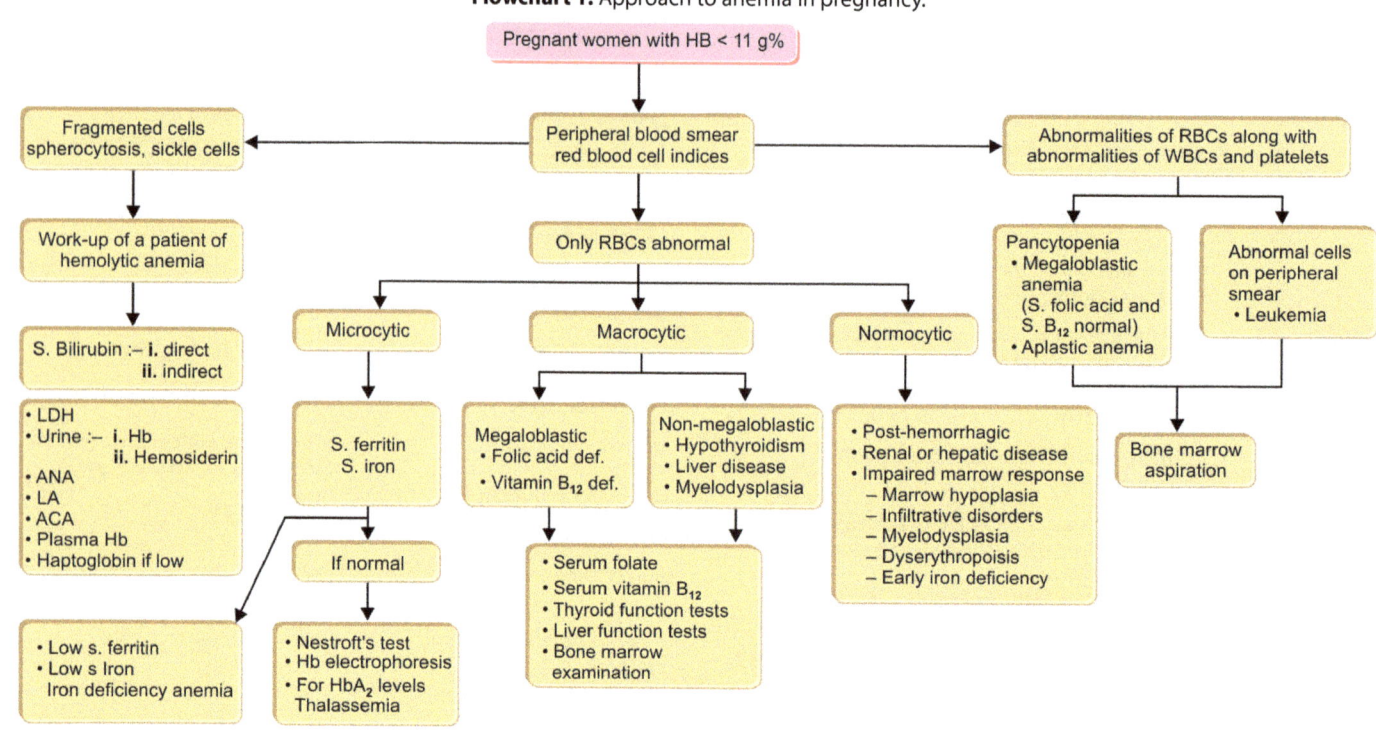

Flowchart 1: Approach to anemia in pregnancy.

(ACA: anticentromere antibody; ANA: antinuclear antibody [Anti-SS-B (Anti-Sjögren Syndrome B) antibody]; def.: deficiency; LA: lupus anticoagulant; LDH: lactate dehydrogenase; RBC: red blood cell; WBC: white blood cell)

consequent to augmented erythropoiesis and growing fetus and placenta. IDA develops over a period and has three stages. Stage 1 is when the iron stores are depleted but hemoglobin is unaffected. Stage 2 when supply of iron to bone marrow is affected with restricted erythropoiesis and is reflected by fall in serum ferritin, plasma iron levels, and transferrin saturation but hemoglobin is unaffected. Stage 3 where hemoglobin falls.[16] Women with normal hemoglobin levels but poor iron stores manifest as overt IDA during pregnancy.

## Etiopathogenesis

Iron deficiency is consequent to factors such as dietary deficiency, malabsorption, increased iron demand, infections, and blood loss. Dietary deficiency can result from poor iron content of diet due to factors like poverty, lack of knowledge of iron rich food and intake of vegetarian diet rich in phytates, and inhibitors of iron absorption. This is further aggravated by factors like malabsorption syndromes, infections like hookworm infestation, amebiasis, tuberculosis, malaria, etc., and poor iron stores due to excessive blood loss during menstruation and bleeding complications in previous pregnancies. More than 50% of women from developing countries have a negative iron balance in nonpregnant state. With, each pregnancy the women's iron reserves are further depleted. Thus, too many, too soon, and too early pregnancies result in a high prevalence of IDA in developing countries.

## Diagnosis

The diagnosis of IDA is largely based on the reports of complete blood count, red blood cell indices, and peripheral smear (Table 8). CBC showing microcytic hypochromic RBC indices with raised red blood cell distribution width (RDW) consequent to anisocytosis and poikilocytosis is suggestive of IDA. Raised RDW differentiates IDA from thalassemia and anemia of chronic disease where RDW is normal. Serum iron studies are indicated in women not responding to iron therapy. Serum iron is decreased, and total iron binding capacity of transferrin is increased in IDA. Of these total iron-binding capacity (TIBC) is more reliable due to lesser diurnal changes.

Bone marrow aspiration shows absent iron stores but is usually not indicated for IDA as it is an invasive procedure. Serum ferritin estimation is an excellent noninvasive tool for assessing the iron stores. It is the first investigation to be affected in IDA, even before hemoglobin levels fall. It has the advantage of not being affected by recent iron intake. A serum ferritin level of less than 30 µg/L is diagnostic of IDA with sensitivity of 90%, and specificity of 85%.[10] However, it is an acute phase reactant, and its level are raised in presence of infections. Simultaneous measurement of the C-reactive protein (CRP) may be helpful in explaining high levels of ferritin. Certain new parameters such as reticulocyte hemoglobin content (CHr) which measures hemoglobin in young RBCs and percentage of hypochromic cells (%HRC) are useful for early diagnosis of iron deficiency.

**TABLE 8:** Laboratory profile of iron deficiency anemia.[17]

| Investigation | Normal value | Iron deficiency anemia |
|---|---|---|
| RBC count | $4.0–5.2 \times 10^{12}/mm^3$ | $< 4.0 \times 10^{12}/mm^3$ |
| MCV | 80–100 fL | < 80 fL |
| MCH | 27–34 pg | < 27 pg |
| MCHC | 33–37 g/dL | < 33 g/dL |
| RDW | 11.5–14.5% | >14.5% |
| Peripheral smear | Normocytic normochromic RBC | Microcytic hypochromic RBC with anisocytosis, target cells |
| *Serum iron studies:* | | |
| Serum iron | 60–170 µg/dL | Reduced |
| TIBC | 250–400 µg/dL | Raised |
| Transferrin saturation (%) | 16–50% | Reduced |
| Soluble transferrin receptor | 2.8–8.5 mg/L | Increased |
| Free erythrocyte protoporphyrin/Zinc protoporphyrin | 30–50 µg/dL | Increased |
| Serum hepcidin | 17–286 ng/mL | Reduced |
| Serum ferritin | 15–200 µg/L | Reduced |
| Bone marrow iron | Present | Absent |

(MCV: mean corpuscular volume; MCHC: mean corpuscular hemoglobin content; RBC: red blood cell; RDW: red blood cell distribution width; TIBC: total iron-binding capacity)

## Prevention and Treatment

*Prevention of IDA:* The various strategies to prevent IDA should aim at improving the diet, increasing the bioavailability of dietary iron, prevention, and treatment of infections like hookworm infestation and malaria, and iron and folic acid supplementation in young girls and pregnant women. Food fortification with iron and genetic modification of food is also being evaluated.

The GOI has been addressing the problem of anemia through the National Nutritional Anemia Prophylaxis Program since 1970. Under this program all pregnant women, lactating women, contraceptive acceptors, and children (1–11 years) were provided iron and folic acid supplements. Then in 2007 GOI launched a 12 by 12 initiative to address anemia in adolescent girls, which included weekly IFA supplementation to adolescent girls, deworming every 6 months, health education and counseling. The counseling included dietary modifications and general hygiene.

The diet should be balanced and contain all nutrients such as folic acid, iron, ascorbic acid, vitamin A, etc. Iron in diet is present in two forms heme and nonheme iron. Heme iron is present in animal food and is better absorbed. The absorption of nonheme iron from vegetarian diet is influenced by iron absorption enhancers and inhibitors. Bioavailability of iron from vegetarian diet can be increased by taking iron rich diet with iron absorption enhancers like citrus fruit, rich in vitamin C and avoiding iron absorption inhibitors like phytates, phosphates, oxalates and calcium present in tea, coffee, eggs, cereals, etc. Diet rich in iron includes jaggery, green leafy vegetables like spinach, mustard leaves, fenugreek leaves (methi), cereals, sprouts and pulses. Moreover, cooking in iron utensils also seems to increase the iron content of the food.

In 2013 National Iron Plus Initiative (NIPI)[18] was launched which followed a life cycle approach and more recently "Anaemia Mukt Bharat" strategy Intensified National Iron Plus Initiative (I-NIPI) has been proposed in 2018 which is a $6 \times 6 \times 6$ strategy which includes targeting six groups of beneficiaries with six interventions and by six institutional mechanisms.[19]

*Iron prophylaxis or iron supplementation:* Iron supplementation is an effective intervention for reducing the prevalence of IDA in pregnant women. Routine iron supplementation during pregnancy has shown to improve maternal and perinatal outcome. WHO recommends universal oral iron supplementation of 60 mg of elemental iron and 400 µg of folic acid once daily for 6 months during pregnancy and for additional 3 months postpartum in all developing countries with prevalence of anemia of more than 40%. In India, currently routine iron prophylaxis is given to all pregnant women with 100 mg elemental iron and 500 µg of folic acid for at least 100 days in second half of pregnancy.

More recently under the "Anaemia Mukt Bharat" Strategy I-NIPI 60 mg of elemental iron and 500 µg folic acid has been recommended for at least 180 days antenatally and 180 days postnatally and deworming with 1 tablet of 400 mg albendazole at least once after first trimester of pregnancy. A recent Cochrane review concluded that intermittent iron supplementation produces similar fetomaternal outcomes as daily supplementation but with better compliance and lesser side effects.[10,20]

*Drug treatment:* The therapeutic dose of elemental iron for treatment of anemia is 180–200 mg per day. Iron can be administered by either oral or parenteral route. The preferred route is oral. However, the route of administration depends on period of gestation, patient's ability to tolerate oral iron, patient's compliance, any associated malabsorption syndromes, and affordability. Oral iron can be given in first trimester, but intravenous (IV) iron is not used during the first trimester, as there are no safety data for first-trimester use.

*Oral iron therapy:* Various oral iron preparations are available in the market. Most preparations contain iron in the form of ferrous salt. Ferrous sulfate, ferrous fumarate, and ferrous ascorbate are the preferred preparations. Ferrous sulfate

**TABLE 9:** Iron content of different salts.

| Salt | Dose of salt in mg | Elemental iron in mg |
|---|---|---|
| Ferrous fumarate | 100 | 30 |
| Ferrous gluconate | 100 | 10 |
| Ferrous glycine sulfate | 100 | 15 |
| Ferrous succinate | 100 | 35 |
| Ferrous sulfate | 100 | 30 |
| Ferrous ascorbate | 100 | 12 |

**BOX 2:** Indication of parenteral therapy.

- Poor tolerance to oral iron therapy
- *Poor absorption:* Malabsorption syndromes
- Noncompliance
- Women with moderate-to-severe anemia near term
- Women on recombinant erythropoietin

is the most used preparation. It is inexpensive and rapidly absorbed but has undesirable gastrointestinal side effects. Ferrous fumarate has lesser side effects. Ferrous ascorbate has an edge over other preparations due to its ascorbate content which enhances iron absorption and possibly protects the gastrointestinal mucosa due to its antioxidant property. It has been shown to have higher bioavailability of iron. Daily dose of each preparation should be decided according to the elemental iron content of each tablet. **Table 9** lists the percentage of elemental iron present in different salts.

The newer preparations like carbonyl iron are better tolerated. This is because pentacarbonyl iron is reduced to fine microspheres of <5 microns in diameter by heating. These are better absorbed and associated with lesser gastrointestinal symptoms.

Sustained release preparations reduce the overall absorption of iron by releasing iron beyond the most actively absorbing regions of the intestines that is the first part of duodenum and hence, excreted. These preparations are more expensive and less effective, hence, should be avoided.[21]

Oral iron intake is associated with side effects like nausea, vomiting, gastritis, abdominal cramps, diarrhea, and sometimes constipation, which affects compliance. For maximizing the iron absorption, women should be advised to take iron tablet either empty stomach or in between two meals with a glass of orange juice or lemon water. To minimize the side effects and improving the compliance, the treatment may be started with a lower dose or prescribing the tablet with meals or given less frequently. Sometimes changing the preparation also helps in reducing side effects.

*Parenteral iron therapy:* The preferred route of administration of iron is oral but in certain conditions parenteral therapy is indicated **(Box 2)**. The main advantage of parenteral iron therapy is the certainty of its administration and possibly early restoration of body stores.

It is available in the market as iron dextran complex, iron sorbitol complex, iron sucrose complex, iron gluconate, and iron carboxymaltose. Iron dextran and iron sorbitol have been largely replaced by iron sucrose and more recently iron carboxymaltose due to decrease in side effects and negligible risk of anaphylactic reactions with it. Cost is the only limiting factor.

Iron dextran by intramuscular (IM) route is associated with pain at injection site, risk of abscess formation, staining of skin, arthralgia, fever, painful lymphadenopathy, etc. It should be administered 100 mg once a day deep IM by Z technique after a test dose of 0.5 mg IM 24 hours before the first dose. Test dose for total dose intravenous (IV) infusion is given by slow IV infusion initially and observing the patient for any adverse reactions like chills, rigors, breathlessness, hypotension, hemolysis, etc. IV administration of Iron dextran can result in severe anaphylactic reaction.

Iron sucrose has largely replaced iron dextran, IM or intravenous (IV) at our institution. Iron sucrose is administered as IV infusion 2–3 times a week in the dose of 200–300 mg per dose to a maximum of 600 mg per week. It can be administered either undiluted 200 mg (4 mL) by slow IV injection at the rate of 20 mg/min after a test dose of 20 mg over 1–2 minutes or alternatively as IV infusion 200 mg (4 mL) diluted in maximum of 200 mL normal saline over 15–20 minutes. The risk of adverse reactions is only 0.5–1.5% compared to 5% with iron dextran. Although anaphylaxis is rare <1/1,000, readiness should be there for treating it and patient should be observed for 30 minutes after the injection or after infusion is over.

Iron carboxymaltose can be administered intravenously either undiluted as slow IV push at the rate of 100 mg (2 mL) per minute or as infusion 1,000 mg FCM added to 250 mL of normal saline over 15 minutes. The concentration of infusion should not be less than 2 mg/mL. This does not require any test dose. The risk of adverse reactions is 3% and risk of anaphylactic reaction is <1/100. Both the drugs should be avoided in first trimester. However, they are safe during lactation. Folic acid and vitamin $B_{12}$ should also be given because increased erythropoiesis may deplete these if already deficient.

The total dose of parenteral iron needs to be calculated carefully to avoid the potential risk of iron overload and side effects. The elemental iron requirement in milligram can be calculated by any of the formulae given below:

- Weight of patient in kg × (Target/normal hemoglobin − patient's hemoglobin in g/dL) × 2.21 + 1,000 mg for stores.
- Weight of patient in pounds × hemoglobin deficit in percentage × 0.3. Add 50% more of the calculated dose, for the stores.
- 200 mg of elemental iron is required for raising the hemoglobin level by 1 g%. Total dose is calculated according to hemoglobin deficit and additional 500 mg is added for stores.

**TABLE 10:** Elemental iron content, route of administration, and food and drug administration category of different preparations of parenteral iron.

| Preparation | Strength | Route of administration | Test dose | Recommended maximum dose |
|---|---|---|---|---|
| Iron dextran complex | • 2 mL ampoule<br>• 50 mg/mL<br>• 10 mL multidose vial | IM or IV | Yes | Multiple doses of 100 mg IM or total dose iron of 1,000 mg IV over 1 hour |
| Iron sorbitol citric acid complex | • 1.5 mL ampoule<br>• 50 mg/mL | IM | No | Multiple doses of 75 mg IM |
| Iron sucrose | • 5 mL ampoule<br>• 20 mg/mL | IV | No | Multiple doses of 200–300 mg over 15 minutes not >600 mg/week |
| Iron gluconate | • 5 mL ampoule<br>• 12.5 mg/mL | IV | No | Multiple doses of 125 mg or 187.5 mg over 1 hour |
| Iron carboxymaltose | • 2 mL and 5 mL vials<br>• 50 mg/mL | IV | No | 2 doses 750–1,000 mg 1 week apart if weight < 50 or >50 kg, respectively each over 15 minutes |
| Iron isomaltoside | 100 mg/mL | IV | No | Single dose 1,000 mg (20 mg/kg) over 15 minutes or 3 doses of 500 mg over 7 days |

The route of administration of parenteral iron can be IM or IV depending upon the preparation used. The elemental iron content and route of administration of different preparation of parenteral iron are given in **Table 10**.

*Assessment of response to therapy:* The response to therapy can be assessed clinically or by hematological indices. Clinically, the woman looks better, feels better and her appetite improves. The reticulocyte count increases within 5–10 days and hemoglobin increase at the rate of 1 g/dL per week. It takes about 4–10 weeks for the hemoglobin levels to be restored to normal.

*Reasons of failure to respond to iron therapy:* The pregnant woman may fail to respond due to any of these causes:
- Noniron deficiency anemia such as thalassemia
- Noncompliance
- Faulty absorption
- Persistent blood loss, e.g., worm infestation, nonsteroidal anti-inflammatory drugs (NSAIDs)
- Coexisting infection
- Concomitant folate or vitamin $B_{12}$ deficiency
- Pyridoxine deficiency.

Recent studies comparing oral iron therapy with parenteral therapy using newer preparations show that parenteral iron therapy with iron sucrose is costly, has no serious side effects, better tolerated; restores iron stores faster and more effectively than oral iron.[22] Recent Cochrane review (2011) concluded that there is insufficient evidence on when and how to treat anemia in pregnancy.[23]

## Folic Acid and Vitamin $B_{12}$ Deficiency Anemia

Folic acid and or vitamin $B_{12}$ deficiency is associated with megaloblastic anemia. The incidence of megaloblastic anemia in pregnant anemic women in developing countries is about 25% compared to only 3–4% in developed world. This type of anemia usually manifests in last trimester of pregnancy when the requirement of folic acid and vitamin $B_{12}$ is significantly increased.

### Etiopathogenesis of Megaloblastic Anemia

Folic acid and vitamin $B_{12}$ are micronutrients required for the synthesis of thymidine, one of the four bases found in DNA during embryogenesis and erythropoiesis. Deficiency or impaired metabolism of folic acid and vitamin $B_{12}$ can affect DNA synthesis resulting in impaired nuclear maturation. As the cytoplasmic maturation is normal there is resultant nuclear cytoplasmic asynchrony with formation of megaloblasts in the bone marrow. These are released in the blood as macrocytes. As many megaloblasts fail to mature they are destroyed in the bone marrow resulting in ineffective erythropoiesis and megaloblastic anemia.

Folic acid deficiency can result from inadequate dietary intake, increased demand, poor absorption, or impaired metabolism. In women from poor socioeconomic status, the dietary folic acid is inadequate to meet the enhanced metabolic demand during pregnancy. This is further aggravated by prolonged cooking, less intake of raw vegetables, pregnancy-induced nausea and vomiting, malabsorption syndromes and vitamin C deficiency. Certain drugs like antiepileptics, pyrimethamine, and trimethoprim and HIV medications can also cause folic acid deficiency. Multiple pregnancies, repeated childbirth, hemoglobinopathies, hemolytic anemia, worm infestation, and bleeding piles, all increase the demand of folic acid. Its requirement is also increased in women with IDA on iron therapy.

The minimum daily requirement of folic acid is during pregnancy is 500 µg. The growing fetus and placenta extract folate from maternal body stores very effectively. Even when mother is severely anemic the fetus is not anemic. Green leafy vegetables, broccoli, spinach, sprouts, beans, liver, kidney, fruits, strawberries, cereals, nuts, etc., are rich sources of folic acid. It is absorbed from duodenum and upper jejunum.

Vitamin $B_{12}$ is a complex organometallic compound known as cobalamin. The absorption of vitamin $B_{12}$ requires intrinsic factor, which is secreted by parietal cells of the mucosa of the fundus of the stomach. Human beings are totally dependent on dietary animal products for their vitamin $B_{12}$ requirements. Plants and vegetables contain little cobalamin except that contributed by microbial contamination. Hence, strict vegetarian or macrobiotic diets do not contain adequate amount of this essential nutrient. Vitamin $B_{12}$ deficiency is common in Indian women presenting in their first trimester as majority of them are vegetarians.[24]

The daily requirement of vitamin $B_{12}$ is about 3 µg in pregnancy. Inadequate intake in the diet as in strict vegans, impaired absorption as in intrinsic factor deficiency, pernicious anemia, gastrectomy, malabsorption, ileal resection, fish tapeworm parasitic infestation, bacterial overgrowth in blind loops and diverticule of bowel and increased requirement as in pregnancy, hypothyroidism, disseminated cancer and chronic infections cause vitamin $B_{12}$ deficiency. Prolonged use of certain drugs such as gastric acid blocking agents like ranatidine, omeprazole, and metformin are also associated with vitamin $B_{12}$ related anemia.

### Diagnosis of Megaloblastic Anemia

The diagnosis is made based on peripheral smear report and red cell indices. The hemoglobin levels are usually < 10 g% and peripheral smear may show macrocytic or normocytic normochromic picture, macroovalocytes, anisocytosis, hypersegmented neutrophils (>5 lobes; normal neutrophils have 4 lobes), giant cell polymorphs, pancytopenia, neutropenia, and thrombocytopenia.

The macroovalocytes present in megaloblastic anemia are different from the macrocytes present in nonmegaloblastic anemia with liver disorders and hypothyroidism as these are not oval.

Serum homocysteine and lactate dehydrogenase (LDH) levels are raised in both folic acid and vitamin $B_{12}$ deficiency. The red cell indices show increased MCV > 100 fL, increased MCH and normal MCHC 33-37 g/dL. The reticulocyte count is low indicating poor erythropoiesis in marrow. This contrasts with hemolytic anemia where the LDH is raised but the reticulocyte count is increased indicating accelerated erythropoiesis consequent to increased destruction of RBCs.

The differentiation between folic acid and vitamin $B_{12}$ deficiency can be done clinically by presence of neurological symptoms in case of vitamin $B_{12}$ deficiency due to the degeneration of the posterior and lateral columns of spinal cord. These include symmetric paresthesia, numbness, impaired vibration, and position sense leading to gait disturbance. The changes are irreversible if prompt therapy is not instituted. These features are absent in folic acid deficiency. Vitamin $B_{12}$ deficiency is associated with hyperpigmentation. Low serum folate levels (<3 ng/mL) and low RBC folate levels < 150 ng/mL are diagnostic of folic acid deficiency.[25] Serum levels of vitamin $B_{12}$ of < 200 pg/mL indicate vitamin $B_{12}$ deficiency.[25] In the absence of availability of these tests, serum methylmalonic acid (MMA) levels can also differentiate between the two, as its levels are raised in vitamin $B_{12}$ deficiency. An increased MMA level is highly sensitive and specific for vitamin $B_{12}$ deficiency. More recently transcobalamin has been suggested as another reliable indicator of vitamin $B_{12}$ deficiency. Examination of bone marrow reveals megaloblastic erythropoiesis. Schilling test to assess the cause of malabsorption of vitamin $B_{12}$ is done in the postpartum period.

### Prevention and Treatment

*Preventive:* Women should be counseled to take diet rich in folic acid like green leafy vegetables, beans, etc. WHO recommends a daily intake of 400 µg of folic acid per day for all pregnant women in antenatal period throughout the antenatal period. It is estimated that this reduces the risk of neural tube defects (NTD) by 36% and if supplemented in a dose of 5 mg/day it reduces the risk by 85%.[26] Ministry of Health and Family Welfare, GoI recommends a daily supplementation of 500 µg of folic acid and 60 mg of elemental iron in antenatal and postnatal period.[19] Periconceptional folic acid supplementation of 400 µg daily in low-risk women and 4-5 mg daily in high risk women with previous pregnancy complicated by NTD from 4 weeks before conception through first trimester of pregnancy is an effective intervention for preventing NTD.[27] However, pregnant women with hemoglobinopathies, on anticonvulsant medications and with multiple pregnancies need a supplementation of 1 mg/day. Routine supplementation of vitamin $B_{12}$ is not recommended but vegetarian women should be encouraged to increase intake of dairy products during pregnancy and lactation.

*Curative:* In megaloblastic anemia due to folic acid deficiency a daily intake of 5 mg of folic acid is sufficient. As most of the patients with vitamin $B_{12}$ deficiency have malabsorption it is preferable to supplement vitamin $B_{12}$ by parenteral route to prevent worsening of peripheral neuropathy. There is no consensus on the dose of vitamin $B_{12}$ for the women with megaloblastic anemia, however a dose of 1,000 µg on alternate day IV or IM for 1-2 weeks followed by 1,000 µg every week for 8 weeks and then once a month. IM route is preferred as significant amount is excreted if administered through IV route. In patients with thrombocytopenia (platelet count < 50,000/mm$^3$) IM injection should be avoided. Oral preparations are also available and are prescribed in the dose of 1,000–2,000 µg per day. Blood transfusion is indicated in women with severe anemia near term. In case both folic acid and vitamin $B_{12}$ deficiency is coexisting, it is important to treat both simultaneously to avoid folate trap because for utilization of folate, vitamin $B_{12}$ is required.

*Response to therapy:* The response to therapy with folic acid and vitamin $B_{12}$ is evident by a fall in LDH levels and an increase in reticulocyte count within 3–5 days. The associated thrombocytopenia also improves within 5–7 days. Total recovery occurs within 6-8 weeks.

## Thalassemia

Thalassemia is the most common monogenetic disorder inherited as an autosomal recessive trait all over the world. It is common in malaria-endemic areas including the Mediterranean area, the Middle East, Southeast Asia, Africa, and the Indian subcontinent. It is a heterogeneous group of genetic disorders of hemoglobin synthesis characterized by absent or decreased synthesis of one or more globin chains. Thalassemia can be classified as α or β, depending on the globin chain affected. In India, β thalassemia comprises 80–90% of all cases of thalassemia and the overall prevalence of beta thalassemia carrier ranges between 2.78 and 4% of general population.[28] The communities commonly affected are Gujaratis, Maharashtrians, Sindhis, Goaneses, Bengalis, and people from northern states such as Haryana, Punjab, UP, and Rajasthan.

### Etiopathogenesis

Hemoglobin is a tetrameric protein compound comprising two pairs of globin chain, each attached to a heme complex. There are various types of globin chains α, β, γ, δ, etc. In adults 95% of circulating hemoglobin is HbA ($\alpha_2 \beta_2$), 2–3% is $HbA_2$ ($\alpha_2 \delta_2$) and < 2 % is HbF ($\alpha_2 \gamma_2$).[25] The genes controlling the synthesis of these chains are located on chromosome 11 and 16. There are 4 genes located on chromosome 16 that control the synthesis of α globin chains. Of these two are derived from each parent. Synthesis of β globin chains is controlled by 2 genes located on chromosome 11, one gene derived from each parent. β thalassemia is a mutation disorder whereas α thalassemia is a deletion disorder resulting in absent or reduced synthesis of globin chains.

The clinical presentation in α thalassemia depends upon the number of genes deleted. The severity of disease increases with an increase in the number of genes deleted. When all the 4 genes are deleted, α globin chains are absent. None of the hemoglobin HbA, $HbA_2$, HbF can be synthesized; instead, tetramers of γ chains known as Hb Bart ($\gamma_4$) are synthesized.[29] This condition is incompatible with life. In β thalassemia, presence of mutant genes results in reduced or absent β globin chains and excess of α globin chains. There is decreased production of HbA ($\alpha_2 \beta_2$) and increased production of $HbA_2$ ($\alpha_2 \delta_2$) and HbF ($\alpha_2 \gamma_2$).[29] The pathophysiology of β thalassemia is depicted in the **Flowchart 2**.

### Clinical Presentation

#### α thalassemia

*α thalassemia trait:* There are normally 4 functioning α globin genes. If one or two of these genes are missing the result is α thalassemia trait. These traits cannot be detected on hemoglobin electrophoresis as no abnormal hemoglobin is synthesized. In addition, there is neither excess nor lack of any normal hemoglobin.

*HbH disease:* Deletion of three α-globin genes results in HbH disease, manifesting as chronic hemolytic anemia with normal life expectancy. This can be detected on Hb electrophoresis. Cholelithiasis is commonly associated with HbH disease. The pregnant women are predisposed to hemolytic crisis in conditions like fever, infection, drug intake, etc.

*Hb Bart's disease:* Deletion of all 4 α-globin genes result in Hb Bart's disease. Tetramers of γ chain known as Hb Bart ($\gamma_4$) are produced. In this condition no α chain is synthesized, so HbF, HbA and $HbA_2$ are not synthesized. This disease is incompatible with life and results in intrauterine hydrops. Serious obstetric complications like preeclampsia, polyhydramnios, placentomegaly, and difficult delivery due to large fetus can occur.

#### β thalassemia

*β thalassemia minor:* In β thalassemia minor, only one mutant gene is present. It is a heterozygous state. The obstetric outcome or complications are the same as that in the general population, but it causes microcytic hypochromic anemia. There is increase in the incidence of anemia and doubtful increase in NTD consequent to relative folate deficiency.

*β thalassemia major:* Women with β thalassemia major have high morbidity and mortality. Although these women are usually subfertile, pregnancies have been reported. Increased incidence of early pregnancy losses, FGR, and prematurity due to maternal anemia and associated chronic placental hypoxia has been reported.[30] Women are predisposed to heart failure, hyper splenic crisis and venous thrombosis (in splenectomized women due to thrombocytosis).[30] These women are small in stature and have small pelvic bones which may be responsible for increased rate of cesarean delivery in these women. Use of iron chelating agents can lead to retardation of bone ossification, vertebral aplasia, and bifurcation or fusion of ribs in the fetus.

### Screening and Diagnosis

Most carriers are asymptomatic, hence, thalassemia should be suspected in pregnant women with following findings:

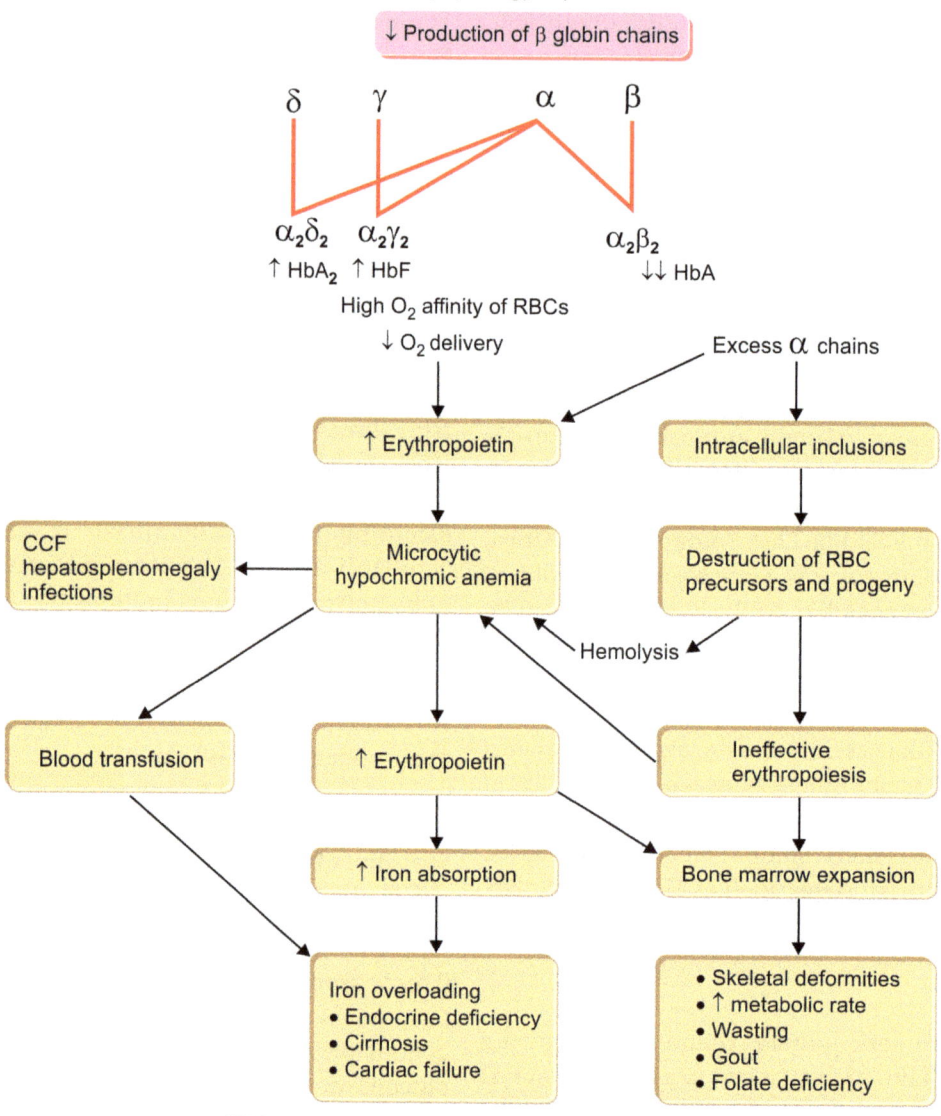

Flowchart 2: Pathophysiology of β-thalassemia.

(CBC: congestive cardiac failure; RBC: red blood cell)

- History of transfusion dependent anemia in self or family.
- Women with mild to moderate microcytic anemia not responding to oral iron.
- Women with a low MCV < 80 fL and or low MCH < 27 pg and normal MCHC.
- Disparity between the hemoglobin levels, and RBC count, i.e., if hemoglobin level is low, but RBC count is normal or high.
- α thalassemia should be suspected in pregnant women with mild anemia with low MCV, not responding to oral iron and with normal hemoglobin electrophoresis.

The diagnosis of β thalassemia is confirmed by hemoglobin electrophoresis or automated high-performance liquid chromatography (HPLC), which show raised $HbA_2$ levels of >3.5% of total hemoglobin and higher HbF sometimes. In some β carriers $HbA_2$ may be normal (False negative). This happens in very mild carriers, in α and β cocarriers where production of both globin chains is equally reduced and δβ thalassemia carrier where production of β globin is also reduced and in hereditary persistence of fetal haemoglobin (HPFH). In case $HbA_2$ is normal HbF should be used to differentiate between α carriers, δβ thalassemia carrier and HPFH. It is normal in α carriers and increased in δβ thalassemia carrier (4–18%) and HPFH (3–30%).[31,32]

α thalassemia trait cannot be diagnosed by hemoglobin electrophoresis or HPLC and requires molecular genetic testing for detecting α globin gene deletion. The iron studies usually show normal serum iron and serum ferritin levels. There may be evidence of hemolysis in thalassemia major.

## Recommendations for Screening for Thalassemia in Pregnancy

The following recommendations are based on good and consistent scientific evidence:[33]

- Complete blood count and hemoglobin electrophoresis are appropriate laboratory tests for screening for hemoglobinopathies. Red cell indices such as MCH < 27 pg and MCV < 80 fL are good measures to select women for HPLC. Routine screening should be offered to all pregnant women with red cell indices. Hemoglobin electrophoresis should be added in populations with increased risk for being carriers of hemoglobinopathies like in populations with high prevalence of thalassemia or those with abnormal red cell indices (low MCH, low MCV). If the woman is screen positive, then her partner needs to be screened as the chances of the carrier couple giving birth to a baby with thalassemia major is 25%.

- Couples at risk for having a child with thalassemia major should be offered genetic counseling to review prenatal testing and reproductive options with them.

Delhi government has implemented thalassemia screening program which includes subjecting all pregnant women to NESTROFT (naked eye single tube rapid osmotic fragility test) with 0.36% buffer solution. In this test 2 mL of 0.36% buffered saline is taken in one tube (10 cm × 1 cm diameter) and 2 mL distilled water is taken in another. A drop of blood is added to each of the tubes, which are left undisturbed for half an hour at room temperature. A positive NESTROFT indicates that all red cells in the tested sample have not undergone lysis in 0.36% buffered saline. These unlysed red cells result in the hazy appearance of the contents of the tube and render the line on the paper indistinct. These red cells also sediment as a button at the bottom of the tube, when it is left undisturbed for some time. Thus, a positive NESTROFT indicates decreased red cell osmotic fragility and increased resistance to osmotic lysis. NESTROFT does not require any specialized equipment, expertise, or rigid conditions, and can be used in field conditions. NESTROFT compares favorably with MCV from the point of view of sensitivity and specificity. The sensitivity of Nestroft test ranges between 95 and 100%, specificity between 66 and 95%, positive predictive value from 33 to 87% and negative predictive value from 97 to 100%.[34] Woman testing positive are followed by hemoglobin electrophoresis and husband's blood for CBC and NESTROFT.

## Prenatal Diagnosis

The couple at risk of giving birth to a thalassemia major baby is offered prenatal counseling and a definite genetic diagnosis of major thalassemia by invasive diagnostic procedures like chorionic villous biopsy or amniocentesis for obtaining fetal samples for genetic testing. In cases where the diagnosis is confirmed, termination of pregnancy can be offered.[35] Next generation sequencing of the fetal cell free DNA circulating in maternal plasma, a noninvasive alternative for the diagnosis of thalassemia major is under study.

In couples with α thalassemia carrier state, it is reasonable to avoid invasive diagnostic procedure if parents wish as ultrasonic surveillance is an effective tool in detecting α thalassemia major cases by detecting evidence of fetal anemia by increased middle cerebral artery peak systolic velocity (MCA-PSV), increased placental thickness, cardiomegaly, increased fetal cardiothoracic ratio of ≥50%, pleural effusion or ascites.[36]

## Preimplantation Diagnosis

For thalassemia carrier couples who wish to avoid the risk of prenatal invasive diagnosis and termination of pregnancy preimplantation genetic diagnosis (PGD) is a viable alternative. In this, in vitro fertilization is followed by selection of healthy embryos using single cell biopsy from the embryo and its transfer into the uterus. The healthy embryos can be cryopreserved. The accuracy is more than 99% but the chance of giving birth to a healthy baby is only 30% per embryo transfer.[37]

## Management of Pregnancy with Thalassemia

*α thalassemia trait:* Pregnancy is well-tolerated. Folate supplementation is recommended for all women during pregnancy, however, iron supplementation should be advised only if iron deficiency is documented. Parenteral iron is contraindicated. Genetic screening of partner should be done. If both parents are carriers of heterozygous α 0 thalassemia trait (--/α α) there is a 25% chance of the fetus being affected by Hb Bart's disease. Prenatal diagnosis should be offered and MTP is advised if fetus is affected by Hb Bart's disease. In case both parents are homozygous α + thalassemia trait (-α /-α), there is no risk of HbH and Bart's disease and fetal testing is not required.

*HbH disease:* Women with HbH disease are likely to have acute exacerbation of chronic anemia during pregnancy. Periconception high dose folate supplementation (5 mg/day) is recommended. Iron supplementation is advised only in presence of iron deficiency. Blood transfusion is indicated in the presence of severe anemia. The partner should be subjected to genetic screening for a carrier state. If the partner tests positive for carrier state, prenatal diagnosis should be offered to the women for early diagnosis of fetus with HbH or Hb Bart's disease and medical termination of pregnancy is offered accordingly.

*β thalassemia minor:* In pregnant women with β thalassemia minor, screening of partner should be advised. If the partner is a carrier, prenatal diagnosis (CVS, amniocentesis, cordocentesis) should be offered. In couples who are heterozygous carriers of β thalassemia has a 25% chance of having a baby with thalassemia major and 50% chance of having a baby with thalassemia minor. Folate supplementation is recommended for all pregnant women and iron supplementation in women with documented iron deficiency. Blood transfusion is indicated if the hemoglobin level is < 8 g% near term.

*β thalassemia major:* In women with thalassemia major, the partner is screened. Prenatal diagnosis is offered if partner is a carrier. These women should undergo a baseline cardiac, liver, and endocrine evaluation including pancreas and thyroid gland before pregnancy for their fitness for pregnancy. Their medical condition should be optimized before they are advised to conceive. This is again repeated at the initial visit after conception and then in the second and third trimesters. As these women have been receiving repeated transfusions, they are at risk of alloimmunization. They should be tested for ABO and full blood group genotype and antibody titers. They are also screened for hepatitis B surface antigen and hepatitis C status. Those positive for antibodies should have cross-matched blood available for delivery. Chelation with desferrioxamine should be stopped as soon as pregnancy is confirmed or in the midcycle when ovulation induction is being done due to its teratogenic effects. However, in women with myocardial dysfunction the risk of stopping chelation therapy outweighs the risk of teratogenicity on continuing the drug. The women are subjected to complete blood count every 2 weeks and transfusion therapy is continued to maintain hemoglobin levels at 10 g%. These women need antenatal checkup every 4 weeks till 28 weeks and there after every 2 weeks by a multidisciplinary team. An ultrasound should be offered at 7–9 weeks for dating, viability, and multiple pregnancies followed by a 11–14 weeks and 18–20 weeks scan and then serial growth scans from 24 weeks.[38]

Regular folate 5 mg per day is recommended. Women who have undergone splenectomy or have a platelet count of 600,000/dL should be offered thromboprophylaxis with low dose aspirin 75 mg/day and those with both should be offered thromboprophylaxis with low dose aspirin 75 mg/day and low-molecular weight heparin as these women are predisposed to thrombosis due to presence of abnormal RBC fragments. These fragments combined with high platelet count increase the risk of thrombosis.[38]

## Sickle Cell Anemia

Sickle cell anemia is an inherited chronic hemolytic anemia due to presence of abnormal hemoglobin S (HbS). The clinical manifestations are because of polymerization of HbS and deformation of RBCs into a characteristic sickle shape. It has highest prevalence in tropical Africa. In India it is prevalent in the tribal population of central India, northern Kerala, and Tamil Nadu.[39] The sickle cell trait provides survival benefit in areas endemic for falciparum malaria. The sickle hemoglobin containing red cells inhibit proliferation of *Plasmodium falciparum* and the infected cells are more likely to become deformed and removed from circulation.

### Etiopathogenesis

It is caused by a point mutation of the β globin gene on chromosome 11 that produces an amino acid change at position 6, changing glutamic acid to valine acid and results in production of HbS. When the gene is heterozygous it is known as sickle cell trait and when it is homozygous it is called sickle cell disease (SCD). In SCD polymerization of Hb S in the deoxygenated state is increased and leads to sickling and increased rigidity of RBCs. Sickle cells exhibit abnormal adherence to vascular endothelium and lead to vaso-occlusion, sickling-induced membrane fragmentation and complement-mediated lysis causing intravascular hemolysis. Poorly deformable sickle cells get entrapped extravascularly and phagocytosed by macrophages and monocytes and results in extravascular hemolysis.

### Investigations

The diagnosis is made based on peripheral smear report which shows sickle cells, target cells, cigar-shaped cells and ovalocytes. The reticulocyte count is raised due to increased bone marrow activity consequent to hemolysis. Mean reticulocyte count is 10% with average ranging between 4 and 24%. Due to hemolysis, indirect bilirubin and LDH may be increased and haptoglobin decreased. The diagnosis is confirmed by identification of HbS by high performance liquid chromatography.

### Management

Preconceptional counseling is important for partner screening, baseline assessment of woman as regards any end organ damage, iron load, updating of the vaccination status (influenza, Pneumococcus, meningococcal) of the woman. Review drugs like hydroxycabamide, angiotensin converting enzyme inhibitors, angiotensin receptor blockers, iron chelators which should be stopped, and advice should be given regarding prevention of crisis. Penicillin prophylaxis should be continued, and folic acid is started. The couple is counseled about increased risk of obstetrical, fetal, and SCD related medical complications during pregnancy. This is an opportunity to discuss various options like use of donor sperm, PGD, adoption and prenatal diagnosis. Noninvasive detection of fetal SCD by evaluation of cell-free DNA in maternal plasma is still under investigation.

At the first antenatal visit, a detailed history particularly with respect to prior sickle cell crises, their nature, frequency, and management is noted. Baseline blood pressure, complete blood count, reticulocyte count, serum iron levels, pulmonary, renal, and liver function tests are obtained. Woman is screened for HIV, hepatitis B and C and alloantibodies. The woman's partner should be screened for presence of sickle cell trait. If partner is positive for sickle cell trait, prenatal diagnosis is offered in the form of CVS or amniocentesis. Folic acid supplementation 5 mg/d is given to all women. Routine iron supplementation is given in the absence of any iron overload.

Patients are counseled regarding the importance of maintaining good hydration and prevention of infections, as dehydration and infections precipitate sickle cell crisis. Opioids are preferred over NSAIDs for the management of painful vaso-occlusive crisis especially after 32 weeks of gestation. Early diagnosis and prompt treatment of infections should be done. Persistent vomiting in early pregnancy can cause dehydration and precipitate sickle cell crisis, these women should be counseled to seek early help to prevent complications. Prophylaxis with low dose aspirin 150 mg per day should be considered to prevent preeclampsia from 12 weeks onward.

Pregnancy is carefully supervised for early detection of complications like preeclampsia, abruption, FGR, preterm labor or any SCD activity. These women are offered a growth scan and mid-stream urine examination every 4 weeks in addition to routine antenatal checkups. Blood transfusion therapy is considered on individual basis. The use of prophylactic transfusion versus selective transfusion is debatable. Waiting for spontaneous onset of labor till 40 weeks is reasonable. Induction of labor or elective cesarean section may be offered, if obstetrically indicated.[39]

During labor, IV fluids and oxygen supplementation help in preventing dehydration and maintaining an adequate circulation. Vaginal delivery is preferred. General anesthesia is avoided due to the risk of hypoxia associated with it; regional block is preferred.

In the postpartum period early mobilization is encouraged. Analgesics are given for pain relief and breastfeeding is encouraged. Postpartum thromboprophylaxis is recommended with low-molecular-weight heparin in the pregnant woman whenever hospitalized, for 7 days following vaginal delivery and 6 weeks following cesarean section.

## SEVERE ANEMIA IN PREGNANCY

The WHO defines severe anemia as Hb level of <7 g% and ICMR further categorizes very severe anemia when Hb < 4 g%. A pregnant woman with severe anemia may present in three stages; compensated, decompensated in congestive cardiac failure, and in circulatory failure. It is reported that the fetal oxygenation is adversely affected with a maternal Hb of <6 g% hence blood transfusion should be considered if Hb is <6 g%.

The treatment of severe anemia depends upon the hemodynamic status, gestational age, severity of anemia, and cause of anemia in the pregnant woman. Blood transfusion is indicated as per indications in **Table 11**.[40]

Definitive treatment depends upon the cause of anemia. In IDA if the POG at presentation is <30 weeks oral iron can be started in therapeutic dose in addition to supplementation of other erythropoietic factors, deworming, and dietary advice. The patient is closely observed for response to treatment and can be switched to parenteral therapy, if she is noncompliant

**TABLE 11:** Indications of blood transfusion during pregnancy.

| < 36 weeks | > 36 weeks |
|---|---|
| • Hb ≤ 5 g/dL<br>• Hb between 5 and 7 g/dL with:<br>  – Signs of cardiac failure or hypoxia<br>  – Any serious bacterial infection like pneumonia, pyelonephritis<br>  – Malaria | • Hb ≤ 6 g/dL<br>• Hb between 6 and 8 g/dL with:<br>  – Signs of cardiac failure or hypoxia<br>  – Any serious bacterial infection, like pneumonia, pyelonephritis<br>  – Malaria |

or intolerant to oral iron. If the POG is in between 30 and 36 weeks parenteral therapy should be considered as first line to ensure compliance to treatment. If pregnancy is >36 weeks, blood transfusion should be considered especially if the woman is likely to have cesarean section, induction of labor or likely to bleed as with APH, preeclampsia, and previous cesarean section.

The management of folic acid deficiency is with oral folate 5 mg/day and that of vitamin $B_{12}$ deficiency with oral tablet of 1,000–2,000 µg per day or parenteral 1,000 µg every day or every other day for 5–7 doses followed by 1,000 µg every week for 1–2 months. It is important to supplement all erythropoietic factors to prevent deficiency due to accelerated erythropoiesis.

## MANAGEMENT OF LABOR

The management of labor in a pregnant woman with severe anemia is challenging. The relatives are counseled about the high risk to the mother and fetus and an informed high-risk consent is taken. Adequate blood, preferably packed blood cells is arranged. The woman is nursed in a propped-up position and administered intermittent oxygen by mask. IV access is established but IV fluids are avoided. Prophylactic antibiotics are given. In women who are decompensated, diuretics like furosemide 40 mg is given intravenously and packed cells may be started under diuretic cover. The flow rate should not exceed 15–30 drops per minute. Maternal and fetal condition and progress of labor is carefully monitored. The labor is usually easy and short in anemic women. The woman is observed for any signs of cardiac decompensation due to increased cardiac load during labor. Cardiac decompensation is suspected if pulse rate is > 100/min, respiratory rate > 24/min, JVP is raised and there are fine basal crepts in lungs.

The second stage may be cut short by application of ventouse or outlet forceps to avoid cardiorespiratory embarrassment. The third stage is managed actively with 10 U of oxytocin intramuscularly immediately after delivery of baby. Injection methergine is contraindicated in women with congestive cardiac failure and per rectal misoprostol 800 µg is preferred. In case of PPH concentrated infusion of oxytocin 20 units in 500 mL of RL is administered at the rate of no more than 125 mL per hour, i.e., 30 drops per minutes. Delayed cord clamping is desirable to provide additional blood to the newborn to build iron stores.

Women with severe anemia tolerate the blood loss poorly and even the normal blood loss in third stage can amount to PPH in these women. The blood loss should be promptly replaced by packed blood cells transfusion.

These women are likely to go into failure immediately after delivery due to increased cardiac load consequent to release of pressure of the gravid uterus from the inferior vena cava and return of blood from the placental bed. These women should be kept propped up and observed carefully for any signs of decompensation immediately after delivery. Diuretics, furosemide 40 mg intravenously may be administered immediately after delivery of placenta to reduce the cardiac load.

In women with mild or moderate anemia, the general principles of management of labor are essentially the same as that of non-anemic women. Extra precautions need to be taken to prevent infection and minimize the blood loss in third stage of labor. Strict aseptic precautions are observed and per vaginum examinations should be kept to a minimum. Blood is kept cross matched and the third stage of labor is managed actively.

## POSTNATAL CARE AND CONTRACEPTION

Women with severe anemia are predisposed to infections and other complications. They need to be carefully observed for complications like subinvolution of uterus, puerperal sepsis, congestive cardiac failure, thromboembolism, and lactation failure. Early ambulation is encouraged. Breastfeeding is not contraindicated.

Blood transfusion is avoided even with severe anemia, if the woman is compensated except if there is any associated sepsis. Oral hematinic therapy is continued in therapeutic dose till the hemoglobin level is more than ≥ 12 g%. It is continued for another 3 months after this for replenishing the iron stores. The woman and her relatives are counseled regarding the importance and need for continuing hematinic preparations.

Anemic women are counseled to avoid pregnancy for at least 2 years. A combination of lactational amenorrhea method (LAM) and barrier contraception is a good option for the first 6 months along with continued hematinic therapy. Once her hemoglobin levels are restored to normal any contraceptive can be advised. Progestin only pills can also be started after 3 weeks of delivery and continued for first 6 months and then switched over to combined oral contraceptive pills. IM depot medroxyprogesterone acetate (DMPA) injection (Antara) 150 mg every 3 months can be started after 6 weeks in breastfeeding mothers and immediately after delivery in those who are not breastfeeding. Centchroman (Chayya) is another good postpartum contraceptive option. Copper intrauterine contraceptive device (IUCD) is avoided till the anemia is corrected for the risk of associated menorrhagia however, progesterone containing IUCD can be given. If she has completed her family, sterilization may be done provided her hemoglobin is 8 g% or more as per eligibility criteria laid down by GOI.

## KEY POINTS

- Anemia is the most common medical disorder in pregnancy.
- Prevalence of anemia in pregnancy ranges from 20% in developed countries to 50–90% in developing countries.
- Nutritional IDA is the most common type of anemia in pregnancy.
- Anemia is associated with an increase in maternal and perinatal morbidity and mortality.
- The clinical presentation of anemia may vary from a completely asymptomatic woman with mild anemia to a severely decompensated woman with severe anemia.
- Overall improvement in diet is an important intervention to tackle nutritional anemia.
- Routine iron and folic acid supplementation is recommended for all pregnant women in antenatal and postnatal period in countries with a high prevalence of anemia.
- The cause of anemia should be systematically identified and treated.
- Labor should be carefully supervised, observing strict asepsis and third stage is managed actively to minimize blood loss.
- Patient is counseled to continue hematinic therapy in the postpartum period and avoid next pregnancy for at least 2 years.
- In all women with anemia due to hemoglobinopathies-thalassemia, sickle cell anemia, it is essential to do a preconceptional counseling, partner screening, and baseline assessment of the woman for her fitness to conceive.
- Those with a carrier partner should be offered prenatal diagnosis and termination if the fetus is a thalassemia major or has SCD.
- These patients have to be managed by a multidisciplinary team during their pregnancy.

## REFERENCES

1. Ezzati M, Lopez AD, Rodgers AA, Murray CJL. Comparative quantification of health risks: global and regional burden of disease attributable to selected major risk factors. Geneva, Switzerland: World Health Organization; 2004.
2. Abou Zahr C, Royston E. Maternal mortality. A global factbook. Geneva: World Health Organization; 1991.
3. Beard JL. Why iron deficiency is important in infant development. J Nutr. 2008;138: 2534-6.

4. Milman N. Anaemia still a major health problem in many parts. Ann Hematol. 2011;90(4):369-77.
5. World Health Organization (WHO). WHO recommendations on antenatal care for a positive pregnancy experience. Luxembourg: World Health Organization; 2016.
6. Centres for Disease Control. Criteria for anemia in children and childbearing aged women. MMWR. 1989;38:400-4.
7. Good Clinical Practice Recommendations for Iron Deficiency Anemia in Pregnancy (IDA) in Pregnancy in India. J Obstet Gynaecol India. 2011;61(5):569-71.
8. Bothwell TH. Iron requirements in pregnancy and strategies to meet them. Am J Clin Nutr. 2000;72(1 Suppl):257S-64S.
9. American College of Obstetricians and Gynecologists ACOG Practice Bulletin No. 95: Anemia in pregnancy. Obstet Gynecol. 2008;112(1):201-7.
10. Pavord S, Daru J, Prasannan N, Robinson S, Stanworth S, Girling J, et al. UK guidelines on the management of iron deficiency in pregnancy. Br J Haematol. 2020;188(6):819.
11. Arnold DL, Williams MA, Miller RS, Qiu C, Sorensen TK. Maternal iron deficiency anaemia is associated with an increased risk of abruption placentae – a retrospective case control study. J Obstet Gynaecol Res. 2009;35:446-52.
12. Patra S, Pasrija S, Trivedi SS, Puri M. Maternal and perinatal outcome in patients with severe anemia in pregnancy. Int J Gynaecol Obstet. 2005;91(2):164-5.
13. Sharma JB, Shankar M. Anemia in pregnancy. JIMSA. 2010;23(4):253-61.
14. Lops VR, Hunter LP, Dixon LR. Anemia in pregnancy. Am Fam Physician. 1995;51:1189-97.
15. Perez EM, Hendricks MK, Beard JL, Murray-Kolb LE, Berg A, Tomlinson M, et al. Mother infant interactions and infant development are altered by maternal iron deficiency anemia. J Nutr. 2005;135:850-5
16. Burke RM, Leon JS, Suchdev PS. Identification, prevention, and treatment of Iron deficiency anaemia in first 1000 days. Nutrients. 2014;6(10):4093-114.
17. Dacie JV, Lewis SM. Davis and Lewis Practical Haematology, 11th edition. China: Elsevier Churchill Livingstone; 2012.
18. National Iron Plus Initiative, GoI (2013). Guidelines for Control of Iron deficiency Anemia. [online]. Available from: http://nhm.gov.in/images/pdf/programmes/child-health/guidelines/Control-of-Iron-Deficiency-Anaemia.pdf [Last accessed July, 2021].
19. MOHFW GoI (2018). Anemia Mukt Bharat—Intensified National Iron Plus Initiative. [online]. Available from: https://anemiamuktbharat.info/wp-content/uploads/2019/09/Anemia-Mukt-Bharat-Brochure_English.pdf. [Last accessed July, 2021].
20. Pena-Roses JP, De-Regil LM, Gomez malave H, Flores-Urrutia MC, Dowswell T. Intermittent oral iron supplementation during pregnancy. Cochrane Database Syst Rev. 2015;(10):CD009995.
21. Kaushansky K, Lichtman MA, Prchal JT, Levi MM, Press OW, Burns LJ, Caligiuri M. Williams Hematology, 9th edition. New York: McGraw-Hill Education; 2015.
22. Govindappagari S, Burwick RM. Treatment of iron deficiency anemia in pregnancy with intravenous versus oral iron: Systematic review and meta-analysis. Am J Perinatol. 2019;36(4):366.
23. Reveiz L, Gyte GM, Guervo LG, Casasbuanes A. Treatments for anemia in pregnancy thought to be due to iron deficiency. Cochrane Database Syst Rev. 2011;(10):CD003094.
24. Mishra J, Tomar A, Puri M, Jain A, Saraswathy KN. Trends of folate, vitamin B12, and homocysteine levels in different trimesters of pregnancy and pregnancy outcomes. Am J Hum Biol. 2020;32(5):e23388.
25. Devalia V, Hamilton MS, Molloy AM; British Committee for Standards in Haematology. Guidelines for the diagnosis and treatment of Cobalamin and Folate disorders. Br J Haematol. 2014;166:496-513.
26. Wald NJ, Law MR, Morris JK, Wald DS. Quantifying the effect of folic acid. Lancet. 2001;358(9298):2069-73.
27. Cheschier N. ACOG Committee on Practice Bulletins Obstetrics. ACOG practice bulletin Neural tube defects Number 44, July 2003. Int J Gynaecol Obstet. 2003;83(1):123-33.
28. Mohanty D, Colah RB, Gorakshakar AC, Patel RZ, Master DC, Mahanta J, et al. Prevalence of β-thalassemia and other haemoglobinopathies in six cities in India: A multicentre study. J Community Genet. 2013;4:33-42.
29. Shang X, Xu X. Update in the genetics of Thalassemia: What clinicians need to know. Best Pract Res Clin Obstet Gynaecol. 2017;41(3):174-9.
30. Leung TY, Lao TT. Thalassemia in pregnancy. Best Pract Res Clin Obstet Gynaecol. 2012;26(1):37-51.
31. Cao A, Melis MA, Galanello R, Angius A, Furbetta M, Giordano P, et al. Delta beta (F) thalassemia in Sardinia. J Med Genet. 1982;19(3):182-92.
32. Forget BG. Molecular basis of hereditary persistence of fetal haemoglobin. Ann NY Acad Sci. 1998;850:38-44.
33. Committee Opinion No. 691: Carrier Screening for Genetic Conditions. Obstet Gynecol. 2017;129(3):e41-55.
34. Piplani S, Manan I, Lalit M, Manjari M, Bhasin T, Bawa J. NESTROFT—A valuable, cost effective screening test for beta thalassemia. Trait in north Indian Punjabi population. J Clin Diagn Res. 2013;7(12):2784-7.
35. Li DZ, Yang YD. Invasive prenatal diagnosis of fetal thalassemia. Best Pract Res Clin Obstet Gynaecol. 2017;39:41-52.
36. Leung KY, Cheong KB, Lee CP, Chan V, Lam YH, Tang M. Ultrasonographic prediction of homozygous alpha 0 thalassemia using placental thickness, fetal cardiothoracic ratio, and middle cerebral artery Doppler: alone or in combination? Ultrasound Obstet Gynecol. 2010;35(2):149-54.
37. Traegar-Synodius J. Preimplantation genetic diagnosis. Best Pract Res Clin Obstet Gynaecol. 2017;39:74-88.
38. RCOG. Management of beta thalassemia in pregnancy RCOG Green Top Guideline no. 66. London: Royal College of Obstetricians and Gynaecologists; 2014.
39. RCOG. Management of sickle cell disease in pregnancy. RCOG Green Top guideline no. 61. London: Royal College of Obstetricians and Gynaecologists; 2011.
40. World Health Organization (2002). The clinical use of Blood 2002 [online]. Available from: www.who.int/bloodsafety/clinical_use/en/Manual_EN.pdf. [Last accessed July, 2021].

# Hypertensive Disorders of Pregnancy

*Swati Agrawal, Monika Bhatia, Shubha Sagar Trivedi*

## INTRODUCTION

Hypertension is a common medical disorder that affects up to 10% of all pregnancies and covers a spectrum of conditions namely gestational hypertension, preeclampsia, chronic hypertension, and preeclampsia superimposed on chronic hypertension. They along with hemorrhage and infection contribute greatly to both perinatal and maternal morbidity and mortality worldwide. Approximately, 30% of hypertensive disorders in pregnancy are due to chronic hypertension and 70% are due to gestational hypertension, preeclampsia.[1] The spectrum of gestational hypertension-preeclampsia ranges from mildly elevated blood pressures (BP) with minimal clinical significance to severe hypertension and multiorgan dysfunction. There is no single, reliable, cost-effective screening test for prediction of gestational hypertension-preeclampsia and there are no well-established measures for primary prevention. Delivery remains the ultimate treatment, but expectant management may be chosen depending on gestational age, fetal status, and severity of maternal condition at the time of evaluation. Access to prenatal care, early detection of the disorder, careful monitoring and appropriate management are crucial elements in the prevention of hypertension related morbidity and mortality. This chapter presents the most widely accepted and current understanding on maternal and fetal risks and the management of hypertension in pregnancy.

## DEFINITION

### Hypertension

Hypertension is defined as a diastolic BP of ≥ 90 mm Hg or a systolic BP of ≥ 140 mm Hg or both, documented twice, 4 hours apart. Severe hypertension is defined as systolic BP of ≥160 or diastolic BP ≥ 110 mm Hg, or both, measured on two occasions; and in order not to delay antihypertensive treatment, the BP in the same range after an interval of 15 minutes confirms the diagnosis of severe hypertension.

It is important to take an accurate reading of the BP observing certain precautions as enumerated further.

### Measurement of Blood Pressure[2,3]

- Properly validated and calibrated BP measuring apparatus should be used.
- A range of cuff sizes should be available. Too small a size will overestimate BP; too large will underestimate it.
- Appropriate size cuff with length 1.5 times upper arm circumference or a cuff with a bladder that encircles 80% or more of the arm should be used.
- Measurements should be taken with the patient in a sitting position after a 10-minute or longer period of rest with the arm supported at the heart level. In the recumbent position, BP can be taken in left lateral decubitus position with cuff at the heart level.

### Proteinuria

Abnormal proteinuria in pregnancy is defined as excretion of 300 mg or more protein in urine in 24 hours. The protein excretion may vary through the day. The most accurate measurement of proteinuria is obtained with a 24 hours collection. Another less cumbersome and preferred way of assessing proteinuria is to measure the urinary protein: creatinine ratio or albumin: creatinine ratio. A value of ≥0.3 mg protein/mg creatinine or 8 mg albumin/mmol creatinine have high sensitivity and specificity in diagnosing proteinuria. When semiquantitative dipstick measurement is used, which is less accurate, a value of 1+ or greater signifies proteinuria. Recent NICE guidelines (2019) recommend that if dipstick screening is positive (1+ or more), protein: creatinine (PCR) or albumin: creatinine ratio (ACR) should be done to quantify proteinuria. First morning sample is reported to give a lower diagnostic accuracy and therefore, should not be tested for proteinuria.[4]

Care should be taken to collect a clean sample because blood, vaginal secretions, and bacteria can increase the amount of protein in the urine. Others causes of a false-positive test by dipstick include contamination of the urine by chlorhexidine preparations, very alkaline urine or very concentrated urine (specific gravity > 1.030). On the other hand very dilute urine (specific gravity < 1.010) may produce false-negative results.

## Edema

Though edema has been eliminated as a diagnostic criterion by the modified classification systems because it is very common during pregnancy in the dependent parts, but nondependent edema on face and arms is mostly pathologic. Pregnant woman should be told to report if edema appears on face, abdomen, or hands or it increases suddenly on feet.

## CLASSIFICATION

The classification system of hypertension in pregnancy was proposed originally by the ACOG committee on Terminology in 1972. Further modifications by National High Blood Pressure Education Program (NHBPEP) working group in 2000 arrived at the classification scheme we use today.[5] It was based on four important features—(1) hypertension, (2) proteinuria, (3) onset of hypertension, and (4) persistence of hypertension beyond 12 weeks postpartum. ACOG formulated evidence for hypertension in pregnancy by forming a task force on hypertension, which stressed on multisystemic nature of preeclampsia characterized by hypertension and involvement of one or more other organ systems and or the fetus. The task force has thus eliminated the dependence of proteinuria in the diagnosis of preeclampsia. In the absence of proteinuria, preeclampsia is diagnosed as hypertension in association with thrombocytopenia, impaired liver function tests, new development of renal insufficiency, pulmonary edema, or new onset cerebral or visual disturbances.[6]

The classification is presented in **Box 1**.

Preeclampsia is further classified into mild or nonsevere preeclampsia and preeclampsia with severe features (also called severe preeclampsia). Mild preeclampsia, however, can rapidly progress to the severe form **(Table 1)**.

According to ACOG task force recommendations, massive proteinuria has been eliminated from the consideration of preeclampsia as severe. Oliguria has also been removed as an indicator of severity. As fetal growth restriction is managed similarly in pregnant women with or without preeclampsia, it has been removed as a finding indicative of severe preeclampsia.[6]

## ETIOPATHOGENESIS

The etiologic agent responsible for the development of preeclampsia is unknown. Several theories have been proposed, which include:
- Abnormal cytotrophoblast invasion
- Abnormal or increased immune response
- Endothelial cell injury
- Genetic predisposition
- Abnormal coagulation or thrombophilia
- Alterations in prostaglandin activity
- Alterations in nitric oxide levels
- Increased oxygen-free radicals
- Abnormal calcium metabolism
- Dietary deficiencies.

The condition is characterized by vasospasm, hemoconcentration, and ischemic changes in the placenta, kidney, liver, and brain. Recent studies have suggested that excess secretion of naturally occurring antiangiogenic molecules of placental origin referred to as soluble fms-like tyrosine kinase-1 may contribute to the pathogenesis of

---

**BOX 1:** Classification of hypertension in pregnancy.[2,3]

*Gestational hypertension:* Systolic BP ≥ 140 mm Hg or a diastolic BP ≥ 90, or both on two occasions at least 4 hours apart for the first time after 20 weeks of gestation.
- Distinguished from preeclampsia by the absence of proteinuria and absence of end organ dysfunction
- Working diagnosis only during pregnancy
- Gestational hypertension resolves by 12 weeks postpartum

*Preeclampsia:*
- Hypertension that occurs after 20 weeks of gestation in a woman with previously normal BP. Systolic BP ≥ 140 mm Hg or diastolic BP ≥ 90 mm Hg on two occasions, 4–6 hours apart and
- Proteinuria: Excretion of ≥ 0.3 g protein in a 24 hours urine sample or urine protein: creatinine ratio >0.3 mg/mg or albumin: creatinine ratio > 8 mg/mmol or 1+ on dipstick testing
Or in absence of proteinuria, new onset hypertension with the new onset of any of the following:
  - Thrombocytopenia
  - Renal insufficiency; S. creatinine >1.1 mg/dL or a doubling creatinine in absence of renal disease
  - Impaired liver function: Liver enzymes, ALT, AST, increased more than twice the normal level or right upper quadrant or epigastric pain
  - Pulmonary edema
  - New onset headache not responsive to medication

*Chronic hypertension:*
- Hypertension with onset before pregnancy or before 20 weeks of gestation
- Persistence of hypertension beyond 12 weeks postpartum

*Superimposed preeclampsia-eclampsia:* Preeclampsia or eclampsia that occurs in a woman with pre-existing chronic hypertension

---

**TABLE 1:** Classification of preeclampsia.

| Mild preeclampsia | Preeclampsia with severe features[2] |
|---|---|
| • Blood pressure ≥ 140/90 mm Hg but < 160/110 mm Hg on two occasions at least 4 hours apart<br>• Proteinuria ≥ 300 mg/24 hours<br>• Asymptomatic<br>• No severe features | • Systolic blood pressure ≥ 160 or diastolic ≥ 110 on two occasions 4 hours apart<br>• Thrombocytopenia: (platelets < 100 × 10$^9$/L)<br>• Renal insufficiency: S. creatinine >1.1 mg/dL or a doubling creatinine in absence of renal disease<br>• Impaired liver function, (rise in liver enzymes > 2 times normal) right upper quadrant or epigastric pain<br>• Pulmonary edema<br>• New onset headache not responsive to medication<br>• Visual disturbances |

preeclampsia.[7] This leads to angiogenesis imbalance further leading to failure of trophoblast invasion and physiological remodeling of uterine spiral arteries hampering their normal physiological vasodilatation with resultant placental hypoxia which leads to further increase in fms-like tyrosine kinase-1 and maternal endothelial dysfunction. The vascular endothelium is known to supply all organ systems, and this explains the widespread aspects of the syndrome.

The sequence of events is summarized in **Flowchart 1**.

The pathologic changes seen in various organ systems due to widespread endothelial damage and vasoconstriction are as follows:[8]

- *Brain:* Fibrinoid necrosis, thrombosis, microinfarcts, petechial hemorrhage, cerebral edema, subarachnoid hemorrhage, and intraventricular hemorrhage.
- *Liver:* Sinusoidal fibrin deposition in periportal areas with surrounding hemorrhage and portal capillary thrombi, centrilobular necrosis, and subcapsular hematoma.

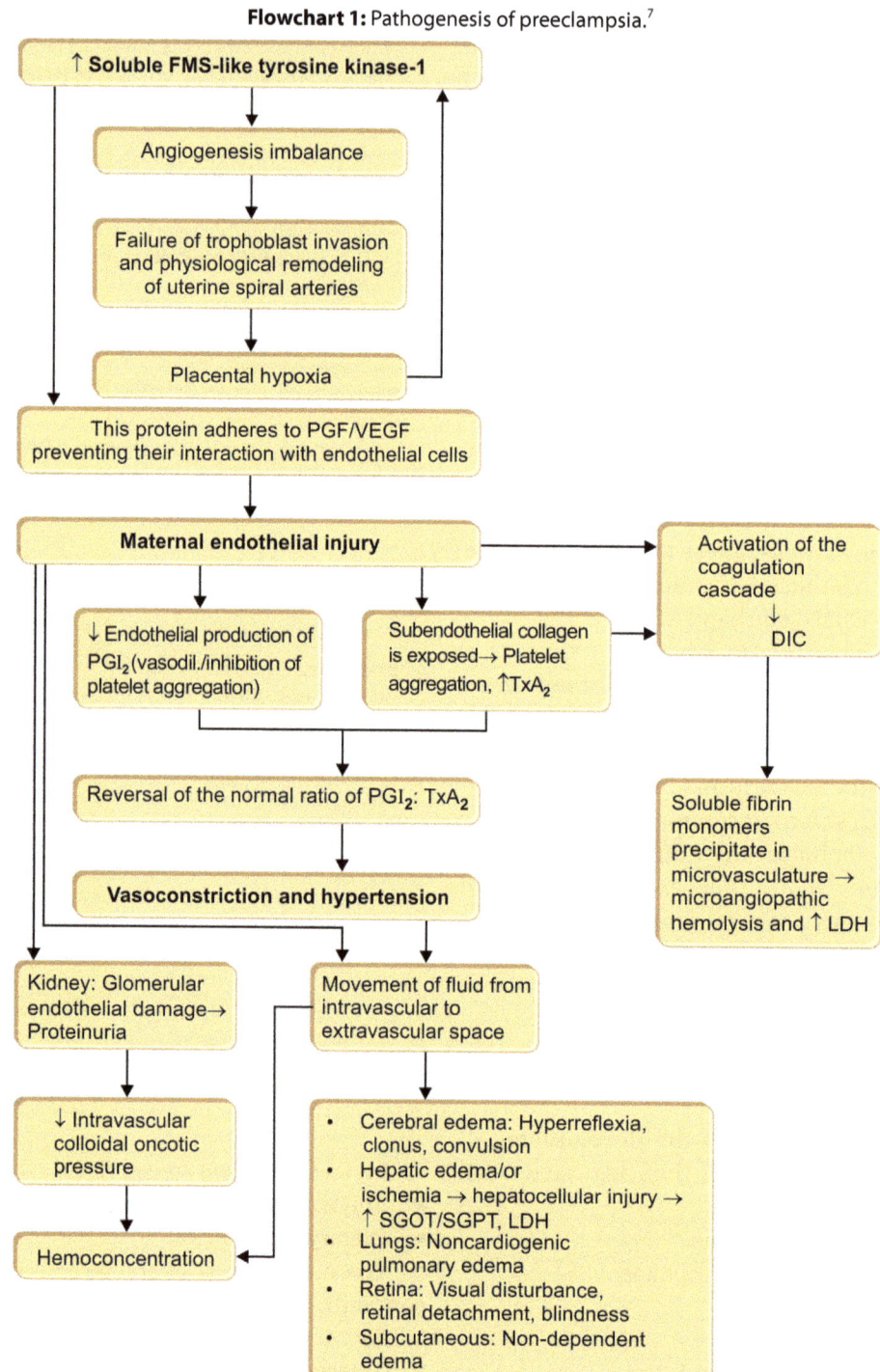

**Flowchart 1:** Pathogenesis of preeclampsia.[7]

(DIC: disseminated intravascular coagulation; LDH: lactic acid dehydrogenase; PGF: prostaglandin F; $PGI_2$: prostacyclin; SGOT: serum glutamic-oxaloacetic transaminase; SGPT: serum glutamic pyruvic transaminase; vasodil.: vasodilation; VEGF: vascular endothelial growth factor)

- *Kidney:* Glomerulo-endotheliosis, i.e., swelling and enlargement of glomerular capillary endothelial cells.
- *Eyes:* Retinal vasospasm, retinal edema, retinal detachment.
- *Cardiovascular system:* Absence of normal intravascular volume expansion, hemoconcentration, and loss of normal refractoriness to endogenous vasopressors including angiotensin II.
- *Uteroplacental circulation:* Acute atherosis, endothelial cell damage, basement membrane disruption, mural thrombi, and increase in smooth muscle cells with vasospasm that leads to a decreased vessel lumen.

## PREDICTION

Many clinical, biophysical, hematological, and biochemical tests have been used for prediction of preeclampsia. An ideal predictive test should be simple, noninvasive, rapid, inexpensive, easy to perform early in pregnancy and reproducible with high sensitivity and predictive value. Currently there is no single screening test for preeclampsia that is reliable, valid, and cost effective.[6] An accurate and thorough maternal history with identification of risk factors (**Box 2**) is a cost-effective screening method.

The various tests which have been used for prediction are as follows:

### Biophysical Tests

- Roll over test
- Angiotensin II infusion test
- Isometric exercise
- Uterine artery Doppler
- Mid-pregnancy mean arterial pressure (MAP).

### Hematological and Biochemical

- Increased maternal serum uric acid
- Elevated second trimester MSAFP/ß-hCG
- Decreased urinary calcium excretion
- Higher fasting insulin levels
- Serum placental growth factor (PLGF).

A recent FIGO initiative on preeclampsia suggests routine first trimester screening by maternal factors and MAP in all pregnancies, and if found to be at high risk for preterm preeclampsia and resources permit, PLGF and uterine artery pulsatility index (UTPI) may be measured at 11–14 weeks of gestation. The risk calculator is available free at https://fetalmedicine.org/research/assess/preeclampsia.[9]

## PREVENTION

The observed alteration in the ratio of vasoconstrictive and vasodilatory prostaglandins in preeclampsia led

> **BOX 2:** Risk factors for preeclampsia.
> - History of preeclampsia in previous pregnancies
> - Diabetes mellitus
> - Obesity
> - Renal disease
> - Thyroid disease
> - Collagen vascular disease
> - Antiphospholipid syndrome
> - Thrombophilia
> - Fetal triploidy
> - Poor outcome in previous pregnancy like fetal growth restriction, intrauterine death
> - History of placental abruption
> - Multiple gestations
> - Chronic hypertension
> - Trophoblastic disease
> - Age < 20 years or > 40 years
> - Maternal body mass index > 35 kg/m$^2$
> - Nulliparity
> - Family history of preeclampsia

the investigators to study different approaches for the prevention of preeclampsia including use of low-dose aspirin, calcium, and magnesium supplements, a low-salt diet and antioxidants. Calcium is essential in the synthesis of nitric oxide, a potent vasodilator believed to contribute to the maintenance of reduced vascular tone in pregnancy. Calcium supplementation may offer protection for calcium-deficient women, but there is no benefit in patients with adequate daily calcium intake.[10] According to the latest SOGC guidelines, calcium supplementation of at least 1 g/day, orally is recommended for women with low-dietary intake of calcium (< 600 mg/day).[11] Low-dose aspirin, which reverses the imbalance between vasoconstrictor thromboxane A2 and the vasodilator prostacyclin have been tried but there has been conflicting evidence regarding its use. A recent systematic review concluded that there is a small to moderate benefit of low aspirin in preventing preeclampsia in women at high risk such as those with a history of chronic hypertension and preeclampsia in a previous pregnancy.[12]

The FIGO recommends aspirin prophylaxis commencing at 11 to $14^{+6/7}$ weeks of gestation at a dose of ~150 mg in women found to be at high risk following first-trimester screening for preterm PE.[9]

The NICE advocates 75–150 mg aspirin daily from 12 weeks until birth of the baby if high-risk factors for preeclampsia are present.[4]

The ACOG (2020) recommends low dose aspirin, 81 mg/day between 12 and 28 weeks, preferably before 16th week of pregnancy till delivery in a woman with any of the high-risk factors such as preeclampsia in previous pregnancy, multifetal pregnancy, renal disease, autoimmune disease, diabetes mellitus, type 1 or type 2, chronic hypertension or with more than one moderate risk factor like first pregnancy, maternal age of 35 years or older, body mass index of >30, family history of preeclampsia.[2]

Initial promising data related to a potential benefit of antioxidants (vitamins C and E) is not supported by the Cochrane review.[13]

## MANAGEMENT

The only definitive therapy for gestational hypertension/preeclampsia is delivery.

In case of preterm pregnancies, the main objective of expectant management is to improve neonatal outcome if the risks for the mother and child remain acceptable. The decision between delivery and expectant management depends on fetal gestational age, fetal status and severity of maternal condition at the time of evaluation. Management plan for mild and severe preeclampsia has been illustrated in **Flowcharts 2 and 3**, respectively.

### Goals of Management

- Prevention of convulsions.
- Prevention of complications like cerebrovascular hemorrhage, pulmonary edema, renal failure, placental abruption, intrauterine death of fetus.
- Delivering a surviving baby with minimal maternal trauma.

### Assessment

Women with hypertension ≥140/90 with or without proteinuria should be admitted to the hospital and evaluated for the severity of new onset hypertension. After serial assessment, the setting for continued management can be determined. Those with mild gestational hypertension/preeclampsia who are remote from term, outpatient management may be an option. Among those with severe disease remote from term, some women will stabilize and would be eligible for expectant management. Conversely, some others will have rapid deterioration of the maternal/fetal condition that will necessitate expeditious delivery regardless of the gestational age.

After admission, the first step is to evaluate the maternal and fetal status.

#### Maternal Evaluation

Includes taking a complete history including evaluation of end organ damage if any, general physical examination, obstetric examination, laboratory evaluation including hematocrit, platelet count, liver function tests, serum creatinine, uric acid, coagulation studies, 24 hours urinary protein and fundus examination.

#### Fetal Evaluation

History of decreased fetal movements and on obstetric examination, evaluation of symphysio-fundal height, abdominal girth, amount of liquor, estimated fetal weight, and fetal heart sounds is done. Nonstress test (NST), biophysical profile (BPP) (after 28–30 weeks of gestation), USG for fetal weight and amount of liquor, umbilical artery Doppler waveform in suspected fetal growth restriction are done to assess the fetus.

### Expectant Management

In patients diagnosed with gestational hypertension/preeclampsia at term, i.e., with gestational period ≥37 weeks, the general consensus is to deliver the woman. For the patient who is preterm (<37 weeks), controversy arises regarding management with respect to the level of activity allowed, hospitalization, administration of antihypertensive medication and anticonvulsants. Usually, patients with mild disease do not require immediate delivery and expectant management is advocated.

Patients with severe preeclampsia at 23–34 weeks gestation receive individualized treatment, including timing of delivery based on their assessment.

### Outpatient Management/Hospitalization

Most of the women with preeclampsia are admitted to hospital. Hospitalization of the woman allows rapid intervention in case of fulminant progression to hypertensive crisis, eclampsia, or abruption placentae. These complications are, however, rare in women who have mild disease. Outpatient management at home or at a day care unit has been evaluated as an option for monitoring women with mild gestational hypertension or mild preeclampsia remote from term. A number of studies suggest that there is a place for ambulatory management in carefully selected women.[14] Thus, women with mild disease who are compliant, asymptomatic, have normal laboratory results and have readily available round the clock transportation facility can be managed in an ambulatory setting. Such management should include frequent maternal and fetal evaluation and access to health care providers. At the time of initial and subsequent visits, the women should be educated and instructed to immediately report to the hospital in case they develop any of the warning symptoms like nausea, vomiting, persistent severe headache, right upper quadrant pain, epigastric pain, scotoma or blurred vision, decreased fetal movements, bleeding or leaking per vaginum or labor pains.

Indicators of disease progression evident on BP records and laboratory tests or on fetal surveillance such as fetal compromise like fetal growth restriction or oligohydramnios, are not suitable for ambulatory management.

Hospitalization is indicated in patients with severe gestational hypertension/preeclampsia and management is best accomplished in a tertiary care setting.

### Surveillance

During expectant management close monitoring of both mother and fetus is initiated by evaluating the clinical symptoms, signs and laboratory findings and the decision to continue pregnancy must be re-evaluated daily. The frequency of testing depends on the severity of disease and its progression.

*Maternal surveillance:* Includes monitoring for clinical symptoms like headache, blurring of vision, epigastric pain, nausea, vomiting, decrease in urine output, and shortness of breath. Blood pressure should be measured every 4–6 hours. Daily fluid intake output should be recorded. Serial assessment of complete blood count, liver function tests, and kidney function test should be performed weekly in case of mild disease with no progression, sooner if the disease progression is questionable and every other day or daily in case of severe disease. Clotting studies are not required if platelet count is more than 100,000/mm$^3$ and liver enzymes are normal.[15]

*Fetal surveillance:* The woman is instructed to keep a daily fetal movement count. Weekly symphysio-fundal height and abdominal girth is charted. NST for fetal well-being is done weekly in mild disease, twice weekly for suspected growth restriction or oligohydramnios and alternate day or daily for severe disease depending upon the progression of the disease with weekly amniotic fluid index (AFI) determinations. Ultrasound examination for fetal growth is done every 3–4 weeks in mild disease and every 2–3 weeks in severe disease. Umbilical artery Doppler is done depending upon the presence and severity of fetal growth restriction.

## Antenatal Steroids

In attempts to enhance fetal lung maturation glucocorticoids have been administered to women with severe hypertension who are <34 weeks of gestation. If early birth is anticipated, within 7 days, in women with preeclampsia, antenatal corticosteroids should be offered.[4] A course of corticosteroids for fetal lung maturity does not worsen maternal hypertension and a reduction in the incidence of respiratory distress and intraventricular hemorrhage and improved fetal survival has been found.[16]

## Bed Rest

Complete or partial bed rest for the duration of pregnancy was recommended in the past for women with gestational hypertension/preeclampsia. However, various studies have shown that strict bed rest in the hospital for pregnant women with preeclampsia does not appear to lower rates of perinatal morbidity and mortality including preterm birth, endotracheal intubations, or neonatal intensive care unit (NICU) admissions.[17] On the other hand prolonged bed rest for the duration of pregnancy increases the risk of thromboembolism. Thus, women with proteinuric or non-proteinuric hypertension are instructed to restrict their activity, not complete bedrest.

## Antihypertensives

Antihypertensive therapy is used to protect the mother from effects of severe hypertension such as cerebrovascular hemorrhage, cardiac failure, abruption, and eclampsia.

There has been a clear consensus that antihypertensives should be prescribed when systolic BP is ≥ 160 mm Hg or diastolic BP is ≥ 110 mm Hg.[2-4] It has also been observed that antihypertensive therapy in women with BP below the severe range or MAP < 125 mm Hg decreases the maternal risk.[18]

The value of antihypertensives in mild to moderate disease (diastolic BP 90–109 mm Hg) has not been very clear. Maternal death and stroke are rare and eclampsia is unusual in these women. Various researchers have used antihypertensive drugs for mild hypertension.

As per SOGC (2014) clinical practice guidelines, in women with non-severe hypertension without comorbidities antihypertensive drug therapy may be used to keep systolic BP at 130 to 155 mm Hg and diastolic BP at 80–105 mm Hg, and in women with nonsevere hypertension with comorbidities to less than 140/90 mm Hg.[11]

An updated Cochrane systemic review (2018) concluded that antihypertensive drug therapy for mild to moderate hypertension during pregnancy reduces the risk of severe hypertension but the effect on other clinically important outcomes remains unclear.[19]

The CHIPS publications have provided evidence that women with non-severe pregnancy hypertension should receive "tight" BP control achieved by a simple algorithm.[20]

Recent NICE (2019) guidelines advocate that antihypertensives should be offered if BP remains above 140/90 mm Hg and aim should be to keep the BP at 135/85 mm Hg or less.[4]

A step-wise approach to the use of antihypertensives is required.
- First line can be labetalol
- Second line is usually nifedipine
- Third line is methyldopa.

A suitable regime is labetalol, 100–200 mg twice daily, increasing to 300 mg four times daily if required. If BP is not controlled, then nifedipine is added. Such therapy is usually sufficient; if BP is not adequately controlled on this combination, the disease is usually sufficiently advanced to warrant delivery. However, occasionally a third line agent is required. In this situation, methyldopa is added at a dose of 250 mg two to three times daily increasing up to 500 mg four times a day. ACE inhibitors and adrenoreceptor blockers (ARBs) must not be used antenatally especially during second and third trimester. Reported complications with ACE inhibitors include oligohydramnios, fetal growth restriction, bony malformations, limb contractures, persistent patent ductus arteriosus, pulmonary hypoplasia, respiratory distress syndrome, prolonged neonatal hypertension, and neonatal death.[21]

| TABLE 2: Antihypertensive drugs for nonemergency oral treatment. | | | | |
|---|---|---|---|---|
| BP medication | Dosage | Maximum dose | Benefits | Adverse effects |
| Labetalol (α and β) blocker-reduction in cardiac output) | 100 mg po bid | 2400 mg/24 h | Effective BP control; lowers BP without altering cerebral autoregulation; lower risk of arrhythmia than with vasodilatory agents | • Fetal bradycardia, neonatal hypoglycemia, impaired fetal response to hypoxia, decreased uteroplacental flow<br>• Labetalol should be avoided in patients with:<br>  – Asthma<br>  – Heart disease<br>  – Heart block, bradycardia<br>  – Congestive heart failure |
| Nifedipine (calcium channel blocker-inhibits extracellular calcium influx into cells through slow calcium channels) | 10–20 mg oral q 4–6 hours | 120–180 mg/24 h | Effective for refractory hypertension, potent tocolysis in preterm labor; lowers BP without effects on blood flow in the umbilical artery | Maternal side effects—flushing headache palpitations; interaction with magnesium-sulfate: profound hypotension; no increased risk of congenital malformations |
| Methyldopa ($\alpha_2$-Adrenergic agonists- central inhibition of sympathetic drive) | 250–500 mg po q 6–12 h | 2–3 g/24 h | Proven to be safe, and efficacious; decreased second-trimester fetal losses | Maternal fatigue, depression, orthostatic hypotension, xerostomia, elevated liver enzymes (5–10%) |

The **Table 2** summarizes the various antihypertensive drugs used for long-term non-emergency oral treatment.

## Treatment of Acute Severe Hypertension

Oral or intravenous therapy can be decided on the basis of the presentation.

Antihypertensive treatment should be initiated as soon as possible for acute-onset severe hypertension (systolic BP of ≥ 160 mm Hg or diastolic BP of ≥ 110 mm Hg or both) that is confirmed as persistent (repeat BP taken 15 minutes or more later).[2]

Rapid but controlled reduction in BP using intravenous medication is required. The objective of treating acute severe hypertension is to prevent potential cerebrovascular and cardiovascular complications such as encephalopathy, hemorrhage and congestive heart failure. Agents used for treatment of acute severe hypertension should be initiated at low doses, given that women with preeclampsia are intravascular volume depleted and are at increased risk for hypotension. Acute-onset, severe hypertension that is persistent for 15 minutes or more is considered a hypertensive emergency and can cause central nervous system injury.

The aim of treatment is not to lower the BP to normal, but to bring it in a range of 140-150/90-100 mm Hg so as to prevent repeated, prolonged exposure to severe systolic hypertension, which can cause loss of cerebral vasculature autoregulation.[22]

Acute severe hypertension may be treated with parenteral labetalol or hydralazine or oral nifedipine. Oral nifedipine is useful as it can be given immediately in absence of an intravenous line. Immediate release oral nifedipine should not be given sublingually because of risk of hypotension. Nifedipine has been associated with an increase in maternal heart rate, and less risk of overshoot hypotension. Intravenous nitroglycerin (glyceryl trinitrate) is recommended as the first-line choice for treatment of pulmonary edema associated with preeclampsia.[23]

**Table 3** depicts the therapeutic options in the treatment of acute severe hypertension.

Regimes have been described with parenteral labetalol, parenteral hydralazine, and oral nifedipine as first line drugs, respectively.[3]

- In case the BP remains uncontrolled despite giving all the medications in either of the regimens, emergent consultation with an anesthesiologist, maternal-fetal medicine subspecialist, or critical care subspecialist is done to discuss second-line intervention.
- Second-line agents to consider in such emergencies include nicardipine or esmolol by infusion pump or IV enalapril.[3]
- Induction of general anesthesia and intubation should not be undertaken without first taking steps to eliminate or minimize the hypertensive response to intubation.[22]
- The BP and pulse rate should initially be monitored every 5 minutes till BP is in range of 140-150/90-100 and then every 10 minutes for 1 hour, every 15-30 minutes for 2 hours and then every hour for 4 hours.
- Parenteral antihypertensive therapy may be needed initially for acute control of BP, and if expectant management is to be continued then oral medications is used for control of BP.

Oral labetalol and calcium channel blockers can be used. One approach is to begin an initial regimen of labetalol at 200 mg orally every 12 hours and increase the dose up to 800 mg orally every 8-12 hours as needed (maximum total 2,400 mg/d). If the maximum dose is inadequate to achieve

**TABLE 3:** Treatment of acute severe hypertension.

| Medication | Onset of action | Dosage | Adverse effects |
|---|---|---|---|
| Labetalol | 5 minutes | 20 mg IV bolus then 40 mg after 10 minutes, then 80 mg every 10 minutes up to a maximum total dose of 300 mg, a continuous infusion of 1–2 mg/min may also be used | See **Table 2** |
| Nifedipine | 10 minutes | 10 mg orally can be repeated in 30 minutes, then 10–20 mg q4–6 h with a maximum dose of 180 mg/24 hours[22] | See **Table 2** |
| Nitroglycerin | 1–3 minutes | Initial infusion rate of 10 µg/min and titrated to the desired pressure by doubling the dose every 5 minutes | Methemoglobinemia may result from high dose IV infusion |
| Hydralazine | 10–20 minutes | 5–10 mg IV every 15–20 minutes until a desired response is obtained (Consider using up to 500 mL crystalloid fluid before or at the time of first dose of hydralazine in antenatal period)[10] | Profound maternal hypotension and oliguria, fetal distress; maternal pyridoxine-responsive polyneuropathy and drug-induced lupus, neonatal thrombocytopenia and lupus |
| Sodium nitroprusside* | 0.5–5 minutes | 0.2–5 µg/kg/min infusion; for use in refractory hypertension | Fetal cyanide and thiocyanate toxicity |

*ACOG (2019)[22] recommends that sodium nitroprusside should be reserved for extreme emergencies and used for the shortest amount of time possible because of concerns about cyanide and thiocyanate toxicity in the mother and fetus or newborn, and increased intracranial pressure with potential worsening of cerebral edema in the mother.

the desired BP goal, or the dosage is limited by adverse effect, then short-acting oral nifedipine can be added gradually.[2]

## Anticonvulsants

Magnesium sulfate is the drug of choice to treat and prevent convulsions in women with eclampsia/preeclampsia. The rate of seizures in women with mild preeclampsia not receiving magnesium sulfate is very low, about 1 in 200 and as such the benefit to risk ratio does not support the routine use of magnesium sulfate in mild preeclampsia. Women with severe preeclampsia and those with features of imminent eclampsia are the best candidates to receive magnesium sulfate prophylaxis as the number needed to be treated to prevent one case of eclampsia is 36. Most authorities now recommend prophylactic magnesium sulfate in all women with severe preeclampsia once a delivery decision has been made and in the immediate postpartum period especially if there is concern about the risk of eclampsia.[2,13] As per NICE Guidelines (2019), magnesium sulfate treatment should be considered if there is ongoing or recurring severe headaches, visual scotomata, nausea or vomiting, epigastric pain, oliguria or severe hypertension or deterioration in laboratory parameters such as thrombocytopenia rise in liver enzymes or creatinine. Serum magnesium levels need to be monitored if serum creatinine is more than 1 mg/dL.

The various regimens are discussed in section on eclampsia.

## Delivery: Indications and Timing

### Mild Disease

In general, women with mild disease developing at 37 weeks gestation or later have a pregnancy outcome similar to that found in normotensive pregnancy. Thus, those who have a favorable cervix should undergo induction of labor and delivery. In addition, cervical ripening with prostaglandins and induction of labor can be used in women with an unfavorable cervix at 37 weeks or more because the mother is at slightly increased risk for development of abruptio placentae and progression to severe disease. ACOG (2019) recommends delivery at 37 week gestation or later, if diagnosed later.[24] Earlier delivery is indicated, if there is nonreassuring fetal status, worsening preeclampsia or hypertension or there is rupture of membranes.

### Severe Disease

The presence of severe disease mandates immediate hospitalization. The maternal and fetal condition is assessed, and a decision is made regarding the need for delivery. Patients with gestational age below 23 weeks should be counseled and offered termination of pregnancy in view of poor prognosis. Patients at 33–34 weeks are given corticosteroids and then delivered after 48 hours. Patients with gestational ages of 23–32 weeks should receive individualized treatment based on their clinical response during 24 hours observation period. If BP is adequately controlled and fetal tests are reassuring, the patients are observed closely in the antepartum high-risk ward until 34 weeks gestation or till development of a maternal or fetal indication for delivery as enumerated in **Box 3**.[25]

### Mode of Delivery

In women with gestational hypertension/preeclampsia without contraindications to labor, vaginal delivery is the preferred approach. Cervical ripening agents and oxytocin are used as needed. BP stabilization prior to induction should be done. The decision to perform cesarean delivery

> **BOX 3:** Indications for delivery in severe preeclampsia.
>
> *Maternal indications:*
> - Uncontrolled severe hypertension
> - Eclampsia
> - HELLP syndrome
> - Persistent oliguria
> - Abruptio placentae
> - Platelet count < 100,000/mm$^3$
> - Elevated liver enzymes with or without epigastric pain or right upper quadrant tenderness
> - Pulmonary edema
> - Persistent severe headache or visual changes
> - Fetal death
> - Spontaneous labor
> - Rupture of membranes
> - Gestational age ≥ 34 weeks
>
> *Fetal indications:*
> - Repetitive decelerations
> - Biophysical score < 4 on two occasions 4 hours apart
> - Estimated fetal weight < 5th percentile
> - Reversed end diastolic flow
> - Severe oligohydramnios
>
> (HELLP: hemolysis, elevated liver enzymes, low platelet count)

should be individualized and based on gestational age, maternal and fetal condition, presence of labor, and Bishop score. Cesarean section is reserved for cases in which the maternal and fetal conditions are adverse and deteriorating and for patients with preterm gestation and an unripe cervix. Regional anesthesia is preferred in the absence of coagulopathy. General anesthesia increases the risk of aspiration and failed intubation due to airway edema and is associated with marked increase in systemic and cerebral pressures during intubation and extubation. If general anesthesia is given, then antihypertensive therapy should be used before intubation to prevent further increase in BP during intubation.[15]

### Intrapartum Management

The goals of treatment of women with gestational hypertension/preeclampsia are early detection of fetal heart rate abnormalities, early detection of progression from mild to severe disease and prevention of maternal complications. Therefore, all these women should receive continuous fetal heart rate monitoring with special attention to hyperstimulation and development of vaginal bleeding during labor. BP should be recorded every hour and in cases with severe hypertension, every 10-15 minutes until BP is less than 160/110 mm Hg.

Women should be assessed about the new onset of symptoms suggesting severe disease. Maternal pain relief during labor and delivery can be provided by systemic analgesics or epidural analgesia. A strict intake output record should be maintained, and rate of intravenous fluids should not exceed 100 mL/hour to avoid pulmonary edema. Invasive hemodynamic monitoring may be used in women with preeclampsia who have severe cardiac/renal disease, pulmonary edema, refractory hypertension or oliguria not responding to fluid challenge. The control of acute severe hypertension and use of magnesium sulfate during labor and 24 hours postpartum in all women with severe preeclampsia has been discussed earlier.

Third stage of labor should be actively managed with oxytocin 5 units intravenous or 10 units intramuscularly and ergometrine should not be given to woman with any hypertensive disorder.[11]

## CARE FOLLOWING DELIVERY

During the immediate postpartum period, women with preeclampsia should receive close monitoring of BP and those with symptoms consistent with severe disease and imminent eclampsia, accurate measurements of fluid intake and urine output is indicated as there is mobilization of extracellular fluid leading to increased intravascular volume for the first 24–48 hours. As a result, these women especially those with abnormal renal function and capillary leaks are at increased risk for pulmonary edema and exacerbation of severe hypertension. In general, most women with gestational hypertension become normotensive during the first week following delivery whereas those with preeclampsia take a longer time to resolve. The antihypertensive regime used antenatally can be continued and dose adjusted, and a second line agent is introduced as required to control the BP. As the BP settles, the drugs are gradually tapered and then withdrawn under supervision usually as an outpatient. Calcium channel blockers are most commonly used as methyldopa has unwanted side effects like postpartum depression. Methyldopa should be stopped within 2 days of delivery and an alternative antihypertensive should be given, if necessary.[4]

Blood pressure is monitored 1-2 times per week. If hypertension persists beyond 12 weeks postpartum, the patient is classified as having chronic hypertension and referred to a specialist for investigation to rule out any underlying medical condition such as renal disease and followed up accordingly. The women have to be explained about the risk of recurrence. The earlier preeclampsia is diagnosed during index pregnancy the greater the likelihood of recurrence. The risk in nullipara where diagnosis is made before 30 weeks it is up to 40%, it is 23% if diagnosis is made at 37 weeks and in HELLP syndrome it is 5-26%.[26]

## LONG-TERM COMPLICATIONS

The long-term cardiovascular prognosis depends on whether preeclampsia has occurred in nulliparous or multiparous women, as the risk of chronic hypertension and death related to hypertension has been found to be increased in multiparous women. Those with recurrent pregnancy induced hypertension are at increased risk for chronic

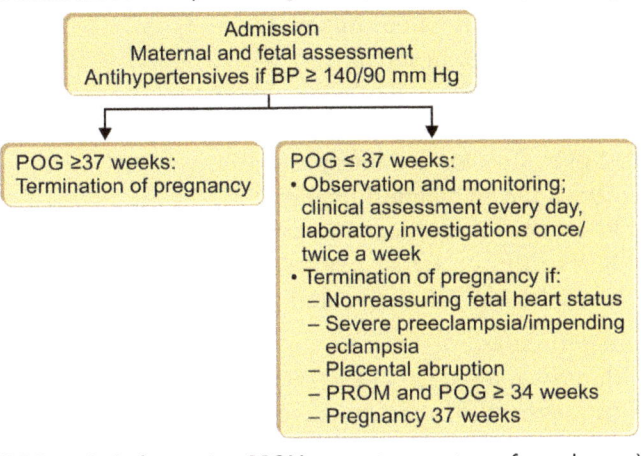

**Flowchart 2:** Summary of management protocol of mild preeclampsia.

(POG: period of gestation; PROM: premature rupture of membranes)

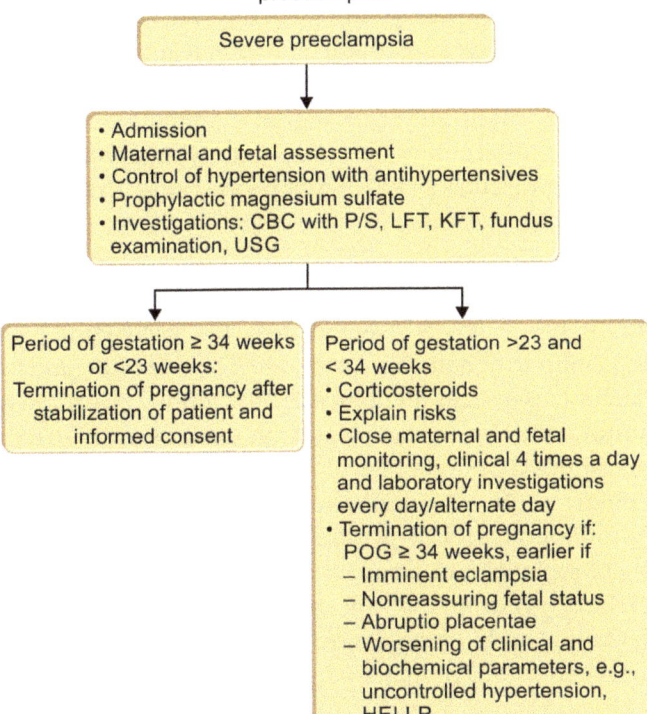

**Flowchart 3:** Summary of management protocol of severe preeclampsia.

(CBC: complete blood count; LFT: liver function test; KFT: kidney function test; HELLP: hemolysis, elevated liver enzymes, low platelet count; POG: period of gestation; USG: ultrasonography)

hypertension whereas those who remained normotensive during subsequent pregnancy are at decreased risk.[26]

## SUMMARY OF MANAGEMENT PROTOCOLS

Summary of management protocols of mild and severe gestational hypertension/preeclampsia is presented in **Flowcharts 2 and 3**.[27]

## ECLAMPSIA

Eclampsia is defined as the development of convulsions and/or unexplained coma during pregnancy or postpartum in patients with signs and symptoms of preeclampsia. The estimated incidence of eclampsia is 1–3 per 1,000 preeclamptic patients. It continues to be a major cause of maternal and perinatal morbidity and mortality worldwide. The maternal mortality rate is 4.2%. The perinatal mortality rate is higher ranging from 13 to 30%. It occurs more commonly near term. Eclampsia can occur antepartum (50%), intrapartum (25%), or postpartum (25%) but when the first convulsion occurs more than 48 hours postpartum, other causes should be excluded.

### Clinical Course

The usual clinical presentation is development of classical prodrome of headache, epigastric pain, visual disturbance followed by convulsions on a background of variable signs and symptoms of preeclampsia. However, the signs and symptoms of preeclampsia are not necessary for the development of convulsions. Complications include placental abruption, neurological deficits, aspiration pneumonia, pulmonary edema, cardiopulmonary arrest, acute renal failure, and maternal death.

### Differential Diagnosis

Other causes of convulsions which are enumerated below must be considered in the differential diagnoses depending upon the clinical presentation:
- Epilepsy
- Intracranial hemorrhage
- Meningitis
- Encephalitis
- Thrombosis
- Rupture of cerebral aneurysm
- Cerebral tumor.

### Management

Definitive treatment of eclampsia includes the following:
- *Avoidance of injury:*
  - Padded bedside rails
  - Physical restraints
  - Padded tongue blade
- *Maintenance of oxygenation to mother and fetus:*
  - Oxygen at 8–10 L/min by face mask.
  - Monitor oxygenation by transcutaneous pulse oximetry and metabolic status with arterial blood gas measurement.
- *Minimize aspiration:*
  - Lateral decubitus position
  - Suctioning of vomitus and oral secretion
- *Initiate magnesium sulfate treatment to prevent recurrent seizures*
- *Control severe hypertension*
- *Stabilize maternal condition*
- *Initiate the delivery process.*

Vaginal delivery is the preferred route after an eclamptic seizure. Cesarean delivery should be performed for obstetric indications only. Induction of labor should be performed with oxytocin or prostaglandins. Magnesium sulfate is the drug of choice and has been shown to be superior to both phenytoin and diazepam for the prevention of eclamptic seizures.[28] The exact mechanism of action is unclear but it appears to have a peripheral action at the neuromuscular junction.

Magnesium sulfate dosing schedules which are used for severe preeclampsia and eclampsia include:

*Continuous intravenous infusion:*
- Give 4-6 g loading dose of magnesium sulfate diluted in 100 mL of IV fluid administered over 15-20 minutes.
- Begin 1-2 g/hour in 100 mL of IV maintenance infusion.
- Measure serum magnesium level at 4-6 hours and adjust infusion to maintain levels between 4 and 7 mEq/L (4.8-8.4 mg/dL).
- Magnesium sulfate is discontinued 24 hours after delivery.

*Intermittent intramuscular injections:*
- Give 4 g of magnesium sulfate ($MgSO_4 \cdot 7H_2O$ USP) as a 20% solution intravenously at a rate not to exceed 1 g/min.
- Follow promptly with 10 g of 50% magnesium sulfate solution, one half (5 g) injected deeply in the upper outer quadrant of both buttocks through a 3 inch long, 20 gauge needle (addition of 1.0 mL of 2% lignocaine minimizes discomfort).
  - If convulsions persist after 15 minutes, give 2 g more intravenously as a 20% solution at a rate not to exceed 1 g/min. If the woman is large, up to 4 g may be given slowly.
  - Every 4 hours thereafter, give 5 g of a 50% solution of magnesium sulfate injected deeply in the upper outer quadrant of alternate buttocks, but only after ensuring that:
    - Patellar reflex is present
    - Respiration is not depressed
    - Urine output in the last 4 hours exceeded 100 mL
    - Magnesium sulfate is discontinued 24 hours after delivery or after the last fit, whichever is later.

Patients receiving magnesium sulfate are at increased risk of postpartum hemorrhage due to uterine atony. This should be anticipated and blood should be cross matched. Patients should be monitored for signs of magnesium toxicity throughout the course of administration. The serum magnesium levels and associated clinical findings are as given below:

- 4.8-8.4 mg/dL: Therapeutic level
- 8-12 mg/dL: Loss of patellar reflex
- 15-17 mg/dL: Respiratory depression
- 30-35 mg/dL: Cardiac arrest.

If a patient develops signs of magnesium toxicity the following steps should be initiated:
- Stop magnesium sulfate
- Begin supplemental oxygen administration
- Give calcium gluconate, 10 cc of 10% calcium gluconate, (1 g) by slow intravenous push
- Check serum magnesium level
- Repeat calcium gluconate administration, if necessary
- If respiratory arrest occurs, begin cardiopulmonary resuscitation, intubation and ventilation.

*Refractory cases:*
- Rarely a patient may be refractory to magnesium sulfate, i.e., she continues to have convulsions even after 20-30 minutes of loading dose or has more than two recurrences.
- In such cases, under careful monitoring, administration of sodium amobarbital, (250 mg IV in 3 minutes) or thiopental, or phenytoin, (1,250 mg IV at a rate of 50 mg/min) has been advocated.[2] Endotracheal intubation and assisted ventilation in the intensive care unit is required in these cases. Full neurological examination should be done as there may be some underlying pathology, or cerebrovascular accident may be the cause. Urgent head imaging is indicated in these cases.

## HELLP SYNDROME

HELLP syndrome is used to describe preeclampsia in association with hemolysis, elevated liver enzymes, and low platelet count. The incidence is 10% among pregnancies complicated by preeclampsia. It is a severe form of preeclampsia and may develop in patients with only mild to moderate BP elevations and occasionally in the absence of proteinuria. HELLP syndrome develops antepartum in 70% of patients and postpartum in the rest. The hallmark of HELLP syndrome is liver involvement that may lead to liver failure and in most severe cases, liver rupture, which is associated with high maternal and fetal mortality rates.

### Criteria for Diagnosis of HELLP Syndrome[29]

- *Hemolysis:*
  - Abnormal peripheral smear
  - Lactate dehydrogenase > 600 U/L
  - Serum bilirubin >1.2 mg/dL
- *Elevated liver enzyme levels:* Serum aspartate aminotransferase >70 U/L
- *Low platelets:* Platelet count < 100,000/mm$^3$.

### Clinical Features

The clinical picture is highly variable, the signs, and symptoms include the following:[30,31]
- Right upper quadrant pain or epigastric pain (86-90%)
- Nausea or vomiting (45-84%)
- Headache (50%)

- Right upper quadrant tenderness on palpation (86%)
- Diastolic BP ≥ 110 mm Hg (67%)
- Proteinuria greater than 2+ on dipstick (85-96%)
- Edema (55-67%).

Hypertension may be absent in as many as 20% of patients. HELLP syndrome is associated with an increased risk of many adverse outcomes including complications like abruption, pulmonary edema, adult respiratory distress syndrome, ruptured liver hematoma, acute renal failure, disseminated intravascular coagulation (DIC), eclampsia, intracerebral hemorrhage, and maternal death. It needs to be differentiated from other conditions which might have overlapping features as given below.

## Differential Diagnosis of HELLP Syndrome[29]
- Acute fatty liver of pregnancy
- Appendicitis
- Cerebral hemorrhage
- Diabetes insipidus
- Gallbladder disease
- Gastroenteritis
- Glomerulonephritis
- Hemolytic uremic syndrome
- Hyperemesis gravidarum
- Idiopathic thrombocytopenia
- Pancreatitis
- Pyelonephritis
- Systemic lupus erythematosus
- Thrombophilias
- Thrombotic thrombocytopenic purpura
- Viral hepatitis including herpes.

## Management

The clinical course of women with HELLP syndrome is usually characterized by progressive and sometimes sudden deterioration in maternal and fetal condition. Therefore, patients with suspected diagnosis of HELLP syndrome should be hospitalized immediately.

Management includes the same principles of treatment as for severe preeclampsia.
- The first priority is to assess and stabilize the maternal condition particularly coagulation abnormalities.
- Fetal assessment
- Control of hypertension
- Initiation of magnesium sulfate
- Plan the delivery process.

Patients at ≥ 34 weeks gestation should be delivered immediately. In patients less than 34 weeks and without proven lung maturity, glucocorticoids can be given for fetal benefits and delivery planned within 48 hours provided no worsening of maternal or fetal status occurs. Patients with a favorable cervix, regardless of the length of gestation should undergo induction of labor with either oxytocin or prostaglandins. Elective cesarean section should be considered in patients with very early gestation who have an unfavorable cervix. In addition, the following precautions should be taken for a patient with HELLP syndrome requiring cesarean section.[8]

- General anesthesia is preferred if platelet count is <75,000/mm$^3$
- Platelets 5-10 units should be transfused before surgery if platelet count is <50,000/mm$^3$
- Vesicouterine peritoneum should be left open
- Subfascial drain should be put
- Secondary closure of skin incision or subcutaneous drain may be put
- Postoperative transfusions should be given as needed
- Close monitoring for at least 48 hours postpartum.

For pain management during labor, intravenous narcotics can be given to achieve analgesia. Local infiltration can be used during vaginal deliveries and vaginal repairs. Pudendal block should be avoided due to potential for unrecognized bleeding into this area. Regional anesthesia should be used with caution in patients with low platelet count. In the postpartum period, these patients require close hemodynamic monitoring for 48 hours and serial laboratory evaluation for worsening of abnormalities. The platelet count, and hematocrit may continue to fall during first 24-48 hours after delivery and then recovery starts and most of the cases show recovery within 7 days. If liver enzymes continue to rise and platelets continue to fall even after 4 days, it may not have been HELLP and other diagnosis must be considered.

## Subcapsular Liver Hematoma

The clinical features include referred pain from phrenic nerve, hepatomegaly, and features of peritoneal irritation. Pain to the pericardium, peritoneum, pleura, shoulder, gallbladder and esophagus are consistent with referred pain from the phrenic nerve.[8] Diagnosis is confirmed by the use of ultrasound, CT scan, or MRI. A hemodynamically stable patient (unruptured hematoma) requires close hemodynamic monitoring, serial evaluation of coagulation profile, and serial evaluation of the size of hematoma and can be kept on conservative management. Whereas on the other hand, a patient with suspected rupture or a hemodynamically unstable patient requires immediate intervention in the form of an emergency laparotomy with a multidisciplinary approach involving the general surgeon and the vascular surgeon. These patients require correction of coagulopathy, massive blood transfusions, packaging, and drainage. Despite immediate intervention maternal and fetal mortality is high.

## CHRONIC HYPERTENSION

Chronic hypertension is an important risk factor for many adverse pregnancy outcomes. In a large study from US, it has been reported to be present in 1.8% of delivery hospitalizations.[32] Chronic hypertension is characterized by a history of high BP before pregnancy, elevation of BP during first 20 weeks of pregnancy or high BP that lasts longer than 12 weeks after delivery. It is classified as:[33]

*Mild:* Systolic BP 140–159 mm Hg diastolic BP 90–109 mm Hg.

*Severe:* Systolic BP ≥ 160 mm Hg or diastolic BP ≥ 110 mm Hg or both. About 86–89% cases of chronic hypertension antedating pregnancy are cases of essential hypertension, i.e., of unknown cause and 11–14% are the cases of secondary hypertension, i.e., because of some underlying pathology such as renal, vascular, or endocrine abnormality.[32]

In women with chronic hypertension an attempt should, therefore, be made to look for any underlying disorder by appropriate history, physical examination and laboratory test. **Box 4** describes the causes of chronic hypertension.[34]

### Evaluation for End Organ Damage

Next step is to evaluate the woman for any evidence of end-organ damage to eyes, kidneys and heart as described below.
- *Abnormal renal function:* Proteinuria > 300 mg/24 hour, > 1 + dip stick, >30 mg/dL; protein: creatinine ratio of > 30 mg protein/mmol creatinine; creatinine clearance < 110 mL/min, serum creatinine > 0.8 mg/dL
- Cardiac involvement
- Left ventricular hypertrophy
- Retinopathy.

---

**BOX 4:** Etiology of chronic hypertension.

*Idiopathic:* Essential hypertension
*Vascular disorders:*
- Renovascular hypertension
- Aortic coarctation

*Endocrine disorders:*
- Diabetes mellitus
- Hyperthyroidism
- Pheochromocytoma
- Primary hyperaldosteronism
- Hyperparathyroidism
- Cushing's syndrome

*Renal disorders:*
- Diabetic nephropathy
- Chronic renal failure
- Acute renal failure
- Tubular necrosis
- Cortical necrosis
- Chronic pyelonephritis
- Chronic glomerulonephritis
- Nephrotic syndrome
- Polycystic kidney

*Connective tissue disorders:* Systemic lupus erythematosus

---

### Maternal and Fetal Risks

Pregnancy complicated with chronic hypertension may be associated with several adverse outcomes including premature birth, fetal growth restriction, fetal demise, placental abruption, superimposed preeclampsia, worsening or malignant hypertension, cerebral hemorrhage, cardiac decompensation, renal deterioration or failure, and cesarean delivery. The incidence of these potential adverse effects is related to the degree and duration of hypertension and associated end-organ damage. The outcome is usually good in patients with mild chronic hypertension and no other complication, but the outlook is less favorable in women with severe hypertension early in pregnancy and in those with evidence of end-organ compromise.

To make the diagnosis of superimposed preeclampsia, the patient should have increasing or difficult to control BP, HELLP syndrome, symptoms such as headache, right upper quadrant pain, visual disturbances, new onset proteinuria, or significant increase in preexisting proteinuria.

### Management

Ideally women with chronic hypertension should be evaluated before conception so that BP is optimized and lifestyle changes are initiated. Once the pregnancy is confirmed the management is individualized. The general guidelines are:

#### Lifestyle Modifications

The patient is advised to adopt a healthy lifestyle and maintain an ideal body weight. She should also be advised to avoid alcohol, tobacco, and restrict sodium intake to 2–3 g/day.

#### Low Dose Aspirin

For women with chronic hypertension, it is recommended to initiate daily low-dose aspirin between 12 and 28 weeks of gestation, preferably before 16 weeks, and to continue it until delivery.[3]

#### Antihypertensives

As per recent NICE (2019) guidelines, women with chronic hypertension who are already on antihypertensive treatment should continue it unless systolic blood pressure remains <110 mm Hg or diastolic pressure remains <70 or if there is symptomatic hypotension.[4]

Women who are on angiotensin-converting enzyme inhibitor or on angiotensin receptor blockers, should discontinue these and should be started on antihypertensives that are safe in pregnancy (*see* **Table 2**).

Antihypertensive treatment should be offered to pregnant women with chronic hypertension who are not already on treatment and have sustained systolic BP of

140 mm Hg or higher or diastolic BP of 90 mm Hg or higher, and the aim should be to keep the BP at around 135/85.[4] In women with acute-onset, severe hypertension, (systolic blood pressure ≥ 160 mm Hg or diastolic blood pressure ≥ 110 mm Hg, or both) that is confirmed to be persistent (15 minutes or more) antihypertensive treatment should be initiated expeditiously[3] (*see* **Table 3**).

Choice of antihypertensives is same as discussed in section on preeclampsia.

Labetalol or nifedipine are preferred over other antihypertensives and can be given when treatment is required for long-time during pregnancy. Methyldopa can also be given if labetalol and nifedipine are not suitable.

### Antenatal Visits

Women with mild hypertension should be seen every 2–4 weeks till 34 weeks and weekly thereafter whereas, women with severe disease need to be seen every 2–3 weeks till 28 weeks and weekly thereafter. At each visit the woman is inquired about symptoms of preeclampsia and her BP, urine protein and fetal growth is checked. Antepartum fetal surveillance is started at 32–34 weeks with weekly NST or BPP and USG for fetal growth every 4 weeks, for women with mild hypertension. For women with severe hypertension USG is generally recommended every 4 weeks after 26 weeks and weekly NST/BPP after 28 weeks.

### Hospitalization

The patient needs to be hospitalized if BP is uncontrolled or she develops superimposed preeclampsia.

*Superimposed preeclampsia:* Superimposed preeclampsia should always be suspected in cases of chronic hypertension where BP rises, especially to severe range. To differentiate transient increase in BP in chronic hypertension from superimposed preeclampsia, particularly with severe-range BPs, complete evaluation is required, and the woman should be hospitalized.

BP monitoring can distinguish between acute and serious increases in BP from transient hypertension.

Elevated hematocrit, serum creatinine, liver enzymes, new-onset or worsening proteinuria, thrombocytopenia, and especially hyperuricemia are indicative of preeclampsia.

Placental growth factor (PlGF)-based testing may also be done to help rule out preeclampsia between 20 and 35 weeks of gestation.[4] Although not recommended yet, triage PlGF test and the immunoassay sFlt1/PlGF ratio are being investigated to help diagnose (rulein) preeclampsia in women presenting with suspected preeclampsia between 20 and $34^{+6/7}$ weeks.

### Delivery[3]

- For women with uncomplicated, isolated chronic hypertension, not on medication, pregnancy should be continued till 38 weeks and delivery is recommended at $38–39^{+6/7}$ weeks; but if BP is difficult to control requiring frequent medication modifications, the delivery is then advised between 36 and 38 weeks.
- In women with superimposed preeclampsia without severe features and with stable maternal and fetal condition, expectant management with close maternal and fetal monitoring is suggested up to 37 weeks followed by delivery.
- Expectant management in a tertiary care center with intensive maternal and neonatal facilities can be given to selected cases with less than 34 weeks gestation and superimposed preeclampsia with severe features but not beyond 34 weeks.
- Immediate delivery after maternal stabilization is recommended at any gestational age in women with superimposed preeclampsia if there is uncontrollable severe hypertension, eclampsia, pulmonary edema, DIC, new or increasing renal insufficiency, placental abruption or nonreassuring fetal status.

## KEY POINTS

- Hypertension is a common medical disorder and covers a spectrum of conditions namely gestational hypertension, preeclampsia, chronic hypertension and preeclampsia superimposed on chronic hypertension.
- Gestational hypertension is new onset hypertension, with systolic BP ≥ 140 mm Hg or diastolic BP ≥ 90 mm Hg on two occasions at least 4–6 hours apart that occurs after 20 weeks of gestation and resolves by 12 weeks postpartum.
- Preeclampsia is new onset hypertension, systolic BP ≥ 140 mm Hg or diastolic BP ≥ 90 mm Hg or both, on two occasions at least 4 hours apart along with proteinuria and/or end organ dysfunction.
- In the absence of proteinuria, preeclampsia is diagnosed as hypertension in association with thrombocytopenia, impaired liver function tests, new development of renal insufficiency, pulmonary edema, or new onset cerebral or visual disturbances.
- It is suggested that excess secretion of naturally occurring antiangiogenic molecules of placental origin referred to as soluble fms-like tyrosine kinase-1 may contribute to the pathogenesis of preeclampsia.
- Currently, there is no single screening test for predicting preeclampsia that is reliable, valid and cost effective, so an accurate and thorough maternal history with identification of risk factors is the most cost-effective screening method.
- Low dose aspirin is recommended for the prevention of preeclampsia in high-risk women.
- The only definitive therapy for gestational hypertension/preeclampsia is delivery. In case of preterm pregnancies, the main objective of expectant management is to

- improve neonatal outcome if the risks for the mother and child remain acceptable.
- Women with overt hypertension, ≥ 140/90, with or without proteinuria should be admitted to the hospital to evaluate the severity of new onset hypertension.
- The decision between delivery and expectant management depends on fetal gestational age, fetal status, and severity of maternal condition.
- Expectant management up to 37 weeks of gestation is given in cases of gestational hypertension or preeclampsia without severe features. Frequent maternal and fetal evaluation and monitoring is required. Ultrasonography for fetal growth is done every 3-4 weeks and amniotic fluid assessment once a week. NST is done one-to-two times per week.
- Antihypertensive therapy is used to protect the mother from effects of severe hypertension such as cerebrovascular hemorrhage, cardiac failure, placental abruption and eclampsia.
- Antihypertensives are used with an aim to keep BP under 135/85 mm Hg; labetalol, nifedipine or methyldopa can be used.
- Acute severe hypertension may be treated with parenteral labetalol or hydralazine or oral nifedipine. Immediate release oral nifedipine should not be given sublingually because of risk of hypotension. Nifedipine has the advantage that it can be given orally in absence of an intravenous line.
- Magnesium sulfate is the drug of choice for the prevention and treatment of seizures in women with preeclampsia with severe features or eclampsia.
- Timing of delivery depends on the severity of hypertension, presence of complications, period of gestation and fetal condition.
- Vaginal delivery is the preferred approach. Regional anesthesia is preferred if cesarean section is undertaken.
- Intrapartum management includes early detection of fetal heart rate abnormalities, early detection of progression from mild to severe disease and prevention of maternal complications.
- Close monitoring of BP is essential in immediate postpartum period.
- Eclampsia is defined as the development of convulsions and/or unexplained coma during pregnancy or postpartum in patients with signs and symptoms of preeclampsia.
- Immediate management of eclampsia is basically supportive and consists of prevention of injury, aspiration and maternal and fetal complications. Administration of antihypertensives, magnesium sulfate, and termination of pregnancy is required.
- HELLP syndrome is used to describe preeclampsia in association with hemolysis, elevated liver enzymes, and low-platelet count.
- Management consists of immediate hospitalization followed by maternal and fetal assessment, control of hypertension and delivery of the baby.
- Chronic hypertension is characterized by a history of high BP before pregnancy, elevation of BP during first 20 weeks of pregnancy or high BP that lasts longer than 12 weeks after delivery.
- The outcome is usually good in patients with mild chronic hypertension and no other complication, but the outlook is less favorable in women with severe hypertension early in pregnancy and in those with evidence of end-organ compromise.
- The timing of delivery depends on the development of confounding complications; women with uncomplicated chronic hypertension of a mild degree generally can be delivered vaginally at 38–40 weeks, whereas women with chronic hypertension not well-controlled should be delivered at 36–38 weeks.

# REFERENCES

1. Sibai BM. Chronic hypertension during pregnancy. In: Sciarra J (Ed.). Gynecology and Obstetrics. Philadelphia: JB Lippincott; 1989. pp. 18.
2. Gestational Hypertension and Preeclampsia: ACOG Practice Bulletin, Number 222. Obstet Gynecol. 2020;135(6):e237-60.
3. American College of Obstetricians and Gynecologists. Committee on Practice Bulletins—Obstetrics. ACOG Practice Bulletin No. 203: Chronic Hypertension in Pregnancy. Obstet Gynecol. 2019;133(1):e26-50.
4. NICE guidelines (2019). Hypertension in pregnancy: diagnosis and management. [online]. Available from: https://www.nice.org.uk/guidance/ng133/resources/hypertension-in-pregnancy-diagnosis-and-management-pdf-66141717671365. [Last accessed July, 2021].
5. Report of the National High Blood Pressure Education Program Working Group on Pregnancy. Am J Obstet Gynecol. 2000;183:S1-22.
6. Hypertension in pregnancy. Report of the American College of Obstetricians and Gynecologists' Task Force on Hypertension in Pregnancy. Obstet Gynecol. 2013;122(5):1122-31.
7. Bdolah Y, Karumanchi SA, Sach's BP. Recent advances in understanding of preeclampsia. Croat Med J. 2005;46:728-36.
8. Moldenhauer JS, Sibai BM. Hypertensive disorders of pregnancy. In: Gibbs RS, Karlan BY, Haney AF, Nygaard Y (Eds). Obstetrics and Gynecology, 10th edition. Philadelphia: Lippincott Williams and Wilkins.
9. Poon LC, Shennan A, Hyett JA, Kapur A, Hadar E, Divakar H, et al. The International Federation of Gynecology and Obstetrics (FIGO) initiative on pre-eclampsia: A pragmatic guide for first-trimester screening and prevention. Int J Gynaecol Obstet. 2019;145(Suppl 1):1-33.
10. Levine RJ, Hauth JC, Curet LB, Sibai BM, Catalano PM, Morris CD, et al. Trial of calcium to prevent preeclampsia. N Engl J Med. 1997;337:69.
11. Magee LA, Pels A, Helewa M, Rey E, von Dadelszen P; Canadian Hypertensive Disorders of Pregnancy Working Group. Diagnosis, evaluation, and management of the

hypertensive disorders of pregnancy: Executive summary SOGC clinical practice guideline No. 307, 2014:416-38.
12. Ruano R, Fontes RS, Zugaib M. Prevention of preeclampsia with low-dose aspirin—a systematic review and meta-analysis of the main randomized controlled trials. Clinics (Sao Paulo). 2005;60(5):407-14.
13. Rumbold A, Duley L, Crowther CA, Haslam RR. Antioxidants for preventing preeclampsia. Cochrane Database Syst Rev. 2008;(1):CD004227.
14. Barton JR, Witlin AG, Sibai BM. Management of mild preeclampsia. Clin Obstet Gynecol. 1999;42:465-9.
15. Barron WM, Heckerling P, Hibbard JU, Fisher S. Reducing unnecessary coagulation testing in hypertensive disorders of pregnancy. Obstet Gynecol. 1999;94:364-70.
16. Haddad B, Sibai BM. Expectant management of severe preeclampsia: proper candidates and pregnancy outcome. Clin Obstet Gynecol. 2005;48(2):430-40.
17. Cabrera ML, McDiarmid T, Mackler L. Does bed rest for preeclampsia improve neonatal outcomes? J Family Prac. 2007;56:938-9.
18. Von Dadelszen P, Magee LA. Antihypertensive medications in management of gestational hypertension, preeclampsia. Clin Obstet Gynecol. 2005;48(2):441-59.
19. Abalos E, Duley L, Steyn DW, Gialdini C. Antihypertensive drug therapy for mild to moderate hypertension during pregnancy. Cochrane Database Syst Rev. 2018;10(10):CD002252.
20. Magee LA, Rey E, Asztalos E, Hutton E, Singer J, Helewa M, et al. Management of non-severe pregnancy hypertension-A summary of the CHIPS Trial (Control of Hypertension in Pregnancy Study) research publications. Pregnancy Hypertens. 2019;18:156-62.
21. Greer IA. Pregnancy induced hypertension. In: Chamberlain G, Steer PJ (Eds.). Turnbull's Obstetrics, 4th edition. Edinburgh: Churchill Livingstone; 2005. pp. 333-53.
22. ACOG. ACOG Committee Opinion No. 767: Emergent Therapy for Acute-Onset, Severe Hypertension During Pregnancy and the Postpartum Period. Obstet Gynecol. 2019;133(2):e174-80.
23. Melchiorre K, Sharma R, Thilaganathan B. Cardiovascular implications in preeclampsia: an overview. Circulation. 2014; 130(8):703-14.
24. ACOG. ACOG Committee Opinion No. 764: Medically Indicated Late-Preterm and Early-Term Deliveries. Obstet Gynecol. 2019;133(2):e151.
25. Shennan A. Hypertensive disorders. In: Edmond K (Ed). Dewhurst's Textbook of Gynecology and Obstetrics, 7th edition. NewYork: Blackwell Publishing; 2007. pp. 227-35.
26. Hypertensive Disorders in Pregnancy. In: Cunningham G, Leveno KJ, Bloom SL, Dashe JS, Hoffman BL, Casey BM, Spong CY. Williams Obstetrics, 25th edition. NewYork: McGraw Hill; 2018. pp. 1086-153.
27. Sibai BM. Diagnosis and management of gestational hypertension and preeclampsia. Obstet Gynecol. 2003;102:181-92.
28. Eclampsia Trial Collaborative Group. Which anticonvulsant for women with eclampsia? Evidence from the collaborative eclampsia trial. Lancet. 1995;345:1455-63.
29. Sibai BM. The HELLP syndrome (Hemolysis, elevated liver enzymes and low platelets): much ado about nothing? Am J Obstet Gynecol. 1990;162:3111-6.
30. Weinstein L. Preeclampsia/eclampsia with hemolysis, elevated liver enzymes, and thrombocytopenia. Obstet Gynecol. 1985;66:657-60.
31. Sibai BM, Taslimi MM, El-Nazer A, Amon E, Mabie BC, Ryan GM. Maternal perinatal outcome associated with the syndrome of hemolysis, elevated liver enzymes and low platelets in severe preeclampsia-eclampsia. Am J Obstet Gynaecol. 1986;155(3):501-9.
32. Bateman BT, Bansil P, Hernandez-Diaz S, Mhyre JM, Callaghan WM, Kuklina EV. Prevalence, trends, and outcomes of chronic hypertension: a nationwide sample of delivery admissions. Am J Obstet Gynecol. 2012;206(2):134.e1-348.
33. Ferrer RL, Sibai BM, Mulrow CD, Chiquette E, Stevens KR, Cornell J. Management of mild chronic hypertension during pregnancy: a review. Obstet Gynecol. 2000;96:849-60.
34. Miller DA. Hypertension in pregnancy. In: Decherney AH, Nathan L, Goodwin TM, Laufer N (Eds). Current Diagnosis and Treatment: Obstetrics and Gynecology, 10th edition. New York: McGraw Hill; 2007.

# CHAPTER 18

# Diabetes Mellitus in Pregnancy

*Kazila Bhutia, Qiu Ju Ng, Manju Puri*

## INTRODUCTION

Diabetes mellitus (DM) is a metabolic disorder secondary to decrease in insulin secretion, increase in insulin resistance or both, with resultant abnormalities of carbohydrate, protein, and lipid metabolism. DM in pregnancy is associated with an increased maternal and fetal morbidity and mortality. It is classified broadly into 2 types; pregestational, also called pre-existing DM and gestational diabetes mellitus (GDM). Pregestational DM can be type 1 insulin-dependent DM or it can be type 2 noninsulin-dependent DM. Majority of patients with DM in pregnancy (DIP) are GDM. Pre-existing diabetes is associated with a much higher risk of maternal and perinatal complications as compared to GDM. There has been a significant increase in the prevalence of GDM as well as type 2 DM globally over the past few decades. This rise reflects a changing demography of the modern society including pregnancies at an advanced age, increase in body mass index (BMI), and a sedentary and stressful lifestyle.

Pregnant women with DM must be managed by a multidisciplinary team consisting of an obstetrician, endocrinologist, neonatologist, and dietician. However, it is essential for all obstetricians to have an adequate knowledge of this disorder so as to provide optimal care and treatment to pregnant women with DM in all health care settings.

## PREVALENCE OF DIABETES MELLITUS

The epidemic of diabetes is now spreading to become a pandemic affecting people from both developed and developing countries. This increase in prevalence is consequent to obesity, a sedentary lifestyle, and increasing life expectancy. The global prevalence of DM in 2000 was 2.8% which is likely to increase to 4.4% in 2030.[1] The reported incidence of DIP varies worldwide and among various racial and ethnic groups, generally in parallel with the prevalence of type 2 DM. The overall incidence is reported to be between 5 and 7% of all pregnancies.[2] As per the International Diabetes Federation, it is estimated that about one in six live births (16.8%) occur in women with hyperglycemia in pregnancy.[3] Of all cases of DM complicating pregnancy, GDM accounts for 88%.[4] In India, the prevalence of GDM ranges from 3.8 to 17.9%.[5-7] Women with GDM in their previous pregnancies have a 33.5% likelihood of recurrence in a subsequent pregnancy, and almost half of them have a risk of progression to diabetes in future.[8]

## CLASSIFICATION OF DIABETES MELLITUS IN PREGNANCY

The classification of diabetes mellitus in pregnancy and the definition of GDM have been evolving. Both the World Health Organization (WHO) and the American Diabetes Association (ADA) have endorsed a classification based on etiology.[9,10]

**Flowchart 1** shows the WHO 2013 classification of diabetes in pregnancy which classifies hyperglycemia in pregnancy into either DIP or as GDM. Hyperglycemia that is diagnosed in pregnancy and does not meet the criteria for DIP is defined as GDM. GDM is usually diagnosed between 24 and 28 weeks of gestation.

Pregestational DM affects the women before pregnancy, whereas GDM develops during pregnancy and resolves after delivery. Pregestational DM can be type 1 insulin-dependent DM or type 2 noninsulin-dependent DM. It may be either diagnosed before pregnancy or diagnosed for the first time during pregnancy as part of screening. Secondary DM is also a form of pregestational DM but due to causes such as pancreatitis, cystic fibrosis, hemochromatosis, pancreatotomy, neoplasm, hyperthyroidism, Cushing's syndrome, or Klinefelter's syndrome. GDM is of 2 types; GDM controlled on medical nutritional therapy alone, class A1 GDM, and that controlled on insulin or antihyperglycemic agents, class A2 GDM.

## PATHOPHYSIOLOGY

### Carbohydrate Metabolism in Pregnancy[11]

Pregnancy is a diabetogenic condition due to hormone-related changes in carbohydrate metabolism **(Flowchart 2)**. First trimester is associated with reduced blood glucose levels due to pregnancy related increase in renal clearance of glucose and decreased gluconeogenesis, thereby predisposing women with type 1 DM to an increased risk of hypoglycemia.

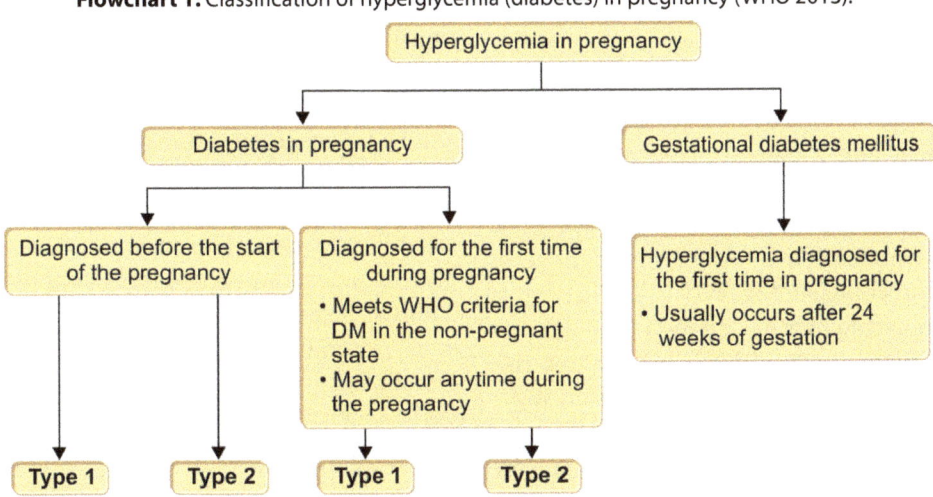

Flowchart 1: Classification of hyperglycemia (diabetes) in pregnancy (WHO 2013).[10]

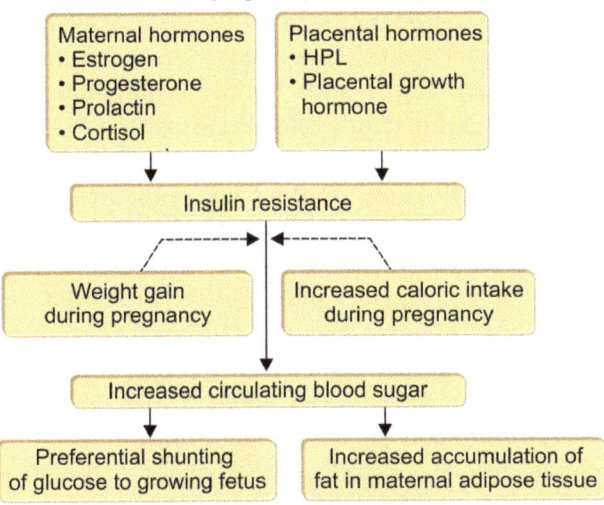

Flowchart 2: Effect of pregnancy on carbohydrate metabolism.

(HPL: human placental lactogen)

Development of insulin resistance is a major change as the pregnancy progresses. There is an approximately 50% reduction in insulin sensitivity by the third trimester. This change is due to the increase in levels of several hormones of maternal and placental origin. Maternal hormones are estrogen, progesterone, prolactin, and cortisol while placental hormones are human placental lactogen (HPL) and placental growth hormone variant. Other factors contributing to insulin resistance are an increase in calorie intake and increased body weight during pregnancy. Development of insulin resistance serves to shunt nutrients preferentially to the growing fetus, while simultaneously allowing for the accumulation of caloric storage in maternal adipose tissue.

During fasting, two important changes in maternal carbohydrate metabolism occur, i.e., decrease in plasma glucose concentration and increase in fat catabolism. This decrease in plasma glucose further accelerates preferential shunting of nutrients to the fetomaternal unit even at low circulating levels of plasma glucose. Simultaneously, fat catabolism or lipolysis is stimulated to ensure adequate nutrient supply to the mother. Hence, this ultimately ensures adequate nutrient supply both to the mother and fetus but predisposes the pregnant woman to ketosis at the time of starvation.

## Carbohydrate Metabolism in Diabetic Pregnancy[11]

Women, who fail to sufficiently increase insulin secretion from the pancreas to overcome pregnancy-induced insulin resistance, will develop hyperglycemia and subsequently GDM. This occurs as the insulin resistance state in pregnancy imposes an additional burden on the already depleted insulin secreting beta cells to prevent overt hyperglycemia in nonpregnant state. Any pre-existing insulin-resistance associated conditions such as obesity, polycystic ovarian syndrome, or metabolic syndrome predispose the women to a higher chance of developing GDM. Similarly, in pregnant women with pre-existing DM, carbohydrate tolerance deteriorates early and they require more insulin to maintain glycemic control. There is a threefold increase in insulin requirement in women with type 1 DM in late pregnancy to counteract the physiological changes. In pregnant women with type 2 DM who already have pre-existing insulin resistance, there is a further deterioration due to pregnancy-related insulin resistance and most of these women require insulin early in pregnancy.

## GESTATIONAL DIABETES MELLITUS

### Screening and Diagnosis

Despite decades of research, there is no consensus regarding the optimal approach for screening for GDM. The major issues include whether screening should be universal or selective, timing of screening, and method of screening.

## Universal or Selective Screening/Testing for GDM

In response to HAPO (The Hyperglycemia and Adverse Pregnancy Outcome) study 2008, the International Association of Diabetes and Pregnancy Study Group and International Federation of Gynecology and Obstetrics (FIGO) recommend universal screening.[3,12] Similar universal screening is also recommended by American College of Obstetricians and Gynecologists (ACOG)[13] and Society of Obstetricians and Gynaecologists of Cananda (SOGC),[14] as majority of pregnant women would have at least one risk factor of glucose impairment in pregnancy. However, WHO and NICE (UK) guidelines recommend a selective screening strategy based on risk assessment for GDM.[4,10] As Asians are at risk of DM, universal screening for DM during pregnancy is recommended in India.

In selective screening, risk assessment is done for all women at first prenatal visit and those at high risk are offered screening. Risk factors of DM are listed in **Box 1**.

### Timing of Testing

In India, universal screening is recommended by Ministry of Health and Family Welfare Government of India (GOI) at registration visit, and repeat screening at 24–28 weeks if the pregnant woman is screen negative at registration visit.[15] In the absence of early screening or testing, universal screening is performed at 24–28 weeks of gestation or later, whenever the woman registers.

### Methods of Screening[3]

Screening for GDM can be done either by one-step or two-step approach.

*One-step approach:* Perform diagnostic oral glucose tolerance test (OGTT) without prior glucose challenge test (GCT). This approach is simple and cost-effective in high-risk patients or populations. Ideally test should be done in the morning after an overnight fast of more than 8 hours after at least 3 days of unrestricted diet, consuming more than or equal to 150 g of carbohydrate per day. Patients should not smoke before the test and should remain seated during the test. This is to avoid carbohydrate depletion, which could cause spurious values on the OGTT. A fasting blood glucose sample is drawn. The pregnant woman is given 75 g of glucose in water and the blood samples drawn at 1 hour and 2 hours. Test is interpreted as per WHO criteria or ADA "one step" criteria given in **Table 1**. However, in DIPSI test, the woman is given 75 g glucose irrespective of her fasting status and a single blood sample is drawn after 2 hours.[15]

*Two-step approach:* In this approach, the first step is to subject all women to a glucose challenge test and if glucose value crosses threshold value then OGTT is performed as a second step.

In first step, pregnant woman is administered 50 g of glucose irrespective of the time of last meal and the blood sample is drawn after 1 hour. Women with blood glucose value exceeding the cutoff value are subjected to OGTT. A cutoff value of plasma blood glucose of ≥140 mg/dL (7.8 mmol/L) identifies 80% of all women with GDM whereas a value of ≥130 mg/dL (7.2 mmol/L) identifies 90% of all women with GDM. It is important to note that if the GCT value is >200 mg/dL (11.1 mmol/L), OGTT should not be done.

The second step, a diagnostic OGTT is performed on the subset of women with GCT value of more than the threshold value. A fasting blood glucose sample is drawn. The pregnant woman is given 100 g of glucose in water and the samples drawn at 1, 2, and 3 hours. The test is interpreted as per Carpenter and Coustan or the National Diabetes Data Group (NDDG) criteria given in **Table 2**.

Screening for gestational diabetes using glucose in urine, random blood sugar or, fasting blood sugar is not recommended. Testing for glycosuria has a poor sensitivity. Random blood sugar has sensitivity of about 40% in detecting gestational diabetes.

### Diagnostic Threshold for GDM[9,12,16,17]

The diagnostic thresholds for GDM have been determined by consensus agreement of various national and international professional organizations **(Table 1)**. All values mentioned above depict plasma blood sugar levels. For converting the blood sugar values in mmol/L to mg/dL the value in mmol/L is multiplied by 18, e.g., 10 mmol/L = 180 mg/dL. Measurement of blood glucose level in capillary blood by glucometer has made screening test easy and simple as it can be done in an office setting and does not require elaborate laboratory facilities. It is important to know that capillary blood glucose levels are comparable to venous blood glucose levels during fasting state but are higher after meals.[18]

---

**BOX 1:** Risk factors for diabetes mellitus in pregnancy.

- Obesity (BMI > 30 kg/m$^2$)
- Family history of diabetes (first degree relative with diabetes)
- Family origin with high prevalence of diabetes (e.g., South Asian, Black Caribbean, Middle Eastern)
- Increasing maternal age >25 years
- Medical conditions:
  – PCOS
  – Current use of glucocorticosteriod
  – Metabolic syndrome
- Pregnancy factors:
  – Multiple pregnancy
  – History of GDM, macrosomic baby (≥4.5 kg), unexplained perinatal loss, birth of malformed baby, or polyhydramnios in previous pregnancy
  – Persistent glycosuria

(BMI: body mass index; GDM: gestational diabetes mellitus; PCOS: polycystic ovarian syndrome)

**TABLE 1:** Diagnostic criteria for gestational diabetes mellitus (GDM).

| Test | Method | Screen positive | Diagnostic test | Threshold level for diagnosing GDM |
|---|---|---|---|---|
| WHO (2013) | One step | NA^ | 75 g OGTT | • Fasting: 5.1–6.9 mmol/L (92–125 mg/dL)<br>• 1-hour post 75 g oral glucose load >=10.0 mmol/L (≥180 mg/dL)#<br>• 2 hours post 75 g glucose 8.5–11.0 mmol/L (153–199 mg/dL) |
| DIPSI* | One step | NA^ | 75 g OGTT (irrespective of fasting status) | 2 hours ≥7.8 mmol/L (≥140 mg/dL) |
| ACOG | Two steps:<br>*Step one:* Glucose challenge screening test (GCT) with 50 g glucose, irrespective of fasting status<br><br>*Step two:* (100 g OGTT for screen positive cases) | 1 hour value ≥7.8 mmol/L (140 mg/dL)<br>**Or**<br>≥7.5 mmol/L (130 mg/dL)<br>Lower threshold for populations with higher prevalence of GDM | 100 g OGTT | Fasting ≥5.3 mmol/L (≥95 mg/dL)<br>1 hour ≥10.0 (≥180 mg/dL)<br>2 hours ≥8.6 mmol/L (≥155 mg/dL)<br>3 hours ≥7.8 mmol/L (≥140 mg/dL)<br><br>≥2 abnormal value needed for diagnosis |
| ADA 2020** | One step | NA^ | 75 g OGTT | • Fasting ≥5.1 mmol/L (≥92 mg/dL)<br>• 1 hour ≥10.0 mmol/L (≥180 mg/dL)<br>• 2 hours ≥8.5 mmol/L (≥155 mg/dL)<br>One abnormal value needed for diagnosis |
| | Two steps:<br>*Step one:* Do 50 g GCT<br><br>*Step two:* If plasma glucose level after 1 hour GCT is ≥ 140 mg/dL (≥7.8 mmol/L), do 100-g OGTT | 1 hour GCT ≥ 140 mg/dL (≥7.8 mmol/L), | 100 g OGTT | • Fasting ≥5.3 mmol/L (≥95 mg/dL)<br>• 1 hour ≥10.0 mmol/L (≥180 mg/dL)<br>• 2 hours ≥8.6 (≥155 mg/dL)<br>• 3 hours ≥7.8 (≥140 mg/dL)<br>≥2 abnormal values needed for diagnosis |
| IADPSG | One step | NA^ | 75 g OGTT | Fasting ≥5.1 mmol/L (≥92 mg/dL)<br>1 hour ≥10.0 mmol/L (≥180 mg/dL)<br>2 hour ≥8.5 mmol/L (≥153 mg/dL)<br>One abnormal value needed for diagnosis |
| SOGC[14] | Two steps (preferred):a<br>*Step one:* 50 g GCT<br><br>*Step two:* If GCT value is ≥7.8 mmol/L and <11.1 mmol/dL | GCT value ≥11.1 mmol/L<br><br>GCT value is ≥7.8 mmol/L and <11.1 mmol/dL | No further test<br><br>75 g OGTT | • GDM diagnosed if on 50 g GCT 1 hour value ≥11.1 mmol/La<br><br>• One abnormal value needed for diagnosis of GDM<br>– Fasting ≥5.3 mmol/L (≥95 mg/dL)<br>– 1 hour ≥10.6 mmol/L (≥191 mg/dL)<br>– 2 hours ≥9 mmol/L (≥160 mg/dL) |
| | One step test (Alternate)a | NA^ | 75 g OGTT | • GDM diagnosed if one value is met or exceededa<br>– FPG ≥5.1 mmol/L<br>– 1-hour PG ≥10.0 mmol/L<br>– 2-hour PG ≥8.5 mmol/L |

#There are no established criteria for diagnosis of diabetes based on 1-hour postload value[10]
*DIPSI diabetes in pregnancy study group India.
**American Diabetes Association.
^NA: not applicable.
a Different diagnostic thresholds for the "preferred" and "alternate" strategies have been adopted by committee[14] for aligning with Diabetes Canada guidelines (SOGC clinical practice guideline no. 393)
(ADA: American Diabetes Association; DIPSI: Diabetes in Pregnancy Study Group; OGTT: oral glucose tolerance test; IADPSG: International Association of Diabetes and Pregnancy Study Group; SOGC: Society of Obstetricians and Gynaecologists of Cananda)

**TABLE 2:** Carpenter and Coustan/NDDG criteria.

| Approach | Criteria | Fasting mg/dL | One-hour mg/dL | Two-hour mg/dL | Three-hour mg/dL |
|---|---|---|---|---|---|
| Two step (100 g load) | Carpenter and Coustan | 95 (5.3 mmol/L) | 180 (10.0 mmol/L) | 155 (8.6 mmol/L) | 140 (7.8 mmol/L) |
| | NDDG | 105 (5.8 mmol/L) | 190 (10.6 mmol/L) | 165 (9.2 mmol/L) | 145 (8.0 mmol/L) |

(NDDG: National Diabetes Data Group)

# MANAGEMENT OF PREGNANCY WITH GESTATIONAL DIABETES MELLITUS[4,8,12,17]

Women should be offered information and education including the role of diet, lifestyle changes, and exercise. Most women respond to changes in diet and exercise. Around 10–20% of women will need insulin therapy if diet and exercise are not effective in optimizing diabetic status. The management of pregnant women with GDM is by a multidisciplinary team comprising of an endocrinologist and obstetrician.

## Medical Nutrition Therapy

Adequate understanding of the importance of medical nutrition therapy (MNT) or dietary therapy by the patient is important, especially the association between certain types of carbohydrates and glucose excursions. Patient should receive nutritional counseling by a dietician upon diagnosis and be placed on appropriate diet.

The aim of dietary therapy is to achieve optimal glycemic control without ketosis and providing adequate weight gain based upon the woman's BMI. The diet should consist of 30–35 kcal/kg/day in the form of three major meals and two to three minor meals. The diet should consist of 50% to 60% carbohydrates, with a minimum of 175 g carbohydrate per day, 20–25% proteins, less than 30% fat and adequate amount of dietary fiber. Complex carbohydrates and foods with low glycemic index are advocated. According to ADA, the daily caloric intake by a pregnant diabetic woman can be calculated according to the proportion of the current body weight of the woman to prepregnancy ideal body weight for her height. For a woman with current body weight as 80–120% of ideal body weight, the calorie requirement is 30 kcal/kg, compared to 36–40 kcal/kg in women who are <80% of the desirable body weight, 24 kcal/kg for those who are 120–150% and 12–18 kcal/kg for those who are more than 150% of desirable body weight.

## Lifestyle Modifications

Regular physical exercise within tolerable limits should be encouraged. Moderate exercise of at least 30 minutes per day such as walking, swimming, or yoga is suggested. Cochrane Database Systemic Review 2017 reported that lifestyle interventions (education, diet, and exercise) in women with GDM were associated with reduced risk of large for gestational age baby and reduced neonatal adiposity. In addition, women were less likely to have postnatal depression and more likely to achieve postnatal weight goal.[19]

## Medical Treatment

Medical therapy is initiated if diet and lifestyle modification fail to optimize blood glucose level within 1–2 weeks. Women with grossly abnormal glucose level may be started on insulin on diagnosis. ACOG and ADA recommend fasting target of ≤5.3 mmol/L (95 mg/dL) and 1 hour postmeal ≤7.8 mmol/L (140 mg/dL) and 2 hours postmeal value of ≤6.7 mmol/L (120 mg/dL).

The NICE recommends targets of fasting blood glucose 4–5.9 mmol/L (72–106 mg/dL), 1 hour postmeal <7.8 mmol/L (140 mg/dL), and 2 hours postmeal <6.4 mmol/L (115 mg/dL).

## Blood Sugar Monitoring

Women should be instructed on how to do home monitoring of blood glucose. Frequency of monitoring and targets for blood glucose control are similar to women with pre-existing diabetes. A 5-sample glucose profile includes a fasting sample, 3 postmeal samples, and one 2 AM sample. Whereas, 7-sample glucose profile includes 2 additional premeal samples, i.e., prelunch and predinner. Women on home-based monitoring can be advised to do their blood testing in a staggered way, e.g., postbreakfast sample one day, postlunch the next day, and postdinner the next day.

## Drug Therapy[3,18,20-22]

Insulin is the first line of drug therapy and used to be the only available medical treatment. There are studies done which showed that metformin and glyburide are relatively safe and effective treatment for GDM. However, these are currently not licensed for use in pregnancy. Metformin is category B drug and glyburide is category C drug. Metformin appears to be more effective than glyburide. There are also no long-term data on the safety of oral antihyperglycemic or oral antidiabetic agents (OAD). Hence, ACOG advises insulin to be the first line of therapy due to its long-term safety data in pregnancy and insulin does not cross the placenta. Oral antihyperglycemic agents are favored among patients as they are more convenient and easier to administer as compared to insulin.

## Oral Antihyperglycemic Agents

### Metformin

Metformin is a biguanide analog which is an insulin sensitizer. It inhibits gluconeogenesis in the liver, reduces glucose absorption in the gastrointestinal tract, and stimulates uptake of glucose by the peripheral tissues. Even though metformin needs insulin to potentiate its effect, it does not increase insulin secretion and hence, it is not associated with hypoglycemic episodes. The usual starting dose is 500 milligrams (mg) at night and can be increased up to a maximum dose of 2,500–3,500 mg, divided into 2–3 doses. The common side effects are nausea, diarrhea, dyspepsia, and abdominal discomfort. It is contraindicated in patient with renal disease.

Metformin crosses the placenta and is transferred in breast milk but it has not been shown to increase risk of congenital anomalies or serious maternal or neonatal morbidity.

### Glyburide

Glyburide, also called glybenclamide, is a second generation sulfonylurea which acts by enhancing insulin secretion and peripheral tissue sensitivity to insulin. The usual starting dose of glyburide is 2.5 mg orally daily, which can be increased by 2.5 mg in the following week and thereafter by 5 mg weekly up to a maximum of 20 mg per day to achieve glycemic control. The onset of action is within 2 hours, with a maximal decrease in blood sugar occurring between 3 and 4 hours. The blood glucose lowering effect lasts for 24 hours following a single morning dose in nonfasting diabetic patient. Its absorption is not affected by food. Its main side effect is hypoglycemia which is dose related. Other side effects are nausea, heart burn, muscle pain, joint pain, and allergic skin reactions including angioedema.

It has been shown to cross the placenta but levels are low enough to be considered safe. However, there was a meta-analysis[22] which showed that glyburide as compared to insulin was associated with about a 100 g higher birth weight, twice the rate of neonatal hypoglycemia, and more than twice the macrosomia rate. Castillo et al.[21] conducted a retrospective study which found that newborns of women treated with glyburide as compared to insulin were at higher risk of neonatal intensive care (NICU) admission, respiratory distress, hypoglycemia, and large for gestational age (LGA). In light of these studies, ACOG advised glyburide not to be used to replace insulin as treatment.

### Insulin

The insulin used in the treatment of DM is mostly biosynthetic human insulin. Insulin is recommended as first-line for women with GDM who are likely to fail on oral antihyperglycemic therapy or have risk factors such as diagnosed with diabetes at less than 20 weeks of pregnancy, fasting blood glucose >95 mg/dL, 1 hour postmeal level >140 mg/dL, or 2 hours postmeal levels >120 mg/dL after maternal nutrition therapy and physical exercise.

The various types of insulin available are short-acting insulin (regular), rapid-acting insulin (insulin analogs like insulin lispro, insulin aspart, insulin glulisine), long-acting insulin (i.e., NPH, insulin glargine, insulin detemir, lente, or ultralente) and mixtard containing 30% short-acting insulin and 70% intermediate-acting insulin. The onset and duration of each of these types are listed in **Table 3**.[18]

Short- or rapid-acting insulin is administered before meals to reduce glucose excursions associated with the meal and allow utilization of consumed fuels, whereas longer acting insulin is basal insulin, used to restrain hepatic gluconeogenesis in between meals and in the fasting state.

## How to Initiate Insulin Therapy?

In GDM, management should start with dietary therapy and exercise, those who fail to maintain optimum blood sugar levels should be started on insulin therapy. As there is endogenous insulin secretion which is capable of providing some coverage for the meal time calorie intake, insulin is started at a lower dose as compared to type 1 DM. The starting dose of insulin is decided on the degree of derangement of blood sugar profile of the pregnant woman. To compensate for postprandial hyperglycemia, short-acting or rapid-acting insulin can be used. Approximately 1 U of insulin is required for every 30 mg/dL (1.6 mmol/L) rise in blood glucose level above the normal expected level. For example, if a patient's 1 hour postprandial blood glucose level is 200 mg/dL (11 mmol/L), she needs approximately 2 units of insulin before

**TABLE 3:** Description of various types of insulin available.

| Types | Onset of action (hour) | Peak of action (hour) | Duration of action (hour) |
|---|---|---|---|
| **Rapid acting** | | | |
| Lispro | <0.25 | 0.5–1.5 | 3–4 |
| Insulin aspart | <0.25 | 0.5–1.5 | 3–4 |
| **Short-acting** | | | |
| Regular | 0.5–1.0 | 2–3 | 3–6 |
| **Intermediate acting** | | | |
| NPH (Neutral protamine Hagedon) | 2–4 | 6–10 | 10–16 |
| Lente combinations | 3–4 | 6–12 | 12–18 |
| 70/30: 70% NPH, 30% regular | 0.5–1 | dual | 10–16 |
| 50/50: 50% NPH, 50% regular | 0.5–1 | dual | 10–16 |
| **Long acting** | | | |
| Insulin glargine | 1–2 | No pronounced peak | 24 hours |
| Insulin detemir | 1–2 | 3–9 | 6–23 hours (dose dependent) |

the meal to bring her closer to the desired level of 140 mg/dL (7.8 mmol/L).[22] It is prudent to start the woman on smaller doses and then titrate it according to the blood sugar levels.

A method for deciding initial insulin dose is based on the anticipated carbohydrate content of the meal (carbohydrate counting), the blood glucose reading before and after meal, and any anticipated activity level after the meal.

Various insulin regimens have been used; however, none has reproduced the precise insulin secretory pattern of the pancreatic islet. One commonly used regimen consists of twice daily injections of intermediate insulin mixed with short-acting insulin before the morning and evening meal. This regimen prescribes two-thirds of the daily insulin dose in the morning (two-thirds as intermediate acting and one third as short-acting) and one-third before the evening meal (one half given as intermediate and one half as short-acting).[22]

It is best for the patient to take the insulin at the same site each day to reduce the site-specific variation in absorption of insulin. Absorption is most rapid from the abdomen (15–30 minutes) compared to arm (30–45 minutes) and thigh (45–60 minutes). The patient can be advised to take her breakfast dose on abdomen, lunch and dinner on her arms, and her bed time injection on her thigh. The best treatment regimen is mixtard insulin, a mixture of short-acting and intermediate- or long-acting insulin that is administered once or twice a day and premeal short-acting regular insulin or rapidly acting analogs as required.

Insulin analogs such as insulin lispro which is rapidly acting insulin, are also available. They have considerable advantage over regular insulin. It can be injected at the start of a meal and the peak effect corresponds to the highest glucose excursion after a meal. This is as compared to regular insulin that must be taken 30 minutes before a meal and has its peak effect after 2–4 hours of injection. Regular insulin also has a longer duration of action 6–8 hours increasing the likelihood of hypoglycemia long after its injection. So, patient's compliance with insulin lispro injections is 100% as compared to 60% with regular insulin. However, insulin analogs are more expensive than regular insulin.[22] Long-acting insulins such as insulin glargine and detemir provide continuous insulin release and are associated with lower risk of hypoglycemia as compared to NPH.[3,23] Glargine is safe and well-tolerated based on limited studies but there are no long-term data available as of now.

## How to Titrate Insulin?

Insulin dose should be adjusted according to glycemic trends every 2–3 days as assessed by glucose profile. A 5–7 sample glucose profile is done every 2–3 days. The dose of insulin is adjusted till an optimum control is obtained. If the control is unsatisfactory, potential sources of the problem such as noncompliance to diet, concurrent medication, intercurrent illness or infections, stress, lack of exercise, and poor lifestyle need to be explored and rectified. For a single abnormal blood glucose value, dietary readjustment or 15 minutes of exercise after the meals is advisable.

## Obstetric Management

Ultrasound monitoring of fetal growth and amniotic fluid volume should be performed every 4 weeks between 28 and 36 weeks.

With regards to antenatal fetal surveillance, there is no data from randomized trials to make specific evidence-based recommendation on type, initiation, or frequency of testing. Many institutions initiate routine fetal surveillance at or near term. However, daily fetal movement count or fetal kick count is an inexpensive and easy way to evaluate fetal wellbeing in the third trimester. Perception of more than 10 movements by mother in a 12-hour period is generally reassuring. Some authors suggest that daily kick count should be started by 26–28 weeks of gestation in pregnancies complicated by DM and those with decreased fetal activity should be evaluated by fetal nonstress testing or biophysical profile (BPP).

Fetal nonstress test (NST) should be done twice a week from 34 weeks onwards. It has a positive predictive value of 50–70%. Biophysical profile does not carry as much significance in monitoring pregnant woman with DM as in a nondiabetic pregnant woman as oligohydramnios may be difficult to assess in the presence of hydramnios associated with DM. The current evidence suggests the use of Doppler flow studies in patients with DM who have pregnancies complicated by hypertensive disease, fetal growth restriction (FGR), or vasculopathy. It is not recommended as a routine method of fetal surveillance.

## Timing of Delivery[4,9]

The primary goal of timed delivery is to prevent stillbirth. The risk of unexplained intrauterine death and stillbirth increases after 36 weeks of gestation in pregnant women with DM. At 36 weeks of gestation, the timing, mode, and management of delivery should be discussed taking into account both maternal and fetal factors. However, elective delivery has to be weighed against the risk of delayed lung maturity and respiratory distress syndrome.

### Insulin-treated Diabetes

Elective delivery after 38 weeks is recommended with the primary intention of reducing the risk of stillbirth, however, there are some other additional advantages like reduced risk of macrosomia and associated lower rate of shoulder dystocia and cesarean section.

The RCOG recommends antenatal steroids for women undergoing elective cesarean section before 39 weeks of gestation to reduce risk of respiratory distress. If steroids are given, consider admitting the woman to monitor and manage the blood glucose levels as steroids result in hyperglycemia.

Delivery may be carried out even without documented fetal lung maturity if maternal or fetal compromise places the life of mother or fetus at significant risk. This includes maternal factors like severe preeclampsia, eclampsia and other factors where maternal well-being is compromised by continuing the pregnancy and severe fetal compromise such as FGR with absent or reversed diastolic flow on Doppler and nonreassuring fetal heart rate pattern at a time when fetal survival after delivery is considered possible.

### Mild Gestational Diabetes on Diet Control

In these women, the risk of stillbirth is not increased. The decision for elective labor induction depends on estimated fetal weight. Based on Cochrane database, there is little evidence to support elective labor induction. Elective labor induction does not increase maternal and fetal risk, however, the benefits of this practice also remain unclear. These women can carry their pregnancies to term, i.e., 40 weeks.

The ACOG recommends delivery between 39 and 39 weeks 6 days for women whose diabetes is well controlled on medication and at 37–38 weeks 6 days for those with poorly controlled diabetes. Delivery as early as 34 weeks and up to 36 weeks 6 days could be considered on an individualized basis among patients with poor inpatient glycemic control or abnormal fetal testing.

## Mode of Delivery

Vaginal delivery is preferable unless there is an obstetric or medical contraindication. Elective cesarean section should be considered for macrosomic fetuses to prevent the potential risk of shoulder dystocia and birth trauma. ACOG considers elective cesarean delivery if estimated fetal weight is more than 4,500 g in a diabetic mother. In women with diabetes and previous history of shoulder dystocia, elective cesarean section should be strongly considered. In those with estimated baby weight between 4,000 and 4,500 g, elective cesarean delivery remains controversial. Diabetes is not a contraindication for vaginal birth after cesarean section (VBAC); however, the success rate may be lower in women with macrosomic babies (birth weight >4,000 g).[24]

## Intrapartum Considerations

As diabetic women are predisposed to infections, strict aseptic technique is to be maintained during labor. The number of per vaginum examinations should be restricted. It is essential to carefully watch for progress of labor and maintain a partogram. The likelihood of diabetic woman to have cephalopelvic disproportion due to fetal macrosomia is high. Cephalopelvic disproportion should be suspected if the dilatation of cervix slows down in late first stage, and the cervix is not well applied to the presenting part or if there is arrest of second stage. An early decision for cesarean section should be taken. Obstetricians should be well versed and well prepared with the management of shoulder dystocia and take strict aseptic precautions while delivering a diabetic woman. Continuous electronic fetal monitoring is recommended during labor as there is an increased risk of fetal distress.

## Glycemic Control during Labor[10,25-27]

A strict glycemic control during labor is important to prevent neonatal hypoglycemia after birth. Insulin requirement during labor is less than the routine daily requirement due to fasting status of the mother and use of energy during labor. It is important to reduce or omit the dose of long-acting insulin on the day of planned delivery or if the woman goes into spontaneous labor. The morning fasting blood sugar sample is sent and further management planned accordingly.

Various protocols for maintaining good glycemic control in diabetic women on insulin during labor are described in literature.[26] There is no clinical evidence to support one intrapartum management protocol over another.

One can start with intravenous fluids based on the fasting blood glucose levels. An infusion of 5% dextrose or dextrose saline is started at the rate of 125 mL/hour if the blood sugar level is <100 mg/dL, no insulin is required. If the fasting blood sugar level is more than 140 mg/dL, the patient is started on normal saline or Ringer's lactate instead of 5% dextrose. If blood sugar level is between 100 and 140 mg/dL, insulin infusion is given by a calibrated pump or microdrip set at a rate of 1 U/h. Insulin infusion rate is further increased by 0.5 U for each increase of blood glucose level by 40 mg/dL. The solution is prepared by adding 25 U of regular insulin in 250 mL of normal saline which contains 1 U of insulin/10 mL. Blood glucose level must be checked hourly during intravenous infusion and maintained at 72–126 mg/dL (4–7 mmol/L) as per NICE guidelines and between 70–110 mg/dL (3.9–6.1 mmol/L) according to ACOG.[17] Urine sugar and ketone should be checked 2–4 hourly for any evidence of ketonuria. In case of nonavailability of infusion pump, it is advisable to give insulin infusion in a diluted solution (10 units in 100 mL of normal saline that is 1 U/10 mL). Insulin may also be administered by a subcutaneous infusion pump.

## Glycemic Management of Diabetes during Cesarean Section[28]

Elective cesarean section should be scheduled as the first case on the morning list. The usual dose of intermediate insulin or antidiabetic medication is given on the night prior to surgery. The patient is kept fasting after midnight and her usual morning dose of insulin is withheld. Regional anesthesia is preferred because an awake patient permits earlier detection of hypoglycemia. A fasting blood sample for blood glucose levels and serum electrolytes is sent.

The blood sugar levels are maintained between 70 and 140 mg/dL (3.9 and 7.8 mmol/L) during surgery. Hyperglycemia during surgery should be avoided to minimize the risk of wound infection, neonatal hypoglycemia, and maternal metabolic complications like diabetic ketoacidosis (DKA).

## Management of Preterm Labor

The commonly used beta mimetic agents like terbutaline, ritodrine, etc., as tocolytic agents can lead to maternal hyperglycemia. However, drugs like nifedepine and magnesium sulfate can be used safely. Nifedipine can be administered in a dose of 10 mg orally every 20 minutes up to 4 doses followed by a maintenance dose of 20 mg every 4-8 hourly to a maximum of 120-180 mg per 24 hours. Magnesium sulfate can be used as a loading dose of 4-6 g intravenously and then maintained by an infusion at the rate of 2 g/h. Corticosteroids used for accelerating fetal lung maturity can also cause maternal hyperglycemia and increase the risk of ketoacidosis. The blood sugar level starts rising within 6-12 hours and may persist up to 5 days. As corticosteroids are indicated in women with DM and preterm labor, it is important to monitor the blood glucose levels closely and use an appropriate dose of insulin according to sliding scale if necessary.

## Postpartum Care[29]

In women with GDM, insulin or hypoglycemics are stopped after delivery but blood sugar testing is done to rule out persistent hyperglycemia. All delivered women with diabetes, should be hydrated adequately in the postpartum period irrespective of the route of delivery. After surgery, the glucose levels are monitored every 2 hours. There is marked decrease in insulin requirement during the first 24-48 hours postpartum; hence, the dose of insulin needs to be titrated carefully to prevent hypoglycemia.

Patients who have type 1 DM will remain insulin dependent even after delivery so insulin is restarted at approximately 0.5-0.6 U/kg postpartum weight. Postpartum glycemic target can be relaxed to fasting and postprandial level of 100 and 150 mg/dL, respectively. Postpartum calorie requirements are approximately 25 kcal/kg per day and higher (27 kcal/kg per day) in lactating women.

Patients who have type 2 DM may not require any medication during the first 24-48 hours postpartum. They can be started on oral agents such as metformin or glyburide or insulin after 24-48 hours after delivery as per their prepregnancy requirements.

They should be encouraged to breastfeed immediately postdelivery to reduce risk of neonatal hypoglycemia. Breastfeeding for at least 6 months postnatally can reduce the risk of childhood obesity in the baby and risk of hyperglycemia in the mother in the future.[30,31] A significant fall in blood glucose level may occur during breastfeeding; therefore the mother should be encouraged to test her blood sugar before and after breastfeeding, so that requirement of maintaining higher blood glucose level during breastfeeding can be ascertained. For breastfeeding mothers, insulin is preferred, although WHO states that oral hypoglycemic agents are not contraindicated in a lactating mother. In patients on metformin, monitoring of baby for hypoglycemia is required as it is secreted in the milk. Glipizide and Glibenclamide are not detected in breast milk and hence are safe for breastfeeding.

## Postnatal Advice and Follow-up after Birth[32,33]

In women with GDM, most women have adequate glycemic control immediately following delivery. An oral GTT at 6 weeks postpartum with 75 g glucose is recommended to determine whether glucose tolerance has normalized and should be repeated in 1 year and then at a minimum of every 3 years thereafter. Patient should be counseled regarding the likelihood of recurrence of GDM in approximately 50% of subsequent pregnancies and a 50-60% lifetime risk for developing type 2 DM. They should be advised for early OGTT at 16-18 weeks of gestation in next pregnancy and repeat at 24-28 weeks if results are normal.

After the pregnancy, the woman should be encouraged to reduce weight, continue positive lifestyle modification, and dietary habits. They should be encouraged to maintain normal glucose levels and informed that this will prevent or slow down the rate of progression of diabetic complications. Exercise programs should be initiated depending upon patient's health status, age, physical fitness, and feasibility.

Postpartum depression is more common among both pregestational and gestational postnatal diabetic women as compared to nondiabetic women, hence screening is warranted.

## Contraception

It is important to discuss contraception before discharging the patient from hospital. There is no evidence that any of the contraceptive methods available are contraindicated in women with diabetes. ACOG[24] recommends use of combined low-dose OCPs in those diabetic women who do not smoke, are less than 35 years old, and who do not have hypertension or vasculopathy. Progestin only pill is recommended which has a minimal effect on glycemic control, lipid metabolism, and cardiovascular risk factors. Barrier contraceptive is also a good method of contraception if acceptable to couple. Intrauterine contraceptive device (IUDs) have no systemic side effects and metabolic effects, hence they are an ideal method for diabetic women with vascular disease such as hypertension, retinopathy, or hyperlipidemia. No studies have found any evidence of increase in rate of pelvic infection or decreased efficacy with use of IUDs in women with DM.[29]

## Neonatal Management[3,12]

A newborn infant of diabetic mother may develop one or more of the following complications. Thorough evaluation to look for earliest symptoms and signs needs to be done.
- Hypocalcemia
- Hypomagnesmia
- Hyperbilirubinemia
- Polycythemia
- Macrosomia
- Birth trauma injury
- Respiratory distress
- Hyaline membrane disease
- Hypertrophic cardiomyopathy
- Hypoglycemia.

Most of these infants display transient hyperinsulinism and are consequently at risk of hypoketonemic hypoglycemia. Screening should be undertaken for at least the first 24 hours of life and the blood glucose concentration maintained at >2.6 mmol/L (47 mg/dL). Testing may be discontinued once satisfactory blood glucose concentrations are maintained without supplementary feeds or intravenous therapy. If a newborn is unwell or shows signs of hypoglycemia manifested by apnea, cyanosis, jitteriness, or convulsions ("symptomatic hypoglycemia"), blood glucose should be measured urgently. If it is below 2.6 mmol/L, 10% glucose infusion should be administered as soon as possible intravenously at the rate of 2 mL/kg over 2–3 minutes. Subsequently, the blood glucose needs to be monitored and the rate of infusion adjusted accordingly. Blood glucose level should be maintained at 70–100 mg/dL. Early feeding should be initiated within 30 minutes after delivery and then at intervals of 2–3 hours thereafter.

## Implications for the Offspring[3,12,25,31]

Diabetes during pregnancy has long-term implications on the child in infancy and adult life. Studies have shown that obesity, impaired glucose tolerance, and type 2 DM are more prevalent in those who were exposed to hyperglycemic state during their fetal development. Long-term life-style modification may minimize the risk of diabetes for all family members.

## PREGESTATIONAL DIABETES MELLITUS

Women with pregestational DM may have difficulties conceiving and pregnancy may worsen the diabetes and precipitate certain complications. Fetuses born to diabetic mothers are at increased risk of congenital malformations, stillbirth, macrosomia, metabolic, and developmental problems. Pregnant women with DM must be managed by a multidisciplinary team consisting of an obstetrician, endocrinologist, neonatologist, and dietician.

## Effect of Pregnancy on Diabetes

Various microvascular complications coexisting with pregestational diabetes may get exacerbated during pregnancy. There is a risk of progression of maternal diabetic complications, such as retinopathy and nephropathy, especially if there is coexisting hypertension. Women with diabetic nephropathy may experience deterioration in renal function and the degree of proteinuria. Hypoglycemia may be more common in pregnancy and women may experience "hypoglycemia unawareness." Pregnancy is poorly tolerated by women who have severe autonomic dysfunction and those with pre-existing coronary artery disease.[32] Early pregnancy nausea and vomiting, infections, such as urinary tract infection and use of antenatal steroids may precipitate DKA. These complications can cause morbidity and poor perinatal outcomes among women with pre-existing diabetes.

### Retinopathy

The prevalence of retinopathy in diabetes depends upon the duration of the disease. The prevalence was found to be 17% in those where diabetes was diagnosed before the age of 30 years and duration of disease was 5 years. This progressively increased to 90% with increase in duration of disease to 15 years.[33] There are two well-characterized stages of retinopathy: nonproliferative or background retinopathy and proliferative retinopathy. In pregnancy, the progression of retinopathy depends on factors such as duration of diabetes, severity of pre-existing disease, presence of hypertensive disorders, degree of metabolic control, and retinal blood flow. Some women may only develop retinopathy during pregnancy, while those who had pre-existing diabetic retinopathy have a two-fold risk of progression during pregnancy.[32] Risk of progression of retinopathy in pregnancy is thought to be mainly due to rapid normalization of glycemic control and increased retinal blood flow during pregnancy. Hence, preconception evaluation of retinopathy is mandatory for all diabetic women who are planning a pregnancy, to initiate timely management before conception. Evaluation for presence of any high-risk factors should also be done, so that intensive monitoring during the pregnancy can be arranged.

### Nephropathy[34]

Diabetic nephropathy is associated with an increased risk of preeclampsia, decline in renal function, preterm delivery, and adverse fetal outcome. If prepregnancy renal assessment has not been carried out, it should be arranged at the earliest. Referral to nephrologist should be done if serum creatinine is ≥120 mmol/L (1.4 mg/dL) or total protein excretion exceeds 2 g/day. In patients with chronic renal failure or advanced proteinuria, the glomerular filtration rate (GFR) may decline rapidly during pregnancy. Patients on

ACE inhibitors should be switched over to methyldopa or labetalol after confirmation of pregnancy due to possible teratogenic effects of ACE inhibitors. Thromboprophylaxis should be considered if proteinuria is >5 g/day.

### Neuropathy[34]

Pregnancy does not worsen neuropathy, except in women with pre-existing carpel tunnel syndrome and those with advanced autonomic neuropathy and severe gastroparesis. The occurrence of gastroparesis manifesting as chronic nausea and vomiting is the most worrisome aspect of diabetic neuropathy, as this is associated with severe maternal and fetal morbidity and needs special consideration during preconception period. Preeclampsia, hypoglycemic attacks, ketoacidosis, congenital malformations, polyhydramnios, FGR, preterm delivery, fetal loss, and perinatal mortality were found to be almost double in these patients as compared to controls. Hence, pregnancy is a relative contraindication in patients with severe gastroparesis.

### Cardiovascular Disease[34]

All diabetic women with proven pre-existing macrovascular disease should undergo extensive cardiovascular evaluation by a cardiologist before conception. Revascularization by bypass graft should be considered if significant myocardial ischemia is detected which may significantly improve maternal and perinatal outcomes. Even though a recent review of literature on diabetic pregnancies with arteriosclerotic heart disease has not suggested a very poor prognosis, pregnancy should still be considered a relative contraindication in these patients due to the associated high mortality until more evidence is available regarding safety of pregnancy in these women.

## Effect of DM on Pregnancy

The abnormal metabolic environment created by hyperglycemia has a profound impact on both the mother and the fetus.

## Maternal Effects

### Obstetric Complications[32]

In women with poorly controlled pregestational DM, fertility is impaired and risk of miscarriage is high. Complications such as preeclampsia, polyhydramnios, preterm labor, and infections are common during pregnancy.

### Hypertension and Preeclampsia

The incidence of preeclampsia is directly proportional to the severity of the diabetes and the presence of proteinuria at the onset of pregnancy. Insulin resistance appears to increase the risk of preeclampsia, even in the absence of overt diabetes. There is some evidence that poor glycemic control increases the risk of developing preeclampsia.

### Polyhydramnios

Diabetic pregnancies are often complicated by polyhydramnios. This is probably due to fetal polyuria resulting from fetal hyperglycemia.

### Preterm Delivery

Iatrogenic and spontaneous preterm delivery is higher among pregnant women with diabetes as compared to nondiabetics. This increased incidence of preterm labor may be attributed to preeclampsia, polyhydramnios, poor glycemic control, and infections.

### Infections

Diabetic pregnant women are more prone to infections, especially with poor glycemic control or end organ damage, which is partly related to impaired neutrophil function. Infections increase the risk of developing preterm labor and preterm prelabor rupture of membranes. It also predisposes the woman to DKA which can cause fetal death in addition to maternal morbidity. Any suspected infection in pregnancy or postpartum period namely urinary tract infection, cesarean section wound or episiotomy infection, and endometritis should be treated promptly with appropriate antibiotic.

### Delivery Morbidity

As a result of fetal macrosomia from poorly controlled diabetes, mothers are at risk of traumatic vaginal deliveries and a higher risk of instrumental deliveries and caesarean sections. There is a higher risk of postoperative or postpartum infection and hemorrhage.

## Fetal Effects

### Congenital Malformations

The congenital malformations are seen in 4–10% of diabetic pregnancies and occurs in women with pre-existing diabetes. The incidence is three to five times higher than in the general population and accounts for about 50% of all perinatal deaths in this population.

Malformations often involve the heart and central nervous system and are potentially lethal. The congenital heart defects include tetralogy of Fallot, transposition of the great arteries, septal defects, anomalous pulmonary venous return, and various defects causing left or right outflow obstruction. Caudal regression syndrome, although very rare, is seen almost exclusively in diabetic pregnancies, and is sometimes associated with failure of femur to develop normally. Central nervous system defects include anencephaly, spina bifida, encephalocele, and hydrocephaly. The risks of limb defects, hypospadias, and orofacial clefts are also increased.

HbA1c values of greater than 8% are associated with three to six times greater risk of congenital malformations in the fetus than when maintained at less than this cut off point.[35]

Hence, a value of HbA1c below 48 mmol/mol (6.5%) is advisable for a diabetic woman planning to conceive.[4]

High dose folic acid supplementation (5 mg/day) preconceptionally and during organogenesis can decrease the risk of some neural tube defects, and possibly other congenital anomalies.

Thus, optimizing diabetic control before conception is essential to lower the rate of congenital malformations and miscarriages to that of the background population.

## Miscarriage[36]

Women with long-standing diabetes complicated by vascular complications have an increased risk of miscarriage. However, well-controlled diabetes is not associated with an increased risk.

## Macrosomia and Fetal Growth Restriction[37]

Fetuses who are exposed to chronic maternal hyperglycemia are macrosomic (birth weight > 4 kg) consequent to fetal hyperglycemia, beta cell hyperplasia, and hyperinsulinemia. Fetal macrosomia is seen in 40–50% women as compared with 8–9% in controls. The risk of shoulder dystocia and operative intervention is increased with fetal macrosomia and is associated with an increase in perinatal asphyxia, acidosis, and birth trauma. On the contrary, diabetic vasculopathy, maternal hypertension, superimposed preeclampsia, nephropathy, and excessively tight control of DIP have been linked to FGR.

## Polyhydramnios

Polyhydramnios occurs especially in diabetic pregnant women with poor glycemic control and large for gestational age fetuses, although the pathophysiology is poorly understood. Polyhydramnios can cause maternal abdominal discomfort and increase the risk of fetal death and preterm delivery.

## Intrauterine Fetal Death and Stillbirth[38]

The incidence of intrauterine fetal death and unexplained stillbirths is also higher, usually after 36 weeks of gestation and particularly in women with poor glycemic control. It is probably due to poor placental perfusion consequent to villus edema.

## Neonatal Effects[38]

Babies born to diabetic mothers are at increased risk of neonatal metabolic complications such as hypoglycemia, hyperbilirubinemia, hypocalcemia, and hypomagnesemia. Respiratory distress syndrome (RDS) happens more commonly in babies born to diabetic mothers compared with gestational age-matched infants born before 38.5 weeks. The long-term effects include DM in later life, neurological deficits, childhood obesity, and metabolic syndrome **(Table 4)**.

**TABLE 4:** Maternal and fetal morbidity associated with diabetes mellitus.[3]

| Maternal complications | Fetal, neonatal, or child complications |
|---|---|
| *Pregnancy:*<br>• Spontaneous miscarriages<br>• Gestational hypertension/preeclampsia<br>• Excessive fetal growth: Large for gestational age, macrosomia<br>• Polyhydramnios<br>• Urinary tract infection<br>• Candidiasis<br>*Intrapartum and postpartum:*<br>• Preterm labor<br>• Prolonged labor<br>• Instrumental delivery<br>• Traumatic delivery: Perineal trauma, obstetric anal sphincter injuries<br>• High cesarean section rate<br>• Postpartum hemorrhage<br>• Infections<br>• Thromboembolism<br>• Failure to initiate and/or maintain breastfeeding<br>*Long-term risks and outcomes:*<br>Weight retention<br>• Future overt diabetes mellitus<br>• Future cardiovascular disease | *Pregnancy:*<br>• Congenital fetal anomalies<br>• Stillbirth<br>• Fetal growth restriction<br>*Delivery:*<br>• Shoulder dystocia<br>• Birth trauma, e.g., Erb's palsy<br>*Postnatal:*<br>• Respiratory distress syndrome<br>• Cardiomyopathy<br>• Neonatal hypoglycemia<br>• Neonatal polycythemia<br>• Neonatal jaundice<br>• Neonatal electrolyte abnormalities, e.g., hypocalcemia<br>• Neonatal death<br>*Long-term outcomes:*<br>Programming and imprinting: Fetal origins of diseases like diabetes mellitus, obesity, hypertension, metabolic syndrome |

## Diagnosis of Pregestational DM

Diagnosis of pre-existing DM may be revealed by the woman during history taking. Symptoms of diabetes mellitus should be enquired into and high-risk factors of DM should be looked for in all antenatal cases. Screening for DM should be performed in the first prenatal visit if there is a high index of suspicion that the pregnant woman has undiagnosed type 2 diabetes, e.g., BMI > 30 kg/m², prior history of gestational diabetes or known impaired glucose metabolism or polycystic ovarian syndrome (PCOS). There are no validated criteria for selecting high-risk pregnant women for early screening. GOI guidelines, however, recommend screening all women for DM at their first antenatal visit, this facilitates early identification of women with undiagnosed pregestational diabetes.

Diagnosis of overt DM is made if following a 75 g oral glucose load fasting plasma glucose is ≥126 mg/dL (7.0 mmol/L) and 2 hours plasma glucose is ≥200 mg/dL (11.1 mmol/L) or Hb1Ac is ≥ 6.5% or random plasma glucose ≥11.1 mmol/L (200 mg/dL) in the presence of signs and symptoms of DM (WHO). In asymptomatic patients the elevated values are confirmed by a repeat test preferably the same.

## Management of Pregnancy with Pregestational Diabetes[16,25,34,35,39]

### Preconception Counseling

Goal of preconception counseling is to optimize the fetomaternal outcome of pregnancy in a women with DM before pregnancy. Preconception counseling and management should include the following:

- Emphasis that it is a high-risk pregnancy.
- Explain to the couple the need to plan the pregnancy with good glycemic control before conception and throughout pregnancy so as to minimize the risk of miscarriage, congenital malformation, maternal, and fetal morbidity and mortality such as stillbirth and neonatal death.
- Women should be informed about how pregnancy affects the diabetes and how diabetes affects the pregnancy.
- Lifestyle modification in the form of weight management, daily exercise, cessation of smoking, and alcohol intake is advised.
- Effect of nausea and vomiting in pregnancy on glucose control.
- Risk of hypoglycemia and education about signs and symptoms of hypoglycemia.
- Increased risk of baby being larger for gestational age, thereby increasing the risk of shoulder dystocia, birth trauma, induction of labor, and cesarean section.
- Risk of neonatal hypoglycemia, hence need for good glycemic control during labor and early feeding of the baby.
- Risk of baby developing childhood obesity, type 2 DM in later life.
- Need for regular follow up and compliance to treatment.
- Evaluation of end organ damage at the first visit.

The various investigations advised for evaluation of end organ damage are listed here:

- *Diabetic retinopathy:* Offer fundoscopy at the first appointment (unless assessment was done within the previous 6 months) and annually thereafter if no diabetic retinopathy. Ophthalmologic follow-up during the first year postpartum is also advised since retinopathy can be aggravated anytime during pregnancy or postpartum.
- *Diabetic nephropathy*: Offer renal assessment including 24-hour urinary protein, creatinine clearance, blood urea nitrogen (BUN), and urine culture. If serum creatinine is abnormal (≥120 mmol/L or 1.4 mg/dL) or estimated GFR is <45 mL/min/1.73 m², consider referral to nephrologist before stopping contraception. Nephropathy is associated with high risk of preeclampsia, preterm delivery and growth restriction.
- *Cardiovascular system*: Blood pressure is recorded. Any suspicion of presence of coronary artery disease should be further evaluated by ECG, echocardiography, stress test, etc., and referred to the cardiologist. Those with pre-existing diabetes of more than 10 years and presence of hypertension or vasculopathy should be offered evaluation.
- *Autonomic dysfunction*: Presence of excessive nausea, vomiting, lack of awareness of hypoglycemia, and orthostatic hypotension should prompt further evaluation.

Potential contraindications to pregnancy in diabetic women include coronary artery disease, untreated proliferative retinopathy, serious renal insufficiency or proteinuria, and severe gastroenteropathy. These women should be advised against planning a pregnancy.

- *Glycemic control*: Explain to the couple the need to plan pregnancy with a good glycemic control so as to minimize the risk of congenital anomalies in the newborn. Women should be strongly advised against getting pregnant if HbA1c is >10%. Offer monthly HbA1c measure and self-monitoring of blood sugar. Aim to maintain HbA1c below 48 mmol/mol (6.5%) before planning to conceive.[4] The reduction of HbA1c toward target 6.5% is likely to reduce risk of congenital malformation.
- When pregnancy is planned in a patient on oral hypoglycemic agents, patient may continue their medications if safe in pregnancy or switch to insulin therapy. It is essential that all medications should be checked and discontinued if not essential.
- Folic acid supplementation in the dose of 5 mg daily for the prevention of neural tube defects is prescribed for 3 months prior to conception.

## Management during Pregnancy[4,12,17,40,41]

### Antepartum Considerations

Patient should book with her obstetrician as early as possible and attend antenatal clinic regularly. The frequency of follow-up depends on the glycemic control and any coexisting obstetric complications.

In the first visit, the patient should be thoroughly evaluated for any end organ damage particularly retinopathy and nephropathy.

- Pre-existing moderate to severe retinopathy may progress to sight threatening retinopathy during pregnancy. Patient should be offered retinal assessment following first antenatal visit and again at 28 weeks if first examination is normal. If any diabetic retinopathy is present, repeat assessment should be done at 16–20 weeks. Laser treatment is safe during pregnancy. The presence of retinopathy should not be considered contraindication for a vaginal delivery or rapid optimization of glycemic control.
- Baseline renal function, overnight or 24 hours urine sample for albuminuria or an albumin/creatinine ratio to screen for nephropathy. Patients with pre-existing microalbuminuria are more likely to develop

preeclampsia.[40] Low dose 150 mg aspirin should be commenced in the first trimester to reduce the risk of preeclampsia and continue till delivery. If serum creatinine ≥120 μmol/L or total protein excretion >2 g/day, consider referring to the nephrologist. Consider starting thromboprophylaxis if proteinuria >5 g/day.
- ECG to screen for ischemic heart disease especially in women with hypertension. Significant coronary artery disease should be treated before pregnancy.
- Thyroid function should be measured in all women with type 1 DM as thyroid abnormalities are common (up to 40%) in diabetics and may adversely affect pregnancy outcome. The possibility of any other coexistent autoimmune diseases (e.g., coeliac disease) in women with type 1 DM should also be considered.

## Assessing Glycemic Control[4,8,24,25]

Self-monitoring of blood sugar is advised (four to seven times per day). Patients are advised to test their blood sugar early morning fasting, premeal and then 1 hour after each meal. One hour postprandial monitoring is found to be associated with tighter glucose control and better outcome as compared to 2 hours postprandial monitoring.

### Metabolic Goal during Pregnancy

*NICE recommends:* Fasting blood glucose <106 mg/dL (5.9 mmol/L) and a 1 hour postprandial <140 mg/dL (7.8 mmol/L).
*ACOG recommends:*
- Fasting blood glucose concentrations ≤95 mg/dL (5.3 mmol/L)
- Preprandial blood glucose concentrations no higher than 100 mg/dL (5.6 mmol/L)
- One-hour postprandial blood glucose concentrations no higher than 140 mg/dL (7.8 mmol/L)
- Two-hour postprandial blood glucose concentrations no higher than 120 mg/dL (6.7 mmol/L)
- Mean capillary glucose 100 mg/dL (5.6 mmol/L) and HbA1C ≤6%
- During the night, blood glucose levels should not decrease to less than 60 mg/dL (3.3 mmol/L).

In pregnant women with type 1 DM and type 2 DM, insulin requirement continues to increase as the pregnancy progresses due to metabolic changes associated with pregnancy which have already been described.

## Dietary Therapy

Adequate understanding of the importance of dietary therapy by the patient is important, especially the association between certain types of carbohydrates and glucose excursions. Patient should receive nutritional counseling by dietician upon diagnosis and be placed on appropriate diet.

Diet modification is as described under the management of GDM.

## Lifestyle Modifications

Regular physical exercise within tolerable limits should be encouraged. Moderate exercise of at least 30 minutes per day such as walking, swimming, or yoga is suggested.

## Oral Antihyperglycemic Agents

Oral antihyperglycemic agents are ideal in treating early stages of type 2 DM and GDM patients. The details are described under the section of medical therapy for GDM. An ideal patient for starting glyburide is a normal weight or an obese diabetic woman who has been hyperglycemic for less than 5 years and willing to follow strict dietary regimen. NICE guideline states that metformin may be used for women with pregestational diabetes as an adjunct or alternative to insulin. This is a class B drug and crosses the placenta.

## Insulin Therapy

In the women with pregestational diabetes, insulin is the mainstay of therapy. The details regarding type of insulin and how to initiate and titrate insulin dose are similar to that in GDM.

Pregnant women with pregestational type 1 DM lack endogenous insulin secretion so administration of basal exogenous insulin is essential for regulating glycogen breakdown, gluconeogenesis, lipolysis, and ketogenesis. Before conception the daily insulin requirement is approximately 0.5 U/kg body weight.[18] In 1st trimester insulin requirement increases to 0.7 U/kg pregnant weight of patient, by 2nd trimester it rises to 0.8 U/kg which further goes up to 0.9 to 1 U/kg pregnant weight per day in the 3rd trimester.[3,17]

Insulin pump therapy, also known as continuous subcutaneous insulin infusion (CSII), is becoming increasingly popular among women with diabetes. It helps with flexibility as well as precise dosing, thus reducing the risk of hypoglycemic episodes. Moreover, it helps the woman to avoid multiple insulin injections as the pump catheter needs to be changed only once every 2–3 days.

The NICE currently recommends the use of insulin pump in women who are unable to achieve satisfactory blood glucose control with insulin injections without having severe hypoglycemia. However, insulin pump use can be associated with higher risks of complications if there is a pump malfunction or poor patient compliance. More studies need to be conducted to compare between insulin pumps and regular insulin injections.[4,42]

## Antepartum Fetal Surveillance[4,24]

- First trimester dating scan should be arranged to document viability and accurate dating as many of these pregnancies undergo elective delivery.
- Offer first trimester prenatal screening for Down syndrome as per general population. However, if second

trimester serum screening test for Down syndrome is performed (e.g., Quadruple test), adjustment needs to be done since serum alfafetoprotein (MSAFP), and unconjugated estriol levels are reduced in women with diabetes.

- Pregestational DM is associated with high risk of neural tube defect. Either ultrasound alone or in combination with MSAFP may be used to screen for neural tube defect.
- Detailed routine anomaly scan along with four chamber view and outflow tract examination at 18–20 weeks to identify any fetal malformations is indicated. Routine detailed specialist cardiac scan is not recommended unless an abnormality is detected during routine anomaly scan.
- A follow-up ultrasound scan at 28 weeks, 32 weeks, and 36 weeks is recommended to identify fetal macrosomia and polyhydramnios or growth restriction.
- Due to the threat of late stillbirths, enhanced fetal surveillance in the form of DFMR, is done after 32-34 weeks pregnancy.

## INTRAPARTUM AND POSTPARTUM MANAGEMENT, CONTRACEPTION, AND CARE OF NEONATE

All details as regards timing and mode of delivery, intrapartum and postpartum management, contraception, and care of neonate are discussed under management of a pregnant woman with GDM.

## DIABETIC KETOACIDOSIS[43]

Diabetic ketoacidosis is an obstetric emergency that can result in life-threatening complications for both the mother and the fetus. This is due to physiological changes in pregnancy that predispose them to DKA. Some of these changes are:

- A state of respiratory alkalosis and lower bicarbonate levels in pregnancy.
- Relative insulin resistance due to gain in weight.
- Hormonal changes that decrease maternal insulin sensitivity.

The overall prevalence of DKA is difficult to evaluate. Various studies report a prevalence ranging from 1 to 10%. DKA is more common in type 1 than type 2 DM and is rare in GDM. If it presents with GDM, the possibility of unrecognized pre-existing diabetes should be suspected. The obstetrician must be aware of various factors that precipitate DKA, so that adequate preventive measures can be taken to prevent DKA from happening. The various risk factors include hyperemesis gravidarum, underlying infection, use of beta sympathomimetic drugs, corticosteroids, poor patient compliance, insulin pump failure, or an error in clinical judgment.

Diabetic ketoacidosis has classical clinical findings; hence, there is no better substitute for a detailed history and physical examination for diagnosing DKA. Patient's presentation is similar to that in nonpregnant women with symptoms of nausea, vomiting, polyuria, hyperventilation, altered mental status, weakness, and dehydration. This clinical presentation can be further confirmed with laboratory findings. There is hyperglycemia at a level of >200 mg/dL (11.1 mmol/L), acidosis (pH < 7.3), an elevated anion gap, elevated base deficit on blood gas analysis, increased serum ketone level ≥3.0 mmol/L or urinary ketones more than 2+, electrolyte abnormalities, and decreased serum bicarbonate level (<15 mEq/L). BUN and serum creatinine level may be elevated if there is dehydration and renal failure.

Maternal hyperglycemia results in fetal hyperglycemia and fetal osmotic diuresis. Maternal acidemia decreases uterine blood flow with a resultant decrease in placental perfusion leading to decreased oxygen delivery to the fetus. Fetal oxygen delivery is further compromised by the leftward shift of the maternal oxyhemoglobin dissociation curve caused by acidemia. High ketone levels present in maternal circulation easily cross the placenta and cause fetal heart rate abnormality including late deceleration and reduced or absent variability. However, this abnormality gets corrected with the stabilization of maternal status. Hence, immediate delivery is not indicated and the mother should always be stabilized first.

### Treatment of Diabetic Ketoacidosis[43]

Treatment involves aggressive fluid and electrolyte management, intravenous insulin administration, and identification and treatment of precipitating factor. The initial fluid used for replacement is normal saline. Overall fluid deficit can be calculated as 100 mL/kg body weight. Isotonic normal saline should be administered at rate of 1,000–2,000 mL/hour for first 1–2 hours followed by 250–500 mL/hour, so that 75% of fluid deficit can be corrected over a 24 hours period. Isotonic normal saline can be used till glucose level is <200 mg/dL (11.1 mmol/L), following which 5% dextrose with 0.45% NaCl at 150–250 mL/hour should be started.

Regular insulin infusion should be started at a rate of 0.1 U/kg/hour, not exceeding 15 U/hour. If glucose level does not fall by 54 mg/dL/hour (3 mmol/L/hour), then the hourly infusion rate should be doubled. The other metabolic targets are decreasing the serum ketones by 0.5 mmol/L/hour and improvement of venous bicarbonate by 3 mmol/L/hour. The IV insulin infusion can be stopped when the DKA has resolved and after 30–60 minutes from the first dose of subcutaneous rapid-acting insulin.

Dyselectrolytemia should be corrected. Serum potassium level should be maintained at 4–5 mEq/L. The need for replacement of other electrolytes like magnesium and calcium is debatable. Role of administration of bicarbonate for correction of metabolic acidosis in DKA is also debatable.

## KEY POINTS

- DM in pregnancy is associated with increased maternal and perinatal morbidity and mortality.
- Pregnancy is a diabetogenic condition due to alteration in carbohydrate metabolism due to maternal hormones.
- As per GOI guidelines screening for DM should be done at first antenatal visit, and if normal, should be repeated between 24 and 28 weeks.
- As per WHO (2013) criteria GDM is diagnosed in pregnancy if fasting plasma glucose is 5.1–6.9 mmol/L (92–125 mg/dL) and 2-hour post 75 g oral glucose load it is 8.5–11.0 mmol/L (153–199 mg/dL).
- Gestational diabetes is hyperglycemia that develops during pregnancy, resolves after delivery and usually responds to MNT and exercise.
- Insulin therapy is recommended when nutritional therapy fails to maintain plasma fasting glucose <105 mg/dL and 2 hours postprandial blood glucose <130 mg/dL.
- Insulin dosage should be adjusted as per blood sugar.
- Metformin and glyburide are also used but there are no long-term data on safety.
- The goal during pregnancy is to maintain premeal plasma blood glucose level of 95 mg/dL (5.3 mmol/L), plasma level of 140 mg/dL (7.8 mmol/L) at 1 hour postprandial, and 120 mg/dL (6.7 mmol/L) at 2 hours postprandial. Levels should be kept above 4 mmol/L (72 mg/dL) to avoid hypoglycemia.
- Self-monitoring of blood sugar is advocated.
- Hypoglycemia should be prevented. Woman should recognize the symptoms of hypoglycemia and should take glucose immediately.
- Healthy diet and exercise such as half an hour walk after meals should be continued. The diet should consist of 30–35 kcal/kg/day in the form of three major meals and two to three minor meals and the composition should be of 50–60% carbohydrates, 20–25% proteins, less than 30% fat with adequate amount of dietary fiber. Complex carbohydrates and low glycemic foods are advised.
- Complications of GDM such as macrosomia, shoulder dystocia, traumatic delivery, and hypoglycemia in newborn are prevented by strict control of blood sugar level.
- Regular antenatal checkups and care is provided. Ultrasound monitoring of fetal growth and amniotic fluid volume is carried out every 4 weeks from 28 to 36 weeks.
- Fetal surveillance is done by DFMR and fetal heart monitoring.
- ACOG recommends delivery between 39 and 39 weeks 6 days for women whose diabetes is well controlled on medication and at 37–38 weeks 6 days for those with poorly controlled diabetes. Delivery as early as 34 weeks and up to 36 weeks 6 days could be considered on an individualized basis among patients with poor inpatient glycemic control or abnormal fetal testing.
- Capillary plasma glucose is checked every hour during labor and is maintained between 4 and 7 mmol/L.
- Newborns must be assessed carefully and managed by pediatrician, they are at risk of hypoglycemia and other complications. Feeding should be started within half an hour and blood sugars monitored.
- In women with GDM, insulin and other hypoglycemics are stopped following delivery.
- Fasting blood sugar should be tested before discharge and again at 6–13 weeks to exclude diabetes. HbA1c done after 13 weeks can also be used to exclude DM. Annual HbA1C estimation should be advised to women with GDM.
- Contraception, life style modification including advice regarding diet, exercise, and weight control is given. Risk of GDM in next pregnancy and development of type 2 diabetes is explained.
- Pre-existing diabetes in pregnancy is diagnosed if there is history of DM or if OGTT or HbA1C confirms DM. As per WHO criteria overt DM is diagnosed if fasting plasma glucose is ≥126 mg/dL (7.0 mmol/L) and 2 hour plasma glucose ≥200 mg/dL (11.1 mmol/L) following a 75 g oral glucose load or Hb1Ac is ≥6.5%. Random plasma glucose ≥11.1 mmol/L (200 mg/dL) in the presence of diabetes symptoms is also diagnostic of DM (WHO).
- The incidence of obstetric complications like spontaneous abortions, preeclampsia, polyhydramnios, and preterm delivery is increased in women with pre-existing diabetes.
- There is risk of progression of diabetic complications like proliferative retinopathy and nephropathy in pregnancy.
- The fetal and neonatal effects of diabetes include increased risk of congenital malformations involving the heart and central nervous system, macrosomia, FGR, intrauterine fetal death, unexplained stillbirths, shoulder dystocia, operative intervention, birth trauma, and perinatal asphyxia.
- Babies born to diabetic mothers are at increased risk of neonatal metabolic complications such as hypoglycemia, hyperbilirubinemia, hypocalcemia, and hypomagnesemia.
- Preconception optimization of blood sugar with aim of HbA1C below 6.5% minimizes the risk of congenital malformations. Evaluation of end organ involvement, review of drugs, lifestyle changes, dietary modifications, and folic acid supplementation is part of preconception care in a diabetic woman.

- Multidisciplinary team consisting of obstetrician, dietician, endocrinologist, and pediatrician should be involved in management.
- Patient should be registered as early as possible and advised to attend antenatal clinic regularly. The frequency of follow up depends on the glycemic control and any coexisting obstetric complications.
- Self-monitoring of blood sugar is advocated (four to six times per day). Target sugar values are same as for GDM but risk of hypoglycemia should be understood by the woman and the family and immediate action should be taken by glucose administration, if hypoglycemia develops.
- The HbA1c concentration should be monitored every 4–6 weeks with the goal of maintaining it at a normal level (<6%).
- The risk of ketoacidosis is higher in pre-existing diabetes but rarely it can occur in GDM.
- Diabetic ketoacidosis is one of the life-threatening complications for both the mother and the fetus.
- The conditions that can precipitate DKA include hyperemesis gravidarum, underlying infection, use of beta sympathomimetics, steroids, poor patient compliance, insulin pump failure, and error in clinical judgment.
- In DKA, there is increased plasma blood glucose level of ≥300 mg/dL (16.7 mmol/L) sometimes it may occur at >200 mg/dL (11 mmol/L), there is acidosis (pH < 7.3), anion gap with acidosis, elevated base deficit on blood gas analysis; there is presence of serum and urinary ketones, electrolyte derangements, and decreased serum bicarbonate level (<15 mEq/L).
- Treatment of DKA involves aggressive fluid management, insulin administration, and identification and treatment of precipitating factor.
- In insulin treated diabetics, elective delivery is indicated at 38–39 weeks with the primary intention of reducing the risk of stillbirth. Early delivery may be considered on an individualized basis among patients with poor glycemic control or abnormal fetal testing.
- Vaginal delivery is preferable unless there is an obstetric or medical contraindication.
- A strict glycemic control during labor is important to prevent neonatal hypoglycemia after birth.
- There is marked decrease in insulin requirement during the first 24–48 hours postpartum; hence, the dose of insulin needs to be titrated carefully.
- It is important to discuss contraception before discharging the patient from hospital. The ACOG recommends use of combined low-dose OCPs in those diabetic women who do not smoke, are less than 35 years old, and who do not have hypertension or vasculopathy. No method of contraception is contraindicated; progestin only pill, IUCD or barrier contraceptives, all can be used by women with DM.
- Counseling on the long-term implications and outcomes of pre-existing DM are essential so that women can embark on measures to reduce the risks and progression of diabetic complications.

## REFERENCES

1. Wild S, Roglic G, Green A, Sicree R, King H. Global prevalence of diabetes: estimates for the year 2000 and projecting for 2030. Diabetes care. 2004;27:1047-53.
2. Caissutti C, Berghella V. Scientific evidence for different options for GDM screening and management: controversies and review of the literature. Bio Med Res Int. 2017;1-12.
3. Hod M, Kapur A, Sacks DA, Hadar E, Agarwal M, Di Renzo GC, et al. The International Federation of Gynecology and Obstetrics (FIGO) Initiative on gestational diabetes mellitus: a pragmatic guide for diagnosis, management, and care. Int J Gynaecol Obstet. 2015;131(Suppl 3):S173-S211.
4. National Institute for Health and Care Excellence. Diabetes in pregnancy: management of diabetes and its complications from preconception to the postnatal period. NG3. August 2015. [online] Available from www.nice.org.uk/guidance/ng3. [Last accessed July, 2021].
5. Raja MW, Baba TA, Hanga AJ, Bilquees S, Rasheed S, Haq IU, et al. A study to estimate the prevalence of gestational diabetes mellitus in an urban block of Kashmir valley (North India). Int J Med Sci Public Health. 2014;3:191-5.
6. Bhatt AA, Dhore PB, Purandare VB, Sayyad MG, Mandal MK, Unnikrishnan AG. Gestational diabetes mellitus in rural population of Western India – results of a community survey. Indian J Endocrinol Metab. 2015;19:507-10.
7. Seshiah V, Balaji V, Balaji MS, Sanjeevi CB, Green A. Gestational diabetes mellitus in India. J Assoc Physicians India. 2004;52:707-11.
8. Aroda VR, Christophi CA, Edelstein SL, Zhang P, Herman WH, Barrett-Connor E, et al. The effect of lifestyle intervention and metformin on preventing or delaying diabetes among women with and without gestational diabetes: the diabetes prevention program outcomes study 10-year follow-up. J Clin Endocrinol Metab. 2015;100(4):1646-53.
9. American Diabetes Association. Classification and Diagnosis of Diabetes: Standards of Medical Care in Diabetes-2020. Diabetes Care. 2020;43(Suppl 1):S14-S31.
10. World Health Organization. Diagnostic Criteria and Classification of Hyperglycaemia First Detected in Pregnancy. (2013) [online] Available at: http://apps.who.int/iris/bitstream/10665/85975/1/WHO_NMH_MND_13.2_eng.pdf. [Last accessed July, 2021].
11. Lain KY, Calalano PM. Metabolic changes in pregnancy. Clin. Obstet. Gynaecol. 2007;50(4):938-48.
12. Metzger BE, Gabbe SG, Persson B. International Association of Diabetes and Pregnancy Study Groups recommendations on the diagnosis and classification of hyperglycemia in pregnancy. Diabetes Care. 2010;33:676-82.
13. Danilenko-Dixon DR, Van Winter JT, Nelson RL, Ogburn PL Jr. Universal versus selective gestational diabetes screening: application of 1997 American Diabetes Association recommendations. Am J Obstet Gynecol. 1999;181:798.

14. Berger H, Gagnon R, Sermer M. Guideline No. 393-Diabetes in Pregnancy. J Obstet Gynaecol Can. 2019;41(12):1814-25.e1.
15. Government of India. National Guidelines for Diagnosis and Management of Gestational Diabetes Mellitus. Maternal Health Division, Ministry of Health and Family Welfare, Government of India; December, 2014. [online] Available from: http://nhm.gov.in/images/pdf/programmes/maternal-health/guidelines/ National_ Guidelines_ for_Diagnosis_ and _Management_of_Gestational_Diabetes_Mellitus.pdf. [Last accessed July, 2021].
16. Seshiah V, Das AK, Balaji V, Joshi SR, Parikh MN, Gupta S. Gestational diabetes mellitus—guidelines for Diabetes In Pregnancy Study Group (DIPSI). JAPI. 2006;54:622-8.
17. Committee on Practice Bulletins—Obstetrics. ACOG Practice Bulletin No. 190: Gestational Diabetes Mellitus. Obstet Gynecol. 2018;131(2):e49-e64.
18. Kelley KW, Carroll DG, Meyer A. A review of current treatment strategies for gestational diabetes mellitus. Drugs Context. 2015;4:212282.
19. Brown J, Alwan NA, West J, Brown S, McKinlay CJ, Farrar D, et al. Lifestyle interventions for the treatment of women with gestational diabetes. Cochrane Database Syst. Rev. 2017;5(5):CD011970.
20. Gui J, Liu Q, Feng L. Metformin vs insulin in the management of gestational diabetes: a meta-analysis. PLoS One. 2013;8(5):e64585.
21. Camelo Castillo W, Boggess K, Sturmer T, Brookhart MA, Benjamin DK Jr, Funk MJ. Association of adverse pregnancy outcomes with glyburide vs insulin in women with gestational diabetes. JAMA Pediatr. 2015;169:452-8.
22. Bishop KC, Harris BS, Boyd BK, Reiff ES, Brown L, Kuller JA. Pharmacologic treatment of diabetes in pregnancy. Obstet Gynecol Surv. 2019;74(5):289-97.
23. Balsells M, García-Patterson A, Solà I, Roqué M, Gich I, Corcoy R. Glibenclamide, metformin, and insulin for the treatment of gestational diabetes: a systematic review and meta-analysis. BMJ. 2015;350:h102.
24. American College of Obstetricians and Gynecologists' Committee on Practice Bulletin-Obstetrics. ACOG Practice Bulletin No 205: vaginal birth after cesarean delivery. Obstet Gynecol. 2019;133(2):e110-e127.
25. Patel N, Hameed A, Banerjee A. Pre-existing type I and type II diabetes in pregnancy. Obstet Gynaecol Reprod Med 2014;24(52):129-34.
26. Royal College of Obstetricians and Gynaecologists (RCOG). Antenatal corticosteroids to prevent respiratory distress syndrome. Clinical Green Top Guidelines. Royal College of Obstetricians and Gynaecologists, 2004.
27. American College of Obstetricians and Gynecologists. ACOG committee opinion no. 560: Medically indicated late-preterm and early-term deliveries. Obstet Gynecol. 2013;121:908.
28. Kalra P, Anakal M. Peripartum management of diabetes. Indian J Endocrinol Metab. 2013;17(Suppl 1):S72-6.
29. Kjos SZ, Brehanan TA. Postpartum management, lactation and contraception. In: Reece EA, Consten DR, Garbe SG (Eds). Diabetes in Women, 3rd edition. Philadelphia: Lippincott, Williams and Wilkins; 2004. pp. 441-2.
30. Gunderson EP, Hedderson MM, Chiang V, Crites Y, Walton D, Azevedo RA, et al. Lactation intensity and postpartum maternal glucose tolerance and insulin resistance in women with recent GDM: the SWIFT cohort. Diabetes Care. 2012;35:50e6.
31. Schaefer-Graf UM, Hartmann R, Pawliczak J, Passow D, Abou-Dakn M, Vetter K, et al. Association of breast-feeding and early childhood overweight in children from mothers with gestational diabetes mellitus. Diabetes Care. 2006;29:1105e7.
32. Nielsen-Piercy C. Handbook of Obstetric Medicine, Fifth edition. Florida: CRC Press; 2019.
33. Klein R, Klein BE, Moss SE, Davis MD, DeMets DL. The Wisconsin epidemiologic study of diabetic retinopathy. Diabetic macular edema. Ophthalmology. 1984;91(12):1964-74.
34. Ballard JZ, Rosenn B, Khoury JC, Miodovnik M. Diabetic fetal macrosomia; significance of disproportionate growth. J Pediatr. 1993;122(1):115-9.
35. Leguizamon G, Igarzabal ML, Reece A. Preconceptional care of women with diabetes. Obstet Gynaecol Clin N Am. 2007;34:225-39.
36. Ylinen K, Aula P, Steinman UH, Kesäniemi-Kuokkanen T, Teramo K. Risk of minor and major fetal malformations in diabetes with high hemoglobin A1c values in early pregnancy. Br Med J (Clin Res Ed). 1984;289(6441):345-6.
37. Jovanovic L, Knopp RH, Kim H, Cefalu WT, Zhu XD, Lee YJ, et al. Elevated pregnancy losses at high and low extremes of maternal glucose in early normal and diabetic pregnancy: evidence for a protective adaptation in diabetes. Diabetes Care. 2005;28:1113.
38. Robert MF, Neff RK, Hubbell JP, Taeusch HW, Avery ME. Association between maternal diabetes and the respiratory distress syndrome in the newborn. N Engl J Med. 1976;294(7):357-60.
39. Institute of Medicine. Dietary Reference Intakes: Energy, Carbohydrate, Fiber, Fat, Fatty Acids, Cholesterol, Protein, and Amino Acids. Washington: National Academies Press; 2002.
40. Hunt KF, Whitelaw BC, Gayle C. Gestational diabetes. Obstet Gynaecol Reprod Med. 2014;24(8):238-44.
41. Schroder W, Heyl W, Hill-Grasshoff B, Rath W. Clinical value of detecting microalbuminuria as a risk factor for pregnancy induced hypertension in insulin treated diabetic pregnancies. Eur J Obstet Gynaecol Reprod Biol. 2000;91(2):155-8.
42. Kesavadev J. Insulin pump therapy in pregnancy. J Pak Med Assoc. 2016;66(9 Suppl 1):S39-S44.
43. Mohan M, Baagar KAM, Lindow S. Management of diabetic ketoacidosis in pregnancy. The Obstet. Gynaecol. 2017;19:55-62.

# Thyroid Disorders in Pregnancy

*Kiran Aggarwal*

## INTRODUCTION

Thyroid disorder is a common endocrine disease in women of reproductive age group, being second only to diabetes. It can affect reproductive performance of a woman. Thyroid dysfunction is difficult to diagnose in pregnancy because physiological changes and symptoms of pregnancy are very similar to those of thyroid disorders.

This chapter highlights the maternal and fetal thyroid physiology, various thyroid dysfunctions, their treatment, and screening for thyroid disease in pregnancy.

## MATERNAL PHYSIOLOGY

Thyroid gland is made up of follicles. Each follicle has a lumen for storage of thyroglobulin. Thyroglobulin is a glycoprotein needed for thyroid hormone synthesis. Thyroid actively traps iodine from extracellular pool which compensates for dietary fluctuations. This is potentiated by thyroid stimulating hormone (TSH).

Thyroid peroxidase enzyme helps in formation of thyroxin (T4) and triiodothyronine (T3) which are the active hormones. T3 is three times more potent than T4 and most of it is produced by peripheral deiodination of T4.[1]

Thyroid function is regulated by hypothalamus-pituitary-thyroid feedback mechanism. TSH is a glycoprotein with alpha and beta subunits. Alpha subunit is shared with other pituitary hormones but beta subunit is unique. It has some similarity to the beta subunit of human chorionic gonadotropin.

The TSH increases synthesis and release of thyroid hormones, both T4 and T3.

Major fraction of T3 and T4 in circulation is protein bound. Only small unbound portions are the active form of the hormone. The binding proteins for thyroid hormones are thyroid binding globulin (TBG), albumin and transthyretin.

The TBG has the greatest affinity for T4 and T3 and 75% of the thyroid hormones are bound to it. Only 0.04% of T4 and 0.5% of T3 are free.[1]

## CHANGES IN THYROID PHYSIOLOGY DURING PREGNANCY

- The high estrogen status of pregnancy increases the half-life of TBG and decreases its clearance. TBG production begins to increase in first 2 weeks of pregnancy and reaches a peak by 20 weeks of gestation. It plateaus for rest of the pregnancy at double the baseline values. Thus, total T4 and T3 production is increased during pregnancy to compensate for this rapid increase in extra thyroid pool of thyroxine. Maternal iodine requirements are increased for production of this extra pool of hormones **(Table 1)**.[1]
- Increase in glomerular filtration rate from early first trimester of pregnancy causes increased renal loss of iodide.[2] This causes decrease in circulatory iodine.
- Fetal thyroid activity starts in early second trimester. Transport of iodide to fetus causes further decrease in the maternal pool of iodine.
- In dietary iodine deficiency, thyroid increases its uptake of iodide from circulation and if this is not sufficient, maternal hypothyroxinemia and enlargement of thyroid occurs. Goiter may be seen in both mother and fetus.[3]
- In iodine-deficient areas, iodine-deprived goiter may take up iodide preferentially over placenta thus causing cretinism in the child.

During first trimester, fetus is dependent on maternal T4. Increased production of T4 occurs for transport to fetus thus maternal iodine requirement increases.

A part of beta subunit of human chorionic gonadotropin (hCG) has thyrotropic activity. It stimulates TSH receptors causing increase in free T4 levels and a decrease in TSH level

**TABLE 1:** Changes in thyroid physiology in pregnancy.

| Thyroid binding globulin (TBG) | Iodine requirements | Human chorionic gonadotropin (hCG) |
|---|---|---|
| • Increased thyroid binding globulin<br>• 10–15% increase in the size of the thyroid gland<br>• Increased total T4 and T3 | Increased iodine requirement because of:<br>• Increased renal loss of iodine<br>• Transport of iodine to fetus<br>• Increased maternal requirement of total T4 and T3<br>• Increased iodine uptake by the thyroid gland | Placental hCG stimulates thyroid receptors:<br>• Increases thyroid hormone secretion<br>• Maternal TSH decreases from first trimester |

by negative feedback mechanism, maximally seen at the end of the first trimester which is the time for peak circulating hCG.[4]

This may be nature's mechanism to provide sufficient thyroxin to fetus.

## ASSESSMENT OF THYROID FUNCTION IN PREGNANCY

The TBG and T4 levels increase from late first trimester and reach a peak by 16 weeks of gestation, after which, levels remain high till delivery.[5] hCG stimulates thyroid receptors and the levels of T4 and T3 increase. Following this, because of negative feedback TSH levels decrease. Maximum decrease in TSH occurs in first trimester and then serum TSH gradually rises in second and third trimester but remains lower than the nonpregnant women.[6,7]

For evaluation of serum TSH levels, population-based trimester-specific ranges should be used. These values are not readily available to most populations.[8]

As per American Association of Thyroid Disorders Guidelines 2017, following trimester-specific ranges and cutoffs should be used when local assessments and trimester-specific ranges are not available

In the first trimester, the lower reference range of TSH can be reduced by approximately 0.4 mU/L, while the upper reference range is reduced by approximately 0.5 mU/L. For the typical patient in early pregnancy, this corresponds to a TSH upper reference limit of 4.0 mU/L. This reference limit should generally be applied beginning with the late first trimester, weeks 7–12, with a gradual return toward the nonpregnant range in the second and third trimesters.[8]

The serum FT4 values are affected by pregnancy, methods used to measure it, and by various labs. If measured in pregnant women, assay method-specific and trimester-specific pregnancy reference ranges should be applied.[8]

Pregnant women with TSH concentrations >2.5 mU/L should be evaluated for TPOAb status.[8]

A maternal TSH concentration that is low but detectable is likely not clinically significant.[9]

## FETAL THYROID PHYSIOLOGY

The fetal thyroid gland develops at 5 weeks of pregnancy and begins concentrating iodine from 10–12 weeks onward. Fetal free and total T3, T4, TSH, and TBG can be detected in fetal blood from 12 weeks of gestation and increase with advancing gestation, reaching adult levels by 36 weeks of gestation.[10] For first 10–12 weeks of pregnancy, fetus is totally dependent on mother for thyroid hormones (T4). By end of first trimester hormone production starts, but fetus is dependent on mother for ingestion of enough iodide to make sufficient thyroid hormones. The fetal thyroid gland comes under control of fetal pituitary by 20 weeks of gestation.

Maternal T3 and TSH do not cross placenta but maternal T4, TRH, iodine, thyroid receptor stimulating antibodies, antithyroid antibodies, and antithyroid drugs cross the placenta readily. The peripheral conversion of T4 to T3 which accounts for most adult T3 is not active in fetus except in fetal brain.[11]

Human fetal brain has T3 receptors from late first trimester, whereas other tissues including liver, heart, and lung have only T4 receptors throughout second trimester. Maternal T3 cannot cross placenta. Fetal brain T3 arises by conversion from T4 which is available only from the mother in the first trimester.[12] This requires increased maternal production of T4 and increased requirement of iodine by the mother.

In areas of chronic iodine deficiency, if maternal hypothyroxinemia occurs, it adversely affects fetal brain development. Fetal and neonatal hypothyroidism may also occur.[3] Where maternal T4 is low but T3 is preserved, the fetal brain may be adversely affected. These are the areas where endemic cretinism occurs due to fetal thyroid dysfunction.[13]

Maternal thyroxine is transferred to fetus throughout pregnancy. It is important for fetal brain development more so before development of fetal thyroid gland function which starts at 12 weeks of gestation. Even after 12 weeks of gestation, maternal thyroxine is important as 30% of thyroxine in fetal serum at term is maternal.

## IODINE NUTRITION IN PREGNANCY

Iodine requirement increases during pregnancy. Lactating women also have increased dietary iodine requirements.[14] Iodine requirement for the infant is met through its secretion in breast milk. Women with adequate pre pregnancy stores of iodine have no added risks.

Maternal iodine deficiency and hypothyroxinemia causes fetal hypothyroidism.[15] Hypothyroxinemia in mother causes stimulation of TSH production from pituitary causing goiter in adults and cretinism in newborns.

Severe iodine deficiency in pregnant women has been associated with increased rates of pregnancy loss, stillbirth, and increased perinatal, and infant mortality.[16]

Children whose mothers are severely iodine deficient during pregnancy may exhibit cretinism, characterized by profound intellectual impairment, deaf-mutism, and motor rigidity.

Women with mild-to-moderate iodine deficiency during pregnancy are at increased risk for the development of goiter and thyroid disorders.[17] Mild-to-moderate maternal iodine deficiency has also been associated with attention deficit and hyperactivity disorders in children.[18]

The recommended dietary intake for iodine in adults and children above the age of 12 years is 150 μg/day.

In pregnancy and breastfeeding mothers, 200–300 μg/day of dietary iodine is recommended.[19]

All pregnant women should ingest approximately 250 µg iodine daily. Different strategies may be required to provide a total of 250 µg iodine ingestion daily.[8]

Universal salt iodization is the most cost-effective way of delivering iodine and improving maternal and infant health.[20] If salt supplementation is not there, oral iodine supplement as potassium iodide 100–200 µg/day or incorporating it in multivitamin tablet especially for pregnancy can be done.

In severely iodine-deficient area, iodine administration to women before conception till second trimester was shown to help improve neurological status and protecting fetal brain.[21]

In many regions with mild-to-moderate iodine deficiency, women during pregnancy and preconception period are advised to supplement their diet with a daily oral supplement that contains 150 µg of iodine in the form of potassium iodide. This is to be started 3 months prior to pregnancy.[8] During lactation, breast milk provides approximately 100 µg of iodine daily to the infant, it is recommended that the breastfeeding mother should continue to take 250 µg/day of iodine.

If salt iodization or daily iodine supplements are not feasible, single dose of iodized oil containing 400 mg of iodine can take care of iodine requirement for 1 year.[22]

Women who are already taking levothyroxine (LT4) regularly do not need supplemental iodine because the substrate is no longer needed for hormone formation.[8]

Excess intake of iodine by mother causes suppression of thyroid hormone synthesis induced by high concentrations of intrathyroid iodine. Pregnant women should avoid taking cough remedies or eye drops with iodine because it will cause fetal hypothyroidism. Iodine intake during pregnancy and breastfeeding should not exceed twice the daily recommended for iodine, i.e., 500 µg/day.

## HYPERTHYROIDISM IN PREGNANCY

Hyperthyroidism is over activity of thyroid gland. Thyrotoxicosis is the clinical manifestation seen as increased metabolic activity and hyperactivity.

Hyperthyroidism is seen in 0.2% of pregnant women. The most common causes are:
- Gestational transient hyperthyroidism
- Graves' disease
- Toxic multinodular goiter
- Solitary toxic nodule
- Acute thyroiditis (de Quervain's or postpartum)
- Subacute thyroiditis
- Well-differentiated thyroid carcinoma
- Hyperfunctioning ovarian teratoma
- TSH-producing adenoma
- hCG-producing tumor
- Overdosing of thyroid hormones.

### Gestational Transient Hyperthyroidism

Gestational hyperthyroidism is seen in later part of the first trimester of pregnancy. It occurs due to stimulation of thyroid receptors by beta subunit of hCG. This causes elevated thyroid hormones and low TSH levels. Variable clinical presentation of hyperthyroidism is seen in these cases. Antithyroid antibodies are absent.[23] It is seen in 2–15% of women in early pregnancy.[24]

Gestational hyperthyroidism is associated with hyperemesis gravidarum which is associated with increased hCG levels. 30–60% of patients with hyperemesis gravidarum have elevated free thyroid hormone concentration with suppressed TSH possibly due to thyroid receptor stimulating activity of hCG.

A small proportion of these patients have clinical hyperthyroidism.[25,26] hCG-induced thyrotoxicosis may also be seen in clinical situations with high levels of hCG like multiple gestation, hydatidiform mole, and choriocarcinoma.

All patients with low TSH levels should have total and free serum T4, and total T3 levels done. Most patients with gestational hyperthyroidism are asymptomatic for hyperthyroidism and levels of hormones return to normal by second half of pregnancy. Management of hyperemesis comprises supportive treatment for dehydration, vomiting, and electrolyte imbalance. Normally antithyroid drugs are not needed for transient hyperthyroidism.[27] A beta-blocker may be given if needed. Antithyroid therapy to patients with symptomatic hyperthyroidism and severely elevated T4 and T3 should be given. Therapy often can be discontinued if hyperemesis subsides by midgestation.

### Graves' Disease

Graves' disease is the most common cause of hyperthyroidism in the reproductive age group. It is an autoimmune disease characterized by diffuse hypertrophic and hyperplastic goiter. There is presence of IgG thyrotropin receptor stimulating antibodies which are specific to Graves' disease. Other thyroid autoantibodies like antiperoxidase antibodies may be present.

Clinical course of Graves' disease follows the levels of thyrotropin receptor stimulating antibodies which increase in the first trimester, fall in the second and third trimesters, and again rise in the puerperium. In the initial part of pregnancy, the symptoms worsen, but with decreasing antibodies in second half of pregnancy they may improve.[28] Graves' disease remits in second and third trimesters with decreasing antibodies and the doses of the antithyroid medications need to be reduced or discontinued in 30% of cases.[28] Symptoms may worsen in puerperium.[29] Labor, cesarean section, and infections may aggravate hyperthyroidism and even trigger thyroid storm.[30] Pregnancy does not influence long-term course of hyperthyroidism.

## Postpartum Thyroiditis

Postpartum thyroiditis is the most common cause of thyrotoxicosis in postpartum period. It may be mild. Severe cases are associated with higher levels of TPO antibody and are often followed by a period of hypothyroidism. The majority of women return to euthyroidism by 1 year postpartum.[31]

The postpartum increase in thyroid autoimmunity is also associated with a 3- to 4-fold increase in the incidence of new Graves' disease.[32]

## Effect of Hyperthyroidism on Pregnancy

If thyrotoxicosis is well-controlled before and throughout pregnancy the outcomes for both mother and baby are generally good. If uncontrolled, thyrotoxicosis may be associated with adverse outcomes for the mother as it increases the risk for preeclampsia, heart failure, and thyroid storm. Cardiac failure is more common and occurs because of cardiomyopathy resulting from long-term myocardial effects of T4. It is precipitated by hypertension, infections, and anemia.[33]

Fetal and neonatal risks of maternal hyperthyroid disease are related to the disease itself and or to the medical treatment of the disease. Inadequately treated maternal thyrotoxicosis is associated with an increased risk of miscarriage, growth restriction, premature labor, placental abruption, and increased perinatal mortality.[34,35] In addition, over treatment of the mother with thionamides can result in iatrogenic fetal hypothyroidism.

## Diagnosis of Hyperthyroidism

Thyrotoxicosis usually presents in late first and early second trimester. Clinical diagnosis of mild hyperthyroidism in pregnancy is difficult because symptoms like fatigue, anxiety, emotional liability, heat intolerance, sweating, warm extremities, etc. may also be reported by normal euthyroid pregnant women. Failure to gain weight particularly in presence of a good appetite and maternal tachycardia greater than 100 beats per minute helps in the diagnosis. Symptoms that persist beyond 20 weeks gestation, symptoms that occur before onset of pregnancy, and presence of thyroid stimulating antibodies suggest true hyperthyroidism.[36]

In early pregnancy, if there are features suggestive of hyperemesis and hyperthyroidism, trophoblastic disease should be ruled out. Eye signs like exophthalmos and lid lag, significant goiter, and presence of thyroid stimulating antibodies may indicate Graves' disease. The diagnosis is confirmed by elevated free-T4 or free-T3 levels with suppressed TSH level. The levels should be interpreted after keeping in mind the fluctuations of hormone levels in normal pregnancy. Thyroid receptor antibodies should also be measured. T3-toxicosis is when only serum T3 levels are raised and cause hyperthyroidism infrequently.

## Management

### Prepregnancy

Patients with thyrotoxicosis should have a stable euthyroid state for 3 months before conception. Patients who have received radioactive iodine should not conceive for 6 months after last treatment. It is contraindicated in pregnancy.[37] Well-controlled thyrotoxicosis has a low-risk of adverse obstetric outcome. Preconception counseling should review the risks and benefits of all treatment options. Risk of birth defects and the patient's desired timeline to conception should be considered.[8]

Antithyroid drugs (ATDs) should be avoided in early first trimester of pregnancy (gestation 6–10 weeks). When necessary propylthiouracil (PTU) is preferred. After first trimester PTU can be stopped and methimazole started. This decreases risk of liver failure in mother.

## Antenatal Management of Hyperthyroidism

### Medical Therapy

Medical management is the first treatment option. The aim of the treatment is to maintain euthyroid state and a free T4 level at the upper nonpregnant reference range.[38] Lowest possible dose of medication should be used so that risk of fetal hypothyroidism is minimized **(Box 1)**.

Antithyroid drugs like propylthiouracil, methimazole (MMI), and carbimazole are used during pregnancy. They inhibit thyroid hormone synthesis via reduction of iodine organification and iodotyrosine coupling. They also have an immunosuppressive effect reducing the titer of TSH receptor antibody.[39]

Onset of action of drug is delayed until preformed hormones are depleted which can take 3–4 weeks. PTU crosses placenta less readily than methimazole and is hepatotoxic.[29] The effect on fetal and neonatal thyroid appears to be similar for two agents. Available evidence suggests that methimazole may be associated with fetal congenital anomalies like esophageal atresia and aplasia cutis.

If the patient is on low doses of ATDs after confirmation of pregnancy it may be tried to stop the drugs in first trimester and thyroid functions may be followed closely at 1–2 weekly intervals. This is to avoid teratogenic effect of the drugs.

---

**BOX 1:** Therapeutic options for treatment of hyperthyroidism.

*Medical treatment*
- *Thionamides:* Propylthiouracil, carbimazole, and methimazole
- *Beta-blockers:* Propranolol
- Iodides
- Radioactive iodine

*Surgical treatment*
- Subtotal thyroidectomy

If medication has to be given then PTU should be used as a first-line drug especially in first trimester, that is, during organogenesis.[29] If PTU is not available or patient cannot tolerate PTU then methimazole may be prescribed.[29,40] PTU in first trimester and methimazole in rest of pregnancy may be given but this may cause poor control of thyroid function so some follow with PTU only.

### Dosage of Drugs

Newly diagnosed patients should be given PTU 400 mg daily or carbimazole 40 mg daily for 4–6 weeks and then the dose can be reduced gradually. It takes 7–8 weeks after starting therapy for the patient to become euthyroid.

The dose of the medication is titrated against maternal wellbeing and biochemical assessment of thyroid status. Aim of the treatment is to maintain thyroid hormone levels slightly above or in high normal range while TSH may remain suppressed.[29]

The initial dose of ATD depends on the severity of the symptoms and the degree of hyperthyroxinemia.

In general, initial doses of ATDs during pregnancy are as follows: MMI, 5–30 mg/d (typical dose in average patient 10–20 mg); carbimazole, 10–40 mg/d; and PTU 100–600 mg/d (typical PTU dose in average patient 200–400 mg/d). The equivalent potency of MMI to PTU is approximately 1:20. (e.g., 5 mg MMI = 100 mg of PTU).[41-43]

### Monitoring

Maternal TT4/FT4 and TSH (and in cases of severe hyperthyroidism, also serum T3) should be measured approximately every 2–4 weeks following initiation of therapy, and every 4–6 weeks after achieving the target value.[44,45] When trimester-specific FT4 values are not available, use of the reference range for nonpregnant patients is recommended. Separately, a TT4 measurement with reference value 1.5 times the nonpregnancy range may be used in second and third trimesters. Overtreatment should be avoided because of the possibility of inducing fetal goiter and or fetal hypothyroidism.[46]

Liver function tests should be monitored in pregnant women on PTU every 3–4 weeks and patients are encouraged to promptly report any new symptoms like fever or sore throat. This may indicate agranulocytosis.[37]

### Side Effects

Drug-induced agranulocytosis and hepatitis may occur with PTU which is idiosyncratic and with carbimazole, it is dose related. Patients are asked to report sore throat and fever immediately. Total leukocyte count should be performed and if neutropenia is there, treatment should be discontinued. Nausea, vomiting, and diarrhea may also occur. Drug rash and urticaria are seen in 1–5% of cases.[37] Fetal side effects of MMI include aplasia cutis, choanal or esophageal atresia, and other defects.[47] PTU-associated birth defects appear less severe than MMI-associated birth defects but occur with similar incidence.[8]

### Beta-Blockers

Propranolol should be used for tremors or tachycardia. It is used to treat symptoms of acute hyperthyroid state and for preoperative preparation. There are no significant teratogenic effects of propranolol reported in humans or in animals. Dose of 10–40 mg every 6–8 hours may be used for controlling hypermetabolic symptoms until patients have become euthyroid on ATD therapy. Dose may be reduced and later stopped as indicated clinically.

Long-term treatment with beta-blockers has been associated with fetal growth restriction, fetal bradycardia, and neonatal hypoglycemia.[48]

### Iodides

Iodides should not be used as a first-line therapy for women with Graves' disease, but they could be used transiently if needed in preparation for thyroidectomy.

Radioactive iodine diagnostic tests or therapy is contraindicated during pregnancy and lactation. Fetal thyroid uptake of iodine commences after 12 weeks of gestation, exposure to maternal radioactive iodine (RAI) before the 12th week is not associated with fetal thyroid dysfunction.[49] Treatment after 12 weeks leads to significant radiation to the fetal thyroid, multiple instances of exposure causing fetal thyroid destruction, and hypothyroidism have been reported.

### Follow-up

A well-controlled patient is followed at 4–6 weekly intervals. At follow-up, she should be examined, and thyroid functions performed. However, if the patient is newly diagnosed or if there is a relapse, more frequent follow-ups should be done. Patient should be followed in puerperium where increase in dosage may be needed.

## Surgical Treatment

Subtotal thyroidectomy during pregnancy as therapy for maternal Graves' disease is considered in following situations:
- If a serious adverse reaction to antithyroid therapy occurs.
- If very high doses of drugs are required (over 30 mg/day of MMI or 450 mg/day of PTU).[17,29]
- In women who develop stridor, respiratory distress, and dysphagia because of the disease.

Beta-blocker and potassium iodide should be given preoperatively.

Surgery should be performed only when deemed to be medically necessary for the mother's health.[50] It is the safest in the second trimester. Morbidity and mortality rates are increased when surgery is done in pregnancy.

## Thyroid Storm

Thyroid storm is an uncommon life-threatening crisis which requires immediate medical treatment. It carries a mortality of 10%. It is characterized by acute exacerbation of thyrotoxicosis in a patient of hyperthyroidism. It may get precipitated by labor, delivery, infection, anesthesia, and withdrawal of antithyroid drugs.

Patient may present with extreme symptoms of thyrotoxicosis, pyrexia, and changes in the mental state. There may be tachycardia, arrhythmias, and cardiac failure. Gastrointestinal symptoms like nausea and vomiting may also be present. Diagnosis is clinical. Thyroid functions may be as in uncomplicated hyperthyroidism. Increased total leucocyte count and increased liver enzymes may be present.

Management of thyroid storm consists of supportive therapy like intravenous fluids, controlling infections, treating fever, and removing precipitating factors. A large loading dose of 1000 mg of PTU is given followed by 150–300 mg 6 hourly. One to two hours after PTU, Lugol's iodine 500 mg 6 hourly should be given to further inhibit release of thyroid hormones from the thyroid gland. Propranolol, digoxin, diuretics, and steroids may be needed as required.[24]

Prolonged maternal hypoxia and dehydration may affect fetus but cesarean section is dangerous in presence of fulminating thyroid storm. Correcting metabolic insult to the mother helps fetus to recover.

## Breastfeeding and Postnatal Care

Breastfeeding is safe with a daily dose of PTU of 50–300 mg or less and carbimazole less than 15 mg daily for periods ranging from 3 weeks to 8 months.[51,52] 0.07% of maternal dose of PTU and 0.5% of carbimazole is excreted in breast milk.[36] No adverse effect on neonates thyroid function has been reported with these doses. Drugs should be given after feeding. Monitoring of the infant's thyroid function should be done. Graves' disease can flare postnatally, and maternal antibodies may rise. In patients who have stopped taking medication during pregnancy, restarting the drugs in 2–3 months after delivery may be required.

Management of hyperthyroidism in pregnancy is summarized in **Box 2**.

## Fetal Effects of Maternal Antithyroid Drugs

Thyroid receptor stimulating antibodies, antithyroid drugs, and most maternal thyroid hormones can cross the placenta.[8] Fetal thyroid can be stimulated by antibodies and maternal hyperthyroxinemia to produce more hormones causing fetal thyrotoxicosis. All antithyroid drugs given to mother also affect fetal thyroid function

---

**BOX 2:** Management of hyperthyroidism in pregnancy.

- Maternal monitoring should include pulse, blood pressure, and thyroid size
- Levels of serum TT4/FT4 and TSH should be done every 2–4 weeks till stabilization and then at 4–6 weeks interval. Dosage of antithyroid drugs should be changed accordingly
- In first trimester propylthiouracil is preferred to methimazole
- The treatment should consist of the lowest dose of antithyroid drugs to maintain serum TSH concentrations between 0.1 and 0.4 mU/L. Patient may remain slightly hyperthyroid
- Antepartum fetal surveillance should be strictly done after 28 weeks
- If TSH receptor antibody titer is positive in early pregnancy, fetal thyrotoxicosis should be ruled out
- If positive in late gestation neonatal thyrotoxicosis should be looked for
- Beta-blockers like propranolol may be needed before surgery like cesarean section
- Thyroid storm is a serious complication which occurs in labor and may cause maternal mortality
- The postpartum period should be carefully monitored as patient may worsen and the drugs may need to be started again or dose may need to be increased
- Surgery in the form of subtotal thyroidectomy is indicated if patient is not able to tolerate antithyroid drugs or very high doses are needed

---

Antithyroid drugs should be given to the mother ensuring that the fetal thyroid function is minimally affected. Transplacental passage of antibodies and drugs varies. Current maternal thyroid status rather than antithyroid dose may be the most reliable marker for titration of therapy to avoid fetal hypothyroidism.[29] If the maternal serum free T4 concentration is either elevated or maintained in the upper third of the normal nonpregnant reference range, serum free T4 levels are normal in more than 90% of the neonates.[38]

High doses of antithyroid medication may cause fetal hypothyroidism in 10–20% of patients on thionamides but rarely goiter. Neonatal hypothyroidism usually resolves spontaneously by day 5 of life.[53]

Umbilical cord blood sampling should be considered only if the diagnosis of fetal thyroid disease is not reasonably certain from the clinical data and the information gained would change the treatment.[29]

The treatment for fetal hypothyroidism resulting from medical treatment of maternal Graves' disease includes decreasing or stopping maternal treatment and considering intra-amniotic thyroxine. For fetal hyperthyroidism, treatment includes modulation of maternal antithyroid medication.

## Fetal Effects of Hyperthyroidism

Fetal or neonatal thyrotoxicosis can occur because of transplacental passage of maternal antibodies associated with Graves' disease though it is rare (0.05% of pregnancies). Fetal thyrotoxicosis may lead to fetal tachycardia (>160 beats/min), fetal goiter, premature delivery, heart failure, hepatosplenomegaly, thrombocytopenia, and fetal growth restriction.

Antibodies should be measured by 22 weeks gestational age in mothers with:
- Current Graves' disease
- History of Graves' disease and treatment with radioactive iodine or thyroidectomy before pregnancy
- Previous neonate with Graves' disease
- Previously elevated thyroid receptor antibodies (TRAb).

Fetal thyroid dysfunction should be screened for during the fetal anatomy ultrasound (18th–22nd week) in women with TRAb or with thyroid-stimulating Ig elevated at least 2- to 3-fold the normal level, and in women treated with ATD. Growth restriction, hydrops, presence of goiter, advanced bone age or cardiac failure are suggestive of fetal thyroid dysfunction. Assessment should be repeated every 4–6 weeks or as clinically indicated along with frequent clinical and laboratory monitoring. Women who have a negative TRAb and do not require antithyroid drugs have a very low risk of fetal or neonatal thyroid dysfunction.[29]

Fetal thyrotoxicosis can be treated in utero by giving the mother increased doses of antithyroid medication and mother may be subsequently given thyroxine which does not cross placenta. In the neonate, thyrotoxicosis may cause jaundice, poor feeding, and poor weight gain.

If high titers are found in late pregnancy, then cord blood and neonatal sampling on days 3–4 and 7–10 for thyroid function tests should be performed. Symptomatic neonatal thyrotoxicosis should be treated.

## HYPOTHYROIDISM

Primary overt maternal hypothyroidism is defined as the presence of an elevated TSH and a decreased serum free T4 concentration during gestation, with both concentrations outside the (trimester-specific) reference ranges.[8]

Subclinical hypothyroidism has elevated TSH but normal FT4. Isolated hypothyroxinemia is a condition where FT4 concentration is in the lower 2.5th–5th percentile of a given population in conjunction with a normal maternal TSH concentration.

The prevalence of overt hypothyroidism in pregnancy is 0.3–1%. Subclinical hypothyroidism is seen in 2–3%. The various causes of hypothyroidism are:
- Hashimoto's thyroiditis
- Iatrogenic hypothyroidism following intake of drugs: lithium, amiodarone, antithyroid drugs
- Following treatment of hyperthyroidism with radioactive ablation or surgery
- Following thyroid surgery for tumors
- Iodine deficiency
- Postpartum thyroiditis (transient).

Most common cause of hypothyroidism in pregnancy in iodine replete areas is Hashimoto's thyroiditis. In this antibodies against thyroid peroxidase are seen with atrophy, fibrosis, and destruction of gland. Regeneration occurs after atrophy and goiter results. Antibodies against thyroid receptors may also be present.

Other causes of thyroid insufficiency include treatment of hyperthyroidism with radioiodine ablation or surgery. Worldwide most important cause of hypothyroidism is iodine deficiency.

### Clinical Features

Clinical presentation of normal pregnancy may have an overlap with those of hypothyroidism. Features which help in the diagnosis are cold intolerance, slow pulse rate, delayed tendon reflexes, hair loss, and dry skin. Others like drowsiness and constipation may also be seen. Many women with hypothyroidism are asymptomatic.

### Diagnosis

Serum TSH determines maternal thyroid status and should be used to guide treatment decisions and goals.

In the 2011 ATA guidelines, the upper reference limit for serum TSH concentration during pregnancy was defined as 2.5 mU/L in the first trimester, and 3.0 mU/L in the second and third trimesters

It has recently been seen that substantial variation exists in TSH levels between populations, with different ethnicities and iodine levels. Many recent investigations confirm a more liberal upper TSH reference range in healthy pregnant women with no thyroid disease.[54]

Elevations in serum TSH concentrations during pregnancy should ideally be defined using pregnancy- and population-specific reference ranges.[8]

If these population or pregnancy-specific TSH reference ranges are not available, an upper reference limit of 4.0 mU/L may be used. For most assays, this limit represents a reduction in the nonpregnant TSH upper reference limit of 0.5 mU/L.[8]

Recent studies demonstrate TPOAb positivity plays an important role on maternal thyroid status. Thyroid autoantibodies can be detected in approximately 30–60% of pregnant women with an elevated TSH concentration.[55,56]

There appears to be a greater risk for adverse events in women who are TPOAb positive compared to those who are TPOAb negative, even when thyroid function is identical. Even euthyroid women who are TPOAb-positive are also at increased risk for adverse clinical outcome.[55]

Pregnant women with TSH concentrations >2.5 mU/L should be evaluated for TPOAb status.[8]

Decisions about levothyroxine (LT4) treatment must be based upon both, measurement of thyroid function and TPOAb status.

## Maternal Concerns

Hypothyroidism is related to decreased fertility. When hypothyroid patient becomes pregnant, there is an increased risk for early and late complications like abortion, anemia, gestational hypertension, placental abruption, and postpartum hemorrhage.

Women with overt hypothyroidism carry a higher risk of fetal loss with inadequate treatment. Gestational hypertension is also seen more frequently in pregnant women with overt maternal hypothyroidism.[57-59]

## Fetal Concerns

Maternal iodine levels should be adequate to prevent fetal and maternal hypothyroidism. Overt hypothyroidism is associated with premature birth, low birth weight, and neonatal respiratory distress. In subclinical hypothyroidism, risk of preterm delivery increases.[9]

### Neurological Development of the Fetus and the Neonate

Thyroid hormone is important for normal fetal brain development.[60,61] At early gestation when fetal thyroid is not functional fetal hormone requirement is met with from transfer of maternal thyroid hormones to fetal compartment. Only T3 is required for fetal brain development which is made available by conversion of maternal T4 received by fetus, to T3 by deiodinases I and II present in fetal brain tissue.[62] Maternal hypothyroxinemia or maternal iodine deficiency at this time may cause mental retardation in the baby.

Cretinism (deaf mutism, spastic motor disorder, and hypothyroidism) is a distinct and severe form of brain damage caused by severe maternal iodine deficiency. Neonatal or fetal hypothyroidism as a result of transplacental transfer of maternal autoantibodies is extremely rare.[63]

## Management

### Prepregnancy

Thyroid disease should be suspected in patients with fertility problems and menstrual irregularities.

If hypothyroidism has been diagnosed before pregnancy, adjustment of the preconception thyroxine dose should be done so that TSH level is not higher than 2.5 mU/L before pregnancy. Woman with hypothyroidism should be counseled to delay pregnancy till good control of thyroid function has been achieved.

The TPOAb-positive euthyroid women who are newly pregnant, if given LT4 will have an improved outcome is not clear. However LT4 may be given to TPOAb-positive euthyroid pregnant women with a prior history of loss. This may be considered given its potential benefits in comparison with its minimal risk. In such cases, 25–50 µg of LT4 may be given in the beginning.[8]

### Antenatal Management

Baseline thyroid function tests should be done as soon as the woman becomes pregnant. Pregnant women with TSH concentrations >2.5 mU/L should be evaluated for TPOAb status.[8]

Thyroxine supplementation is not recommended in TPOAb-negative women with a normal TSH (TSH within the pregnancy-specific reference range or <4.0 mU/L if reference range unavailable).[8]

Patient on thyroxine preconceptionally, need the dose to be altered at 4–6 weeks of gestation so that the euthyroid state is achieved, which is better for pregnancy outcome.

The recommended treatment of maternal hypothyroidism is administration of oral levothyroxine (LT4). Other thyroid preparations such as T3 or desiccated thyroid should not be used in pregnancy.

*Dose:* The dose in pregnancy needs to be increased on an average by 30–50% above preconception dosage because of rapid rise in TBG levels because of estrogen, increased placental transport and metabolism of maternal T4.[1] One can administer two additional tablets weekly of the patient's current daily LT4 dosage.

*Target range:* If hypothyroidism has been diagnosed during pregnancy, thyroid functions should be normalized as soon as possible. Thyroxine doses should be titrated to rapidly reach and maintain serum TSH concentrations to less than 2.5 mIU/L in first trimester and 3 mIU/L in the second and third trimester by increasing doses of l-thyroxine by 25–50 µg.

*Monitoring:* Women with overt and subclinical hypothyroidism (treated or untreated) or those at risk for hypothyroidism (e.g., patients who are euthyroid but TPOAb or TgAb positive, posthemithyroidectomy, or treated with radioactive iodine) should be monitored with a serum TSH measurement approximately every 4 weeks until midgestation and at least once near 30 week gestation.[8]

In the care of women with adequately treated hypothyroidism, no other maternal or fetal testing (such as serial fetal ultrasounds, antenatal testing, and/or umbilical blood sampling) is recommended beyond measurement of maternal thyroid function unless needed due to other circumstances of pregnancy. An exception to this is women with Graves' disease effectively treated with [131]I ablation or surgical resection, which require TRAb monitoring.[8]

### Intrapartum Management

If adequately controlled, no extra-measures are needed but large goiter may have anesthetic or surgical concerns.

### Postnatal Management

After delivery, dose in most patients needs to be decreased over a period of 4 weeks postpartum. Following delivery, LT4 should be reduced to the patient's preconception dose.

> **BOX 3:** Management of hypothyroidism in pregnancy.
>
> - Baseline thyroid function tests to be done as soon as possible
> - If thyroid functions show hypothyroidism in pregnancy, rapidly normalize the levels by starting thyroxine to maintain serum TSH concentrations to less than 2.5 mIU/L in first trimester and 3 mIU/L in second and third trimesters
> - Repeat thyroid function tests every 4 weeks till controlled and then 6 weekly
> - After delivery, dose may need to be decreased

Additional thyroid function testing should be performed at approximately 6 weeks postpartum. Patient with autoimmune etiology may develop postpartum thyroiditis so monitoring should be done for at least 6 months postdelivery.[64] The management of hypothyroidism in pregnancy is summarized in **Box 3**.

## SUBCLINICAL HYPOTHYROIDISM

It is seen in 2–5% of pregnant women.[24] This is characterized by serum TSH concentration above the upper limit of the reference range with a normal free T4. It has been reported to be associated with an adverse outcome for both the mother and offspring.[9] Thyroxine treatment has been shown to improve obstetrical outcome, but has not been proved to modify long-term neurological development in the offspring.

Subclinical hypothyroidism in pregnancy should be approached as follows[8]:

- LT4 therapy is recommended for
  - TPOAb-positive women with a TSH greater than the pregnancy-specific reference range
  - TPOAb-negative women with a TSH greater than 10.0 mU/L.
- LT4 therapy may be considered for
  - TPOAb-positive women with TSH concentrations >2.5 mU/L and below the upper limit of the pregnancy-specific reference range.
  - TPOAb-negative women and TPOAb-negative women with TSH concentrations greater than the pregnancy specific reference range and below 10.0 mU/L.
- LT4 therapy is not recommended for
  - TPOAb-negative women with a normal TSH (TSH within the pregnancy-specific reference range or <4.0 mU/L if unavailable).

In women at risk for hypothyroidism (TPOAb or TgAb positive, posthemithyroidectomy, and/or postradioactive iodine) increased surveillance is recommended. Based on findings extrapolated from investigations of treated hypothyroid women from early pregnancy onwards,[65] it is reasonable to evaluate these women for TSH elevation approximately every 4 weeks during pregnancy. Serial testing is preferably continued through midpregnancy because the increased T4 demand continues throughout the first half of gestation.[8]

## THYROID NODULES AND THYROID CARCINOMA

Thyroid nodules, solitary toxic nodules, or adenomas are found in 2% of pregnant women[66] and usually cause hyperthyroidism. They increase with increasing parity. Thyroid cancers are rare but most of them present as thyroid nodules. In iodine insufficiency, pre-existing nodules are prone to increase in size during pregnancy. All women with a thyroid nodule should have a TSH measurement.[67]

Thyroid cancer is seen in 14.4/100,000 of pregnancies. Papillary cancer is the most frequent pathological type.[68] Thyroid function tests are usually normal in women with thyroid cancer. Functional nodules are rarely malignant. Serum Calcitonin levels may be useful in medullary carcinoma. Radionuclide scanning of thyroid is contraindicated in pregnancy which is used to distinguish cold (malignant) from hot (benign) nodules outside pregnancy. In pregnancy, diagnosis is dependent on ultrasound and fine needle aspiration biopsy.[69,70] 5–20% of thyroid nodules in pregnancy are found to be malignant. Fine needle aspiration should be done based on ultrasonographic findings and risk of cancer. FNAC is done for any single dominant nodule >1 cm[71] and rapidly enlarging nodules.

### Preconception

If patient comes before pregnancy, thyroid nodule should be evaluated and treatment should be given before pregnancy. Pregnancy should be delayed for minimum of 6 months and preferable for 1 year if therapeutic radioactive iodine has been used.[72]

### Pregnancy

Most of thyroid nodules are cytologically benign and do not need surgery. In the absence of rapid growth, nodules with biopsies that are benign do not require surgery during pregnancy.[73]

If suspicious or positive for thyroid carcinoma, gestational age, tumor stage, and personal inclination of patient should be considered.

If FNAC is highly suggestive of papillary or medullary carcinoma, surgery should be performed without interrupting pregnancy.[74]

In follicular neoplasm risk of malignancy is 10–15% and surgery can be delayed because it is minimally invasive and well capsulated. If the cytology is indeterminate one should wait till delivery. If nodule is found in third trimester further workup and treatment can be delayed until after delivery.[75] Surgery should be done in a rapidly growing lesion or if anaplastic tumor is present.

### Postnatal

Radioactive iodine can be used after delivery but breastfeeding is contraindicated.

## POSTPARTUM THYROIDITIS

Postpartum thyroiditis is the occurrence of thyroid dysfunction, excluding Graves' disease, in the first postpartum year in women who were euthyroid prior to pregnancy.[76] It may present as hyperthyroidism, hypothyroidism, and/or hyperthyroidism followed by hypothyroidism in the first year postpartum in women without overt thyroid disease before pregnancy. Its incidence varies between 5% and 10% of pregnancies.[77] Postpartum thyroiditis (PPT) occurs almost exclusively in women who are thyroid antibody positive.

Women with other autoimmune disorders have an increased risk of PPT. Specifically, the prevalence of PPT is 3-4 times higher in women with diabetes mellitus type 1 compared to unselected populations.[78]

In the classic form, transient thyrotoxicosis is followed by transient hypothyroidism with a return to the euthyroid state by the end of the initial postpartum year.[79]

The condition usually occurs 3-4 months postpartum but has been reported up to 6 months after delivery. Lymphocytic infiltration of the gland is seen. These subjects have a subclinical autoimmune thyroiditis which exacerbates after delivery.

It is believed to be caused by an autoimmunity induced discharge of preformed hormone from the thyroid which causes hyperthyroidism. After few months, it causes hypothyroidism as stores of preformed hormone are depleted and gland is destroyed. The thyrotoxic phase of postpartum thyroiditis is twenty times more common than postpartum Graves' disease. Symptoms during PPT are milder than Graves' disease. About 95% of women with Graves' disease are TSH receptor stimulating antibody positive and may also present with a bruit and exophthalmos. In contrast to Graves' disease PPT is characterized by 0% radioactive iodine uptake. Fifty percent of women who are thyroid antibody positive in first trimester will develop postpartum thyroiditis.[50]

## Management

The hypothyroid phase of PPT is more frequently symptomatic. Symptoms during the hypothyroid phase of PPT may include cold intolerance, dry skin, fatigue, impaired concentration, and paresthesias.[80] Most cases resolve spontaneously. In the hyperthyroid phase of the disease propranalol should be given to relieve symptoms. The duration of therapy does not usually exceed 2 months.

Treatment for women in hypothyroid phase depends on degree of the disease and plan to conceive. Asymptomatic patients not planning a pregnancy and whose TSH level is between 4 and 10 mIU/L do not require intervention and should be evaluated again in 4-8 weeks' time. Women with TSH between 4 and 10 mIU/L who are either symptomatic or attempting to become pregnant should be treated with thyroxine. All women with levels of TSH above 10 mIU/L should be treated with thyroxine. This dysfunction is transient but 20-64% of women may develop permanent hypothyroidism during long-term followup.[81,82]

Women known to be thyroid peroxidase antibody (TPO-Ab)-positive should have a TSH tested at 3 and 6 months postpartum. Women with a history of PPT have a markedly increased risk of developing permanent primary hypothyroidism in the 5- to 10-year period following the episode of PPT. An annual TSH level should be performed in these women.

### Neonatal Concerns

Neonatologist should be informed about the maternal thyroid diagnosis, treatment, and thyroid antibody status. All newborns should be screened for hypothyroidism by blood spot analysis typically 2-5 days after birth. Subclinical and overt hypothyroidism should be treated in lactating women because these may affect lactation. The use of $^{131}I$ is contraindicated during lactation. The lowest effective dose of antithyroid drugs should be used. All breastfeeding women should ingest approximate 250 µg of dietary iodine daily.

## SCREENING FOR THYROID DYSFUNCTION DURING PREGNANCY

Universal screening is not recommended but the association of thyroid abnormalities and untoward outcomes during pregnancy and postpartum is impossible to ignore.

American Thyroid Association and American Association of Clinical Endocrinologists uniformly recommend screening only those at increased risk during pregnancy.[29]

Although, the benefits of universal screening for hypothyroidism may not be justified by current evidence, targeted case findings should be done.

Targeted screening is recommended for women as listed below who have an increased incidence of thyroid disease and in whom treatment for thyroid disease if found, would be warranted.

- Age >30 years
- Morbid obesity (BMI >40 kg/m$^2$)
- Women with a history of hyperthyroid or hypothyroid disease, postpartum thyroiditis or thyroid lobectomy
- Women with a goiter
- Women with thyroid antibodies
- Women with symptoms or clinical signs suggestive of thyroid under function or over function including anemia, elevated cholesterol, and hyponatremia
- Women with type I diabetes or other autoimmune disorders
- Women with infertility should have screening with TSH as part of their infertility workup
- Women planning artificial reproductive techniques
- Women with prior therapeutic head or neck irradiation
- Women with a prior history of miscarriage or preterm delivery

- Residing in an area of known moderate to severe iodine insufficiency
- Screening should consist of a TSH measurement done before pregnancy when possible or at first prenatal visit and appropriate tests should be done accordingly.

## KEY POINTS

- Thyroid disorders are common endocrine disorders in young women and difficult to diagnose clinically in pregnancy because of overlap of normal signs and symptoms of pregnancy with those of thyroid diseases.
- Human chorionic gonadotropin has some thyrotrophic function, so it stimulates thyroid receptors causing increase in free T4 levels and decrease in TSH levels particularly in first trimester.
- For thyroid functions in pregnancy, total/free T4, T3, and TSH should be done and trimester specific range should be considered.
- Pregnant women with TSH concentrations >2.5 mU/L should be evaluated for TPOAb status.
- During first trimester, fetus is dependent on maternal T4 for its requirements as fetal thyroid is not active and maternal hypothyroxinemia or iodine deficiency at this time can affect fetal brain development.
- In pregnancy and lactation, 200–300 µg/day of iodine is needed.
- Medical treatment is of choice in hyperthyroidism. Propylthiouracil and methimazole both can be used but former is used in first trimester preferably.
- In hyperthyroidism, maternal levels of free T4 should be maintained in the upper nonpregnant reference range with treatment.
- Both maternal and fetal hypothyroidism are known to have serious adverse effects on the fetus.
- Autoimmune thyroiditis is the most common cause of hypothyroidism in pregnancy.
- If hypothyroidism is first detected in pregnancy, rapid institution of thyroxine should be done to normalize thyroid levels otherwise neurological functions of the fetus are jeopardized.
- In subclinical hypothyroidism, treatment with thyroxine improves obstetrical outcome.
- Fine needle aspiration cytology should be performed for single or dominant thyroid nodule larger than 1 cm in pregnancy.
- If these nodules are found to be malignant or rapidly growing, surgery should be offered in the second trimester without interrupting pregnancy.
- Women known to be thyroid peroxidase antibody positive should have a TSH performed at 3 and 6 months postpartum.
- Universal screening for thyroid disease is not recommended at present but case finding in the high-risk group for thyroid dysfunction should be done.

## REFERENCES

1. Glinoer D. The regulation of thyroid function in pregnancy: pathways of endocrine adaptation from physiology to pathology. Endocr Rev. 1997;18:404-33.
2. Glinoer D. The regulation of thyroid function during normal pregnancy: importance of the iodine nutrition status. Best Pract Res Clin Endocrinol Metab. 2004;18:133-52.
3. Hetzel BS. Iodine deficiency disorders and their eradication. Lancet. 1983;2:1126-9.
4. Pekonen F, Alfthan H, Stenman JH, Ylikorkala O. Human chorionic gonadotrophin and thryroid function in early human pregnancy: circadian variation and evidence for intrinsic thyrotropic activity of HCG. J Clin Endocrinol Metab. 1988;66:853-6.
5. Weeke J, Dybkjaer L, Granlie K, Eskjaer Jensen S, Kjaerulff E, Laurberg P, et al. A longitudinal study of serum TSH, and total and free iodothyronines during normal pregnancy. Acta Endocrinologica. 1982;101:531.
6. Baloch Z, Carayon P, Conte-Devolx B, Demers LM, Feldt-Rasmussen U, Henry JF, et al. Laboratory medicine practice guidelines. Laboratory support for the diagnosis and monitoring of thyroid disease. Thyroid. 2003;13:3-126.
7. Soldin OP, Tractenberg RE, Hollowell JG, Jonklaas J, Janicic N, Soldin SJ. Trimester-specific changes in maternal thyroid hormone, thyrotropin, and thyroglobulin concentrations during gestation: trends and associations across trimesters in iodine sufficiency. Thyroid. 2004;14:1084-90.
8. Alexander EK, Pearce EN, Brent GA, Brown RS, Chen H, Dosiou D, et al. Guidelines of the American Thyroid Association for the diagnosis and management of thyroid disease during pregnancy and the postpartum. Thyroid. 2017; 27(3):315-89.
9. Casey BM, Dashe JS, Wells CE, McIntire DD, Leveno KJ, Cunningham FG. Subclinical hyperthyroidism and pregnancy outcomes. Obstet Gynecol. 2006;107:337-41.
10. Thorpe-Beeston JG, Nicolaides KH, Felton CV, Butler J, McGregor AM. Maturation of the secretion of thyroid hormone and thyroid-stimulating hormone in the fetus. N Engl J Med. 1991;324:532-6.
11. Santini F, Chiovato L, Ghirri P, Lapi P, Mammoli C, Montanelli L, et al. Serum iodothyronines in the human fetus and the newborn: evidence for an important role of placenta in fetal thyroid hormone homeostasis. J Clin Endocrinol Metab. 1999;84:493-8.
12. Bernal J, Pekonen FD. Ontogenesis of nuclear 3,5,3'-triiodothyronine receptor in the human fetal brain. Endocrinology. 1984;11:577-9.
13. Vulsma T, Gons MH, de Vijlder JJ. Maternal-fetal transfer of thyroxine in congenital hypothyroidism due to a total organification defect or thyroid agenesis. N Engl J Med. 1989;321:13-6.
14. Azizi F, Smyth P. Breastfeeding and maternal and infant iodine nutrition. Clin Endocrinol (Oxf). 2009;70:803-9.
15. World Health Organization. Assessment of Iodine Deficiency Disorders and Monitoring Their Elimination: A Guide for Program Managers, 2nd edition. Geneva: WHO; 2001. pp. 7-8.
16. Delange FM, Dunn JT. Iodine deficiency. In: Braverman LE, Utiger RD (Eds). Werner and Ingbar's The Thyroid: A Fundamental and Clinical Text, 9th edition. Philadelphia: Lippincott, Williams and Wilkins; 2005. pp 264-88.

17. Moreno-Reyes R, Glinoer D, Van Oyen H, Vandevijvere S. High prevalence of thyroid disorders in pregnant women in a mildly iodine-deficient country: a population-based study. J Clin Endocrinol Metab. 2013;98:3694-701.
18. Vermiglio F, Lo Presti VP, Moleti M, Sidoti M, Tortorella G, Scaffidi G, et al. Attention deficit and hyperactivity disorders in the offspring of mother exposed to mild-moderate iodine deficiency: a possible novel iodine deficiency disorder developed countries. J Clin Endocrinol Metab. 2004;89:6054-60.
19. Glinoer D. Fetomaternal repercussions of iodine deficiency during pregnancy: An update. Ann Endocrinol (Paris). 2003;64:37-44.
20. Zimmermann MB. The effects of iodine deficiency in pregnancy and infancy. Paediatr Perinat Epidemiol. 2012;26(Suppl 1):108-17.
21. Cao XY, Jiang XM, Dou ZH, Rakeman MA, Zhang ML, O'Donnell K, et al. Timing of vulnerability of the brain to iodine deficiency in endemic cretinism. N Engl J Med. 1994;331:1739-44.
22. Chaouki ML, Benmiloud M. Prevention of iodine deficiency disorders by oral administration of lipiodol during pregnancy. Eur J Endocrinol. 1994;130:547-51.
23. Rotondi M, Mazziotti G, Sorvillo F, Piscopo M, Cioffi M, Amato G, et al. Effects of increased thyroxine dosage pre-conception on thyroid function early pregnancy. Eur J Endocrinol. 2004;151:695-700.
24. Fitzpatrick D, Russel M. Diagnosis and management of thyroid disease in pregnancy. Obstet Gynecol Clin North Am. 2010;37;173.
25. Goodwin TM, Montoro M, Mestman JH. Transient hyperthyroidism and hyperemesis gravidarum: clinical aspects. Am J Obstet Gynecol. 1992;167:648-52.
26. Tan JY, Loh KC, Yeo GS, Chee YC. Transient hyperthyroidism of hyperemesis gravidarum. BJOG. 2002;109:683-8.
27. American College of Obstetricians and Gynecologists. Thyroid disease in pregnancy. Practice Bulletin No. 37. Washington, DC: ACOG; 2013.
28. Mestman JH. Hyperthyroidism in pregnancy. Curr Opin Endocrinol Diabetes Obes. 2012;19:394.
29. Bahn RS, Burch HB, Cooper DS, Garber JR, Greenlee MC, Klein I, et al. Hyperthyroidism and other causes of thyrotoxicosis: management guidelines of the American Thyroid Association and American Association of Clinical Endocrinologists. Endocr Pract. 2011;17(3):456.
30. Sheffield JS, Cunningham FG. Thyrotoxicosis and heart failure that complicate pregnancy. Am J Obstet Gynecol. 2004;190:211-7.
31. Stagnaro-Green A. Postpartum thyroiditis. Best Pract Res Clin Endocrinol Metab. 2004;18:303-16.
32. Andersen SL, Olsen J, Carle A, Laurberg P. Hyperthyroidism incidence fluctuates widely in and around pregnancy and is at variance with some other autoimmune diseases: a Danish population-based study. J Clin Endocrinol Metab. 2015;100:1164-71.
33. Glinowe D, Soto MF, Bourdux P, Lejeune B, Delange F, Lemone M, et al. Pregnancy in patients with mild thyroid abnormalities: maternal and neonatal repercussions. J Clin Endocrinol Metab. 1991;73:421-7.
34. Davis LE, Lucas MJ, Hankins GD, Roark ML, Cunningham FG. Thyrotoxicosis complicating pregnancy. Am J Obstet Gynecol. 1989;160:63-70.
35. Millar LK, Wing DA, Leung AS, Koonings PP, Montoro MN, Mestman JH. Low birth weight and preeclampsia in pregnancies complicated by hyperthyroidism. Obstet Gynecol. 1994;84:946-9.
36. Krasas G. Thyroid disease and female reproduction. Fertil Steril. 2000;74:1063-70.
37. Brent GA. Graves' disease. N Engl J Med. 2008;358:2594.
38. The Endocrine Society. Management of thyroid dysfunction during pregnancy and postpartum: an Endocrine Society Clinical Practice Guideline. Chevy Chase (MD): The Endocrine Society; 2007.
39. Ratanachaiyavong S, Mc Gregor AM. Immunosuppressive effects of antithyroid drugs. Clin Endocrinol Metab. 1985;14:449-66.
40. Di Gianantonio E, Schaefer C, Mastroiacovo PP, Cournot MP, Benedicenti F, Reuversm M, et al. Adverse effects of prenatal methimazol exposure Teratology. 2001;64:262-6.
41. Nicholas WC, Fischer RG, Stevenson RA, Bass JD. Single daily dose of methimazole compared to every 8 hours propylthiouracil in the treatment of hyperthyroidism. South Med J. 1995;88:973-6.
42. Kallner G, Vitols S, Ljunggren JG. Comparison of standardized initial doses of two antithyroid drugs in the treatment of Graves' disease. J Intern Med. 1996;239:525-9.
43. Nakamura H, Noh JY, Itoh K, Fukata S, Miyauchi A, Hamada N. Comparison of methimazole and propylthiouracil in patients with hyperthyroidism caused by Graves' disease. J Clin Endocrinol Metab. 2007;92:2157-62.
44. Patil-Sisodia K, Mestman JH. Graves hyperthyroidism and pregnancy: a clinical update. Endocr Prac. 2010;49(16):118-29.
45. Glinoer D. Thyroid hyperfunction during pregnancy. Thyroid. 1998;8:859-64.
46. Bliddal S, Rasmussen AK, Sundberg K, Brocks V, Feldt-Rasmussen U. Antithyroid drug-induced fetal goitrous hypothyroidism. Nat Rev Endocrinol. 2011;7:396-406.
47. Yoshihara A, Noh J, Yamaguchi T, Ohye H, Sato S, Sekiya K, et al. Treatment of Graves' disease with antithyroid drugs in the first trimester of pregnancy and the prevalence of congenital malformation. J Clin Endocrinol Metab. 2012;97:2396-403.
48. Rubin PC. Current concepts: beta-blockers in pregnancy. N Engl J Med. 1981;305:1323-6.
49. Magee LA, Elran E, Bull SB, Logan A, Koren G. Risks and benefits of beta receptor blockers for pregnancy hypertension: overview of randomized trials. Eur J Obstet Gynecol Repro Biol. 2000;88:15-26.
50. Stagnaro-Green A, Pearce E. Thyroid disorders in pregnancy. Nat Rev Endocrinol. 2012;8:650.
51. Azizi F, Hedayati M. Thyroid function in breast-fed infants whose mothers take high doses of methimazole. J Endocrinol Invest. 2002;25:493-6.
52. Momotani N, Yamashita R, Yoshimoto M, Noh J, Ishikawa N, Ito K. Recovery from fetal hypothyroidism: evidence for the safety of breastfeeding while taking propylthiouracil. Clin Endocrinol (Oxf). 1989;31:591-5.
53. Cheron RG, Kaplan MM, Larsen PR, Selenkow HA, Crigler JF Jr. Neonatal thyroid function after propylthiouracil therapy for maternal Graves disease. N Engl J Med. 1981;304:525-8.

54. Medici M, Korevaar TI, Visser WE, Visser TJ, Peeters RP. Thyroid function in pregnancy: what is normal? Clin Chem. 2015;61:704-13.
55. Allan WC, Haddow JE, Palomaki GE, Williams JR, Mitchell ML, Hermos RJ, et al. Maternal thyroid deficiency and pregnancy complications: implications for population screening. J Med Screen. 2000;7:127-30.
56. Casey BM, Dashe JS, Spong CY, McIntire DD, Leveno KJ, Cunningham GF. Perinatal significance of isolated maternal hypothyroxinemia identified in the first half of pregnancy. Obstet Gynecol. 2007;109:1129-35.
57. Korevaar TI, Schalekamp-Timmermans S, de Rijke YB, Visser WE, Visser W, de Muinck Keizer-Schrama SM, et al. Hypothyroxinemia and TPO-antibody positivity are risk factors for premature delivery: the generation R study. J Clin Endocrinol Metab. 2013;98:4382-90.
58. Leung AS, Millar LK, Koonings PP, Montoro M, Mestman JH. Perinatal outcome in hypothyroid pregnancies. Obstet Gynecol. 1993;81:349-53.
59. Sahu MT, Das V, Mittal S, Agarwal A, Sahu M. Overt and subclinical thyroid dysfunction among Indian pregnant women and its effect on maternal and fetal outcome. Arch Gynecol Obstet. 2010;281:215-20.
60. Calvo RM, Jauniaux E, Gulbis B, Asuncion M, Gervy C, Contempre B, et al. Fetal tissues are exposed to biologically relevant free thyroxine concentrations during early phases of development. J Clin Endocrinol Metab. 2002;87:1768-77.
61. Iskaros J, Pickard M, Evans I, Sinha A, Hardiman P, Ekins R. Thyroid hormone receptor gene expression in first trimester human fetal brain. J Clin Endocrinol Metab. 2000;85:2620-23.
62. Kester MH, Martinez de Mena R, Obregon MJ, Marinkovic D, Howatson A, Visser TJ, et al. Iodothyronine levels in the human developing brain: major regulatory roles of iodothyronine deiodinases in different areas. J Clin Endocrinol Metab. 2004;89:3117-31.
63. Brown RS, Bellisario RL, Botero D, Fournier L, Abrams CA, Cowger ML, et al. Incidence of transient congenital hypothyroidism due to maternal thyrotropin receptor-blocking antibodies in over one million babies. J Clin Endocrinol Metab. 1996;81:1147-51.
64. Caixas A, Albareda M, Garcia-Patterson A, Rodriguez-Espinosa J, de Leiva A, Corcoy R. Postpartum thyroiditis in women with hypothyroidism antedating pregnancy? J Clin Endocrinol Metab. 1999;84:4000-05.
65. Alexander EK, Marqusee E, Lawrence J, Jarolim P, Fischer GA, Larsen PR. 2004 Timing and magnitude of increases in levothyroxine requirements during pregnancy in women with hypothyroidism. N Engl J Med. 2004;351(3):241-9.
66. Mazzaferri EL. Evaluation and management of common thyroid disorders in women. Am J Obstet Gynecol. 1997;176:507-14.
67. Bennedbaek FN, Perrild H, Hegedus L. Diagnosis and treatment of the solitary thyroid nodule. Results of a European survey. Clin Endocrinol (Oxf). 1999;50:357-63.
68. Smith LH, Danielsen B, Allen ME, Cress R. Cancer associated with obstetric delivery: results of linkage with the California cancer registry. Am J Obstet Gynecol. 2003;189:1128-35.
69. Choe W, McDougall IR. Thyroid cancer in pregnant women: diagnostic and therapeutic management. Thyroid. 1994;4:433-5.
70. Glinoer D. Thyroid nodule and cancer in pregnant women. Ann Endocrinol (Paris). 1997;58:263.
71. Hamburger JI. Thyroid nodules in pregnancy. Thyroid. 1992;2:165-8.
72. Auala C, Navarro E, Rodriguez JR, Silva H, Venegas E, Astorga R. Conception after iodine-131 therapy for 424 differentiated thyroid cancer. Thyroid. 1998;8:1009.
73. American Thyroid Association (ATA) Guidelines Taskforce on Thyroid Nodules and Differentiated Thyroid Cancer, Cooper DS, Doherty GM, Haugen BR, Kloos RT, Lee SL, et al. Revised American Thyroid Association management guidelines for patients with thyroid nodules and differentiated thyroid cancer. Thyroid. 2009;19:1167-214.
74. Sam S, Molitch ME. Timing and special concerns regarding endocrine surgery during pregnancy. Endocrinol Metab Clin North Am. 2003;32:337-54.
75. Tan GH, Gharib H, Goellner JR, van Heerden JA, Bahn RS. Management of thyroid nodules in pregnancy. Arch Intern Med. 1996;156:2317-20.
76. Amino N, Mori H, Iwatani Y, Tanizawa O, Kawashima M, Tsuge I, et al. High prevalence of transient post-partum thyrotoxicosis and hypothyroidism. N Engl J Med. 1982;306:849-85.
77. Stagnaro-Green A. Recognizing, understanding and treating postpartum thyroiditis. Endocrinol Metab Clin North Am. 2000;29(2):417-30.
78. Gerstein HC. Incidence of postpartum thyroid dysfunction in patients with type I diabetes mellitus. Ann Intern Med. 1993;118:419-23.
79. Qaseem A, Snow V, Owens DK, Shekelle P. The development of clinical practice guidelines and guidance statements of the American College of Physicians: summary of methods. Ann Intern Med. 2010;153:194-9.
80. Hayslip CC, Fein HG, O'Donnell VM, Friedman DS, Klein TA, Smallridge RC. The value of serum antimicrosomal antibody testing in screening for symptomatic postpartum thyroid dysfunction. Am J Obstet Gynecol. 1988;159:203-9
81. Lazarus JH. Clinical manifestations of postpartum thyroid disease. Thyroid. 1999;9:685-9.
82. Azizi F. The occurrence of permanent thyroid failure in patients with subclinical postpartum thyroiditis. Eur J Endocrinol. 2005;153:367-71.

# Heart Disease in Pregnancy

*Shalini Malhotra, Reva Tripathi, Monika Bhatia, Divya Verma*

## INTRODUCTION

Heart disease is among the leading causes of maternal mortality during pregnancy. It complicates approximately 0.8% of pregnancies.[1] The various types of heart diseases complicating pregnancy include congenital and acquired. Rheumatic heart disease (RHD) accounts for most of the heart disease cases in pregnancy in developing countries compared to congenital heart disease in the developed countries. Due to an increasing number of successful surgical corrections of congenital defects, a larger proportion of women are reaching childbearing age in developing countries also. Significant hemodynamic alterations occur during normal pregnancy to supply blood to the fetoplacental unit. Such cardiovascular adaptations are well-tolerated by healthy women but can significantly compromise women with abnormal or damaged hearts. These women are at increased risk of complications such as heart failure, pulmonary edema, arrhythmias, thromboembolism, hypoxemia, infective endocarditis (IE), angina, stroke, and sudden cardiac death. The care of pregnant women with heart disease requires a multidisciplinary approach involving the obstetrician, cardiologist, and anesthetist. These women should preferably be seen in a specialized antenatal cardiac clinic to minimize the number of visits and maximize care. Knowledge of the pregnancy-associated risks and complications specific to each type of heart disease allows the physician to choose management options that optimize the pregnancy outcome. This chapter reviews the current literature on the diagnosis and management of pregnancy complicated by various types of cardiac diseases.

## HEMODYNAMIC CHANGES DURING PREGNANCY

### During Pregnancy

Normal pregnancy entails significant changes in cardiovascular physiology. These changes create hemodynamic burden even on a normal maternal heart and may cause symptoms and signs like those of heart disease. Women with pre-existing cardiac disease may become symptomatic for the first time during this period or show evidence of clinical deterioration in cases diagnosed earlier. The plasma volume begins to rise as early as 5–6 weeks of gestation, increasing until mid-pregnancy when it is 50% higher than the prepregnancy levels. The red blood cell volume increases only by about 25–30%, resulting in physiologic anemia. Cardiac output starts to increase by 10 weeks gestation, plateauing early in third trimester, to about 30–50% higher than the prepregnancy value. The increase in cardiac output is achieved by increase in stroke volume and heart rate and remains constant from mid-pregnancy to term. Heart rate increases, peaking in third trimester. It increases by 10–20 beats per minute and is the reason for the increased risk of arrhythmias during pregnancy. The stroke volume increases by 30–50% by the end of second trimester. The peripheral vascular resistance falls by about 20% due to relaxation of smooth muscles on the arterial side because of progesterone, circulating prostaglandins, endothelial nitric oxide, and low resistance vascular bed of placenta. The systemic arterial pressure falls during the second trimester, reaching a nadir at 24–28 weeks, and again reaches the nonpregnant levels at term. The reduction in diastolic pressure (10–15 mm Hg) is more than the reduction in systolic pressure (5–10 mm Hg) leading to a widening of pulse pressure.

The colloid oncotic pressure decreases throughout pregnancy. In addition, there is an accompanying increase in capillary pressure which favors peripheral edema especially in late pregnancy, complicating the diagnosis of cardiac decompensation. The same mechanism also makes the pregnant women susceptible to pulmonary edema.

In late pregnancy, the pressure of the gravid uterus on the inferior vena cava (IVC) in supine position may cause a reduction in venous return to the heart and a consequent fall in stroke volume and cardiac output called the supine hypotension syndrome. Pregnant women should therefore be advised to rest in the left lateral position. The hypercoagulability of pregnancy may pose additional problems for women with prosthetic valves.

### Labor and Postpartum Period

During labor, the uterine contractions pump an additional 300–500 mL of blood with each contraction, further augmenting the cardiac output which increases by 30% during first stage of labor and by 45% during the second stage of labor. The cardiac output during this time is influenced by the maternal position, pain, anxiety, maternal vascular volume, and the method of pain relief.

Immediately following delivery, the blood volume increases further due to the removal of caval compression coupled with autotransfusion from the contracted uterus which results in further increase in cardiac output to almost 60% of prepregnancy levels. These changes predispose the woman to decompensation in the immediate postpartum period. This increase is only marginally offset by the third stage blood loss unless it is large in amount.

Most of these changes revert to prepregnancy levels by 2 weeks postpartum, as there is loss of placental circulation, the peripheral vascular resistance increases and at the same time, extravascular fluid is mobilized. **Box 1** describes the critical periods for a woman to get decompensated during pregnancy and postpartum period.

## ■ PRECONCEPTION COUNSELING

A thorough evaluation of the woman with pre-existing heart disease should ideally be initiated before the pregnancy is planned. This includes preconception risk assessment, evaluation, and counseling.

### Preconception Risk Assessment

This involves assessing the risk of pregnancy, based on cardiac lesion present, functional status of heart, using New York Heart Association (NYHA) functional classification **(Box 2)** and identifying any additional risk factors such as anemia, thyrotoxicosis, etc. The associated conditions need to be treated prior to conception to optimize the fetomaternal outcome.

### Evaluation

This aims at optimizing the timing of conception in consultation with cardiologist. Her cardiac status needs to be optimized by the medical and surgical teams by completion of diagnostic procedures prior to pregnancy and replacing teratogenic drugs such as ACE inhibitors, warfarin, etc., with safer alternatives.

### Counseling

The counseling includes advise on modifying domestic and work responsibilities so that she can optimize her physical ability to care for a child after delivery. Counsel the woman of the increased risk of maternal mortality due to certain cardiac lesions before she conceives **(Box 3)**.

Explain the risk of having a child with same or different cardiac lesion. Counsel the woman about the possibility of developing complications in pregnancy based on prepregnancy assessments **(Box 4)**. Presence of two or more of the enlisted factors predict a cardiac complication rate of 66% as compared to only 30% when one factor is present and 3% when none of the factors is present at the beginning of pregnancy. Counsel regarding conditions which add high risk to the life of the patient and thus could be considered contraindications to pregnancy. There is a need to prescribe reliable contraception in these cases **(Box 5)**

---

**BOX 1: Critical periods for decompensation.**

- Early pregnancy when the hemodynamic changes of pregnancy begin
- Between 28 and 32 weeks of gestation when the hemodynamic changes of pregnancy peak and cardiac demand is at its maximum
- During labor and delivery due to sudden and frequent variation in the cardiac output with each uterine contraction
- Imediate postpartum period (48–72 hrs)

---

**BOX 2: New York Heart Association cardiac functional classification.**

- *Class I:* No limitations of physical activity; ordinary physical activity does not cause undue fatigue, palpitation, dyspnea or anginal pain
- *Class II:* Slight limitation of physical activity; ordinary physical activity results in fatigue, palpitation, dyspnea or anginal pain
- *Class III:* Marked limitation of physical activity; less than ordinary activity causes fatigue, palpitation, dyspnea or anginal pain
- *Class IV:* Inability to perform any physical activity without discomfort; symptoms of cardiac insufficiency or anginal syndrome may be present, even at rest; any physical activity increases discomfort

---

**BOX 3: Risk categories of cardiac lesions in pregnancy.**

*Low risk (0–1%)*
- Atrial and ventricular septal defects previously repaired without pulmonary hypertension
- Pulmonary or tricuspid disease
- Mitral valve prolapse
- Patent ductus arteriosus
- Corrected congenital heart disease without residual cardiac dysfunction
- Mitral stenosis: NYHA Class I and II
- Bioprosthetic valve
- Fallot tetralogy, corrected

*Moderate risk (5–15%)*
- Mitral stenosis Class III or IV or with atrial fibrillation (AF)
- Aortic stenosis
- Artificial valve
- Moderate to severe systemic ventricular dysfunction
- History of peripartum cardiomyopathy with no residual ventricular dysfunction
- Coarctation of aorta, uncomplicated
- Tetralogy of Fallot; uncorrected or with residual disease
- Previous myocardial infarction
- Marfan's syndrome with normal aorta

*High risk (25–50%)*
- Pulmonary hypertension
- Coarctation of aorta, complicated
- Marfan's syndrome with aortic involvement
- History of peripartum cardiomyopathy with residual ventricular dysfunction

> **BOX 4:** Predictors of adverse cardiac events during pregnancy.
>
> New York Heart Association grade >II
> *Obstructive lesions of left heart*
> - Mitral valve <1.5 cm²
> - Aortic valve <1.5 cm²
> - Gradient peak >30 mm Hg
>
> *Prior cardiac event before pregnancy*
> - Heart failure
> - Arrhythmia
> - Transient ischemic attack
> - Stroke
>
> Ejection fraction <40%

> **BOX 5:** Contraindications to pregnancy due to high risk of maternal mortality.
>
> - Primary or secondary pulmonary hypertension
> - Aortic coarctation with valvular involvement
> - Marfan's syndrome with aortic involvement

> **BOX 6:** Predictors of cardiac complications.
>
> - New York Heart Association (NYHA) class III or more; cyanosis
> - Valvular and outflow tract obstruction
> - Aortic valve area <1.5 cm²
> - Mitral valve area <1 cm²
> - Left ventricular outflow tract peak gradient >30 mm Hg
> - Ejection fraction <40%

For each patient, the prepregnancy cardiovascular status as assessed by NYHA functional classification should be used as a reference for assessing any pregnancy-related changes in cardiac function, although, it does not necessarily prognosticate pregnancy outcome. Any deterioration during pregnancy should prompt a thorough evaluation and aggressive management. Ninety percent or more of patients are categorized as having class I or II disease. Although few patients have class III or IV disease, historically, nearly 85% of maternal deaths occur in these groups. These women should also be counseled that risk of cardiovascular complications such as heart failure, arrhythmias, thromboembolism, angina, hypoxemia, infective endocarditis, pulmonary edema, stroke, or sudden cardiac death are increased if they have had prior cardiac events such as heart failure, arrhythmia, transient ischemic attack, or stroke **(Box 6)**.

## Congenital Inheritance Risk

The risk of congenital heart disease in the baby of a woman with congenital heart disease varies from 3 to 50% depending on the specific lesion in the mother.[2] Risk increases if the previous sibling or the father is also affected. In conditions such as Marfan's syndrome with autosomal inheritance there is a 50% risk of occurrence in the offspring.

## DIAGNOSIS AND WORKUP

The physiological changes of normal pregnancy may mimic a cardiac problem making an accurate diagnosis of heart disease difficult. Many of the potentially significant cardiac lesions which may be previously asymptomatic are unmasked in pregnancy due to pregnancy-related physiological changes. Nonetheless, the diagnosis of heart disease and the specific cardiac lesion are essential to determine the associated maternal and fetal risk and develop a therapeutic plan.

## History

The common findings encountered during a normal pregnancy such as fatigue, decreased exercise tolerance, lightheadedness, syncope, palpitations, and breathlessness on exertion are due to the hyperdynamic changes in pregnancy and, may mimic the symptoms of heart disease. However, progressive dyspnea or orthopnea, nocturnal cough, hemoptysis, recurrent attacks of syncope or chest pain, mandate a thorough investigation for heart disease. It is also essential to enquire about the history of rheumatic fever, cyanosis during early childhood, family history of congenital heart disease, history of palliative or corrective surgery and history of sudden death in family members.

## Physical Examination

The hyperdynamic circulation of pregnancy causes alterations in the physical findings in the cardiovascular system which simulates heart disease. The common findings in a normal pregnancy include distended neck veins, brisk and displaced left ventricular impulse, palpable right ventricular impulse, loud S1, exaggerated splitting of S2, third heart sound or mid systolic soft ejection murmurs over the sternal borders or the pulmonary area. These may be confused with disease states. However, a diastolic murmur or additional heart sounds such as fourth heart sound, ejection click, opening snap or presence of precordial thrill strongly suggests heart disease as also do other clinical findings like presence of cyanosis, clubbing, persistent neck vein distention, systolic murmur grade 3/6 or greater, cardiomegaly, persistent arrhythmia, persistent split-second sound and features of pulmonary hypertension.

## Evaluation

- *ECG:* Some common pregnancy-induced changes include QRS axis deviation, small Q and inverted P waves in Lead III, sinus tachycardia and premature atrial/ventricular beats. However, significant arrhythmias or heart blocks should be evaluated for underlying heart disease.
- *Chest radiography:* The amount of radiation received by the fetus during a maternal chest X-ray is minimal and it should not be withheld if clinically indicated. Straightening of the left heart border, horizontal position of the heart and prominent lung markings are some of the changes which are seen in normal pregnancy.

- *Echocardiography:* It is the investigation of choice not only to define the cardiac anatomy but also to describe ventricular function and estimate intracardiac pressure gradients. There is no radiation hazard, it is noninvasive, and the information provided allows an accurate diagnosis. Transesophageal echocardiography is also safe, and it can provide better visualization of the left atrium and mitral valve. Some normal changes seen during pregnancy include enlargement of all cardiac chambers and mild physiologic regurgitation of mitral, tricuspid, and pulmonary valves.

It must be reiterated that a diagnosis of heart disease first made during pregnancy could be erroneous even after echocardiography as the distinction between normal and diseased state could be confounding even to an experienced physician unless the disease is of an advanced nature. This would therefore mandate a cardiology review once the puerperium is over irrespective of course of pregnancy.

## MANAGEMENT

### General Principles

*Antenatal*

Between 15 and 52% of cardiac abnormalities are first diagnosed during pregnancy on routine antenatal examination or due to symptoms precipitated by the physiological changes of pregnancy.[3] Therefore, the cardiovascular system of all pregnant women should be thoroughly evaluated in the first antenatal visit with a high index of suspicion. Once the diagnosis of heart disease is confirmed by appropriate investigations, the patients' functional cardiac status should be established according to the NYHA classification system. These women are evaluated for risk of maternal cardiac complications which include pulmonary edema, symptomatic arrhythmias, stroke, transient ischemic attack, congestive heart failure, thromboembolism, and sudden cardiac death. The predictive indicators of complications are given in **Box 7**.

The main aim of management is to keep the patient within her cardiac reserve and thus, the patient is instructed to restrict physical activity. The degree of physical restriction requires individualization. Dietary advice is given to restrict sodium intake to less than 2 g/day. The patient should be assessed by the cardiologist for requirement of cardiac drugs, diuretics, and anticoagulants.

**BOX 7:** Indications for hospitalization during antenatal period.
- New York Heart Association (NYHA) class III/IV irrespective of period of gestation
- Symptoms and signs suggestive of complications
- When patients on oral anticoagulants are switched over to heparin, i.e., from 6 weeks or earlier to 12 weeks and again at 36 weeks till delivery
- NYHA class I/II at 38 weeks for safe confinement

The antenatal management of these patients varies with the functional class. Patients belonging to class I and II are advised routine obstetric evaluation and fetal monitoring. In the antenatal clinic special attention must be paid to weight gain, vitals and signs or symptoms of cardiac failure. These women are instructed to avoid contact with persons with respiratory infections and report if there is any evidence of infection. Other factors which increase the risk of heart failure include anemia, obesity, hypertension, arrhythmias, and hyperthyroidism which should be identified and vigorously treated. They should also be advised to avoid smoking and drug abuse if applicable.

Patients in NYHA class III and IV must be managed as in-patients initially till the class improves. Management includes limitation of physical activity and judicious use of drugs to decrease preload and to increase inotropic activity of heart. Medical management of the woman's cardiac condition should be optimized, surgery is best avoided during pregnancy. However, failure of medical management and significant risk of recurrence of pulmonary edema are justifiable indications for surgery.

Maternal complications of heart disease include congestive heart failure, pulmonary edema, arrhythmias, and sudden cardiac arrest. The fetal morbidity in these women is contributed by premature labor, premature rupture of membranes, intrauterine growth restriction and congenital heart disease (4.5% vs. 0.6% in general population).[4]

Fetal assessment of growth should be monitored clinically, and fetal echocardiogram performed between 18 and 22 weeks especially in patients with congenital heart disease. Antenatal testing for fetal wellbeing may be required in some cases. The timing of initiation of monitoring needs individualization and the frequency of testing depends upon the maternal functional class. Expectedly, the higher the NYHA class, earlier the monitoring is to be started. Patients should receive RHD prophylaxis as routine and endocarditis prophylaxis when a planned procedure likely to produce bacteremia is contemplated.

*Labor and Delivery*

Spontaneous onset of labor is awaited in these women and induction of labor or elective cesarean delivery are reserved for obstetric indications only. Delivery must be conducted in a tertiary care center. If induction with vaginal prostaglandin is used, it is probably wise to start with a low dose because acute uterine hyperstimulation requiring either tocolysis or an urgent delivery is particularly risky in a woman with significant cardiac disease. During labor, the mother should be nursed in a semirecumbent position with lateral tilt to avoid aortocaval compression and possible hypotension. Intermittent oxygen inhalation is provided. Fluid balance necessitates careful and expert attention as these women may easily develop pulmonary edema. Adequate pain control can be achieved with parenteral analgesics or epidural analgesia. However, it is important to avoid hypotension while administering regional anesthesia. The risk of cardiac overload must be avoided during preload prior to regional analgesia hence the services of an experienced anesthesiologist are required.

Maternal vital signs pulse, BP, respiratory rate, and oxygen saturation are frequently monitored for early signs of congestive heart failure. Chest is auscultated intermittently for basal crepitations suggestive of pulmonary edema. The frequency of monitoring depends on the maternal condition. Progress of labor is monitored as usual by maintaining a partogram. The number of per vaginal examinations must be strictly restricted to bare minimum to reduce the risk of infection.

Vaginal delivery is preferred for patients with heart disease as hemodynamic fluctuations and blood loss are more common with cesarean section and its attendant anesthesia requirements. Cesarean section increases the risk of infection, thromboembolism, and postoperative complications. Cesarean delivery should be reserved for standard obstetric indications.

During second stage, the patient should be propped up. Intravenous access must be secured. Vitals should be frequently monitored with intermittent chest auscultation for basal crepts. High-flow oxygen inhalation intermittently must continue throughout. Shortening of second stage with operative vaginal delivery may be considered, However, second stage should be routinely shortened in patients with NYHA class III and IV, maternal decompensation and for obstetric indications.

During third stage, careful monitoring of vitals such as oxygen saturation, blood pressure, and respiratory rate is done. Pain relief and or sedation must be provided. Intravenous furosemide 20–40 mg should be given if systolic blood pressure is more than 100 mm Hg. This will minimize preload and thus prevent pulmonary edema which is a frequent occurrence at this time due to increase in circulating blood volume because of shift of blood from the uteroplacental circulation. Methylergometrine is contraindicated and intramuscular oxytocin is preferred. Prostaglandin (PG) F2α is best avoided.

## Postnatal

The immediate postpartum period is critical for these patients. During the first 48–72 hours significant fluid shifts occur and features of decompensation can appear. Hence, careful monitoring of pulse, blood pressure, respiratory rate, and urine output is required. It is especially important in women who have progressive reduction in oxygen saturation monitored by pulse oximetry. This often heralds the onset of clinical pulmonary edema.

> **BOX 8:** High-risk cases requiring infective endocarditis prophylaxis.
>
> - History of previous endocarditis
> - Prosthetic valve
> - Unrepaired cyanotic congenital heart disease
> - Repaired congenital heart disease with residual shunt or regurgitation at the site of prosthetic patch or shunt
> - Bicuspid aortic valve and mitral valve prolapse

> **BOX 9:** Antibiotic regimens for women with heart disease.
>
> - *Standard regimen:* Amoxicillin 2 g orally or Ampicillin 2 g IV or IM or cefazolin or ceftriaxone 1 g IM or IV 30 to 60 minutes before procedure
> - *Penicillin allergic standard regimen:* Clindamycin 600 mg orally, IM or IV 30–60 minutes before procedure or Vancomycin 15–20 mg/kg (maximum 2 g) IV 120 minutes before procedure

## Infective Endocarditis Prophylaxis

The current guidelines, including recommendations from the American Heart Association do not recommend routine IE prophylaxis for patients with RHD as they suggest that the risk of adverse events related to antibiotic prophylaxis such as antibiotic resistance exceeds the benefits.[5]

Pregnant women who are at high-risk for IE should receive antibiotic prophylaxis before certain dental, oral, or upper respiratory tract procedures but do not usually need antibiotic prophylaxis before a normal vaginal delivery, gastrointestinal surgery, or genitourinary surgery. In this context, an episiotomy or repair of a vaginal tear is not considered to be a complication, unless there is an extension involving the rectal mucosa. Routine antibiotic prophylaxis is recommended in women undergoing cesarean section and those at high risk of endocarditis **(Box 8)**.

Various antibiotic regimens to be used in patients with heart disease are described in **Box 9**.

## SPECIFIC LESIONS

### Rheumatic Heart Disease

*Mitral Stenosis*

Mitral stenosis is the most common lesion in women with RHD. Symptoms include fatigue and dyspnea on exertion which may progress to dyspnea at rest, paroxysmal nocturnal dyspnea, and hemoptysis. Dizziness and symptoms of low cardiac output like syncope may also be present.

The stenotic mitral valve impairs left ventricular filling and limits any increase in cardiac output. Chronic left atrial outflow obstruction leads to severe pulmonary venous congestion, pulmonary hypertension, and later right ventricular failure. Pregnancy-mediated cardiovascular changes, especially increased intravascular volume, and increased heart rate, can exacerbate the impaired filling and lead to decompensation during pregnancy and especially during labor, delivery and puerperium when circulating blood volume rises sharply within a short-time period.

On physical examination, there is loud first heart sound, an opening snap, and a low frequency diastolic murmur at the apex with or without presystolic accentuation. The murmur is best heard in the left lateral position with the bell of the stethoscope. Accentuated pulmonic component of the second heart sound and other features of pulmonary hypertension may be present.

Echocardiography is the investigation of choice to confirm the diagnosis and is used to define the valvular anatomy, degree of stenosis as denoted by functional valvular area, associated regurgitation, other valvular anomalies, and presence of pulmonary arterial hypertension. ECG is often normal or may indicate left atrial enlargement, right axis deviation, right ventricular hypertrophy, and left atrial p-waves. Chest X-ray shows straightening of left heart border with prominent left atrial appendage, pulmonary congestion, and edema.

Goals of management include optimizing the cardiac output, preventing tachycardia, avoiding decrease in systemic vascular resistance, and reducing the stress on right ventricle by minimizing increase in blood volume and avoiding situations in which pulmonary artery pressures are increased such as hypercarbia, hypoxia, or acidosis.

Serious complications are more common in severe mitral stenosis (mitral valve area <1 cm$^2$), moderate or severe symptoms prior to pregnancy and in those diagnosed late in pregnancy. Pulmonary edema can develop because of tachycardia, injudicious use of fluids during third stage of labor leading to an increase in intravascular volume. A rapid heart rate in mitral stenosis prevents ventricular filling decreasing the time for left atrial emptying leading to increase in left atrial pressure and pulmonary edema. This leads to more tachycardia and a vicious cycle. Thus, beta-blockers are indicated if HR >90/min.

Labor imposes an additional stress and congestive heart failure (CHF) may develop for the first-time during labor in a previously well-controlled patient. Hence, bedside cardiac monitoring is necessary. Also, central hemodynamic monitoring is required if the patient is class III or IV or a valve diameter is <2.5 cm$^2$. For pain relief, epidural analgesia can be used but care should be taken to avoid fluid overload. If general anesthesia becomes necessary, agents that produce tachycardia such as atropine and ketamine should be avoided.

Sometimes, balloon mitral valvotomy or percutaneous mitral commissurotomy may be required in antenatal patients with severe symptomatic disease. Initially, this was considered an extreme procedure but over the years it has achieved greater acceptance due to minimal complications. Rarely, mitral valve replacement along with elective cesarean during the same anesthesia may be considered in patients with severe symptomatic disease complicated by mitral regurgitation as well.

## Mitral Regurgitation

This lesion has various etiologies such as rheumatic, floppy mitral valve in association with mitral valve prolapse (MVP), papillary muscle dysfunction and ruptured chordae tendinae. Due to the fall in systemic vascular resistance and reduced left ventricular afterload, this condition is well-tolerated in pregnancy. Women in NYHA class I and II need to be managed by rest. If ventricular failure develops, it should be managed with digoxin, diuretics, and afterload reduction. Any rise of blood pressure could worsen regurgitation and should be avoided.

## Aortic Stenosis

Aortic stenosis (AS) can be congenital, rheumatic, or due to age-related calcification. The most common cause in women of childbearing age is congenital bicuspid valve. Aortic stenosis of rheumatic origin is less common in women of childbearing age group as it is a progressive condition. This usually occurs in conjunction with mitral valve disease. Pregnancy outcome depends on the degree of stenosis. Women with severe AS (aortic valve area <0.7 cm$^2$, mean gradient >50 mm Hg) should be advised to delay conception until after surgical correction as patients tend to respond poorly to the physiological increase of circulating blood volume.

Fluid management is an important component of intrapartum care as volume overload can lead to pulmonary edema and hypovolemia can cause sudden death. Patients should labor in lateral position to avoid aortocaval compression. Spinal and epidural blocks are contraindicated due to vasodilatory effect; however, narcotic epidural can decrease the chances of hypotension.

If a pregnant woman becomes symptomatic or is so when pregnancy is confirmed, bed rest and valve replacement should be considered. However, open heart surgery and cardiac bypass should be avoided due to 1.5% maternal mortality rate and 16–33% fetal mortality rates irrespective of gestational age.[6]

Antepartum aortic balloon valvuloplasty is not as commonly performed as for mitral valve lesions but may be occasionally considered as a palliative procedure deferring valve replacement after delivery.

## Aortic Regurgitation

This regurgitant lesion of the aortic valve is not common. Etiological factors may be rheumatic, Marfan's syndrome or syphilitic aortitis. Pregnancy is well-tolerated as the increased heart rate of pregnancy causes decreased time for regurgitation and the decreased systemic vascular resistance promotes forward flow, both of which are physiologically helpful. Severe lesions may require drug therapy.

## Mitral Valve Prolapse

Mitral valve prolapse may be sporadic or inherited as a dominant condition in some families with variants of Marfan's syndrome. The prevalence of MVP is 2-4% in general population and it is almost twice more common in females. Here, one or more mitral valve leaflets extend above the plane that separates atria and ventricles due to myxomatous degeneration of the valve leaflets, annulus, or the chordae tendinae. Most women are asymptomatic and are diagnosed incidentally. On echocardiography the mitral valve is seen prolapsing into the left atrium. Complications are rare as pregnancy-induced hypervolemia improves the alignment of mitral valve. These include severe mitral regurgitation, infective endocarditis, cerebral ischemia, embolism, and sudden death. The risk of complications is increased if there is associated mitral regurgitation or valvular damage. These women should avoid caffeine, alcohol, tobacco, and beta-mimetic drugs. Symptomatic women are given beta-blockers to reduce the sympathetic tone and relieve symptoms.

## Prosthetic Heart Valves

Many women with severe valvular heart disease now survive and become pregnant because of surgical valve replacement. There are two types of valves—mechanical and bioprosthetic. Porcine tissue valves are safer during pregnancy as anticoagulation is not required but valvular dysfunction and heart failure are more common. Moreover, they are not as durable as mechanical valves and generally require repeat valve replacement in 10-15 years. Pregnancy does not appear to shorten this interval.

Prosthetic or mechanical valves are longer lasting but require anticoagulation for life. American College of Obstetricians and Gynecologists (ACOG) recommends full anticoagulation throughout pregnancy with prosthetic valves. Warfarin has the advantage of oral administration but can lead to warfarin embryopathy (6%) if used between 6 and 9 weeks. Another disadvantage is that anticoagulant effect cannot be readily reversed. Warfarin embryopathy is characterized by nasal hypoplasia and stippled epiphysis. The risk is higher if the daily dose exceeds 5 mg/day. Warfarin has also been found to increase the risk of miscarriage (32%) and stillbirth (7%). Also, since warfarin crosses the placenta it causes fetal anticoagulation and intracerebral bleeding particularly if used within 2 weeks of labor. On the other hand, heparin does not cross the placenta and its effects are rapidly reversible but are associated with increased risk of valve thrombosis, embolic events and retroplacental hemorrhage. Unfractionated heparin needs to be administered parenterally, has a short duration of action, narrow therapeutic index and in high doses can lead to osteoporosis. Though low molecular weight heparins have been found to have better safety profile in pregnancy, these are not recommended as anticoagulants in patients with prosthetic heart valves by ACOG as there have been reports of valvular thrombosis in women who have been apparently anticoagulated with low molecular weight heparin (LMWH).[7,8] On the other hand American College of Chest Physician has recommended use of any regimen that includes unfractionated heparin (UFH) or LMWH.

Though, the optimal agent for anticoagulation during pregnancy is not available, the most used regime is to stop warfarin and give high dose unfractionated heparin from 6 to 12 weeks gestation to avoid warfarin embryopathy and then switch back to warfarin from 12 to 37 weeks. Near term warfarin is substituted by heparin till the onset of labor. The target INR is 2.5-3.5 for warfarin and monitoring of the patients on UFH is done by aPTT (target aPTT twice normal). Heparin is restarted 6 hours after normal vaginal delivery and 24 hours after cesarean section. Warfarin is started concomitantly, and heparin stopped after 3 days. If a patient fully anticoagulated with warfarin requires urgent delivery, the effects are reversed with fresh frozen plasma and vitamin K and the effects of heparin are reversed with protamine sulfate.

## Congenital Heart Disease

With the relative decline of rheumatic heart disease especially in the developed countries, this group now represents majority of women with heart disease during pregnancy. A study showed that the number of delivery hospitalizations with congenital heart disease increased significantly from 6.4 to 9 per 10,000 deliveries from 2000 to 2010 and that these deliveries had a greater than expected rate of medical and obstetric complications.[9] A review reported that congenital heart disease now comprises 80% of all pregnancies in women with heart conditions in the Western world.[10] Asymptomatic acyanotic women with simple defects usually tolerate pregnancy well whereas women with cyanotic lesions are likely to fare poorly. These women are at increased risk of having a baby with congenital heart disease (CHD) for which genetic counseling and fetal echocardiography is recommended at 18-22 weeks.

## Left to Right Shunts

### Atrial Septal Defect

It is the second most common congenital cardiac lesion among adults after bicuspid aortic valve. Ostium secundum type accounts for 70% of all atrial septal defects (ASDs) and is more common in women. Most are asymptomatic until third or fourth decade. The defect should be repaired if discovered in adulthood. Complications of uncorrected lesions are more common after 40 years of age and include supraventricular arrhythmias, paradoxical emboli following right ventricular heart failure, pulmonary hypertension, and mitral regurgitation caused by mitral leaflet prolapse in 15%. These complications should ideally be identified before pregnancy and managed appropriately. Pulmonary hypertension if present before pregnancy is a contraindication to conception. Pregnancy and labor are generally tolerated well but acute blood loss is tolerated poorly as it can increase systemic vascular resistance and the left to right shunt leading to a precipitous fall in left ventricular output, blood pressure, coronary blood flow and even cardiac arrest. Epidural analgesia is preferred during labor as it reduces the systemic vascular resistance and the left to right shunt. Early ambulation is encouraged in the postpartum period to reduce the risk of deep vein thrombosis and paradoxical embolization. A paradoxical embolism, also called a crossed embolism, is a form of arterial thrombosis caused by embolism of a thrombus of venous origin through an opening in the heart, such as ASD or ventricular septal defect (VSD). The risk of having a baby with congenital heart disease varies from 3 to 10% in these women.[11,12]

## Ventricular Septal Defect

It is an uncommon lesion in adults as most are identified and repaired in childhood and small defects close spontaneously. Repaired defects usually do not present with problems. Maternal morbidity in an uncorrected lesion depends on the size of the lesion and presence and severity of pulmonary artery hypertension. In general, if the defect is smaller than 1.25 cm$^2$ pulmonary arterial hypertension (PAH) and congestive heart failure do not develop. Pregnancy is usually well-tolerated. These women should be evaluated pre-pregnancy for PAH and if present, pregnancy is discouraged. Complications include congestive heart failure, pulmonary artery hypertension, paradoxical systemic embolization, and bacterial endocarditis. It is advisable to avoid hypotension during labor which can lead to shunt reversal. Risk of congenital heart disease in the baby varies from 6 to 10%.

## Pulmonary Artery Hypertension and Eisenmenger Syndrome

Pulmonary artery hypertension is extremely dangerous in pregnancy and is associated with high maternal mortality (50%). It can be primary or secondary. Primary type is a rare idiopathic condition which occurs in the absence of intracardiac or aortopulmonary shunt. It is more common in women and mean survival from diagnosis is 2 years. The criteria for diagnosis of primary PAH include mean pulmonary arterial pressure (MPAP) > 25 mm Hg at rest or >30 mm Hg with exertion in the absence of heart disease, chronic thromboembolic disease, underlying pulmonary disease or other secondary causes. Secondary PAH can be due to several cardiac, respiratory, or embolic causes. Eisenmenger physiology occurs when the increased pulmonary vascular blood flow due to left to right shunt produces a right-sided pressure greater than the left side and hence reversal of shunt occurs and subsequently cyanosis develops. The pulmonary vascular resistance in PAH is fixed and cannot fall in response to pregnancy and consequently pulmonary blood flow cannot increase resulting in refractory hypoxemia. Elective termination of pregnancy carries a 7% risk of mortality and hence the importance of avoiding pregnancy and even considering permanent sterilization for these women if they come for prepregnancy counseling. If pregnancy is encountered termination should be offered. Treatment of pregnant women who are symptomatic requires a multidisciplinary care and includes limitation of activity, avoidance of supine position in late pregnancy, diuretics, supplemental oxygen, elective admission for bed rest, vasodilators, thromboprophylaxis with LMW heparin, and avoiding increase in pulmonary vascular resistance.[12] Use of calcium channel blockers has been reported to improve outcome. Sildenafil which is a phosphodiesterase inhibitor has shown a beneficial effect in patients with severe pulmonary artery hypertension. Heparin is given in the dose of 5,000/10,000 IU subcutaneously twice daily. During labor, these women are at the greatest risk of dying because of diminished venous return and right ventricular flow. Spontaneous labor is preferred but when indicated, induction with PGE2 gel and oxytocin can be used. Cesarean section is reserved for obstetric indication which is associated with an increased risk of maternal morbidity and mortality. Epidural catheter is placed early in labor, but it is important to avoid hypotension. Oxygen is given at 5–6 L/min and oxygen saturation is monitored. These patients should ideally have invasive cardiac monitoring during delivery. Placement of Swan-Ganz catheter and arterial line is to be considered for frequent blood sampling. If it is not possible at least a CVP catheter is inserted early in labor and an adequate preload is maintained. Intravenous prostacyclin and inhaled nitric oxide have also been used during labor as these drugs can cause vascular dilatation and inhibition of platelet aggregation and have been shown to improve oxygenation, decrease pulmonary vascular resistance and the risk of thromboembolism. Fluid shifts in the postpartum period because of excessive blood loss and right heart failure can result in sudden death.

## Coarctation of Aorta

Coarctation of aorta is a relatively uncommon condition as most of these conditions are corrected during childhood. Other cardiovascular abnormalities which may be associated with coarctation of aorta include bicuspid aortic valve (20%), aneurysm of the circle of Willis, intercostal arteries, and distal aorta; patent ductus arteriosus (PDA), ASD and Turner's syndrome. Unrepaired lesions can lead to maternal hypertension in the upper extremity but normal or reduced blood pressure in the lower extremity. Ideally, if identified preconceptionally the lesion should be repaired. The patient should be thoroughly investigated for associated abnormalities and elective surgery considered accordingly as these associated abnormalities put the patient at risk of significant morbidity. The major complications in a pregnant patient with an uncorrected lesion include congestive heart failure, subacute bacterial endocarditis of the bicuspid aortic valve, aortic dissection, rupture, and cerebral hemorrhage from aneurysm in the circle of Willis. Maternal mortality has been reported to be 3–9% and fetal death as high as 20%. During pregnancy, hypertension is controlled by beta-blockers. During labor and delivery, hypertension should be controlled and use of epidural analgesia is encouraged as it controls pain and reduces the systemic vascular resistance. Though, it was previously thought that a cesarean section is best for these women, the current available evidence suggests that cesarean delivery should be limited to obstetric indications. It is sometimes indicated in pregnant women with hemodynamically unstable women in advanced heart failure. The risk of congenital heart disease in the fetus is 4–7%.

## Cyanotic Heart Lesions

### Tetralogy of Fallot

This is the most common type of cyanotic congenital heart disease characterized by large subaortic VSD, subvalvular pulmonary stenosis, right ventricular hypertrophy and overriding aorta that receives blood from both right and left ventricles. The magnitude of shunt varies inversely with systemic vascular resistance. During pregnancy when systemic vascular resistance decreases, the shunt increases, and hypoxemia and cyanosis worsen leading to rise in hematocrit. Pregnancy in a woman with an uncorrected lesion carries high-risk of maternal and fetal mortality. Women who have undergone repair and in whom cyanosis does not reappear, do well in pregnancy. Complications include supraventricular tachycardia, right ventricular failure, pulmonary embolism, pulmonary hypertension, and progressive right ventricular dilatation. Preconception evaluation includes assessment of right and left ventricular function, severity of pulmonary insufficiency and stenosis, and consideration for repair of severe pulmonary insufficiency before pregnancy. Certain risk factors that worsen the prognosis are prepregnancy hematocrit exceeding 65%, a history of congestive heart failure or syncope, cardiomegaly, right ventricular pressure exceeding 120 mm Hg or strain pattern on electrocardiogram or oxygen saturation <80%. Epidural or spinal anesthesia should be avoided as any decrease in systemic vascular resistance can be life-threatening. Neonatal outcome is poor in patients with uncorrected lesion because of increased rates of spontaneous abortion, prematurity, and growth restriction.[13]

In cases where mother has tetralogy of Fallot, congenital heart disease affects approximately 5% of infants.

## PERIPARTUM CARDIOMYOPATHY

Peripartum cardiomyopathy (PPCM) is a global congestive heart failure characterized by dilatation of all four chambers of the heart, low cardiac output, and pulmonary edema. The criteria used for diagnosis include:
- Development of cardiac failure in the last month of pregnancy or within 5 months of delivery
- The absence of an identifiable cause for cardiac failure
- Absence of recognizable heart disease prior to last month of pregnancy
- Left ventricular systolic dysfunction demonstrated by classic echocardiographic criteria such as reduced ejection fraction.

Peripartum cardiomyopathy is a type of dilated cardiomyopathy and is a diagnosis of exclusion. Women usually present with heart failure at the end of pregnancy or more commonly during puerperium. It occurs in 1 in 1,300 to 1 in 15,000 deliveries.[14]

These women are generally older than 30 years of age, multiparous, with recognized risk factors such as pre-eclampsia, gestational hypertension, and multiple gestation. The pathogenesis is unknown and various immunologic and infective etiologies have been proposed. Studies are also ongoing to consider a genetic cause or predilection. These women present with signs and symptoms of congestive heart failure. ECG shows tachycardia and arrhythmias. Chest X-ray is consistent with cardiomegaly with varying number of pulmonary infiltrates and pleural effusion. On echocardiography, the left atrium and ventricle are seen to be enlarged, ejection fraction is less than 45% or fractional shortening less than 30% or both and an end diastolic dimension >2.7 cm/m$^2$. The complications include life-threatening arrhythmias and pulmonary or systemic embolization.[15] Management consists of aggressive treatment of heart failure with bed rest, sodium restriction, diuretics, digoxin, prophylactic heparin and afterload reduction with hydralazine or other vasodilators. Immunosuppressive therapy with prednisolone and azathioprine has been used to improve left ventricular function. Cautious use of beta-blockers can be done if tachycardia persists and cardiac output is preserved well. Recently, bromocriptine or its derivative cabergoline, has been recommended as a successful treatment modality after it was shown that the cause of PPCM was a result of unbalanced oxidative stress following a dysregulation of vascular and hormonal factors. Treatment is now summarized using the acronym BOARD for Bromocriptine, Oral heart failure therapies, Anticoagulants, Vasorelaxing agents and Diuretics.[16] Those who are seriously ill, need intubation and ventilation and use of ventricular assist device. Heart transplantation can be lifesaving in severe cases. Fifty percent of patients make spontaneous and full recovery and for those who do not, 85% mortality in 4–5 years is reported. Persistent cardiac dysfunction is seen in 45–90% of patients. The prognosis is poor. Maternal mortality is as high as 25–50% but likely to be lesser if correctly diagnosed and treated timely in a specialized tertiary level center.

The risk of recurrence in a subsequent pregnancy is close to 80%. It depends on normalization of left ventricular function within 6 months of delivery. Those women with severe myocardial dysfunction, defined as left ventricular diastolic dimension more than 6 cm and fractional shortening less than 21% are unlikely to regain normal cardiac function on follow-up. Those in whom left ventricular function and size do not return to normal within 6 months and prior to a subsequent pregnancy are at significant risk of worsening heart failure (50%) and death (25%) or recurrent PPCM in next pregnancy. Pregnancy is strongly discouraged in women with prior history of PPCM and especially those with residual cardiac dysfunction. If pregnancy occurs, termination should be offered to those with persistent echocardiographic abnormalities. However, if pregnancy is continued, decreased activity and bed rest along with symptomatic treatment is given. During labor and delivery, these women must be closely watched for congestive heart failure and pulmonary embolism. Pulmonary artery catheterization for hemodynamic monitoring may be considered. Vaginal delivery is preferred, and cesarean section is reserved for obstetric indications. Postnatally, these patients can be given ACE inhibitors for afterload reduction. Reliable contraception should be provided.

## Hypertrophic Cardiomyopathy

Most cases of hypertrophic cardiomyopathy are familial and inherited as autosomal dominant trait. It is characterized by left ventricular hypertrophy without chamber dilatation. The older names for this condition such as idiopathic hypertrophic subaortic stenosis and hypertrophic obstructive cardiomyopathy have been replaced as there is no left ventricular outflow obstruction in most cases. Women may be asymptomatic and diagnosed because of family screening or may experience syncope or "angina-like" chest pain. Pregnancy in asymptomatic women is well-tolerated while cases with severe symptoms or heart failure before pregnancy are at a risk of symptomatic progression, atrial fibrillation, syncope, and maternal death.[17] Clinical risk factors for sudden death include a family history of sudden cardiac death, previous syncope and documented ventricular tachycardia.

## ■ MYOCARDIAL INFARCTION

Myocardial infarction (MI) is an uncommon event in women of childbearing age. However, as the birth rate for women older than 40 years has increased in recent years in some countries such as the United States, MI in pregnant women is likely to become more common. In a study from USA acute MI occurred in 1 of every 12,400 hospitalizations during pregnancy and postpartum; 20.6% occurred in the antepartum period, 23.7% during the labor and delivery hospitalization, and 53.4% in the postpartum period. The rate of MI increased over time even after adjustment for age and race/ethnicity. The mortality rate was 4.5%.[18]

## Causes of Myocardial Infarction in Pregnancy

These include atherosclerosis, thrombosis, or vasospastic disease. Pregnant women with coronary artery disease commonly have classic risk factors such as diabetes, smoking, hypertension, hyperlipidemia, and obesity. However, no cardiac risk factors are present in 40% of the cases. Associated risk factors include administration of oxytocic agents, drug abuse (crack cocaine), embolism due to mitral stenosis and or infective endocarditis.

## Diagnosis

Diagnosis is usually difficult because the index of suspicion is low and physiologic changes during pregnancy may mimic symptoms. The patient presents with chest pain and clinical examination reveals pericardial friction rub. The diagnosis is supported by typical ECG changes. Acute MI is present when there is a rise and/or fall of cardiac troponin and the presence of one of the following: ischemic signs; new Q waves, significant ST-segment-T wave changes, or new left bundle branch block on the ECG; or intracoronary thrombus on angiography.

Troponin-I should be used to document acute MI because myoglobin and creatine kinase are increased two-folds during labor and delivery. Creatine kinase-MB isoenzyme is also used for the diagnosis of MI during pregnancy.

## Management

Bed rest is given to minimize cardiac workload and myocardial oxygen consumption. Aspirin, nitrates, calcium channel blockers, and beta-blockers have been found to be safe during pregnancy. Coronary angiography and percutaneous transluminal coronary angioplasty and stenting all have been successfully performed in pregnancy. Pregnancy is a relative contraindication to thrombolytic therapy because of theoretical increased risk of maternal and fetal bleeding. Spontaneous vaginal delivery should be allowed. Cesarean section is empirically advocated in patients who start laboring within 4 days of acute MI. Epidural analgesia should be provided during labor and delivery along with supplemental oxygen and left lateral tilt position. Oxytocin infusion is used rather than ergometrine which can cause coronary artery spasm. Patients are advocated not to become pregnant for at least 1 year after acute MI, after which prepregnancy cardiac evaluation should be done including echocardiography and stress testing before a pregnancy can be planned cautiously in future if there is no residual cardiac dysfunction.

## Complications in Pregnancy

In a study of over 100 cases of myocardial infarction (MI) in pregnant women[19] the complications noted were heart failure or cardiogenic shock in over 38%, ventricular arrhythmias in about 12%, recurrent angina, or MI in nearly 20% with left ventricular ejection fraction ≤40% in almost 64%, ≤30% in 24%, and ≤20% in 9% of the women.

## Prognosis

The in-hospital maternal mortality was between 4.5 and 7% in published studies.[19] The highest risk for maternal death exists when MI occurs in the late third trimester.

## CARDIAC ARRHYTHMIAS

Arrhythmias are the most common cardiac complications encountered during pregnancy in women with and without structural heart disease.[20] In the United States, the incidence of pregnancy-related hospitalizations with arrhythmias has increased between 2000 and 2012 primarily due to increases in the incidence of ventricular tachycardia.[21]

Arrhythmias may manifest for the first-time during pregnancy, and in other cases, pregnancy can trigger exacerbations in women with pre-existing arrhythmias.[20,21] Women with established arrhythmias or structural heart disease or those with corrected congenital heart lesions, are at highest risk of developing arrhythmias during pregnancy (**Box 10**).

Atrial and ventricular premature beats are frequently present during pregnancy and have no adverse effects on the mother or fetus and thus, require no further investigations. The most common arrhythmia seen during pregnancy is supraventricular tachycardia (SVT).[19] Atrial fibrillation and atrial flutter are rare.

## Management in Pregnancy and Labor

Early treatment, either with conversion to sinus rhythm or ventricular rate control is important because of the risk of thromboembolism and detrimental effect on the fetus. Initial treatment should be the vagal maneuver but 50% of SVTs do not respond to vagal maneuvers. Intravenous adenosine, propranolol and verapamil have been safely used for acute termination of SVTs. Initial therapy with lidocaine or procainamide should be considered in hemodynamically stable women. Amiodarone is contraindicated as it is associated with fetal hypothyroidism, growth restriction, and prematurity. Beta-blockers can be used. Electrical cardioversion is safe in pregnancy and may be done in all women with tachyarrhythmias who are hemodynamically stable. Airway management is essential and supine position should be avoided.

## HEART BLOCK IN PREGNANCY

Heart block is an unusual complication of pregnancy. By itself complete heart block rarely creates any obstetric problems, so prophylactic placement of a permanent pacemaker is not indicated in all asymptomatic patients. Fetal growth restriction (FGR) and polycythemia have been reported with complete heart block.[22] Labor in these patients may be complicated by syncope and convulsions caused by slowing of the heart rate during the Valsalva maneuver exercised at the time of forceful contractions of the second stage of labor which should be shortened by using forceps. Management involves use of cardiac pacemaker,[23,24] which should be implanted before pregnancy (or whenever heart block is diagnosed in pregnancy) to maintain cardiac function. For symptomatic patients in the first and second trimester, permanent pacemaker implantation is the therapy of choice. In symptomatic women who present at or near term, temporary pacing followed by induction of labor should be done at the earliest possible time to prevent complications of prolonged temporary pacing. Overall maternal and neonatal outcome is unaffected in such cases.

## PREGNANCY AFTER HEART TRANSPLANT

The last decade has shown better survival among both the congenital and adult transplant recipients, with an increased number of female patients of childbearing age desiring pregnancy, and many publications of successful pregnancies in such women reported though with limited long-term outcome data. It is hence recommended that multidisciplinary team input is considered regarding the optimal timing and management of pregnancy in postcardiac transplant patients.

## Preconception

### Risk Assessment

Assessment of overall risk to both mother and fetus is done preconceptionally. Baseline electrocardiogram and graft function should be assessed since a successful pregnancy is most likely to occur in a cardiac transplant recipient with normal graft function and no evidence of rejection. If clinically indicated, dobutamine stress echocardiography or left and right heart catheterization with subsequent endomyocardial biopsy should be performed prior to pregnancy.

---

**BOX 10:** Reasons for increase in arrhythmias in pregnancy (even in the absence of documented cardiac lesions).

- Hormonal changes
- Alterations in autonomic tone
- Increased hemodynamic demand
- Mild hypokalemia, with the highest risk during labor and delivery

Review of potential teratogenic immunosuppressive or other medications must be performed with a plan to alter these medications prior to pregnancy. Mycophenolate mofetil has been shown to be teratogenic and counseling is needed regarding same. Immunization status should be reviewed. The patient should be vaccinated against influenza, Pneumococcus, hepatitis B, and tetanus. However, live viruses should not be administered to any postcardiac transplant patient since vaccination of an immunosuppressed patient with an attenuated live virus may result in systemic sepsis or even death.[24]

### Counseling

Counseling must include information on the risk of acute rejection, graft dysfunction, infection, and the possible teratogenic effects of immunosuppressive medications. The risk of allograft rejection during conception is worth a discussion. At some centers, fathers undergo human leukocyte antigen (HLA) testing, as if the female cardiac transplant recipient's donor and the father share the same antigen, (and particularly if the recipient already has donor specific antibodies to this HLA locus) then conception could provoke allograft rejection and the patient is counseled about the heightened risk to her graft.[25]

Evaluation of risks of transmitting disease which necessitated transplant, should be done by a genetic counselor, as most causes could be genetic. If a cardiac transplant recipient chooses to conceive then the patient is counseled to delay pregnancy until at least 1-year postcardiac transplant by when normal graft function and absence of rejection has been established.

## Antenatal Care

Immunosuppressive medication levels must be closely monitored. For example, cyclosporine metabolism is often increased during pregnancy. As such cyclosporine dose may need to be increased during pregnancy and subsequently decreased postdelivery. Immunosuppressive medication levels should be closely monitored and adjusted in patients with hyperemesis gravidarum.

If pregnancy occurs, the risk of spontaneous abortion in the pregnant postcardiac transplant patient is approximately 15–20%. With regards to graft rejection, some authors have reported a higher risk in pregnancy, with few reporting rejection episodes in 21% of patients. At least 40% of these reported rejections were mild and required no treatment.[25] Once a patient is pregnant, frequent blood pressure assessments along with baseline renal and liver function tests should be obtained. Screening for asymptomatic urinary tract infections with routine urine culture is warranted.

### Maternal Complications

Hyperemesis gravidarum poses a particular problem in the cardiac transplant recipient since immunosuppressive medications may not be properly absorbed, placing the patient at increased risk of rejection. Hypertension is the most common maternal complication in the pregnant postcardiac transplant patient with associated fetal growth restriction and preterm delivery. Urinary tract infections are the second most frequent maternal complication in the pregnant postcardiac transplant patient and are reported in up to 11% of pregnancies in the National Transplantation Pregnancy Registry (NTPR) data.

Venous thromboembolism and pulmonary embolism are known risks in pregnant women throughout the pregnancy and postpartum period and a high index of suspicion should be maintained in pregnant cardiac transplant recipient presenting with shortness of breath. If thromboembolic disease is confirmed, appropriate anticoagulation that is safe to use in pregnancy should be initiated.

## Intrapartum and Postpartum Care

Decisions regarding mode of delivery in the pregnant post-cardiac transplant patient do not differ when compared to the general population. Patients should be closely monitored for arrhythmias via continuous electrocardiogram, with invasive hemodynamic monitoring via Swan-Ganz catheter if significant rejection with graft dysfunction has occurred during pregnancy. The cardiac transplant patient is at highest risk during the immediate postpartum period, due to postpartum hemodynamic changes and volume shifts which are well tolerated in a patient with normal graft function. There is a slight increased risk of infection with cesarean delivery in patients on immunosuppressive medications and this should be taken into consideration.

In the absence of clear evidence, some authors recommend the use of epidural analgesia since it is well tolerated and provides effective pain control while minimizing the pain-induced sympathetic response. Postpartum patients are also at risk of postpartum thromboembolism and need active vigilance. From a cardiovascular perspective, use of prophylactic antibiotics should be in accordance with the 2008 ACC/AHA guidelines where prophylactic antibiotics as routine are not recommended (**Box 11**).

## Breastfeeding

All immunosuppressive medications are secreted through breast milk, and their long-term effects of exposure on infants are unknown. As such, the International Society of Heart and Lung Transplantation (ISHLT) recommends against breastfeeding.

---

**BOX 11:** Indications of antibiotics in transplanted patients.

- Women who have had prior episodes of infective endocarditis in the graft
- Presence of significant valvopathy in the transplanted graft
- Presence of residual patches from prior cardiothoracic surgeries

## Contraception

Both barrier methods and combined hormonal contraception are acceptable methods of contraception in cardiac transplant patients. Prior to the use of combination hormonal contraception, patients need screening for risk factors for a hypercoagulable state, hypertension, severe cardiac allograft vasculopathy, active liver disease, and estrogen-sensitive cancers.

Both intrauterine devices (IUDs) and depot-medroxyprogesterone acetate are contraindicated in cardiac transplant recipients due to increased risk of pelvic inflammatory disease and decreased bone density which has been associated with the long-term use of depot-medroxyprogesterone acetate.[26]

## Vaccination Schedule in Postpartum Period

Maintaining an appropriate vaccination schedule postpartum for both mother and child will be essential in decreasing risk of overall infection. The transplant recipient should discuss the type of vaccination administered with the newborn's pediatrician during the postpartum period. Special attention should be made to avoid live vaccinations which can be substituted with inactivated vaccinations such as the influenza and polio vaccines.

If live vaccines must be administered to the child, the transplant recipient should minimize contact including diaper changes (for children receiving rotavirus) while other household members assume the role of care provider. Occasionally, immunocompromised patients should avoid changing diapers for 4 weeks after a child is vaccinated against rotavirus.

## CONTRACEPTION

Unplanned pregnancies need to be avoided in cardiac patients as pregnancy with heart disease is associated with higher maternal morbidity and mortality. Appropriate use of contraceptive measures should be encouraged to avoid these complications. Barrier method for spacing and vasectomy as permanent method are the preferred contraceptive methods. The WHO chart for Medical Eligibility Criteria (MEC) must be consulted and followed.

## KEY POINTS

- Cardiac disease complicates approximately 0.8% of pregnancies and is among the leading causes of maternal mortality during pregnancy.
- The physiologic cardiovascular adaptations of pregnancy are well-tolerated by healthy women but the same can significantly compromise women with heart disease.
- A thorough evaluation of the woman with pre-existing heart disease should ideally be initiated before pregnancy.
- For each patient, the prepregnancy cardiovascular status should be established and used as a reference in assessing any pregnancy-related changes.
- It is important to counsel the woman about the risk of maternal mortality and morbidity due to the specific cardiac lesion before conception.
- Any additional risk factors which might worsen the outcome such as anemia, thyrotoxicosis, etc., should be evaluated and corrected before conception to optimize the fetomaternal outcome.
- The risk of the congenital heart disease in the baby of a woman with congenital heart disease varies from 3 to 50% depending on the specific lesion.
- The hyperdynamic circulation of pregnancy causes alterations in the physical findings in the cardiovascular system which can mimic heart disease and therefore heart disease diagnosed for the first-time during pregnancy needs to be viewed with caution and confirmed postnatally.
- Women with heart disease should be seen in a multidisciplinary antenatal clinic with special focus on the gestational weight gain and signs or symptoms of imminent cardiac failure together with close attention to factors which may increase the risk of heart failure including anemia, obesity, hypertension, and arrhythmias.
- Women with cardiac disease and their close family members need good counseling to help minimize risk of worsening of cardiac status in a woman planning pregnancy.
- Labor, delivery and postpartum are periods of hemodynamic instability and require intensive monitoring and ideally should be conducted in a tertiary level center.
- Vaginal delivery is preferred for patients with cardiac disease as hemodynamic fluctuations and blood loss are more common with cesarean delivery.
- Intrapartum antibiotic prophylaxis should be used according to standard recommendations.

## REFERENCES

1. Siu SC, Sermer M, Colman JM, Alvarez AN, Mercier LA, Morton BC, et al. Prospective multicenter study of pregnancy outcomes in women with heart disease. Circulation. 2001;104:515-21.
2. Uebing A, Steer PJ, Yentis SM, Gatzoulis MA. Pregnancy and congenital heart disease. BMJ. 2006;332(7538):401-6.
3. Canobbio MM, Warnes CA, Aboulhosn J, Connolly HM, Khanna A, Koos BJ, et al. Management of Pregnancy in Patients With Complex Congenital Heart Disease: a Scientific Statement for Healthcare Professionals From the American Heart Association. Circulation. 2017;135:e50.
4. RCOG. Cardiac Disease and Pregnancy. RCOG Good practice No. 13. 2011.

5. Allen U. Infective endocarditis: updated guidelines. Can J Infect Dis Med Microbiol. 2010;21(2):74-7.
6. Parry AJ, Westaby S. Cardiopulmonary bypass during pregnancy. Ann Thorac Surg. 1996;61:1865-9.
7. Leyh RG, Fischer S, Ruhparwar A, Haverich A. Anticoagulation for prosthetic heart valves during pregnancy: is low-molecular-weight heparin an alternative? Eur J Cardiothorac Surg. 2002;21:577-9.
8. ACOG. Pregnancy and Heart Disease. ACOG Practice Bulletin No. 212. Obstet Gynecol. 2019;33(5):320-56.
9. Thompson JL, Kuklina EV, Bateman BT, Callaghan WM, James AH, Grotegut CA. Medical and obstetric outcomes among pregnant women with congenital heart disease. Obstet Gynecol. 2015;126:346.
10. Elkayam U, Goland S, Pieper PG, Silverside CK. high-risk cardiac disease in pregnancy: Part II. J Am Coll Cardiol. 2016;68(5):502-16.
11. Burn J, Brennan P, Little J, Holloway S, Coffey R, Somerville J, et al. Recurrence risks in offspring of adults with major heart defects: results from first cohort of British collaborative study. Lancet. 1998;351:311-6.
12. Van Mook WN, Peeters L. Severe cardiac disease in pregnancy, part II: impact of congenital and acquired cardiac diseases during pregnancy. Curr Opin Crit Care. 2005;11:435-48.
13. Stout KK, Daniels CJ, Aboulhosn JA, Bozkurt B, Broberg CS, Colman JM, et al. Guideline for the Management of Adults With Congenital Heart Disease: Executive Summary: a Report of the American College of Cardiology/American Heart Association Task Force on Clinical Practice Guidelines. J Am Coll Cardiol. 2019;73(12):1494.
14. Veille JC. Peripartum cardiomyopathies: a review. Am J Obstet Gynecol. 1984;148:805-18.
15. Pearson GD, Veille JC, Rahimtoola S, Hsia J, Oakley CM, Hosenpud JD, et al. Peripartum cardiomyopathy: National Heart, Lung, and Blood Institute and Office of Rare Diseases (National Institutes of Health) workshop recommendations and review. JAMA. 2000;283(9):1183-8.
16. Sliwa K, Blauwet L, Tibazarwa K, Libhaber E, Smedema JP, Becker A, et al. Evaluation of bromocriptine in the treatment of acute severe peripartum cardiomyopathy: a proof-of-concept pilot study. Circulation. 2010;121(13):1465-73.
17. Autore C, Conte MR, Piccininno M, Bernabo P, Bonfiglio G, Bruzzi P, et al. Risk associated with pregnancy in hypertrophic cardiomyopathy. J Am Coll Cardiol. 2002;40:1864-9.
18. Smilowitz NR, Gupta N, Guo Y. Acute myocardial infarction during pregnancy and the puerperium in the United States. Mayo Clin Proc. 2018;93:1404.
19. Elkayam U, Jalnapurkar S, Barakkat MN. Pregnancy-associated acute myocardial infarction: a review of contemporary experience in 150 cases between 2006 and 2011. Circulation. 2014;129:1695.
20. Drenthen W, Pieper PG, Roos-Hesselink JW, van Lottum WA, Voors AA, Mulder BJ, et al. Outcome of pregnancy in women with congenital heart disease: a literature review. J Am Coll Cardiol. 2007;49:2303.
21. Vaidya VR, Arora S, Patel N, Badheka AO, Patel N, Agnihotri K, et al. Burden of arrhythmia in pregnancy. Circulation. 2017;135:619.
22. Sharma JB, Malhotra M, Pundit P. Successful pregnancy outcome with cardiac pacemaker after complete heart block. Int J Gynecol Obstet. 2000;68:145-6.
23. Jaffe R, Gruber A, Fejgin M, Altaras M, Ben-Aderet N. Pregnancy with an artificial pacemaker. Obstet Gynecol Survey. 1987;42:137-9.
24. Marwah A, Donna M. Management of pregnancy in the post-cardiac transplant patient. Semin Perinatol. 2014;38(5):318-25.
25. O'Boyle PJ, Smith JD, Danskine AJ, Lyster HS, Burke MM, Banner NR. De novo HLA sensitization and antibody mediated rejection following pregnancy in a heart transplant recipient. Am J Transplant. 2010;10(1):180-3.
26. Costanzo MR, Dipchand A, Starling R, Anderson A, Chan M, Desai S, et al. The International Society of Heart and Lung Transplantation Guidelines for the care of heart transplant recipients. J Heart Lung Transplant. 2010;29(8):914-56.

# Jaundice in Pregnancy

*Chitra Raghunandan, Swati Agrawal, Manoj Kumar Sharma*

## INTRODUCTION: MAGNITUDE OF PROBLEM

Jaundice in pregnancy is characterized by yellow discoloration of sclera, conjunctiva, skin, and mucosa, along with rise in serum bilirubin above 1.2 mg/dL. Jaundice may be due to pregnancy specific conditions such as obstetric intrahepatic cholestasis (IHC), acute fatty liver of pregnancy (AFLP); hemolysis, elevated liver enzymes, and low platelets (HELLP) syndrome, and hyperemesis gravidarum or it may be due to coincidental causes such as viral hepatitis and cholelithiasis.

There is a global variation in the incidence of this medical disorder. It is more often seen in developing than developed countries and affects 0.4–0.9/1,000 women. Jaundice during pregnancy can result in high maternal (30%) and perinatal mortality (61.76%).[1-3] At Lady Hardinge Medical College and Associated Hospitals, which is a tertiary care referral center, it has been among the top in the list of causes of maternal deaths and was found to cause 29% of all maternal deaths.[4] An Indian Council of Medical Research (ICMR) task force study reported anemia and jaundice as the most prevalent indirect causes of maternal deaths (17.4%) in seven districts of Uttar Pradesh.[5] In a recent study from tertiary care hospital in Bhopal, maternal mortality of 4.33% and perinatal mortality of 36% have been reported[6] with jaundice. In urban slums in Mumbai, a high incidence of 3–5% cases of jaundice in pregnant women has been reported with a fatality of 40%.[7] Acute viral hepatitis E (AVH) has been reported as the leading cause of jaundice and associated mortality in these studies. In a tertiary care hospital in Bangladesh, the prevalence of jaundice was 1.3% among all obstetric patients. Maternal mortality was 8.7%, perinatal mortality 6.4%, and hepatitis E viral infection was the main cause.[8] Mortality rates of 0–25% have been reported from developed countries. These are influenced by the cause of liver disease, degree of laboratory abnormalities, and delay in delivery, mainly with AFLP and HELLP syndrome.[9-12] Acute hepatic dysfunction in these conditions leads to hepatic encephalopathy, disseminated intravascular coagulopathy, hepatorenal failure, gastric hemorrhage or postpartum hemorrhage (PPH) and these can result in maternal mortality.

## PHYSIOLOGICAL CHANGES AND LIVER FUNCTIONS IN PREGNANCY

The anatomic and physiologic changes that accompany pregnancy alter physical findings and liver biochemistry. Yet, normal pregnancy does not significantly affect liver metabolism or function.[13]

### Anatomic Changes

Pregnancy does not affect the liver size and in the third trimester, the uterus displaces the liver superiorly and posteriorly. Therefore, a palpable liver in pregnancy suggests significant hepatomegaly and underlying liver disease. Spider angiomas, palmar erythema, and peripheral edema are findings that usually suggest chronic liver disease, but they can occur in pregnancy due to high levels of circulating estrogen.

### Physiological Changes

These include increase in plasma volume by 20% and increase in cardiac output by 30–50%. This increase is shunted to the placenta, with the hepatic blood flow being unaltered. This results in a proportional decrease in cardiac output being delivered to liver by 10% leading to reduction in the clearance of various compounds from blood especially during the latter half of pregnancy.

Histologic changes in liver include nonspecific findings such as lymphocytic infiltration in portal areas and increase in glycogen and fat.

### Liver Functions in Pregnancy

The liver in the human body performs important functions of protein synthesis, its metabolism, and excretion. It also inactivates many metabolites. Normal pregnancy may affect these functions and may interfere and overlap with alterations consequent to liver diseases. Liver function tests (LFTs) were studied in 103 pregnant women and compared with nonpregnant women not taking oral contraceptive pills (OCPs), following changes were observed:[14]

- Alteration in serum proteins.
- Total serum proteins decrease by 20%.

- Serum albumin decreases. This is due to the dilutional effect of increased plasma volume and increased catabolism.
- Serum globulin levels show slight decline.
- Serum fibrinogen and coagulation factors VII, VIII, IX, and X increase.
- Prothrombin time (PT) is unchanged.
- Serum ceruloplasmin and serum transferrin increase.
- Hormone binding proteins of thyroxine, corticosteroids increase.
- Serum bilirubin is slightly reduced.
- Serum alkaline phosphatase (ALP) levels increase and is maximum in the third trimester. The increase is up to 2–4 times the normal, but if it is more than four times the normal, it is usually indicative of pathology. It normalizes in 2–3 months postdelivery. The rise in ALP is mainly due to ALP of placental origin.
- Serum alanine transaminase (ALT) and aspartate aminotransferase (AST) levels are not altered.
- 5′ nucleotidase is raised significantly.
- Gamma-glutamyl transpeptidase (GGT) is normal or slightly decreased.

Hence, any increased value of ALT, AST, PT, international normalized ratio (INR), GGT or bile acids level should be considered pathologic and warrant further evaluation.

## CAUSES OF JAUNDICE IN PREGNANCY

The causes of jaundice in pregnancy can be either unique to pregnancy or coincidental with pregnancy. **Table 1** describes the various causes.

## WORK-UP OF A PREGNANT WOMAN WITH JAUNDICE

Jaundice in pregnancy is a manifestation of a wide spectrum of liver diseases with many diagnostic possibilities. It has adverse fetomaternal effects, hence it is important to have awareness of typical clinical presentations and the course of disease in various conditions, so that a reasonable presumptive diagnosis can be made, and optimum management is carried out. As in the nonpregnant patient, a practical approach for evaluating suspected hepatobiliary disease involves a systematic search for patterns that are characteristic of a particular disease, and judicious diagnostic testing to exclude other causes.

## History Taking

The patient may present with vague upper abdominal discomfort and pain, fatigue, malaise, low-grade fever, loss of appetite, nausea, vomiting followed by appearance of jaundice, clay-colored stools, pruritus, swelling of feet, headache, diminished urine output, blurring of vision, and altered sensorium. It is important to assess socioeconomic status, geographic location, water supply, etc. Daily dietary intake needs to be assessed correctly. Menstrual date, obstetric performance including period of gestation and any other clinical history associated with pregnancy needs to be enquired. History of jaundice, liver disease, gallstones and related surgery, drug intake, and blood transfusion in the past needs to be taken in detail.

## Clinical Examination

*General physical and systemic examination includes:*
- Level of consciousness and response to verbal commands
- Vital signs including temperature, pulse, and blood pressure (BP)
- Icterus of skin, sclera, and conjunctiva
- Presence of anemia, rash, signs of bleeding diathesis such as petechiae, purpura, and ecchymosis
- Swelling of feet.

Per abdomen examination should include looking for enlarged tender liver, enlarged spleen, ascites, venous distention, bruit or rub, and reduced liver dullness. The height of the uterus, fetal presentation, and fetal heart sound should be assessed.

## Initial Laboratory Tests

*Hematological investigations:* Hemoglobin (Hb), total leukocyte count (TLC), differential leukocyte count (DLC), platelet count, and peripheral smear.

Prothrombin time and activated partial thromboplastin time (aPTT).

*Biochemical liver function tests:*
- Total bilirubin (direct/indirect)
- Serum ALP and AST/ALT

Serum total protein and albumin:globulin ratio.

*Other tests:*
- Urine examination—albumin, sugar, bile pigment, bile salts, and microscopy
- Serum cholesterol
- Blood sugar fasting
- Serum creatinine, uric acid, and electrolytes.

**TABLE 1:** Causes of jaundice during pregnancy.

| Causes unique to pregnancy | Coincident causes in pregnancy | Causes probably related to pregnancy |
|---|---|---|
| Hyperemesis gravidarum | Hemolysis | Biliary tract abnormalities |
| Acute fatty liver of pregnancy | Acute viral hepatitis | |
| Pre-eclampsia/Eclampsia/HELLP syndrome | Cholelithiasis | Budd–Chiari syndrome |
| Intrahepatic cholestasis of pregnancy | Drug induced | |

(HELLP: hemolysis, elevated liver enzymes, low platelet count)

*Serum viral markers:*

- Hepatitis A immunoglobulin M (IgM)
- Hepatitis B—surface antigen (HBsAg), IgM and HB core Ab, hepatitis B virus (HBV) DNA, hepatitis B e antigen (HBeAg), and hepatitis B e antibody (HBeAb)
- Hepatitis C—Ab
- Hepatitis E—Ag/Ab
- Human immunodeficiency virus (HIV), herpes simplex virus (HSV), cytomegalovirus (CMV), and Epstein-Barr virus (EBV).

## Special Investigations

- Ultrasound is used to diagnose fatty liver, cholelithiasis, and subcapsular hemorrhage. Routine use of pulsed Doppler imaging in the first trimester is not advisable due to the concern for higher energy intensity and the need to keep the beam in a fixed position. If further imaging is required, magnetic resonance imaging (MRI) is the preferred modality in all trimesters. However, gadolinium contrast should be avoided as it crosses the placenta and there is risk of fetal exposure. The most radiation exposure to the developing fetus results from a computerized tomography (CT) scan of the abdomen and pelvis. Usually, radiation exposure through radiography or a CT scan is at a dose much lower than the exposure associated with fetal harm. Therefore, if these techniques are necessary in addition to ultrasonography (USG) or MRI or are more readily available for the diagnosis in question, they should not be withheld from a pregnant patient.[15] Liver biopsy and histopathology can be done only if coagulation profile is not deranged. Technical difficulties due to displacement of liver by enlarged uterus need to be kept in mind. However, liver biopsy is rarely done during pregnancy.

### Approach to Clinical Diagnosis of Pregnancy-related Liver Disease

Gestational age can guide to the differential diagnosis of pregnancy related liver disease **(Table 2)**. Furthermore, while specific diseases are typically confined to a particular trimester, there may be exceptions.

Differential diagnosis of liver diseases is carried out based on:

- Timing, nature, and course of disease
- Liver function tests
- Hematological tests
- Immunological tests.

Liver function tests may overlap in a wide range of conditions, but help in arriving at a clinical diagnosis, in assessing adequacy of treatment, and in evaluating the course of disease.

## ACUTE FATTY LIVER OF PREGNANCY

Acute fatty liver of pregnancy is defined as acute hepatic failure in the absence of other causes such as viral hepatitis, IHC, etc. It is also referred to as acute yellow atrophy of liver in pregnancy, acute fatty metamorphosis of liver, and reversible peripartum liver failure. It is a rare, potentially lethal disease and manifests usually in third trimester of pregnancy but may present after delivery. It involves maternal microvascular fat deposition in liver cells leading to rapid hepatic dysfunction.[16]

### Incidence

Acute fatty liver of pregnancy is reported to occur in 1 in 7,000–15,000 pregnancies. It is an inherited genetic defect with variable presentation in different ethnic groups. It is more common in primigravida, in women with multiple pregnancies, male fetus, and low body mass index (BMI < 20 kg/m$^2$). It can be associated with pre-eclampsia and HELLP syndrome. It is reported to recur in subsequent pregnancies.

### Etiology

Molecular biology suggests that AFLP may be the result of mitochondrial dysfunction. There is an inherited defect in the fetus of long-chain-hydroxyacyl co-enzyme A dehydrogenase (LCHAD) deficiency, resulting in a relative insufficiency of the oxidation pathway of fatty acids. This is needed to meet the high energy demands of the maternal fetal unit during the advanced pregnancy. Mothers may be carriers of LCHAD deficiency. This enzyme is part of mitochondrial transfunctional protein or mitochondrial trifunctional protein (MTP). G1528C and E447Q mutation of MTP are said to cause LCHAD deficiency.[17] The fatty acids from the fetal liver traverse the placenta and overwhelm the mother's mitochondrial capacity for fatty acid oxidation and this results in fat accumulation in maternal liver cells and their dysfunction.[18]

### Diagnosis

Polydipsia with or without polyuria is a prominent early symptom. Diuresis is due to abnormally high levels of placental vasopressinase. It typically presents between 30 and 38 weeks of pregnancy but has been reported in early pregnancy and in postpartum patients as well. Initially, vague symptoms of nausea, vomiting, headache, malaise, and upper abdominal pain appear. It may rapidly progress to signs and symptoms of acute liver failure (ALF) including jaundice, hypoglycemia, ascites, encephalopathy, and disseminated intravascular coagulation (DIC). Many patients (20–40%) also show features of pre-eclampsia and HELLP syndrome. Acute renal failure, acute pancreatitis,

## Jaundice in Pregnancy

**TABLE 2:** Characteristics of pregnancy related liver diseases.

| Disease | Trimester | Aminotransferase, (IU/L) | Total bilirubin, (mg/dL) | Other laboratory tests | Differential diagnosis |
|---|---|---|---|---|---|
| HELLP syndrome | Mid 2nd, 3rd trimesters and postpartum | Usually <500, may be more if hepatic infarction | May have deep jaundice | Platelets low (<100,000) LDH > 600 | • Acute fatty liver of pregnancy<br>• Gastroenteritis<br>• Viral hepatitis<br>• Pyelonephritis<br>• Cholelithiasis<br>• Appendicitis<br>• Idiopathic<br>• Thrombocytopenic purpura<br>• Hemolytic uremic syndrome |
| Acute fatty liver of pregnancy | 3rd trimester and postpartum | Usually <500, may be as high as 1,000 occasionally | May be deep jaundice | • ↑WBC; prolonged prothrombin time/INR<br>• ↓Platelets<br>• ↓Blood glucose<br>• ↑Uric acid | • HELLP syndrome<br>• Drug hepatotoxicity<br>• Acute liver failure |
| Hyperemesis gravidarum | 1st and early 2nd trimester | Usually <200, may be as high as 1,000 | Usually <4 | | • Gastroenteritis<br>• Cholecystitis<br>• Intestinal obstruction<br>• Peptic ulcer<br>• Pancreatitis<br>• Appendicitis<br>• Diabetic ketoacidosis<br>• Hyperthyroidism<br>• Hyperparathyroidism<br>• Drug toxicity |
| Cholestasis of pregnancy | 3rd trimester and postpartum | Usually <500, may be >1,000 occasionally | Usually <6 | ↑ Bile acids; ALP 4 × ULN (out of proportion to GGT) | • Cholelithiasis<br>• Viral hepatitis<br>• Primary biliary cirrhosis<br>• Primary sclerosing cholangitis<br>• Drug hepatotoxicity |

(ALP: alkaline phosphatase; HELLP: hemolysis, elevated liver enzymes and low platelets; INR: international normalized ratio; LDH: lactate dehydrogenase; GGT: gamma-glutamyltransferase; ULN: upper limit of normal; WBC: white blood cell)

upper gastrointestinal (GI) bleeding, and multiorgan failure may follow. Clinical improvement occurs slowly, 1–4 weeks after delivery.

*Abnormalities in laboratory investigations include:*

- Hyperbilirubinemia up to 5–15 mg/dL and it is mostly due to conjugated bilirubin.
- ALT shows moderate elevation but is usually <1,000 IU/mL.
- Alkaline phosphatase is increased to 3–4 times the normal but is nonspecific.
- Prolonged PT, partial thromboplastin time with kaolin (PTTK), and INR.
- Decrease in serum fibrinogen.
- Low serum glucose.
- Elevated serum creatinine and uric acid.
- Elevated blood urea nitrogen and ammonia levels.
- Leukocytosis up to 20,000–30,000 with shift to left.
- Blood smear shows hemolytic features like fragmented red blood cells (RBCs) in DIC. Platelets are usually normal but may be low due to DIC or overlap with HELLP syndrome.
- Proteinuria.
- Viral markers for hepatitis are negative.

Role of imaging liver with ultrasound, CT, and MRI is uncertain in AFLP. Ultrasound may be helpful in ruling out biliary tract disease. Liver biopsy is not required for diagnosis of AFLP. It is only required in rare cases of AFLP where diagnosis is in doubt and it affects management of patients especially in persistent hepatic failure, needing liver transplant.

Histopathological examination shows foaming cytoplasm in the hepatocytes in centrilobular zones due to microvacuolar fat deposition. No inflammation or necrosis is seen. Diagnosis is by clinical presentation and laboratory parameters. The LFTs deteriorate with rapidity in aggressive phase of disease, which is often diagnostic as it is not observed in IHC or HELLP syndrome.

Swansea diagnostic criteria for AFLP have been proposed in 2002. The presence of six or more of the following: vomiting, abdominal pain, polydipsia/polyuria, encephalopathy, elevated transaminases (AST or ALT >42 IU/L), elevated bilirubin (>0.8 mg/dL), hypoglycemia (<72 mg/dL), leukocytosis (>11 × 10⁶/L), elevated uric acid

(>5.7 mg/dL), elevated ammonia (>42 IU/L), ascites or bright liver on ultrasound, renal impairment (creatinine > 1.7 mg/dL), coagulopathy (PT > 14 seconds or PTT > 34 seconds), or microvesicular steatosis on biopsy, in the absence of another cause, are highly correlated with a clinical diagnosis of AFLP **(Table 3)**. The Swansea criteria have been demonstrated to have 100% sensitivity, 57% specificity, 85% positive predictive value, and 100% negative predictive value in the diagnosis of AFLP.[19]

To simplify and facilitate early suspicion of AFLP, a "simplified" criteria has been proposed for diagnosis of AFLP by investigators at the Christian Medical College (CMC), Vellore, India. According to this, we should consider AFLP in all women presenting in late pregnancy (i.e., late 2nd or 3rd trimester) with unexplained ALF (i.e., jaundice with coagulopathy and/or encephalopathy and/or hypoglycemia) **(Box 1)**. Presence of coagulopathy is a sine qua non (present in almost all the patients), and encephalopathy/hypoglycemia is noted in a few patients. The time required to evaluate other etiologies of liver failure has to be balanced against the urgency of delivery. Other causes such as history of ingestion of potentially hepatotoxic drugs, malaria, and AVH should be ruled out before a diagnosis of AFLP is entertained. **Flowchart 1** shows an algorithmic approach to a pregnant woman presenting in late pregnancy with jaundice.

The ultimate management of this condition is termination of pregnancy and the endeavor should be to urgently deliver these patients.

The other major condition that must be excluded is the HELLP syndrome, which is characterized by hemolysis, elevated liver enzymes, and a low platelet count. There is a large clinical overlap between AFLP and HELLP syndrome and it may be difficult, even impossible, to differentiate them. However, evidence of hepatic insufficiency such as hypoglycemia or encephalopathy are suggestive of AFLP. Imaging tests are primarily used to exclude other diagnoses, such as a hepatic infarct or hematoma.

**TABLE 3:** "Swansea" diagnostic criteria for acute fatty liver of pregnancy.

*In late pregnancy; presence of 6 of the 14 criteria in absence of alternate explanation*

| Symptoms | Laboratory parameters | Radiology and histology |
|---|---|---|
| • Abdominal pain<br>• Vomiting<br>• Polydipsia/polyuria<br>• Encephalopathy | • Hyperbilirubinemia<br>• Raised aminotransferase<br>• Hypoglycemia<br>• Coagulopathy<br>• Deranged renal function<br>• Hyperuricemia<br>• Hyperammonemia<br>• Leukocytosis | • Ascites/bright liver on ultrasound<br>• Diffuse/perivenular microvesicular steatosis on liver biopsy |

**BOX 1:** "Simplified" CMC Vellore criteria for diagnosis of acute fatty liver of pregnancy.

*Presence of all three criteria is required for the presumptive diagnosis of AFLP:*
1. *Setting:* Late pregnancy (late 2nd or 3rd trimester)
2. *Acute liver failure:* Jaundice with coagulopathy and/or hypoglycemia and/or encephalopathy
3. No other explanation for liver failure (No history of ingestion of hepatotoxic drugs, negative hepatitis viral serology, peripheral smear negative for malarial parasite, etc.)

(AFLP: acute fatty liver of pregnancy; CMC: Christian Medical College)

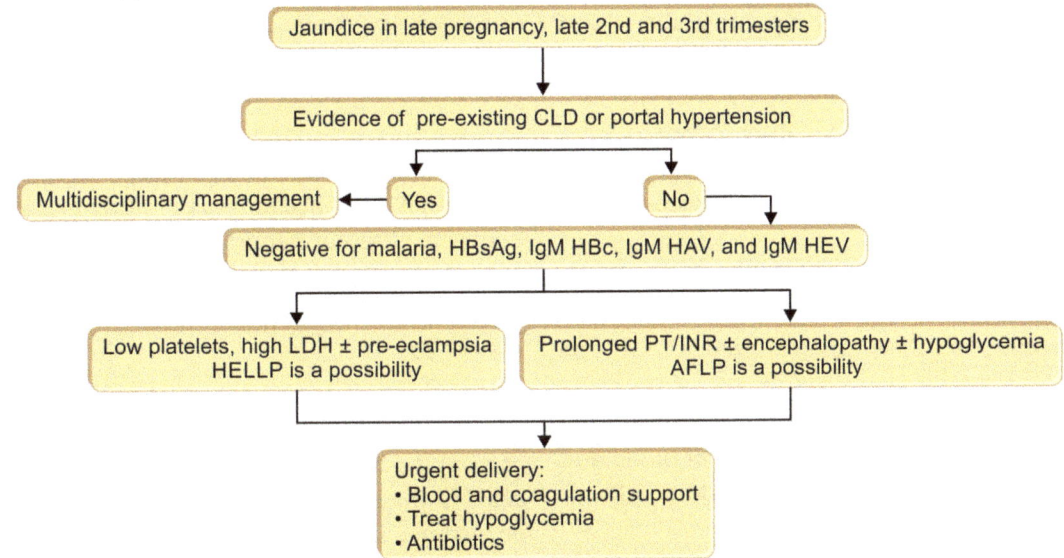

**Flowchart 1:** Approach to a pregnant woman presenting in late pregnancy with jaundice (late 2nd and 3rd trimesters).

(AFLP: acute fatty liver of pregnancy; CLD: chronic liver disease; HEV: hepatitis E virus; HBsAg: hepatitis B surface antigen; HAV: hepatitis A virus; HELLP: hemolysis, elevated liver enzymes, low platelet count syndrome; IgM: immunoglobulin M; LDH: lactate dehydrogenase; PT: prothrombin time; INR: international normalized ratio)

Recovery occurs gradually in most patients following delivery. The initial sign of recovery is decrease in PT. Full clinical and laboratory recovery occurs over 1–4 weeks. Even after delivery, the disease may progress and starts resolving only after a few days but no recovery has been reported without resorting to immediate delivery.

## Management

- The optimal management of AFLP is prompt delivery of the fetus irrespective of its gestational age after stabilization of maternal condition. Treatment is mainly supportive and is directed toward management of liver insufficiency and complications.
- The difficulty faced in distinguishing severe pre-eclampsia and HELLP syndrome from AFLP should not delay delivery. Both require termination of pregnancy.
- Patients with encephalopathy and coagulopathy should be transferred without any delay to advanced facility with intensive care unit (ICU) and availability of liver transplantation.
- A multidisciplinary team of senior obstetrician, neonatologist, medical internist, hepatologist, anesthetist, and hematologist should be available.
- Monitoring of hypoglycemia every 6–8 hours and continuous infusion of 10% glucose to maintain plasma glucose above 65 mg/dL.
- The most sensitive indicator of hepatic dysfunction is coagulopathy which is monitored every 4–6 hours with PT and INR.
- Blood and blood components should be available.
- Prompt delivery is planned, and route of delivery is based on the probability of successful vaginal birth and severity and rate of maternal and fetal decompensation.
- Labor induction with cervical ripening agent and oxytocin can be carried out to achieve successful vaginal birth.
- Coagulopathy should be simultaneously corrected, fresh frozen plasma (FFP) is administered in doses of 10–15 mL/kg body weight (one unit increases plasma factors by 5%).
- Traumatic delivery, episiotomy, and regional anesthesia are to be avoided.
- In postpartum period, intensive care should be continued.
- Advanced support such as mechanical ventilation, dialysis for acute renal failure, transfusion of blood and its components for continued hemolysis, atonic PPH or for postoperative bleeding may be needed.
- Baby delivered of mother with AFLP should be managed in the neonatal ICU, especially to watch for hypoglycemia or features of fatty acid oxidation defect.
- In severe cases with fulminant hepatic failure, liver transplantation is the only alternative. Hence, close liaison with an advanced gastroenterology department which has a transplantation unit is required.

Acute fatty liver of pregnancy has been associated with significant maternal and fetal mortality. Maternal mortality is due to hepatic encephalopathy, DIC, acute respiratory distress syndrome (ARDS), renal failure, acute pancreatitis, hypoglycemia, and PPH. Recent reviews of case series have however, reported improved outcome for mother and baby.

Babies may have deficiency of LCHAD and need to be genetically screened along with mothers for G1528C mutation. If the baby has LCHAD deficiency, the recurrence of AFLP in mother is 15–25% in subsequent pregnancy. Prenatal diagnosis is possible in next pregnancy by chorionic villous sampling or by amniocentesis if previous baby is affected. Acute fatty liver can recur in subsequent pregnancy even if LCHAD mutation is negative.[20]

## INTRAHEPATIC CHOLESTASIS OF PREGNANCY

Intrahepatic cholestasis of pregnancy (IHCP) is the most common hepatobiliary disease associated with pregnancy. It is characterized by cholestasis with rise in bile acid and serum transaminases and occasionally bilirubin. It manifests mainly as pruritus during second and third trimester of pregnancy and disappears spontaneously after delivery. It frequently recurs in subsequent pregnancy in 45–70% of the cases. More importantly, it represents a spectrum of disease which is associated with severe adverse pregnancy outcome including fetal distress, meconium-stained liquor (MSL), spontaneous or iatrogenic preterm births, and still births. There is no established pharmacotherapy to avert this. Antenatal fetal monitoring has not been helpful in accurately guiding timing of delivery to prevent still births, at the same time avoid late preterm or early term deliveries with likely short-term and long-term adverse effects on health of the newborn.

## Incidence

The overall incidence ranges from 0.02 to 2.4% with variation between different geographical locations. The incidence varies from 1.2 to 1.5% in Indian Asians.[21]

## Etiology

The pathogenesis of IHC involves pregnancy hormones which affect the gallbladder function resulting in slowing or stopping of the flow of bile. This leads to build up of bile acids in the liver, which can spill into the blood stream. Its occurrence in some pregnant women suggests hereditary hepatic sensitivity to estrogens leading to exaggerated liver response to estrogens. It may be due to high estrogen levels as in multiple pregnancy. Progesterone has also been associated with IHC as treatment with progesterone in the third trimester increases the risk of development of IHC. Mutation ABCB4 and ABCB11 in the hepatocellular phospholipids transporter and bile salt export pump (BSEP) is said to be present in the cases with IHC.[22] A familial predisposition is also seen, and it is more common in those whose mother or sister had cholestasis. Previous liver damage also predisposes to IHC.

## Diagnosis

Symptoms of IHC typically manifest in third trimester of pregnancy but can occur as early as 10 weeks of gestation. Pruritus is the most dominant and most disturbing clinical feature and is seen in 70% cases of IHC in the third trimester. It occurs particularly on the hands and feet and is more severe at night. Dark colored urine occurs shortly after the onset of pruritus. There may be steatorrhea. Severe pruritus can lead to insomnia, fatigue, depression, and other mental disturbances.[23] Jaundice is seen in 10% of cases. It is usually mild and develops 1-4 weeks after pruritus. Right upper quadrant pain, biliary colic, nausea, anorexia, vomiting, fever, and arthralgia are usually absent. Urinary tract infection may be associated, therefore it should be actively sought for in a patient with IHC. Physical examination reveals evidence of scratching and rarely slight tender hepatomegaly may be present. IHC is frequently associated with cholelithiasis and cholecystitis in women.

## Laboratory Findings

- Rise in serum bile acids is the earliest and the most consistent change. There is a 10-100 fold rise in serum cholic acid. Chenodeoxycholic acid also increases but less than serum cholic acid. Therefore ratio of cholic acid to chenodeoxycholic acid is high. Fasting serum total bile acid concentration is a specific test for diagnosis of cholestasis during pregnancy (>10 µmol/L).[24] The rise may occur up to 15 weeks after the onset of pruritus. Therefore, repeat testing is required if pruritus persists.
- Alkaline phosphatase increases above the normal elevation but is not much helpful in diagnosis.
- ALT and AST are increased 2-10 folds and may exceed 1,000 U/L, but it is important to rule out viral hepatitis when the rise is excessive.
- Hyperbilirubinemia occurs in 20% of women and is almost exclusively direct reacting. Bilirubin levels are usually between 2 and 5 mg/dL.
- Serum cholesterol increases 2-4 times. Triglyceride levels may be normal or increase to about 2 fold above normal. Phospholipid and low-density lipoprotein (LDL) levels also increase.
- Prothrombin time is usually normal unless there is malabsorption.
- A new marker of hepatocellular damage plasma glutathione S-transferase alpha helps in differentiating between pruritus gravidarum and obstetric cholestasis much before the rise in bile acids and transaminases. It rises in IHC, 9 weeks before rise in bile acids and transaminases.[25]
- Fasting serum bile acid is >10 µmol/L and there is increase in liver transaminases.
- Serum viral markers are negative.

Intrahepatic cholestasis is a diagnosis of exclusion and is confirmed by resolution of the symptoms and biochemical abnormalities postpartum. Imaging of liver by USG is not helpful in diagnosing IHCP, but can rule out extrahepatic biliary obstruction. Gallstones may be seen which are usually asymptomatic.

Liver biopsy is not required for diagnosis. It may be rarely required to exclude parenchymal liver disease. Biopsy shows dilated centrilobular bile canaliculi and bile plugs but these changes are not diagnostic of IHCP. Inflammation, necrosis, or bile duct injury is not seen.

## Clinical Course

Pruritus can be a distressing symptom. It begins to decline a few hours after delivery and usually disappears in a few days following delivery. Pruritus as a rule persists longer than jaundice. Resolution occurs within 2-3 weeks after delivery. Liver failure and hepatic encephalopathy do not occur, if liver failure sets in, the diagnosis of IHCP must be reviewed. The conditions with a similar presentation include skin disease specifically dermatosis of pregnancy. Biochemical abnormalities normalize in a few weeks following delivery. If biochemical abnormalities persist for >3 months after delivery, investigations to rule out chronic liver disease [chronic hepatitis, primary biliary cirrhosis (PBC), primary sclerosing cholangitis (PSC)] must be carried out.[26]

Intrahepatic cholestasis of pregnancy leads to an increased cesarean section rate (25-36%). PPH occurs in 20-22% cases (due to prolonged PT).

The risk of preterm delivery is 15-60%. Perinatal mortality is 35-70/1,000 live births. Sudden intrauterine fetal death occurs in 0.4-4.1% cases. Fetal distress occurs in one-third of cases. Fetal bradycardia occurs in 14% and MSL in 35% cases.[27] Toxic effects of bile acids on fetal myocardium is thought to be responsible for sudden fetal death.[28] Hence, close fetal monitoring is warranted. These outcomes are more likely if disorder begins early in pregnancy and with severe pruritus. Higher fetal complications were seen with fasting serum bile acid level of >40 µmol/L

Contrary to the previously suggested cut off of maternal fasting serum bile acid level of 40 µmol/L, a recent meta-analysis has shown that the highest risk group is women with total bile acids ≥100 µmol/L. Levels of bile acids in mother and fetus correlate, supporting a causal relationship between bile acid levels and fetal complications.[29]

There is a risk of developing gallstones after pregnancy. There is also a risk of recurrence in next pregnancy and with usage of OCP. Therefore, these women should avoid estrogen containing OCPs.

In a population-based cohort study from Sweden analyzing ~ 11,000 women with IHC, it was found to be associated with later liver and biliary tree cancer [HR: 3.61, 95% confidence interval: (CI) 1.68–7.77, and 2.62, 95% CI: 1.26–5.46, respectively]. It was also associated with later immune-mediated diseases (HR: 1.28, 95% CI: 1.19–1.38), specifically diabetes mellitus (HR 1.47, 95% CI: 1.26–1.72), thyroid disease (HR: 1.30, 95% CI: 1.14–1.47), psoriasis (HR: 1.27, 95% CI: 1.07–1.51), inflammatory polyarthropathies (HR: 1.32, 95% CI: 1.11–1.58), and Crohn's disease (HR: 1.55, 95% CI: 1.14–2.10), but not ulcerative colitis (HR 1.21, 95% CI 0.93–1.58). Women with IHC also had a small increased risk of later cardiovascular disease (HR: 1.12, 95% CI: 1.06–1.19).[30]

## Management

*Ursodeoxycholic acid (UDCA)*: It relieves distressing pruritus by decreasing the concentration of bile acids in the blood and it also improves biochemical abnormalities. It is given in a dose of 10–20 mg/kg/day. It acts by improving impaired hepatocellular secretion by mainly posttranscriptional stimulation of canalicular expression of key transport proteins. It also restores the impaired maternal-placental bile acid transport across the trophoblast. It is well-tolerated. UDCA at first increases fasting bile acids therefore if UDCA is given, follow-up should be done with serum transaminases. However, in the largest randomized, placebo-controlled study of UDCA in women with IHCP (24% with baseline total serum bile acids ≥40 μmol/L) (n = 306 UDCA and 300 placebo), there was no difference between groups in the primary composite outcome of perinatal death, preterm delivery, and neonatal ICU stay for ≥4 hours: 23% UDCA group versus 27% placebo group (adjusted risk ratio, 0.85; p = 0.28). Thus, UDCA is regarded as a safe first-line therapy for management of pruritus and liver test abnormalities but has not been shown to reduce fetal complications.[31]

- *Corticosteroids*: Dexamethasone in a dose of 12 mg/day for 1 week, improves biochemical abnormalities but does not improve pruritus. However, it is less effective as compared to UDCA.[32]
- *S-adenosyl methionine*: It has been seen to improve pruritus. It decreases the negative effects of estrogen on bile acid secretion.
- *Cholestyramine*: It binds to bile acids in the gut and relieves pruritus. It increases the risk of vitamin K deficiency thus increasing the risk of PPH. Therefore, monitoring of PT is essential with the use of this drug. Side effects are nausea, anorexia, and bloating.
- Conventional antepartum testing does not predict fetal mortality as sudden fetal death is due to acute hypoxia.
- Until recently, it was believed that when bile acids level are above 40 μmol/L fetal complications develop. A weaker but significant association with higher ALT levels was suggested too. However, more recent systematic review on perinatal outcome has identified an increased risk of still birth in IHCP only when serum bile acid concentration exceeded 100 μmol/L. The current opinion is that women can be reassured that incidence of stillbirth is similar to the general population as long as the total bile acid concentrations is <100 μmol/L. However, it is advisable to get repeat weekly testing done till delivery.[29]
- Currently delivery is recommended at 37–38 weeks, in pregnancy associated with IHC, an intervention with clearly demonstrated benefits.

## HELLP SYNDROME

HELLP syndrome, i.e., hemolysis, elevated liver enzymes, and low platelets, is usually a manifestation of liver involvement in severe pre-eclampsia or eclampsia. It generally occurs in the latter half of pregnancy, usually the third trimester (between 28 and 36 weeks of gestation). In 30% cases it may have its onset after delivery. It occurs in 0.2–0.6% of all pregnancies and 10–15% of cases of severe pre-eclampsia/eclampsia, and is associated with high maternal mortality of up to 25%.

## Pathogenesis

The HELLP syndrome is a microangiopathic hemolytic anemia associated with vascular endothelial injury. It involves vasospasm of the vascular system due to imbalance between vasoconstrictors (thromboxane and endothelin) and vasodilators (prostacyclin and nitric oxide). Thrombocytopenia is thought to result from platelet activation and consumption. In liver, segmental vascular spasm leads to vascular injury, release of thromboplastins with consequent platelet aggregation, and fibrin deposition. Decreased liver perfusion leads to endothelial damage, hemorrhage, and hepatocellular necrosis.

## Clinical Features

Right upper quadrant, epigastric or right sided chest pain may occur. Not all patients diagnosed with this disease have hypertension and proteinuria at the time of presentation.

## Laboratory Changes

Liver function changes are mostly suggestive of hepatocellular damage.
- Serum bilirubin may be normal or slightly increased. Clinical jaundice occurs in cases with severe hemolysis.
- AST and ALT show a modest elevation but can sometimes be high (up to several thousand) when associated with subcapsular hematoma and hepatocellular necrosis or liver rupture.

- Prothrombin time is usually normal unless DIC occurs.
- Fibrinogen levels are normal.
- Platelets are low < 100,000/dL.
- Peripheral smear shows features of hemolysis.
- LDH is increased.
- Ultrasound or CT of the liver may show intraparenchymal hemorrhage, subcapsular hematoma or infarction.

Liver biopsy shows unique features, but biopsy is not needed to confirm the diagnosis. There is localized involvement of liver. Periportal hemorrhage and fibrin deposition, peliotic collection of red cells and necrosis of hepatocytes, steatosis, and neutrophilic infiltration adjacent to areas of hemorrhage is seen. There is no correlation between the severity of the histologic involvement and the degree of abnormality of aminotransferases and platelet count.

The HELLP syndrome is classified based on severity of observed thrombocytopenia, liver enzyme elevation, and hemolysis. According to Mississippi triple classification, Class 1 includes severe thrombocytopenia (platelets ≤ 50,000/μL), evidence of hepatic dysfunction (AST and/or ALT ≥ 70 IU/L), and evidence suggestive of hemolysis (serum LDH ≥ 600 IU/L); class 2 includes similar criteria except thrombocytopenia is moderate (>50,000 to <100,000/μL); and class 3 includes mild thrombocytopenia (platelet count >100,000 to <150,000/μL), mild hepatic dysfunction (ALT and AST ≥ 40 IU/L), and hemolysis (serum LDH > 600 IU/L). Tennessee classification categorizes HELLP syndrome into complete and partial HELLP syndrome. The Mississippi protocol has described the pharmacological intervention.[33]

## Course

Delivery is indicated for all cases. After delivery, most women recover, and platelet count returns to normal within 7 days. Failure to deliver the patient may lead to eclampsia, worsening of the liver disease, hepatic hematoma or hepatic rupture. Serum uric acid >7.8 mg/dL is associated with increased maternal and fetal morbidity and mortality.

## Differential Diagnosis

- *Viral hepatitis*: Serology for viral markers is useful to differentiate but takes time. History of symptoms such as malaise, nausea, vomiting, or fever are present in viral hepatitis and hypertension is absent.
- *Acute fatty liver of pregnancy*: It is difficult to exclude this condition as it is often associated with pre-eclampsia but unlike HELLP syndrome, there is true hepatic failure leading to coagulopathy, hypoglycemia, and encephalopathy in AFLP.
- Various other causes of thrombocytopenia.
- *Thrombotic thrombocytopenic purpura (TTP)*: Involvement of central nervous system (CNS) and renal system may mimic HELLP syndrome but hypertension is absent and fever is present. Features of TTP, HELLP, and hemolytic-uremic syndrome are summarized in **Table 4**.
- Idiopathic thrombocytopenic purpura (ITP).
- Antiphospholipid antibody syndrome.
- Incidental thrombocytopenia of pregnancy.

**TABLE 4:** Comparison of frequency of signs, symptoms, and laboratory findings in TTP, HUS, and HELLP.

| | TTP | HUS | HELLP |
|---|---|---|---|
| Abdominal pain, nausea, and vomiting | ++ | ++ | ++ |
| Fever | + | – | – |
| Headache or visual disturbance | ++ | – | ++ |
| Hypertension | ++ | ++ | ++ |
| Jaundice | – | – | + |
| Elevated transaminases | –/+ | –/+ | ++ |
| Elevated LDH | ++++ | ++ ++ | ++ |
| Anemia | ++ | ++ | + |
| Thrombocytopenia | ++ | ++ | ++ |
| Proteinuria | +/Hematuria | ++ | ++ |
| von Willebrand factor | ++ | ++ | – |
| ADAMST13 activity | ++ | – | – |

(HELLP: hemolysis, elevated liver enzymes and low platelets; HUS: hemolytic-uremic syndrome; TTP: thrombotic thrombocytopenic purpura; LDH: lactate dehydrogenase)

## Management of HELLP Syndrome

- Stabilize maternal condition.
- Control hypertension. Systolic BP to be kept < 160 mm of Hg and diastolic < 100 mm of Hg with antihypertensive drugs.
- Antiseizure prophylaxis with magnesium sulfate in cases with severe pre-eclampsia and impending eclampsia.
- Intravenous dexamethasone may be given to increase platelet count.
- Planning of delivery.
- Ultrasonography, if subcapsular hematoma is suspected
- Assessment of fetal well-being.
- *Definitive therapy is delivery of the baby* as conservative therapy is associated with risks of eclampsia, abruptioplacentae, pulmonary edema, renal failure, and maternal and perinatal death. Delivery is indicated in all cases irrespective of gestational age. In case of fetal immaturity, delivery can be carried out after 48 hours following steroid administration under close maternal and fetal monitoring.

## Mode of Delivery

Vaginal delivery is preferred. In patients with favorable cervix, induction of labor is carried out. In cases where cesarean section is contemplated following points are to be taken care of:

- General anesthesia is administered if platelet count <75,000/mm³.
- 5-10 units of platelets should be arranged and transfused prior to surgery if platelet count is <40,000/mm³.
- Vesicouterine peritoneum is left open with subfascial drain.
- Subcutaneous drain is placed or secondary closure of skin incision may be done.
- Postoperative transfusions as per requirement.
- Intensive monitoring for 48 hours postpartum.
- After delivery most women recover and platelet count returns to normal within 7 days.
- Liver transplant may be needed in hepatic decompensation despite medical therapy and in hepatic hematoma and rupture.[34]
- If abdominal pain, shoulder pain or hypotension develop, urgent imaging must be performed to rule out hepatic hemorrhage, rupture or infarction, which can occur in up to 45% of patients. Hepatic hemorrhage or rupture is associated with increased mortality. Management includes coagulation support, antibiotics, and transfusion. Urgent angiography and hepatic artery embolization or surgical intervention (packing of the liver, hepatic artery ligation, or resection) is indicated if supportive measures are unsuccessful.[15]

## Prognosis

The maternal mortality is 2-25% and perinatal mortality can be as high as 30%. The risk of recurrence in subsequent pregnancies is 25%.[35] Clinical features and abnormal LFT resolve rapidly in puerperium. There is no evidence of permanent liver damage after recovery from this disorder. Platelet count decreases immediately after delivery and starts to rise from third postpartum day. If no rise in platelet count occurs even after 96 hours of delivery, it indicates severe disease with high possibility of life-threatening complications.

## HYPEREMESIS GRAVIDARUM

Hyperemesis gravidarum is characterized by intractable nausea and vomiting resulting in dehydration and ketosis and may lead to liver dysfunction. Hyperemesis is the extreme of the spectrum of morning sickness. Jaundice may appear if liver dysfunction occurs. It is more common in obese, nulliparous women, and in twin pregnancy. Its prevalence varies between 0.3 and 2% of pregnancies. The exact etiology remains uncertain. The various factors implicated include psychological, hormonal and genetic factors, abnormal gastric motility, specific nutrient deficiencies, alterations in lipid levels, and changes in autonomous nervous system. There may be high density *Helicobacter pylori* infection in these cases.

Liver injury may be due to multiple factors including dehydration, starvation, and placental derived cytokines including tumor necrosis factor-α (TNF-alpha).[36]

## Clinical Features

Its onset is in the first trimester usually by 10-12th weeks of gestation and resolves by 20th week in most cases. In 15-20%, it continues till third trimester and in 5% till delivery. The symptoms include persistent nausea and vomiting, dehydration, ketosis, weight loss of >5% of body weight, electrolyte derangements such as hypokalemia and metabolic alkalosis. Rarely, Wernicke's encephalopathy and severe malnutrition may occur. Hyperthyroidism, hyperparathyroidism, and hypercalcemia may also occur. There are no long-term sequelae.

## Liver Involvement

Abnormality in liver enzymes occurs in 50% of the patients. ALT is the most sensitive test and may increase up to 1,000 IU/mL.[37] Hyperbilirubinemia is usually mild, and jaundice is rare.

## Differential Diagnosis

It includes various GI disorders such as gastroenteritis, hepatitis, pancreatitis, cholelithiasis, diabetes mellitus, psychological disorders, and drug toxicity.

## Management

Improvement in symptoms and laboratory abnormalities occurs with supportive therapy, which involves correction of dehydration and electrolyte imbalance.

Antiemetics such as metoclopramide, promethazine, and ondansetron are safe in pregnancy and can be given. Patient is given folic acid and thiamine supplements. However, a watch should be kept for complications such as Wernicke's encephalopathy, osmotic demyelination syndrome, and thromboembolism. The woman should eat frequent, small, low fat and high carbohydrate meals and should avoid triggers that aggravate nausea. This condition mostly resolves by 20th week of gestation.

## ACUTE VIRAL HEPATITIS IN PREGNANCY

Viral hepatitis is the most common cause of jaundice in pregnancy in our country and can lead to high maternal morbidity and mortality. It is caused by hepatitis viruses A, B, C, and E apart from CMV, HSV, and HIV viruses. The acute manifestation of these viral infections is similar, but they differ in terms of viral structure, modes of transmission, epidemiology, and their propensity to lead to chronic hepatitis and liver cancer.[38]

In a study done at tertiary level hospital from Delhi; a total of 220 patients of AVH with pregnancy were treated

| TABLE 5: Types of viral hepatitis found in pregnancy.[39] | |
|---|---|
| Total pregnant patients with hepatitis | 220 |
| Hepatitis E virus (HEV) | 133 (60%) |
| Hepatitis B virus (HBV) | 72 (33%) |
| Hepatitis C virus (HCV) | 11 (5%) |
| Hepatitis A virus (HAV) | 1 (0.7%) |
| Coinfection (HCV + HBV) and (HBV + HEV) | 3 (1.3%) |

from 2003–2005. There were 91 patients (40%) of fulminant hepatic failure and 27% maternal deaths.[39]

Various types of viral hepatitis found in pregnancy in the study are given in **Table 5**.

## Hepatitis A Virus

Hepatitis A virus is a global disease. Outbreaks occur frequently in areas of crowding or poor sanitation. Causative agent is a picornavirus and transmission is through orofecal contamination. The incubation period is 15–40 days. It is a self-limiting condition but may occasionally lead to fulminant hepatitis. It does not lead to a chronic carrier state and there is no risk of increased severity in pregnancy. The clinical condition is characterized by initial period of fever, anorexia, nausea, malaise, fatigue, and weight loss. Jaundice appears in the second week of disease. Palpable hepatomegaly and liver function abnormalities with elevated ALT are found in this condition.

Hepatitis A virus infection is infrequently reported among pregnant women; hence, there is little data on the incidence and outcome of HAV infection during pregnancy. However, the available evidence supports that HAV infection during pregnancy is generally not associated with adverse maternal or fetal outcomes.

Increased risk of preterm birth with hepatitis A has been reported.[40] The virus is not teratogenic in nature and there is negligible risk of fetal transmission. No intervention is required for hepatitis A infection as anti-HAV IgG antibodies generated during HAV infection cross the placenta and protect the baby after delivery. Breastfeeding is not contraindicated in HAV infection. HAV infection should be prevented by observing good hygiene and avoiding food contamination. Pre-exposure vaccination involves use of inactivated HAV vaccine which is safe to use in pregnancy. Postexposure immunoglobulin should be given within 2 weeks of exposure of HAV and is safe in pregnancy.

## Hepatitis B Virus

Hepatitis B infection is endemic in Asia and Africa. India has 40–50 billion chronic HBV infected subjects. All pregnant women should be tested for HBsAg and HBV DNA testing performed if HBsAg is positive. Prevalence of hepatitis B in pregnant women worldwide is 2.5–15%, whereas, in India it is 0.2–7.7%.[41] In Lady Hardinge and associated hospitals, incidence was 0.6% among 6,000 pregnant women screened.

Hepatitis B infection is caused by a DNA virus. It leads to acute hepatitis and may also have serious sequelae in the form of cirrhosis and hepatocellular carcinoma. Hepatitis B infection is transmitted through blood, blood products, and sexual contact. Mother to child transmission (MTCT) and early childhood acquisition of HBV are the modes of transmission in 50% individuals who develop chronic HBV infection. It can coexist with HIV infection. Health personnel, homosexual, hemophiliacs, and intravenous drug abusers are particularly prone to the hepatitis B infection. The infection is often chronic and asymptomatic and diagnosed during prenatal screening of women.[42] During acute infection, nausea, vomiting, and abdominal pain may be present. There is infrequent transplacental transmission of viral infection to fetus in early half of pregnancy. The vertical transmission of infection is mainly in third trimester and the peripartum period through infected vaginal secretions as well as breast milk.

*Hepatitis B virus antigen and antibodies are classified in three groups:*
1. Surface antigen and antibodies (HBsAg and anti-HBs)
2. Core antigen and antibodies (HBcAg and anti-HBc)
3. "e" or precore antigen and antibodies (HBeAg and anti-HBe).

HBsAg is detected in the serum from several weeks before the onset of symptoms, may persist for months and is an indicator of infectivity. Anti-HBs appears during recovery and is indicator of resolution of the disease and is diagnostic of acute HBV infection. Anti-HBc (IgG) appears during convalescence and persists for a lifetime. Presence of HBeAg indicates high infectivity and it is likely that 90% of babies born to women who are HBsAg and HBeAg positive will be infected. Anti-HBe appears after anti-HBc and signifies reduced infectivity.

Women with chronic hepatitis B infection can be highly infectious (HBeAg positive) to rarely infectious (anti-HBe positive). It is estimated that 10% of adults and >90% of infected babies will go on to develop chronic infection with long-term complications such as cirrhosis and hepatocellular carcinoma.[43] Obstetric outcomes are not significantly affected by HBV infection. Premature births can occur as in hepatitis A infection.

Acute infection with hepatitis B during pregnancy is not associated with increased mortality or teratogenicity. Thus, infection during pregnancy should not prompt consideration of termination of the pregnancy.

In acute infection, there may be transplacental transmission. 10% of fetuses may be infected in first trimester but in 80–90% cases, infection occurs in third trimester. Cesarean delivery does not reduce risk of transmission of infection to the child and hence should be used for obstetrical indications only. Similarly, breastfeeding is not contraindicated as infants are protected by vaccination and hepatitis B immunoglobulin (HBIG).[44]

For the prevention of MTCT, immunoprophylaxis with Hepatitis B immunoglobulin and first dose of HBV vaccine within 12 hours of birth is recommended and is highly effective. However, mothers with HBV DNA >200,000 IU/mL are at risk of failure of this strategy. In these mothers, antiviral therapy in the third trimester is associated with a 70% reduction in HBV transmission to child compared to no antiviral therapy (although this is more applicable to mothers with chronic HBV infection). The preferred drug is tenofovir disoproxil fumarate (TDF), which is started at 28–32 weeks of gestation.[44]

## Hepatitis C Virus

The infection carries a very high-risk of chronic liver disease and hepatocellular carcinoma. The prevalence of hepatitis C infection in pregnancy is 2.3–17%. Hepatitis C virus (HCV) infection presenting as acute hepatitis causing jaundice is rare. It can rarely cause acute fulminant hepatitis. After infection with HCV, antihepatitis C antibodies are not detected for long periods. Even if antihepatitis C antibodies are present, 86% cases are still infected with virus. Vertical transmission is said to occur in 3–6% cases especially if it is a persistent disease. Vertical perinatal transmission is dependent on viral load (HCV viral load >100,000 is associated with increased risk) and HIV status. There is no role of elective cesarean delivery for prevention of perinatal transmission and is not recommended even if the viral load is high. It is however recommended that fetal scalp blood monitoring is avoided due to reports of increased risk of HCV transmission.[45] HCV therapy consists of direct-acting antiviral (DAA) drugs ribavirin and interferon. The safety of the currently recommended DAAs has not been extensively studied in pregnant women and hence treatment of HCV during pregnancy is not routinely recommended.[15] Currently, there are no vaccines or immunoglobulins and there is no method to prevent fetal transmission at birth. Universal screening of all pregnant women for hepatitis C is emphasized by American Association for the Study of Liver Diseases (AASLD) and Infectious Diseases Society of America. As with HBV, the HCV-infected women may breastfeed, as postpartum risk of HCV transmission is negligible.

## Hepatitis E Virus

Hepatitis E virus is endemic in India and causes AVH in sporadic and epidemic settings. The attack rates during epidemic are 3–30% among young adults with mortality of <1% due to fulminant hepatic failure. HEV as the cause of AVH is significantly more common in pregnant females than in males and nonpregnant females.[46] It is believed that reduced toll-like receptor (TLR) 3 and 7 in pregnant women make them susceptible to hepatic failure induced by HEV.[47] The mechanism of severe liver injury in pregnancy remains a mystery. It may be related to several factors such as differences in hormonal, immunological, genetic, environmental, and nutritional factors in developing countries. Maternal malnutrition is also seen as a precipitating factor.

Hepatitis E is enterically transmitted. The clinical features include vague malaise, anorexia, nausea, fever, and upper abdominal pain. There may be diarrhea, arthralgia, rash, and pruritus. Vertical transmission to the fetus occurs through transplacental route. Fetal loss is high due to abortions, still births, and neonatal deaths.

Detection of HEV IgM antibodies by enzyme-linked immunosorbent assay (ELISA) kits helps to clinch the diagnosis but these tests have high-false positive and false-negative rates. Serological tests for HEV RNA may be required for confirmation of diagnosis.[48]

Acute viral hepatitis due to HEV is mostly self-limiting. The management of acute HEV infection is symptomatic and supportive.

Vigilance is required for any evidence of ALF the fatality of which can be very high, up to 15–25%. It is more common in third trimester of pregnancy. The onset of encephalopathy, coagulopathy, high levels of serum bilirubin, liver enzymes, and raised INR above 1.5 indicate severe illness. These women require intensive care support in highly specialized unit with facilities for liver transplantation. Management of ALF is the same as ALF due to any other cause. There is little data to support termination of pregnancy to improve the maternal outcome. For the improvement of fetal outcomes, the decision to deliver the baby needs to be individualized. Ribavirin and interferon alpha, although effective therapy for HEV, are contraindicated in pregnancy. If the mother is not critically ill, there is no evidence to support stopping breastfeeding to prevent transmission. However, if the mother has fulminant hepatic disease or an increased viral load, breastfeeding may be unsafe. There is no evidence of pre- or postexposure prophylaxis being useful. Recombinant vaccine to HEV has been found to be successful in China but it is not licensed for use anywhere except in China.[49] Improved sanitation, safe food and drinking water, safe disposal of human excreta, and good personal hygiene are the main preventive measures to save pregnant women from HEV infection.

## Herpes Simplex Hepatitis

Hepatitis due to primary systemic infection with HSV may be severe when occurring in the third trimester. Fulminant herpetic hepatitis may also occur. Affected patients may have a prodrome of fever and upper respiratory tract symptoms. Despite marked abnormalities in serum aminotransferases and the PT, they are usually anicteric at presentation.

A vesicular eruption, if present, should suggest the diagnosis. Culture of the vesicular fluid, serologic testing, and liver histology help to distinguish herpetic hepatitis from other severe liver disorders associated with pregnancy, such as AFLP and pre-eclamptic liver disease. In contrast to those diseases, delivery is usually unnecessary and therapy with acyclovir is often successful.

## Hepatitis due to Other Viral Infections

Cytomegalovirus, EBV, and adenoviruses can cause hepatitis in association with systemic infection, which are usually self-limited, requiring only supportive care. However, transmission to the fetus can occur.

## Acute Hepatic Failure

Acute liver failure (ALF) in pregnancy is rare, but it negatively affects both maternal and fetal outcomes. It is important to have a high index of suspicion for pregnant women presenting with altered mental status, deranged LFTs, and coagulopathy. The treating doctor must consider pregnancy related as well as nonpregnancy-related causes of ALF.

It is often difficult to differentiate pre-eclamptic liver dysfunction, HELLP syndrome, and AFLP in a patient, as the diagnostic criteria for more than one condition is fulfilled in majority of them. Though liver biopsy may help differentiate these conditions, it is usually neither needed nor feasible in most cases. Hypoglycemia, prolonged PT, and encephalopathy are more commonly seen in AFLP as compared to HELLP syndrome and severe renal dysfunction and hypertension are more commonly noted in HELLP syndrome. In clinical practice, majority of patients with AFLP fulfill the diagnostic criteria for HELLP or partial HELLP syndrome **(Table 6)**. At this stage, this differentiation might not be so essential as the treatment for all conditions remain urgent delivery. But with enhanced understanding of the pathogenesis of these conditions in future, newer therapeutic targets might be uncovered and then a rapid diagnosis may prove necessary.

At present, there are few evidence-based recommendations for managing the pregnant women with ALF. Therefore, management of ALF should broadly be guided by the same principles followed for the management of nonpregnant patients with ALF. Management protocol should be individualized for each case, keeping in mind the risk versus benefit to both mother and fetus. Management of ALF in pregnancy requires a combined and coordinated effort by the obstetrician, intensivist, hepatologist, neonatologist, and the liver transplant surgeon. For the patient with ALF not recovering, a liver transplant may be essential. The evaluation and determination of the need for liver transplantation is generally made according to criteria as those for the nonpregnant patient. Delivery before transplant is likely to be recommended regardless of gestational age because fetal loss during liver transplantation is high.[44]

**TABLE 6:** Differential diagnosis of acute hepatic dysfunction in pregnancy.

| Features | AFLP | HELLP | AVH |
| --- | --- | --- | --- |
| Symptoms | Nausea, vomiting, abdominal pain, jaundice, and coma | Asymptomatic nausea, vomiting, abdominal pain, and jaundice | Nausea, vomiting, abdominal pain, coma, and jaundice |
| Other features | High BP, edema, and proteinuria | High BP, edema, and proteinuria | Normal BP |
| Hematological investigation | | | |
| Platelet | Normal | Low | Normal |
| PT and PTTK | Prolonged | Normal | Prolonged |
| Hemolysis | Nil | Present | Rare |
| Leukocytosis | Marked | Nil | Variable |
| LFT | | | |
| Serum bilirubin | 2–10 mg/day | 1–6 mg/dL | 10–30 mg/dL |
| SGOT | <1,000 | <500 | 500–3,000 |
| Serum fibrinogen | Low | Normal | Normal/low |
| Serum glucose | Low | Normal | Normal |
| Serum uric acid | High | High | Normal |
| Serum ammonia | High | Normal | High |
| Liver biopsy (if possible) | Centrilobular fat particles | Periportal hemorrhage with necrosis, and fibrin deposition | Multilobular hepatic cell necrosis and collapse |
| Viral markers | Negative | Negative | Positive |
| Treatment | Prompt delivery with fresh frozen plasma (FFP) transfusions | Control of BP and convulsions. Prompt delivery with platelet transfusion | Correction of coagulation defects, delivery for obstetric indications |

(AFLP: acute fatty liver of pregnancy; AVH: acute viral hepatitis; BP: blood pressure; HELLP: hemolysis, elevated liver enzymes, and low platelets; LFT: liver function tests; PTTK: partial thromboplastin time with kaolin; PT: prothrombin time; SGOT: serum glutamic oxaloacetic transaminase)

## AUTOIMMUNE HEPATITIS

In pregnant women, autoimmune hepatitis (AIH) activity is found to be variable from 30 to 50%.[50] The flares are seen more in women who are currently not on therapy or who did have flares in the year before pregnancy. These are probably due to pregnancy induced altered immunological responses. Women who have AIH related cirrhosis are prone to severe maternal decompensation and fetal complications.[51] Observational data show that immune suppression with corticosteroid and azathioprine in women with AIH should be continued throughout pregnancy and in postpartum period.

## NON-ALCOHOLIC FATTY LIVER DISEASE

This is now known to occur in childbearing age and in pregnant women due to metabolic syndrome of obesity, insulin resistance, and altered lipid metabolism. Nonalcoholic fatty liver disease (NAFLD) in pregnancy is associated with gestational diabetes, pre-eclampsia, preterm birth, and low-birth weight babies.[52] Prepregnancy counseling and screening can reduce its impact.

## CIRRHOSIS AND PORTAL HYPERTENSION

Pregnancy is rare in this condition but adversely affects the condition of the woman with cirrhosis and portal hypertension. Rise in portal pressure in pregnancy can cause esophageal varices, hemorrhage, and ascites.[53] Obstetric complications include placental abruption, low-birth weight, preterm birth, and increased cesarean section rate. Management of esophageal varices is same as in nonpregnant women. Endoscopy is preferably done in second trimester of pregnancy.[54] Data on transjugular intrahepatic portosystemic shunt (TIPS) is limited.

### Pregnancy in Women with Underlying Cirrhosis

Causes of portal hypertension can be cirrhotic or noncirrhotic. In general, there is a low prevalence of cirrhosis in women of reproductive age and there is reduced fertility in women with cirrhosis. Sometimes patients with underlying chronic liver disease or cirrhosis can get pregnant and present with jaundice during pregnancy.

Pregnant women with cirrhosis should ideally be managed in a multidisciplinary setting with obstetrics along with hepatology. With current therapeutic advances and intensive care monitoring, these complicated pregnancies can have favorable outcomes.

### Diagnosis of Cirrhosis

The preliminary diagnosis of cirrhosis is often made by history, physical examination, and laboratory findings. A careful history may reveal a cause of cirrhosis such as prior transfusion, exposure to hepatotoxins, a systemic autoimmune disorder or alcohol or intravenous drug abuse. On physical examination of a patient with cirrhosis signs may be absent, subtle, or may include obvious spider angiomas, ascites, liver nodularity, splenomegaly, prominent abdominal wall vessels, or encephalopathy. The laboratory findings in cirrhosis are variable, but often hypoalbuminemia, a prolonged PT, and thrombocytopenia are present. Ultrasonography can be used to support the diagnosis of cirrhosis. Specific etiologies of cirrhosis should be investigated accordingly.

Cirrhosis needs to be distinguished from disorders that can cause portal hypertension in the absence of cirrhosis, i.e., noncirrhotic portal hypertension (NCPH).

Noncirrhotic portal hypertension comprises diseases having an increase in portal pressure due to intrahepatic or prehepatic lesions, in the absence of cirrhosis. The two diseases that are common in India are noncirrhotic portal fibrosis (NCPF) and extrahepatic portal vein obstruction (EHPVO).

The diagnosis of EHPVO is based upon the presence of portal hypertension and normal or near normal liver enzymes and liver function; portal vein obstruction, presence of intraluminal thrombus in the portal vein, and/or portal vein cavernoma on Doppler ultrasound (US); and grossly noncirrhotic liver.

The diagnosis of NCPF is based upon the presence of portal hypertension and normal or near normal liver enzymes and liver function; patent hepatic and extrahepatic portal vein; grossly noncirrhotic liver; portal fibrosis without diffuse nodule formation on liver biopsy. Child's A cirrhosis may mimic NCPF, but tests of liver function, viral serology, and histology (lobular disarray, pseudolobule formation) can distinguish between the two. Moreover, a disproportionately large spleen with a dilated and thickened portal vein favors the diagnosis of NCPF.

### Management of Pregnancy with Cirrhosis

Such patients ideally should be managed at centers with facilities for high-risk obstetric care, perinatal intensive care, and expertise with hepatology.

## HEMOLYTIC JAUNDICE

Excessive destruction of RBCs results in hyperbilirubinemia which is mainly due to the rise in unconjugated bilirubin. There are no changes in the level of transaminases. The causes of hemolytic anemia include thalassemia, sickle cell disease, hereditary spherocytosis, etc.

About 50% of pregnant women may experience worsening of jaundice. The serum transaminases remain normal and the reticulocyte count is increased. In Crigler-Najjar syndrome, there is absence of UDP transferase due to autosomal dominant trait that results in severe unconjugated hyperbilirubinemia and jaundice which may be seen at birth.

Dubin Johnson syndrome (autosomal recessive) and Rotor syndrome are similar conditions caused by mutations in multidrug resistance associated proteins that result in the failure of transfer of bilirubin across hepatocytes. The jaundice is usually mild and fluctuating.

## EXTRAHEPATIC BILIARY OBSTRUCTION

A rare cause of jaundice in pregnant women is cholelithiasis. There is usually a history of biliary colic, fever, jaundice, and recurrent episodes of acute cholecystitis. USG of the upper abdomen will be helpful in diagnosing gallstones, distended gallbladder, or hepatobiliary canaliculi.

### Budd–Chiari Syndrome

It is a rare condition caused by obstruction of hepatic veins by clots. There is portal hypertension, ascites, and esophageal varices. It is associated with polycythemia, thrombasthenia, sickle cell disease, and irritable bowel syndrome (IBS) in pregnancy. It is diagnosed by color and pulse Doppler ultrasound. Treatment includes anticoagulation and minimal access surgery such as angioplasty of hepatic vein, TIPS, and even liver transplantation.

## CONGENITAL HYPERBILIRUBINEMIA

In this condition, there is either defective conjugation of bilirubin as in Gilbert's disease caused by deficiency of UDP transferase. This familial benign disease is probably due to a gene mutation. It is usually asymptomatic or there may be intermittent jaundice. **Flowchart 2** shows diagnostic approach to congenital hyperbilirubinemia.

## DRUG-INDUCED HEPATIC INJURY

Drug-induced liver injury (DILI) may lead to acute syndromes that resemble viral hepatitis, fatty liver of pregnancy, and obstructive jaundice, as well as to several chronic syndromes. Pregnancy is a high-risk factor. Hepatic injury induced by large single overdose of intrinsically toxic drugs (e.g., acetaminophen, ferrous salts) develops within 24–72 hours of intake and is usually accompanied by renal failure. Regular intake of some toxic drugs leads to slowly evolving chronic disease. Liver damage due to hypersensitivity-type idiosyncrasy usually appears after 1–5 weeks of taking the drug unless there has been previous exposure in which case it is accompanied by systemic features that are hallmarks of hypersensitivity. Hepatic injury attributable to metabolic idiosyncrasy may appear after weeks to months of taking the drug and usually presents without systemic features.

Common drugs causing severe liver injury are anabolic steroids, OCP, antitubercular and antifungal agents, nonsteroidal anti-inflammatory drugs, antiemetics, chlorothiazides, antidepressants, alpha-methyldopa, propylthiouracil, nevirapine cimetidine, ranitidine, acetaminophen, and antiarrhythmics.[55] The morphological changes vary from hepatitis, cholestasis, fatty liver, granulomatous hepatitis, periportal inflammation to fibrosis with cirrhotic alterations, vascular lesions, and tumors. The prerequisite for specialized treatment of drug-induced adverse hepatic reactions is establishing the diagnosis which is obtained by a thorough medical history taken by an experienced physician with special emphasis on drug or toxin exposure. Clinical criteria for the diagnosis are based on appearance of the disease, regression of symptomatology when the drug is interrupted, and recurrence when it is administered again. Definite treatment may be available in only a minority of cases. Therefore, the main aim is to prevent chronic liver damage through early diagnosis and cessation of treatment and substitution with another drug. Increase in the serum concentration of aminotransferases might be the only biochemical disturbance and it might be overlooked if not investigated.

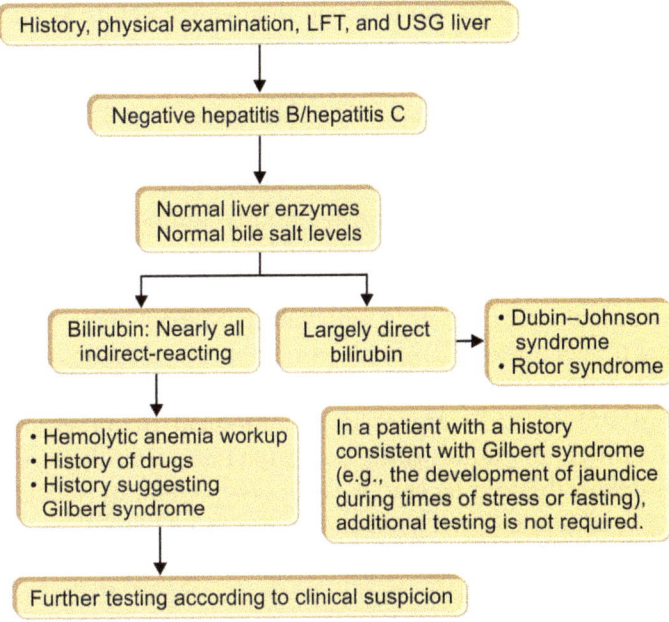

**Flowchart 2:** Diagnostic approach to congenital hyperbilirubinemia.

(LFT: liver function test; USG: ultrasonography)

### Management of Acute Hepatic Failure

Acute liver disease and its injury in severe form leads to acute hepatic failure in pregnant women. ALF is characterized by encephalopathy and defective synthetic function of coagulation factors leading to increase in PT and INR above 1.5. This acute form of disease may occur in acute fatty liver in pregnancy, pre-eclampsia and HELLP syndrome and AVH E. Other chronic liver diseases that become acute in pregnancy are hepatitis B, autoimmune hepatitis, and Wilson's disease.

American association for the study of liver diseases and European association of study of liver diseases have issued guidelines for the management of ALF.[56,57] The pregnant women with ALF should be managed in centers which have facility for liver transplantation. There should be transfer of patients to such centers well in advance before severe coagulopathy and acute cerebral edema sets in.[58]

Serial biochemical tests are to be done to assess the progress of the disease and its complications. Serum bilirubin and aminotransferases are to be done daily. Complete blood count, coagulation parameters, metabolic panel, and arterial blood gases are to be done 4–6 hourly and monitoring of serum glucose is done after every 6 hours.[59]

Underlying cause should be treated promptly. Termination of pregnancy and delivery of the fetus in AFLP and in severe pre-eclampsia and/or HELLP syndrome is life-saving. High-risk labor management, atraumatic delivery, and PPH control are essential. Medical management is aimed at maintaining hemodynamic stability with judicious fluid replacement, vasopressors, and in selected cases of septic shock glucocorticoid may be administered. Lactulose administration is not found to be associated with improved outcome. It might cause abdominal distension and electrolyte imbalance. Patient must be intubated in grade 3/4 encephalopathy.[60] Coagulopathy should be treated to prevent bleeding. Prophylactic administration of FFP is not recommended as it may interfere with assessment of liver function and cause fluid overloading.[61] GI bleeding warrants stress ulcer prophylaxis with H2 blocker or proton pump inhibitor. Infection surveillance and prevention involves cultures of urine, blood, sputum, and ascitic fluid. Prophylactic antibiotics are not recommended especially those which are hepatotoxic or nephrotoxic. If needed, piperacillin/tazobactam or fluroquinolone can be administered.[62] Nutrition support can be enteral in grade I/II encephalopathy or parenteral in intubated cases of grade III/IV encephalopathy.

Complications include metabolic abnormalities, hepatic encephalopathy, cerebral edema, and raised intracranial pressure. Acute renal failure and pulmonary complications develop which warrant highly specialized unit acting together. Approximately 40% of patients of acute hepatic failure recover spontaneously with supportive care. Prognostic model such as Kings college criteria and model of end-stage liver disease (MELD) have been devised to help in selecting those cases who are unlikely to improve spontaneously as the decision to proceed with liver transplantation depends in part upon the probability of spontaneous hepatic recovery.[63,64]

## Liver Transplantation

Prognostic models are used to screen for those patients likely to require liver transplantation after ruling out probability of spontaneous recovery.

The most important determining factor for spontaneous recovery is degree of hepatic encephalopathy.[65]

- In grade I and II recovery occurs in 65–70%
- In grade III it is 40–45%
- Grade IV it is <20%.

Patients with age between 20 and 40 years, i.e., pregnant women have better survival following spontaneous recovery.

Variables such as PT/INR, ammonia level, and liver histopathology do not affect outcome.

*Liver support* are the different approaches to undertake function of liver which will help in delay or obviate the need for liver transplantation. These are artificial hepatic assist devices, hepatocyte transplant, auxiliary liver transplant, xenotransplantation, high volume plasma exchange, and granulocyte colony-stimulating factor (G-CSF) administration.[66] Following liver transplantation 1 year survival rate is reported to be 80%.

## KEY POINTS

- Jaundice in pregnancy is a clinical sign of an array of hepatobiliary diseases. It is one of the leading causes of maternal mortality in our country and is associated with serious fetal complications.
- Hepatobiliary diseases may present as disorders that are unique to pregnancy. These include hyperemesis gravidarum, pre-eclampsia/eclampsia and HELLP syndrome, AFLP, and IHC. Hepatic diseases incidentally associated with pregnancy include AVH and other chronic form of hepatic disorders including AIH, drug induced hepatitis, nonalcoholic fatty liver in pregnancy, and cirrhosis. They all affect maternal and fetal outcome.
- Acute fatty liver is peculiar to pregnancy and leads to sudden progression to hepatic failure, encephalopathy, and coagulopathy with high-risk of maternal and perinatal mortality.
- Pre-eclampsia and eclampsia with HELLP syndrome as part of systemic vascular disorder and liver dysfunction is associated with similar high-risk to mother and fetus.
- Clinical picture of both, AFLP and HELLP, may overlap and lead to diagnostic dilemma. But, management of both conditions is prompt delivery of the fetus irrespective of fetal age. Correction of coagulopathy, intensive care, and multidisciplinary approach improves the prognosis.
- A close collaboration between medical internist, hepatologist, anesthesiologist, obstetrician, and pediatrician is of paramount importance. The newborn babies born to mothers with AFLP need genetic screening along with their mothers.
- Recently significant advances have come across in the development and implementation of various noninvasive tests and scoring system for diagnosis, staging, and prediction of outcome of liver diseases in pregnancy. The MELD is one such score that directs the team for liver transplantation as life-saving procedure in the event of acute hepatic failure.
- Intrahepatic cholestasis of pregnancy is associated with distressing pruritus and mild jaundice. The rise in serum bile acids is associated with substantial risk to the fetus in utero and warrants termination of pregnancy before or at 37 weeks.

- In our country, AVH A and E are the most common cause of jaundice in pregnant women. Serological tests for viral markers help to clinch the diagnosis. Hepatitis E during pregnancy carries a high-risk of maternal and perinatal mortality.
- Generating public awareness about jaundice; imparting health education about its prevention through personal hygiene, safe water, food, and clean sanitary conditions for pregnant women is crucial.
- Hepatitis B though asymptomatic and chronic is not uncommon and carries serious threat of MTCT. All pregnant women need to be screened for hepatitis B and C. All babies born to HbsAg positive mothers are given passive immunization with immunoglobulin at birth along with active immunization. Antiviral drugs are being administered to pregnant women to reduce the viral load.

## REFERENCES

1. Jayanti K, Anuradha M. Jaundice in pregnancy, maternal and fetal outcome. Int J Reprod Contracept Obstet Gynecol. 2016;5:2541-5.
2. Rathi U, Bapat M, Rathi P, Abraham P. Effect of liver diseases on maternal and fetal outcome: a prospective study. Indian J Gastroenteral. 2007;26(2):59-63.
3. Mohan NL, Kushla P, Devindra K. Matrernal and fetal outcome among pregnant women with Jaundice Attending A Tertiary Care Institute in Northern India. Int J Recent Sci Res. 2019;10(04):31793-6.
4. Trivedi SS, Goyal U, Gupta U. A study of maternal mortality due to viral hepatitis. J Obstet Gynecol Ind. 2003;53(6):551-3.
5. Gupta N, Kumar S, Saxena NC, Nandan D, Saxena BN. Maternal mortality in seven districts of Uttar Pradesh—ICMR task force study. Indian J of Public Health. 2006;50(3):173-8.
6. Richa T, Prachi K, Archana M. Analytical study to determine the impact of Jaundice in pregnancy on maternal and perinatal outcome. Adv Human Biol. 2020:10(3)153-7.
7. Pradnya C, Niranjan C, Neha R, Priyanka G. An observational study to evaluate maternal and fetal outcomes in pregnancies complicated with Jaundice. J Obstet Gynaecol India. 2019;69(1):31-6.
8. Praveen T, Begum F, Akhter N. Feto-maternal outcome of jaundice in pregnany in a tertiary care hospital. Mymensingh Med J. 2015;24(3):528-36.
9. Ellington SR, Flowers L, Legardy-Williams JK, Jamiesons DJ, Kourtis AP. Recent trends in hepatic diseases during pregnancy in United States, 2002-2010. Am J Obstet Gynecol. 2015;212(4):524.e1-7.
10. Nelson DB, Yost NP, Cunningham FG. Acute fatty liver in pregnancy. Clinical outcomes and expected duration of recovery. Am J Obstet Gynecol. 2013;209(5):456.e1-7.
11. Murali AR, Devarbhavi H, Venkatachala PR, Singh R, Sheth KA. Factors that predict I month mortality in patients with pregnancy specific liver disease. Clin Gastroenterol Hepatol. 2014;12(1):109-13.
12. Reau N. Finding the needle in the haystack: predicting mortality in pregnancy related liver disease. Clin. Gastroenterol Hepatol. 2014;12(1):114-6.
13. Gonzalez-Brown V, Frey HA. The hepatobiliary system: an overview of normal function and diagnostic testing in pregnancy. Clin Obstet Gynecol. 2020;63(1):122-33.
14. Bacq Y, Zarka O, Brechot JF, Mariotte N, Vol S, Tichet J, et al. Liver function tests in normal pregnancy. A prospective study of 103 pregnant women and 103 match controls. Hepatology. 1996;23(5):1030-4.
15. Sarkar M, Brady CW, Fleckenstein J, Forde KA, Khungar V, Molleston JP, et al. Reproductive Health and Liver Disease: Practice Guidance by the American Association for the Study of Liver Diseases. Hepatology. 2021;73(1):318-65.
16. Knight M, Nelson-Piercy C, Kurinczuk JJ, Spark P, Brocklehurst P. A prospective National Study on acute fatty liver of pregnancy in the UK. Gut. 2008;57(7):951-6.
17. Brady CW. Liver diseases in pregnancy, what is new. Hepatol Commun. 2020;4(2):145-56.
18. Ko H, Yoshida EM. Acute fatty liver in pregnancy. Can J Gastroenterol. 2006;20(1):25-30.
19. Goel A, Ramakrishna B, Zachariah U, Ramachandran J, Eapen CE, Kurian G, et al. How accurate are Swansea criterion to diagnose acute fatty liver of pregnancy in predicting hepatic microvascular steatosis? Gut. 2011;60(1):138-9.
20. Bacq Y, Assor P, Gendrot C, Perrotin F, Scotto B, Andres C. [Recurrent acute fatty liver in pregnancy]. Gastroenterol Clin Biol. 2007;31(12):1135-8.
21. Kumar S, Puri P, Gujral K. Intrahepatic cholestasis of pregnancy. Current Medicine Research and Practice. 2018;8(6):230-4.
22. Floreani A, Gervasi MT. New insights on intrahepatic cholestasis of pregnancy. Clin Liver Dis. 2016;20(1):177-89.
23. Beuers U, Pusl T. Intrahepatic cholestasis of pregnancy—a heterogeneous group of pregnancy related disorder? Hepatology. 2006;43(4):647-9.
24. Laatikainen T, Tulenheimo A, Maternal Serum Bile acid levels and fetal distress in Cholestatasis of pregnancy. Int J Gynaecol Obstet. 1984;22(2):91-4.
25. Joutsiniemi T, Leino R, Timonen S, Pulkki K, Ekblad U. Hepatocellular enzyme glutathione S-transferase alpha and intrahepatic cholestasis of pregnancy. Acta Obstet Gynecol Scand. 2008;87(12):1280-4.
26. Kenyon AP, Girling JC. "Obstetric Cholestasis". In: Studd J (Ed). Progress in Obstetrics and Gynaecology: volume 16. Edinburgh: Churchill Livingstone; 2004. pp. 37-56.
27. Heinonen S, Kirkinen P. Pregnancy outcome with intrahepatic cholestasis. Obstet Gynecol. 1999;94(2):189-93.
28. Samhal CY, Kara O, Yucel A. Can fetal left ventricular modified myocardial performance index predict adverse perinatal outcomes in IHCP? J Matern Fetal Neonatal Med. 2017;30(8):911-16.
29. Ovadia C, Seed PT, Skiaveunos A, Geenes V, Di Ilio C, Chamber J, et al. Association of adverse perinatal outcome of IHCP with biochemical marker: results of aggregate and individual patient data meta-analyses. Lancet. 2019;393(10174):899-909.
30. Wikström Shemer EA, Stephansson O, Thuresson M, Thorsell M, Ludvigsson JF, Marschall HU. Intrahepatic cholestasis of pregnancy and cancer, immune-mediated and cardiovascular diseases: a population-based cohort study. J Hepatol. 2015;63:456-61.
31. Chappell LC, Bell JL, Smith A, Linsell L, Juszczak E, Dixon PH, et al. Ursodeoxycholic acid versus placebo in women

with intrahepatic cholestasis of pregnancy (PITCHES): a randomised controlled trial. Lancet. 2019;394(10201):849-60.
32. Glantz A, Marshall HU, Lammert F, Mattsson LA. IHC-A randomised contolled trial comparing dexamethesone and UDA. Hepatology. 2005;42(6):1399-405.
33. Martin JN Jr, Owens MY, Keiser SD, Parrish MR, Tam Tam KB, Brewer JM, et al. Standardized Mississippi Protocol. Treatment of 190 patients with HELLP syndrome: slowing disease progression and preventing new major maternal morbidity. Hypertens Pregnancy, 2012;31(1):79-90.
34. Zarrinpar A, Farmer DG, Ghobrial RM, Lipshutz GS, Gu Y, Hiatt JR, et al. Liver transplantation for HELLP syndrome. Am Surg. 2007;73(10):1013-6.
35. Chabbra S, Qureshi A, Datta N. Prenatal outcome with HELLP complicating hypertensive disorders of pregnancy. An Indian Rural experience. J Obstret Gynaecol. 2006;26(6):531-3.
36. Kaplan PB, Gucer F, Sayin NC, Yuksel M, Yuce MA, Yardim T. Maternal serum cytokine levels in women with hyperemesis gravidarum in the first trimester of pregnancy. Fertil Steril. 2003;79(3):498-502.
37. Conchillo JM, Pijnenborg JM, Peeters P, Stockbrugger RW, Fevery J, Kock GH. Liver enzyme elevation induced by hyperemesis gravidarum: Actiology diagnosis and treatment. Neth J Med. 2002;60(9):374-8.
38. Mathew. Jaundice in pregnancy. Obstetrics and Gynaecology for postgraduates. New Delhi: Jaypee Brothers Medical Publishers; 1993. pp. 73-7.
39. Patra S, Kumar A, Trivedi SS, Sarin SK. Maternal and fetal outcome in pregnant women with acute hepatites E virus infection. Ann Inter Med. 2007;147(1):28-33.
40. World Health Organization. (2016). Hepatitis A [online]. Available from https://www:who.int/news-room/fact-sheets/detail/hepatitis-a [Last accessed, July 2021].
41. Gill HH, Majumdar PD, Dhunjibhoy KR, Desai HG. Prevalance of hepatitis B e antigen in pregnant women and patients with liver disease. J Assoc Physicians India. 1995;43(4):247-8.
42. Jonas MM, Reddy RK, De Medina M, Schiff ER. Hepatitis infection in Large Municipal population: Characterization and prevention of perinatal transmission. Am J Gastroenterol. 1990;85(3):277-80.
43. World Health Organization. (2008). Hepatitis B-fact sheet- No 204 [online]. Available from htpp/www.whoint/mediacenter/factsheet fs 204/en/index html [Last accessed, July 2021].
44. Arora A, Kumar A, Anand AC, Puri P, Dhiman RK, Acharya SK, et al. India National Association for the study of the liver-federation of obstetrics and gynaecological societies of India position statement on management of liver diseases in pregnancy. J Clin Exp Hepatol. 2019;9(3):383-406.
45. Mast EE, Hwang LY, Seto DS, Nolte FS, Nainen OV, Wurtzek H, et al. Risk factors for perinatal transmission of hepatitis C virus (HCV) and natural history of HCV infection acquired in Infancy. J Infect Dis. 2005;192(11):1880-9.
46. Bi Y, Yang C, Yu W, Zhao X, Zhao C, He Z, et al. Pregnancy serum facilitates hepatitis E virus replication in vitro. J Gen Virol. 2015;96(Pt 5):1055-61.
47. Navaneethan U, Al Mohajer M, Shata MT. Hepatitis E and pregnancy: understanding the pathogenesis. Liver Int. 2008;28(9):1190-9.
48. Clayson ET, Myint KS, Snitbhan R, Vaughn DW, Innis BL, Chan L, et al. Viremia fecal shedding, and IgM and IgG responses in patients with hepatitis E. J Infect Dis. 1995;172(4):927-33.
49. Zhang J, Zhang XF, Huang SJ, Wu T, Hu YM, Wang ZZ, et al. Long-term efficacy of a hepatitis E vaccine. N Engl J Med. 2015;372(10):914-22.
50. Schramm C, Herkel J, Beuers U, Kanzler S, Galle PR, Lohse AW. Pregnancy in autoimmune hepatitis outcome and risk factors. Am J Gastroenterol. 2006;101(3):556-60.
51. Westbrook RH, Yeoman AD, Kriese S, Heneghan MA. Outcome of pregnancy in women with AIH. Autoimmune. 2012;38(2-3):239-44.
52. Hagstrom H, Hoijer J, Ludvigsson JF, Bottai M, Ekbom A, Hultcrantz R, et al. Adverse outcomes of pregnancy in women with non-alcoholic fatty liver disease. Liver Int. 2016;36(2):268-74.
53. Russell MA, Criago SD. Cirrhosis and portal hypertension in pregnancy. Semin Perinatal. 1998;22(2):156-65.
54. Garcia Tsao G, Abraldes JG, Berzigotti A, Bosch J. Portal hypertensive bleeding in cirrhosis: risk stratification, diagnosis, and management: 2016 practice guidance by the AASLD. Hepatology. 2017;65(1):310-35.
55. Lao TT. Drug induced liver injury in pregnancy. Best Pract Res Clin Obstet Gynaecol. 2020;68:32-43.
56. Lee WM, Stravitz RT, Larson AM. Introduction to the revised American Association for the study of Liver diseases Position paper on acute liver failure 2011. Hepatology. 2012;55(3):965-7.
57. Wendon J; Panel members, Cordoba J, Dhawan A, Larsen FS, Manns M, Samuel D, et al. EASL clinical practical guidelines on the management of acute (Fulminant) liver failure. J Hepatology. 2017;66(5):1047-81.
58. Goldberg E, Chopra S, Rubin JN. Acute liver failure Management and Prognosis. In: Brown RS Jr, Robson KB, (Eds). UpToDate [online]. Available from: https://www.uptodate.com/contents/acute-liver-failure-in-adults-management-and-prognosis [Last accessed, July 2021].
59. Stravitz RT, Kramer DJ. Management of acute liver failure. Nat Rev Gastroenterol Hepatol. 2009;6(9):542-53.
60. Alba L, Hay JE, Lee WM. Lactulose therapy in acute liver failure. J. Hepatology. 2002;36(1):33.
61. Munoz SJ, Stravitz RT, Gabriel DA. Coagulopathy of acute liver failure. Clin Liver Dis. 2009;13(1):95-107.
62. Karvellas CJ, Cavazos J, Battenhouse H, Durkalski V, Balko J, Sanders C, et al. Effects of antimicrobial prophylaxis and blood stream infections in patients with acute liver failure: a retrospective cohort study. Clin Gastroenterol Hepatol. 2014;12(11):1942-9.e1.
63. McPhail MJ, Wendon JA, Bernal W. Meta-analysis of performance of Kings College Hospital Criterion in prediction of outcome in nonparacetamol induced acute liver failure. J Hepatol. 2010;53(3):492-9.
64. Zaman MB, Hoti E, Qasim A, Maguire D, McCormick PA, Hegarty JE, et al. MELD score as a prognostic model for listing acute liver failure in patients for liver transplantation. Transplant Proc. 2006;38(8):2097-7.
65. O'Grady JG, Alexander GJ, Hayllar KM, Williams R. Early indicators of prognosis in fulminant hepatic failure. Gastroenterology. 1989;97(2):439-45.
66. Liu JP, Gluud LL, Als-Nielsen B, Gluud C. Artificial and bioartificial support system for liver failure. Cochrane Database Syst Rev. 2004;2004(1):CD003628.

# Renal Disease in Pregnancy

*Pakhee Aggarwal, Suneeta Mittal*

## INTRODUCTION

Renal disease in pregnancy represents an alteration beyond physiological limits in renal structure and function that may result in a detrimental maternal and fetal or neonatal outcome. Renal disease may antedate pregnancy and may be exacerbated by the physiological alterations in pregnancy or it may arise de novo and progress during pregnancy. Management is best done by a multidisciplinary team consisting of obstetrician, pediatrician, nephrologist, and urologist.

To evaluate renal disorders in pregnancy, it is important to know:
- The effect of pregnancy on renal structure and function and
- The effect of underlying renal disease on the outcome of pregnancy.

## EFFECT OF PREGNANCY ON RENAL STRUCTURE AND FUNCTION

Physiological adaptations to pregnancy include:[1-4]
- Increase in kidney size by 1-1.5 cm, due to increased blood flow, such that they appear enlarged on ultrasound.
- Dilatation of the renal collecting system due to progesterone effects as well as mechanical compression at pelvic brim.
- Increased risk of pyelonephritis, especially in women with asymptomatic bacteriuria (ASBU).
- Increase in glomerular filtration rate (GFR) and renal plasma flow (RPF): GFR increases from the luteal phase of menstrual cycle by 10-20% and if pregnancy is established, reaches maximum in mid-trimester (55%). Renal blood flow reaches a maximum of 70-80% in mid-trimester and falls to 45% above non pregnant levels at term. These are mediated through vasodilators such as relaxin (produced by the corpus luteum) and nitric oxide.
- Fall in serum creatinine (20%) due to increased GFR, thus levels normal for a non-pregnant woman (0.8 mg/dL) may indicate renal impairment in pregnancy.
- Fall in blood urea nitrogen levels (8-10 mg/dL), due to increased GFR and reduced hepatic synthesis.
- Proteinuria up to 200 mg in 24 hours is normal.
- Fall in serum albumin by 5-10 g/L, this can increase free levels of protein bound drugs in pregnancy.
- Rise in serum cholesterol.
- Gestational glucosuria due to reduced tubular re-absorption.
- Bicarbonaturia due to metabolic acidosis compensating the respiratory alkalosis of pregnancy due to hyperventilation.
- Plasma osmolality falls by 10 mOsm/kg, with a proportionate decrease in serum sodium levels by 4-5 mEq/L.
- Increased plasma renin, erythropoietin, and vitamin D levels.
- Bacteriuria is more common in pregnancy due to dilated collecting system, urinary stasis and vesicoureteral reflux (VUR), leading to increased incidence of urinary infections.
- Lower urinary tract symptoms of frequency, urgency, nocturia and stress incontinence are common during pregnancy, while bladder atony and urinary retention are common in the postpartum period.

## EFFECT OF RENAL DISEASE ON PREGNANCY

The prognosis for fetomaternal outcome depends on the nature of renal disease, level of underlying renal impairment, degree of hypertension, other coexisting conditions such as infection and proteinuria. Some diseases such as renal scleroderma or polyarteritis nodosa contraindicate pregnancy as deterioration is the rule, while in others like systemic lupus erythematosus and mesangiocapillary glomerulonephritis, deterioration may occur despite normal function prior to pregnancy.[2] The diagnosis of pregnancy may be doubtful and confirmed late, as women with chronic kidney disease have irregular cycles and impaired fertility. In addition, blood hCG levels are usually elevated in the presence of renal failure making the diagnosis of pregnancy uncertain. Specific renal diseases will be discussed subsequently, but certain features which are common to all renal pathologies in general include:[1]

- *Isolated mild renal dysfunction (Serum creatinine up to 1.5 mg%):* Low risk of worsening during pregnancy.

- *Moderate dysfunction (Serum creatinine 1.5–2.4 mg%):* Up to 40% may worsen in pregnancy and in about half of these the deterioration persists in the postpartum period.
- *Severe dysfunction (Serum creatinine >2.5 mg%):* 33–45% progress to end stage renal disease in the postpartum period.

The normal gestational increment in GFR is attenuated in women with moderate renal impairment and is absent in those with serum creatinine > 2.3 mg/dL (200 mmol/L). Similarly, the gestational increase in blood volume and erythropoiesis is inversely related to the pre-conception serum creatinine.[4]

Chronic hypertension and preconception proteinuria usually worsen in the third trimester and may have an accelerated decline postpartum. Asymptomatic proteinuria (>500 mg/day) detected in early pregnancy often reveals underlying renal impairment. Such women should be followed up postpartum until proteinuria disappears or a diagnosis is made.[2]

In terms of fetal prognosis, there is increased incidence of spontaneous abortions, preterm labor—both spontaneous and iatrogenic, low birth weight and growth restricted infants (secondary to hypertension and uremia), dehydration (due to osmotic diuresis caused by high blood urea levels), osteomalacia (due to maternal disturbance of calcium metabolism) and a higher perinatal mortality.[5] Fetal outcome also correlates with level of renal dysfunction:[1]

- *Mild dysfunction:* Overall good fetal outcome with 95% live birthrate, 20% preterm and 25% small for gestational age (SGA), 10% superimposed preeclampsia (SPE)
- *Moderate dysfunction:* 7–16% perinatal mortality, 30–60% preterm delivery rate, 35% SGA, 40% SPE
- *Severe dysfunction:* 73–86% preterm delivery, 43–57% SGA, 80% SPE.

A cesarean section rate of around 60% is a consistent finding in most series with women who have markedly impaired renal function.[2] In a large systematic review, renal disease was associated with higher risk of preeclampsia [odds ratio (OR) 10.4], premature delivery (OR 5.7), small for gestational age/low birth weight (OR 4.9), cesarean delivery (OR 2.7) and pregnancy failure (OR 1.8)[5]

## GENERAL PRINCIPLES OF ANTEPARTUM MANAGEMENT

*Preconception care:* Ideally, pregnancy in chronic renal disease should be planned to ensure optimal maternal and fetal outcomes. Baseline evaluation for fetotoxic medication, vaccination, blood pressure, liver kidney function, complete blood counts, urinalysis, blood glucose, HbA1C and disease activity in lupus should be done prior to planning conception. Until conception is planned, reliable long-term contraception like Copper IUCD and levonorgestrel intrauterine system (LNG-IUS) should be offered. depot-medroxy-progesterone-acetate (DMPA) and progesterone only pills may be suited in some cases, while combined pills are generally avoided.

After conception, management should be multidisciplinary in a tertiary care center. Initial baseline renal function helps in detecting the degree of renal impairment as well as superimposed preeclampsia. These tests include serum creatinine and its clearance, blood urea nitrogen, serum albumin and cholesterol, serum electrolytes, uric acid levels, SGOT and SGPT, lactate dehydrogenase (LDH), prothrombin time, partial thromboplastin time, platelet count, 24-hour protein excretion, urine analysis for casts and culture.[6] These tests may detect renal insufficiency in an asymptomatic patient without known dysfunction, in which case, infection, inflammation and renal toxic exposures, such as nonsteroidal anti-inflammatory drug (NSAID) overdose or abuse should be ruled out.[1]

### Maternal Surveillance

Folic acid 400 μg daily should be started periconceptionally and continued up to 12 weeks' gestation. With pre-existing kidney disease, diagnosis of pregnancy should be confirmed by early ultrasound as it helps in accurate dating of the pregnancy.

Because of the risk for preterm delivery, an increased frequency of antepartum visits is recommended for women with renal dysfunction. Some authorities suggest 2-week intervals until 28 weeks and then weekly till delivery.[1] After baseline investigations serum creatinine can be repeated every 4–6 weeks. Proteinuria should be checked by dipstick at each visit. Notable increase in proteinuria should prompt testing for 24-hour urine protein.

Blood pressure (diastolic) <90 mm Hg is a reasonable target, although it should be maintained between 120/80 and 140/90 mm Hg throughout pregnancy. Women who are hypertensive at conception or in early pregnancy have a 10 times higher relative risk of fetal loss as compared to normotensive women with the same level of renal dysfunction.[4] Regarding antihypertensive agents, calcium channel blockers (nifedipine), beta-blockers (labetalol), and alpha-methyldopa are safe and can be continued if the patient is taking them pre-pregnancy. Thiazide diuretics may attenuate gestational plasma volume expansion and are associated with an increased risk of fetal growth restriction (FGR), thus they are better avoided. If a woman conceives on angiotensin-converting-enzyme (ACE) inhibitors and angiotensin receptor blockers (ARB), they should be changed as soon as pregnancy is diagnosed, due to their teratogenic action at later gestations.[4]

Treatment for anemia using erythropoietin is similar to non-pregnant chronic kidney disease. Treatment is recommended if Hb is <10 g/dL, provided that transferrin saturation is >25% and ferritin is >200 ng/mL. Dose is titrated to maintain Hb between 10 and 11.5 g/dL. Due to its large molecular weight, erythropoietin does not cross the placenta.[6] Oral and intravenous iron sucrose is supplemented as needed to maintain stores.

Other specific risks of renal disease in pregnancy include gestational diabetes mellitus and infections, exacerbated by the use of immunosuppressive agents and glucocorticoids.

Some authorities recommend prophylactic low-dose aspirin (50–150 mg/day) on confirmation of pregnancy to prevent glomerular capillary thrombosis, preserve maternal renal function and reduce the risk of preeclampsia.[4]

Pregnant women with proteinuria (>1 g/day), whether due to nephrotic syndrome or preeclampsia, are at increased risk of venous thrombosis and should receive thromboprophylaxis with low-molecular-weight heparin (LMWH)—enoxaparin 40 mg SC daily, until 6 weeks postpartum. Twice the non-pregnant thromboprophylaxis dose is required due to increased renal clearance of heparin in pregnancy.[3,4]

## Fetal Surveillance

Fetal surveillance begins with the first-trimester nuchal screen and maternal serum screen (combined test). However, due to the variations in hCG as explained earlier, false positive screen can occur. Due to the advanced age as well, assessment of cell-free fetal DNA may be necessary.[6] A detailed anomaly scan is carried out between 18 and 20 weeks.

Fetal growth may be compromised in pregnancies complicated by renal disease, thus it is prudent to monitor it by ultrasonography every 2 weeks. Umbilical artery Doppler can be used to detect compromise early in the growth restricted fetus. Monitoring of fetal wellbeing should start at 26 weeks' gestation when the fetus begins to have a reasonable chance of survival outside the uterus. Timing, mode and place of delivery is decided by the degree of fetal compromise and iatrogenic preterm delivery may be required. Vaginal delivery is preferred if there are no obstetric contraindications. Increasing proteinuria alone is not an indication for delivery, since after correction for prematurity, massive proteinuria (>10 g/day) has no significant effect on neonatal outcome.[4]

## ACUTE RENAL DYSFUNCTION IN PREGNANCY

Other than women who have pre-existing renal pathology, acute deterioration in renal function can occur during pregnancy. Common causes during early gestation are prerenal azotemia (due to hyperemesis or excessive bleeding during abortion), acute tubular necrosis (due to volume depletion as mentioned before or sepsis), renal cortical necrosis, thrombotic thrombocytopenic purpura (TTP) and pyelonephritis. Similarly, certain disorders arising late in pregnancy can also cause acute renal compromise. These include preeclampsia, acute fatty liver of pregnancy and hemolytic-uremic syndrome (HUS). Other causes could be obstructive uropathy (due to polyhydramnios, fibroids or kidney stones), nephrolithiasis and acute lupus. Sometimes kidney dysfunction occurs for the first time postpartum, occurring several days or weeks following a normal delivery. This can be in the form of severe hypertension, hemolytic anemia, thrombocytopenia and kidney failure. This may be related to HELLP syndrome, HUS or retained placental bits.

## SPECIFIC RENAL PATHOLOGY IN PREGNANCY

Special problems associated with renal impairment influencing pregnancy outcome include:
- Preeclampsia
- Lupus nephritis
- Glomerulonephritis and IgA nephropathy
- Asymptomatic bacteriuria and acute pyelonephritis
- Reflux nephropathy
- Upper urinary tract obstruction
- Acute renal failure/renal cortical necrosis
- Hepatorenal syndrome
- HUS and TTP
- Diabetic nephropathy
- Polycystic kidney disease
- Renal calculi
- Dialysis
- Post-renal transplant.

### Preeclampsia

The ultrastructural pathology characteristic of preeclampsia is, "glomerular capillary endotheliosis", characterized by enlargement of the glomeruli with maintenance of normal amounts of stroma and cells. This affects the kidney both functionally and morphologically, causing increased protein excretion and decreased blood flow.[7]

More importantly, preeclampsia is more common in women who have underlying renal disease, especially when associated with chronic hypertension. In fact, in one report, women who had gestational proteinuria or preeclampsia before 30 weeks' gestation were more likely to have underlying renal disease.[8] The diagnosis of preeclampsia may be difficult if there is chronic hypertension and proteinuria, as these two parameters usually worsen in late pregnancy. However, the presence of raised hepatic transaminases, thrombocytopenia and hyperuricemia support the diagnosis of preeclampsia.[2] HELLP syndrome distinguished from other microangiopathic hemolytic diseases by mild to moderately reduced levels of *ADAMTS13*, which is severely deficient in TTP.

### Lupus Nephritis

Pregnancy outcomes are favorable when systemic lupus erythematosus (SLE) has been in remission for at least 6 months.

Best outcomes are seen in:[4]
- Women with quiescent lupus nephritis,
- Absent antiphospholipid (APL) antibodies,
- Normal or near normal renal function (serum creatinine < 1.4 mg/dL),
- Proteinuria < 500 mg/day and
- Controlled hypertension for at least 6 months before conception.

However, pregnancy or puerperium can provoke exacerbations of lupus. Paracetamol is the first-choice analgesic and antirheumatic agent in pregnancy. NSAID should be avoided in the third trimester as they may induce premature closure of the ductus arteriosus.[9] A flare of lupus nephritis during pregnancy usually needs treatment with intravenous methylprednisolone 500 mg daily for 3 days and an increase of oral prednisolone to around 60 mg daily. Hydroxychloroquine and azathioprine have also been safely used in pregnancy.[2] Steroid resistant and progressive lupus nephritis has been successfully treated during pregnancy with cyclophosphamide.[4]

Additional treatment includes antihypertensive medication to control blood pressure and thromboprophylaxis with low-dose aspirin and LMW heparin, especially in the presence of APL antibodies and proteinuria of >1 g/day.

Even though flares are more common postpartum, there is a consensus not to enhance steroid therapy prophylactically in the peripartum period in the absence of signs of disease activity. Flares of SLE are more common in pregnant women who have had more than three flares before pregnancy, have antiphospholipid antibodies, C3 hypocomplementemia and hypertension.[3] A relapse of SLE during pregnancy may be difficult to distinguish from preeclampsia, but the following should be kept in mind:[2,4]
- *Features in favor of lupus:* Consumption of complement (C3 and C4), active urinary sediment with hematuria and red cell casts, extra-renal manifestations affecting the skin and joints, rising titer of dsDNA antibodies.
- *Features in favor of preeclampsia:* Associated low platelet counts, elevated liver enzymes and uric acid.

Sometimes a renal biopsy may be required to distinguish between the two as the treatment options are very different.

There is increased risk of early pregnancy loss, FGR, preterm delivery, preeclampsia and perinatal and maternal mortality. Women with anti-Ro and anti-La antibodies are at risk of having an infant affected by congenital lupus. Neonatal lupus may be associated with transient liver dysfunction (25%), congenital heart block (1–2%) or cutaneous lupus.

## Glomerulonephritis

The histological type of primary glomerulonephritis (GN) does not affect pregnancy outcome as much as the clinical parameters of hypertension, proteinuria and reduced GFR.[2] Nevertheless, rarely a kidney biopsy may be required to settle the diagnosis and exclude a steroid responsive glomerular disease, especially if there is sudden renal impairment (serum creatinine >1.4 mg/dL) or new onset heavy proteinuria (>5 g/day) or an active urinary sediment with red cell casts occurring before 30–32 weeks' gestation in the absence of preeclampsia.[4] Some authorities, however, advise against a renal biopsy in pregnant women with a rapidly deteriorating renal function and swollen kidneys, severe preeclampsia or any kind of severe renal disease due to increased risk of complications.[10] IgA nephropathy is the most common pattern of chronic primary glomerulonephritis in young people and therefore quite common in pregnant women. Pregnancy outcomes are not different significantly.[4] Acute nephritic syndrome is defined as the abrupt onset of hematuria, proteinuria, reduced glomerular filtration rate, salt retention and arterial hypertension. Nephrotic proteinuria is defined as protein excretion of 3.5 g/day or greater. Non-nephrotic proteinuria is protein excretion between 0.31 and 3.5 g/day.[11] Nephrotic syndrome needs to be managed in conjunction with a nephrologist. Management includes low dose aspirin, anticoagulation and immunosuppressive agents.

## Asymptomatic Bacteriuria (ASBU) and Acute Pyelonephritis

About 5% of all pregnant women have ASBU. Untreated infection can ascend the urinary tract to cause acute pyelonephritis in 25% of these patients (about 1% of all pregnancies).

Clinical presentation is with backache/flank pain, fever with chills, nausea/vomiting and costovertebral angle tenderness, in the presence or absence of urinary symptoms. Most common pathogen is *Escherichia coli* and 15–20% may have bacteremia with endotoxic shock. It occurs most commonly in the second trimester.

Patients are often dehydrated from nausea and vomiting and require intravenous crystalloids. Impaired renal function, thrombocytopenia, hemolysis and ARDS are more common than in non-pregnant women.[2] Treatment involves intravenous broad-spectrum beta-lactam antibiotics with gram negative cover until antibiotic sensitivity is determined. If patient does not respond within 48–72 hours, underlying structural abnormality must be excluded by ultrasound which can also help to exclude stones. If adequate response is seen with parenteral antibiotics, (afebrile for 48 hours), patient can be switched to oral therapy which is continued for 10–14 days. Following successful treatment, urine culture is repeated after 7–10 days and screening for infection is done every 4–6 weeks, as relapse is common. In addition, untreated bacteriuria has been associated with low birth weight infants. Acute pyelonephritis can trigger preterm labor, but the use of tocolytics, especially beta-mimetics should be judicious as it may precipitate pulmonary edema in patients with endotoxemia.

## Reflux Nephropathy

It is characterized by renal scarring, reduced GFR, recurrent urinary tract infections (UTI), proteinuria and hypertension. Vesicoureteric reflux (VUR) leading to reflux nephropathy is one of the most common renal diseases in women of childbearing age.[2] Acute pyelonephritis is twice as common in women with persistent VUR compared with those who have had spontaneous or surgical resolution of VUR.[4]

Certain guidelines have been proposed for management of reflux nephropathy in women planning conception.[12]

### Preconception Counseling

- Consider surgical correction of reflux prior to conception in cases with recurrent episodes of upper urinary tract infection despite careful prophylaxis.
- Discourage pregnancy when the serum creatinine level exceeds 0.22 mmol/L (2.5 mg/dL).
- There is considerable maternal morbidity when serum creatinine values exceed 0.16 mmol/L (2 mg/dL), especially when hypertension is also present.

### Management of Pregnancy

- Every patient should be frequently screened (every 4–6 weeks) for bacteriuria and treated for urinary tract infection.
- Following one UTI, low-dose prophylactic antibiotics, chosen according to the sensitivity of the most recent urine culture, will reduce the risk of further UTI and may therefore preserve renal function.
- In women with impaired renal function, the following are required:
  - Close cooperation between the obstetrician and the physician or the nephrologist
  - A monthly determination of the serum creatinine concentration, creatinine clearance, proteinuria and blood pressure
  - Active antihypertensive treatment
  - Treatment of anemia by subcutaneous recombinant erythropoietin
  - Initiation of dialysis if serum creatinine > 0.4 mmol/L (5 mg/dL) and/or blood urea > 20 mmol/L (120 mg/dL)
  - Reinforced fetal monitoring and preterm delivery when necessary, according to fetal status
  - Prolonged surveillance of maternal renal function and blood pressure after delivery.

Pregnancy is uneventful whenever renal function is normal or near normal and hypertension is absent at conception.

## Upper Urinary Tract Obstruction

Ultrasonography of the renal pelvis at the end of first trimester provides a useful baseline. The right pelvicalyceal system normally dilates by a maximum of 0.5 mm each week from 6 to 32 weeks, reaching a maximum diameter of approximately 20 mm (90th centile), which is maintained until term. The left pelvicalyceal system reaches a maximum diameter of 8 mm (90th centile) at 20 weeks of gestation.[4] A repeat ultrasound scan is indicated whenever there is renal pain suggestive of obstruction, persistent infection or a rise in serum creatinine in a woman with a single kidney. Monitoring during pregnancy involves serial assessment of renal function, urine culture, and blood pressure. Hydronephrosis can be managed symptomatically by insertion of pigtail catheter to drain the distended kidneys with good outcome.[13]

## Acute Renal Failure/Renal Cortical Necrosis

Acute renal failure (ARF) in pregnancy is uncommon, occurring in only one in 10,000 pregnancies.[14] Usually, it is associated with septic abortion, preeclampsia or uterine hemorrhage from placenta previa or placental abruption. Other rare causes may be hyperemesis gravidarum,[15] post-streptococcal glomerulonephritis,[16] bilateral ureteral obstruction, cocaine associated rhabdomyolysis,[17] hemolytic uremic syndrome (HUS), thrombotic thrombocytopenic purpura, amniotic fluid embolism and disseminated intravascular coagulation. Placental abruption is reported to be the most frequent precipitating event in developed nations, however, in India, septic abortion may be a more important cause. Acute tubular necrosis is a more likely diagnosis but renal cortical necrosis should be suspected if anuria persists for longer than a week. Acute tubular necrosis is suspected if granular casts are present in the urine. A definitive diagnosis can be made with renal biopsy. Selective renal angiography will also confirm the diagnosis.[2] Renal cortical necrosis is a rare cause of severe acute kidney injury, although it is more commonly associated with pregnancy, especially in older multiparous women and multiple gestations. It presents as gross hematuria, flank pain, and severe oliguria/anuria. The diagnosis can usually be confirmed by demonstrating a radiolucent rim in the cortex on CT. Recovery is poor and takes months.[18]

Renal failure has been classified as pre-renal, renal and post-renal in causation. Pre-renal ARF occurs due to hypovolemia and hypoperfusion, intrinsic renal failure occurs due to renovascular obstruction, diseases of glomeruli or renal vasculature, tubular necrosis and interstitial nephritis, while post-renal failure is due to obstruction of the urinary tract. It is important to distinguish pre-renal from intrinsic renal azotemia as the former responds to a fluid challenge, while in the latter fluids should be restricted if kidney damage has already occurred. The rate of fluid replacement should be based on central venous pressure, hourly urine output and insensible losses. Low-dose dopamine infusion and furosemide have been used to maintain renal flow and defer hemodialysis.

**TABLE 1:** Parameters to distinguish prerenal and renal failure.

| Parameter | Prerenal | Renal |
| --- | --- | --- |
| Urine osmolality | >500 mOsm/kg | <350 mOsm/kg |
| Urinary sodium (mmol/L) | <20 | >40 |
| Urinary urea/plasma urea nitrogen ratio | >8 | <3 |
| Urinary creatinine/plasma creatinine ratio | >40 | <20 |
| Fractional excretion of Na (%) | <1 | >1 |
| Urinary sediment | Hyaline casts | Muddy brown granular casts |

Prerenal and renal failure can be distinguished by certain blood and urine parameters (**Table 1**).[19]

## Hepatorenal Syndrome

It is defined as the development of renal failure in patients with severe acute or chronic liver disease in the absence of any identifiable cause of renal pathology. Hepatorenal syndrome is a diagnosis of exclusion. It is diagnosed only when all other causes of renal failure such as dehydration, nephrotoxic agents, sepsis and organic renal diseases have been excluded.[20] It usually develops in the third trimester and resolves within 1–2 weeks postpartum.

## Hemolytic Uremic Syndrome and Thrombocytopenic Purpura

These represent a spectrum of disease including microangiopathic hemolytic anemia, thrombocytopenia and acute kidney injury. While TTP is more common in second and third trimesters, HUS commonly presents postpartum. Treatment for the former is plasmapheresis and high dose corticosteroids and only plasmapheresis for the latter.

## Diabetic Nephropathy

It affects about 30% of all patients with insulin dependent diabetes mellitus. The characteristic glomerular lesion is Kimmelstiel Wilson lesion. Unlike the increased GFR of normal pregnancy, the hyperfiltration of early diabetic nephropathy is damaging to the glomeruli, as it is mediated by an increase in glomerular capillary pressure. Pregnancy in women with IDDM does not lead to an increased risk of diabetic nephropathy and established diabetic nephropathy with preserved renal function does not progress more rapidly in pregnancy. However, women with diabetic nephropathy and moderate-to-severe renal impairment have considerable maternal and fetal morbidity as a consequence of pregnancy.[2] Although ACE inhibitors are the standard drugs used outside pregnancy, their use in pregnancy is contraindicated. Microalbuminuria in early pregnancy increases during the third trimester and is associated with an increased incidence of preeclampsia and preterm delivery.[4]

## Autosomal Dominant Polycystic Kidney Disease

Those who have normal renal function and blood pressure usually have a successful outcome of pregnancy. Complications during pregnancy can be severe hypertension, anemia, hemorrhage into the cysts and peritonitis. There is a 50% chance of their offspring being affected.

## Renal Calculi

The most common nonobstetric cause of abdominal pain requiring hospitalization during pregnancy is renal colic.[21] Symptomatic renal calculi are more common in Caucasians compared with African-Americans and in multigravidae compared with primigravidae. Renal colic is also more common in the second and third trimesters.[4]

Despite renal tract dilatation, urinary stasis, partial obstruction, and hypercalciuria, symptomatic renal stone disease is not more common in pregnancy. This is because inhibitors of stone formation such as magnesium, citrate and nephrocalcin (an acidic glycoprotein) are excreted in greater concentrations in the urine during pregnancy.[2] Physiological alkalinization of the urine during pregnancy usually prevents precipitation of uric acid and cysteine stones. Struvite stones are associated with infection rather hypercalciuria and have a higher frequency of urological surgery and contralateral stone formation.

A good history and physical examination can point toward renal calculi in the symptomatic patient. Specific points to be asked are: age at onset of stone disease, family members with stone disease, diet and medications, prior urinary tract infections, results of previous abdominal radiographs and other medical disorders or prior surgeries. Ultrasound can identify renal calculus in about 50% cases. In women with a normal ultrasound, plain X-ray KUB and single shot intravenous urogram (IVU) can identify the rest.

Indications for an IVU during pregnancy include:[21]
- Symptoms of calculi unresponsive to conservative therapy.
- A decline in renal function in association with symptoms of kidney stones.
- Severely symptomatic pyelonephritis refractory to antibiotics, especially in a patient with a past history of nephrolithiasis.

Standard excretory urograms usually deliver less than 1.5 rad to the fetus. To decrease fetal radiation exposure, one should film only the involved side, shield the maternal pelvis and limit the number of films obtained.

To avoid even a small dose of radiation to the fetus, magnetic resonance urography has been used to differentiate physiological urinary tract dilatation and obstruction due to calculi.[4]

Up to 75% of pregnant women with renal stones will pass their stones spontaneously with conservative management, which consists of adequate hydration, antibiotics, and pain relief with either pethidine or NSAID prior to the third trimester.

Specific indications for interventions during pregnancy include:[21]
- Persistent infection proximal to an obstructing stone
- Intractable pain
- Renal colic precipitating premature labor that is refractory to drug therapy
- Worsening renal function with a persistent obstruction
- Obstruction in a solitary kidney.

The options are ureteral stenting (which requires X-ray guidance), percutaneous nephrostomy (which has to be maintained for the entire duration of pregnancy) and the most recent holmium laser lithotripsy, which delivers direct stone crushing energy up to within 0.5 mm of the laser fiber tip using a ureteroscope. This technique has been successfully and safely used in all stages of pregnancy.[4]

The increased frequency of UTI with symptomatic renal stones is associated with an increased risk of preterm rupture of membranes. UTIs associated with renal stones should be treated for longer time and followed up with antibiotic prophylaxis. During pregnancy, xanthine oxidase inhibitors for uric acid stones and D-penicillamine for cysteine stones should be avoided.[2]

Stone disease should always be evaluated postpartum using the following tests:[21]
- Serum calcium, phosphorus, uric acid, creatinine
- Spot urine for urinalysis and culture, pH
- 24 hour urine for creatinine, uric acid, calcium, phosphorus, oxalate, citrate
- Stone analysis (if stone is available)
- X-ray KUB and intravenous pyelography.

## Patients on Dialysis

In the past, pregnancy was discouraged as fetal outcome was poor and maternal complications were almost universal. Today, almost 60% of reported pregnancies result in a live birth, although 80% of these are preterm (around 32 weeks) or small for gestational age. Urea crosses the placenta and a high fetal urinary urea causes osmotic diuresis, which leads to polyhydramnios and preterm labor. Premature rupture of membranes and maternal hypertension are other causes for preterm delivery.

Although the focus should be on contraceptive counseling, if an unintentional conception occurs, termination of pregnancy is no guarantee that the decline in renal function will be reversed.[4]

In addition, the spontaneous abortion rate for pregnant women who require dialysis is approximately 50%. For pregnancies that continue, however, the fetal survival rate is as high as 71%.[18] It is a common practice to begin dialysis in the pregnant woman before it becomes necessary for her health. In this circumstance, the normal hyperfiltration of pregnancy is mimicked with daily dialysis.

Women on peritoneal dialysis are less likely to conceive than women on hemodialysis (HD). Furthermore, as pregnancy progresses it is increasingly difficult for peritoneal dialysis to meet the physiological demands of pregnancy, and a switch to hemodialysis may be necessary. Frequent dialysis should aim to keep the pre-dialysis blood urea nitrogen (BUN) <50 mg/dL (serum urea <17 mmol/L). It will also reduce the need for large fluid shifts, which may compromise uteroplacental blood flow.[4] Daily dialysis reduces the fetal azotemic environment, prevents polyhydramnios, ensures optimal fluid and electrolyte balance and allows easier control of hypertension. Careful uterine and fetal monitoring is required during dialysis to watch for dialysis induced hypotension, uterine contractions or fetal compromise. If peritoneal dialysis is employed it often becomes difficult to tolerate large exchange volumes in late pregnancy. Thus, the volume of each exchange is reduced (say from 2 to 1.5 L) and compensated by increased exchange frequency (4–6 sessions/week or long nightly dialysis).[9] Hypokalemia may become a problem requiring potassium supplementation. Metabolic acidosis and hypocalcemia should also be corrected. Also, the dialysate sodium and bicarbonate levels should fall with the gestational reduction in these levels.[22]

Nutrition for women on dialysis is modified to daily protein intake of 1.5–1.8 g/kg/day, doses of water-soluble vitamins are doubled, folate increased to 5 mg/day and dietary phosphate is not restricted. Assessment of dry weight is done to ensure weight gain of 2–4 lbs/week in first trimester and 1 lb/week in second and third trimesters.

The preferred modality in pregnant women requiring dialysis is hemodialysis, due to better fetal outcomes. In a systematic review of case series, the prevalence of small for gestational age infants was less than half with hemodialysis as compared to peritoneal dialysis.[23] HD may be required 5–6 times/week, and frequent and/or longer dialysis decreases risk of polyhydramnios, controls blood pressure and improves birth outcomes.

Anemia and hemorrhage are common in the dialysis population. Blood iron, total iron binding capacity and serum ferritin should be monitored monthly and the patient treated with intravenous iron and erythropoietin as needed along with folic acid. The dose of erythropoietin usually has to increase by 50–100% in pregnancy. It does not appear to cross the placenta and consequently, there have been no reports of teratogenicity or polycythemia in the infant.[21]

The long-acting erythropoietin stimulating protein darbepoetin has also been used in a transplant patient during pregnancy, but more information regarding its safety is needed before widespread use can be recommended.[4]

## Post-transplant Patient

Ovarian dysfunction, anovulatory vaginal bleeding, amenorrhea, high prolactin levels, and loss of libido are the causes of infertility in women with chronic renal failure. After renal transplantation, endocrine function generally improves after recovery of renal function. Following transplantation, libido and fertility usually return rapidly to normal. Conception is usually not recommended in the context of severe renal impairment or dialysis-dependent renal failure.

The ideal method of contraception in transplant recipients should be individualized. Oral contraceptive pills interfere with the metabolism of some immunosuppressive agents and may also aggravate hypertension. There is increased risk of bacterial pelvic infection associated with the use of an intrauterine device. Barrier contraception is safe, effective and the method of first choice in this group of patients.[9] Vaccinations for *Pneumococcus*, influenza, hepatitis B and any others should ideally be given pretransplant, but if not given then should be given prepregnancy. Live vaccines are contraindicated post-transplant.

Following kidney transplantation, worldwide experience of successful pregnancies is increasing. Preconception counseling with a transplant physician and obstetrician should be encouraged in all transplant recipients who are contemplating pregnancy. Approximately 20% of pregnancies will end in spontaneous abortion in early pregnancy, but of those that go beyond the first trimester, at least 90% will end successfully. These pregnancies are, however, more likely to be complicated by preterm labor (30–50%), preeclampsia (30–37%), and FGR (20–33%).[4] The overall incidence of congenital anomaly is similar to the background population. Although vaginal delivery is not contraindicated, over 50% deliver by cesarean, the risk of cesarean is 5-fold higher than general population, due to fetal compromise or deteriorating renal function.[24] The location of the transplanted kidney, donor ureter and recipient bladder in relation to the gravid uterus should be confirmed on ultrasound to avoid unintentional injury during cesarean.

Criteria for advising pregnancy post-transplantation:[9]
- At least 2 years post-transplantation (or 1 year if a living related donor)
- Good general health
- Stable renal function with serum creatinine <0.18 mmols/L (<2 mg/dL)
- On maintenance immunosuppression regimen
- Absence of ongoing rejection episodes
- Blood pressure controlled (<135/85 mm Hg)
- 24-hour protein excretion < 500 mg
- Drugs contraindicated in pregnancy have been withdrawn (e.g., angiotensin receptor blockers, mycophenolate mofetil, sirolimus).

A shorter interval between transplantation and conception is associated with an increased risk of very low-birth-weight infants and neonatal death. Perinatal outcome is good if renal function is preserved (creatinine clearance >60–70 mL/min) and blood pressure is normal. However, hypertension in early pregnancy and impaired renal function are associated with a poor perinatal outcome and premature labor.[2]

The common pregnancy complications in transplant recipients are infection, preeclampsia, premature delivery, premature rupture of the membranes, intrauterine growth retardation, low birth weight, still birth, gestational diabetes, and graft rejection.[25] Pregnancy does not appear to affect the rate of rejection, provided the graft was functioning well prior to pregnancy.[22]

Kidney transplant recipients are also at higher risk for ectopic pregnancy because of previous surgical procedures and continuous ambulatory peritoneal dialysis. Owing to immunosuppression, prophylactic antibiotics are essential for all surgical interventions. During labor, the pelvic kidney seldom obstructs, therefore, vaginal delivery should be the aim. Prophylactic antibiotics and careful wound closure cannot be over emphasized in these immunosuppressed women. Furthermore, the dose of steroids should be temporarily increased at this time.[2]

Human studies have reported that compared to a normal population, infants delivered by kidney transplant recipients have higher rates of low birth weight, prematurity, jaundice, respiratory distress syndrome and aspiration.[25]

Prednisolone at doses of 20 mg/day rarely causes problems for the neonate, as only small amounts cross the placenta (maternal: cord blood ratio is 10:1). Azathioprine crosses the placenta, but it is not converted to its active metabolite, 6-mercaptopurine by the immature fetal liver and appears to be safe. Women taking cyclosporine appear to have small for gestational age babies compared with women who take prednisolone and azathioprine. However, it is otherwise well tolerated in pregnancy with no increased risk of teratogenesis.[22] Drugs used for immunosuppression, their class, dose and pregnancy category are given in **Table 2**.

In women on maintenance immunosuppression, very small amounts of prednisolone, cyclosporine and azathioprine are excreted in breast milk, and had not been associated with any adverse effects. Insufficient data on long term effects of mycophenolate and balacept in breast milk suggests that breastfeeding should be discouraged.[24]

## KEY POINTS

- Gestational changes in renal physiology can both mimic and mask renal disease.
- Renal disease with preserved renal function carries a good prognosis for the mother and baby.
- In general, the worse the baseline renal function and more the associated complications (proteinuria, hypertension, UTI, poor glycemic control), the more likely is an adverse pregnancy outcome for the mother and fetus.
- Women with a baseline serum creatinine >0.18 mmol/L (2 mg/dL) have a one in three chance of an accelerated

**TABLE 2:** Drugs used for immunosuppression, their class, dose, and pregnancy category.

| Drug | Class | Use in transplant recipient | Maintenance dose | FDA category |
|---|---|---|---|---|
| Prednisolone | Corticosteroid | Maintenance | 5–10 mg/day | B |
| Methylprednisolone | Corticosteroid | Induction; acute rejection | | B |
| Azathioprine | Purine antagonist | Maintenance | 1.5–2 mg/kg/day | D |
| Mycophenolate mofetil | Purine antagonist | Maintenance; refractory rejection | 1–2 g/day | C |
| Cyclosporine | Calcineurin antagonist | Maintenance | 3–6 mg/kg/day (depending on serum levels) | C |
| Tacrolimus | Calcineurin antagonist | Maintenance; refractory rejection | 0.1–0.2 mg/kg/day (depending on serum levels) | C |
| Rapamycin | Macrolide | Maintenance; refractory rejection | 2–5 mg/day | C |

decline in renal function that is unlikely to recover postpartum.
- Assessment of intravascular volume is a critical part of peripartum management of women with renal disease, especially if complicated by preeclampsia.
- Invasive monitoring with a central venous pressure line or pulmonary artery catheter is necessary if there is more than mild renal impairment, pulmonary edema or severe preeclampsia.

## REFERENCES

1. Sanders CL, Lucas MJ. Renal disease in pregnancy. In: Medical complications of pregnancy. Obstet Gynecol Clin N Am. 2001;28(3):593-600.
2. Williams DL. Renal disease in pregnancy. Curr Obstet Gynaecol. 1997;7:156-62.
3. UpToDate. Maternal adaptations to pregnancy: renal and urinary tract physiology. [online] Available from: https://www.uptodate.com/contents/maternal-adaptations-to-pregnancy-renal-and-urinary-tract-physiology. [Last accessed July, 2021].
4. Williams DL. Renal disease in pregnancy. Obstet Gynaecol Reprod Med. 2007;17(5):147-53.
5. Zhang JJ, Ma XX, Hao L, Liu LJ, Lv JC, Zhang H. A systematic review and meta-analysis of outcomes of pregnancy in CKD and CKD outcomes in pregnancy. Clin J Am Soc Nephrol. 2015;10(11):1964-78.
6. UpToDate. Pregnancy in women with nondialysis chronic kidney disease. [online] Available from: https://www.uptodate.com/contents/pregnancy-in-women-with-nondialysis-chronic-kidney-disease. [Last accessed July, 2021].
7. Gaber LW, Spargo BH, Lindheimer MD. Renal pathology in preeclampsia. Baillière's Clin Obstet Gynaecol. 1987;1(4):971-95.
8. Murakami S, Saitoh M, Kubo T, Koyama T, Kobayashi M. Renal disease in women with severe preeclampsia or gestational proteinuria. Obstet Gynecol. 2000;96(6):945-9.
9. Marsh JE, Maclean D, Pattison JM. Drugs in pregnancy. Renal disease. Best Pract Res Clin Obstet Gynaecol. 2001;15(6):891-901.
10. Wide-Swensson D, Strevens H, Willner J. Antepartum percutaneous renal biopsy. Int J Gynecol Obstet. 2007;98(2):88-92.
11. Moroni G, Quaglini S, Banfi G, Caloni M, Finazzi S, Ambroso G, et al. Pregnancy in lupus nephritis. Am J Kidney Dis. 2002;40(4):713-20.
12. Jungers P. Reflux nephropathy and pregnancy. Baillière's Clin Obstet Gynaecol. 1994;8(2):425-42.
13. Fainaru O, Almog B, Gamzu R, Lessing JB, Kupferminc M. The management of symptomatic hydronephrosis in pregnancy. BJOG. 2002;109(12):1385-7.
14. Jena M, Mitch WE. Rapidly reversible acute renal failure from ureteral obstruction in pregnancy. Am J Kidney Dis. 1996;28(3):457-60.
15. Hill JB, Yost NP, Wendel GD Jr. Acute renal failure in association with severe hyperemesis gravidarum. Obstet Gynecol. 2002;100(5 Pt 2):1119-21.
16. Fervenza F, Green A, Lafayette RA. Acute renal failure due to postinfectious glomerulonephritis. During Pregnancy. Am J Kidney Dis. 1997;29(2):273-6.
17. Lampley EC, Williams S, Myers SA. Cocaine-associated rhabdomyolysis causing renal failure in pregnancy. Obstet Gyneco. 1996;87(5 Pt 2):804-6.
18. MedScape. Kidney disease and pregnancy. [online] Available from: URL: http://emedicine.medscape.com/article/246123-overview. [Last accessed July, 2021].
19. Brady HR, Brenner BM. Acute renal failure. In: Braunwald E, Hauser SL, Fauci A, Longo DL, Kasper DL, Jameson JL (Eds). Harrison's Principles of Internal Medicine, 15th edition. New York: McGraw Hill; 2001. pp. 1541-51.
20. Wong F, Blendis L. Hepatorenal failure. Clin Liver Dis. 2000;4(1):169-89
21. Maikranz P, Coe FL, Parks JL, Lindheimer MD. Nephrolithiasis and gestation. Baillière's Clin Obstet Gynaecol. 1987;1(4):909-19.
22. Levidiotis V, Chang S, McDonald SJ. Pregnancy and maternal outcomes among kidney transplant recipient. Am Soc Nephrol. 2009;20(11):2433-40.
23. Piccoli GB, Minelli F, Versino E, Cabiddu G, Attini R, Vigotti FN, et al .Pregnancy in dialysis patients in the new millennium: a systematic review and meta-regression analysis correlating dialysis schedules and pregnancy outcomes. Nephrol Dial Transplant. 2016;31(11):1915-34.
24. Bramham K, Nelson-Piercy C, Gao H, Pierce M, Bush N, Spark P, et al. Pregnancy in renal transplant recipients: a UK national cohort study. Clin J Am Soc Nephrol. 2013;8(2):290-8.
25. Basaran O, Emirolu R, Seçme S, Moray G, Haberal M. Pregnancy and renal transplantation. Transplant Proc. 2004;36(1):122-4.

# CHAPTER 23: Pregnancy with Epilepsy

*Monika Madaan*

## INTRODUCTION

Epilepsy is a common neurological disorder and has a prevalence of 5.25 per 1,000 pregnancies.[1] Globally around 15 million women with epilepsy belong to reproductive age group. Majority of women with epilepsy have uneventful pregnancy outcome, at the same time antiepileptic drugs (AED) are associated with fetal risks such as growth restriction, major congenital malformations and neurocognitive abnormalities in the offspring.

Thus, managing women with epilepsy requires knowledge of such risks as well as an understanding of effect of pregnancy on seizure control and of gestational effects on AED disposition.

## DIAGNOSING EPILEPSY

The diagnosis of epilepsy should be made by a physician with expertise in epilepsy or a neurologist. International League against Epilepsy (ILAE) has given a revised classification of epilepsy in 2017. According to this classification seizures are broadly divided into three types based upon area of onset **(Fig. 1)**.

### Focal Seizures

This type of seizure starts in a particular area of the brain. It can be motor or non-motor.
- *Focal motor seizure:* In focal motor seizure, some type of movement occurs during the event such as twitching, jerking, or stiffening movements of a body part or automatic movements such as licking lips, rubbing hands, etc.
- *Focal non-motor seizure:* This type of seizure involves changes in sensation, emotions, thinking, or experiences.

### Generalized Onset Seizures

Generalized onset seizure starts in both hemispheres of the brain. It can be motor or non-motor.
- *Generalized motor seizure:* In this type of disorder there is stiffening (tonic) and jerking (clonic) movements

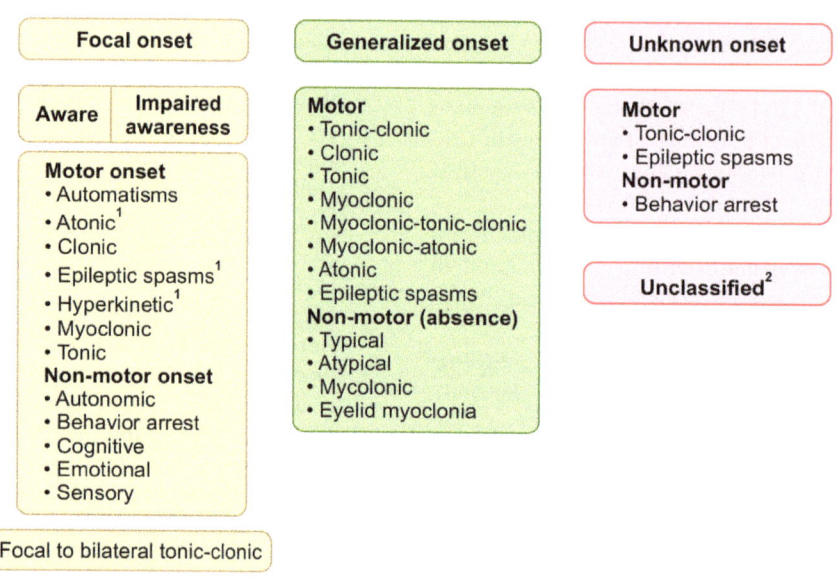

**Fig. 1:** International League against Epilepsy 2017 Classification of seizure types expanded version.
[1]Degree of awareness usually is not specified
[2]Due to inadequate information or inability to place in other categories
*Source:* Fisher et al. Instruction manual for the ILAE 2017 operational classification of seizure types. Epilepsia doi: 10.1111/epi.13671

of the body (generalized tonic-clonic seizure). Earlier this type of epilepsy was called grand mal epilepsy. It is associated with fetal hypoxia. It also has the highest risk of sudden unexpected death in epilepsy (SUDEP), i.e., sudden unexpected death in epilepsy. SUDEP is defined as "sudden, unexpected, witnessed or unwitnessed, nontraumatic and non-drowning death in patients with epilepsy, with or without evidence for a seizure and excluding documented status epilepticus, in which postmortem examination does not reveal a toxicological or anatomical cause of death."[2,3]

- *Generalized non-motor seizure:* These are primarily absence-seizures and previously it was called petit mal. These seizures involve brief changes in awareness, staring, and some may have automatic or repeated movements like lip smacking.

## Unknown Onset Seizures

When the beginning of a seizure is not known, then it is classified under this category.

## DIFFERENTIAL DIAGNOSIS

It is important to rule out other conditions when the woman presents for the first time in pregnancy without any past history of epilepsy. In the second half of pregnancy, any seizure without previous history of epilepsy should be considered as eclampsia until proved otherwise and managed accordingly. Other conditions which may lead to seizures include space occupying lesions, cerebral venous sinus thrombosis, syncope, hypoglycemia, dyselectrolytemia and last but not the least pseudoseizures.

## EFFECT OF PREGNANCY ON EPILEPSY

Approximately one-third of women experience an increase in seizure frequency during pregnancy.[4] In about 1–2% of women there is seizure deterioration during labor and delivery.[5] This is attributed to physiological changes of pregnancy leading to altered AED clearance. The disposition of many AEDs may change during pregnancy, reflected in declining plasma drug concentrations. The causes are:

- Nausea and vomiting may cause missed doses.
- Gastrointestinal absorption decreases because of decreased intestinal motility and use of antacids.
- Increased hepatic and renal clearance of most AEDs.
- Expanded intravascular volume lowers serum drug levels.
- Decreased albumin levels in pregnancy leading to lower total drug levels.
- Poor compliance often due to fear of teratogenicity.

In pregnancy, the increased clearance of newer antiepileptics such as lamotrigine, levetiracetam and oxcarbazepine results in lower drug levels thereby leading to increased seizure frequency if their dosages are not increased.[6] Sleep deprivation, anxiety and psychological stress associated with pregnancy also contributes to seizure aggravation. The control of epilepsy achieved before pregnancy directly affects the number of seizures occurring in pregnancy. The fewer the number of seizures occurring in 9 months before pregnancy, the less the risk of seizures during pregnancy.[7]

These changes reverse postpartum resulting in prepregnancy drug levels.

## EFFECT OF EPILEPSY ON PREGNANCY

Generalized tonic-clonic seizures during pregnancy are associated with risks to both woman and fetus. They may lead to maternal and fetal hypoxia and acidosis. Falls associated with seizures may also lead to blunt trauma to the uterus and may cause abortion or abruption. Focal seizures may lead to growth restriction in the fetus.

### Fetal Effects

- *Small-for-gestational-age (SGA) and microcephaly:* Various studies have shown increased risk of fetal growth restriction and small head circumference associated with AED monotherapy or polytherapy with carbamazepine, valproate, phenobarbitone, zonisamide and primidone.[8,9] Topiramate has been consistently found to be associated with SGA in all the studies thereby cautioning its use in pregnancy if other alternative drugs are available.[10]
- *Teratogenicity:* Majority of AEDs belong to category C and D. Women with epilepsy have a risk of bearing children with a congenital malformation that is approximately twice that of general population.[11] Polytherapy with AEDs is associated with increased risk of congenital malformations than monotherapy.[11] With monotherapy, highest risk of congenital malformation is seen with valproate and its inclusion in polytherapy amplifies the risk.[12] Lamotrigine, levetiracetam and carbamazepine in lower doses are associated with least risk of major congenital malformations.[12-14]

Several of these drugs cause fetal antiepileptic drug syndrome characterized by craniofacial anomalies (mildly dysmorphic face and fingers with stubby distal phalanges), finger nail hypoplasia, developmental delay, cardiac defects and facial clefts.

*Specific teratogenesis of various antiepileptic drugs are:*
*Valproate:* The absolute risk of major congenital malformations associated with valproate is 6–10% and is three-fold greater than other AEDs. Its use is associated with major anomalies such as spina bifida and hypospadias.[15] The risk of congenital malformations is dose related and increase in the risk of around 20% is seen when the dose is 1,500 mg/day or more.[16] Thus, its use should be avoided in women with childbearing potential.

*Phenobarbitone:* The use of phenobarbitone must also be avoided in pregnancy as it is significantly associated with major congenital malformations, most commonly cardiac anomalies.[12]

*Carbamazepine:* Carbamazepine use in pregnancy is associated with increased risk of spina bifida, although the risk is 80% lower than valproate. Doses at or below 400 mg/day are associated with low risk of congenital malformations of around 2% as compared to 7.7% with doses exceeding 1,000 mg/day.[17]

*Levetiracetam:* Recent studies show low risk of teratogenesis with use of levetiracetam in pregnancy, around 2.4%. The effect is dose related, with normal doses showing favorable outcome and high doses being associated with inguinal hernia and reflux.[12]

*Topiramate:* The use of topiramate in pregnancy is associated with increased incidence of facial clefts.[12,14] Therefore in March 2011, United States Food and Drug Administration (US FDA) has changed the pregnancy label of topiramate from category C to category D.

Other factors may contribute to the risk of teratogenicity include genetic predisposition, concomitant diseases such as diabetes mellitus, occupational exposure to teratogens, excessive prepregnancy weight and various nutritional deficiencies. It has been observed that there is increased risk of congenital malformation in the baby if previous pregnancy resulted in major congenital malformation. This effect was more pronounced with valproate. The maternal genetic factors might predispose to teratogenicity and compound the risk.

Thus, probably safest AEDs in pregnancy are carbamazepine, lamotrigine, levetiracetam and phenytoin. Drugs with safety profile better than valproate are oxcarbazepine, zonisamide and gabapentin. AED's with highest risk are valproate, phenobarbitone and topiramate.

Available evidence does not suggest that epilepsy per se is associated with major increase in risk of congenital malformations.[18]

**Table 1** summarizes the congenital malformations associated with commonly used AEDs.

Coagulopathy has been seen with drugs such as phenobarbitone, primidone and phenytoin as they cause functionally defective neonatal vitamin K dependent clotting factors II, VII, IX, and X.

- *Cognitive abnormalities:* In utero exposure of valproic acid leads to poor brain development in the baby. Valproic acid is also associated with cognitive abnormalities such as poor attention, lower IQ, memory and learning difficulties. Its use also leads to increased risk of autism in the offspring.[19] Even low doses of Valproic acid of less than 400 mg/day are associated with neurodevelopmental abnormalities **(Box 1)**.[20] Carbamazepine, lamotrigine, levetiracetam and phenytoin do not appear to cause cognitive abnormalities in babies of women exposed to these drugs in pregnancy although data pertaining to newer AEDs like levetiracetam is limited but reassuring.[21]

**TABLE 1:** Teratogenic side effects of antiepileptic drugs (AEDs).

| Drug | Teratogenesis |
| --- | --- |
| Phenytoin | Fetal hydantoin syndrome, craniofacial anomalies, fingernail hypoplasia, growth deficiency, developmental delay, cardiac defects, facial clefts |
| Carbamazepine | Fetal AED syndrome, spina bifida |
| Valproate | Neural tube defects, hypospadias, brain malformations, facial clefts, limb defects, cognitive abnormalities, autism |
| Trimethadione, paramethadione | Craniofacial anomalies, including cleft palate, V-shaped eyebrows, microcephaly, growth deficiency, mental retardation, speech disturbance, cardiac defects |
| Phenobarbital | Clefts, cardiac anomalies, urinary tract malformations |
| Lamotrigine | Fetal AED syndrome |
| Topiramate | Facial clefts, cardiac defects |

**BOX 1:** Antiepileptic drugs (AEDs) use in pregnancy.

- Valproate is associated with the highest risk of causing major congenital malformation and the risk is dose dependent
- The risk of major congenital malformation is lowest with levetiracetam and lamotrigine
- In utero exposure of valproate is also associated with cognitive and neurodevelopmental problems in children
- Carbamazepine and lamotrigine do not appear to cause neurodevelopmental abnormalities in children
- Some AEDs are associated with intrauterine growth restriction (IUGR)
- Topiramate is consistently associated with IUGR

# MANAGEMENT IN PREGNANCY

## Preconception Care

The treatment of women with epilepsy has to be done in conjunction with a neurologist. Women who have been seizure free for more than 2 years can be considered for withdrawal of AEDs. In women where drug cannot be withdrawn the common treatment strategy is to use the appropriate AED as monotherapy in the lowest effective dosage throughout pregnancy, the objective being to use AEDs in such a way that seizures are avoided but with a minimized risk to the fetus, the newborn and the breastfed infant. The patient's seizures should be well controlled. Valproic acid should be avoided if possible. Any major change in the treatment of women with epilepsy should ideally be done before conception. An individual therapeutic level of the drug must be obtained prior to conception.

Folic acid supplementation in the dose of 5 mg/day should be started 3 months before conception as it is associated with significant risk reduction of congenital anomalies of around 50% in the offspring. Royal College of Obstetricians and Gynecologists (RCOG) endorses daily folic acid supplementation of 5 mg/day in women on AEDs both during preconception and till first trimester of pregnancy.[22]

Couple should be made to understand the importance of compliance regarding AEDs for seizure control and the associated risk of fetal congenital malformations. It is important to screen for anxiety disorders and depression.

## Antepartum Care

Management of pregnancy in women with epilepsy requires close coordination between obstetrician, neurologist, patient herself and her family and in some cases psychologist.

Regular intake of drug needs to be emphasized in the antenatal period to achieve optimal drug levels. Re-evaluation of AED dosage is required if not done recently. Nausea and vomiting needs to be treated in the first trimester. Emphasize on adequate diet, sleep and refraining from activity that can provoke seizures should be given during each antenatal visit. It is important to screen for anxiety disorders and depression.

High levels of estrogen and progesterone in pregnancy causes induction of antiepileptic drug metabolism in the liver which results in decreased levels of the drug. There is induction of glucuronidation of lamotrigine and oxcarbazepine in pregnancy which results in the formation of inactive metabolites of these drugs. This is the main reason for increase in frequency of seizures seen in pregnant patients taking these two drugs. Thus, frequent monitoring and dose adjustments are required when women are taking lamotrigine and oxcarbazepine.

The levels of carbamazepine do not change much in pregnancy. The levels of valproate and topiramate change from 10 to 30% in pregnancy whereas the levels of phenytoin, phenobarbitone, zonisamide and levetiracetam decline approximately 40–70% in pregnancy.[23]

The need of drug level monitoring depends upon the type of AED being used and her seizure control. Thus, in ideal situation, the therapeutic level of the drug at which woman is well controlled must be documented before pregnancy and then drug levels are monitored monthly in pregnancy.[23]

Another practical approach is to get AED levels every 4 weeks when using drugs such as lamotrigine, levetiracetam, oxcarbabazepine, phenobarbitone, phenytoin and zonisamide as these drugs are associated with increased clearance in pregnancy and also if clinically indicated, in case of poor seizure control and concerns about compliance of drugs. The idea here is to achieve seizure control as there is seizure worsening if levels fall by more than 35% of baseline nonpregnant levels.[6]

Monitoring for fetal malformations begins toward the end of first trimester with biochemical screening combined with detailed first trimester ultrasound. Maternal serum alpha fetoprotein (AFP) levels are elevated in open neural tube defects. The levels should be interpreted carefully according to the gestational age and considering other factors that might result in high values such as twins, placental hemorrhage, etc. Detailed ultrasonography at 18–20 weeks has become an integral part of antenatal checkup in women with epilepsy. Amniocentesis and cord blood sampling may be required in selected cases where fetal karyotype is needed. Serial ultrasounds may be performed in late second and third trimester if there is suspicion of growth restriction. There is no role of routine cardiotocography (CTG) in antenatal monitoring of these women. There is no need of alteration in dose of steroids in women taking enzyme inducing AEDs who are at risk of preterm delivery.

## Intrapartum Management

The delivery of women with epilepsy should be conducted in tertiary care setting. Most patients can have normal vaginal delivery. Special attention is required for pain management, maintaining adequate hydration and supportive care during labor. Pethidine should not be used for analgesia as it is metabolized to norpethidine which can provoke seizures.

Routine dose of AEDs should be continued in labor and if required may be given parenterally.

Monitoring of patients with epilepsy during labor is same as that of normal pregnant women. Continuous CTG monitoring is required following intrapartum seizures, and in women who are at high risk of seizures. There is no role of induction of labor or elective cesarean section in women with epilepsy apart from obstetric reasons.

Cesarean section, however, is indicated in the following circumstances:
- Patients refractory to treatment during third trimester.
- Status epilepticus as it may cause fetal asphyxia and intrauterine death (IUD).
- Repeated psychomotor or absence seizures, which limit maternal awareness and ability to cooperate.

If seizures occur during labor, lorazepam (a short-acting benzodiazepine) is given in 4 mg bolus and can be repeated in 10–15 minutes. Diazepam 5–10 mg slow IV may also be used.

### *Status Epilepticus*

Status epilepticus is a life-threatening medical emergency. In status epilepticus, seizures continue for more than 30 minutes or there are recurrent seizures without full recovery of consciousness between the seizures. Causes include uncontrolled epilepsy, eclampsia, encephalitis, meningitis, tumor, trauma, sudden drug withdrawal, metabolic derangements and cardiovascular disease.

*Maternal effects*
- Metabolic acidosis
- Acute renal failure
- Irreversible brain damage.

*Fetal effects*
- Fetal hypoxia and asphyxia may result in fetal death
- Preterm labor
- Rupture of membranes
- Abruption.

*Management*
*Resuscitation:*
ABC of resuscitation is followed. This involves:
- Securing patient's airway
- Supplemental oxygenation
- Left lateral position
- Intravenous fluids to avoid hypotension.

*Investigations:* Investigations to find the underlying cause are performed simultaneously. These include complete blood count, liver and kidney function tests, serum electrolytes, AED levels in blood and cerebral spinal fluid (CSF) analysis, if indicated.

*Control of seizures:*
- For acute control of seizures, either lorazepam 0.1 mg/kg IV bolus repeated after 10 minutes or diazeparm 5–10 mg slow intravenously are given.
- If seizures are not controlled, phenytoin is started at a loading dose of 18 mg/kg in 100 mL normal saline given over half an hour.
- This regimen can control seizures in 75–85% of cases. In cases where seizures persist additional 5 mg/kg of phenytoin can be added.
- In refractory cases last resort is to perform elective intubation.

## Care of Newborn

There is insufficient evidence to support or refute a benefit of prenatal vitamin K supplementation for reducing the risk of hemorrhagic complications in the newborns of women with epilepsy. Thus, newborns exposed to AEDs in utero routinely receive vitamin K 1 mg intramuscular at delivery, as is the routine practice for all newborns.[7]

## Postpartum Care

The incidence of seizures occurring in women with epilepsy is slightly higher postpartum. Seizures occurring for the first time in postpartum period require complete evaluation to rule out intracranial hemorrhage, cortical venous thrombosis, infections and eclampsia.

Supportive care is required so as to prevent sleep deprivation; and also stress and pain. AEDs are continued postnatally. It is also prudent to screen these women for depression and provide treatment where indicated.

As physiological alterations caused by pregnancy revert postpartum, the drug levels increase. This may necessitate decreasing the drug levels to prepregnancy levels if the dose has been increased in pregnancy.

Most of the AEDs pass in the breast milk in inverse relation to their protein binding. Newer AEDs cross to a greater extent than the older ones. Because the benefits of breastfeeding far outweigh the risks, it is not contraindicated in women with epilepsy. The general, recommendation is to continue breastfeeding, but the infant must be carefully monitored for any untoward side effect attributable to AEDs.[8]

Management of epilepsy is summarized in **Box 2**.

## Contraception

Contraception counseling should be done for all women with epilepsy. The choice of contraception offered depends

**BOX 2:** Management of epilepsy before, during and after pregnancy.

*Preconception:*
- Review current seizure frequency and severity. If seizures persist, consider further seizure management before endorsing pregnancy
- The potential teratogenic effects of antiepileptic drugs (AEDs) need to be carefully weighed against the efficacy of the drug to control seizures
- Consider gradual withdrawal of treatment before pregnancy if epilepsy is in remission and the patient is willing to take the risk
- Review history for congenital malformations with previous pregnancies or family history of such malformations
- Should congenital malformations be present, discuss the higher risk of malformations, consider genetics consultation, consider a switch from the AED used in previous pregnancy that resulted in malformations, and encourage more intensive monitoring in future pregnancies
- Review all medications. If the patient is taking valproate, change in medication should be considered
- Try out the lowest effective dose of single drug. Avoid polytherapy
- If the patient is taking the lowest effective dose of an appropriate AED, obtain serum level preferably on two occasions weeks apart
- Recommend 5 mg of folic acid per day
- All changes in AED therapy should be completed and fully evaluated before conception

*Antepartum:*
- Continue folic acid throughout pregnancy
- Avoid changes in AEDs unless prompted by poor maternal seizure control. Avoid AED withdrawals during pregnancy
- Monitor for seizure occurrence regularly
- Where methods are available, obtain serum AED levels at the time of pregnancy confirmation and at regular intervals throughout pregnancy
- Monitor for vomiting in pregnancy, and if it is occurring, consider methods to reduce vomiting
- Fetal screening with level ultrasounds in first and second trimesters for a detailed view of fetal structures
- If a malformation is recognized in ultrasonography, more detailed evaluation with confirmatory tests such as fetal MRI, amniocentesis is to be done
- If seizures occur late in pregnancy with therapeutic AED levels, monitor for preeclampsia

*Postpartum:*
- If the patient is stable and the dose has been increased during pregnancy, decrease the AED dose over the first 10 days after delivery to a dose slightly above prepregnancy maintenance dose
- Advocate breastfeeding but indicate that adverse effects could occur occasionally if the mother is taking phenobarbital
- Counsel the patient about getting adequate sleep and to report adverse mood effects

upon the type of AED woman is taking. Broadly it can be classified as here:

- *Contraceptive choices for women taking enzyme inducing AEDs:* Women should be explained that hormonal contraceptive failure may occur with phenobarbitone, primidone, phenytoin carbamazepine, oxcarbazepine, topiramate and eslicarbazepine because of induction of hepatic microsomal enzymes. The efficacy of all hormonal contraceptives such as combined oral contraceptive pills, transdermal implants, vaginal rings, progesterone only pills, progesterone only implants may be affected in women taking these drugs.

  Copper IUDs, levonorgestrel intrauterine systems, depot medroxyprogesterone injections are the preferred choices for contraception in these women. Similarly, copper IUDs are indicated for emergency contraception in contrast to levonorgestrel and ulipristal acetate.

- *Contraceptive choices for women taking nonenzyme inducing AEDs:* All methods of contraception are suitable for women on non-enzyme inducing AEDs such as valproate, levetiracetam, gabapentin, vigabatrin, pregabalin, zonisamide, ethosuximide, clobazam, and tiagabine.

- *Contraceptive choices for women taking lamotrigine:* Estrogen containing oral contraceptives are not indicated in women on lamotrigine as estrogen induces uridine diphosphate glucuronosyl transferase in the liver leading to metabolism of lamotrigine thereby causing reduction in serum levels and precipitation of seizures. Lamotrigine levels are not affected by progesterone containing contraceptives.

Lastly, on discharge advice regarding general safety measures as regards mother and baby needs to be given to the couple and family. This includes advice regarding not to let the mother alone bathe the baby and drive alone with the baby and not to let mother bathe alone with locked door.

Women with epilepsy have several special problems related with pregnancy, which need careful attention from the attending neurologists and obstetricians. Majority of these women can have safe pregnancy and childbirth. Fetal malformations attributable to exposure to AEDs occur in a small proportion of cases only and appropriate preconception management can probably reduce this risk.

## KEY POINTS

- Management of epilepsy in pregnancy requires an understanding of optimal dose of AEDs for seizure control and their associated risk of fetal congenital malformation.
- Seizure control before pregnancy is as important as their control in pregnancy.
- Women with AEDs have twice the risk of fetal congenital malformations compared to general population.
- Polytherapy is associated with major risk of congenital malformation than monotherapy.
- Valproate is associated with dose dependent increase in risk of congenital malformation especially at doses above 800–1,000 mg/day.
- Valproate is also associated with cognitive impairment and developmental delay in babies born to mothers on AEDs.
- Changes in AED therapy, if required, should be done before conception.
- Folic acid supplementation is a must in women on AEDs.
- Counseling of the couple regarding compliance of drugs and risk of teratogenicity must be done.
- Fetal evaluation for congenital malformations is a must in women on AEDs.
- Lorazepam and/or diazepam are the drugs of choice in a woman with seizures during labor or if the woman goes in status epilepticus.
- The levels of many AEDs change (decline) during pregnancy and these changes revert postpartum necessitating change in drug dosage.

## REFERENCES

1. Koehler P, Bruyn G, Pearee JMS. Neurological Eponyms. New York: Oxford University Press; 2000.
2. Fisher RS, Cross JH, French JA, Higurashi N, Hirsch E, Jansen FE, et al. Operational classification of seizure types by the international league against epilepsy: position paper of the ILAE Commission for Classification and Terminology. Epilepsia. 2017;58:522-30.
3. Nashef L. Sudden unexpected death in epilepsy: terminology and definitions. Epilepsia. 1997;38(Suppl 11):S6-8.
4. Thomas SV, Syam U, Devi JS. Predictors of seizures during pregnancy in women with epilepsy. Epilepsia. 2012;53(5):e85-8.
5. Battino D, Tomson T, Bonizzoni E, Craig J, Lindhout D, Sabers A, et al. Seizure control and treatment changes in pregnancy: Observations from the EURAP epilepsy pregnancy registry. Epilepsia. 2013;54(9):1621-7.
6. Voinescu PE, Park S, Chen LQ, Stowe ZN, Newport DJ, Ritchie JC, et al. Antiepileptic drug clearances during pregnancy and clinical implications for women with epilepsy. Neurology. 2018;91(13):e1228-36.
7. Vajda FJ, Hitchcock A, Graham J, O'Brien T, Lander C, Eadie M. Seizure control in antiepileptic drug-treated pregnancy. Epilepsia. 2008;49:172-6.
8. Harden CL, Meador KJ, Pennell PB, Hauser WA, Gronseth GS, French JA, et al. Management issues for women with epilepsy-focus on pregnancy (an evidence-based review): II. Teratogenesis and perinatal outcomes: Report of the Quality Standards Subcommittee and Therapeutics and Technology Subcommittee of the American Academy of Neurology and the American Epilepsy Society. Epilepsia. 2009;50(5):1237-46.
9. Pennell PB, Klein AM, Browning N, Baker GA, Clayton-Smith J, Kalayjian LA, et al. Differential effects of antiepileptic drugs on neonatal outcomes. Epilepsy Behav. 2012;24(4):449-56.

10. Hernandez-Diaz S, Mcelrath TF, Pennell PB, Hauser WA, Yerby M, Holmes LB. Fetal growth and premature delivery in pregnant women on antiepileptic drugs. Ann Neurol. 2017;82(3):457-65.
11. Battino D, Tomson T. Management of epilepsy during pregnancy. Drugs. 2007;67(18):2707-46.
12. Hernandez-Diaz S, Smith CR, Shen A, Mittendorf R, Hauser WA, Yerby M, et al. North American AED Pregnancy Registry. Comparative safety of antiepileptic drugs during pregnancy. Neurology. 2012;78(21):1692-9.
13. Weston J, Bromley R, Jackson CF, Adab N, Clayton-Smith J, Greenhalgh J, et al. Monotherapy treatment of epilepsy in pregnancy: congenital malformation outcomes in the child. Cochrane Database Syst Rev. 2016;11:CD010224.
14. Veroniki AA, Cogo E, Rios P, Straus SE, Finkelstein Y, Kealey R, et al. Comparative safety of anti-epileptic drugs during pregnancy: a systematic review and network meta-analysis of congenital malformations and pre-natal outcomes. BMC Med. 2017;15(1):95.
15. Jentink J, Loane MA, Dolk H, Barisic I, Garne E, Morris JK, et al. EUROCAT Antiepileptic Study Working Group. Valproic acid monotherapy in pregnancy and major congenital malformations. N Engl J Med. 2010;362:2185-93.
16. Vajda FJ, Graham J, Roten A, Lander CM, O'Brien TJ, Eadie M, et al. Teratogenicity of the newer antiepileptic drugs—the Australian experience. J Clin Neurosci. 2012;19(1):57-9.
17. Tomson T, Battino D, Bonizzoni E, Craig J, Lindhout D, Sabers A, et al. EURAP study group. Dose-dependent risk of malformations with antiepileptic drugs: an analysis of data from the EURAP epilepsy and pregnancy registry. Lancet Neurol. 2011;10(7):609-17.
18. Perucea E. Birth defects after prenatal exposure to antiepileptic drugs. Lancet Neurol. 2005; 4(11):781-6.
19. Meador KJ, Baker GA, Browning N, Cohen MJ, Bromley RL, Clayton-Smith J, et al. NEAD Study Group. Fetal antiepileptic drug exposure and cognitive outcomes at age 6 years (NEAD study): a prospective observational study. Lancet Neurol. 2013;12(3):244-52.
20. Baker GA, Bromley RL, Briggs M, Cheyne CP, Cohen MJ, García-Fiñana M, et al. IQ at 6 years after in utero exposure to antiepileptic drugs: a controlled cohort study. Neurology. 2015;84(4):382-90.
21. Bromley R, Weston J, Adab N, Greenhalgh J, Sanniti A, McKay AJ, et al. Treatment for epilepsy in pregnancy: neurodevelopmental outcomes in the child. Cochrane Database Syst Rev. 2014;(10): CD010236.
22. Royal College of Obstetricians and Gynaecologists. Epilepsy in Pregnancy. Green-top Guideline No. 68. London: RCOG; 2016.
23. Tomson T, Landmark CJ, Battino D. Antiepileptic drug treatment in pregnancy: changes in drug disposition and their clinical implications. Epilepsia. 2013;54(3):405-14.

# Autoimmune Disorders in Pregnancy

*Kiran Guleria, Bindiya Gupta, Sneha Shree*

## INTRODUCTION

Autoimmune diseases are one of the most common causes of chronic illness, and a principal cause of morbidity in women in the developed countries.[1] Autoimmunity results from the failure of immune system to recognize self-antigens or failure of the regulatory mechanisms that maintain self-tolerance. Various conditions, such as maternal disease activity, circulating antibodies, and drug treatment have an impact on fetal outcome in autoimmune diseases. In general, autoimmune diseases carry a higher risk for adverse fetal outcome as compared to others. Lately, with good antenatal care, multidisciplinary approach and improved treatment, the prognosis for fetal outcome has improved in these women.

The best known condition of maternal transmission of IgG antibodies to the fetus is neonatal lupus syndrome which is due to the transmission of anti-Ro and/or anti-La antibodies to the fetus from a mother with systemic lupus erythematosus (SLE). Neonatal thrombocytopenia is also well recognized as a result of the transmission of antiplatelet antibodies from the mother to the fetus. However, the disease in the neonate usually resolves over 3–6 months as maternal antibodies are gradually destroyed in the infant.

Most autoimmune diseases occur more frequently in women than in men, with female: male ratios ranging from 3:1 in rheumatoid arthritis (RA) to 10:1 in SLE and up to 12:1 in anti-phospholipid antibody syndrome (APAS).[2]

## SYSTEMIC LUPUS ERYTHEMATOSUS

It is a multisystem autoimmune disorder that usually affects women in reproductive years, characterized by periods of remission and relapse. SLE may affect numerous organ systems, most commonly the joints, skin, kidneys, lungs, and nervous system.

### Epidemiology

Systemic lupus erythematosus affects women of child-bearing age and the incidence varies among populations. It is approximately two to four times higher in African Americans and Hispanics.[3] The prevalence in Asian countries usually ranges from 30 to 50 per 100,000 and the incidence varies from 0.9 to 3.1 per 100,000.[4]

### Pathophysiology

Lupus is an autoimmune disease characterized by the production of antinuclear antibodies which lead to inflammation, immune complex deposition, and vasculitis. The exact etiology of the disease is not known.

### Diagnosis

Both clinical and immunologic criteria are considered mandatory in order to establish a definitive diagnosis of SLE, according to the Systemic Lupus International Collaborating Clinics (SLICC) group.[5] According to the SLICC rule, an SLE patient must satisfy at least 4 criteria, including at least one clinical criterion and one immunologic criterion **(Box 1)**.

### Maternal Risks

The risk of flare-ups is increased, especially in the puerperium. Also, there is an increased risk of preeclampsia and placental abruption during pregnancy.

### Fetal Risks

There is an increased risk of miscarriages, premature delivery, premature rupture of membranes, fetal growth restriction (FGR), intrauterine fetal death, and neonatal lupus syndrome. Women with anti-Ro or anti-La antibodies may transplacentally transfer these antibodies leading to congenital heart block in the neonate. Also, transient skin lesions may appear in neonate in the first few weeks of life.

### Preconception Counseling

Conception should be advised ideally after achieving a disease remission for at least 6 months as it reduces the risk of flare-ups during pregnancy. Counseling of patients about the various maternal and fetal risks needs to be done. Obstetric history should be reviewed, especially history of pregnancy losses, preeclampsia, small for gestational age fetus, and preterm birth.

> **BOX 1:** Clinical and immunological criteria used in the Systemic Lupus International Collaborating Clinics classification system.[5]
>
> *Clinical criteria:*
> - Acute cutaneous lupus, including lupus malar rash, bullous lupus, toxic epidermal necrolysis variant of systemic lupus erythematosus, maculopapular lupus rash, photosensitive lupus rash, or subacute cutaneous lupus (psoriasiform or annular polycyclic lesions, or both)
> - Chronic cutaneous lupus, including classic discoid rash (localized and generalized), hypertrophic lupus, lupus panniculitis, mucosal lupus, lupus erythematosus tumidus, chilblains lupus, and discoid lupus/lichen planus overlap
> - Oral or nasal ulcers
> - Nonscarring alopecia
> - Synovitis involving two or more joints and at least 30 minutes of morning stiffness
> - Serositis
> - Renal [urine protein-to-creatinine ratio (or 24 h urine protein) representing 500 mg protein per 24 h or red blood cell casts]
> - *Neurological:* Seizures, psychosis, mononeuritis multiplex, myelitis, peripheral and cranial neuropathy, acute confusional state
> - Hemolytic anemia
> - Leukopenia (<4,000 cells per µL at least once) or lymphopenia (<1,000 cells per µL at least once)
> - Thrombocytopenia (<100,000 cells per µL at least once)
>
> *Immunological criteria:*
> - Antinuclear antibody concentration greater than laboratory reference range
> - Antidouble-stranded DNA antibody concentration greater than laboratory reference range (or two-fold the reference range if tested by ELISA)
> - *Anti-Sm:* Presence of antibody to Sm nuclear antigen
> - *Antiphospholipid antibody positivity as determined by any of the following:* Positive test result for lupus anticoagulant, false-positive test result for rapid plasma reagin, medium-titer or high-titer anticardiolipin antibody concentration (IgA, IgG, or IgM), or positive test result for anti-β2-glycoprotein I (IgA, IgG, or IgM)
> - Low complement C3, C4, and $CH_5O$
> - Positive direct Coombs' test in the absence of hemolytic anemia

Besides routine preconception tests, a maternal and fetal risk assessment should be done based on the blood pressure, renal function tests, liver function test, thyroid function test, antiphospholipid status [lupus anticoagulant (LA), immunoglobulin G (IgG) and IgM anticardiolipin (aCL) antibodies, and IgG and IgM anti-beta2-glycoprotein (GP) I antibodies], anti-Ro/SSA and anti-La/SSB antibodies and anti-double-stranded deoxyribonucleic acid (dsDNA) antibodies. Medications should be reviewed and dose adjusted to achieve good disease control.

## Monitoring Disease Severity during Pregnancy

It is difficult to diagnose flare-ups during pregnancy as the symptoms such as fatigue, joint aches and anemia, mimic changes in normal pregnancy. Fall in complement C3 levels and a rise in anti-DNA levels may be used as an objective index for assessment of disease activity. Women with preexisting renal disease should have frequent serum creatinine measurements, ds-DNA titers, complement levels (C3 and C4) as well as monthly 24 h urine collection for creatinine clearance and proteinuria.

Various factors such as active disease, preexisting lupus nephritis, hypertension, presence of antiphospholipid antibodies (aPL) are associated with poor prognosis, particularly in primigravida.

## Neonatal Lupus

Neonatal SLE is associated with maternal anti-Ro and anti-La antibodies. Neonatal lupus rash manifests as annular inflammatory lesions similar to those of adult cutaneous SLE, usually on the face and scalp, which appears after sun or ultraviolet light exposure in the first 2 weeks of life. The rash disappears spontaneously within 6 months. The most severe complication is congenital heart block which is between 18 and 30 weeks, and fetal echocardiography should be performed over this period for early detection.

## Management

Management of SLE requires a multidisciplinary approach. It is important to continue drugs on which remission is achieved, such as hydroxychloroquine, as discontinuation can lead to flare-ups. Flare-ups should be managed by short course of intravenous pulses of methylprednisolone. Details of other medications safe to be used in pregnancy is given in the next segment on RA. Calcium supplementation and antiplatelet therapy in the form of low dose aspirin (LDA) should be started in all patients. Antihypertensives safe to use in pregnancy, such as alpha methyldopa and labetalol, may be needed in patients developing hypertension.

### Postpartum Period

Some women can have disease flare up in the postpartum period. Complete blood count, renal function, urine protein/urine creatinine ratio; anti-dsDNA and complement (CH50, or C3 and C4) should be tested after 1 month in uncomplicated cases.

Breastfeeding is encouraged for most women in SLE. The safety of medications in lactation should be reviewed, especially in preterm babies. HCQ, prednisone, cyclosporine, azathioprine and tacrolimus are relatively safer. Breastfeeding should be avoided in patients on methotrexate, mycophenolate mofetil, cyclophosphamide and leflunomide.[6]

## RHEUMATOID ARTHRITIS

Autoimmune rheumatic disorders are predominantly seen in young women of childbearing age. Both pregnancy and lactation modulate immune functions and affect rheumatic disease by either triggering the onset of a rheumatic disease in the postpartum period or by modifying disease activity of established rheumatic disease.

## Pathophysiology

Rheumatoid arthritis is a systemic autoimmune disease which primarily affects the joints. The fetal cells persisting in the maternal circulation play an important role in the aggravation of RA in pregnancy. The disease activity is inversely related to the amount of fetal DNA detected in maternal circulation.

## Epidemiology

The incidence of new onset RA in immediate postpartum period ranges from 13 to 37% in various population based studies from different countries.[7,8] In contrast, the risk of developing disease during pregnancy is reduced.

## Maternal Risks

Pregnancy has a beneficial effect on RA and 48–62% show symptomatic improvement while 16–27% may show complete remission in the antepartum period.[9,10] Increase in estrogen and progesterone; and HLA incompatibility between the mother and the fetus play an important role in amelioration of disease in pregnancy. However, flare-ups are common in the puerperium.

## Fetal Risks

There are usually no adverse effects on the fetus unless the woman is anti-Ro positive or has aPL.

## Preconception Counseling

The counseling of the patient is the same as described under the section on SLE.

## Management

Various drugs which may be used in the management of RA in pregnancy are described here:

### Corticosteroids

Steroids such as prednisolone, hydrocortisone and cortisone are category B drugs while dexamethasone and betamethasone are considered category C as they cross the placenta. Reports of cleft lip and palate have been seen after systemic steroid therapy and higher doses of prednisone (1–2 mg/kg/day) should be omitted in the first trimester.[11] Maternal complications of steroid therapy include diabetes and hypertension. Fetal complications include conditions such as intrauterine growth restriction, low birthweight and theoretical risk of fetal adrenal gland dysfunction.

Corticosteroid therapy can be started or continued during pregnancy, at any gestational age and in the standard dosages. When the treatment is continued until delivery, neonatal monitoring of urine output, blood glucose, and body weight is desirable.[12] Ensure optimum calcium and vitamin D supplementation to avoid osteoporosis. Stress doses of corticosteroids are recommended during labor followed by gradual tapering in the postpartum period.

### Nonsteroidal Anti-inflammatory Drugs

Nonsteroidal anti-inflammatory drugs (NSAIDs) are category B drugs but they may lead to premature closure of ductus arteriosus, fetal pulmonary hypertension, fetal hemorrhage (due to impaired platelet aggregation), and oligohydramnios. Cyclooxygenase-2 (COX-2) inhibitors have similar side effects but are considered to be category C drugs.

It is recommended that the drugs should not be used beyond 24 weeks and even before 24 weeks restricted usage is recommended.[10] NSAIDs are approved for use during lactation, but they increase the risk of neonatal jaundice due to the potential to displace bilirubin.

### Hydroxychloroquine (HCQ)

It is widely used in treatment of autoimmune diseases such as RA, SLE and other connective tissue disorders. It is a category C drug and has a long half-life (approximately 8 weeks). The recommended dosage is 200–600 mg/day. No documented teratogenic effects are known and it is a safe drug in pregnancy.

### Sulfasalazine

It is a dihydrofolate reductase inhibitor. The colonic bacteria metabolize it into 5-aminosalicylic acid (5 ASA) and sulfapyridine. Sulfasalazine and sulfapyridine cross the placenta; however, no teratogenic effects have been documented. It is a category B drug and can be safely used in pregnancy with folate supplementation.[12]

### Azathioprine

It is a category D drug and reports are available of its association with prematurity, immunosuppression, and superimposed infections such as cytomegalovirus and theoretical risk of malignancy. Despite this it is used if necessary for disease control, the drug can be continued under close obstetrical and neonatal monitoring (especially to rule out infections). It is suggested to decrease the dose at 32 weeks.[12]

### Cyclosporine

It is a category C drug and may be used if required for disease control. It is mainly associated with the risk of immunosuppression and consequent infections like cytomegalovirus.

### TNF-alpha Antagonists

TNF-alpha antagonists include infliximab, etanercept, and adalimumab. Infliximab readily crosses the placenta while etanercept rarely crosses the placenta.[13] The major concern is the immunosuppressive effect of the drug leading to infections such as cytomegalovirus, Listeria and Toxoplasma.

They may be used in women who require these medications for the maintenance or establishment of control of active disease during pregnancy. It is highly debatable whether these medications should be stopped in the late second or early third trimester.[14]

If benefits outweigh risks, treatment can be individualized. Infliximab should be stopped at 16th week and adalimumab, etanercept, and golimumab should be discontinued, if possible, by the third trimester. Certolizumab can be given, if necessary, throughout pregnancy. Infants of these mothers should avoid live vaccines during the first 6 months (rotavirus and Bacillus Calmette-Guérin).[14,15] However, they are not contraindicated during breastfeeding.

Drugs which are not recommended in the management are:

### Methotrexate

It is a dihydrofolate reductase inhibitor and has a strong teratogenic potential. It is associated with various cranial malformations, limb defects and central nervous system abnormalities like hydrocephalus. It is recommended to stop the drug at least 4 months prior to conception.[16]

The drug has a strong teratogenic potential and due to extensive enterohepatic circulation of the drug it remains in the circulation for up to 2 years. If the drug needs to be eliminated, it is recommended to take cholestyramine 8 g three times a day for 11 days and conception should be avoided for at least 3 months after stopping the drug.[17] In case of pregnancy, alternative drugs can be started or it can be continued with serial anomaly scans to detect anomalies stated in animal studies.

### Mycophenolate

It is associated with a high teratogenic and immunosuppressive potential. Teratogenic effects are defects of external and middle ear (microtia or anotia with atresia or absence of the external auditory canals and abnormal ossicles) and sporadic abnormalities of heart, kidney, corpus callosum agenesis and diaphragmatic hernia.[18-21] Patients on this drug are advised appropriate contraception and the drug should immediately be discontinued if the patient becomes pregnant.

### Anti-CD20 Antibodies (Rituximab)

It is not recommended in pregnancy due to limited evidence.

## ANTIPHOSPHOLIPID SYNDROME

Antiphospholipid antibody syndrome (APS) is a form of autoantibody induced thrombophilia characterized by recurrent thrombosis and pregnancy complications. It is now a well-recognized and an easily manageable cause of recurrent pregnancy loss (RPL).

### Epidemiology

Recurrent miscarriage occurs in about 10–15% women with APS in contrast to 1% in general population.[22] About 5–10% of all pregnancies in women with APS are complicated by preeclampsia or placental insufficiency (FGR), or both, and up to three-fourths result in induced preterm births.[23] Patients with SLE who have aPL and/or lupus antibodies have a 40% higher risk of thrombosis than others.[24]

### Pathogenesis

Antiphospholipid antibody syndrome is an autoimmune disease characterized by the presence of aPL in the circulation, of which the most common are the aCL antibodies and LA. It is a prothrombotic condition and carries a high risk of arterial and venous thrombosis as well as other pregnancy related complication. aPL appears to have a direct effect on human placental trophoblast function[25] decreasing trophoblast viability, syncytialization, and capacity for invasion, alteration in the production of hormones and signaling molecules by trophoblast cells.[26]

### Diagnostic Criteria

The diagnosis of APS is made by the presence of one clinical criteria and one laboratory criteria which must be positive on two occasions 6 weeks apart (Sapporo criteria).[27] This is because transient positive results for APA may occur due to infections, drugs, etc.

In 2006, two revisions were made in which anti-beta-2-glycoprotein was added to the laboratory criteria and the time between two positive determinations was increased from 6 to 12 weeks.[28] The clinical criteria for diagnosis of APS include vascular thrombosis and pregnancy morbidity.

### Vascular Thrombosis

One or more clinical episodes of arterial, venous, or small vessel thrombosis in any tissue or organ should be present. Thrombosis should be supported by objective validated criteria, i.e., findings of appropriate imaging studies or histopathology.

### Pregnancy Morbidity

- One or more unexplained deaths of a morphologically normal fetus >10 weeks of gestation documented by ultrasound or direct examination.
- One or more preterm births at or before 34 weeks of gestation due to severe preeclampsia or placental insufficiency (evidenced by presence of abnormal or nonreassuring fetal surveillance tests, low score on a biophysical profile, abnormal Doppler waveform,

oligohydramnios, birth weight <10th percentile for the gestational age).
- Three or more consecutive abortions before 10 weeks gestation with no maternal hormonal, anatomic or chromosomal abnormalities and other causes of recurrent losses being ruled out.

The *laboratory criteria* for the diagnosis of APS include:
- LA present in plasma on two or more occasions 12 weeks apart.
- Anticardiolipin antibody of IgG or IgM subtype should be present in medium or high titers in serum or plasma that is >40 GPL units or MPL units, or >the 99th centile on two or more occasions 12 weeks apart.
- Anti-beta-2-glycoprotein I antibody of IgG and/or IgM isotype in serum or plasma (in titer >the 99th centile), present on two or more occasions at least 12 weeks apart.

## Maternal Risks

This condition is associated with recurrent and late fetal loss, increased risk of development of preeclampsia and placental abruption. The association of aPL antibodies with preeclampsia and abruption is less stronger than recurrent pregnancy loss.

## Fetal Risks

Intervillous thrombosis leads to diffuse infarction of the placenta. The resultant decrease in uteroplacental blood flow causes FGR, oligohydramnios, fetal hypoxia, and sometimes fetal demise.

## Preconception Counseling

The maternal and fetal risks associated with the condition should be explained to the patient. She must be counseled about the need to take daily injections of antithrombotic therapy and careful surveillance as soon as pregnancy is diagnosed and continue it throughout the duration of pregnancy.

## Management

For women with APS with RPL (≥3 pregnancy losses before 10 weeks of gestation), antenatal administration of heparin combined with LDA is recommended throughout pregnancy. For women with APS and a history of preeclampsia or FGR, LDA is recommended.[29]

Aspirin prevents thrombosis and prevents damage to trophoblast. It is started as soon as pregnancy is detected. It has been found to be ineffective when used alone. The live birth rate has been seen to be much greater in the heparin plus LDA group compared to those who received LDA alone.[29] Heparin reduces the binding of aPL facilitating implantation and inhibiting complement activation. Heparin is available in two forms—(1) unfractionated heparin (UFH) and (2) low molecular weight heparin (LMWH). UFH is associated with complications such as bleeding, thrombocytopenia, and osteoporosis. Platelet counts must be done 1 week after commencement of therapy and then monthly in all patients on UFH therapy. However, it has the advantage of a shorter half-life than LMWH and a near complete reversal with protamine sulfate. LMWHs are the agents of choice for thromboprophylaxis. LMWHs inhibit factor Xa and also act on antithrombin III and factor IIa, which lead to its anticoagulant activity. Advantages of LMWH include lower risk of bleeding, thrombocytopenia, and osteoporosis. The efficacy is comparable to UFH. Monitoring of platelet count or anti-Xa levels are not advocated with use of LMWH. Enoxaparin in the dose of 20–40 mg/day subcutaneously has been used successfully in pregnancy. LMWHs are safe in breastfeeding women; however, their dose needs to be reduced in women with renal impairment.

The standard treatment to prevent adverse pregnancy outcomes in pregnant women with APS includes prophylactic dose of antithrombotic agents for patients with no prior thrombosis. This includes 0.5 mg/kg/day of LMWH (enoxaparin) or 5,000 U twice daily UFH + low dose (81 mg) aspirin. The anti-factor Xa is checked 4 hours after last dose of LMWH once or twice during treatment and a level of 0.2–0.6 U/mL is adequate.

In those with prior thrombosis a full dose of anticoagulants is desirable that is 1 mg/kg every 12 hours of enoxaparin or 10–12,000 units of UFH every 12 hours. The anti-factor Xa activity is checked after 4 hours of the last dose, since PTT is usually abnormal in patients with LAC. Target value of serum anti-factor Xa levels 4 hours after last dose for 0.5–1.1 U/mL if the dosing is twice a day or 1.0–2.0 U/mL if the dosing is once a day.

Combination of LDA and LMWH injections improves both fetal and maternal outcomes, thus, without treatment, the chances of successful pregnancy are around 30%, 50% with LDA alone, and up to 70% with both molecules. Treatment begins at conception and continues for 6–12 weeks postpartum if there is no history of thrombosis; and indefinitely if there is history of thrombosis.[30]

Women receiving antenatal LMWH should be advised to withhold any further injections if they have any vaginal bleeding or labor pains start. They should report to the hospital and decision regarding further doses should be taken by medical staff. Regional techniques should be avoided if possible until at least 12 hours after the last prophylactic dose of LMWH and 24 hours if the patient is on therapeutic dose. Women receiving antenatal LMWH having an elective cesarean section should receive a thromboprophylactic dose of LMWH on the day prior to delivery and, the morning dose on the day of delivery should be omitted and the operation performed that morning. The first thromboprophylactic dose of LMWH should be given as soon as possible usually after

6–12 hours after delivery provided there is no postpartum hemorrhage and regional analgesia has not been used. The Royal College of Obstetricians and Gynaecologists (RCOG) recommends that women with previous thrombosis and APS should be offered both antenatal and 6 weeks of postpartum thromboprophylaxis. Women with persistent aPL with no previous venous thromboembolism (VTE) but with other risk factors for thrombosis may also be considered for antenatal or postnatal thromboprophylaxis.[31]

### Immunosuppressive Agents

Corticosteroid in combination with LDA was used in the past. Although the live birth rates reported with this regime was as high as 75%, it is not used now because of high rate of complications such as hypertension, diabetes, osteoporosis, steroid psychosis, preterm rupture of membranes and preterm labor.

### Intravenous Immunoglobulin

Several reports exist on successful pregnancy outcome and fewer pregnancy complications when high dose intravenous immunoglobulin (IVIG) was used with prednisone, heparin, LDA or alone.[32]

However, a 2010 meta-analysis concluded that IVIGs do not improve pregnancy outcome in women with APS and immunotherapy is expensive and has potentially serious adverse effects including transfusion reaction, anaphylactic shock, and hepatitis.[33]

### Future Therapies

These include combination antiaggregant therapy (LDA plus clopidogrel or dipyridamole), oral antifactor-Xa drugs (rivaroxaban, apixaban), direct thrombin inhibitors (dabigatran), statins (fluvastatin, rosuvastatin), hydroxychloroquine, B-cell depletion (rituximab). These are still experimental in both pregnant and nonpregnant population.[34] Paternal cell immunization, third party donor leukocytes, trophoblast membranes are other immunotherapy options but still in the experimental phase.

## Management of Women with APS Planning In Vitro Fertilization

Of late, autoimmunity is not considered a likely cause of infertility, except when it leads to drug-induced ovarian failure, or amenorrhea due to severe flare or subfertility related to renal insufficiency.[35,36] Most recent studies have underlined the relative safety of assisted reproductive technology (ART) procedures in patients with SLE and/or APS, which include ovarian stimulation, oocyte retrieval, in vitro fertilization (IVF), and transfer of the fertilized embryo into the uterus.[37] There has been inconsistent rise in the incidence of lupus flare or thrombosis in patients with SLE and/or APS undergoing ARTs contrary to prior understanding.[38] The risk of thrombosis is actually increased only in women with thrombophilia or a history of a thromboembolic event.[39]

In women with SLE or APS undergoing ART, the risks ascribed to ovulation induction and controlled ovarian hyperstimulation have been observed as a result of elevated serum 17β-E2 concentrations, irrespective of the method,[39] which in turn exacerbates SLE. Few anecdotal cases have reported complications such as transverse myelopathy, pulmonary embolism, venous and arterial thrombosis, all attributing these thromboembolic complications to ovarian hyperstimulation syndrome (OHSS), hence all focus should be directed to OHSS preventing strategies.[40,41] To summarize in brief, approach should include mild stimulation protocols, cycle cancellation, coasting, administration of lower doses of hCG or GnRH agonists, embryo freezing, single embryo transfer, selection of natural estrogen and progesterone over synthetic ones, preference of vaginal and transdermal routes over oral, and addition of luteal phase support. Aims should target on preventing ovarian hyperstimulation syndrome and addition of adjuvant therapy (anticoagulation, corticosteroids, immunosuppressants) whenever warranted to prevent thrombosis or lupus flares.[42]

The American College of Rheumatology Guideline 2020 conditionally recommends against an empiric dosage increase of prednisone during ART procedures in patients with SLE.[43] In patients with treated thrombotic APS, ART with anticoagulation is recommended. Prophylactic anticoagulation with heparin or low molecular weight heparin in women with APS, therapeutic anticoagulation in women with thrombotic APS, during ART procedures is strongly recommended.[43]

### Neonatal APS

About 30% of children born to mothers with aPL are said to passively acquire these autoantibodies; but the occurrence of thrombosis is rare in these babies. The prospective ongoing studies of children born to APS patients found the general health of these babies to be good although some data suggest that learning difficulties might occur, possibly related to in utero exposure to aPL.[44]

## VASCULITIS

During pregnancy, immune and endocrine systems undergo dramatic transformation, and seem to favor Th-2 cytokine polarization at the fetomaternal and systemic level. Such immunological changes may suggest a natural improvement of primarily Th1-mediated vasculitis [mainly Takayasu arteritis (TA) and Behçet disease (BD), which are the most prevalent vasculitis during pregnancy] and a worsening of Th2-driven ones, such as Wegener granulomatosis or Churg-Strauss syndrome.[28]

## Takayasu's Arteritis

It is a granulomatous vasculitis which affects large vessels such as aorta, its major branches, and the pulmonary arteries. Severe hypertension and/or preeclampsia, low birthweight and fetal growth restriction (FGR), preterm delivery and fetal loss are the most common complications. In case of disease relapse during pregnancy, treatment consists of prednisolone. In refractory cases the use of azathioprine and rituximab is recommended.

## Behçet's Disease

It is a chronic, relapsing, multisystemic, inflammatory process characterized by recurrent oral and genital ulcers, ocular, gastrointestinal, neurological manifestations, and thrombosis. Fetomaternal complications include hypertension/preeclampsia, prematurity, FGR and fetal losses. Corticosteroids are the treatment of choice.

## Polyarteritis Nodosa

Polyarteritis nodosa (PAN) is a disorder characterized by necrotizing inflammation of medium size or small arteries. In patients with PAN prevalent features are general symptoms, musculoskeletal, skin and gastrointestinal manifestations, and peripheral neuropathy, especially mononeuritis multiplex. Most common complication seen in pregnancy is premature rupture of membranes (PROM) which results in preterm delivery.

## Wegener Granulomatosis

It is an uncommon, small-vessel, necrotizing vasculitis which usually affects upper respiratory tract, lungs, and kidney. Premature delivery and spontaneous abortions are its effects in pregnancy.

## Microscopic Polyangiitis

Microscopic polyangiitis (MPA) is a systemic, pauci-immune, necrotizing, and small-vessel vasculitis. Patients with MPA developed severe renal disease and pulmonary hemorrhage. Apart from low birthweight and prematurity, the occurrence of an MPA-like syndrome in the newborn has been described, which could be due to the transfer of maternal ANCA through the placenta.

Other rare vasculitides reported in pregnancy are Henoch-Schönlein's Purpura, Churg–Strauss syndrome, cryoglobulinemia and Cogan's syndrome.

## KEY POINTS

- Autoimmune diseases are the principal cause of morbidity in women in the developed countries and are not uncommon in young women in reproductive age group.
- Pregnancy with autoimmune diseases is associated with a higher risk of adverse fetal outcome due to factors such as maternal disease activity, circulating antibodies, and drug treatment.
- SLE, RA, APS are some common autoimmune disorders in women.
- The approach to pregnancy in the autoimmune diseases has undergone great evolution in the past few decades with a significant improvement in fetal outcome.
- Preconceptional counseling has played a major role in this evolution.
- The fetomaternal outcome improves significantly by a multidisciplinary approach involving a rheumatologist, obstetrician and a neonatologist.
- Preconception counseling involves apprising the couple about the maternal and fetal risks, assessing the woman for any evidence of disease activity, any end organ damage and review of the drugs she is taking.
- SLE is a multisystem disorder characterized by remissions and relapses and conception is best advised 6 months after remission to reduce the risk of any flare ups during pregnancy.
- The treatment on which remission has been achieved needs to be continued during pregnancy and the woman has to be carefully observed for any flare up during pregnancy.
- There is an increased risk of congenital heart block, premature delivery, premature rupture of membranes, FGR, intrauterine fetal death and neonatal lupus syndrome in the fetus. Echocardiography is indicated between 18 and 30 weeks.
- RA is an autoimmune disease mainly involving joints of young women. Due to pregnancy related immune modulation the disease is triggered in postpartum period. However, during pregnancy patients have symptomatic improvement and may go into remission.
- Women need to be informed about potential risks related to the disease or to the presence of particular autoantibodies.
- Women should be made aware that treatment should be continued during pregnancy in order to prevent disease flares that may be harmful to both the mother and the baby.
- APS is acquired antibody induced thrombophilia associated with recurrent thrombosis and pregnancy complications such as recurrent abortions, late pregnancy loss, early onset preeclampsia, uteroplacental insufficiency manifesting as FGR and oligohydramnios. Antenatal administration of LDA and LMWH is recommended to prevent adverse fetal outcome.

## REFERENCES

1. Thomas SL, Griffiths C, Smeeth L, Rooney C, Hall AJ. Burden of mortality associated with autoimmune diseases

among females in the United Kingdom. Am J Pub Health. 2010;100(11):2279-87.
2. Borchers AT, Naguwa SM, Keen CL, Gershwin ME. The implications of autoimmunity and pregnancy. J Autoimmun. 2010;34:287-99.
3. Kotzin BL. Systemic lupus erythematosus. Cell. 1996;85:303-6.
4. Osio-Salido E, Manapat-Reyes H. Epidemiology of systemic lupus erythematosus in Asia. Lupus. 2010;19:1365-73.
5. Petri M, Orbai AM, Alarcón GS, Gordon C, Merrill JT, Fortin PR, et al. Derivation and validation of the Systemic Lupus International collaborating clinics classification criteria for systemic lupus erythematosus. Arthritis Rheum. 2012;64:2677-86.
6. TOXNET. Drugs and lactation database (LactMed) of the United States National Library of Medicine. [online] Available from: https://www.nlm.nih.gov/toxnet/index.html. [Last accessed July, 2021].
7. Davidson L. The Scientific Advisory Committee of the Empire Rheumatism Council. A controlled investigation into the aetiology and clinical features of rheumatoid arthritis. BMJ. 1950;8:799-809.
8. Oka M. Effect of pregnancy on the onset and course of rheumatoid arthritis. Ann Rheum Dis. 1953;12(3):227-9.
9. Barrett JH, Brennan P, Fiddler M, Silman AJ. Does rheumatoid arthritis remit during pregnancy and relapse postpartum? Results from a nationwide study in the United Kingdom performed prospectively from late pregnancy. Arthritis Rheum. 1999;42:1219-27.
10. de Man YA, Dolhain RJ, van de Geijn FE, Willemsen SP, Hazes JM. Disease activity of rheumatoid arthritis during pregnancy: results from a nationwide prospective study. Arthritis Rheum. 2008;59:1241-8.
11. Park-Wyllei L. Birth defects after maternal exposure to corticosteroids. Teratology. 2000;62:385-92.
12. Temprano KK, Bandlamudi R, Moore TL. Antirheumatic drugs in pregnancy and lactation. Semin Arthritis Rheum. 2005;35:112-21.
13. Treacy G. Using an analogous monoclonal antibody to evaluate the reproductive and chronic toxicity potential for a humanized anti-TNF alpha monoclonal antibody. Human Exp Toxicol. 2000;19:226-8.
14. Götestam Skorpen C, Hoeltzenbein M, Tincani A, Fischer-Betz R, Elefant E, Chambers C, et al. The EULAR points to consider for use of antirheumatic drugs before pregnancy, and during pregnancy and lactation. Ann Rheum Dis. 2016;75:795.
15. Sheibani S, Cohen R, Kane S, Dubinsky M, Church JA, Mahadevan U. The effect of maternal peripartum anti-TNFa use on infant immune response. Dig Dis Sci. 2016;61(6):1622-7.
16. Kremer JM. Toward a better understanding of methotrexate. Arthritis Rheum. 2004;50:1370-82.
17. Brent RL. Teratogen update: reproductive risks of leflunomide (Arava): a pyrimidine synthesis inhibitor: counseling women taking leflunomide before or during pregnancy and men taking leflunomide who are contemplating fathering a child. Teratology. 2001;63:106-12.
18. Armenti VT, Moritz MJ, Davison JM. Drug safety issues in pregnancy following transplantation and immuno-suppression: effects and outcomes. Drug Saf. 1998;19:219-32.
19. Armenti VT, Radomski JS, Moritz MJ, Gaughan WJ, Philips LZ, McGrory CH, et al. Report from the National Transplantation Pregnancy Registry (NTPR): outcomes of pregnancy after transplantation. Clin Transpl. 2001;97-105.
20. Pergola PE, Kancharla A, Riley DJ. Kidney transplantation during the first trimester of pregnancy: immunosuppression with mycophenolate mofetil, tacrolimus, and prednisone. Transplantation. 2001;71:994-7.
21. Le Ray C, Coulomb A, Elefant E, Frydman R, Audibert E. Mycophenolate mofetil in pregnancy after renal transplantation: a case of major fetal malformations. Obstet Gynecol. 2004;103(5 Pt 2):1091-4.
22. Stirrat GM. Recurrent miscarriage: definition and epidemiology. Lancet. 1990;336:673-5.
23. Branch DW, Scott JR, Kouchenour NK. Obstetric complications associated with lupus anticoagulant. N Engl J Med. 1985;313:1322-6.
24. Gharavi AE, Pierangeli SS, Levy RA, Harris N. Mechanisms of pregnancy loss in antiphospholipid syndrome. Clin Obstet Gynecol. 2001;44:11-9.
25. Abrahams VM, Chamley LW, Salmon JE. Emerging treatment models in rheumatology: antiphospholipid syndrome and pregnancy: pathogenesis to translation. Arthritis Rheumatol. 2017;69:1710.
26. Matrai CE, Rand JH, Baergen RN. Absence of distinct immunohistochemical distribution of annexin A5, C3b, C4d, and C5b-9 in placentas from patients with antiphospholipid antibodies, preeclampsia, and systemic lupus erythematosus. Pediatr Dev Pathol. 2019;22:431.
27. Wilson WA, Gharavi AE, Koike T, Lockshin MD, Branch DW, Piette JC, et al. International consensus statement on preliminary classification criteria for definite antiphospholipid syndrome: report of an international workshop. Arthritis Rheum. 1999;42:1309-11.
28. Miyakis S, Lockshin MD, Atsumi T, Branch DW, Brey RL, Cervera R, et al. International consensus statement on an update of the classification criteria for definite antiphospholipid syndrome (APS). J Thromb Haemost. 2006;4:295-306.
29. Keeling D, Mackie I, Moore GW, Greer IA, Greaves M; British Committee for Standards in Haematology. Guidelines on the investigation and management of antiphospholipid syndrome. Br J Haematol. 2012;157:47-58.
30. Bates SM, Greer IA, Middeldorp S, Veenstra DL, Prabulos AM, Vandvik PO. VTE, thrombophilia, antithrombotic therapy, and pregnancy—antithrombotic therapy and prevention of thrombosis, 9th edition: American college of chest physicians evidence-based clinical practice guidelines. Chest. 2012;141(2 Suppl):e691S-e736S.
31. Royal College of Obstetricians and Gynaecologists. Thrombosis and Embolism during Pregnancy and the Puerperium, Reducing the Risk. Greentop Guideline 37a. 2015.
32. Vaquero E, Lazzarin N, Valensise H, Menghini S, Menghini S, Di Pierro G, et al. Pregnancy outcome in recurrent spontaneous abortion associated with antiphospholipid antibodies: a comparative study of intravenous immunoglobulin versus prednisone plus low-dose aspirin. Am J Reprod Immunol. 2001;45:174-9.
33. Stephenson MD, Kutteh WH, Purkiss S, Librach C, Schultz P, Houlihan E, et al. Intravenous immunoglobulin and idiopathic secondary recurrent miscarriage: a multicentered

33. randomized placebo-controlled trial. Human Reprod. 2010;25:2203-9.
34. Ruiz-Irastorza G, Crowther M, Branch W, Khamashta MA. Antiphospholipid syndrome. Lancet. 2010;376:1498-1509.
35. Lockshin MD. Autoimmunity, infertility and assisted reproductive technologies. Lupus. 2004;13:669-6.
36. Bertsias G, Ionnadis JPA, Boletis J, et al. EULAR recommendations for the management of systemic lupus erythematosus. Report of a Task Force of the EULAR Standing Committee for international clinical studies including therapeutics. Ann Rheum Dis. 2008;67:195-205.
37. Huong LT, Wechsler B, Piette JC. Induction d'ovulation et lupus. Ann Med Interne. 2003;154:45-50.
38. Levine AB, Lockshin MD. Assisted reproductive technology in SLE and APS. Lupus. 2014;23:1239-41.
39. Shulman A. Safety of IVF under anticoagulant therapy in patients at risk for thrombo-embolic events. Reprod Biomed Online. 2006;12:354-8.
40. Chan WS, Dixon ME. The "ART" of thromboembolism: a review of assisted reproductive technology and thromboembolic complications. Thromb Res. 2008;121:713-26.
41. Girolami A, Scandellari R, Tezza F, et al. Arterial thrombosis in young women after ovarian stimulation: case report and review of the literature. J Thromb Thrombolysis. 2007;24:169-74.
42. Bellver J, Pellicer A. Ovarian stimulation for ovulation induction and in vitro fertilization in patients with systemic lupus erythematosus and antiphospholipid syndrome. Fertil Steril. 2009;92:1803-10.
43. Lisa R, Sammaritano LR, Bermas BL, Chakravarty EE, et al. 2020 American College of Rheumatology Guideline for the Management of Reproductive Health in Rheumatic and Musculoskeletal Diseases. Arthritis Care & Research. 2020;72(4):461-88.
44. Tincani A, Rebaioli CB, Andreoli L, Lojacono A, Motta M. Neonatal effects of maternal antiphospholipid syndrome. Curr Rheumatol Rep. 2009;11:70-6.

# Thromboembolism in Pregnancy

*Sarita Singh, Swaraj Batra, Reena Jain*

## INTRODUCTION

Venous thromboembolism (VTE) comprises deep vein thrombosis (DVT) and pulmonary embolism (PE). 75-80% cases of VTE in pregnancy are contributed by DVT and 20-25% are due to PE.[1] The risk of VTE is increased during pregnancy, its risk increases as the gestational age increases, the increased VTE risk persists in postpartum period and is highest in first 3-6 weeks of postpartum period.[2,3]

The estimated incidence of VTE in western studies is 0.5-2.2/1,000 pregnancies.[4-6] Population based studies are lacking in India; the incidence of VTE in pregnant females was 0.1% in a single center study.[7]

Venous thromboembolism is the leading cause of maternal mortality in developed countries, being 13.8% of all maternal deaths while in developing countries it is 3.1% of all maternal deaths.[8] Mortality in VTE is primarily due to massive PE; most common source of pulmonary embolus is a thrombus embolizing from veins of lower extremities. Risk of PE is greater with thrombosis of iliofemoral veins as compared to calf veins and the former is more common in pregnancy.[9] VTE can also have long-term sequelae including pulmonary hypertension, right heart failure, and post-thrombotic syndrome (PTS). The women with history of VTE may also suffer from poor pregnancy outcomes such as recurrent pregnancy losses, fetal growth restriction (FGR), stillbirths, early-onset severe preeclampsia, and abruptio placenta.

Guidelines that have been published for management and prevention of VTE are largely based on studies among nonpregnant females and high quality studies among pregnant females addressing management and prevention of VTE are lacking.[10-19]

## PATHOPHYSIOLOGY

Hemostasis is a normal physiological process comprising four major steps occurring in following order:
- *Step 1*: Vasoconstriction
- *Step 2*: Activation and aggregation of platelets
- *Step 3*: Formation of fibrin clot
- *Step 4*: Dissolution of clot by fibrinolysis.

Pregnancy is a prothrombotic state and all the three components of Virchow's triad that predispose to thrombosis are present in pregnancy and these are:
1. Hypercoagulability
2. Venous stasis
3. Vascular damage

*Hypercoagulability:* The physiological changes occurring during pregnancy result in hypercoagulability thus, increasing the risk of VTE[20] **(Table 1)**.

*Stasis:* The raised levels of progesterone induce venous stasis. Gravid uterus compresses pelvic and lower limb veins thus, resulting in slowing of venous flow.

*Endothelial injury:* It can occur at the time of delivery and can initiate the thrombus formation.

## RISK FACTORS FOR VENOUS THROMBOEMBOLISM

Besides the physiological changes of pregnancy predisposing to VTE mentioned above, there are other risk factors which also increase the risk of developing VTE in pregnant females **(Table 2)**.

### Thrombophilia

The acquired and inherited thrombophilia result in hypercoagulability and increase the risk of VTE.[17,21-23] About 20-50% of females who have VTE can have underlying thrombophilia.[24]

**TABLE 1:** Physiological changes in coagulation factors during pregnancy.

| Coagulant factors | Levels in pregnancy |
|---|---|
| • Procoagulants: | |
| – Factors VII, VIII, X, and fibrinogen | Increased |
| – von Willebrand factor | Increased |
| – Plasminogen activator inhibitor 1 and 2 | Increased |
| – Factor II, V, and X | Not changed |
| • Anticoagulants: | |
| – Protein S | Decreased |
| – Protein C and antithrombin III | Not changed |

**TABLE 2:** Risk factors for venous thromboembolism (VTE) in pregnancy.

- History of estrogen provoked VTE
- Unprovoked VTE in past
- Family history of VTE in first degree relative
- Inherited thrombophilia
- Antiphospholipid antibodies
- Age > 35 years
- Obesity
- Smoking
- Pregnancy following ART and IVF
- Ovarian hyperstimulation syndrome
- Medical conditions, e.g., active lupus and sickle cell disease
- Surgical procedure
- Systemic infection
- Anemia
- Hyperemesis
- Dehydration
- Gross varicose veins
- Prolonged bed rest
- Long distance travel
- Multifetal gestation
- Parity > 3
- Preeclampsia
- Prolonged labor
- Cesarean section
- Peripartum hysterectomy
- Postpartum hemorrhage
- Puerperal infection
- Still birth

(ART: assisted reproduction therapy; IVF: in vitro fertilization)

The screening for thrombophilia is recommended in patients with a history of VTE, unexplained fetal loss at 20 weeks of gestation or later, hypertension, HELLP (hemolysis, elevated liver enzymes, low platelet count) at <34 weeks gestation, unexplained FGR, family history of VTE or a first degree relative with specific mutation in genes of coagulant factors.[17,23,25]

The thrombophilia screening should not be done during the pregnancy, during VTE episode, and while patient is on treatment with anticoagulants because levels of procoagulant factors are altered during these conditions affecting the results of screening tests.[26]

## PREVENTION OF DEEP VEIN THROMBOSIS (THROMBOPROPHYLAXIS)

It is recommended that all women should undergo assessment of risk for VTE in early pregnancy or prepregnancy and assessment should be repeated if the woman is admitted to hospital for any reason or develops other intercurrent problems and should be assessed again in the postpartum period.[15]

The Royal College of Obstetricians and Gynaecologists (RCOG) guidelines stratifies risk of VTE in antenatal and postnatal period on the basis of pre-existing risk factors, pregnancy related risk factors, and transient risk factors. The thromboprophylaxis recommendations are based on the risk stratification using these risk factors[15] **(Table 3)**.

## DEEP VEIN THROMBOSIS

Any pregnant woman with clinical suspicion of DVT should be evaluated urgently as 15–24% of untreated DVT patients can have PE and it is fatal in 15% of them and 66% of deaths occur within 30 minutes of the embolic event.[14]

**TABLE 3:** Risk stratification and thromboprophylaxis during pregnancy and postpartum period.

| Risk stratification | Thromboprophylaxis |
|---|---|
| **Antepartum** | |
| *High-risk:* Any previous venous thromboembolism (VTE), except single VTE related to major surgery | Antenatal prophylaxis with low-molecular-weight-heparin (LMWH) |
| *Intermediate risk* <br>• Single VTE—surgery related <br>• High-risk thrombophilia$ with no VTE <br>• Medical comorbidities# <br>• Surgical procedure <br>• Ovarian hyperstimulation syndrome (first trimester) | Antenatal prophylaxis with LMWH to be considered |
| *Risk factors:*## <br>• ≥4 risk factors | • Prophylaxis with LMWH from first trimester |
| • 3 risk factors | • Prophylaxis with LMWH from 28 weeks |
| *Low-risk:* <br>• <3 risk factors## <br>• Transient risk factors (hyperemesis, long distance travel, and systemic infection) | • Early ambulation <br>• Early ambulation |
| **Postpartum** | |
| *High-risk:* <br>• Previous VTE <br>• High-risk thrombophilia$ <br>• Low-risk thrombophilia* with family history <br>• Already receiving LMWH | LMWH: At least for 6 weeks |
| *Intermediate risk:* <br>• Cesarean section <br>• BMI ≥ 40 kg/m² <br>• Medical comorbidities# <br>• Admission >3 days <br>• Surgical procedure in puerperium except perineal repair <br>• ≥2 risk factors### | LMWH: At least 10 days |
| *Low-risk:* <2 risk factors### | Early ambulation |

$High-risk thrombophilias: Homozygous for factor V Leiden, homozygous for prothrombin gene *G20210A* mutation, protein C or S deficiency and antithrombin deficiency.
*Low-risk thrombophilias: Heterozygous for factor V Leiden; heterozygous for prothrombin *G20210A* mutation.
#Cancer, heart failure, active SLE, IBD, Type I DM with nephropathy, sickle cell disease, and nephrotic syndrome.
##Obesity, age >35 years, parity ≥3, smoker, gross varicose veins, PIH, immobility, VTE family history, low-risk thrombophilias, multiple pregnancy, in-vitro fertilization or assisted reproduction.
###Age >35 years, BMI ≥ 30 kg/m², smoker, elective cesarean section, parity ≥3, low-risk thrombophilia, VTE family history, active infection, gross varicose veins, immobility, multiple pregnancy, PIH, preterm delivery, still birth, operative delivery, PPH or blood transfusion, and prolonged labor.
(BMI: body mass index; SLE: systemic lupus erythematosus; IBD: inflammatory bowel disease; DM: diabetes mellitus; PIH: pregnancy-induced hypertension; PPH: postpartum hemorrhage)

## Signs and Symptoms

The clinicians should have a high index of suspicion for DVT because symptoms and signs of DVT can be taken as normal physiological changes of pregnancy. In pregnant women, 90% of DVTs are in left lower limb. The probable causes are compression of the left iliac vein by the right iliac and the ovarian arteries that cross the vein on left side (May-Thurner syndrome/iliac vein compression syndrome), and compression on the left pelvic veins by the presenting part due to dextrorotation of the uterus.[27] The DVT is categorized into proximal and distal, distal DVT is thrombosis below the knee, and includes DVTs of the paired peroneal, posterior tibial, anterior tibial, and/or the deep calf muscle veins; proximal DVT is thrombosis of femoral and iliac veins. In pregnant women proximal thrombosis is more common (72%), as compared to nonpregnant females (9%). The most common symptoms of DVT are swelling in leg, pain or discomfort in extremity, other symptoms which can be seen are difficulty in walking and erythema. The symptoms of isolated iliac vein thrombosis are abdominal pain, back pain, and/or swelling of the entire leg. The signs of DVT are change in limb color, difference in limb circumference of >2 cm and calf pain on squeezing or stretching Achilles tendon (Homan's sign). The LEFt clinical rule comprises three variables, left leg presentation (L), calf circumference difference of at least 2 cm (E for edema), and first trimester presentation (Ft), this clinical rule has high negative predictive value, however, its clinical utility is limited as it can be used only in first trimester of pregnancy.[27]

## Diagnostic Tests

The diagnostic tests for DVT include Doppler venous ultrasound, magnetic resonance venography (MRV), computed tomography (CT), and D-dimer assay.

### Doppler Venous Ultrasound (Fig. 1)

Real-time duplex compression ultrasonography (CUS) with color Doppler is the first investigation for diagnosing DVT in pregnant women.[28] CUS has been well studied for diagnosing DVT in pregnancy and has various advantages.

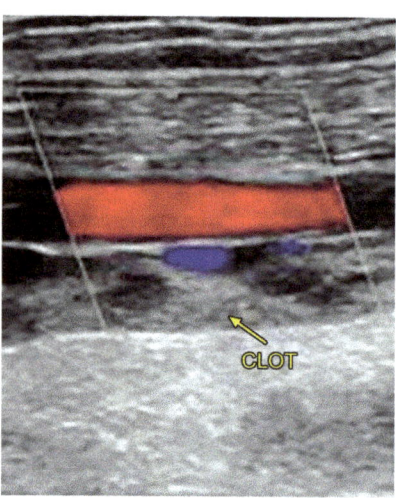

**Fig. 1:** Doppler venous ultrasound.

It is safe, rapid, noninvasive and can be done at the bedside. Noncompressibility of the venous lumen is the most accurate diagnostic criteria for venous thrombosis. In patient with high suspicion of DVT and initial negative CUS, serial CUS can be done over a 7 days period, on 3rd and 7th day.[29] The serial CUS with Doppler imaging has high sensitivity (94.1%) and high negative predictive value (99.5%) for diagnosing DVT.[29] The CUS with Doppler is first investigation during the pregnancy for suspected iliac vein thrombosis also, as iliac vein thrombi are extensive in pregnant females.

### Computed Tomography and Magnetic Resonance Imaging

Computed tomography and magnetic resonance imaging (MRI) are alternative modalities to establish the diagnosis of DVT and are indicated when there is a strong clinical suspicion of DVT and CUS findings are equivocal or negative. The CT is not indicated during pregnancy due to obvious risk of radiation exposure to the fetus, MRI has shown to be sensitive, specific, and highly reproducible for the diagnosis of DVT in nonpregnant patients, also the true extent of a DVT into the pelvis/abdomen can be determined.[30,31] The imaging protocols of MRI without gadolinium, magnetic resonance direct thrombus imaging (MRDTI) are used in pregnancy as these protocols are safe for fetus.[32] The high signal intensity within a vein on T1 images (methemoglobin in the thrombus) is diagnostic of acute venous thrombus in MRI, other features that suggest acute thrombus are enlargement of the vein and perivascular inflammation.[33]

### D-dimer Assay

The D-dimer is product of fibrin degradation formed by plasmin. D-dimer utility in diagnosis of DVT in pregnant women is limited due to physiologically increased levels during pregnancy. The D-dimer alone is not recommended in pregnant or postpartum patients for diagnosing DVT or PE.[34]

### Diagnostic Algorithm for Deep Vein Thrombosis

The CUS with Doppler screening for all veins of lower limb is first investigation for diagnosing DVT in pregnancy. Imaging of the iliac veins should also be done if there is high index of suspicion and CUS is negative for lower limb veins including femoral vein. The serial CUS with Doppler imaging can be performed over a 7-day period if initial CUS is negative; CUS is usually repeated on day 3 and day 7. In women with high clinical suspicion of isolated iliac vein thrombosis (swelling of the entire leg and flank, buttock, or back pain) in whom CUS is negative or nondiagnostic, MRDTI can be done if available, if MRI is not available then depending on the clinical suspicion one can start anticoagulation empirically if risk of bleeding is not high and follow-up is done with serial CUS (**Flowchart 1**).[14]

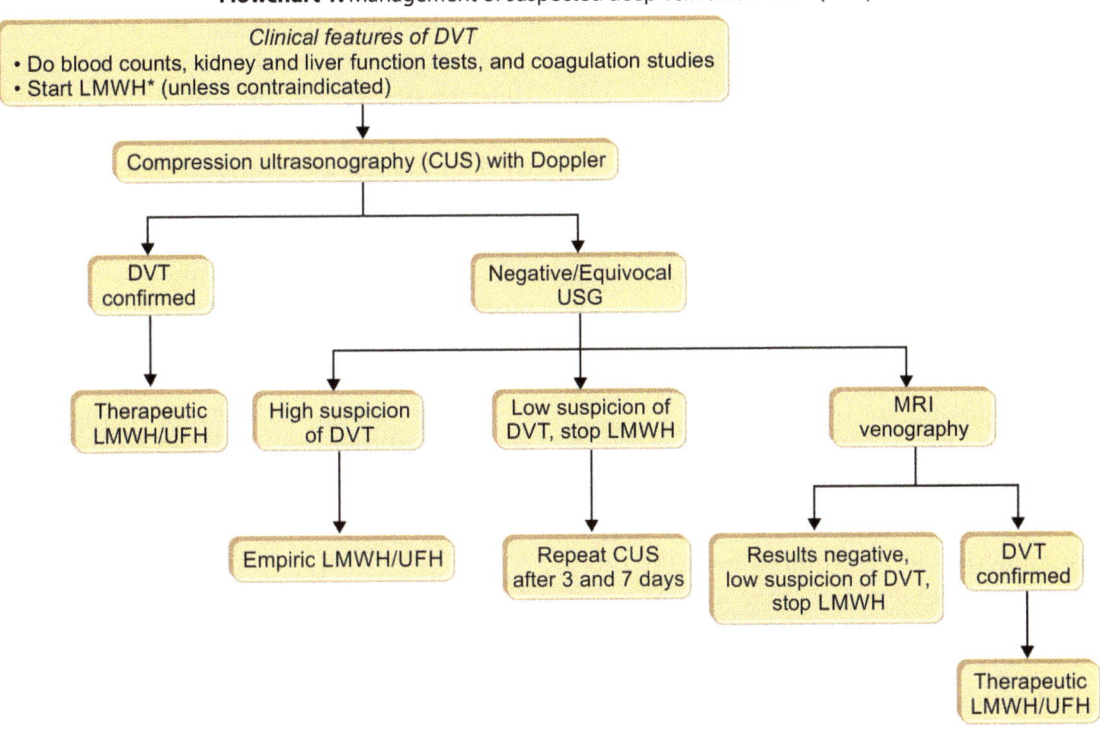

**Flowchart 1:** Management of suspected deep vein thrombosis (DVT).

*LMWH (Low molecular weight heparin) preferred over UFH (unfractionated heparin)
(MRI: magnetic resonance imaging; USG: ultrasonography)

## Management of Deep Vein Thrombosis

The initial management of DVT is leg elevation and anticoagulation. The limb elevation and graduated elastic compression stocking help in reducing edema. Early mobilization is advocated. Meta-analysis of randomized controlled trials (RCTs) have shown that early ambulation with graduated elastic compression stockings results in faster recovery from pain and swelling and it does not increase the risk of PE.[35]

The mainstay in management of DVT is prompt anticoagulation. Anticoagulation should be started if there is high index of clinical suspicion, until the diagnosis is excluded by testing, unless anticoagulation use is strongly contraindicated.[14]

### Classification of Anticoagulants

*Indirect thrombin inhibitors*
- Unfractionated heparin (UFH)
- Low molecular weight heparins (LMWHs): Enoxaparin, nadroparin, dalteparin, reviparin, and tinzaparin
- Heparnoids-danaparoid and lepirudin
- Fondaparinux.
  *Vitamin K antagonists:* Warfarin and acenocoumarol.

*Thrombin inhibitors:* Dabigatran.

*Anti-Xa inhibitors:* Rivaroxaban, apixaban, edoxaban, and betrixaban.

### Unfractionated Heparin

It is a mixture of polysaccharide chains ranging in molecular weight from 3,000 to 30,000 daltons. It binds to antithrombin III (AT-III) and forms a complex which inhibits factors IIa, IXa, and Xa.

### Low Molecular Weight Heparins

Low molecular weight heparins are produced by enzymatic or chemical depolymerization of UFH. LMWHs bind to AT-III and this complex selectively inhibits factor Xa. Each LMWH is a distinct molecule and cannot be used interchangeably.

*Danaparoid:* Danaparoid is a heparinoid, it is administered by intravenous (IV) or subcutaneous (SC) injection.

*Lepirudin:* Lepirudin is a direct thrombin inhibitor used in management of patients of heparin induced thrombocytopenia.

### Fondaparinux

Fondaparinux is a synthetic pentasaccharide that functions as an anticoagulant through specific inhibition of factor Xa via antithrombin.

### Oral Anticoagulants

Warfarin is a vitamin K antagonist. It inhibits production of factors II, VII, IX, and X.

## Anticoagulants for Venous Thromboembolism in Pregnancy

The anticoagulants of choice for treating VTE in pregnancy are LMWHs or UFH due to their established efficacy and safety in treating VTE.[36,37] LMWHs are more effective than UFH for treatment and prevention of VTE in pregnant females.[36,37] Also, the LMWHs are safer than UFH as the risk of obstetrical hemorrhage, heparin-induced thrombocytopenia (HIT), and osteoporosis is lower with LMWH than UFH.[38,39] Thus, at present LMWH is preferred over UFH for VTE management in pregnancy unless there are cost constraints. In pregnancy enoxaparin and dalteparin have established safety and efficacy.[40,41] The reviparin, tinzaparin, and nadroparin have not been widely used in pregnant women for treating VTE. However, UFH is preferred over LMWH in massive PE, when delivery or surgery is imminent, thrombolysis will be required for VTE, there is renal dysfunction (creatinine clearance <30 mL/min) and when there is cost constrain in using LMWH.

The UFH or LMWH are used in therapeutic or adjusted dose regimen for treating acute VTE or when there is high-risk of VTE (history of recurrent VTE or mechanical heart valves). The therapeutic or adjusted doses of LMWHs are based on the maternal weight though it is still not clear whether to use early pregnancy, prepregnancy, booking or current maternal weight for determining LMWHs dose. Maternal weight at time of booking or in early pregnancy can be used for calculating therapeutic dose of LMWHs.[14] LMWHs therapeutic doses can be given once daily or twice daily, the twice daily regimen is recommended by American College of Obstetricians and Gynecologists (ACOG), other guidelines do not recommend one over other due to lack of evidence.[11,12,14,18] Main advantage of once daily dose is that it improves compliance by simplifying treatment. The UFH therapeutic or adjusted dose regimen of UFH is to achieve activated partial thromboplastin time (APTT) in range of 1.5-2.5 of patient as compared to control value, UFH can be given by SC or IV route depending on urgency of need of anticoagulation.

The full blood count, coagulation screen, renal functions, electrolytes, and liver function tests should be done before starting treatment with LMWH/UFH.[14,42] The doses of LMWHs (enoxaparin and dalteparin) are reduced if the creatinine clearance is <30 mL/min or <20 mL/min with tinzaparin or else one can use UFH.[43]

The routine monitoring to confirm adequate dosing of LMWHs is not recommended, monitoring is recommended only in pregnant women with extreme body weight (<50 kg or ≥90 kg), having underlying renal disease or recurrent VTE.[11,14] The monitoring for adequate dosing of LMWHs is done by measuring anti-Xa level, anti-Xa levels are measured 4 hours after the dose, the therapeutic anti-Xa levels are between 0.6-1.0 and 1.0-2.0 U/mL for twice-daily and once-daily regimens, respectively.[11,14] The periodic monitoring with APTT is required to confirm the adequate dosing of UFH, dose of UFH is titrated to achieve APTT 1.5-2.5 times of control value. APTT is measured 6 hours after the last dose of UFH and in cases of heparin resistance the anti-Xa levels are used for titrating UFH dose. Pregnant women on UFH have low-risk of developing HIT (<1%) thus do not need platelet count monitoring. The postoperative cases have increased risk of HIT, hence, it is recommended that in postoperative obstetric patients, platelet count monitoring should be done starting from day 4 till patient is on UFH, platelet count can be repeated every 3rd or 4th day.[44]

Duration of treatment after acute VTE is with therapeutic doses of LMWH for rest of the pregnancy and is to be continued in postpartum period for at least 6 weeks; a total minimum treatment period of 3-6 months is recommended.[11,14,17] The American College of Chest Physicians (ACCP) guidelines suggest that one can reduce the intensity of therapy after an initial therapeutic dosing as pregnant women are at high-risk of complications from therapeutic dose regimen.[17] A reasonable approach is to individualize the treatment duration on basis of risk stratification depending on patient medical and obstetric risk factors for recurrence of VTE and risk of PE or propagation due to present episode depending on location and size of thrombus.

The prophylactic or intermediate doses (75% of therapeutic dose) of LMWHs are prespecified doses depending on type of LMWH being used, UFH prophylactic or intermediate doses are also prespecified doses as per trimester of pregnancy. The prophylactic or intermediate doses of LMWHs/UFH are used in pregnant females for prevention of VTE or after 3-6 months of treatment of acute VTE episode.[11]

The danaparoid and fondaparinux are second line anticoagulants and are considered only when there is severe allergic reaction or HIT with LMWH/UFH use, danaparoid is preferred over fondaparinux if available.[11,14,45,46]

The oral anticoagulants are listed as category D drug in pregnancy because of known teratogenic effects. They are also associated with still births and increased risk of fetal bleeding. The patients who are on warfarin should have preconceptional counseling and should be switched to LMWH as soon as they conceive. Warfarin can be restarted after 13 weeks in women with cardiac valve replacement who were on warfarin before pregnancy and it can be continued till the time of anticipated labor.[47] Monitoring is required while using oral anticoagulants, INR (international normalized ratio) is measured for monitoring and target is to maintain INR in range of 2.0-3.0.

Direct thrombin inhibitors and anti-Xa inhibitors should be avoided in pregnancy and lactation as there is insufficient data regarding safety during pregnancy for fetus and breastfeeding neonate **(Table 4)**.[12,48]

**TABLE 4:** Anticoagulants dose, side effects, and monitoring.

| Drug | Adjusted (Therapeutic) dose | Intermediate dose | Prophylactic dose | Side effects | Monitoring | Reversal agents |
|---|---|---|---|---|---|---|
| UFH | 10,000 U SC every 12 hours adjust dose to target APTT of 1.5–2.5 of control 6 hours after administration | - | • 1st trimester 5,000 U–7,500 SC 12 hours<br>• 2nd trimester 7,500–10,000 U 12 hours<br>• 3rd trimester 10,000 U 12 hours | • Bleeding<br>• Thrombocytopenia usually after 10 days of therapy<br>• Osteoporosis usually after 2–3 months of therapy Hypersensitivity<br>• Increase AST/ALT | • APTT<br>• Platelet count | Protamine sulfate |
| LMWH | • Enoxaparin 1 mg/kg 12 hourly<br>• Dalteparin 100 U/kg 12 hourly or 200 U/kg once daily<br>• Tinzaparin 175 U/kg once daily | • Enoxaparin 40 mg/kg SC, 12 hourly<br>• Dalteparin 5,000 U/kg SC, 12 hourly | • Enoxaparin 40 mg SC OD<br>• Dalteparin 5,000 U OD<br>• Tinzaparin 4,500 U OD<br>• Nadroparin 2,850 U OD | • Bleeding Thrombocytopenia Increased AST/ALT | Anti-Xa Platelet count | Partial reversal by protamine sulfate |
| Danaparoid | 2,000 U SC 12 hourly | | 750 U SC 12 hourly | • Bleeding<br>• Asthma exacerbation | Anti Xa (monitoring usually not required) | None |
| Warfarin | Dosage according to INR | | Dosage according to INR | • Bleeding. Congenital anomalies<br>• Miscarriage<br>• Still birth<br>• Fetal-bleeding Neurological sequelae in neonates | INR | • Vitamin K<br>• Fresh frozen plasma |

(AST/ALT: aspartate transaminase/alanine transaminase (alanine aminotransferase); UFH: unfractionated heparin; LWWH: low molecular weight heparin; SC: subcutaneous; INR: international normalised ratio; APTT: activated partial thromboplastin time; OD: once daily)

## PULMONARY EMBOLISM

Pulmonary embolism is a potentially fatal condition and requires prompt management. Any case of suspected PE with clinical features suggestive of VTE should be started on LMWH till the simultaneous diagnostic workup can exclude it.

## Clinical Features

Signs and symptoms of PE depend on the site and extent of embolus. The common presenting symptoms are breathlessness, cough, pleuritic chest pain, hemoptysis, syncope, anxiety, and diaphoresis. The common signs are sudden dyspnea, tachycardia, hypotension, cyanosis, and new murmur. Woman with massive PE may present in shock.

The severity of PE as per American Heart Association (AHA) and ACCP guidelines is:[49]
- *Massive PE*: Persistent hypotension with systolic blood pressure (SBP) < 90 mm Hg lasting >15 minutes or requiring inotropic support, pulselessness, or bradycardia (heart rate < 40 beats/min).
- *Submassive PE*: Right ventricular (RV) dysfunction without systemic hypotension. RV dysfunction is diagnosed on either imaging (transthoracic echocardiogram or computed tomography pulmonary angiography, CTPA) or elevated biomarkers [brain natriuretic peptide (BNP), N-terminal pro-BPN (NT-pro-BNP), or elevated troponin].
- *Low-risk PE*: No hemodynamic instability or RV dysfunction.

## DIAGNOSTIC TESTS

The early diagnosis of PE is essential to improve maternal and fetal outcomes. The patients of PE should be evaluated on urgent basis. In suspected cases of PE, it is recommended that the diagnostic workup should be completed within 1 hour of presentation.

The investigations which are done in patients suspected of PE are given here.

## Arterial Blood Gas Analysis

Hypoxia and hypocapnia are usually seen with massive PE, however, normal $PO_2$ does not exclude the diagnosis.[50]

## Electrocardiogram

Electrocardiogram (ECG) may show tachycardia, right axis deviation, P-pulmonale, nonspecific T-wave inversions, and classic S wave in lead I, Q in lead III, T in lead III. Right axis deviation and right bundle branch block are suggestive of significant cardiac compromise. Up to 40–60% of patients can have these ECG changes.[51]

## Chest X-ray

The most common findings in chest X-ray (CXR) are atelectasis, pleural-based opacity, and pleural effusion. Classic wedge shape infiltrate, decreased vascularity, and enlarged right descending pulmonary artery may be seen.[52] It is helpful in excluding other diagnoses with similar clinical presentation, e.g., pneumonia, pneumothorax, pleural effusion, and pulmonary edema.[52] The radiation dose to the fetus from a CXR performed at any stage of pregnancy is negligible (<0.01 mSv). The CXR is helpful in deciding for the next investigation, normal CXR increases the likelihood of definitive V/Q result, and in case CXR is abnormal and clinical possibility of PE is high CTPA has better diagnostic yield.[52]

## Echocardiography

Echocardiographic abnormalities of right ventricle function and size are seen with a large embolus. Typical findings are dilated and hypokinetic right ventricle and tricuspid regurgitation. Echocardiography (ECHO) helps in planning management, stratifying risk, and delineating the prognosis.

## Ventilation and Perfusion Scan (V/Q)

It is a well-established diagnostic modality for confirming PE in pregnant patients. Patients are categorized into different diagnostic probability categories, including high, intermediate, low, and normal on the basis of V/Q scan results. The V/Q scan is modified in pregnancy and V component is only done if Q is abnormal to reduce radiation exposure. In patients other than normal or high probability categories, further evaluation is required. Main drawbacks of V/Q scan are that it is time consuming, not available routinely, and sensitivity depends on the clinical suspicion of PE **(Figs. 2A and B)**.

## Computed Tomography Pulmonary Angiography (CTPA)

Computed tomography pulmonary angiography is highly sensitive (94%) and specific (100%) investigation for PE with very high negative predictive value (99.1%). The normal CTPA essentially rules out the diagnosis of PE.

### V/Q Scan or Computed Tomography Pulmonary Angiography for Diagnosis of Pulmonary Embolism

The main advantages of CTPA over V/Q scan is that it can be done rapidly, more widely available, CTPA delivers a low radiation dose to the fetus, and also rules out other similar medical conditions, e.g., pneumonia, pulmonary edema,

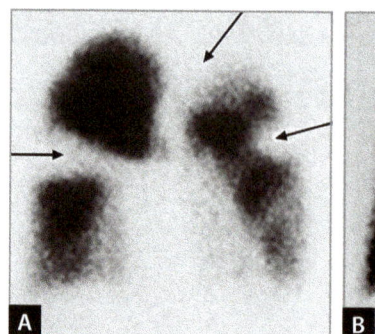 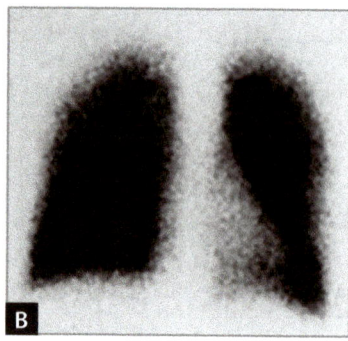

**Figs. 2A and B:** (A) Perfusion scan: Pulmonary emboli; (B) Normal.

and aortic dissection.[53,54] The CTPA and V/Q scan radiation doses exposure to fetus are well below accepted thresholds for teratogenicity; fetal death, fetal growth restriction (FGR), and the risk of malignancy in childhood is also very low.[53] The maternal radiation exposure is 20–100 times greater with CTPA than V/Q scan thus concern for increased risk of breast cancer with CTPA. However, the risk of breast cancer with CTPA is very small and it has been overestimated.[55] The radiation doses with CTPA can be reduced by 20–40% by placing the bismuth shields over the breasts.[56] As per recent Cochrane review both V/Q scan and CTPA are reasonable in excluding PE in pregnancy, however overall quality of evidence is low, and which one is more accurate is not clear yet.[57] Thus, choice between V/Q scan or CTPA for definitive diagnosis of PE depends on available modality and expertise.

## Magnetic Resonance Angiography

Newer generation MRI has faster imaging acquisition time and this has made possible to visualize pulmonary vasculature. The studies in nonpregnant females are promising and have high sensitivity and specificity for diagnosing PE. There are no reported studies of MR angiography use in pregnancy at present and its role is yet to be established.

## Arteriography

Pulmonary arteriography was the gold standard test for diagnosis of PE. This procedure is associated with morbidity and mortality primarily due to catheter placement and contrast injection. Complications can occur, i.e., local hematoma, renal failure, respiratory failure, and cardiac perforation. At present it has been replaced by CTPA and V/Q scan for diagnosing PE.

## Diagnostic Approach

The diagnostic approach of PE depends on risk factors for developing VTE, clinical condition of patient, and available investigations. Patients at high-risk of VTE and presenting with clinical features of PE should be started on anticoagulation immediately. CUS of lower limb should be done in patients of PE who also have clinical features of DVT.[58-60]

The patients with clinical features of PE in whom CUS diagnoses DVT can be managed as PE, if CUS is negative, CTPA or V/Q scan are next line of investigation. The CTPA is preferred if CXR is abnormal and V/Q scan if CXR is normal.[60] Patients on whom CTPA or V/Q scan confirm diagnosis of PE are continued on anticoagulation, if CTPA or V/Q scan is negative, PE is rule out. In patients who have high suspicion of PE with indeterminate CTPA or V/Q scan for PE diagnosis, the imaging films should be reviewed by expert if available otherwise either CTPA or V/Q scan whichever was not done earlier is done.[60] Management of suspected case of PE is given in **Flowchart 2**.

## Management of Pulmonary Embolism

Pulmonary embolism, especially massive PE, has high mortality. Patients with PE should be managed expeditiously by multidisciplinary team in intensive care unit.

## Supportive Treatment

- Supplemental oxygen for hypoxia.
- Vasopressors or inotropic support for hypotension.

If required, maternal resuscitation as per standard ABC protocol should be started. In event of cardiac arrest in a pregnant woman, cardiopulmonary resuscitation should be performed with manual left uterine displacement.

## Specific Treatment

### Anticoagulation

Intravenous UFH is used for treatment of PE as it has rapid onset of action, extensive experience with its use in PE, and is rapidly adjustable in case thrombolytic therapy is also required.[58] The UFH is started at loading dose of 80 U/kg, followed by a continuous IV infusion of 18 U/kg/h, in case patient has received thrombolysis then loading dose of UFH is omitted.[61] The dose of UFH is titrated by measuring APTT and it is measured 4–6 hours after the loading dose, 6 hours after any dose change and once therapeutic range is reached at least twice a day. The target is to achieve APTT ratio 1.5–2.5 times the laboratory control value. The anti-Xa level is used for titrating the UFH dose in cases of resistance to UFH, and target range is 0.5–1.2 U/mL for patients with PE.

### Thrombolytic Therapy

At present recommendation of thrombolytic therapy is for patients with severe PE with hemodynamic instability.[49] Patients with massive PE treated with thrombolysis have significant reduction of recurrent PE and death. In a recent systematic review it was concluded that the risk of using thrombolytics in pregnancy is reasonable with encouraging results in majority of cases.[62] The complication rate of thrombolytic treatment was also similar in pregnant and

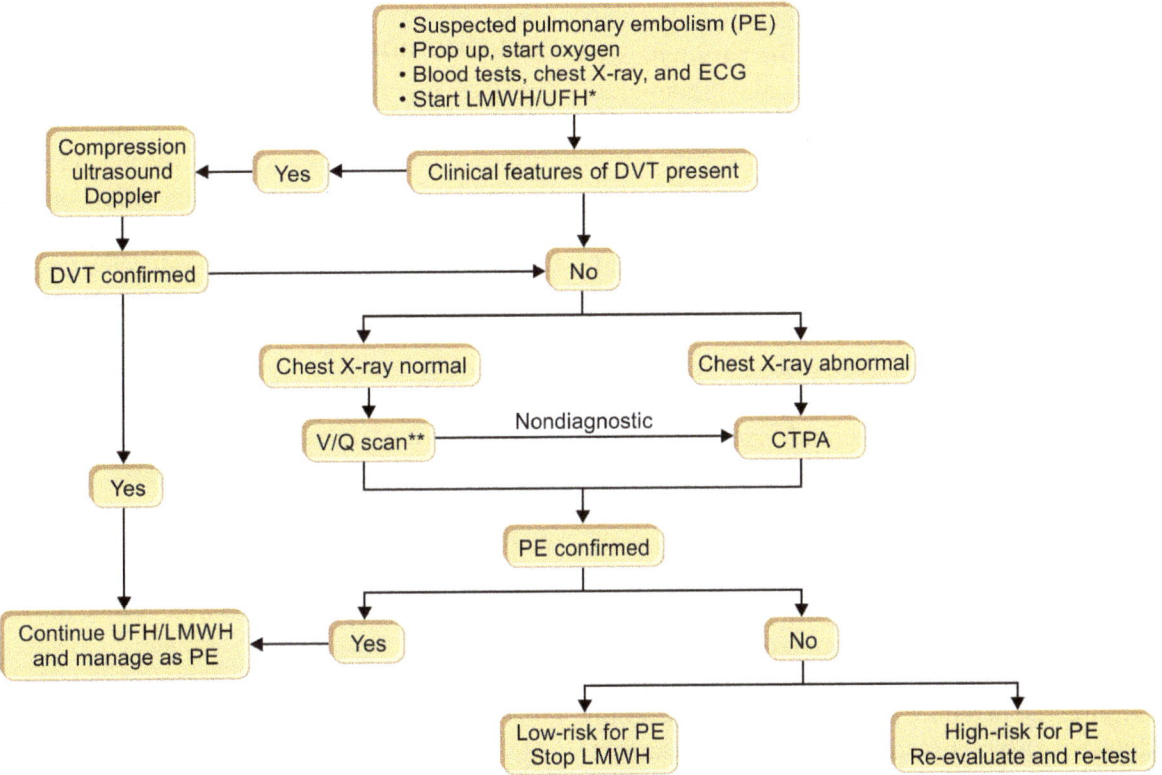

**Flowchart 2:** Management of suspected pulmonary embolism (based on RCOG guidelines).

*LMWH (low-molecular-weight heparin) is preferred over UFH (unfractionated heparin). UFH is preferred in massive pulmonary embolism.[14]
**If V/Q scan (ventilation/perfusion scan) is not available or not diagnostic, perform CTPA (computerized tomography pulmonary angiogram).
(DVT: deep vein thrombosis; RCOG: Royal College of Obstetricians and Gynecologists)

nonpregnant women and poor fetal outcome was found in mothers with poor prognosis.[63] The various thrombolytic drugs, streptokinase, urokinase, recombinant tissue plasminogen activator (rtPA; alteplase), and tenecteplase have been used in pregnant females with PE for thrombolysis.

### Surgical or Catheter Embolectomy

The embolectomy can be done in patients not suitable for thrombolysis or are in a moribund state.[64] Another important indication is, massive PE within 24 hours of delivery due to high-risk of major bleeding with thrombolysis.

### Inferior Vena Cava Filter

The inferior vena cava (IVC) filters are placed temporarily when recurrent VTE occurs despite adequate anticoagulation, or when anticoagulation is contraindicated absolutely (such as the peripartum period).[14] The ACCP or ACOG societies do not have specific recommendations for using IVC filter during pregnancy.[11,17] Thus, use of IVC filter in pregnancy for treating VTE should be based on expected risk/benefit for individual and after discussion with patient.[65] The complications seen with IVC filter are failure to retrieve the filter (26%), perforation of the IVC (7.0%), fracture of filter (5.1%), and thrombosis of the filter (2.3%).[66]

## Intrapartum Management of Patients on Anticoagulants during Pregnancy

For women on anticoagulants, timing of delivery is decided on the basis of obstetric indications. The prophylactic LMWH should be stopped at least 12 hours, and therapeutic LMWH should be stopped at least 24 hours before scheduled induction of labor or cesarean delivery respectively.[67] The SC UFH should be stopped 12 hours and IV UFH should be stopped 6 hours before delivery respectively. The coagulation studies should be done in patients on UFH before invasive and surgical procedures. If any urgent or emergent procedure is anticipated one should switch to IV UFH from LMWH. The regional anesthesia or analgesia should not be given at least 24 hours before the last dose of therapeutic LMWH.[67] Women who undergo active labor shortly after injecting LMWH can be reassured as bleeding complications are very uncommon with LMWH. Women who are receiving therapeutic doses of UFH, monitoring with APTT is recommended and if APTT is markedly prolonged near the time of delivery, protamine sulfate may be required to reduce the risk of bleeding. The pneumatic compression devices can be used during the time when anticoagulation has been discontinued to reduce the risk of VTE. The wound drains (abdominal and rectus sheath) at time of cesarean section can be placed and the skin incision should be closed with interrupted sutures to allow drainage of any hematoma in patients on therapeutic doses of LMWH/UFH.

## Postpartum Management of Patients Anticoagulated during Pregnancy

The anticoagulation therapy can be started 4-6 hours after vaginal delivery or 6-12 hours after cesarean section as this minimizes the risk of bleeding without increasing risk of VTE.[67] Prophylactic LMWH is started at least 4 hours postoperatively and therapeutic LMWH is started after at least 8-12 hours postoperatively. The pregnant women who have received neuraxial anesthesia during delivery, the prophylactic LMWH should be started at least 12 hours after the neuraxial block or at least 4 hours after the epidural catheter removal, whichever is later. The therapeutic LMWH should be started at least 24 hours after the neuraxial block and at least 4 hours after the removal of the epidural catheter. The LMWH, UFH or warfarin, can be used safely in postpartum period as they are not excreted in breast milk. Women in whom long-term postpartum (>6 weeks) anticoagulation therapy is needed, either LMWH or warfarin can be used. Warfarin is usually started once the risk of postpartum bleeding has subsided, it should be started at least 5 days after normal delivery. Warfarin administration is overlapped with LMWH or UFH until INR is in therapeutic range (2.0-3.0) for 2 consecutive days. Women who are on warfarin need routine monitoring with INR to prevent both over and under coagulation.

The pneumatic compression devices should be used until the patient is ambulatory and anticoagulation therapy is restarted.

## Post-thrombotic Syndrome

The PTS manifests as chronic persistent leg swelling, feeling of heaviness, dependant cyanosis, telangiectasis, chronic pigmentation, eczema, associated varicose veins, and in severe cases venous ulceration may be present. The prevalence of PTS is variable and it can be up to 42%; independent predictors of the development of PTS are proximal postnatal thrombosis, smoking, age > 33 years, recurrent ipsilateral DVT, and obesity.[68] In an RCT, a significantly lower rate of PTS was seen in nonpregnant patients who were given prolonged LMWH, on further subanalysis the PTS rates were even lower in proximal DVT patients who received prolonged LMWH.[69] As proximal DVT is more common in pregnant women, a longer duration of LMWH treatment may be useful in preventing PTS. In a meta-analysis, the graduated elastic compression stockings have shown substantial protection against the development of PTS in the nonpregnant females.[70] However, in recent RCT compression stockings compared to a placebo did not prevent the PTS and also did not reduce the severity of PTS.[71]

## KEY POINTS

- Venous thromboembolism is the leading cause of maternal mortality in developed world.

- Pregnant and postpartum women are at increased risk of VTE.
- A high index of suspicion helps in early diagnosis and timely treatment.
- Women with thrombophilia disorders should be counseled about increased risk of thrombosis and adverse outcomes during pregnancy, and should be offered prophylactic antepartum and postpartum anticoagulant therapy.
- If VTE is suspected during pregnancy, treatment should be started on clinical suspicion and should not be withheld until an objective diagnosis is obtained. LMWH is safe, effective, and has a low-risk of bleeding. Treatment can be stopped if test results exclude the diagnosis of VTE.
- The mainstay of treatment for pulmonary thromboembolism in pregnancy is anticoagulation with LMWH for a minimum period of 3 months and until at least 6 weeks postpartum.
- Longer duration of LMWH treatment may be useful in preventing PTS.
- Timely diagnosis and institution of therapeutic and prophylactic anticoagulation are essential for prevention of maternal morbidity and mortality associated with VTE.

## REFERENCES

1. Blanco-Molina A, Rota LL, Di Micco P, Brenner B, Trujillo-Santos J, Ruiz-Gamietea A, et al. Venous thromboembolism during pregnancy, postpartum or during contraceptive use. Thromb Haemost. 2010;103(2):306-11.
2. Pomp ER, Lenselink AM, Rosendaal FR, Doggen CJ. Pregnancy, the postpartum period and prothrombotic defects: risk of venous thrombosis in the MEGA study. J Thromb Haemost. 2008;6(4):632-7.
3. Jackson E, Curtis KM, Gaffield ME. Risk of venous thromboembolism during the postpartum period: a systematic review. Obstet Gynecol. 2011;117(3):691-703.
4. Heit JA, Kobbervig CE, James AH, Petterson TM, Bailey KR, Melton LJ 3rd. Trends in the incidence of venous thromboembolism during pregnancy or postpartum: a 30-year population-based study. Ann Intern Med. 2005;143(10):697-706.
5. Virkus RA, Løkkegaard EC, Bergholt T, Mogensen U, Langhoff-Roos J, Lidegaard Ø. Venous thromboembolism in pregnant and puerperal women in Denmark 1995-2005. A national cohort study. Thromb Haemost. 2011;106(2):304-9.
6. Kane EV, Calderwood C, Dobbie R, Morris C, Roman E, Greer IA. A population-based study of venous thrombosis in pregnancy in Scotland 1980-2005. Eur J Obstet Gynecol Reprod Biol. 2013;169(2):223-9.
7. Vora S, Ghosh K, Shetty S, Salvi V, Satoskar P. Deep vein thrombosis in antenatal period in a large cohort of pregnancies from western India. Thromb J. 2007;5:9.
8. Say L, Chou D, Gemmill A, Tunçalp Ö, Moller AB, Daniels J, et al. Global causes of maternal death: a WHO systematic analysis. Lancet Glob Health. 2014;2(6):e323-33.
9. Chan WS, Spencer FA, Ginsberg JS. Anatomic distribution of deep vein thrombosis in pregnancy. CMAJ. 2010;182(7):657-60.
10. Cantwell R, Clutton-Brock T, Cooper G, Dawson A, Drife J, Garrod D, et al. Saving Mothers' Lives: Reviewing maternal deaths to make motherhood safer: 2006-2008. The Eighth Report of the Confidential Enquiries into Maternal Deaths in the United Kingdom. BJOG. 2011;118(Suppl 1):1-203.
11. American College of Obstetricians and Gynecologists' Committee on Practice Bulletins—Obstetrics. ACOG Practice Bulletin No. 196: Thromboembolism in pregnancy. Obstet Gynecol. 2018;132(1):e1-17.
12. Bates SM, Rajasekhar A, Middeldorp S, McLintock C, Rodger MA, James AH, et al. American Society of Hematology 2018 guidelines for management of venous thromboembolism: venous thromboembolism in the context of pregnancy. Blood Adv. 2018;2(22):3317-59.
13. Linnemann B, Scholz U, Rott H, Halimeh S, Zotz R, Gerhardt A, et al. Treatment of pregnancy-associated venous thromboembolism–position paper from the working Group in Women's health of the Society of Thrombosis and Haemostasis (GTH). Vasa. 2016;45(2):103-18.
14. Royal College of Obstetricians and Gynaecologists. Thrombosis and Embolism during Pregnancy and the Puerperium: Green Top Guideline No. 37b. London (UK): RCOG; 2015.
15. Royal College of Obstetricians and Gynaecologists. Reducing the risk of venous thromboembolism during pregnancy and the puerperium. Green Top Guideline No. 37a. London (UK): RCOG; 2015.
16. Chan WS, Rey E, Kent NE. Venous thromboembolism and antithrombotic therapy in pregnancy. J Obstet Gynaecol Can. 2014;36(6):527-53.
17. Bates SM, Greer IA, Middeldorp S, Veenstra DL, Prabulos AM, Vandvik PO. VTE, thrombophilia, antithrombotic therapy, and pregnancy: Antithrombotic Therapy and Prevention of Thrombosis, 9th ed: American College of Chest Physicians Evidence-Based Clinical Practice Guidelines. Chest. 2012;141(2 Suppl):e691S-736S.
18. Mclintock C, Brighton T, Chunilal S, Dekker G, McDonnell N, McRae S, et al. Recommendations for the diagnosis and treatment of deep venous thrombosis and pulmonary embolism in pregnancy and the postpartum period. Aust N Z J Obstet Gynaecol. 2012;52(1):14-22.
19. Mclintock C, Brighton T, Chunilal S, Dekker G, McDonnell N, McRae S, et al. Recommendations for the prevention of pregnancy-associated venous thromboembolism. Aust N Z J Obstet Gynaecol. 2012;52(1):3-13.
20. Bremme KA. Haemostatic changes in pregnancy. Best Pract Res Clin Haematol. 2003;16(2):153-68.
21. Croles FN, Nasserinejad K, Duvekot JJ, Kruip MJ, Meijer K, Leebeek FW. Pregnancy, thrombophilia, and the risk of a first venous thrombosis: systematic review and bayesian meta-analysis. BMJ. 2017;359:j4452.
22. American College of Obstetricians and Gynecologists' Committee on Practice Bulletins—Obstetrics. ACOG Practice Bulletin No. 197: Inherited thrombophilias in pregnancy. Obstet Gynecol. 2018;132(1):e18-e34.
23. Robertson L, Wu O, Langhorne P, Twaddle S, Clark P, Lowe GD, et al. Thrombophilia in pregnancy: a systematic review. Br J Haematol. 2006;132(2):171-96.

24. James AH. Venous thromboembolism in pregnancy. Arterioscler Thromb Vasc Biol. 2009;29(3):326-31.
25. Baglin T, Gray E, Greaves M, Hunt BJ, Keeling D, Machin S, et al. Clinical guidelines for testing for heritable thrombophilia. Br J Haematol. 2010;149(2):209-20.
26. Said JM, Ignjatovic V, Monagle PT, Walker SP, Higgins JR, Brennecke SP. Altered reference ranges for protein C and protein S during early pregnancy: implications for the diagnosis of protein C and protein S deficiency during pregnancy. Thromb Haemost. 2010;103(5):984-8.
27. Chan WS, Lee A, Spencer FA, Crowther M, Rodger M, Ramsay T, et al. Predicting deep venous thrombosis in pregnancy: out in "LEFt" field? Ann Intern Med. 2009;151(2):85-92.
28. Le Gal G, Kercret G, Ben Yahmed K, Bressollette L, Robert-Ebadi H, Riberdy L, et al. Diagnostic value of single complete compression ultrasonography in pregnant and postpartum women with suspected deep vein thrombosis: prospective study. BMJ. 2012;344:e2635.
29. Chan WS, Spencer FA, Lee AY, Chunilal S, Douketis JD, Rodger M, et al. Safety of withholding anticoagulation in pregnant women with suspected deep vein thrombosis following negative serial compression ultrasound and iliac vein imaging. CMAJ. 2013;185(4):E194-200.
30. Dronkers CE, Srámek A, Huisman MV, Klok FA. Accurate diagnosis of iliac vein thrombosis in pregnancy with magnetic resonance direct thrombus imaging (MRDTI). BMJ Case Rep. 2016;2016:bcr2016218091.
31. Torkzad MR, Bremme K, Hellgren M, Eriksson MJ, Hagman A, Jörgensen T, et al. Magnetic resonance imaging and ultrasonography in diagnosis of pelvic vein thrombosis during pregnancy. Thromb Res. 2010;126(2):107-12.
32. Ray JG, Vermeulen MJ, Bharatha A, Montanera WJ, Park AL. Association between MRI exposure during pregnancy and fetal and childhood outcomes. JAMA. 2016;316(9):952-61.
33. Saha P, Andia ME, Modarai B, Blume U, Humphries J, Patel AS, et al. Magnetic resonance T1 relaxation time of venous thrombus is determined by iron processing and predicts susceptibility to lysis. Circulation. 2013;128(7):729-36.
34. Damodaram M, Kaladindi M, Luckit J, Yoong W. D-dimers as a screening test for venous thromboembolism in pregnancy: is it of any use? J Obstet Gynaecol. 2009;29(2):101-3.
35. Aissaoui N, Martins E, Mouly S, Weber S, Meune C. A meta-analysis of bed rest versus early ambulation in the management of pulmonary embolism, deep vein thrombosis, or both. Int J Cardiol. 2009;137(1):37-41.
36. Bates SM, Middeldorp S, Rodger M, James AH, Greer I. Guidance for the treatment and prevention of obstetric-associated venous thromboembolism. J Thromb Thrombolysis. 2016;41(1):92-128.
37. Romualdi E, Dentali F, Rancan E, Squizzato A, Steidl L, Middeldorp S, et al. Anticoagulant therapy for venous thromboembolism during pregnancy: a systematic review and a meta-analysis of the literature. J Thromb Haemost. 2013;11(2):270-81.
38. Knol HM, Schultinge L, Veeger NJ, Kluin-Nelemans HC, Erwich JJ, Meijer K. The risk of postpartum haemorrhage in women using high dose of low-molecular-weight heparins during pregnancy. Thromb Res. 2012;130(3):334-8.
39. Rodger MA, Kahn SR, Cranney A, Hodsman A, Kovacs MJ, Clement AM, et al. Long-term dalteparin in pregnancy not associated with a decrease in bone mineral density: substudy of a randomized controlled trial. J Thromb Haemost. 2007;5(8):1600-6.
40. Jacobson B, Rambiritch V, Paek D, Sayre T, Naidoo P, Shan J, et al. Safety and efficacy of enoxaparin in pregnancy: a systematic review and meta-analysis. Adv Ther. 2020;37(1):27-40.
41. Hellgren M, Mistafa O. Obstetric venous thromboembolism: a systematic review of dalteparin and pregnancy. J Obstet Gynaecol. 2019;39(4):439-50.
42. Scottish Intercollegiate Guidelines Network (SIGN). Prevention and management of venous thromboembol-ism. SIGN publication no. 122. Edinburgh: SIGN; 2010.
43. National Patient Safety Agency. (2010). Reducing treatment dose errors with low molecular weight heparins. [online] Available from: http://www. nrls.npsa.nhs.uk/alerts/entryid45=75208 [Last accessed July, 2021].
44. Watson H, Davidson S, Keeling D. Guidelines on the diagnosis and management of heparin-induced thrombocytopenia: second edition. Br J Haematol. 2012;159(5):528-40.
45. Magnani HN. An analysis of clinical outcomes of 91 pregnancies in 83 women treated with danaparoid (Orgaran). Thromb Res. 2010;125(4):297-302.
46. De Carolis S, di Pasquo E, Rossi E, Del Sordo G, Buonomo A, Schiavino D, et al. Fondaparinux in pregnancy: could it be a safe option? A review of the literature. Thromb Res. 2015;135(6):1049-51.
47. van Hagen IM, Roos-Hesselink JW, Ruys TP, Merz WM, Goland S, Gabriel H, et al. Pregnancy in women with a mechanical heart valve: Data of the European Society of Cardiology Registry of Pregnancy and Cardiac Disease (ROPAC). Circulation. 2015;132(2):132-42.
48. Burnett AE, Mahan CE, Vazquez SR, Oertel LB, Garcia DA, Ansell J. Guidance for practical management of DOACs in VTE management. J Thromb Thrombolysis. 2016;41(1):206-32.
49. Jaff MR, McMurtry MS, Archer SL, Cushman M, Goldenberg N, Goldhaber SZ, et al. Management of massive and submassive pulmonary embolism, iliofemoral deep vein thrombosis, and chronic thromboembolic pulmonary hypertension: a scientific statement from the American heart association. Circulation. 2011;123(16):1788-830.
50. Rodger MA, Carrier M, Jones GN, Rasuli P, Raymond F, Djunaedi H, et al. Diagnostic value of arterial blood gas measurement in suspected pulmonary embolism. Am J Respir Crit Care Med. 2000;162(6):2105-8.
51. Rodger M, Makropoulos D, Turek M, Quevillon J, Raymond F, Rasuli P, et al. Diagnostic value of the electrocardiogram in suspected pulmonary embolism. Am J Cardiol. 2000;86(7):807-9.
52. Leung AN, Bull TM, Jaeschke R, Lockwood CJ, Boiselle PM, Hurwitz LM, et al. American Thoracic Society documents:an official American Thoracic Society/Society of Thoracic Radiology Clinical Practice Guideline–evaluation of suspected pulmonary embolism in pregnancy. Radiology. 2012;262(2):635-46.
53. Tromeur C, van der Pol LM, Le Roux PY, Ende-Verhaar Y, Salaun PY, Leroyer C, et al. Computed tomography pulmonary angiography versus ventilation-perfusion lung scanning for diagnosing pulmonary embolism during pregnancy: a systematic review and meta-analysis. Haematologica. 2019;104(1):176-88.

54. Righini M, Robert-Ebadi H, Elias A, Sanchez O, Le Moigne E, Schmidt J, et al. Diagnosis of pulmonary embolism during pregnancy: a multicenter prospective management outcome study. Ann Intern Med. 2018;169(11):766-73.
55. Burton KR, Park AL, Fralick M, Ray JG. Risk of early-onset breast canceramong women exposed to thoracic computed tomography in pregnancy or early postpartum. J Thromb Haemost. 2018;16(5):876-85.
56. Hurwitz LM, Yoshizumi TT, Goodman PC, Nelson RC, Toncheva G, Nguyen GB, et al. Radiation dose savings for adult pulmonary embolus 64-MDCT using bismuth breast shields, lower peak kilovoltage, and automatic tube current modulation. AJR Am J Roentgenol. 2009;192(1):244-53.
57. Van Mens TE, Scheres LJ, de Jong PG, Leeflang MM, Nijkeuter M, Middeldorp S. Imaging for the exclusion of pulmonary embolism in pregnancy. Cochrane Database Syst Rev. 2017;1(1):CD011053.
58. National Institute for Health and Clinical Excellence. Venous thromboembolic diseases: the management of venous thromboembolic diseases and the role of thrombophilia testing. NICE clinical guideline 144. Manchester: NICE; 2012.
59. van der Pol LM, Tromeur C, Bistervels IM, Ni Ainle F, van Bemmel T, Bertoletti L, et al. Pregnancy-adapted YEARS algorithm for diagnosis of suspected pulmonary embolism. N Engl J Med. 2019;380(12):1139-49.
60. Cohen SL, Feizullayeva C, McCandlish JA, Sanelli PC, McGinn T, Brenner B, et al. Comparison of international societal guidelines for the diagnosis of suspected pulmonary embolism during pregnancy. Lancet Haematol. 2020;7(3):e247-58.
61. Raschke RA, Gollihare B, Peirce JC. The effectiveness of implementing the weight-based heparin nomogram as a practice guideline. Arch Intern Med. 1996;156(15):1645-9.
62. Martillotti G, Boehlen F, Robert-Ebadi H, Jastrow N, Righini M, Blondon M. Treatment options for severe pulmonary embolism during pregnancy and the postpartum period: a systematic review. J Thromb Haemost. 2017;15(10):1942-50.
63. Sousa Gomes M, Guimarães M, Montenegro N. Thrombolysis in pregnancy: a literature review. J Matern Fetal Neonatal Med. 2019;32(14):2418-28.
64. Hajj-Chahine J, Jayle C, Tomasi J, Corbi P. Successful surgical management of massive pulmonary embolism during the second trimester in a parturient with heparin-induced thrombocytopenia. Interact Cardiovasc Thorac Surg. 2010;11(5):679-81.
65. Crosby DA, Ryan K, McEniff N, Dicker P, Regan C, Lynch C, et al. Retrievable Inferior vena cava filters in pregnancy: risk versus benefit? Eur J Obstet Gynecol Reprod Biol. 2018;222:25-30.
66. Harris SA, Velineni R, Davies AH. Inferior vena cava filters in pregnancy: a systematic review. J Vasc Interv Radiol. 2016;27(3):354-60.
67. Leffert L, Butwick A, Carvalho B, Arendt K, Bates SM, Friedman A, et al. The Society for Obstetric Anesthesia and Perinatology consensus statement on the anesthetic management of pregnant and postpartum women receiving thromboprophylaxis or higher dose anticoagulants. Anesth Analg. 2018;126(3):928-44.
68. Wik HS, Jacobsen AF, Sandvik L, Sandset PM. Prevalence and predictors for post-thrombotic syndrome 3 to 16 years after pregnancy-related venous thrombosis: a population-based, cross-sectional, case-control study. J Thromb Haemost. 2012;10(5):840-7.
69. Hull RD, Liang J, Merali T. Effect of long-term LMWH on post-thrombotic syndrome in patients with iliac/noniliac venous thrombosis: a subanalysis from the Home-LITE study. Clin Appl Thromb Hemost. 2013;19(5):476-81.
70. Musani MH, Matta F, Yaekoub AY, Liang J, Hull RD, Stein PD. Venous compression for prevention of postthrombotic syndrome: a meta-analysis. Am J Med. 2010;123(8):735-40.
71. Kahn SR, Shapiro S, Wells PS, Rodger MA, Kovacs MJ, Anderson DR, et al. Compression stockings to prevent post-thrombotic syndrome: a randomised placebo-controlled trial. Lancet. 2014;383(9920):880-8.

# CHAPTER 26: Psychiatric Disorders in Pregnancy

*Prerna Kukreti, Madhavi Puri*

## INTRODUCTION

Pregnancy is traditionally considered as a time of happiness, but like any other medical illness, it offers no protection from mental illnesses. Rather perinatal period is a high-risk period for developing mental illnesses. As per report of Global Burden of Diseases, Injuries, and Risk Factors Study (GBD) 2016, suicide was the leading cause of mortality in women of child-bearing age in India from 1990 to 2016.[1] In United States, suicide is the leading cause of mortality in postpartum period accounting for 20% deaths in first year after delivery.[2] Mental illnesses during pregnancy have adverse impact on course and outcome of pregnancy and lay detrimental effect on child's development. Pregnant women with major mental disorders are the high-risk pregnancies which pose wide range of clinical, ethical and administrative challenges to obstetricians ranging from poor compliance to antenatal care services to handling acutely agitated patients in labor with limited time for decision making.

## CLASSIFICATION OF PERINATAL MENTAL DISORDERS

"Perinatal mental disorders" refer to the psychiatric illnesses occurring during entire period of pregnancy and postpartum period up to 1 year. Description of postpartum time frame is contentious ranging from 4 weeks to 6 weeks to 1 year.[3] Perinatal mental disorders range from "common mental illnesses" such as depression, anxiety disorders to "severe mental illnesses" such as schizophrenia and bipolar disorders. Two international classification systems classify perinatal mental disorders as follows:

1. International Classification of Mental and Behavioral Disorders (ICD-11) classifies it under as "Mental or behavioral disorders associated with pregnancy, childbirth and the puerperium" and refers to perinatal mental disorders occurring during pregnancy or puerperium (commencing within about 6 weeks after delivery) causing significant socio-occupational dysfunction. It includes three categories:
    i Mental or behavioral disorders associated with pregnancy, childbirth and the puerperium, without psychotic symptoms.
    ii Mental or behavioral disorders associated with pregnancy, childbirth and the puerperium, with psychotic symptoms.
    iii Mental or behavioral disorders associated with pregnancy, childbirth and the puerperium, unspecified.
    iv It does not include any transient condition like "postpartum blues" which does not last long enough to reach diagnostic criteria for depressive disorder.[4]
2. *Diagnostic and Statistical Manual (DSM5):* It does not mention any separate category for perinatal disorders, rather uses specifiers in different disorders such as brief psychotic disorder, depressive disorder or bipolar disorder *"with peripartum onset" if onset of symptoms is during the pregnancy or within 4 weeks postpartum".*[5]

## CLINICAL FEATURES AND COURSE OF MENTAL DISORDERS DURING PERINATAL PERIOD

### Perinatal Depression

Mood disorders include major depressive disorder, bipolar disorder, persistent depressive disorder, cyclothymia and minor depression. Point prevalence of depression during pregnancy is 15.5% in early and mid-pregnancy, 11.1% in the 3rd trimester, and 8.7% in the postpartum period. In postpartum depression, in up to 40% of cases, symptoms begin antenatally. Approximately 20–40% of women experiencing postnatal depression are more likely to relapse in subsequent pregnancies.[6]

### Diagnostic Criteria for Major Depression

For a diagnosis of major depression, a woman should have at least five symptoms from the list given here, of which one must be symptom 1, or symptom 2, occurring on most days in the previous 2 weeks:[5]

1. Depressed mood/irritability.
2. Diminished interest in activities.
3. Significant weight or appetite change.
4. Sleeping problems, e.g., insomnia or hypersomnia.
5. Fatigue.
6. Feelings of worthlessness/guilt.

7. Inability to think clearly or concentrate.
8. Recurrent thoughts of death and/or suicide.
9. Psychomotor agitation and/or retardation.

While the symptoms of a major or minor depressive disorder in the perinatal period are the same as those at any other time of life, the presence of an infant or unborn baby can make depression at this time harder to deal with and also to identify as some of the physical changes associated with motherhood overlap with the symptoms of depression, e.g., changes in sleeping, changes in appetite, etc. Features of depressive disorder in perinatal period are also similar, however, presence of negative thoughts toward child, comorbid anxiety symptoms, and comorbid obsessional ideas is more commonly seen in perinatal depressive disorders. Risk factors include past history of psychiatric illness in self or family, childhood abuse, prior traumatic experiences, domestic abuse, substance use, comorbid medical disorder, pressure for birth of a specific gender of child, or pregnancy losses.

Early identification is important as ongoing depression can leave women, their infants and their families vulnerable to a wide range of negative and lasting consequences.

## Perinatal Anxiety Disorder

It includes generalized anxiety disorder (GAD), obsessive-compulsive disorder (OCD) and panic disorder. Sometimes severity and effect of anxiety symptoms (e.g., worry, avoidance, and obsessions) do not rise to the level of an anxiety disorder diagnosis; nevertheless, they cause at least mild-to-moderate levels of distress and impairment. In most cases, past history of anxiety disorder is a known risk factor for perinatal anxiety disorders. Given the deleterious effects of significant maternal anxiety on the developing fetus, and the way in which it complicates early parenting, the obstetrician should be as alert for anxiety symptoms as for depressive symptoms in the perinatal period. Also 66% of women with major depression in the postpartum period had comorbid anxiety disorders.

Anxiety disorders involve excessive worry and anxiety that the woman finds difficult to control, occurring on most days.

### Diagnostic Criteria for Generalized Anxiety Disorder

It includes anxiety and worry over most days over a number of events/activities that is difficult to control plus three of the following six symptoms:[5]
1. Restlessness or feeling keyed up or on edge.
2. Being fatigued easily.
3. Difficulty concentrating.
4. Irritability.
5. Muscle tension.
6. Sleep disturbance.

### Diagnostic Criteria for Panic Disorder

It is characterized by multiple sudden onset panic attacks comprising following symptoms lasting for minimum of 2 weeks and associated with apprehension of future attacks:[5]
1. Palpitations, pounding heart, accelerated heart rate.
2. Trembling, numbness or tingling sensations.
3. Sensations of shortness of breath.
4. Chills or hot flushes.
5. Feeling dizzy, lightheaded or faint.
6. Fear of losing control.
7. Fear of dying.

Panic disorder is also commonly associated with agoraphobia; a fear and avoidance of being in public or unfamiliar places where escape is not possible or is embarrassing. Panic disorder with agoraphobia has avoidance of visiting such places.

Any first onset episode of panic attack in pregnancy warrants for excluding thyroid disorders, anemia and cardiac arrhythmias before making diagnosis of panic disorder. Prevalence of panic disorder ranges from 1.4 to 9.1% in pregnancy to 0.5 to 2.9% after 6 to 10 weeks of postpartum.[6]

### Perinatal Obsessive–Compulsive Disorder

*Diagnostic criteria:* It refers to a syndrome characterized by presence of obsessions (recurrent, intrusive, unwanted thoughts, images or impulse) and compulsions (standardized stereotypical behavior or thought being done in response to obsessions) lasting at least a month and causing significant distress in persons' social and occupational life.[5]

Prevalence of OCD ranges from 1.2 to 5.2% during pregnancy to 4.0% after 6 months of pregnancy.[6] In peripartum period, it is often associated with unwanted intrusive aggressive obsessive thoughts of "hurting baby" or "extreme concern of psychological well-being of infant" leading to significant distress and is often associated with depressive symptoms. OCD is known to worsen or recur in women with past history of this disorder during perinatal period.[7]

### Perinatal Psychosis

*Diagnostic criteria:* It refers to syndrome characterized by presence of delusions (false firm unshakable belief), hallucinations (perceptions in absence of a real stimulus), markedly disorganized behavior or speech or predominant negative symptoms. Peripartum period up to 3 months postpartum is a high-risk period of developing perinatal psychosis and onset is most common in first 2 weeks after delivery. Its incidence is 1.1–4.0 cases per 1,000 deliveries and in 20–30% cases it is with history of bipolar disorder or affective psychosis.[8] Clinical features are fluctuating; characterized by presence of psychotic symptoms, mood symptoms, thoughts of harm for self and rarely for the infant or catatonic symptoms. Risk factors include past history of similar illness, poor social support, stressful life events and sleep disturbances.[9]

## Postpartum Blues

It refers to constellation of symptoms characterized by presence of sudden onset "blues symptoms" within first week postpartum including dysphoric mood, crying, mood lability, anxiety, insomnia, loss of appetite, and irritability. It is usually transient, self-limiting and symptoms are more common in women with past history of psychiatric disorder and in medically high-risk pregnancies.[10]

## ■ RISK FACTORS

Pregnancy and transition to parenthood is often associated with significant biological, psychological and social changes, which often predispose the vulnerable women at higher risk of developing mental disorders. Psychological risk factors include past history of psychiatric disorders, family history of psychiatric disorder, lifetime use of alcohol or tobacco and poor coping skills. Biological risk factors include sudden reduction in estradiol levels up to 100-fold leading to precipitation of depressive or psychotic symptoms in postpartum phase. Obstetric risk factors include primigravida, comorbid medical disorder, unwanted conception, negative experience during any stage of pregnancy, fear of childbirth and apprehensions about delivery. Social risk factors include poor social support, intimate partner violence, past history of childhood abuse, poor socioeconomic status, and significant negative life events.[11]

## ■ RISK OF UNTREATED PERINATAL MENTAL DISORDERS

"Risks of untreated mental disorder in pregnancy" refers to the risk to mothers and children posed by psychiatric disorder especially when not treated. Most of the time due to concern of fetus safety and absence of reliable data on safety of psychotropics, mothers do not get the due treatment. Importance of the issue is highlighted by a recent analysis revealing that 1 in 25 women, aged 20–25 years who attempt suicide, do so in perinatal time period.[12,13]

- *Risk of relapse:* Pregnancy is not protective against mental illness. Decision to discontinue medications is associated with high risk of relapse. Very high relapse rates are found in depressive disorders, up to 70%[13] and in bipolar disorders up to 86%.[14] Antenatal mental illnesses are predictor of postpartum onset or continuation of symptoms.
- *Impact on antenatal care and family:* Untreated mental disorders may be associated with delayed health seeking for antenatal services, poor follow-ups, poor dietary patterns, self-neglect, smoking, alcohol use, high-risk behaviors such as indiscriminate sex, exposure to sexually transmitted infections, and restrained interpersonal relationships with caregivers.[15]
- *Impact on pregnancy outcome:* Maternal mental illness during pregnancy has been associated with adverse perinatal outcomes, including small-for-gestational-age fetuses, fetal distress, preterm delivery, low birthweight, and neonatal hypoglycemia.[16]
- *Effect on infant development:* Untreated mental illnesses have been associated with detrimental effect on infant's neurodevelopment. This has been partly attributed to effect of uterine environment and fetal programming during critical period of in-utero development. High risk behaviors due to untreated mental illness such as smoking, alcohol use and poor nutrition status may also contribute to it. Poor mother-child bonding and attachment, increased rates of emotional and behavioral problems have been found in children born to mothers with mental disorders.[17] **Table 1** summarizes different psychiatric disorders and impact on pregnancy and neonatal outcome.

## ■ IMPACT OF PSYCHOTROPIC DRUGS ON PREGNANCY AND INFANT

The potential risks of psychotropic drug use in pregnancy include teratogenicity or major malformation (first-trimester

**TABLE 1:** Impact of psychiatric illness on pregnancy and neonatal outcome.

| Illness | Teratogenic effect | Impact on obstetric outcome | Impact on neonatal outcome |
| --- | --- | --- | --- |
| Anxiety disorder | N/A | Increased incidence of forceps deliveries, prolonged labor, precipitate labor, fetal distress, preterm delivery, and spontaneous abortion | Decreased developmental scores and inadaptability; slowed mental development at 2 years of age |
| Depressive disorder | N/A | Increased incidence of low birth weight, decreased fetal growth, and postnatal complications | Increased newborn cortisol and catecholamine levels, infant crying, rates of admission to neonatal intensive care units |
| Schizophrenia | Congenital malformations, especially of cardiovascular system | Increased incidence of preterm delivery, low birth weight, small for gestational age, placental abnormalities, and antenatal hemorrhage | Increased rates of postnatal death |

exposure), neonatal toxicity (third-trimester exposure), longer-term neurobehavioral effects and increased risk of physical health problems in adult life.[18]

The safety of psychotropic drugs in pregnancy cannot be clearly established because robust, prospective trials are obviously unethical. Individual decisions on psychotropic use in pregnancy are therefore based on database studies that have many limitations (e.g., failure to control for the effects of illness, smoking, obesity, other medications, and other confounders).

**Table 2** summarizes the psychotropics, different class they belong to as per old system of FDA to classify psychotropics in pregnancy as category A to X and in lactation, as Hales category of L1 to L4, and current recommendations based on latest regulation of Pregnancy and Lactation Labeling Rule (PLLR).[18-20]

Based on knowledge of psychotropics safety, **Table 3** summarizes different class of psychotropics and management pearls during different stages of pregnancy.[19]

## GENERAL MANAGEMENT GUIDELINES FOR PERINATAL MENTAL DISORDERS

Obstetricians may encounter perinatal mental disorders in following situations:

- *Prepregnancy:* A patient with mental disorders on medications wanting to conceive
- *During pregnancy:* A patient with perinatal mental disorders
  - Acutely symptomatic (first episode or relapse)
  - In remission (with/without medication)
- *Postdelivery:* A patient with perinatal mental disorders
  - Acutely symptomatic (first episode or relapse)
  - In remission (with/without medication).

As a golden dictum, these patients are best managed with a collaborative perinatal mental health team having obstetrician, psychiatrist and neonatologist who are sensitive to needs of such patients, can collaboratively share documented decisions across departments and convey uniform messages about safety of evidence-based therapeutic options to patient and family.

### Management in Preconception Phase

#### General Measures

Any woman with mental disorder planning to conceive can be offered following management:

- *High dose folic acid:* Consider starting such patients on high dose (5 mg) folic acid daily.
- *Healthy lifestyle practices advice:* Work on addressing other modifiable risk factors (if present any) for poor obstetrical outcome, e.g., offering treatment for smoking cessation, alcohol deaddiction, obesity and diabetes.

Refer clients reporting history of domestic violence to social worker.

- *Avoid unplanned pregnancy:* Advise contraception, preferably barrier methods (oral contraceptives may have drug interaction with some psychotropics) and maintain menstrual calendar.

Specific issues in management of mental disorders:

- *Referral to psychiatrist:* Any person with any perinatal mental disorder planning to conceive while on medication should be referred to treating psychiatrist. Such patient can be offered following treatment options:
  - Discontinue the treatment prior to conception,
  - Continue treatment until pregnancy is verified, or
  - Continue treatment throughout the pregnancy.

All these decisions would depend on following variables:

- Frequency and severity of previous episodes
- Past and current levels of functioning or impairment
- Past and recent duration of clinical stability, with and without medication
- The nature of prodromal symptoms that indicate an impending relapse and
- Average time to recovery following re-introduction of treatment.

### Stable Patient/Mild or Infrequent Illness

If there is past history of one or infrequent episodes with long period of remission:

- Pharmacological agents can be tapered off slowly and the woman should be closely monitored for conception and relapse of symptoms, or
- Continue treatment until pregnancy is verified and, then gradually taper off: Uteroplacental circulation is not established until approximately 2 weeks' postconception and hence this strategy reduces the risk of fetal exposure to drugs and extends the protective treatment up to the time of conception. However, it is important to remember that this strategy may lead to relatively abrupt treatment discontinuation, thereby placing the patients at increased risk for relapse.

### Severe Illness with Frequent Episodes or Difficult to Manage Episodes in Past with History of Self Harm

- Consider continuing medication throughout pregnancy
- Prefer to keep patient on monotherapy if possible
- Safer drug should be chosen, but change of medication is usually not advised (except in case of valproate or paroxetine) because it puts patient at increased risk of relapse, and exposes infant to two different psychotropic agents.

**Flowchart 1** summarizes the treatment algorithm for patients on medication wanting to conceive.[21]

**TABLE 2:** Psychotropics and safety recommendations for pregnancy and lactation.

| Class of drugs and generic name | Old system | | New system | Remarks |
|---|---|---|---|---|
| | FDA category* for pregnancy | Hales category# for lactation | PLLR | |
| *Antidepressants* | | | | |
| Fluoxetine | C | L2 in older infant/L3 if used in neonatal period | First trimester fluoxetine use is associated with increased risk of cardiovascular malformations; paroxetine is linked to cardiac malformations (ventricular septal and valve defects) Consideration should be given to either discontinuing paroxetine use or switching to another antidepressant | Sertraline is most preferred molecule |
| Sertraline | C | L2 | | Paroxetine is to be avoided |
| Escitalopram | C | L2 | | |
| Venlafaxine | C | L3 | | |
| Mirtazapine | C | L3 | | |
| Paroxetine | D | L2 | | |
| *Anti-obsessive medication* | | | -- | -- |
| Fluvoxamine | C | L2 | | |
| Clomipramine | C | L2 | | |
| *Benzodiazepine (BZD)* | | | | |
| Clonazepam | D | L3 | Nonteratogenic risks include reports of neonatal flaccidity, respiratory and feeding difficulties, hypothermia, and neonatal withdrawal symptoms during the postnatal period. Use of these drugs is rarely a matter of urgency, so first trimester exposure should almost always be avoided | BZD with short half-life such as lorazepam preferred. If using it in last trimester, observe infant for any withdrawal signs |
| Alprazolam | D | L3 | | |
| Chlordiazepoxide | D | L3 | | |
| Lorazepam | D | L3 | | |
| Diazepam | D | L3/L4 if used chronically | | |
| *Non-BZD sedative* | | | | |
| Zolpidem | B | L3 | -- | ---- |
| *Non-BZD Anxiolytic* | | | | |
| Buspirone | B | L3 | -- | -- |
| *Antipsychotic* | | | | |
| Haloperidol | C | L2 | No teratogenic effects or fetal toxicity have been observed in animal studies involving exposure to clozapine or lurasidone in animals. There are no adequate and well-controlled studies in pregnant women. Third trimester exposure increases risk for neonatal extrapyramidal and/or withdrawal symptoms (EPS) | Women on Olanzapine and clozapine to be worked up for gestational diabetes |
| Chlorpromazine | C | L3 | | |
| Aripiprazole | C | L3 | | |
| Risperidone | C | L3 | | |
| Quetiapine | C | L4C | | |
| Olanzapine | C | L2 | | |
| Clozapine | B | L3 | | |
| *Mood stabilizer* | | | | |
| Lithium | D | L4 | There are no adequate and well-controlled studies in pregnant women Lithium may cause Ebstein's anomaly Carbamazepine is associated with risk to the fetus, including congenital malformations (spinal bifida), and developmental delays Valproate may produce congenital malformations (e.g., neural tube defects) at a rate higher than other drugs and general population Valproate should not be used | Lithium is safest in pregnancy but contraindicated in lactation Carbamazepine is safe in lactation Lamotrigine is a good mood stabilizer for maintenance therapy in pregnancy and lactation Valproate is to be avoided |
| Valproate | D | L2 | | |
| Carbamazepine | D | L2 | | |
| Lamotrigine | C | L3 | | |

*FDA categories: **A** controlled study shows no risk, **B** No evidence of risk in humans, **C** risk cannot be ruled out for humans, **D** possible evidence of risk, **X** contraindicated
#Hales Lactation risk category: L1 safest, L2 safer, L3 moderately safe, L4 possibly hazardous, L5 contraindicated

**TABLE 3:** Psychotropics and management issues in different stages of pregnancy.

| Medication class | Birth defects | Pregnancy | Delivery | Neonatal | Lactation | Preferred medications |
|---|---|---|---|---|---|---|
| Benzodiazepine | Possible increased incidence of cleft lip or palate | Ultrasonography for facial morphology | Floppy infant syndrome | Withdrawal syndrome | Infant sedation reported | Clonazepam Lorazepam Alprazolam |
| Antidepressants | None confirmed | Decreased serum concentrations across pregnancy | None | Neonatal, withdrawal syndrome | None | Fluoxetine Sertraline Paroxetine Citalopram Nortriptyline |
| Lithium | Increased incidence of heart defects | Ultrasonography or fetal echocardiography for heart development or both decreases serum concentrations across pregnancy Intravenous fluids Increased risk for lithium toxicity in m | Intravenous fluids Increased risk for lithium toxicity in mother | Increased risk for lithium toxicity in infant | Monitor infant complete blood count, thyroid stimulating hormone levels, and lithium levels | Sustained release lithium |
| Mood stabilizers | Increased incidence of birth defects | Decreased serum concentrations across pregnancy Folate supplementation, vitamin K for some antiepileptic drugs | None | Neonatal symptoms, vitamin K for some antiepileptic drugs | Monitor infant complete blood count, thyroid-stimulating hormone levels, and lithium levels | Lamotrigine Carbamazepine |
| Antipsychotics | | | None | Possible risk for neuroleptic malignant syndrome and intestinal obstruction | Monitor infant complete blood count, liver enzyme levels, antiepileptic drug levels | Haloperidol |

*Patient with mental disorder on medications having difficulty in conceiving:* Refer to psychiatrist for evaluation for:
- Ruling out depressive disorder or negative symptoms contributing to it
- Ruling out sexual dysfunctions primary or secondary to any psychotropic
- For switching on to use of prolactin sparing medications in cases of drug-induced amenorrhea/other menstrual abnormalities/hyperprolactinemia. **Table 4** mentions psychotropics and effect on ability to conceive.[21]

## Management of Perinatal Mental Disorders during Pregnancy[21]

### General Measures
- *Flag as high-risk pregnancy:* Manage pregnancy among women with severe mental illness as a high-risk pregnancy requiring more intensive monitoring, with close liaison with psychiatrist.
- *High dose folic acid:* Consider starting such patients on high dose (5 mg) folic acid daily.
- *Healthy lifestyle practices advice:* Work on addressing other modifiable risk factors for poor obstetrical outcome, e.g., offering treatment for smoking cessation, alcohol deaddiction, obesity, diabetes. Referral to social worker for clients reporting history of domestic violence.
- *Excessive weight gain and gestational diabetes:* Monitor for excessive weight gain and gestational diabetes, particularly for women on a second-generation antipsychotic (SGA).

Specific issues in management of mental disorders:
- *Psychiatry referral:* For individualized treatment plan to be made weighing risk and benefit based on following clinical situations.

### Patient with Mental Disorder in Remission Conceives
- *Single episode of mild illness, currently in remission:* Can be considered for tapering off medicines

**Flowchart 1:** Treatment planning for persons with mental disorder on medication planning to conceive.

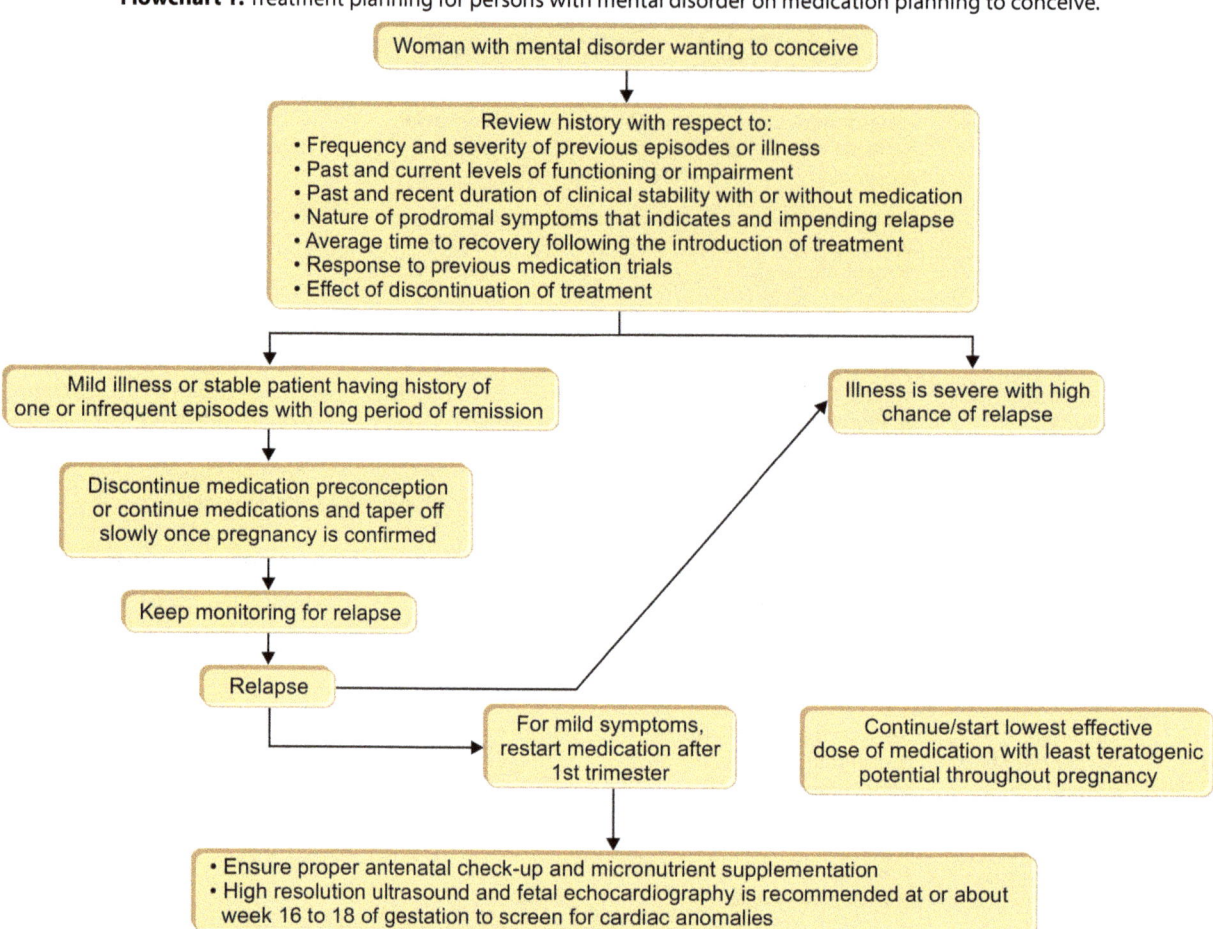

- *If infrequent episodes/mild illness (pregnancy <3 months):* Referral to psychiatrist for tapering off medicines or starting psychotherapeutic options if mild depression or mild anxiety disorders
- *If infrequent episodes/mild illness (pregnancy > 3 months):* Referral to psychiatrist for risk assessment and future treatment
- *Severe illness with frequent episodes or difficult to manage episodes in past with history of self-harm:* Continue medications, psychiatry opinion for assessing safety of psychotropics.

### Symptomatic Patient with Mental Disorder Conceives

- **On treatment:** Refer to psychiatrist for optimizing preexisting treatment. Avoid switching medications unless risk outweighs benefit, e.g., stopping valproate. In rest all cases, consider continuing patient on monotherapy preferably on agent with best response in past
- **First episode/patient off drugs:** Referral to psychiatrist for initiating a medicine safe for peripartum period if symptoms severe, else trying to keep patient on nonpharmacological therapies, e.g., psychotherapy for mild depressive disorder or anxiety disorder

**TABLE 4:** Psychotropics and effect on ability to conceive.

| Medication class | Effect on ability to conceive |
| --- | --- |
| Antidepressants | No effect on the ability of women to conceive, although there is some evidence that they may affect male sperm count and morphology[22] |
| Anxiolytic and hypnotic | No effect |
| Antipsychotics | All FGAs and some SGAs (especially risperidone and amisulpride) can cause hyperprolactinemia and impaired fertility)[23] |
| Lithium | Lithium is not known to have significant effects on female fertility but may inhibit sperm motility[24] |
| Mood stabilizers | Women with epilepsy using valproate have an increased rate of polycystic ovary syndrome/ovaries.[25] Valproate treatment is reported to be associated with adverse spermatogenesis in men[26] |

- *Antipsychotics:* Among first generation antipsychotics (FGAs) haloperidol is preferred, among second generation antipsychotics (SGAs) Quetiapine followed by Olanzapine is preferred
- *Antidepressants:* Selective serotonin reuptake inhibitors (SSRIs) are preferred and most data on safety is concerning sertraline and fluoxetine. Paroxetine is to be avoided.

- *Sedatives and hypnotics*: Prefer using non-BZD derivatives such as zolpidem as hypnotic and buspirone as anxiolytic. If needed to use BZD, consider using BZD with short half-life like lorazepam. Use before delivery should be cautious and minimal to avoid neonatal withdrawal syndrome.
- *Mood stabilizers*: Lithium is safest mood stabilizer but still carries risk of cardiac anomalies, so fetal echocardiography and anomaly scans should be planned well. Valproate is contraindicated and should be avoided as much as possible

## Urgent Mental Health Conditions

Urgent referral to psychiatrist is needed in case of marked agitation or if there is risk of suicide or of harm to others.

**Flowchart 2** summarizes the treatment algorithm for management of patients having active symptoms of common mental illnesses (depression/anxiety/OCD) during pregnancy.

**Flowchart 3** summarizes the treatment algorithm for management of patients having active symptoms of severe mental illnesses (psychosis/schizophrenia/mania) during pregnancy.

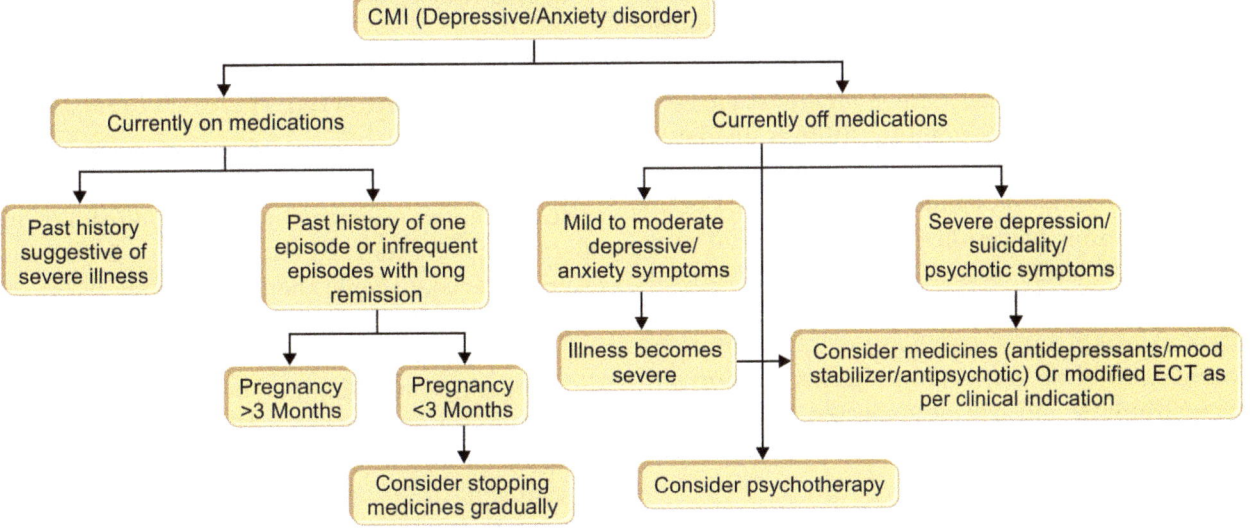

**Flowchart 2:** Management algorithm for persons with symptoms of common mental illnesses (CMI) during pregnancy.

(ECT: electroconvulsive therapy)

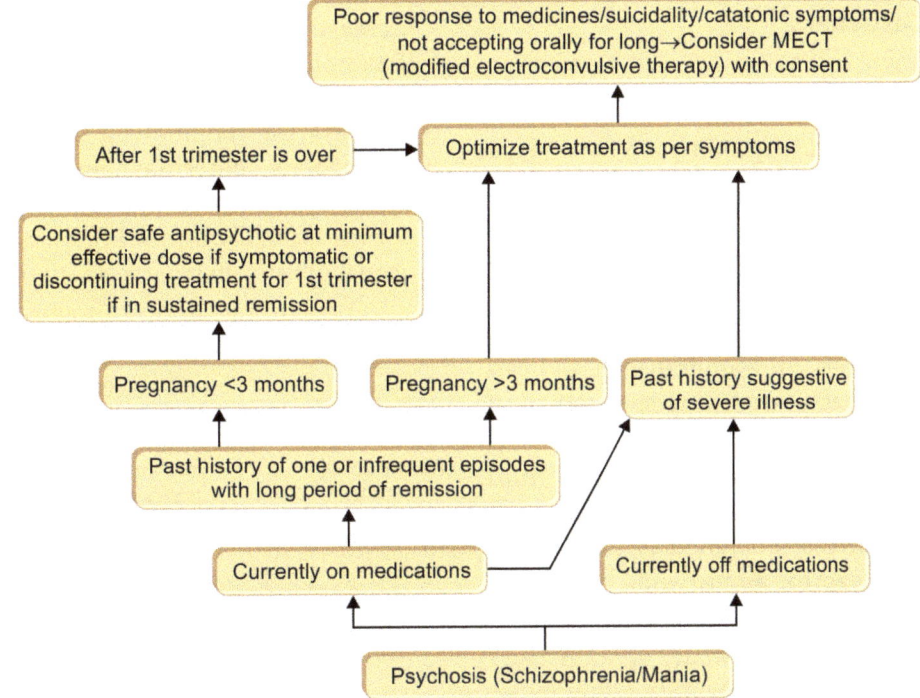

**Flowchart 3:** Management algorithm for persons with symptoms of severe mental illnesses (SMI) during pregnancy.

(MECT: modified electroconvulsive therapy)

## Intrapartum Management of Perinatal Mental Disorders[21]

- In women with a severe mental illness, it is recommended that delivery should be in tertiary care hospital with round the clock psychiatry services.
- With the help of perinatal mental health team, identify potential issues which might arise during intrapartum period.
- Clear orders should be given for medication which needs to be reduced or stopped before labor weighing benefit and risk for example:
  - Considering dose reduction of FGA (like haloperidol) if possible, to reduce chance of extrapyramidal symptoms to neonate or if not possible, inform neonatologist to observe for any such signs[21]
  - National Collaborating Centre for Mental Health suggests reducing or stopping lithium on day of delivery for reducing neonatal complications.[27] Lithium blood levels should be measured 24 hours before and after delivery in mother and lithium levels and Free T4 levels in umbilical cord.[28,29] Hydration should be maintained for preventing lithium toxicity. If cesarean is planned, anesthetist should be informed because Lithium potentiates succinylcholine and pancuronium and can be expected to potentiate effect of other depolarizing and nondepolarizing muscle relaxants.[30]
- Ensure good analgesia and sleep to avoid triggers for relapse or exacerbation of mental illnesses.

## Postnatal Management of Perinatal Mental Disorders[21]

### General Measures

- *Social support:* Encourage mothers with known past or family history of severe mental illness to have social support for care of neonate and mother and ensure adequate sleep to mother.
- *Supportive measures:* Pain and insomnia can be potential triggers for exacerbation, address them well.
- *Assessment of mother:* Be watchful in stable patients also, for postpartum blues, they are transient and can be managed well with assurance, any sustenance of symptoms will warrant psychiatry evaluation
- *Maternal-child dyad:* Encourage mother and child bonding and breast feeding. If due to poor mental health mother is unable to breastfeed in immediate postpartum period, allow her to express breast milk at regular intervals.
- *Adjusting psychotropics:* Take psychiatry opinion again for psychotropic dosages, especially if it's a premature delivery and mother is breastfeeding. Adjust medicines causing excessive sedation as it can hinder baby care and breastfeeding.
- *Neonate care:* Advise mothers against cosleeping with babies if excessively sedated and encourage use of baby crib besides her bed. Monitor the infant for adverse effects such as over sedation and poor feeding.
- *Mental disorders—new episode or exacerbation:* Postnatal period up to 6 weeks is period for likely exacerbation of mental illnesses. Screen women using standardized rating scale. Choose treatments with the lowest known risk for women who are breastfeeding. As in pregnancy, previous treatment response should guide future treatment choices. **Table 5** summarizes psychotropic agents' usage guideline in lactating women.

## USE OF CONTRACEPTIVE MEASURES AND PERINATAL MENTAL HEALTH CONDITIONS

Patients should be encouraged to plan pregnancy while on psychotropics and should be psycho-educated about range of contraceptive measures available. But following drug interactions[31,32] **(Table 6)** and impact on illness should be taken into account while taking a decision:

- *Effect of contraceptives on mental illness:* Progesterone-only pills and high-dose estrogen pills increase serotonin metabolism in brain, thereby lowering serotonin levels and predisposing to depression.
- *Effect of contraceptives on psychotropics:* Synthetic estrogen stimulates protein synthesis, which may affect protein-binding of certain drugs, and inhibits some cytochrome P450 enzymes, both of which can affect blood levels of other medications.
- *Increase metabolism of psychotropics:* Oral contraceptives increase the metabolism of some benzodiazepines (lorazepam and temazepam).
- *Decrease metabolism of psychotropics:* Oral contraceptives decrease the metabolism of some benzodiazepines (alprazolam, chlordiazepoxide and diazepam) and tricyclic antidepressants predisposing to toxicity. It decreases metabolism of FGAs also but the effect has not been replicated in large scale studies.

**TABLE 5:** Psychotropics class and safety profile during lactation.

| Psychotropic class | Safety profile for lactation |
| --- | --- |
| Antidepressants | SSRIs can be used with moderate safety |
| Antipsychotics | Haloperidol, olanzapine and quetiapine are preferred. Clozapine use should be avoided |
| Mood stabilizers | Valproate and carbamazepine are preferred Lithium use to be avoided |
| Sedative and anxiolytic | Benzodiazepines are associated with sedation, lethargy, withdrawal in infant Consider non BZD drugs such as zolpidem for sleep and buspirone for anxiety |

(BZD: benzodiazepine)

**TABLE 6:** Psychotropics and oral contraceptives interaction.

| Psychotropic class | Drug interaction and individual psychotropics | | | |
|---|---|---|---|---|
| | No interaction | Increases metabolism of oral contraceptives/ decreasing contraceptive effectiveness | Oral contraceptives increase metabolism of psychotropic/ decreasing psychotropic effectiveness | Oral contraceptives decrease metabolism of psychotropic/ predisposing to psychotropic toxicity |
| Antidepressant | SSRI | | | TCA |
| Antipsychotics | SGA | | | ± FGA |
| Mood stabilizer | Valproate | Carbamazepine, oxcarbazepine, and topiramate | Lamotrigine | |
| Benzodiazepines | | | Lorazepam and temazepam | Alprazolam, chlordiazepoxide diazepam |

## Effect of Psychotropics on Contraceptives

- *Increases metabolism of contraceptives*: Carbamazepine, oxcarbazepine, and topiramate, mood stabilizers which induce the P450 3A4 pathway can increase the metabolism of oral contraceptives (many of which are substrates of the P450 3A4 pathway), thereby reducing their effectiveness. This effect is also seen with vaginal contraceptive rings, because the hormones contained in these preparations are also metabolized by the liver.

Thus, patient should either change her contraceptive method or change her mood stabilizer. Contraceptive alternatives include the birth control patch (which largely avoids liver metabolism) and barrier methods.

## SCREENING FOR MENTAL DISORDERS IN PERINATAL PERIOD

Considering huge impact of mental illnesses on health of mother, child, family and perinatal care services, it is important to be aware of these disorders and their clinical presentation. Since these disorders are so prevalent yet they go under reported or often undiagnosed and are considered as part of normal pregnancy, so, American College of Obstetrics and Gynecology recommends screening for common mental disorders at least once during perinatal period. Easy to use structured clinical tools as given in **Table 7**, can aid in routine screening.

## KEY POINTS

- Psychiatric disorders during pregnancy are common.
- Severe mental illnesses during pregnancy are high risk pregnancies requiring collaboration between service users (patients and family), and all concerned health care providers (obstetrician, psychiatrist, neonatologist).
- Regular screening for mental disorders can improve detection and following structured operational algorithms can make clinicians provide effective evidence based uniform care.
- Informing the patient and family about current clinical status, course of illness, effects and side effects of medication should govern shared decision making.

**TABLE 7:** Overview of screening tools for common mental disorders in perinatal period.

| Mental disorder screened | Screening instrument | Validated for use in India |
|---|---|---|
| Depression | Edinburg depression rating scale 10 items (EDPS) | Yes, in English and Hindi |
| | Patient health questionnaire 2 items and 9 item (PHQ-2/PHQ-9) | Yes, in English and Hindi |
| | Whooley questions 2 items | Yes, In English |
| Anxiety | Generalized anxiety disorder scale 2 items (GAD2) | Yes, in English and Hindi |
| Depression and anxiety | Kessler psychological distress 10 item (K10) | Yes, in English and Hindi |

- Concerns about effect of psychotropics safety alone should not deny due care needed for women with mental disorders.
- A judicious clinical decision can help reduce burden of maternal mental disorders on mother, infant and family.

## REFERENCES

1. India State-Level Disease Burden Initiative Suicide Collaborators. Gender differentials and state variations in suicide deaths in India: the Global Burden of Disease Study 1990-2016. Lancet Pub Health. 2018;3(10):e478-e489.
2. Campbell J, Matoff-Stepp S, Velez ML, Cox HH, Laughon K. Pregnancy-associated deaths from homicide, suicide, and drug overdose: review of research and the intersection with intimate partner violence. J Womens Health. 2021 30(2):236-44.
3. O'Hara MW, Wisner KL. Perinatal mental illness: definition, description and aetiology. Best Pract Res Clin Obstet Gynaecol. 2014;28(1):3-12.
4. World Health Organization. International Statistical Classification of Diseases and Related Health Problems, 11th edition. Geneva: World Health Organization; 2020.

5. American Psychiatric Association. Diagnostic and Statistical Manual of Mental Disorders, 5th edition. Washington, DC: American Psychiatric Publishing; 2013.
6. Teixeira C, Figueiredo B, Conde A, Pacheco A, Costa, R. Anxiety and depression during pregnancy in women and men. J Affect Disord. 2009:119:142-8.
7. House SJ, Tripathi SP, Knight BT, Morris N, Newport DJ, Stowe ZN. Obsessive-compulsive disorder in pregnancy and the postpartum period: course of illness and obstetrical outcome. Arch Womens Ment Health. 2016;19(1):3-10.
8. Baron EC, Hanlon C, Mall S, Honikman S, Breuer E, Kathree T, et al. Maternal mental health in primary care in five low- and middle-income countries: A situational analysis. BMC Health Serv Res. 2016;16:53.
9. Rai S, Pathak A, Sharma I. Postpartum psychiatric disorders: Early diagnosis and management. Indian J Psychiatry. 2015;57:S216-21.
10. Harsha G, Acharya M. Trajectory of perinatal mental health in India. Indian J Social Psychiatr. 2019;35(1):47.
11. Alipour Z, Kheirabadi GR, Kazemi A, Fooladi M. The most important risk factors affecting mental health during pregnancy: a systematic review. East Mediterr Health J. 2018;24(6):549-59.
12. Kim JJ, Silver RK. Perinatal suicide associated with depression diagnosis and absence of active treatment in 15-year UK national inquiry. Evid Based Ment Health. 2016;19:122.
13. Cohen LS, Altshuler LL, Harlow BL. Relapse of major depression during pregnancy in women who maintain or discontinue antidepressant treatment. JAMA. 2006;295:499-507.
14. Epstein RA, Moore KM, Bobo WV. Treatment of bipolar disorders during pregnancy: maternal and fetal safety and challenges. Drug Health Patient Saf. 2014;7:7-29.
15. Dean BB, Gerner D, Gerner RH. A systematic review evaluating health-related quality of life, work impairment, and healthcare costs and utilization in bipolar disorder. Curr Med Res Opin. 2004;20:139-54.
16. Jablensky AV, Morgan V, Zubrick SR, Bower C, Yellachich LA. Pregnancy, delivery, and neonatal complications in a population cohort of women with schizophrenia and major affective disorders. Am J Psychiatry. 2005;162:79-91.
17. Glover V. Maternal depression, anxiety and stress during pregnancy and child outcome; what needs to be done. Best Pract Res Clin Obstet Gynaecol. 2014;28:25-35.
18. Creeley CE, Denton LK. Use of prescribed psychotropics during pregnancy: a systematic review of pregnancy, neonatal, and childhood outcomes. Brain Sci. 2019;9(9):235.
19. Clinical Management Guidelines for Obstetrician-Gynecologists Use of Psychiatric Medications During Pregnancy and Lactation. ACOG Practice Bulletin, FOCUS 2009 7:3, 385-400
20. Hale TW. Medications in Mother's Milk. Amaraillo (TX): Pharmasoft Publishing, 2004.
21. McAllister-Williams RH, Baldwin DS, Cantwell R, Easter A, Gilvarry E, Glover V, et al. British Association for Psychopharmacology consensus guidance on the use of psychotropic medication preconception, in pregnancy and postpartum 2017. J Psychopharmacol. 2017;31(5):519-52.
22. Akasheh G, Sirati L, Noshad Kamran AR, Sepehrmanesh Z. Comparison of the effect of sertraline with behavioral therapy on semen parameters in men with primary premature ejaculation. Urology. 2014;83:800-4.
23. Haddad PM, Wieck A. Antipsychotic-induced hyperprolactinaemia: mechanisms, clinical features and management. Drugs. 2004;64:2291-314.
24. Raoof NT, Pearson RM, Turner P (1989) Lithium inhibits human sperm motility in vitro. Br J Clin Pharmacol. 1989;28:715-7.
25. Svalheim S, Sveberg L, Mochol M, Taubøll E. Interactions between antiepileptic drugs and hormones. Seizure. 2015;28:12-7.
26. Hamed SA, Moussa EM, Tohamy AM, Mohamed KO, Mohamad ME, Sherif TM, et al. Seminal fluid analysis and testicular volume in adults with epilepsy receiving valproate. J Clin Neurosci. 2015;22:508-12.
27. National Collaborating Centre for Mental Health. Antenatal and postnatal mental health: clinical management and service guidance. London: NICE; 2014.
28. Newport DJ, Viguera AC, Beach AJ, Ritchie JC, Cohen LS, Stowe ZN. Lithium placental passage and obstetrical outcome: implications for clinical management during late pregnancy. Am J Psychiatry. 2005;162(11):2162-70.
29. Poels EMP, Bijma HH, Galbally M, Bergink V. Lithium during pregnancy and after delivery: a review. Int J Bipolar Disord. 2018;6(1):26.
30. Blake LD, Lucas DN, Aziz K, Castello-Cortes A, Robinson PN. Lithium toxicity and the parturient: case report and literature review. Int J Obstet Anesth. 2008;17(2):164-9.
31. Sivertz K, Kostaras X. The use of psychotropic medications in pregnancy and lactation. BC Medical Journal. 2005;47(3):135-8.
32. Berry-Bibee EN, Kim MJ, Simmons KB, Tepper NK, Riley HE, Pagano HP, et al. Drug interactions between hormonal contraceptives and psychotropic drugs: a systematic review. Contraception. 2019;94(6):650-67.

# Tuberculosis in Pregnancy

*Abha Singh, Bhawani Singh*

## INTRODUCTION

Tuberculosis (TB) is an ancient disease that has afflicted mankind since many centuries. TB can involve multiple organs of the body and is classified as pulmonary when it is limited to lungs or extrapulmonary TB (EPTB) when systems outside lungs are involved like lymph nodes, bones, kidneys, abdominal TB, meningeal, and miliary TB. Increasing prevalence of multidrug resistant (MDR) TB or coexisting human immunodeficiency virus (HIV) infection are additional impediments to successful management.

Women of childbearing age are reported to constitute a significant number among TB patients with a slightly higher prevalence of EPTB when compared to men.[1] As per notifications, 75% of TB in India is pulmonary.[2] Latent TB in women is known to become active during pregnancy or in postpartum period. Depressed immunity in pregnancy may also aid acquiring fresh TB infection or reinfection that may proceed rapidly to result in active disease. TB during pregnancy is known to result in fetal growth restriction (FGR), low birth weight, perinatal mortality, maternal morbidity and mortality. In addition, the fetus is at risk of acquiring the infection through blood borne vertical transmission or from intrapartum aspiration of infected amniotic fluid/genital secretions. Inhalation of infected droplets by the newborn in the postpartum period could also result in neonatal TB. Considering, the adverse effects of TB on the fetomaternal outcome, all high-risk pregnant women should be actively screened for TB.

In a study published in Lancet in 2014, India was ranked highest in the estimated number of pregnant women with TB in South East Asian region with more than 44,000 cases and 21% of the global burden.[3] However, in a recent study from a tertiary care center from India 0.02% of 4,203 pregnant women screened were found to have active TB.[4] This number is small in comparison to the incidence of anemia, gestational diabetes or preeclampsia observed in pregnant women and hence becomes a low priority and simultaneously a challenge for the clinician.

## CLINICAL FEATURES

The signs and symptoms of TB in pregnant women are similar to those seen in nonpregnant women and include fever with night sweats, weight loss, cough, and anorexia with general malaise. Almost a quarter of patients may have very few or no symptoms. Diagnosis may be delayed in early stages due to nonspecific symptoms of anorexia, malaise, weight loss, and lethargy.

## DIAGNOSIS

Diagnosis of TB in pregnancy can be particularly challenging as the presentation can range from virtually asymptomatic at one end to a crippling multisystem presentation at the other end. The high-risk factors such as past history or family history of TB, close contact with active case, poor socioeconomic status, HIV infection, intravenous drug abuse, alcohol, and other addictions should be enquired into.

Confirming the suspicion requires obtaining relevant samples and also ascertaining at the very outset the risk of MDR TB. One should also evaluate the patient for coexisting HIV and diabetes. On occasions treatment has to be started on clinical grounds, as proof is not always available. The discussion below, lists various investigation modalities used to confirm TB in all cases including the pregnant women.

### Sputum Direct Examination

This is the most important, readily available tool for confirming pulmonary TB (PTB). Results of acid fast bacilli (AFB) staining are available within hours and can be carried out even in peripheral areas. As per Revised National TB Control Programme (RNTCP) of India two sputum smears on consecutive days should be examined to isolate AFB. Diagnosis of PTB is made, if at least one of the two smear is positive for AFB.

### Microbiology

A mycobacterial culture to evaluate for drug resistance should invariably be sent. Recently, tests based on polymerase chain reaction (PCR) technology to amplify unique nucleic acid of the bacilli, have been found to have higher sensitivity and specificity in detecting TB bacilli when compared to sputum staining. They also detect gene markers of drug resistance and have a short turn-around time. GeneXpert is one such test that has given good results in detecting TB bacilli and rifampicin resistance in samples of sputum, cerebrospinal fluid (CSF), and tissue samples. Since rifampicin resistance most often overlaps with isoniazid (INH) resistance, it points toward MDR TB. Occasionally sputum induction or bronchoscopy may be required if patient is unable to expectorate.

Growth of TB bacilli in culture is the gold standard for diagnosis. It indicates alive, active bacteria and provides material for drug sensitivity studies. Conventional solid media cultures have a long turnaround time of 6–8 weeks and are less sensitive for EPTB. Mycobacteria growth indicator tube (MGIT) cultures are liquid-based culture, have a turnaround time of 4–14 days and can also detect drug resistance.

Wide range of specimens depending on the clinical context like sputum, CSF, urine, blood, body fluids including amniotic fluid, tissue specimens including placenta may be sent for culture.

Nucleic acid amplification technology (NAAT) based tests have further reduced the turnaround time in the detection of TB bacilli and drug resistance to a matter of hours or days. At most reference laboratories, specimens are cultured in both solid and liquid media and are also subjected to tests based on NAAT to detect TB bacilli and drug resistance.

## Radiology

Historically, concerns on the effect of radiation on fetus have limited its use. However, with adequate abdominal protection, it is a safe modality in pregnancy especially after the first trimester. A chest X-ray (CXR) results in fetal exposure of only 0.02 mRad and with computed tomography (CT) chest, it is less than 1 rad, which is considered to be safe.[5] Magnetic resonance imaging (MRI) and ultrasound may also be required during evaluation in some cases of EPTB such as those involving the central nervous system (CNS) and gastrointestinal (GI) tract.

## Histopathology

Caseating granuloma in a tissue biopsy or fine needle aspiration cytology (FNAC) specimen is considered to be suggestive of TB in the clinical context. Tissue can also be subjected to AFB stain and cultures.

## Tuberculin and Interferon Gamma Release Assays Tests

Mantoux test (Tuberculin Skin Test) is done using 1 tuberculin unit PPD RT23 (Purified Protein derivative). A swelling of 10 mm after 48 hours may be considered positive in high risk cases.

Tuberculin or interferon gamma release assays (IGRA) such as Quantiferon TB gold test if positive indicate latent TB in an asymptomatic person but not active disease.

The onus is on the clinician to rule out active disease by clinical and relevant investigative tests like sputum examination or CXR. Tuberculin positivity averages 35–40% in high TB burden countries. Latent TB does not affect fetus but due to the immunosuppression associated with pregnancy can reactivate into active disease in the mother. This needs to be carefully looked for during pregnancy and postnatal period.

## MANAGEMENT

The broad management of TB is similar to that in nonpregnant women. **Flowcharts 1 and 2** summarize the approach for the diagnosis of PTB and EPTB as per RNTCP guidelines of India.[6]

The emphasis is to rapidly confirm the presence of TB bacilli and drug resistance with the use of sputum smear, CBNAAT tests and liquid culture in sequential manner. This results in appropriate management of cases. In pregnant patients a call to use or abstain from CXR in the first trimester may be taken on clinical grounds.

All efforts should be made to collect appropriate specimens from target sites. Other diagnostic tools, either histopathology, which can be confirmatory or radiological modalities like ultrasound, CT, MRI, or biochemical tests such as adenosine deaminase (ADA) estimation in pleural fluid, which can be supportive in the clinical context. The detection rates of CBNAAT tests on biopsy and FNAC specimens from lymph nodes, CSF, other tissues are higher when compared to the gold standard of culture, but are low in pleural, pericardial, ascitic and synovial fluid. A positive CBNAAT test is confirmatory in the right clinical situation but a negative test does not rule out the disease.

## TREATMENT

Drug-sensitive TB is treated with an RNTCP approved 2 months intensive phase daily treatment with rifampicin (R), isoniazid (H), ethambutol (E), (RHE) and pyrazinamide (Z), which is followed by a 4 months continuation phase with RHE. Pyridoxine supplementation is required throughout the treatment. Streptomycin is avoided in pregnancy as it causes fetal deafness. The other drugs mentioned are safe though Center for Disease Control and Prevention (CDC), USA, does not recommend pyrazinamide since its effect on fetus are not known and it is reserved only for cases with drug resistance. In countries where drug resistance is significantly prevalent the use of Z cannot be avoided for good outcome. Breastfeeding is allowed and the mother is instructed to observe cough etiquette. The child should receive supplemental pyridoxine and requires 6 months of H prophylaxis followed by BCG vaccination.

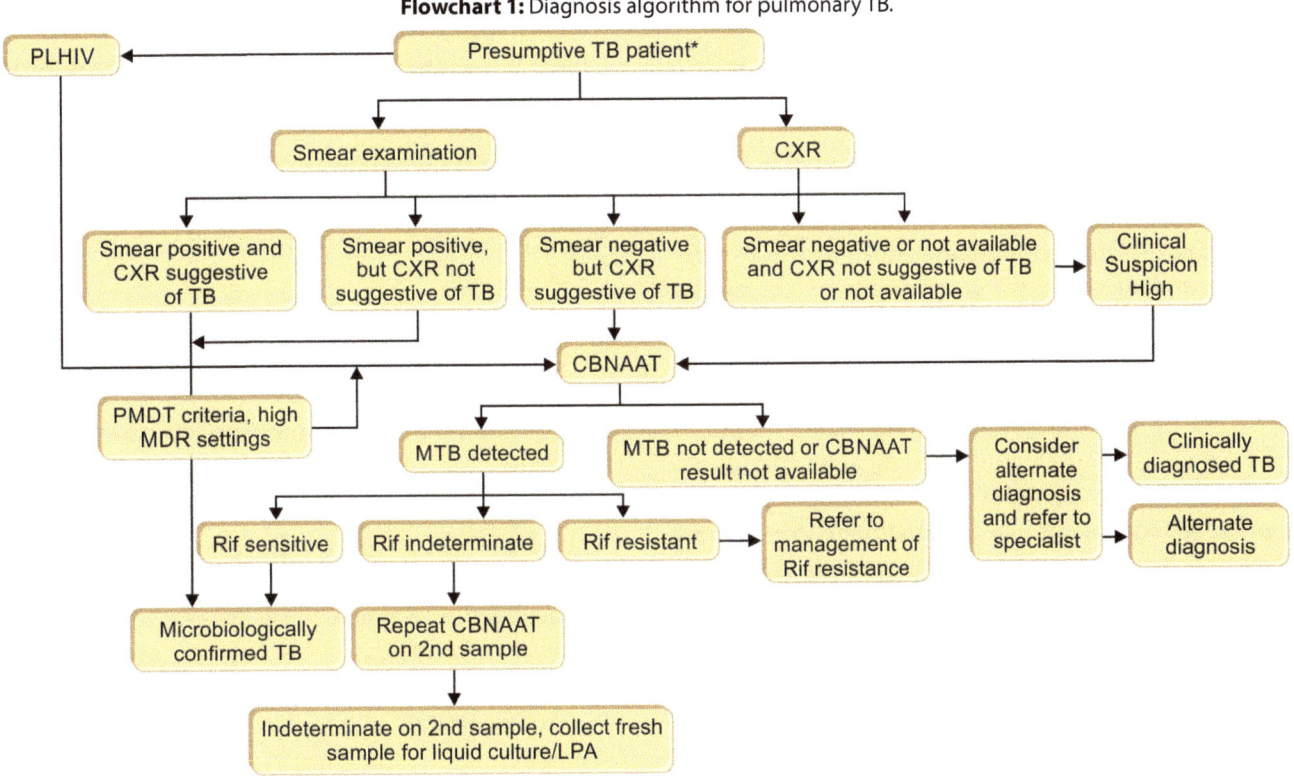

**Flowchart 1:** Diagnosis algorithm for pulmonary TB.

*All presumptive TB cases should be offered HIV counseling and testing: however, diagnostic work up for TB must not be delayed.
(CBNAAT: cartridge based nucleic acid amplification technology based tests; CXR: chest X-ray; PLHIV: people living with HIV; PMDT: programmatic management of drug resistant TB; Rif: rifampicin; LPA: line probe assay; MTB: *Mycobacterium tuberculosis*)

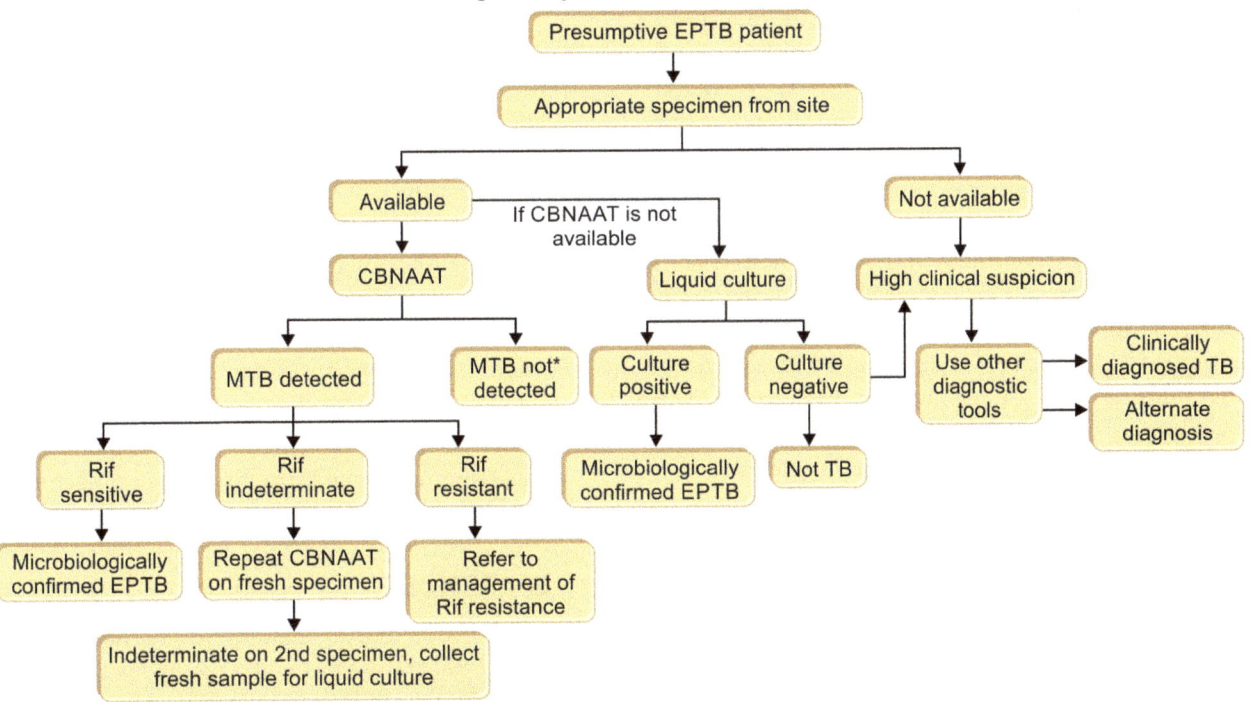

**Flowchart 2:** Diagnosis algorithm for extrapulmonary TB (EPTB).

*If high clinical suspicion then follow high clinical suspicion flow diagram
(CBNAAT: cartridge based nucleic acid amplification technology based tests; Rif: rifampicin; MTB: *Mycobacterium tuberculosis*)

Coinfection with HIV during pregnancy presents clinicians with significant challenges. Treatment of TB may be started as per RNTCP guidelines stated above. Initiation of anti-retroviral therapy (ART) is done as soon as possible in coinfection usually between 2 weeks and 2 months of starting antitubercular treatment (ATT).[7] A low CD4 count is indication for early ART except in TB meningitis where it is advisable to initiate at 2 months because of greater side effects. Patient intolerance to ATT and ART, high pill count, drug interactions and toxicities and possibility of immune reconstitution inflammatory syndrome (IRIS) are situations that demand special care.

Multidrug resistant and extensively drug-resistant (XDR) treatment is associated with greater morbidity, mortality, higher risks of drug toxicity, teratogenicity and treatment failure. Patient should be made aware of the potential risks and benefits of treatment which is long and requires a high degree of compliance with instructions. An assessment of the extent of disease and gestational age is made. In pregnancies of less than 20 weeks, medical termination of pregnancy (MTP), if acceptable to the patient, is indicated. In the remaining patients appropriate treatment on secondary line is started. Kanamycin and ethionamide are substituted with others such as para-aminosalicylic acid (PAS) for the duration of pregnancy. In the postpartum period kanamycin can be added and PAS stopped till the end of continuation phase. In case mother becomes sputum and culture negative at the time of delivery, separation of the child is not required and breast feeding is permissable.[6] Prophylaxis for child would depend on the drug resistance observed in the mother.

Treatment of latent TB with H prophylaxis in high burden areas has been a subject of debate. Adherence to the full course and completion of treatment are important concerns. Isoniazid monotherapy for 6 months is recommended by WHO for treatment of latent TB infection in both adults and children in countries with high and low TB incidence.[8] Baseline liver function tests and monitoring should be done in pregnant women. Pyridoxine (vitamin $B_6$) 50 mg daily is added to prevent peripheral neuropathy. As per CDC, USA, 4-month daily regimen of rifampin or 3 months daily regimen of isoniazid (INH) and rifampicin (3HR) or 6- or 9-month daily regimen of INH (6H or 9H), with pyridoxine (vitamin $B_6$) supplementation can be given if there is high risk of progression from latent infection to TB disease during pregnancy. Shorter duration regimens are preferred because of better adherence and fewer adverse events. In high risk situations such as HIV there is unanimity on treatment for latent TB with appropriate drugs.

## Contraception

Barrier contraceptive method or injection medroxy-progesterone acetate is preferred over oral contraceptive pills while on rifampicin based ATT.

## CONCLUSION

Timely diagnosis of TB in pregnancy and treatment with effective ATT may help in reducing the maternal and perinatal mortality and morbidity associated with the disease.

## KEY POINTS

- India has a high burden of TB with significant MDR and HIV association.
- Latent TB in women is known to become active during pregnancy or in postpartum period.
- Tuberculosis during pregnancy may result in FGR, low birth weight, perinatal mortality, and maternal morbidity and mortality.
- The signs and symptoms of tuberculosis in pregnant women include fever with night sweats, weight loss, cough, anorexia with general malaise.
- Diagnosis of TB in pregnancy can be challenging.
- Sputum examination is the most commonly used diagnostic test used for diagnosis of PTB.
- As per RNTCP of India, two sputum smears on consecutive days should be examined to isolate AFB; diagnosis of PTB is made, if at least one of the two smears is positive for AFB.
- Imaging procedures such as X-ray chest, may be performed safely in pregnancy if done with abdominal shield.
- Growth of tubercle bacilli in culture is the gold standard for diagnosis. MGIT cultures and NAAT-based tests have reduced the turnaround time for culture results.
- Caseating granuloma in a tissue biopsy or FNAC specimen is considered to be suggestive of TB in the clinical context.
- Tuberculin or IGRA such as Quantiferon TB gold test, if positive indicate latent TB in an asymptomatic person but not active disease.
- Drug sensitive TB is treated with a RNTCP-approved 2 months intensive phase daily treatment with RHE, and pyrazinamide (Z), which is followed by a 4 months continuation phase with RHE.
- The neonate should receive supplemental pyridoxine and requires 6 months of H prophylaxis followed by BCG vaccination.
- Barrier contraceptive methods or injection medroxy-progesterone acetate is preferred over oral contraceptive pills while on rifampicin based anti-tubercular treatment.

## REFERENCES

1. Pitre A. A rapid assessment of gender and tuberculosis in India 2018. New Delhi: Central TB Division, MOHFW; 2018.
2. WHO (2019). WHO Global tuberculosis report. [online] Available from: https://www.who.int/teams/global-tuberculosis-programme/tb-reports. [Last accessed July, 2021].
3. Sugarman J, Colvin C, Moran AC, Oxlade O. Tuberculosis in pregnancy: an estimate of the global burden of disease. Lancet Glob Health. 2014;2(12):e710-6.

4. Vijayageetha M, Kumar AM, Ramakrishnan J, Sarkar S, Papa D, Mehta K, et al. Tuberculosis screening among pregnant women attending a tertiary care hospital in Puducherry, South India: is it worth the effort? Glob Health Action. 2019;12(1):1564488.
5. Cunningham FG, Gant NF, Leveno KJ, Larry C. Williams Obstetrics, 21st edition. J Midwifery Women Health. 2010;48(5):369.
6. Central TB division, DGHS, MOHFW. (2016). Technical and operational guidelines for tuberculosis control in India 2016. [online]. Available from: https://tbcindia.gov.in/index1.php?lang=1&level=2&sublinkid=4573&lid=3177. [Last accessed July, 2021].
7. National AIDS Control Organization Ministry of Health and Family Welfare Government of India. National Technical Guidelines on Antiretroviral Treatment 2018. New Delhi: NACO, MOHFW; 2018.
8. WHO Guidelines Approved by the Guidelines Review Committee. Latent tuberculosis infection: updated and consolidated guidelines for programmatic management. Geneva: World Health Organization; 2018.

# CHAPTER 28: Malaria in Pregnancy

*Abha Singh, Bhawani Singh*

## INTRODUCTION

Malaria in pregnancy is a public health problem affecting the antenatal women and neonates. The World Health Organization (WHO) estimated the global burden of malaria to be 228 million cases in the year 2018. Out of these, 93% of cases occurred in Africa and the South-East Asian Region Office (SEARO). India, which is a part of the SEARO region, accounted for 3.4% of the global burden of the disease.[1]

In a study conducted in 2007, it was found that 125.2 million pregnancies occur in areas with *Plasmodium falciparum* and/or *P. vivax* transmission every year and hence are at a high risk of the disease.[2] In endemic areas, 25% of pregnant women are estimated to be infected with malaria. Primigravida, adolescents, those coinfected with human immunodeficiency virus (HIV) and in second trimester are most at risk.[3] Pregnant women infected with malaria are likely to have severe symptoms and adverse outcomes as compared to their nonpregnant counterparts. Higher rates of miscarriage, intrauterine death, premature delivery, low-birth weight neonates, and neonatal death are widely reported. They are also at a higher risk for severe anemia and maternal death.[4]

A study from Jharkhand, India reported a prevalence of 1.8% (43/2,382) in an antenatal clinic cohort of whom 53.5% were *P. falciparum*, 37.2% *P. vivax*, and 9.3% mixed infections.[5] Another study reported a prevalence of 1.3% peripheral parasitemia (35/2,696) at antenatal clinic and 1.9% at delivery units (19/1.025) in Chhattisgarh, India.[6] A study from Bikaner, Rajasthan has reported higher incidence of maternal mortality and complicated course in pregnant women infected with falciparum malaria when compared to nonpregnant women.[7] Similar results in maternal outcome were also observed from central India.[8]

In absolute numbers malaria in pregnancy is not uncommon in India and poses a challenge for the treating clinician.

## LIFE CYCLE OF MALARIAL PARASITE

Malaria is a parasitic infection caused by species of *Plasmodium* that infect humans. *Vivax, falciparum, malariae, ovale* and *knowlesi* are species causing human disease, of which the first two are more common in India. Out of nine anopheline vectors involved in transmitting malaria in India, female *Anopheles culicifacies* is the principal vector in rural areas and *An. stephensi* is the primary urban vector.

Infected female *Anopheles* mosquito bite triggers the exoerythrocytic cycle of parasite development in humans.

Sporozoites are injected in the host that rapidly migrate to the liver and over time mature into schizonts releasing merozoites in about 1–2 weeks. By attacking the red blood cells, merozoites can trigger the symptomatic erythrocytic phase of asexual multiplication of malarial parasite. *P. vivax* and *P. ovale* may persist in the liver for a long time (exoerythrocytic stage) as hypnozoites, capable of causing relapse of the disease even after many months. It must be noted that malaria drugs used to treat acute disease are incapable of eradicating the hypnozoites for which primaquine is required.

The merozoites infect the RBC and use them to mature into greater numbers, ultimately destroying them in a cyclic and repetitive manner resulting in typical symptoms of malaria. This is the stage of its development where most diagnostic and therapeutic efforts are targeted. During this stage few parasites develop into macrogametes (female) and microgametes (male). When ingested by a mosquito they enter the sporogonic phase of its development in the vector to mature into sporozoites that can infect.

Hence, two hosts and two strategic vector bites are required to complete this life cycle.

## PATHOGENESIS

Pregnancy is a state of reduced cell immunity designed to sustain placenta and the fetus. Hormonal changes such as increased cortisol levels also adversely impact immunity. Hence, the parasite finds an easy access in pregnancy. Pregnant women are consequently at greater risk to acquire malaria as well as progress to severe manifestations with adverse outcomes for the mother, fetus and pregnancy. Repeated exposure to the parasite in areas of high transmission produces a level of immunity to the disease that modifies clinical manifestations and outcomes when compared to areas of low transmission and populations with little or no tolerance. Placenta is characterized by sequestration of *P. falciparum*-infected erythrocytes to blood vessels in the intervillous space thereby avoiding the defense mechanism like spleen and resulting invascular injury. Placenta can be riddled with parasite and stained black due to deposition of malarial pigment. Presence of parasites invites inflammatory cells and markers resulting in oxidative stress and changes in the placental morphology, and hormonal changes triggering adverse outcomes. In mother, there can be anemia, metabolic acidosis, jaundice, renal failure, pulmonary edema, respiratory distress, convulsions, coma and death, if left untreated. Malaria is likely to cause abortions, preterm labor, fetal growth restriction (FGR) and intrauterine death (IUD).[9-11]

## CLINICAL FEATURES

The signs and symptoms would depend on malarial transmission in the geographical location as well as the immune status of the individual. Generally in areas of high transmission, women may be asymptomatic with no or minimal parasites in blood. Pregnancy predisposes to a severe course more often when compared to nonpregnant women for reasons discussed above. Primigravida are more susceptible to adverse outcomes. Uncomplicated malaria presents with nonspecific symptoms such as fever, body aches, chills, rigors, diarrhea and headache. History of residence or travel to malaria endemic area may provide a clue to the diagnosis. Since the differential diagnosis is expansive, necessary diagnostic tests should be sent to confirm the diagnosis. In some situations, empirical treatment may be justified if investigations are unavailable or results are delayed.

Severe or complicated malaria should be suspected if the patient presents with altered sensorium, convulsions, severe anemia, jaundice, anuria, abnormal bleeding, and extreme breathlessness. Laboratory results may show hemoglobin less than 7 g/dL, thrombocytopenia, altered kidney or liver function, hypoglycemia, acidemia and hemoglobinuria. Parasite count in blood may exceed >10%. Mortality is higher in pregnant women and approaches 50% with neurological involvement.[12]

## DIAGNOSIS

The microscopic examination of thin and thick smears from peripheral blood (made during fever) remains the gold standard of diagnosis. It allows identification of the malarial species as well as a count of the parasite that aids treatment. Three negative smears at 12-hourly interval argue against the diagnosis. One must consider the use of prophylactic drugs and high background immune status of the patient when peripheral blood is negative (where the placenta may be sequestrated with the parasite). Rapid diagnostic tests (RDTs) to identify *P. falciparum* and *P. vivax* are available and have significant role especially in places where microscopy is not immediately available. The sensitivity of RDT to identify the parasite is lower as compared to microscopy (200 vs. 50/µL) and therefore simultaneous smears should also be tested.[13] RDT also remain positive for a few weeks after cure. Polymerase chain reaction (PCR)-based nucleic acid amplification tests have a very high sensitivity (1/µL) but are not readily available.[13]

Depending on the presentation, other diagnostic tests such as cerebrospinal fluid (CSF) examination, blood cultures, imaging studies and other follow-up studies to evaluate response to treatment and adverse drug reactions may be required.

Placental blood and cord blood samples can also be collected during delivery. Placental specimens can also be examined for the parasite.

## TREATMENT

The aim of the treating clinician is to treat malaria and manage the pregnancy leading to a healthy baby and a healthy mother. Reduced immunity in the pregnant mother is not the only hurdle to achieve this aim. The drug pharmacokinetics in pregnancy is also altered resulting in lower drug levels in the blood and more likely failure of treatment in the nonimmune patient.[14] Drug resistance too, is widely prevalent in malaria. Furthermore, many effective drugs are not considered safe in pregnancy especially during the first trimester. Physiological changes in pregnancy may also complicate decisions such as fluid management. These factors warrant treatment by a multispecialty team comprising an obstetrician, infectious disease specialist and a neonatologist. **Tables 1 and 2** summarize important aspects of drug treatment in a pregnant patient. In case species of parasite is not known, treatment should be given as for uncomplicated falciparum infection.

Artemisinin combination therapy or ACT is currently the treatment of choice in uncomplicated falciparum malaria as it far exceeds efficacy and safety of other drugs and combinations. There are recent recommendations that

**TABLE 1:** Treatment for nonfalciparum species.

| Organism | Drug | Dose |
|---|---|---|
| P. vivax | Chloroquin as base: Each 250 mg tablet contains 150 mg base and each 5 mL of suspension contains 50 mg base Or Artemisinin combination therapy (ACT) in doses as given in text | 600 mg base at diagnosis, 300 mg after 6 hours, then 300 mg at 24 hours and 48 hours. The last two doses can be divided equally into BD at 12 hours interval |
| P. ovale | As above | As above |
| P. malariae | As above | As above |
| P. vivax resistant | As for uncomplicated P. falciparum | See text |

| TABLE 2: Treatment of *falciparum* species and mixed infections. | |
|---|---|
| Type of infection | Treatment |
| Complicated or severe | • *Initial treatment in 2nd and 3rd trimester* drug of choice Artesunate intravenous infusion (IVI) 2.4 mg/kg at 0, 12 and 24 hours, then once daily thereafter. This dose should be diluted as per instructions provided with the pack. Once able to take orally artemisinin-based combination therapy (ACT) for 3 days must be given to complete treatment, prevent relapse and drug resistance. Use in *any stage* of pregnancy is also recommended in severe malaria<br>• *Alternatively and in 1st trimester:* Quinine IVI diluted in 5% dextrose. Dose 20 mg/kg over 4 hours slowly. Further 10 mg/kg IVI TDS over 4 hours. Accompanied by IVI Clindamycin 450 mg TDS. Once patient is fit to take orally tablet Quinine 600 mg and tablet Clindamycin 450 both TDS to complete total 7 days treatment. Modify dosage in case of renal or hepatic dysfunction. Monitor for hypoglycemia. Doxycycline must not be used as an accompanying drug in pregnancy |
| Uncomplicated | ACT is the treatment of choice except in first trimester. The choice of combination prescribed depends on local drug resistance patterns (see text). Alternatively quinine may be used |

**BOX 1:** Preventive or eradicative treatment for non-falciparum species

- 300 mg chloroquine per week during the entire period of pregnancy and lactation
- Primaquine is contraindicated during pregnancy and lactation
- Primaquine may be started after completing lactation and glucose 6-phosphate dehydrogenase (G6PD) estimation

artemisinin-based drugs can be safely used in any stage of pregnancy for severe malaria.[15] Artemisinin are a group of semisynthetic derivatives from the sweet wormwood plant (*Artemisia annua*). Since monotherapy with these derivatives results in rapid development of drug resistance, they are used in combination with other drugs to prevent this. Combination of artesunate with pyrimethamine and sulfadoxine, artemether with lumefantrine, artesunate and amodiaquine and others are available. The presence of accompanying drug prevents the development of resistance and synergizes the primary drug. The combination of artesunate at 4 mg/kg (200 mg maximum) with sulfadoxine at 25 mg/kg (maximum 750 mg) and pyrimethamine at 1.25 mg/kg (maximum 37.5 mg) is recommended for most parts of India. In adults with weight more than 35 kg all three drugs are given on day 1 as per dosage indicated and it is followed by identical dosage of artesunate only on day 2 and 3 to complete the treatment. The combination of artemether with lumefantrine is recommended in North East states of India due to reports of resistance to the above combination.[16] Each tablet contains artemether 20 mg and lumefantrine 120 mg. In adults weighing ≥35 kg, an initial dose of 4 tablets, followed by 4 tablets given at 8, 24, 36, 48, and 60 hours thereafter, to a total of 24 tablets are given over 3 days to complete the treatment. This is a category C drug for pregnancy. These drugs have few adverse reactions in the dosage prescribed with rare cases of neutropenia, hemolytic anemia and deranged liver functions tests.

Mefloquine is preferably avoided in pregnancy because of its association with stillbirths and neuropsychiatric manifestations in the mother. Growing resistance to sulfadoxine and pyrimethamine combination and serious drug toxicity such as Stevens-Johnson reaction has reduced the usage of this previously very effective combination. Tetracyclines should be avoided due to adverse effects on fetal bones. Amodiaquine, chlorproguanil-dapsone, halofantrine, lumefantrine and piperaquine in isolation have not been adequately evaluated in pregnancy to inspire confidence.[15] Quinine administration requires close supervision as it can cause hypoglycemia, hypotension, QT prolongation and auditory nerve damage. Primaquine use is contraindicated in pregnancy. Its use to eradicate the dormant hypnozoites in the liver to prevent relapse, is avoided during pregnancy and till infant is weaned off from mother's milk. In the interim, chloroquine is given as indicated in **Box 1**, to prevent relapse. Before starting primaquine, a G6PD estimation is a must to identify those at the risk of developing hemolysis. The dose is 0.5 mg/kg body weight in a single dose for 14 days. Primaquine is also the only effective drug acting on the gametocytes of *P. falciparum* hence capable of reducing onward transmission. A single dose of 0.25 mg/kg body weight is prescribed along with ACT for this purpose.

## CONGENITAL MALARIA

It can occur in up to 0.1–7% of newborns born to unprotected susceptible women affected by malaria. Normally maternal antibodies cross the placental barrier and protect the fetus. With poor passive immunity, congenital malaria can occur in the fetus with parasites passing through the damaged placenta. Fetal death is usually not due to congenital malaria but maternal hyperpyrexia. Both *falciparum* and *vivax*, present in the newborn with symptoms similar to neonatal sepsis. The diagnosis may be more difficult in areas of high transmission where the mother may be asymptomatic. In areas of chloroquine resistance, treatment should be given with ACT or quinine. *P. vivax* that is not resistant may be treated with chloroquine. Primaquine is avoided in first 6 months and administered after estimating G6PD.

## CHEMOPROPHYLAXIS

In malaria endemic areas, preventive treatment in pregnancy by use of sulfadoxine and pyrimethamine given in three doses at least 1 month apart starting in the second trimester has been found to be effective.[15] Success with this approach is widely reported from Africa. It is found to be more effective than screening, early detection and treatment primarily because of the lower sensitivity of RDTs to detect malaria in pregnancy.[17] Growing drug resistance to this combination has resulted in trials of newer agents such as dihydroartemisinin-piperaquine.[17]

Insecticide treated mosquito nets have also been useful in preventing infection in endemic areas.

## KEY POINTS

- India accounts for 3.4% of the global burden of malaria.
- Malaria in pregnancy is not uncommon in India and poses a challenge for the treating clinician.
- Pregnant women infected with malaria are likely to have more severe symptoms and adverse outcomes as compared to their nonpregnant counterparts. Malaria is likely to cause abortions, preterm labor, FGR and IUD.
- Repeated exposure to the parasite in areas of high transmission modifies clinical manifestations and outcomes when compared to areas of low transmission and populations with little or no tolerance.
- Uncomplicated malaria presents with nonspecific symptoms such as fever, body aches, chills, rigors, diarrhea and headache.
- Severe or complicated malaria should be suspected if the patient presents with altered sensorium, convulsions, severe anemia, jaundice, anuria, abnormal bleeding, extreme breathlessness.
- The microscopic examination of thin and thick smears from peripheral blood remains the gold standard of diagnosis.
- RDTs have significant role especially in places where microscopy is not immediately available.
- Altered drug pharmacokinetics in pregnancy and resistance to antimalarial drugs is a big challenge in the treatment of malaria in pregnancy.
- *Plasmodium vivax, P. ovale* and *P. malariae* are treated with chloroquine while for *P. falciparum*, artemisinin combination therapy (ACT) is preferred for uncomplicated infection and injection artesunate for complicated infection.
- Resistant *P. vivax* is also treated with ACT therapy.
- Congenital malaria can occur in up to 0.1–7% of newborns born to unprotected susceptible women affected by malaria.
- Chemoprophylaxis with sulfadoxine and pyrimethamine in the second trimester may be given in malaria endemic areas.

## REFERENCES

1. World Health Organization. World Malaria Report 2019. Geneva: WHO; 2019.
2. Dellicour S, Tatem AJ, Guerra CA, Snow RW, Kuile FO. Quantifying the number of pregnancies at risk of malaria in 2007: a demographic study. PLoS Med. 2010;7:e100022.
3. Desai M, KuileFO, Nostan F, McGready R, Asamoa K, Brabin B, et al. Epidemiology and burden of malaria in pregnancy. Lancet Infect Dis. 2007;7:93-104.
4. Schantz-Dunn J, Nour NM. Malaria and pregnancy: a global health perspective. Rev Obstet Gynecol. 2009;2(3):186-92.
5. Hamer DH, Singh MP, Wylie BJ, Yeboah-Antwi K, Tuchman J, Desai M, et al. Burden of malaria in pregnancy in Jharkhand State, India. Malar J. 2009;8:210.
6. Singh N, Singh MP, Wylie BJ, Hussain M, Kojo YA, Shekhar C, et al. Malaria prevalence among pregnant women in two districts with differing endemicity in Chhattisgarh, India. Malar J. 2012;11:274.
7. Kochar DK, Thanvi I, Joshi A, Aseri S, Kumawat BL. Falciparum malaria and pregnancy. Indian J Malariol. 1998;35:123-30.
8. Singh N, Shukla MM, Sharma VP. Epidemiology of malaria in pregnancy in Central India. Bull World Health Organ. 1999;77:567-72.
9. WHO. Severe falciparum malaria. Transaction of Roy Soc Trop Med Hyg. 2000;94(Suppl 1):1-90.
10. Sharma L, Shukla G. Placental malaria: a new insight into the pathophysiology. Front Med. 2017;4:117.
11. Fried M Duffy PE. Malaria during pregnancy. Cold Spring Harb Perspect Med. 2017;7:a025551.
12. White NJ, Farrar J. Manson's Tropical Diseases. New York: Elsevier; 2013. pp. 532-600.
13. Mathison BA, Pritt BS. Update on malaria diagnostics and test utilization. J Clin Microbiol. 2017;55;2009-17.
14. Wilby KJ, Ensom MH. Pharmacokinetics of antimalarials in pregnancy. A systemic review. Clin Pharmacokinet. 2011;50:705-23.
15. WHO. Guidelines for the Treatment of Malaria, 3rd edition. Geneva: WHO; 2015.
16. Mishra N. Guidelines for Diagnosis and Treatment of Malaria in India, 3rd edition. New Delhi: National Institute of Malaria Research; 2014.
17. Desai M, Gutman J, L'anzivas A, Otieno K, Juma E, Kariuki S, et al. Intermittent screening and treatment or intermittent preventive treatment with dihydroartemisinin-piperaquine versus intermittent preventive treatment with sulfadoxine and pyrimethamine for the control of malaria in pregnancy in western Kenya: an open label three groups randomized controlled superiority trial. Lancet. 2015;386:2507-19.

# CHAPTER 29: HIV Infection in Pregnancy

*Sudha Salhan*

## INTRODUCTION

Human immunodeficiency virus (HIV) is a virus responsible for causing acquired immune-deficiency syndrome (AIDS), a condition which causes progressive failure of the immune system resulting in life-threatening opportunistic infections (OI) and cancers. French researchers Françoise Barré-Sinoussi and Luc Montagnier first published Human Immuno-deficiency Viral (HIV) infection report in 1983 and were awarded Nobel Prize in 2008. To begin with, HIV/AIDS was considered a disease of male population supposed to be acquired by men having sex with men (MSM). Later on, it was reported in women also. Now in new cases of HIV, women are equally affected, if not more, than men. As per The Joint United Nations Programme on HIV/AIDS (UNAIDS) 2020 data women and girls accounted for about 48% of all new HIV infections in 2019 and, there were 38.0 million people living with HIV; 36.2 million adults and 1.8 million were children (0–14 years).[1]

Women are more vulnerable to this infection than men due to factors such as exposure of larger surface area of vagina to infected secretions; sexual exposure of immature vaginal epithelium as a result of marriage at an early age; little control or negotiation power in their sexual relation and inability to practice safe sex practices (e.g., abstinence during menstrual period, condom use), poor access to healthcare services and lack of knowledge regarding HIV and also due to economic dependence.[2]

In 2017–18, National Aids Control Organization (NACO) reported 9,550 new cases of HIV infected women in India. The National AIDS Control Programme (NACP) launched Prevention of Parent-to-Child Transmission (PPTCT) of HIV Programme in the year 2001–2002 in India **(Table 1)**. With the efforts of world bodies, viz. World Health Organization (WHO), Centers for Disease Control and prevention (CDC) in America, UNAIDS and in India NACO, the prevalence of HIV is steadily declining. **Table 2** shows a 66% decline in new infections from 2000 against a global average decline of 35% in 2015.

Almost all cases of HIV infection in children (91%) are acquired by mother-to-child transmission (MTCT). The perinatal transmission of HIV from mother to child (vertical transmission) can occur during pregnancy, labor or during breastfeeding and the incidence varies from 15 to 45%.[3] Out of about 29 million deliveries every year in India, 35,255 occur in HIV positive mothers. If no intervention is done, 10,361 HIV infected neonates will be born annually (NACO).

As the mother usually gets the infection from the male partner, it is also called parent-to-child transmission (PTCT).

To prevent the HIV transmission to the child by effective interventions including antiretroviral therapy (ART), it is of utmost importance to determine the HIV status of woman in early pregnancy. There are two types of HIV viruses, viz. HIV-1 and HIV-2. HIV-1 is associated with higher MTCT rate (20–35%) compared to 0–4% with HIV-II.

## FACTORS AFFECTING MTCT OF HIV[4]

Vertical transmission of HIV from mother to child (MTCT) is not 100%. If the mother is not treated it is 15–45%. Various factors that affect the MTCT of HIV are listed in **Box 1**.

**TABLE 1:** Age distribution with percentage of HIV patients in India.

| Age group | Percentage |
|---|---|
| <15 years | 3.8 |
| 15–49 years | 88.7 |
| >50 years | 7.5 |

*Source:* National AIDS Control Organization

**TABLE 2:** The steady decline of HIV cases in India.

| Year | National adult HIV prevalence in India (%) |
|---|---|
| 2001–2003 | 0.38 |
| 2007 | 0.34 |
| 2012 | 0.28 |
| 2015 | 0.26 |

*Source:* National AIDS Control Organization.

> **BOX 1:** Factors affecting mother-to-child transmission of HIV.
>
> - *Maternal factors:*
>   - Maternal plasma viral load
>   - Concurrent sexually transmitted infections and other infections
>   - Unprotected sexual intercourse
>   - Maternal CD4 and lymphocyte count
>   - Mother's neutralizing antibody status
>   - Nutritional status
>   - Smoking, illicit drug use
>   - Ruptured fetal membranes
>   - Viral type
>   - Detectable p24 antigen in maternal serum
>   - Placental barrier
>   - Viral load in genital tract
> - Mode of delivery
> - *Fetal factors:*
>   - Genetic makeup
>   - Prematurity
>   - Duration of exposure to maternal secretions
>   - Newborn immune response
>   - Low fetal weight
>   - Breastfeeding

## Maternal Factors

### Viral Load

Viral load in a pregnant woman is maximum just after infection when body's immune response is not developed, and hence virus replicates at a rapid pace and also in advanced stage of the disease. It can be diagnosed by RNA HIV-I PCR test or quantitative culture. In the current era of potent ART knowledge of the base line viral load is very important. Transmission to the fetus is there at all concentrations, but is directly proportional to the maternal viral load. When maternal viral load is below 50 copies/mL, the MTCT is below 0.5%.[5,6]

### Concurrent Reproductive Tract Infections and STI

Sexually transmitted infections (STIs) especially those with ulcers, e.g., syphilis, increase MTCT of HIV. Evidence is accumulating to suggest the role of malaria, tuberculosis, parasitic infestation (hookworm, etc.) in the transmission of HIV. Bacterial vaginosis and *Chlamydia trachomatis* in pregnant women is associated with more MTCT of HIV. Hepatitis C with HIV in pregnancy doubles the MTCT of HIV. Hepatitis B and herpes simplex virus (HSV) is also associated with higher MTCT of HIV.

### Unprotected Sexual Intercourse

Unprotected sexual intercourse during pregnancy increases the risk of transmission to the fetus. Though transmission through a single sexual act is small, if the frequency of the act is high even in pregnancy, the cumulative effect makes it the most common route of infection of HIV. Use of spermicides, e.g., nonoxynol disrupts the membranes of cells in the lining of the vagina making it easy for the HIV to penetrate. Traditional practices such as douching with lime juice, etc., may damage the vaginal lining increasing the susceptibility to acquire HIV infection. Correct and consistent use of condom (male/female) is recommended.

### Maternal CD4 and Lymphocyte Count

It is an independent predictor of prenatal transmission risk. There is an inverse relation, i.e., lower the CD4 and lymphocyte count more is MTCT of HIV.

### Maternal Neutralizing Antibody Status

Maternal neutralizing monoclonal HIV antibodies may have a protective effect in preventing MTCT of HIV.

### Nutritional Status of the Mother

Malnutrition may increase MTCT of HIV. There is weakness in epithelial integrity of the placenta and genital tract and hence associated accelerated transmission of HIV infection. The trace element zinc is involved in many immunologic impairments and may reduce circulating T lymphocytes in HIV positive woman. Low vitamin A level during pregnancy is seen to be associated with higher MTCT of HIV.[7]

### Use of Illicit Drugs

Smoking, use of illicit drugs (cocaine, heroin, etc.) and alcohol consumption may have direct effect on the integrity of placenta. They may adversely affect the developing immune system in the fetus thus increasing MTCT of HIV.

### Status of Fetal Membranes

Both amnion and chorion when intact, reduce MTCT of HIV. A correlation between the time elapsed from rupture of membranes to actual delivery affects the rate of MTCT of HIV. If the membranes are ruptured for more than 4 hours the transmission rate doubles.

### Operative Procedures

Procedures such as episiotomy, forceps or ventouse delivery, fetal scalp blood sampling, amniocentesis, or umbilical cord blood sampling increase MTCT of HIV.

### Type of Virus

The biological phenotype of virus may influence the transmission risk. Monocyte macrophage tropic (M-Tropic) maternal virus is reported to be more likely to be transmitted than maternal isolates of T cell tropic phenotype.

### Placental Barrier

Breaches in the placenta may be associated with mixing of maternal and fetal blood, as occurs in chorioamnionitis, cigarette smoking and in illicit drug users. These are associated with increased MTCT of HIV.

### Viral Load in Genital Tract

Increased viral load in the cervix and vagina will have more MTCT of HIV.

## Mode of Delivery

Vaginal delivery is safe. But it depends on many factors such as viral load, whether the woman is on any treatment, etc. If the pregnant women is on ART throughout pregnancy and the viral load is less than 50 copies/mL, the MTCT is less than 2% (0.5–1.5%).[5,6,8] Hence, cesarean section is not recommended for prevention of MTCT, particularly where women are taking ART for their own health or have had adequate duration of antiretroviral (ARV) prophylaxis for PTCT. NACO guidelines (2013) clearly state that cesarean section in HIV positive women should be performed for obstetric indications only.

## Fetal Factors

### Genetic Makeup

Susceptibility to HIV infection may be different for different fetuses due to variation in genetic makeup.

### Maturity

Immunological maturity is directly proportional to the fetal maturity because of increased expression of CD4+ count as the pregnancy progresses. In preterm neonates, the MTCT of HIV is 3.7 times more than in a term neonate.

### Duration of Exposure to Maternal Secretions

Mother-to-child transmission is directly proportional to duration of exposure of fetal thin skin and mucous surfaces to maternal secretions. It is more with the first twin than second twin (26% vs. 13%).

### Newborn Immune Response

Immune response to HIV has a role in averting MTCT of HIV by cell mediated immunity in the fetus or newborn. It may play a crucial role in protection or clearance of infection.

### Breastfeeding

There is HIV I in both cellular and acellular components of breast milk. There is a 30% independent risk of MTCT of HIV by breastfeeding by HIV infected mother. Therefore, complete avoidance of breastfeeding is the surest way to avoid MTCT of HIV through breastfeeding. The risk of transmission depends on the period of breastfeeding, maternal viral load, HIV disease status (early or terminal stage), associated breast abscess or cracked nipple, use of ART and exclusive/mixed feeding.

## TIMING OF VERTICAL TRANSMISSION

Timing of vertical transmission from mother to the fetus is not clear. Most acquire infection at the time of delivery and rest through breastfeeding. Intrauterine transmission has been documented by identification of HIV in aborted products, placental tissue, fetal blood samples and amniotic fluid. Twenty percent of transmission occurs before 36 weeks, 50% during delivery and 30% through breast milk in postpartum period.[9] Hence, protection at all levels is essential to prevent MTCT.

## POTENTIAL ROUTES OF INFECTION

Known route of infection are mixing of mother and fetal blood, antenatal infection across the placenta, extensive skin and mucous membrane exposure to maternal blood and vaginal secretions during delivery.

## DIAGNOSIS

Centers for Disease Control (CDC), USA and NACO has recommended that all pregnant women be tested for HIV as early as possible during each pregnancy, and in high-risk groups repeat HIV test is performed at 36 weeks of pregnancy. Early diagnosis of HIV infection in the pregnant woman can prevent MTCT of HIV by ARV therapy and other interventions. Partners of the pregnant women should be encouraged to undergo HIV testing when their HIV status is unknown (CDC Guidelines, December 2019).

After pretest counseling (in group) the woman is offered the test for HIV detection.[10] If she agrees ("opts in") her blood sample is drawn. If she refuses ("opts out") her blood sample is not drawn and this fact is mentioned in her clinical record, but she is provided all antenatal and postnatal services available. The counselor may go into the causes of opting out and address them with empathy and eventually may turn her round for "opting-in" to get the test done.

The common test performed is serological test for detection of viral specific antibodies by enzyme linked immunosorbent assay (ELISA). Three different ELISA kits are used on the serum samples, to diagnose an asymptomatic woman. The pregnant woman is called on the subsequent day to collect the report. The importance of collecting the report is emphasized. Before handing over the report, one to one post-test counseling is done. The report is confidential and not told to anyone else without the permission of the woman.

If she comes in labor at odd hours with no previous testing, expedited or rapid test can be offered on whole blood 24 × 7. The result is available within an hour. If positive, the ARV prophylaxis is immediately started to the mother. The confirmation is done in the morning of next working day from the same blood sample by confirmatory tests such as Western Blot or immunofluorescence assay (IFA). Same procedure is to be done for mother and neonate pair who was not tested till delivery. Hence, test is done in immediate postpartum period. This rapid testing and immediate treatment will reduce MTCT of HIV from 25% to 9–13%.

Tests for *Chlamydia trachomatis*, *Neisseria gonorrhoeae* and bacterial vaginosis are carried out. She must also be screened for hepatitis B and C and opportunistic infections (OI) like *Pneumocystis jiroveci* pneumonia (PJP), *Mycobacterium avium* complex (MAC) and cancer of the uterine cervix. Screening for diabetes mellitus is done at 24–28 weeks of pregnancy. Protease inhibitor drugs can cause hyperglycemia and diabetic ketoacidosis.

A baseline CD4 count is done and repeated every 3 months. If possible, plasma HIV RNA is done initially and repeated every 2 months and finally at 36 weeks.

## INTERVENTIONS AIMED AT DECREASING MTCT OF HIV

The risk of MTCT without any intervention is around 15–45%. These recommendations have the potential to reduce the risk of MTCT to less than 5% in breastfeeding populations. Different guidelines are advocated by various countries and groups.[11-13]

The NACO has a four-pronged PPTCT program. Prevention of HIV especially in women of reproductive age group:

1. *Prevention of HIV especially in women of the reproductive age group:* Through voluntary counseling and testing (VCT) centers throughout our country (started by National AIDS Control Programme III of NACO), HIV testing is possible in any female of 15 years or above. If she tests HIV negative, she is advised abstinence or motivated to practice safe sexual behavior (promotion of consistent and constant use of condoms-male and female condoms, developing negotiation skills, encouraging monogamous relations or minimal sex partners, and no sex during menstrual periods). Early diagnosis and treatment of reproductive tract infections (RTI), STI and other infections is done. Advise against sharing needles in intravenous drug users. She is also immunized against hepatitis B. All these will go a long way in preventing HIV. In case of couples who come for testing their fitness for pregnancy (preconceptional counseling) and those who come for treatment of infertility, both partners be tested for their HIV status. If both are HIV positive, they are directed to ART centers where they are given appropriate ART for lifetime and are properly followed up. They are asked to try pregnancy when their viral load is undetectable so that chances of MTCT are minimal. If one partner is HIV positive (discordant couple) she/he is directed for ART therapy. ART taken by HIV infected partner considerably reduces the chances of transmitting this infection to the uninfected partner.

The HIV negative partner is counseled for safe sexual practices and pre-exposure prophylaxis (PrEP). This drug treatment reduces sexually transmitted HIV by 90% and in injection drug user by 70%. Condom use reduces the transmission rate further for the partner. Two drug combonations are available for PrEP:
   i. Emtricitabine + Tenofovir disoproxil fumarate (approved for adolescents and adults) and
   ii. Emtricitabine + Tenofovir alafenamide (not recommended for risk of receptive vaginal sex).

   These drugs are taken daily. Follow-up is done after every 3 months for HIV test and repeating the prescription.[14,15] Dapivirine vaginal ring: The female partner who is HIV negative and is 18 years or older can use this under trial, flexible silicon ring as PrEP. The ring constantly releases this anti-HIV drug for one month.[16]

2. *Prevention of unintended pregnancy:* Reaching out to women before they become pregnant is a very important and cost-effective primary preventive measure for MTCT. Since more than 25% pregnancies are unintended, many HIV positive pregnancies can be averted by contraception. Overall attention to increase contraceptive awareness will be an effective strategy.

3. *Prevention of transmission of HIV from pregnant woman to her child:* The broad principles are an early testing of the pregnant woman for HIV, if HIV positive, she is started on ART. And if she is in early pregnancy she is given the option of medical termination of pregnancy (MTP).

4. *Giving care, support and treatment to women with HIV in reproductive age group, her children and family.*

## MANAGEMENT

### Antenatal Management

The management of HIV positive pregnant woman is a multidisciplinary team approach comprising a counselor, obstetrician, physician, psychiatrist and a pediatrician. After knowing the positive status of the pregnant woman and her decision to continue this pregnancy the following measures are emphasized besides normal routine antenatal care (ANC).

Besides detailed history, any history of ARV drug therapy in the past or present, and any symptoms of opportunistic infection are elicited. First trimester ultrasound is required for exact dating of pregnancy and for measuring nuchal translucency. Double marker test is done at 11–13 weeks of pregnancy. Hemoglobin should be checked from time to time for development of anemia. Liver functions tests (LFT) are performed as a baseline before starting on protease inhibitors (PI). Follow-up with LFT and electrolytes is required from time to time and monthly in last trimester. The need for supportive care such as psychological support, home support, etc., is assessed. Second trimester ultrasound is performed at 18–20 weeks for fetal growth and any detectable congenital abnormality.

She is advised about proper diet and hygiene. Any deficiency in diet is addressed because a well-nourished woman will pass less viral load to the fetus. Any infection, e.g., STI, RTI, tuberculosis, etc., should be looked for and if present should be treated vigorously. Screening for hepatitis B, hepatitis C and cancer cervix should be done.

She is advised to discontinue smoking, drinking alcohol and using illicit drugs. She is made aware of safe sexual practices and is referred to ART center for proper therapy and follow-up. She is encouraged to regularly come for ANC whenever called. Emphasis on institutional delivery is done on each ANC visit. No live vaccination is given.

If she is aware of her HIV status and is on proper ART for her health, she is advised to continue the same. No increase in congenital malformations is proven with this therapy. If she is diagnosed with HIV infection for the first time in this pregnancy, ART is started at the earliest possible and she is made aware of its importance for her health and for prevention of infection in the fetus.

If CD4 count is 250 cell/mm$^3$ or less double strength cotrimoxazole one tablet daily is started and continued throughout pregnancy, labor and breastfeeding to prevent opportunistic infections.

Start counseling about contraceptive choices from early pregnancy so as to prevent or delay next pregnancy.

## Immunological Measures

Maximum transmission of HIV from the mother to the neonate is at or around the time of delivery. Hence, a combination of active and passive immunization will be effective in prevention of this transmission with as is seen in hepatitis B infection. Till date, vaccination, i.e., active immunization is still a dream and passive protection using HIV IgG is under investigation. Protocols to test neutralizing monoclonal antibodies are in the developing stage.

Based on the new guidelines of WHO and NACO,[17-19] it has been decided to provide life-long ART for all pregnant and breastfeeding women living with HIV. A triple drug ART regimen regardless of CD4 count, WHO clinical stage or trimester of pregnancy is recommended, both for their own health and for preventing vertical HIV transmission from mother-to-child (NACO 2015 and 2018 Guidelines). Life-long ART helps in maximizing coverage for those needing treatment, (will keep them alive and healthy), avoids stopping and starting drugs with repeat pregnancies, provides early protection against MTCT in future pregnancies and will avoid drug resistance.

Antepartum, intrapartum and postpartum ARV therapy is essential to reduce MTCT. All HIV infected mothers should start triple drug ARV therapy as soon as they come under the supervision of a hospital and continue treatment lifelong. The same has been adopted by NACO in guidelines issued in 2013, 2015 and 2018.

Antiretroviral drugs are given at ART centers. Recent trend is toward triple drug regime with the use of fixed-dose combination formulations, enabling one-pill a day treatment which is well tolerated and is affordable.

*The ARV drugs act by reducing MTCT by multiple mechanisms detailed as follows:* ARV drugs lower maternal viral load in blood and in genital secretions to undetectable level. Thus, leaving fewer number of viruses to cross the placenta or to reach the milk. ARV drugs also improve health and prolong the survival of the mother.

Some of the drugs cross the placenta and enter the fetus giving adequate systemic levels of drug in fetus. This gives pre-exposure prophylaxis to the fetus during its passage through the birth canal of the mother.

Postexposure prophylaxis is provided by giving ARV drugs to the neonates after birth.

The woman is explained about the necessity of consistent use of these drugs for prevention of emergence of resistant strains and optimizing prevention of MTCT.

## Antiretroviral Therapy in Different Situations

If a pregnant HIV positive woman is receiving ART before pregnancy, it should be continued throughout life. It does not increase congenital abnormalities in the fetus.

If the woman has come for ANC and is diagnosed to be HIV positive for the first time, she is started on triple drug ART after initial laboratory tests. She is also tested for STI, tuberculosis, and if possible CD4 count besides routine tests of pregnancy. If STI is present treatment should be given to both partners.

*The recommended ARV drugs and their dosage for first line ART regimen is:*

Tenofovir (TDF) 300 mg + Lamivudine (3TC) 300 mg + Efavirenz (EFV) 600 mg once a day 2 hours after low fat diet. This regime is given if there is no history of exposure to non-nucleoside reverse transcriptase inhibitors (NNRTI) such as nevirapine (NVP) and efavirenz in this or previous pregnancy. Newer guidelines have recommended the use of EFV in all trimesters of pregnancy.

If the pregnant woman has been exposed to NNRTI previously, the regimen used is TDF (300 mg) + 3TC (300 mg) once daily + Lopinavir 200 mg/ritonavir 50 mg (LPV/r) 2 tablets BD for full effect of the treatment. The dose of LPV is 400 mg twice a day and of ritonavir is 100 mg twice a day.

Other alternative regimens if the first-line regime is not tolerated due to severe side effects are:
- Zidovudine (AZT) + 3TC + EFV
- AZT + 3TC + NVP
- TDF + 3TC + NVP

If the woman has come in labor without any HIV testing or ARV medication, rapid testing for HIV from whole blood (finger prick) test is done and the sample is stored for further testing. If positive, the treatment is started immediately with 3 drugs ART (TDF + 3TC + EFV). The confirmatory test is done as soon as possible by Western blot or IFA. If she is positive, the therapy is continued for life and she is further evaluated at ART center as and when advised. If found to be negative the treatment is stopped.

## Associated Hepatitis B Virus in HIV Positive Women

An elevation in liver enzymes following the initiation of ART may occur in HIV/HBV-coinfected women because of an immune-mediated flare in hepatitis B virus (HBV), particularly in women with low CD4 cell counts. HBV infection may also increase the risk of hepatotoxicity with certain ARV drugs, specifically NVP and PI. Pregnant women with HIV/HBV coinfection should be counseled about signs and symptoms of liver toxicity.

The neonate is administered hepatitis B immunoglobulin (HBIG) and first dose of hepatitis B vaccine within 12 hours of birth. Second and third doses are given at 1 month and 6 months of age respectively.

## Associated Hepatitis C Virus with HIV Positive Pregnancy

No specific changes in treatment are recommended in the adult ART treatment guidelines. Ribavirin and pegylated interferon alpha cannot be given during pregnancy but can be administered after delivery. After birth, the infant is tested for HCV RNA between 2 and 6 months of age and for hepatitis C virus (HCV) antibodies after 15 months of age.

## Associated Tuberculosis

If the pregnant woman reports for the first time and is diagnosed with both HIV and TB, antitubercular treatment (ATT) is started first followed by ART as soon as clinically possible. Rifampicin may be replaced with rifabutin for better effect.

## HIV 2 Infection in Pregnancy

It is very uncommon in India and the transmission risk of infection from mother to child is only 0–4%. Use of 2NRTI + LPV/r is recommended as NNRTI such as NVP and EFV are not effective. However, if the woman is both HIV 1 and 2 positive, she is given the standard ART regime recommended for HIV-1 infection. The infants are given AZT instead of NVP in the dose of 5 mg twice daily for birth weight < 2,000 g, 10 mg twice a day for birth weight 2,000–2,500 g and 15 mg twice a day for birth weight > 2,500 g: for a period of 6 weeks.

## Monitoring of Pregnant Women on ART

Clinical and laboratory monitoring of HIV-1 infected pregnant women on ART should be done as follows (National ART Guidelines—NACO + WHO):

The HIV care and follow-up of pregnant women should be scheduled to coincide with their antenatal visits, as far as possible. Clinical evaluation including general physical examination and obstetrical examination is done every month. Clinical screening for symptoms of tuberculosis and STIs and OI should be done at each visit. Weight of the patient should be checked every month as weight loss is an indicator of progression of the disease.

Injection tetanus toxoid is given. Routine examination of the urine should be done at each visit and hemoglobin is rechecked at 28–32 weeks and at 36 weeks of gestation. Baseline liver and kidney function tests are done and repeated as and when clinically required. Baseline blood sugar and lipid profile should also be done and repeated every 6 months if LPV/r based regimen is being given.

CD4 counts are measured at baseline and every 3–6 months thereafter. Cotrimoxazole prophylactic therapy (CPT) should be initiated if CD4 ≤ 250 cells/mm$^3$. The dose is one tablet every day of a double strength preparation with one folic acid tablet. Baseline total lymphocyte and T lymphocyte count is done.

Resistance to ART drugs is tested by ART physician. Adverse drug reaction is noted and reported to ART center. Viral load is checked at the start of ART and then after 2–4 visits and then every month till it is undetectable and then every 3 months. Advice for contraception, infant feeding and hospital delivery is provided at each ANC visit. She is made aware to report immediately if any warning sign of pregnancy develops.

If ART contains EFV, liver enzymes AST and ALT are checked after 4–6 weeks of starting treatment. When TDF is used check serum creatinine and creatinine clearance every 3–6 months. If PI drug is used blood glucose, total cholesterol and triglycerides are to be checked annually.

Adherence must be monitored at each visit since effective prevention of MTCT is dependent on regular intake of ARV drugs during pregnancy and postpartum. Psychological support is given and any abnormal behavior to be taken seriously. Appropriate nutritional counseling is provided.

## DELIVERY

### Vaginal Delivery

If the viral load at 36 weeks of gestation is 50 copies or less per mL, vaginal delivery can be safely conducted. Due to COVID pandemic we have learnt all to use all the protective gears while conducting delivery **(Fig. 1)**.

During normal vaginal delivery, all ART drugs are continued, which were being used antenatally. Procedures such as artificial rupture of membranes, fetal scalp blood sampling; routine episiotomy and operative vaginal delivery (forceps or ventouse) are avoided unless strongly indicated. There is less fetal trauma with outlet forceps hence it is preferred over ventouse when indicated. Vaginal examinations should

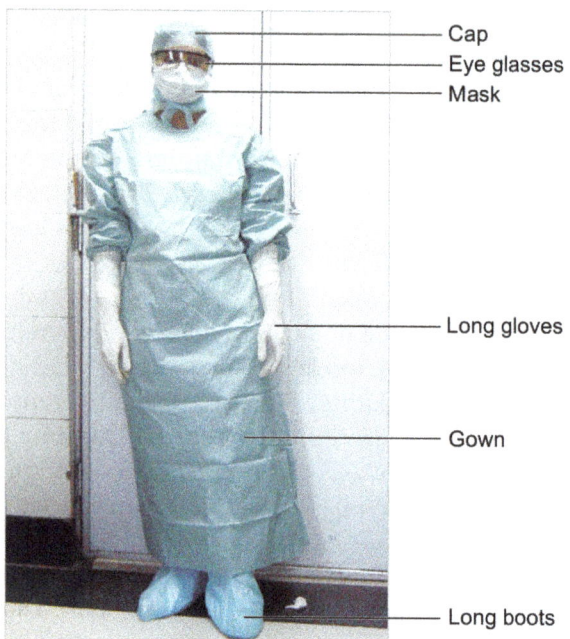

**Fig. 1:** Items to be used during delivery by the obstetrician.

be kept to a minimum and all aseptic precautions should be taken. Chorioamnionitis should be prevented, and if present, treated promptly. Systematic birth canal cleaning has been attempted with betadine, chlorhexidine, etc. without any proven benefit. Vaginal gels which kill the HIV virus are under research. After delivery, umbilical cord is clamped as early as possible. Suctioning the newborn with a nasogastric tube should be avoided unless there is meconium staining of the liquor. Methergine is not used if woman is on PI as it can cause exaggerated vasoconstriction response, however, prostaglandin F2 alpha, misoprostol or oxytocin can be used in the active management of third stage of labor. Post-placental Intrauterine contraceptive device (IUCD) insertion may be safely carried out. Biological waste management guidelines should be followed for disposal of placenta and all universal precautions should be followed for normal delivery as well as cesarean section.

## Cesarean Section

Cesarean section is indicated (besides for obstetric causes) when the viral load is 50–399 copies/mL at 36 weeks of pregnancy (elective section done at 38–39 weeks). If the viral load is 400 or more/mL at 36 weeks of gestation or when viral load is not known the elective cesarean section is done at 38 weeks of pregnancy. For cesarean section, ART drugs are given before starting the operation in addition to prophylactic antibiotics. Use of atraumatic (blunt tip) needle is advised. Use forceps (not hands) for manipulation of needle. HIV positive women have more complications during cesarean section especially sepsis.[20] In case of an emergency cesarean section in pregnant women who are not on ART, the woman is started on triple drug ART prior to the procedure. During cesarean section, wherever possible, the membranes are left intact until the head is delivered through the surgical incision.

The cord should be clamped as early as possible after delivery. Proper hemostasis should be ensured, and judicious use of electrocautery is advocated. Blood less cesarean section, in which the uterus is opened with a staple gun which cuts and prevents bleeding at the same time is shown to have less chances of MTCT of HIV.

## CARE OF THE NEONATE (NACO GUIDELINES PPTCT)

The neonate should be bathed promptly after birth before giving any injections such as hepatitis B and BCG vaccination or vitamin K injection. Oral polio drops are also given at birth. Also do detailed physical examination. After birth, clinical examination for development and growth monitoring is done at 6, 10, and 14 weeks and then at 6, 9, 12 and 18 months of age. Routine immunization schedule is normally followed.

### Investigations

Newborn is tested for anemia, baseline complete blood count and serum biochemistry is done. In 2010 WHO updated on early infant diagnosis (EID):

- PCR test for HIV 1 is done at birth, at 6 weeks of age and repeated at 6 and 12 months after birth.
- A test of HIV antibody at 18 months of age gives final diagnosis. The 3-ELISA test confirmation can be performed 6 weeks after complete stopping of breast feeding.

### Medications

Besides treatment of any illness occurring from time to time the following medication is given to all HIV exposed infants and children:

- The HIV exposed infant is given prophylaxis against PJP after 6 weeks of age with cotrimoxazole prophylactic therapy (CPT) which is continued till 18 months of age.
- All children diagnosed with HIV after the rapid test is positive (before confirmation test) should be immediately started on appropriate ART (without considering CD4 count).

In prophylactic ARV medicine syrup nevirapine (NVP) is given according to the weight of the neonate as early after birth as possible till at least 6 weeks of age, irrespective of type of feeding. If ART during pregnancy is started late in mother, then NVP cover is to be increased to 12 weeks. Nevirapine syrup is given according to weight of infant at birth:

- Birth weight less than 2,000 g dose is 2 mg/kg/day
- Birth weight 2,000–2,500 g give 10 mg/day
- Birth weight > 2,500 g give 15 mg/day.

If mother has taken NVP before, the neonate is given zidovudine (AZT) or LPV (200 mg × 3)/r (100 mg).

## Breastfeeding

As we know that breastfeeding by HIV positive mother causes vertical transmission up to 30% if the mother is not receiving ART. Therefore, complete avoidance of breastfeeding is the surest way to avoid MTCT of HIV through breastfeeding. However, it may not be feasible in lower socioeconomic households in developing countries as the mortality from diarrhea, malnutrition and respiratory illness may be more in these cases than from HIV. Besides mixed feeding before 6 months of age increases MTCT. Hence, WHO/NACO guidelines recommend exclusive breastfeeding as the preferred feeding option for HIV exposed infants <6 months of age. However, in cases of maternal death or severe maternal illness where breastfeeding may not be possible, exclusive replacement feeding can be done. Exclusive replacement feeding is done only when AFASS criteria are fulfilled, that is:

- **A**–affordable
- **F**–feasible
- **A**–acceptable
- **S**–sustainable
- **S**–safe

Mixed feeding in first 6 months of life should not be allowed as it increases MTCT.

If the HIV positive mother, who is adequately covered with ART and if this neonate has appropriate ARV drugs he/she is allowed exclusive breastfeeding for 6 months. But if the mother's ART is started during or immediately after delivery, breastfeeding is not allowed till her confirmative test is negative for HIV. If the mother's confirmatory test is positive, both mother and neonate are started on ART. Decision of exclusive breastfeeding is then taken on individual basis.

If the infant becomes HIV negative, breastfeeding is stopped at 12 months of age. But when HIV status continues to be positive the child is given breast milk till 2 years of age along with complementary feeding as the mother is on lifelong ART.

## POSTPARTUM CARE

At discharge both mother and neonate must be referred to appropriate ART centers for ongoing care. The mother is educated about the benefits of continued ART and ARV prophylaxis for the neonate. Emphasis is given on compliance. She must take adequate rest and balanced diet.

If indicated a mental health checkup and de-addiction of illicit drugs and alcohol should be offered. There is also a need to support the woman physically and psychologically as there is a higher risk of postnatal blues. The family members are counseled accordingly.

She should be screened for cancer cervix, if not screened earlier.

## CONTRACEPTION

Contraceptive counseling is given and need for safe sexual practices is emphasized. An HIV infected woman can use almost all methods of contraception, if clinically well. She is advised to always use condom (male or female) consistently and correctly to prevent further transmission of HIV, for protection from STI and for contraception.

She is advised the use of dual method which means using condom with other methods such as IUD or hormonal methods. Oral contraceptive drug levels may be decreased by ARV drugs like NVP, ritonavir, amprenavir and fosamprenavir as they expedite metabolism but use of condoms will make up for this. NET-EN or depot-medroxy- progesterone acetate (DMPA) does not significantly alter the levels of ARV drugs as the hormone is absorbed in the blood before being metabolized by the liver.[21] IUDs both copper and hormone bearing can be used. An IUD does not need to be removed unless it gets infected later on or she develops AIDS.

The dose of emergency contraceptive is not to be increased. Spermicides are not to be used. The couple can be counseled for non-scalpel vasectomy or sterilization as a permanent method of contraception with additional use of condoms to prevent the spread of disease and STIs. It is important to remember that except condom, no other method of contraception can prevent transmission of STI/HIV.

## EFFECT OF HIV ON PREGNANCY

The HIV positive pregnant women are at more risk of low birth weight newborns and preterm deliveries.[22] Low Apgar score, still birth and FGR are seen with low CD4 counts. Low CD4 counts also correspond to postpartum endometritis. Wound infection is more common in postpartum period.

## EFFECT OF PREGNANCY ON HIV DISEASE PROGRESSION

No major effect is seen in otherwise asymptomatic HIV positive women. Morbidity and mortality is not increased by pregnancy (though CD4 count falls during pregnancy). Chances of acquiring HIV during pregnancy are higher possibly due to hormonal influence or immunosuppression in pregnancy.

Therefore, it is concluded that knowing HIV serostatus of pregnant women is very important in prevention of MTCT of HIV. Contraception also plays a very vital role in preventing the spread of infection.

## KEY POINTS

- There are two types of HIV viruses, viz. HIV-1 and HIV-2. HIV-1 is associated with higher mother to child transmission (MTCT) rate (20–35%) compared to 0–4% with HIV-II.
- Women are more vulnerable to acquire this infection than men.
- Almost all cases of HIV in children (91%) are acquired by mother to child transmission (MTCT).
- Not all babies of HIV positive mothers acquire the infection. The incidence varies from 15 to 45%. Transmission by this route can be prevented if HIV status of mother is detected in early and timely ART and other measures are instituted.
- CDC (USA) and NACO have recommended that all pregnant women be tested for HIV as early as possible, and in high-risk groups repeat HIV test is done at 36 weeks of pregnancy.
- It is important to know the factors which increase the PTCT of HIV.
- Most infected neonates acquire infection at the time of delivery and rest through breastfeeding.
- ARV drugs are given to prevent MTCT of HIV and treating mother for her disease.
- Prophylactic ARV medicines are given to the neonate. NVP 2 mg/kg orally within 72 hours of birth is advised by NACO.
- There is 30% independent risk of PTCT of HIV by breastfeeding by HIV infected mother or wet nurse.
- UNICEF and WHO have recommended exclusive breastfeeding for a shorter duration (6 months).
- No mixed feeding should be given as there is more MTCT of HIV with mixed feeding.
- At discharge both mother and neonate must be referred to appropriate centers for ongoing care.

## REFERENCES

1. UNAIDS. Global HIV and AIDS statistics—2020 fact sheet. [online] Available from: http://www.unaids.org/en/resources/fact-sheet. [Last accessed July, 2021].
2. Salhan S. Women and HIV infection including mother to child transmission. In: Salhan S. Women and HIV, 2nd edition. New Delhi: Jaypee Brothers Medical Publishers; 2013. pp. 93.
3. Conner EM, Sperling RS, Gelber R, Kiselev P, Scott G, O'Sullivan MJ, et al. Reduction of maternal infant transmission of HIV type with Zidovudine treatment. New England J Med. 1994;331:1173.
4. Salhan S. HIV in pregnancy. In: Salhan S (Ed). Textbook of Obstetrics, 2nd edition. New Delhi: Jaypee Brothers Medical Publishers; 2016. pp. 467-78.
5. Townsend CL, Byrne L, Cortina-Borja M, Thorne C, de Ruiter A, Lyall H, et al. Earlier initiation of ART and further decline in mother-to-child HIV transmission rates, 2000-2011. AIDS. 2014;28(7):1049-57.
6. Salters K, Loutfy M, de Pokomandy A, Money D, Pick N, Wang L, et al. Pregnancy incidence and initiation after HIV diagnosis among women living with HIV in Canada. Plos One. 2017;12:eo180524.
7. WHO. WHO guidelines for Vitamin A supplementation during pregnancy for reduction of Parent-to-child transmission of HIV. Geneva: WHO; 2010.
8. Aho I, Kaijo M, Kivela P, Surcel HM, Sutinen J, Heikinheimo O, et al. Most women living with HIV can deliver vaginally-National data from Finland, 1993-2013. Plos one 2018:13. e0194370.
9. Kourtis AP, Bullory M, Nesheim SR. Understanding the timing of HIV transmission from mother to infant. JAMA. 2001;285:709.
10. Salhan S. Voluntary counseling and testing and its rationale for HIV infection. In: Salhan S. Women and HIV, 2nd edition. New Delhi: Jaypee Brothers Medical publishers; 2013. pp. 47.
11. Recommendations for use of anti-retroviral drugs in prevention of HIV 1 infected women for maternal health and intervention to reduce perinatal HIV transmission in the United States. Panel on treatment of HIV infected pregnant women and prevention of perinatal transmission. 2018.
12. Recommendations for use of ARV drugs in pregnant women with HIV infection and interventions to reduce perinatal HIV transmission in the United States. 2020.
13. British HIV association Guidelines for the management of HIV infection in pregnant women. 2018.
14. CDC. Interim guidelines for clinicians considering for the use of pre-exposure prophylaxis for prevention of HIV infection in heterosexually active adults. MMWR Morb Mortal Wkly Rep. 2012;61(31):586-9.
15. Salhan S. Post-exposure prophylaxis and pre-exposure prophylaxis. In: Salhan S. Women and HIV, 2nd edition. New Delhi: Jaypee Brothers Medical Publishers; 2013. pp. 175-88.
16. CDC. Vaginal Ring for HIV prevention. Atlanta, Georgia: Centers for Disease Control and Prevention; 2020.
17. NACO. Prevention of Parent to Child Transmission (PPTCT) of HIV using Multidrug Antiretroviral Regimen in India. New Delhi: NACO; 2013.
18. WHO. WHO update 2017: What is new in treatment monitoring: viral load and CD4 count. Geneva: WHO; 2017.
19. NACO 2018: National technical guidelines on ART. New Delhi: NACO; 2018.
20. Panburana P, Phaupradit W, Tantisirin O, Sriintravanit N, Buamuenvai J. Maternal complications after caesarean section in HIV infected pregnant women. Aust NZ J Obstet Gynaecol. 2003;43:160-3.
21. Cohn SE, Park JG, Watts DH, Stek A, Hitti J, Clax PA, et al. Depo-medroxyprogesterone in women on antiretroviral therapy: contraception and lack of clinically significant interactions. Clin Pharmacol Ther. 2007;81(2):222.
22. Xiao PL, Zhou YB, Chen Y, Yang MX, Song XX, Shi Y, et al. Association between maternal HIV infection and low birth weight and prematurity: a meta-analysis of cohort studies. BMC Pregnancy Childbirth. 2015:15:246.

# TORCH Infections in Pregnancy

*K Aparna Sharma, Deepika Deka*

## INTRODUCTION

"Congenital infection" commonly refers to transplacentally acquired infection by the fetus from an infected mother. Some organisms such as *Toxoplasma gondii* (T), Rubella (R), Cytomegalovirus (C), Herpes simplex virus (H) and others (O—varicella zoster virus, parvovirus, etc.) have several clinical features in common and hence given the acronym "TORCH" group of infections. In the acute (viremic or parasitemic) stage of maternal infection, placental infection is initiated and subsequently fetal infection occurs. Though not common, some organisms may reinfect a person with waning host immunity more than once-causing fetus to be infected, as in re-exposure of immune mothers to cytomegalovirus, toxoplasma and rubella viruses. Microbes may persist as a chronic asymptomatic infection, causing fetal disease such as malaria, *Toxoplasma gondii* (only when the mother is immunocompromised), syphilis, hepatitis, herpes zoster, and HSV.

The incidence varies geographically and socio-economically. Fetal infection has been reported to occur in up to 10% of pregnancies per year.[1-3] In India, there is difficulty in collecting reliable and accurate data because serology is expensive. Magnitude of the problem needs to be studied, so that we can prioritize perinatal problems and avoid focusing attention only on TORCH agents. A study carried out at AIIMS by the author found that 17.8% adolescent girls and 20% pregnant women were seronegative for rubella infection, identifying a group of women at risk for primary rubella infection during pregnancy.

## FETAL EFFECTS OF TORCH INFECTIONS

Infections during pregnancy have been identified as an important cause of spontaneous abortions and perinatal mortality. Unexplained stillbirths have also been attributed to infections.[4] Any infection that occurs in the first 20 weeks of pregnancy can lead to spontaneous abortion due to direct placental damage, endometrial vascular involvement, primary embryonic death or may alter embryogenesis, with resultant congenital malformations (congenital rubella).[5,6] If the infection occurs between 20 and 37 weeks, it can cause preterm labor and delivery. Infections acquired during the birth process result in neonatal morbidity **(Table 1)**.

The classic "clinical triad" of TORCH baby refers to jaundice, petechiae and hepatosplenomegaly. However, every infection has specific distinguishing clinical features allowing specific diagnosis **(Table 2)**.

Infection of the mother during pregnancy can have short- or long-term devastating effects on the newborn as is determined by the period of gestation when infection occurs **(Table 3)** and the immune status of the mother.

Though TORCH infections may occur during pregnancy, maternal symptoms are rarely serious.[7,8] Clinical recognition of maternal infection, a prerequisite for preventive measures, is important. Routine screening by serology is not always possible, because of cost of serology and the low yield.

## INDICATIONS FOR TORCH TESTING IN PREGNANCY

The maternal serological screening for TORCH group of infections should be advised only under special conditions, when the mother has symptoms and signs of these infections or there are USG features of fetal involvement **(Box 1)**. Routine screening is recommended for syphilis, HIV and hepatitis B in pregnancy. Rubella screening in preconceptional period helps to identify women who can be vaccinated against rubella, thereby eliminating risk of rubella infection during pregnancy. In some countries screening for toxoplasmosis is a routine practice because of a widespread prevalence.

## DIAGNOSIS OF MATERNAL INFECTIONS

Paired serological tests are most helpful only when the first sample has been drawn during clinical illness or it is available from the routine antenatal blood sample. The second sample is drawn 4 weeks later and rises in titer or otherwise is used to interpret the test results and diagnosing infection. **Table 3** presents an overview of the serology.

## DIAGNOSIS OF FETAL INFECTION

The fetal infection and fetal affection are two different entities in the context of TORCH infection. An earlier infection in the gestation results in a greater severity of affection **(Table 4)**.

**TABLE 1:** Effect of congenital infection on the fetus and newborn infant.

| Etiological agent | Premature birth | Intrauterine growth restriction | Structural anomalies | Congenital disease | Persistent postnatal infection |
|---|---|---|---|---|---|
| *Toxoplasma gondii* | + | + | - | + | + |
| Rubella | - | + | + | + | + |
| CMV | + | + | + | + | + |
| HSV | + | - | - | + | + |
| Parvovirus B19 | - | - | - | + | - |

**TABLE 2:** Fetal and neonatal features of TORCH infections.

| Organism | Manifestation | Critical factor for clinical manifestations |
|---|---|---|
| Cytomegalovirus | *Eye*: Chorioretinitis (macular sparing), microophthalmia<br>*Brain*: Cerebral calcification, microcephaly<br>*Hematological*: Petechiae, hepatosplenomegaly, *FGR* | Neonatal disease severity is more with primary CMV infection of pregnant women rather than recurrent or reactivation of disease |
| Rubella | *Eye*: Cataract, glaucoma, chorioretinitis; retinopathy,<br>*Heart*: Congenital heart disease<br>*Skeletal system*: Bone lesions<br>*Brain*: Rarely microcephaly<br>*Hematological*: Hepatosplenomegaly, jaundice, purpura, *fetal growth restriction (FGR)* | First trimester infection |
| Herpes simplex | *Eye*: Keratoconjunctivitis in newborn, retinal dysplasia<br>*Brain*: Meningoencephalitis, microcephaly, mental retardation, microophthalmia<br>*Skin*: Skin vesicles | Intrapartum infection |
| Toxoplasma | *Eye*: Chorioretinitis (macular)<br>*Brain*: Microcephaly, hydrocephalus, *stillbirth* | Severity of fetal disease is inversely proportional to gestational age |

In the case of confirmed maternal infection, it is important to test whether the fetus is infected. Prenatal diagnosis should be made as soon as possible since treatment of the mother can minimize fetal sequelae. The prenatal diagnosis of congenital infection is also important to prevent unnecessary termination of pregnancy. Prenatal diagnosis is now possible with use of ultrasonography **(Box 2)** and ultrasound-guided procedures. 3D ultrasound improves detection of fetal anomalies such as cleft lip, brain lesions, limb malformations and structural heart defects associated with fetal infections.

Amniocentesis, chorionic villus sampling and cord blood sampling are used for accurate diagnosis of presence or absence of fetal infection by various laboratory testing **(Table 5)**.[12-15]

Most affected fetuses appear sonographically normal, but serial scanning may reveal evolving findings.[16] However, by the time structural anomalies are visible on ultrasonography (USG), fetal organ damage is considerable.

The fetal infection can be confirmed after a confirmed maternal infection by an amniotic fluid PCR. The amniocentesis should be done at least 6-8 weeks after the maternal infection and at least after 18-20 weeks of gestation when fetal urination is established.

Even if the fetus is found to be infected, the fetus may not have any signs of affection on USG or MRI and would still need to be followed for long term sequelae.

Invasive procedures are relatively safe, but should be carried out in referral centers.[12-16]

**TABLE 3:** Interpretations of TORCH serology.

| IgM positive, IgG negative | Unexposed/Susceptible/Unvaccinated (Rubella) |
|---|---|
| IgM positive, IgG negative | Acute infection or primary infection<br>IgM antibodies known to cross react and hence false positive report can occur<br>(*Repeat serology*: IgM decreasing or negative with IgG positive indicative of acute infection) |
| IgM negative, IgG positive | Past Infection<br>Timing of past infection can be determined by the avidity test<br>*High avidity*: Infection before 3 months<br>*Low avidity*: Infection within 3 months<br>(Depending on the gestational age fetal affection can be predicted) |

**BOX 1:** Indications for maternal TORCH screen during pregnancy.

- Clinical signs and symptoms of maternal TORCH infection or history of exposure
  - Fever, rash
  - Lymphadenopathy, unexplained hematological dyscrasias
- Ultrasound markers for congenital TORCH
- Early onset fetal growth restriction (FGR <24 weeks), severe (<5th centile), symmetrical, and for associated sonographic markers (echogenic bowel, calcifications in brain, liver, hydrops)
- Screening (targeted in high risk group)

## SPECIFIC INFECTIONS

### Rubella

It is also called "German measles" or "red measles". It has an incubation period of 10-14 days from the time of exposure

**TABLE 4:** Perinatal TORCH transmission.[1,2,9-11]

| Infection | | 1st trimester | 2nd trimester | 3rd trimester | Vaginal delivery |
| --- | --- | --- | --- | --- | --- |
| | | *Transplacental* | | | |
| Toxoplasmosis | | | 20–25% (<5% severe) | 60–70% (mild/asymptomatic) | – |
| Rubella | Primary | 60% (4 weeks) | <5% after >20 weeks | | |
| | | 25% (5–8 weeks) | | | |
| | | 15% (9–12 weeks) | Absent | | |
| | Recurrent | Rare | | | |
| CMV | Primary | 30–40% (10% symptomatic, severe = 1st and early 2nd trimester) | | | Rare |
| | Recurrent | 0.2–2% (<1% symptomatic) | | | |
| HSV | Primary | First trimester primary outbreak in the first trimester can be teratogenic and associated with neonatal chorioretinitis, microcephaly, and skin lesions[24] | | | 40–60% |
| | Recurrent | | | | < 5% |
| VZV | | 0.4–0.6% risk of congenital varicella syndrome | 1.4–2% (between 13 and 20 weeks) | No increased risk beyond 20 weeks | |
| Parvovirus | | 10–15% fetal loss | 2–3% fetal loss | | |

(CMV: cytomegalovirus; HSV: herpes simplex virus; VZV: varicella zoster virus)

**BOX 2:** Nonspecific ultrasound markers.

*Cranial abnormalities*
- Ventriculomegaly
- Calcifications
- Intraventricular synechiae
- Cerebellar abnormalities
  - Vermian hypoplasia
  - Cerebellar hemorrhage
  - Calcifications
  - Cysts
- Periventricular pseudocysts
- Malformations of cortical development
  - Lissencephaly-pachygyria
  - Oligo-/pachygyria
  - Polymicrogyria
  - Schizencephaly
- Microcephaly

*Extracranial abnormalities*
- Small-for-gestational age
- Hyperechogenic bowel
- Hepatomegaly
- Splenomegaly
- Liver calcifications
- Ascites
- Pericardial effusion
- Skin edema
- Hydrops or fetal anemia
  - (MCA-PSV > 1.5 MoM) in absence of maternal atypical antibodies

*Placental/amniotic fluid abnormalities*
- Placentomegaly
- Placental calcifications
- Oligohydramnios/anhydramnios
- Polyhydramnios

**TABLE 5:** Prenatal diagnosis of fetal TORCH infections.

| | |
| --- | --- |
| Toxoplasmosis | AF (PCR, mouse inoculation, culture) after 4–5 weeks of infection and not before 18–20 weeks<br>Cord blood (IgM, IgA, hematological parameters)<br>US for features |
| Rubella | AF (PCR)<br>Fetal blood (IgM)<br>CVS<br>US for abnormalities |
| CMV | AF (PCR), CVS, U/S |
| HSV | US<br>AF, fetal blood |
| Parvovirus | US for hydrops<br>Amniocentesis<br>Cordocentesis |
| VZV | US for fetal abnormalities<br>AF PCR for VZV DNA |

(AF: amniotic fluid; CVS: chorionic villus sampling; US: ultrasound; PCR: polymerase chain reaction)

which mostly is through respiratory droplets. A significant "contact" is defined as one being in the same room for over 15 minutes or face-to-face contact. A brief prodromal period with malaise, fever and anorexia may occur before rashes appear. Rashes are maculopapular, beginning in the face and spreading to the trunk and extremities, usually lasting for 3–5 days, hence called the "3 day rash".

There may be fever of low or high grade, mild coryza, conjunctivitis, malaise, lymphadenopathy—posterior auricular, cervical and suboccipital. If present, "Koplik's spots" on the buccal mucosa are pathognomonic. Less commonly, there may be arthralgia and arthritis.

**TABLE 6:** Risk of fetus infection with respect to period of gestation.

| Period of gestation | Risk to fetus (affected) |
|---|---|
| < 12 weeks | 97% |
| 12–16 weeks | 20% |
| 16–20 weeks | Minimal risk of deafness only |
| > 20 weeks | Very small |
| Reinfection | <5% |

## Fetal Affection

Pregnancy outcomes as a result of maternal rubella infection include spontaneous abortion, fetal infection, stillbirths or fetal growth restriction and the congenital rubella syndrome (CRS) with the classical triad of sensorineural deafness, eye abnormalities such as microophthalmia, cataracts and congenital heart disease—especially pulmonary artery stenosis and patent ductus arteriosus.

## Neonatal Affection

About 3–10% of suspected CRS cases are ultimately proven to have confirmed CRS with the aid of laboratory tests. CRS accounts for 10–15% of pediatric cataract.

## Transmission

When maternal infection occurs in the first trimester, fetal infection rates are up to 90%, dropping to <1% after 20 weeks **(Table 6)**.

## Diagnosis

Diagnosis of primary maternal infection during pregnancy should be made by history, clinical examination and serologic tests. A large number of cases, more than 50% of cases are asymptomatic.

A woman seropositive at the first screening test may have been infected a few weeks earlier. A 4-fold rise in rubella IgG antibody titers between acute and convalescent serum specimens suggests rubella infection.

Extra serological investigations especially RV-IgM and RV-IgG avidity testing, should be performed on the earliest serum available especially if there are ultrasound abnormalities, including fetal growth restriction. Rubella RT-PCR in amniotic fluid (AF) confirms the diagnosis.

## Management

If a pregnant woman has not received MMR vaccine and IgG for rubella is negative, she should be educated on signs and symptoms suggestive of a viral infection or exposure to rubella. Infection acquired in first trimester of pregnancy warrants prenatal diagnosis by ultrasound, cord blood sampling or amniocentesis. Decision depends on period of gestation at maternal infection, counseling based on gestational age is as accurate as prenatal diagnosis (PND) and termination of infected fetus is viable option.[17,18] Fetal infection occurring after 20 weeks is usually not of much consequence, deafness may be the only rare effect and pregnancy can be continued.

## Prevention of Rubella

Immunization at least 1 month before conception, universal MMR, vaccination of all children, revaccination of adolescent girls should be emphasized. Vaccination is a cheaper alternative to preconception serology. In India, vaccine action programs and effective prevention guidelines should be promulgated.[19]

In 2011, the World Health Organization (WHO) updated guidelines on the preferred strategy for introduction of rubella-containing vaccine (RCV) into national routine immunization schedules with an initial wide-age-range vaccination campaign that includes children aged 9 months to 15 years. By 2016, 152 out of 194 countries (78%) were using the vaccine and this increased rubella vaccine coverage globally resulted in a decrease in reported rubella cases from 94,277 in 2012, to 22,361 cases in 2016. The WHO Region of the Americas were declared free of rubella and congenital rubella syndrome in 2015, and 33 (62%) of 53 countries in the European Region have now eliminated endemic rubella and congenital rubella syndrome.[20]

## Acute Toxoplasmosis

It goes unrecognized in 80–90% of cases or produces a glandular fever-like illness or fatigue without fever or sore throat, myalgia and maculopapular rash. The disease is self-limiting and lasts for several weeks, though lymphadenopathy may last for several months. Cervical lymphadenopathy may be followed by generalized lymphadenopathy in 20–30% of symptomatic cases, in suboccipital, supraclavicular, axillary and inguinal nodes which are nontender, discrete and firm.

## Fetal Affection

Fetal affections in acute toxoplasmosis are given in **Box 3**.

## Transmission

The overall risk of congenital toxoplasmosis following maternal infection, without treatment, ranges from 20 to 50% **(Table 7)**.

## Diagnosis

Immunoglobulin M is the first antibody to increase with the highest level at about 1 month after infection. It is stable for about 1 more month and then decreases. It is not particularly helpful for timing the infection as it can persist for years.

Immunoglobulin G is detectable after 2 weeks with a maximum level at 3 months. A change in level on repeat testing (usually after 2 weeks) determines the timing of infection **(Fig. 1)**. Serologic assays for toxoplasmosis, however, are not well-standardized and hence the tests should be performed in an experienced reference toxoplasmosis laboratory.

## Treatment

In acute maternal toxoplasmosis, spiramycin therapy is started immediately, 2–3 g/day (6–9 MIU/day) in divided doses, continued until delivery since the placenta remains infected for rest of the duration of pregnancy, with ultrasonographic surveillance to monitor the development of any morphological lesions in the fetus.

If the fetal infection is diagnosed early in pregnancy especially with ultrasonic evidence of abnormalities or prenatal diagnostic techniques, therapeutic abortion is an important option. However, if the pregnancy is continued, drug treatment with sulfonamides and pyrimethamine is started after fetal infection is documented. Sulfadiazine (50–100 mg/kg/day) and pyrimethamine (1 mg/kg/day) act synergistically to antagonize folate synthesis in *T. gondii* and thus arrest the replication of the organism. Because pyrimethamine is a folic acid antagonist, 5 mg of folinic acid should be provided twice each week.

Pyrimethamine is contraindicated in first trimester of pregnancy because of its teratogenic effects. Prenatal therapy does not eliminate the risk of congenital infection but decreases the severity and its sequelae in the neonates and later childhood. Review of studies comparing treatment of toxoplasmosis in pregnancy with no treatment concludes that it is unclear whether antenatal treatment reduces transmission of toxoplasma and it is controversial whether treatment was effective in improving infant outcome.[21,22]

## Prevention

Seronegative women are advised on good hygiene to avoid acute infection. Undercooked or raw red meat should be avoided, the parasites in meat can be killed by cooking at 165 degrees Fahrenheit or frozen for at least 24 hours, smoked or curried. Everybody should avoid handling stray cats and kittens. Seronegative women should not handle cat's stool. Washing hands with soap and water after touching raw meat and after gardening, yard work, and other outdoor activities will help avoid infection. Pet cats should be kept indoors to prevent it from hunting. Feeding the cat only commercial cat food or cooking all meat products thoroughly before giving them to cat will prevent acquiring infection. Washing all fruits and vegetables thoroughly before eating them raw is helpful.[23] Early diagnosis and treatment of toxoplasmosis during pregnancy can significantly reduce congenital toxoplasmosis and its consequences.[24]

## Primary Maternal CMV

Infection may present as a mononucleosis such as syndrome of generalized malaise with profound fatigue as the most

> **BOX 3:** Fetal affections in acute toxoplasmosis.
> - CNS: Microcephaly, hydrocephalus, ventriculomegaly
> - Eyes: Chorioretinitis, blindness
> - Developmental delay, epilepsy and blindness
> - Hepatosplenomegaly, anemia, rash, jaundice and pneumonitis
> Most infected infants do not have clinical signs of infection at birth, up to 90% will develop sequelae later in life

**TABLE 7:** Overall risk of congenital toxoplasmosis.

| GA at maternal seroconversion (weeks) | Risk of congenital infection [% (95% CI)] | Fetal affection in infected offspring [% (95% CI)] |
|---|---|---|
| 13 | 6 (3–9) | 61 (34–85) |
| 26 | 40 (33–47) | 25 (18–33) |
| 36 | 72 (60–81) | 9 (4–17) |

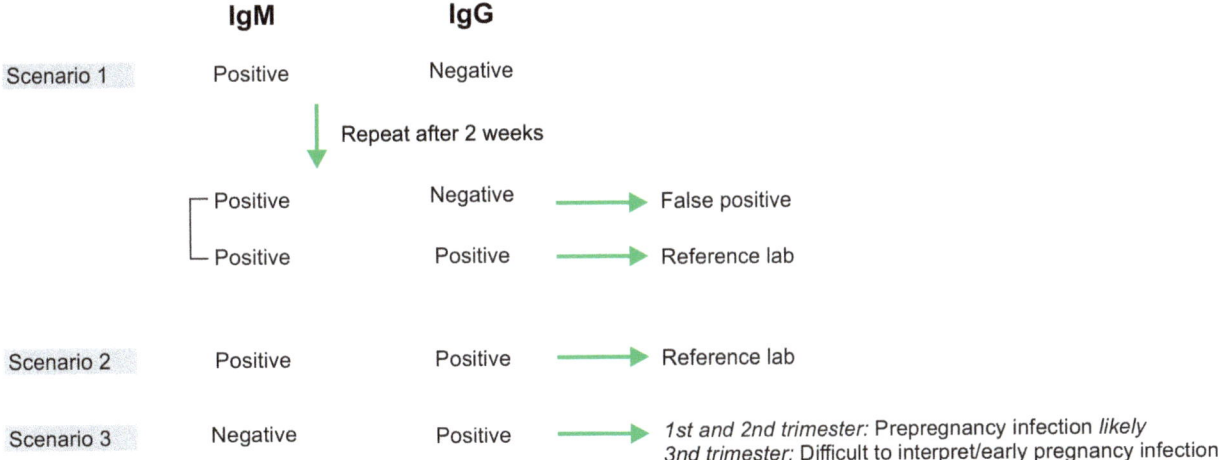

**Fig. 1:** Diagnosis of acute toxoplasmosis.

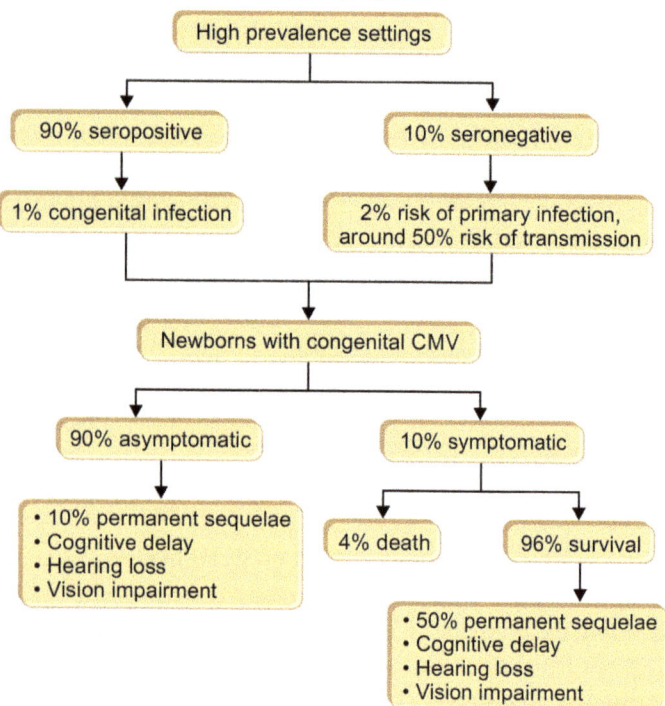

**Flowchart 1:** Relative risk of fetal and neonatal affection in primary maternal CMV.

impressive symptom generally lasting 2–6 weeks. There may be prolonged high fever with chills, myalgia, headache and rarely rashes. Pharyngitis, cervical lymphadenopathy and hepatosplenomegaly may be present. Rarely pneumonitis, retinitis, hepatitis, gastrointestinal ulcerations and Guillain-Barré syndrome complicate CMV and infectious mononucleosis. Most patients recover without any chronic features, but rarely fatigue may persist.

### Fetal Affection and Transmission

The risk of seroconversion in pregnancy is 2–2.5%. Primary infection more commonly is transmitted to the fetus and has a more severe fetal affection as compared to the secondary infections. **Flowchart 1** shows the relative risk of fetal and neonatal affection.[25]

### Management of CMV Infection

In maternal CMV infection, termination of pregnancy has a clear role in the event of definite fetal neurologic involvement by ultrasonography or if fetal infection is diagnosed, despite the poor predictive values of prenatal testing as to whether intrauterine infection has occurred and if the infection would lead to serious neurologic sequelae or not.[26,27]

Currently, maternal CMV infection can be treated with ganciclovir or foscarnet. Several reports of ganciclovir usage in mothers with life-threatening or sight-threatening CMV have been reported. However, the efficacy of treatment of primary CMV with the purpose of preventing or reversing fetal infection is not advisable. Extensive counseling about the possible benefits and toxicity of the drug is mandatory prior to maternal drug therapy. Termination of pregnancy is also offered to affected couples who are unwilling to accept any chance of neurologically affected children in the absence of prenatal diagnosis.

Screening of pregnant women for CMV infection and repeated audiological examinations of infants are necessary because there are infants with delayed-onset sensorineural hearing loss (SNHL) or SNHL caused by asymptomatic congenital CMV infection.[28]

### Prevention

For prevention of CMV infection, frequent hand washing, practicing good hygiene and avoiding exposure to CMV positive toddlers is important. Besides hygienic intervention in those susceptible, CMV immunoglobulin has shown an efficacy of 50% if it is given to pregnant women who have acquired a primary CMV infection during pregnancy.[29]

Two different vaccines have been developed—the gB/MF59 and the DNA vaccine. The gB/MF59 vaccine exhibited a vaccine efficacy of 50% in healthy, postpartum females; and in transplant patients, gB/MF59 and the DNA vaccine TransVax both limited the periods of viremia and consequently the need for antiviral treatment.[30]

## Primary and Recurrent HSV Infection

It is clinically diagnosed based on the appearance of characteristic painful bilateral, widely spaced vesicular lesions and painful erythematous pustules or ulcers on the external genitalia at various stages of progression. Cervix and urethra are involved in 80%. However, one-third of women do not have typical ulcers. Most women have recurrent rather than primary infection. First episode of primary genital herpes is associated with fever, headache, malaise and myalgia more often than in recurrent infection. Symptoms last longer and there are more complications. There may be vaginal/urethral discharge, dysuria, hematuria, pelvic pain and cervical inflammation. Genital infection with HSV-2, though clinically indistinguishable from infection with HSV-1, has 8–10 times increased recurrence rate than HSV-1. Rectal and perianal involvement cause anorectal pain, discharge, tenesmus and constipation. Clinical features of primary orolabial HSV infections are gingivostomatitis and pharyngitis involving tonsils, hard and soft palate, tongue, lips and facial area.

Edema, erythema, pustular or vesicular ulcers on fingers after primary oral or genital herpes, called "herpetic whitlow" may occur.

### Fetal Affection

The HSV-2 infection in pregnancy has been associated with premature delivery, low birth weight infants, fetal malformations, and vertical transmission of the virus during childbirth.[31,32]

## Transmission

While neonatal herpes occurs in less than 1% of prevalent infections, the risk of transmission increases to 25-50% among women infected during pregnancy. In addition, it is estimated that prevalent HSV-2 infection is associated with a 2- to 4-fold increased risk of HIV-1 acquisition.[33]

## Neonatal Affection

Although both HSV-1 and HSV-2 may cause neonatal herpes, HSV-2 is responsible for 70% of cases. Neonatal herpetic infection is defined as infection within 28 days of birth. 90% of infections are perinatally transmitted in the birth canal. HSV infection acquired in this manner carries a 70% risk of dissemination.

Approximately 10% of infections are congenital, usually a consequence of the mother acquiring primary HSV infection during pregnancy and the fetus acquiring the infection transplacentally.

## Management

Active primary herpes can be very effectively treated with oral acyclovir, 200 mg five times a day for 5-7 days. Suppressive therapy in last 4 weeks of pregnancy, 200 mg four times a day may prevent recurrence at term and reduce cesarean section rates.[34-36] The dictum is "no lesion, no cesarean section". Cesarean section if indicated, should be done irrespective of duration of rupture of membranes. There is no role of serial cultures to detect asymptomatic viral shedding.

## Prevention

Safe sexual practices to avoid exposure to herpes virus.

## Varicella Zoster Virus Infection

Varicella zoster virus is a highly contagious DNA virus of the herpes family. Most varicella-zoster (VZ) infections are acquired during childhood and nearly 95% women enter pregnancy with serological evidence of immunity. The incubation period is 10-21 days, and the disease is infectious 48 hours before the rash appears and continues to be infectious until the vesicles crust. The typical maculopapular and vesicular rash is accompanied by fever and constitutional symptoms for 3-5 days. Secondary streptococcal or staphylococcal skin infection is the most common complication. 10-20% of pregnant women with VZ infection may develop pneumonia, this incidence and associated mortality of pneumonia being greater than in nonpregnant women.

## Fetal Infection

The classical congenital varicella syndrome (CVS) results from a transplacental infection of the fetus in the first half of pregnancy. Maternal chickenpox in the first 20 weeks of pregnancy is associated with an incidence of CVS of 0.91%. The features of the syndrome include skin lesions in 70%, and limb hypoplasia in 46-72%. Other abnormalities include neurological abnormalities (microcephaly cortical atrophy, hydrocephaly, mental retardation), eye disorders (microophthalmia, chorioretinitis, and cataracts, muscular hypoplasia), developmental delay and abnormalities of the gastrointestinal, genitourinary and cardiovascular system. The highest risk to the fetus is 1.4-2% between 13 and 20 weeks of gestation. The risk between 2 and 12 weeks is 0.4-0.6% and virtually nil beyond 28 weeks. In seronegative individuals exposed to VZ virus, the fetal infection rate can be as high as 90%.

## Treatment

Every pregnant woman with chickenpox should be started immediately on oral acyclovir (800 mg 5 times daily) or valaciclovir (1 g 3 times daily). If given within 24-72 hours of development of rash, acyclovir is effective in reducing the fetomaternal mortality and morbidity, especially if used intravenously. In cases of progression to varicella pneumonitis, maternal admission to hospital should be seriously considered and intravenous acyclovir can be considered for severe complications in pregnancy in a dose of usually 10-15 mg/kg of BW or 500 mg/m$^2$ IV every 8 h for 5 to 10 days for varicella pneumonitis, and it should be started within 24 to 72 h of the onset of rash. Fetal exposure to the virus just before or during delivery can lead to fulminant neonatal varicella and therefore, it is recommended that VZIG should be administered to the neonate when maternal infection occurs within 5 days, before or after delivery. Despite VZIG administration, 30-40% of newborns still develop infection but the complication and fatality rates are substantially reduced.

## Parvovirus

Parvoviridae are small, single stranded nonenveloped DNA viruses of which human parvovirus B19 is the predominant parvovirus pathogen in humans. It replicates in rapidly proliferating cells such as erythroblast precursors and causes a mild childhood infection known as erythema infectiosum, or Fifth disease. Erythema infectiosum is a common childhood illness and the virus causes only mild infection in adults. Adults have a self-limited infection with a milder rash and symmetrical polyarthralgia that may persist for several weeks. In 20-30% of adults, however, the infection is asymptomatic. Due to the tropism of B19 to erythroid progenitor cells, in women with hemolytic anemia, it causes an aplastic crisis. There is no evidence that the course of parvovirus infection is altered by pregnancy.

### Fetal Infection

There is vertical transmission to the fetus in about one-third of cases with maternal parvovirus infection. The virus attaches to the P antigen on red blood stem cells and suppresses erythropoiesis, resulting in severe anemia and high-output congestive heart failure. This same antigen is also present on fetal myocardial cells, and causes a cardiomyopathy that contributes further to heart failure. The immature immune response of the fetus may render it susceptible to infection, leading to abortion, hydrops fetalis, development of congenital anemia and even fetal death.

Fetal infection develops usually within 10 weeks of maternal infection and, therefore, more than 80% of hydrops cases are found in the second trimester. The overall fetal loss rate is 10–15% when infection occurs before 20 weeks, but only 2–3% after 20 weeks. Fetal infection can be diagnosed by cordocentesis which can aid in detection of parvovirus-specific IgM in fetal blood by enzyme immunoassay, immunofluorescence test, or radioimmunoassay and by detection of viral DNA in fetal blood or amniotic fluid by the polymerase chain reaction technique. When maternal infection is confirmed, the fetus should be evaluated for evidence of anemia by assessment of the middle cerebral artery (MCA) peak systolic velocity via Doppler velocimetry. Regular serial ultrasound examinations to measure MCA-PSV and/or identifying signs of hydrops are indicated and it should be performed every 1–2 weeks for 8–12 weeks after exposure.

### Treatment

Fetal management depends on gestational age and intrauterine transfusion is offered in cases with elevated peak systolic velocity values in the fetal middle cerebral artery (>1.5 MoM) and/or hydrops. There is currently no role of IVIG in pregnancy.

## SCREENING RECOMMENDATIONS

Current routine screening programs in the UK include testing for rubella, syphilis, hepatitis B and human immunodeficiency viruses. Screening for *Toxoplasma* in France and Austria has been available compulsorily for 25 years. In India, except for syphilis, Hepatitis B and HIV, there are no recommendations as regards routine screening for toxoplasmosis, rubella, CMV or HSV infection in antenatal period. Past history of chicken pox, history of MMR vaccination should be enquired into and documented in prenatal visit. Women should be encouraged to report any signs and symptoms of infections. Obstetricians should be able to diagnose these conditions clinically, interpret the laboratory results and manage these women.

## KEY POINTS

- Prevention of congenital infections by health education should be a priority. Frequent hand washing, practicing good hygiene, safe sexual practices and universal vaccination against rubella can avoid many serious congenital infections.
- Early detection of maternal infection, confirmation and early treatment if available (e.g., acyclovir for primary herpes and chickenpox; spiramycin and pyrimethamine-sulfadiazine for toxoplasmosis) will prevent or minimize fetal affection.
- Screening is done if mother is infected or exposed to TORCH infections or ultrasound shows fetal involvement.
- Women should be encouraged to report any signs and symptoms of infections. Obstetricians should be able to diagnose these conditions clinically and interpret the laboratory results.
- For toxoplasmosis in early pregnancy, termination is an option. Spiramycin is used in an effort to prevent congenital infection and if congenital infection is confirmed, sulfadiazine and pyrimethamine are used with careful monitoring for toxic side effects.
- Pregnancies complicated by possible maternal infection should preferably be referred to fetomaternal medicine centers.
- Infants with the suspicion of congenital infection and those born preterm, where infection may have played a role, need careful follow up especially the neurological and auditory follow-up by a competent pediatrician.

## REFERENCES

1. Remington JS. Toxoplasmosis. In: JS Remington, JO Klein (Eds). Infectious Disease of the Fetus and Newborn Infant, 5th edition. Philadelphia: Saunders; 2001.
2. Hanshaw JB. Cytomegalovirus. In: Remington JS, Klein JO (Eds). Infectious Disease of the Fetus and Newborn, 2nd edition. Philadelphia: WB Saunders; 1983. pp. 104.
3. Schendel DE. Infection in pregnancy and cerebral palsy. J Am Med Womens Assoc. 2001;56:105-8.
4. Tolockiene E, Morsing E, Holst E, Herbst A, Ljungh A, Svenningsen N, et al. Intrauterine infection may be a major cause of stillbirth in Sweden. Acta Obstet Gynecol Scand. 2001;80(6):511-8.
5. Vijayalakshmi P, Amala Rajasundari T, Prasad N, Prakash SK, Narendran K, Ravindran M, et al. Prevalence of eye signs in congenital Rubella Syndrome in South India: a role for population screening. Br J Ophthalmol. 2007;91:1418-9.
6. Deka RC, Kumar S, Venkatakarthikeyan C. Neonatal hearing screening. Indian J Otol. 2006;12(3):3-5.
7. American College of Obstetrics and Gynecologists. Perinatal viral and parasitic infections. ACOG Practice Bulletin 20. Washington: ACOG; 2000.
8. Sever JL. Toxoplasmosis: maternal and pediatric findings in 23,000 pregnancies. Pediatrics. 1988;82:181.
9. Stagno S, Pass RF, Dworsky ME, Alford CA. Maternal cytomegalovirus infection and perinatal transmission. Clin Obstet Gynecol. 1982;25:563.

10. Jones JL, Lopez A, Wilson M, Schulkin J, Gibbs R. Congenital toxoplasmosis: a review. Obstet Gynecol Surv. 2001;56(5):296-305.
11. De Santis M, Cavaliere AF, Straface G, Caruso A. Rubella infection in pregnancy. Reprod Toxicol. 2006;21(4):390-8.
12. Tanemura M, Suzumori K, Yagami Y, Kartow S. Diagnosis of fetal infection with reverse transcription and nested polymerase chain reaction: a study of 34 cases diagnosed in fetuses. Am J Obstet Gynecol. 1996;174:578.
13. Jin L, Thomas B. Application of molecular and serological assays to case based investigations of rubella and congenital rubella syndrome J Med Virol. 2007 l;79(7):1017-24.
14. Tang JW, Aarons E, Hesketh LM, Strobel S, Schalasta G, Jauniaux E, et al. Prenatal diagnosis of congenital rubella infection in the second trimester of pregnancy. Prenat Diagn. 2003;23:509-12.
15. Crino JP. Ultrasound and fetal diagnosis of perinatal infection. Clin Obstet Gynecol. 1999;42:71-80.
16. Degani S. Sonographic findings in fetal viral infections: a systematic review. Obstet Gynecol Surv. 2006;61(5):329-36.
17. Bhaskaran P, Ramalakshmi BA, Raju LA Raman L. Need for protection against rubella in India. Indian J Pediatr. 1991;58:811-84.
18. Muller CP, Kremer JR, Best JM, Dourado I, Triki H, Reef S. WHO Steering Committee for Measles and Rubella. Reducing global disease burden of measles and rubella: Report of the WHO Steering Committee on research related to measles and rubella vaccines and vaccination, 2005. Vaccine. 2007;2;25(1):1-9.
19. American College of Obstetricians and Gynecologists. ACOG Committee Opinion: Number 281, December 2002. Rubella vaccination. Obstet Gynecol. 2002;100(6):1417.
20. Grant GB, Reef SE, Patel M, Knapp JK, Dabbagh A. Progress in rubella and congenial rubella syndrome control and elimination—worldwide, 2000–2016. MMWR Morb Mortal Wkly Rep. 2017;66:1256–60.
21. Daffos F, Forestier M, Capella-Pavlovsky M. Prenatal management of 746 pregnancies at risk for congenital toxoplasmosis. N Eng J Med. 1998;318:271-5.
22. Berrebi A, Kobuen We, Bessieres MH. Termination of pregnancy for maternal toxoplasmosis. Lancet. 1994;344:36-9.
23. US Department of Health and Human Services (2000). CDC recommendations regarding selected conditions affecting women's health: Preventing congenital toxoplasmosis. MMWR. 2000;49(RR-2):57-75.
24. Capobiango JD, Mitsuka Breganó R, Navarro IT, Rezende Neto CP, Barbante Casella AM, Ruiz Lopes Mori FM, et al. Congenital toxoplasmosis in a reference center of Paraná, Southern Brazil. Braz J Infect Dis. 2014:S1413-8670(14)00046-4.
25. Manicklal S, Vincent CE, Lazzarotto T, Boppana S, Ravindra KG. The "Silent" Global Burden of Congenital Cytomegalovirus. Clin Microbiol Rev. 2013;1:86-102.
26. Brown H, Abernathy M. Cytomegalovirus infection. Semin Perinatol. 1998;22:260-6.
27. Hagay Z, Biran G, Orney A, Reece E. Congenital cytomegalovirus infection a long standing problem still seeking a solution. Am J Obstet Gynaecol. 1996;174:241-5.
28. Iwasaki S, Yamashita M, Maeda M, Misawa K, Mineta H. Audiological outcome of infants with congenital cytomegalovirus infection in a prospective study. Audiol Neurootol. 2007;12(1):31-6.
29. Adler SP, Nigro G. Prevention of maternal-fetal transmission of cytomegalovirus. Clin Infect Dis. 2013;57(Suppl 4):S189-92.
30. Rieder F, Steininger C. Cytomegalovirus vaccine: phase II clinical trial results. Clin Microbiol Infect. 2014;20(Suppl 5):95-102.
31. Straface G, Selmin A, Zanardo V, De Santis M, Ercoli A, Scambia G. Herpes simplex virus infection in pregnancy. Infect Dis Obstet Gynecol. vol. 2012;385697.
32. Zhang HJ, Patenaude V, Abenhaim HA. Maternal outcomes in pregnancies affected by varicella zoster virus infections: population based study on 7.7 million pregnancy admissions. J Obstet Gynaecol Res. 2015;41:62.
33. Corey L, Wald A, Celum CL, Quinn TC. The effects of herpes simplex virus-2 on HIV-1 acquisition and transmission: a review of two overlapping epidemics. J Acquir Immune Defic Syndr. 2004;35(5):435-45.
34. Sheffield JS, Hollier LM, Hill JB, Stuart GS, Wendel GD. Acyclovir prophylaxis to prevent herpes simplex virus recurrence at delivery: A systematic review. Obstet Gynecol. 2003;102(6):1396-403.
35. Management of Genital Herpes in Pregnancy: ACOG Practice Bulletin Number 220. Obstet Gynecol. 2020;135(5):e193-e202.
36. Hollien LM, Wendel GD. Third trimester antiviral prophylaxis for preventing maternal genital HSV recurrence and neonatal infections. Cochrane database systematic review. 2008;23(1):CD004946.

# Obesity and Pregnancy

*Sirisha Rao Gundabattula*

## ■ INTRODUCTION

Obesity is the major public health issue of our time. The World Health Organization describes obesity as one of the most blatantly visible, yet most neglected public health problems that threaten to overwhelm both more and less developed countries. Obesity is usually defined epidemiologically, using the body mass index (BMI), weight related to height, where >30 kg/m² is considered as obese. A BMI of 18–25 kg/m² is considered a healthy weight with 26–29 kg/m² identified as overweight. Adults with BMI ranging from 30–34.9, 35–39.9 and ≥40 kg/m² are classified as obese classes I, II and III, respectively.[1]

In pregnancy, BMI is calculated using prepregnant weight. If this is unknown, the first weight measurement at prenatal care is used. The BMI is an imprecise estimate of body fat. It does not consider the difference in lean body mass between individuals of the same height and weight, or differences in the distribution of body fat (waist circumference and waist-hip ratio) which are important determinants of the risk of disease. However, BMI is inexpensive, practical and easily applicable in large populations which makes it suitable for epidemiological studies.

The effect of adiposity is evident in nearly every aspect of a woman's reproductive life. This could present as a metabolic or a reproductive complication. Obesity is known to be associated with serious obstetric complications. This chapter will review the obesity-related adverse pregnancy outcomes and discuss the most optimum steps in the care of an obese mother through her pregnancy.

## ■ PREVALENCE AND SIGNIFICANCE

Over the last few decades, the prevalence of overweight and obesity in women has more than doubled. In the Unites States, more than one-third of women are obese, more than one half of pregnant women are overweight or obese and 8% of women in the reproductive age group are extremely obese.[2] The United Kingdom (UK) has seen a sharp increase in the proportion of obese women; as many as 21.3% of antenatal women are obese.[3] In most countries, the prevalence exceeds 15%.[4]

### Indian Scenario

According to the National Family Health Survey (NFHS), the percentage of ever-married women aged 15–49 years who are overweight or obese increased from 13% in NFHS-3 to 21% in NFHS-4.[5] In 2014, India accounted for the largest number of overweight and obese pregnant women (4.3 million) which contributed to 11.1% of the world total.[6]

Pregnancy is associated with permanent weight increase in every BMI category and is a major contributor to the obesity epidemic.[7] There are strong associations between higher BMI and older age, higher parity and higher socioeconomic status.[8] South Asians are more sensitive than Europeans to the effects of obesity and develop diabetes and cardiovascular disease at lower average age and BMI.[9] The UK Confidential Enquiry into. Maternal and Child Health identified that overweight and obesity, was either directly or indirectly the cause of half of maternal mortality.[10]

## ■ OBESITY AND FERTILITY

Obesity reduces fertility and has been shown to affect the health of the oocyte and the quality and development of the embryo early in gestation.[11] At least 40% of women with polycystic ovary syndrome (PCOS) are obese and increasing abdominal obesity is correlated with reduced menstrual frequency and fertility together with greater insulin resistance.[12] A high BMI is related to a lower live birth rate and a higher incidence of early pregnancy loss among women achieving in vitro fertilization (IVF) conceptions.[13]

Obese women respond less well to ovarian stimulation, require higher doses of clomiphene and gonadotropins and are at greater risk of over-response. Further, obesity may affect the safety of procedures due to difficulties encountered in sonographic visualization of ovaries and anesthesia for laparoscopy or oocyte retrieval.[14]

Women who have a BMI of ≥30 kg/m² are likely to take longer to conceive and losing weight (at least 5%–10%) is likely to increase their chance of conception if they have anovulatory cycles. Dietary restriction and exercise together will lead to weight loss and more pregnancies.[15,16] Weight loss in women with PCOS improves the endocrine profile, menstrual cyclicity, rate of ovulation and likelihood of a healthy pregnancy.[17] Metformin appears to be less effective if the BMI is >30.[18]

## OBESITY-RELATED ADVERSE PREGNANCY OUTCOMES

Obesity has a major impact on pregnancy. In the Confidential Enquiries into Maternal Deaths in the UK report (2006-08), 49% of the women who died and for whom BMI was known were either overweight or obese. In terms of the impact of maternal weight on specific causes of death, it was most significant for mortality from thromboembolism followed by cardiac disease (78% and 61% women overweight/obese in these two groups, respectively).[10] **Table 1** enlists the adverse pregnancy outcomes associated with obesity.

## Maternal Complications

It is hypothesized that insulin resistance, low-grade inflammation, dyslipidemia and alteration in systemic microvascular function, all parts of the metabolic syndrome, may predispose to placental vascular dysfunction and account for the association between obesity and maternal complications such as gestational diabetes mellitus (GDM) and pre-eclampsia.[31]

There is a positive correlation between waist-hip ratio and glucose concentrations after an oral glucose tolerance test during pregnancy and postpartum.[32] The ratio of upper-body to lower-body fat is more accurately associated with development of preeclampsia and GDM than total body fat, and with newborn size.[33]

The gain of only 1-2 BMI units increases the risk of GDM, gestational hypertension and large-for-gestational-age (LGA) birth by an average of 20-40% and these risks in relation to interpregnancy weight gain are higher for women with a healthy prepregnancy BMI.[34]

### Gestational Diabetes Mellitus

Approximately 17% of obese women develop GDM during pregnancy.[35] Obese mothers with GDM have twice the risk of delivering children with chromosomal defects.[36] A tight control of blood sugar levels reduces the risk of macrosomia. Apart from a strict dietary regime, insulin therapy is required more often in obese women with GDM than in lean women.[37]

Mothers who develop GDM have a 50% higher risk of developing diabetes during their lifetime[38] with this risk increasing in obese women.[39] Therefore for the obese woman with GDM, pregnancy is a wake-up call for a lifestyle change in terms of exercise, weight loss and in reducing the risk for vascular disease in the long-term.

### Hypertensive Disorders

Most published reports quote between a two- and three-fold increase in risk of pre-eclampsia with a BMI of >30 kg/m². The risk doubles with each 5-7 kg/m² increase in BMI.[40] Waist circumference >80 cm, measured at <16 weeks gestation, is predictive of pregnancy induced hypertension (OR 1.8; 95%

**TABLE 1:** Pregnancy outcomes in obese women (reference category: women with normal BMI) expressed as odds ratio (95% confidence interval).

| | | |
|---|---|---|
| Maternal complications | Gestational diabetes mellitus (GDM) | 3.6 (3.25–3.98)[19]<br>2.6 (2.1–3.4)[20] |
| | Hypertension | 2.5 (2.1–3.0)[20] |
| | Pre-eclampsia | 2.14 (1.85–2.47)[19]<br>1.6 (1.1–2.2)[21] |
| | Thromboembolism | 1.6 (1.01–2.56)[19]<br>5.3 (2.1–13.5) adjusted OR[21] |
| | Antenatal depression | 1.43 (1.27–1.61)[22] |
| | Antenatal anxiety | 1.41 (1.10–1.80)[22] |
| | Genital infection | 1.30 (1.07–1.56)[19] |
| | Urinary tract infection | 1.39 (1.18–1.63)[19] |
| | Wound infection | 2.24 (1.91–2.64)[19] |
| | Postpartum depression | 1.30 (1.20–1.42)[22] |
| Fetal complications | Birth defects | 1.6 (1.0–2.5)[23] |
| | Neural tube defects | 1.8 (1.1–3.0)[24] |
| | Spina bifida | 2.6 (1.5–4.5)[24]<br>3.5 (1.2–10.3)[25]<br>2.8 (1.7–4.5)[26] |
| | Omphalocele | 3.3 (1.0–10.3)[25] |
| | Heart defects | 2.0 (1.2–3.4)[24] |
| | Orofacial clefts | 1.3 (1.11–1.53)[25] |
| | Macrosomia | 2.4 (2.2–2.5)[19] |
| | Birth weight >4,500 g | 2.0 (1.4–3.0)[20] |
| | Birth weight >4,000 g | 1.7 (1.4–2.0)[20] |
| | Shoulder dystocia | 2.9 (1.4–5.8)[25] |
| | Stillbirth | 2.1 (1.5–2.7)[26] |
| | Neonatal death | 2.6 (1.2–5.8)[27] |
| Obstetric complications | Spontaneous miscarriage | 3.05 (1.45–6.44)[28] |
| | Recurrent miscarriage (>3 successive) | 3.51 (1.03–12.01)[29] |
| | Induction of labor | 1.7 (1.64–1.76)[19] |
| | Failure to progress during first stage | 3.1 (2.5–3.8)[30] |
| | Operative vaginal delivery | 1.0 (0.8–1.3)[20] |
| | Cesarean section | 3.2 (2.9–3.5)[30]<br>2.05 (1.86–2.27)[26] |
| | Vaginal birth after cesarean (VBAC) | 0.53 (0.29–0.98)[31]* |
| | Postpartum hemorrhage (PPH) | 1.39 (1.32–1.46)[19] |
| | Breastfeeding | 0.86 (0.56–0.60)[19] |

*Reference category is underweight women.

CI 1.1–2.9) and pre-eclampsia (OR 2.7;95% CI 1.1–6.8).[41] Given the increased risk of pre-eclampsia, obese women should have appropriate surveillance for preeclampsia.[42] The National Institute for Health and Care Excellence (NICE) Clinical Guideline on hypertensive disorders during pregnancy states that women with more than one moderate risk factor may benefit from taking 75–150 mg aspirin daily from 12 weeks' gestation until delivery.[43]

### Thromboembolism

Maternal obesity is associated with a significant risk of thromboembolism during both the antenatal and postnatal period.[44] It is not known whether the association between obesity and venous thromboembolism (VTE) is due to obesity alone, or whether it is due to comorbidities or confounding variables, such as cesarean section. Any effect of obesity on VTE risk is strongly influenced by immobilization.[45] Placement of thromboembolic deterrent stockings before cesarean delivery is recommended for all women. The need for anticoagulants is individualized. Postpartum thromboprophylaxis in these women may be beneficial.[46]

### Infections

Genital tract, wound and urinary tract infections are all significantly more common in women who are obese or overweight.[19] Obesity is an established risk factor for surgical-site infections, nosocomial infections, periodontitis and skin infections. In the absence of sufficient scientific evidence, no dosing guidelines of antimicrobials for obesity have been published.[47]

### Respiratory Complications

Sleep apnea and asthma are associated with obesity in pregnancy. All obese patients should also be assessed for obstructive sleep apnea, because its prevalence correlates with weight.[48] Sahota et al., showed an increased rate of snoring, sleep-related apnea and 4% oxygen desaturation in obese pregnant women compared to nonobese pregnant women.[49]

## Fetal Complications

### Congenital Anomalies

Congenital anomalies with increased prevalence in obese patients include neural tube defects, cardiac defects, orofacial clefts, hydrocephaly, hypospadias, anal atresia, cystic kidney, diaphragmatic hernia and omphalocele.[50] The reasons are poorly understood. One hypothesis suggests an association with undetected type 2 diabetes in early pregnancy or due to lower circulating levels of folate.[51]

The risk of neural tube defects among obese pregnant women is double that of pregnant women of normal weight after correcting for diabetes as a potential confounding factor. In a population-based Swedish study of >1 million live births, risks of major congenital malformations progressively increased with increasing severity of obesity with the greatest relative risk for nervous system malformations.[52] Lower detection rate of fetal anomalies during prenatal ultrasonography is a worrying consequence of maternal obesity.[46]

### Macrosomia

Obesity and excessive weight gain during pregnancy are associated with LGA infants.[46] Fetal hyperinsulinemia and an increased energy flux to the fetus (secondary to increased amino acids in insulin-resistant individuals) may explain the increased frequency of LGA infants seen in women who are obese but not diabetic.

The odds ratio for an obese mother delivering an LGA infant is 1.4–1.8.[53] Macrosomia in turn increases the risk of shoulder dystocia, birth injury and the incidence of low Apgar scores and perinatal death. Kristensen et al., found a significantly ($p<0.0001$) higher incidence of cesarean section (25.8%) among the macrosomic group (>4 kg) compared with the general population (13.1%).[27]

### Neonatal Intensive Care Unit Admissions

In a retrospective analysis, Galtier-Dereure et al. found the percentage of infants requiring neonatal intensive care unit (NICU) admissions was 3.5 times higher when maternal obesity was present.[54] Lower Apgar scores have been reported in the neonates of obese mothers, when compared with those of lean mothers.[53]

The higher incidence of diabetes mellitus and GDM in the obese population may contribute to this effect in view of the need for glycemic control in these infants. Birth trauma due to macrosomia may also increase the rate of perinatal morbidity in them.

### Stillbirths

A gain of 3 or more BMI units is significantly associated with stillbirth independent of other risk factors (63% greater adjusted odds). This association is stronger for term than for preterm stillbirths. The probable explanation could be obesity-mediated inflammation leading to early endothelial dysfunction of the placenta but this warrants further investigation.[34]

## Obstetric Complications

### Miscarriage and Preterm Birth

Obesity is a risk factor for spontaneous miscarriage among women who undergo infertility treatment as well as those who conceive naturally.[29,46] The incidence of spontaneous miscarriages rises as insulin resistance increases. In these women, insulin sensitizing agents, such as metformin, reduce miscarriage rates.[55]

Obesity is associated with PCOS and irregular menses. Obesity also makes sonography technically more challenging.[56] For both these reasons, particular caution should be exercised in making the diagnosis of miscarriage.

The association between maternal obesity and premature birth is a matter of controversy. Some investigators have reported a higher rate of premature delivery for obese women than those of normal weight while others quote a lower rate.[46,54]

## Intrapartum Issues

Women with a booking BMI ≥ 30 kg/m$^2$ should have an informed discussion antenatally about possible intrapartum complications associated with a high BMI, and management strategies considered.[44,46] The inability to obtain an interpretable external cardiotocograph tracing in obese women makes intrapartum monitoring difficult.[46] Consideration should be given to using a fetal scalp electrode early in labor. The labor or operating table needs to be adequate. Experienced personnel trained to lift and transfer obese individuals are a specific requisite.

Obese women have higher rates of induction of labor and cesarean section, and the frequency of both elective and emergency cesarean section is almost doubled.[19] In the absence of other obstetric or medical indications, obesity alone is not an indication for induction of labor.[44] The increase in cesarean section rate may be due to the higher incidence of LGA infants, suboptimal uterine contractions and increased fat deposition in the soft tissues of the pelvis leading to dystocia during labor.[54]

There is difficulty estimating fetal weight even with ultrasonography. Prophylactic cesarean delivery may be considered with estimated fetal weights >5,000 g in women without diabetes and >4,500 g in women with diabetes.[46] The surgical incision should be placed above the panniculus adiposus. A higher dose of preoperative antibiotics should be given for surgical prophylaxis. Suture closure of the subcutaneous layer may be preferable to placement of a subcutaneous drain in order to reduce postoperative wound disruption.[46] There is insufficient evidence to recommend routine use of negative pressure dressing therapy, barrier retractors and insertion of subcutaneous drains.[44]

Obese women are less likely to have a successful VBAC, and the operative and anesthetic risks of emergency cesarean section will be higher for these women. In a study of 1,213 women, obese women were 50% less successful when attempting a trial vaginal delivery after a cesarean section, compared with underweight women. An informed discussion should be held with the woman during the antenatal period and an individualized decision made regarding mode of delivery after consideration of all relevant clinical factors.[44]

## Postpartum Issues

In the puerperium, VTE, endometritis, postpartum hemorrhage (PPH), prolonged hospitalization, wound infection and dehiscence are seen with increased frequency in obese women.[20] They are 30% more frequent. There is a decreased response to suckling in terms of serum prolactin levels.[57] The newborn is often given formula feeds which in turn predisposes to childhood obesity.

## OBESITY AND ANESTHESIA

Obese mothers present difficulties for anesthetists. Blood pressure recording may be inaccurate, peripheral intravenous access is difficult to obtain and the risk of failed epidurals is higher. Intubation may also pose a problem due to excessive tissue and edema.[46] Respiratory complications such as aspiration and pneumonitis are increased.[58]

Epidural or spinal anesthesia is recommended when anesthesia is needed or elected; however, it may be technically difficult because of obscured landmarks, difficult positioning and excessive layers of adipose tissue.[46] The obese mother may require to be monitored postpartum in a high dependency unit and at times in an intensive care unit with the support of a trained team of anesthetists.[58]

## LONG-TERM OUTCOMES

### Fetal Implications

Obesity during pregnancy has been hypothesized to exert long-term health effects on the developing child through "early life programming". Large-for-gestational age infants and those born to diabetic mothers are at increased risk of childhood and adolescent obesity.[46,59] Maternal obesity has been associated with a number of long-term adverse health outcomes in the offspring, including lifelong risk of obesity and metabolic dysregulation with increased insulin resistance, hypertension and dyslipidemia, as well as behavioral problems and risk of asthma.[60]

A multicentric randomized controlled trial was conducted to assess whether a behavioral intervention, based on changing diet (to foods with a lower glycemic index) and physical activity, would reduce the risk of GDM and delivery of a large-for-gestational-age infant and lower the long-term risk of obesity in the offspring.[61] Findings from the UK Pregnancies Better Eating and Activity Trial (UPBEAT) suggest that lifestyle intervention may contribute to a healthier metabolic profile.[62]

### Maternal Consequences

Weight gain during pregnancy is a strong predictor for sustained weight retention and weight gains >9 kg are correlated with the amount of weight retained between two successive pregnancies.[63] Linne et al. reported that both high weight gainers and high weight retainers had higher BMI at the 15-year follow-up and concluded that weight retention at the end of the postpartum year predicts future overweight 15 years later.[64] This can lead to increased mortality and morbidity from coronary heart disease, diabetes, hypertension, stroke, cancers. All of this may also be associated with poor self-esteem and a negative self-image, thus leading to poor mental health.[63]

Gestational diabetes mellitus is a major risk for later type 2 diabetes, the risk being greatest for women who are obese. The most rapid incidence of type 2 diabetes following GDM occurs in the first 5 years after delivery, after correcting for ethnicity.[65] Obese mothers are more likely to experience urinary symptoms such as stress incontinence and urgency.[66] Women who are obese are at increased risk of developing hormone-dependent malignancies such as breast and endometrial cancer (OR 2.5 for both).[67]

## COST IMPLICATIONS

Obesity during pregnancy is associated with increased use of healthcare services, especially when the BMI is ≥35 kg/m$^2$. Galtier-Dereure et al. in a study of 435 women, found that the average cost in terms of antenatal care was five times higher in women with a high prepregnancy BMI. The duration of stay was also 3.9 to 6.2-fold higher.[54]

A higher-than-normal BMI is associated with significantly more antepartum fetal surveillance, ultrasonography and medication use. The length of hospital stay for delivery is significantly greater in women with higher-than-normal BMI and is largely due to increased cesarean rates and obesity-related high-risk conditions.[8]

## PREGNANCY AFTER BARIATRIC SURGERY

- Antiobesity surgery should be considered in young women of reproductive age when all other therapies have failed (BMI >40 kg/m$^2$ or BMI 35–40 kg/m$^2$ plus other disease such as type 2 diabetes); if BMI is >50, bariatric surgery should be considered as first-line therapy.[16]
- Although women who undergo bariatric surgery are advised to avoid pregnancy postoperatively during the early rapid weight-loss phase (12–18 months), there is no evidence to support this theory.[68]
- These women should have consultant-led antenatal care.[44]
- Pregnancies after bariatric surgery are less likely to be complicated by GDM, hypertension, pre-eclampsia and macrosomia than pregnancies of those women who have not undergone such surgery.[69]
- Bariatric surgery has an increased risk of fetal growth restriction and stillbirth.[70]
- These women should be evaluated for nutritional deficiency (iron, vitamin $B_{12}$, folate, vitamin D and calcium) and vitamins supplemented if indicated.[46]
- Adjustment of a gastric band may be needed during pregnancy.[71]
- Bariatric surgery is not an independent indication for cesarean delivery.[72]

## MANAGEMENT PRINCIPLES

- The obese mother must be considered a high risk and should be managed in a perinatal center where a multidisciplinary approach can be offered.
- Care and communications need to be conducted in a sensitive and respectful manner.[73,74]
- Obesity will make ultrasound assessment of anatomy, fetal size and fetal wellbeing more difficult;[19] and some women may require referral to a specialist center for ultrasound assessment.[42]
- The maternity units should ensure circulation space, adequate doorway widths, safe working loads, transportation facilities and appropriately-sized equipment.[44]
- Multiparous, low-risk women can be given a choice of planning birth in midwifery-led units with clear pathways for referral.[44]
- Women with moderate to severe obesity (BMI >34.9 kg/m$^2$) are not suitable for a home birth because of the associated high incidence of comorbidities and the need for early intravenous access, especially for the management of postpartum hemorrhage.[44]

### Care Pathway for Pregnant Women with Obesity[42,44,46,75-78]

*Prepregnancy*

- Provide specific information concerning maternal and fetal risks
- Advise weight loss and aim for BMI between 20 and 25 kg/m$^2$
- Inform women that weight loss between pregnancies decreases the risk of stillbirth, hypertensive complications and macrosomia; and increases the chances of successful VBAC
- Commence 5 mg folic acid daily at least 3 months prior to conception
- Screen for hypertension and carbohydrate intolerance
- Provide psychological support if depressive illness is identified.

*At Booking*

- Calculate and document BMI
- Provide specific information concerning maternal and fetal risks
- Use an appropriate-sized BP cuff (large cuff if mid-arm circumference >33 cm)

| TABLE 2: Gestational weight gain recommendations. | | | |
|---|---|---|---|
| Revised Institute of Medicine Guidelines for gestational weight gain[79] | | | |
| Prepregnancy | BMI (kg/m²) | Range (kg) | Range (lbs) |
| Underweight | (<18.5) | 12.5–18.0 | 28–40 |
| Normal weight | (18.5–24.9) | 11.5–16.0 | 25–35 |
| Overweight | (25.0–29.9) | 7.0–11.5 | 15–25 |
| Obese | (>29.9) | 5.0–9.0 | 11–20 |

Provisional guidelines were made for multiple pregnancies:[42]
- Normal weight women should gain 17–25 kg (37–54 pounds) at term,
- Overweight women should gain 14–23 kg (31–50 pounds) at term, and
- Obese women should gain 11–19 kg (25–42 pounds) at term

There is uncertainty regarding safety of weight loss during pregnancy on neonatal outcomes.[42]

- Educate about recommendations for weight gain **(Table 2)**
- Suggest lifestyle modification **(Box 1)**
- Antiobesity drugs are not recommended
- Continue 5 mg folic acid daily up to 12 weeks of gestation
- Commence 10 mg vitamin D daily throughout pregnancy
- Consider 150 mg aspirin daily from 12 weeks of pregnancy until the birth of the baby if associated with >1 of the following: first pregnancy, maternal age >40 years, family history of pre-eclampsia, multiple pregnancy
- Screen for GDM [75 g oral glucose tolerance test (OGTT)]
- Assess VTE risk and administer thromboprophylaxis if indicated **(Box 2)**.

## Antepartum

- Review recommendations for weight gain periodically **(Table 2)**
- Screen for chromosomal anomalies and consider use of transvaginal scan if it is difficult to obtain nuchal translucency measurements transabdominally
- Perform a detailed scan for fetal anomalies
- Repeat OGTT at 28 weeks if booking OGTT is normal
- Influenza vaccination is strongly recommended
- Screen for mental health problems and refer when appropriate
- Advise regular antenatal visits with blood pressure checks
- Weekly antepartum fetal surveillance beginning at 37 weeks for women with BMI of 35-39 kg/m² and at 34 weeks for women with BMI ≥ 40 kg/m²
- Multiple gestation especially monochorionic gestations require increased surveillance
- Symphysio-fundal height measurements are likely to be inaccurate and external palpation may be technically difficult; hence, ultrasound should be considered for assessment of fetal presentation and serial assessment of fetal size
- Arrange for anesthesiology consultation

**BOX 1:** Lifestyle modifications for obese mothers.

- Observational studies have reported that physical exercise during pregnancy is associated with a decreased risk of pre-eclampsia and GDM and unless there are medical or obstetric contradictions obese women should be encouraged to maintain regular exercise during and after pregnancy[80]
- While significant weight loss *before pregnancy* is rarely practical, guidance to minimize weight gain *during pregnancy* and to achieve weight loss after *delivery* should be offered on an urgent basis Pregnancy may be an especially powerful "teachable moment" and pregnant women are more prone to adopt healthy lifestyles, have better and more frequent access to medical care, and are under close medical supervision[48]
- Combinations of dietary modification and exercise are effective in avoidance of postpartum weight retention. The loss of at least 1 BMI unit reduces the risk of LGA birth and maintains the risk of GDM and gestational hypertension at general population level[34]
- Avoidance of excessive intake of high energy and a healthy diet including fresh meat and fish, low-fat dairy foods, vegetables, high-fiber cereals, fruit and water should be emphasized[80]
- During the antenatal period, a moderate intensity exercise for 30 minutes per day is recommended. If pregnancy and delivery are uncomplicated, a mild exercise program consisting of walking, pelvic floor exercises and stretching may begin immediately. After complicated deliveries or cesarean sections, prepregnancy levels of physical activity should not be resumed until 8–12 weeks postpartum[80]

**BOX 2:** Thromboprophylaxis recommendations for obese mothers.[81]

*Antepartum thromboprophylaxis:*
- *BMI ≥30 and ≥2 additional risk factors for thromboembolism:* Commence prophylactic low molecular weight heparin (LMWH) from 28 weeks of gestation and continue for 6 weeks postpartum but after making postnatal risk assessment
- *BMI ≥30 and ≥3 additional risk factors for thromboembolism:* Commence prophylactic LMWH from the first trimester and continue for 6 weeks postpartum but after making postnatal risk assessment
- *Postpartum thromboprophylaxis:* BMI ≥40 regardless of mode of delivery OR BMI ≥30 with ≥1 additional persisting risk factor for thromboembolism: LMWH for 10 days postpartum. In class III obese women, weight-based dose of LMWH should be considered after cesarean delivery

- Anticipate problems and prepare in terms of equipment and personnel
- Advise regarding benefits, initiation and maintenance of breastfeeding
- Birth plan should be clearly documented
- Decision for induction of labor at term and VBAC should be individualized; planned cesarean section should involve a multidisciplinary approach.

## Intrapartum

- Secure early venous access; site a second cannula if BMI ≥40 kg/m²
- Consider early epidural
- Women with class III obesity should receive continuous midwifery care and measures to prevent pressure sores

- Provide antiembolism stockings and ensure adequate hydration
- Advocate active management of third stage of labor
- Ensure administration of prophylactic antibiotic as per hospital policy.

### Postpartum

- Motivate to mobilize as early as practicable
- Encourage breastfeeding
- Initiate thromboprophylaxis (*see* Box 2)
- Refer for ongoing lifestyle advice (*see* Box 1)
- If pregnancy is complicated by GDM, advise OGTT at 6 weeks postpartum and annual screening for type 2 diabetes
- Advise on long-term risks of obesity, hypertension and diabetes
- Suggest weight loss prior to next pregnancy
- While providing postnatal contraceptive advice, remember that these women are at increased risk of VTE if they take the hormonal contraceptive pill
- Screen for postpartum depression and anxiety.

## KEY POINTS

- Obesity is a rapidly growing health epidemic.
- Pregnancy in an obese mother must be considered a "high risk pregnancy" that needs multidisciplinary care; this mother is at an increased risk of almost every complication of pregnancy.
- Obese mothers are more likely to develop metabolic syndrome later on in life thus posing a significant health and economic burden worldwide.
- Greater awareness is needed by the health professionals who can target obese women of childbearing age, education and advice being the key factors.
- Preventing obesity needs a change in thinking—a societal change. There is an urgent need for active partnership between government, science, business and civil society.

## SUGGESTED READING

1. Denison FC, Aedla NR, Keag O, et al. Care of women with obesity in pregnancy. Green-top Guideline No. 72. BJOG. 2019;126(3):e62-e106.
2. McAuliffe FM, Killeen SL, Jacob CM, Hanson MA, Hadar E, McIntyre HD, et al. Management of prepregnancy, pregnancy, and postpartum obesity from the FIGO Pregnancy and Non-Communicable Diseases Committee: a FIGO (International Federation of Gynecology and Obstetrics) guideline. Int J Gynaecol Obstet. 2020;151 Suppl 1:16-36.
3. Ramsey PS, Schenken RS. Obesity in pregnancy: complications and maternal management. In: UpToDate, Post, CJL, FXP and VAB (Eds). UpToDate, Waltham, MA, 2020.
4. The American College of Obstetricians and Gynecologists. Obesity in Pregnancy. ACOG Practice Bulletin No. 230, Obstet Gynecol. 2021;137(6):e128-e144.
5. The Royal Australian and New Zealand College of Obstetricians and Gynaecologists. Management of Obesity in Pregnancy. College Statement C-Obs 49, March 2017.

## REFERENCES

1. World Health Organization. Obesity: preventing and managing the global epidemic. WHO Technical Report Series. Geneva: WHO; 2000.
2. Flegal KM, Carroll MD, Kit BK, Ogden CL. Prevalence of obesity and trends in the distribution of body mass index among US adults, 1999–2010. JAMA. 2012;307:491-7.
3. NMPA Project Team. National Maternal and Perinatal Audit: Clinical Report 2017. London: RCOG; 2017.
4. Haslam D, James WP. Obesity. Lancet. 2005;366:1197-209.
5. Government of India (MOHFW). India Fact Sheet. National Family Health Survey (NFHS-4), 2015-16. Mumbai: International Institute for Population Sciences; 2020.
6. Chen C, Yu X, Yan Y. Estimated global overweight and obesity burden in pregnant women based on panel data model. PLoS One. 2018;13(8):e0202183.
7. Siega-Riz AM, Viswanathan M, Moos MK, Deierlein A, Mumford S, Knaack J, et al. A systematic review of outcomes of maternal weight gain according to the Institute of Medicine recommendations: birth weight, fetal growth, and postpartum weight retention. Am J Obstet Gynecol. 2009;201(4):339.e1-e14.
8. Chu SY, Bachman DJ, Callaghan WM, et al. Association between Obesity during Pregnancy and Increased Use of Health Care. N Engl J Med. 2008;358:1444-53.
9. Mukhopadhyay B, Forouhi NG, Fisher BM, Kesson CM, Sattar N. A comparison of glycaemic and metabolic control over time among South Asian and European patients with Type 2 diabetes: results from follow-up in a routine diabetes clinic. Diabet Med. 2006;23:94-8.
10. Centre for Maternal and Child Enquiries. Saving Mothers' lives: reviewing maternal deaths to make motherhood safer: 2006–2008. BJOG. 2011;118:1.203.
11. Robker RL. Evidence that obesity alters the quality of oocytes and embryos. Pathophysiology. 2008;15(2):115-21.
12. Balen AH, Conway GS, Kaltsas G, Techatrasak K, Manning PJ, West C, et al. Polycystic ovary syndrome: The spectrum of the disorder in 1741 patients. Hum Reprod. 1995;10:2705-12.
13. Linsten AM, Pasker-de Jong PC, de Boer EJ, Burger CW, Jansen CA, Braat DD, et al. Effects of subfertility cause, smoking and body weight on the success of IVF. Hum Reprod. 2005;20:1867-75.
14. Balen AH. Polycystic ovary syndrome, obesity and reproductive function. In: Baker P, Balen AH, Poston L, Sattar N (Eds). Obesity and Reproductive Health. London; RCOG Press; 2007. pp. 69-80.
15. National Institute for Health and Care Excellence. Fertility: Assessment and treatment for people with fertility problems. NICE clinical guideline 156; 2013.
16. National Institute for Health and Care Excellence. Obesity: guidance on the prevention, identification, assessment and management of overweight and obesity in adults and children. NICE clinical guideline 43; 2006.
17. Norman RJ, Noakes M, Wu R, Davies MJ, Moran L, Wang JX. Improving reproductive performance in overweight/obese

women with effective weight management. Hum Reprod Update. 2004;10:267-80.
18. Tang T, Glanville J, Hayden CJ, White D, Barth JH, Balen AH. Combined life-style modification and metformin in obese patients with PCOS. A randomized, placebo-controlled, double-blind multi-centre study. Hum Reprod. 2006;21:80-9.
19. Sebire NJ, Jolly M, Harris JP. Maternal obesity and pregnancy outcome: A study of 287213 pregnancies in London. Int J Obesity. 2001;25:1175-82.
20. Weiss JL, Malone FD, Emig D, Ball RH, Nyberg DA, Comstock CH, et al. Obesity, obstetric complications and cesarean delivery rate-A population-based screening study. Am J Obstet Gynecol. 2004;190:1091-7.
21. Larsen TB, Sorensen HT, Gislum M, Johnsen SP. Maternal smoking, obesity, and risk of venous thromboembolism during pregnancy and the puerperium: a population-based nested case-control study. Thrombosis Research. 2007;120(4):505-9.
22. Molyneaux E, Poston L, Ashurst-Williams S, Howard LM. Obesity and mental disorders during pregnancy and postpartum: a systematic review and meta-analysis. Obstet Gynecol. 2014;123(4):857-67.
23. Callaway LK, Prins JB, Chang AM, McIntyre HD. The prevalence and impact of overweight and obesity in an Australian obstetric population. Med J Aust. 2006;184(2):56-9.
24. Anderson JL, Waller DK, Canfield MA, Shaw GM, Watkins ML, Werler MM. Maternal obesity, gestational diabetes, and central nervous system birth defects. Epidemiology. 2005;16:87-92.
25. Usha Kiran TS, Hemmadi S, Bethel J, Evans J. Outcome of pregnancy in a woman with an increased body mass index. BJOG. 2005;112:768-72.
26. Chu SY, Kim SY, Schmid CH, Dietz PM, Callaghan WM, Lau J, et al. Maternal obesity and risk of cesarean delivery: a meta-analysis. Obes Rev. 2007;8(5):385-94.
27. Kristensen J, Vestergaard M, Wisborg K, Kesmodel U, Secher NJ. Pre-pregnancy weight and the risk of stillbirth and neonatal death. BJOG. 2005;112:403-8.
28. Mulders AG, Laven JS, Eijkemans MJ, Hughes EG, Fauser BC. Patient predictors for outcome of gonadotrophin ovulation induction in women with mormogonadotrophic anovulatory infertility: a meta-analysis. Hum Reprod Update. 2003;9:429-49.
29. Lashen H, Fear K, Sturdee W. Obesity is associated with increased risk of first trimester and recurrent miscarriage: matched case-control study. Hum Reprod. 2004;19:1644-6.
30. Sheiner E, Levy A, Menes TS, DeFranco E. Maternal obesity as an independent risk factor for caesarean delivery. Pediatr Perinat Epidemiol. 2004;18:196-201.
31. Gate E, Ramsay JE. Antenatal complications of maternal obesity: Miscarriage, fetal abnormalities, maternal gestational diabetes and pre-eclampsia. In: Baker P, Balen AH, Poston L, Sattar N (Eds). Obesity and Reproductive Health. London: RCOG Press; 2007. pp. 127-43.
32. Landon MB, Osei K, Platt M, O'Dorisio T, Samuels P, Gabbe SG. The differential effects of body fat distribution on insulin and glucose metabolism during pregnancy. Am J Obstet Gynecol. 1994;171:875-84.
33. Ijuin H, Douchi T, Nakamura S, Oki T, Yamamoto S, Nagata Y. Possible association of body-fat distribution with preeclampsia. J Obstet Gynaecol Res. 1997;23:45-9.
34. Villamor E, Cnattingius S. Interpregnancy weight change and risk of adverse pregnancy outcomes; a population-based study. Lancet. 2006;368:1164-70.
35. Linne Y. Effects of obesity on women's reproduction and complications during pregnancy. Obes Rev. 2004;5:137-43.
36. Kral JG. Preventing and treating obesity in girls and young women to curb the epidemic. Obes Res. 2004;12:1539-46.
37. Comtois R, Seguin MC, Aris-Jilwan N. Comparison of obese and non-obese patients with gestational diabetes. Int J Obes Relat Metab Disord. 1993;17:605-8.
38. Linne Y, Barkeling B, Rossner S. Natural course of gestational diabetes mellitus: long term follow up of women in the SPAWN Study. BJOG. 2002;109:1227-31.
39. Schranz AG, Sarona-Ventura C. Long-term significance of gestational carbohydrate intolerance: A longitudinal Study. Exp Clin Endocrinol Diabetes. 2002;110:219-22.
40. O'Brien TE, Ray JG, Chan WS. Maternal body mass index and the risk of pre-eclampsia: A systematic overview. Epidemiology. 2003;14:368-274.
41. Sattar N, Clark P, Holmes A. Antenatal waist circumference and hypertension risk. Obstet Gynecol. 2001;97:268-71.
42. The Royal Australian and New Zealand College of Obstetricians and Gynaecologists. Management of Obesity in Pregnancy. College Statement C-Obs 49; 2017.
43. National Institute for Health and Care Excellence. Hypertension in pregnancy: diagnosis and management. NICE guidance 133; 2019.
44. Denison FC, Aedla NR, Keag O, Hor K, Reynolds RM, Milne A, et al. Care of Women with Obesity in pregnancy. Green-top Guideline No. 72. BJOG. 2019;126(3):e62-e106.
45. Jacobsen AF, Skjeldestads FE, Sandset PM. Ante- and postnatal risk factors of venous thrombosis: A hospital-based case-control study. J Thromb Haemost. 2008;6:905-12.
46. The American College of Obstetricians and Gynecologists. Obesity in Pregnancy. ACOG Practice Bulletin No. 230, Obstet Gynecol. 2021;137(6): e128-44.
47. Huttunen R, Syrjanen J. Obesity and the risk and outcome of infection. Int J Obesity. 2013;37:333-40.
48. Artal R, Flick A. Obesity and weight gain in pregnancy. Contemporary Obs Gyn; 2017.
49. Sahota PK, Jain SS, Dhand R. Sleep disorders in pregnancy. Curr Opin Pulmon Med. 2003;9:477-83.
50. Blomberg MI, Kallen B. Maternal obesity and morbid obesity: the risk for birth defects in the offspring. Birth Defects Res A Clin Mol Teratol. 2010;88:35-40.
51. Werler MM, Louik C, Shapiro S, Mitchell AA. Prepregnant weight in relation to risk of neural tube defects. JAMA. 1996;275:1089-92.
52. Persson M, Cnattingius S, Villamor E, Söderling J, Pasternak B, Stephansson O, et al. Risk of major congenital malformations in relation to maternal overweight and obesity severity: cohort study of 1.2 million singletons. BMJ. 2017;357:j2563.
53. Edwards LE, Hellerstedt WL, Alton IR, Story M, Himes JH. Pregnancy complications and birth outcomes in obese and normal – weight women: Effects of gestational weight change. Obstet Gynecol. 1996;87:389-94.
54. Galtier-Dereure F, Boegner C, Bringer J. Obesity and pregnancy: complications and cost. Am J Clin Nutr. 2000;71(Suppl 5):1242S-8S.
55. Stewart FM, Ransay JE, Greer IA. Obesity, impact on obstetric practice and outcome. Obstetn Gynaecol. 2009;11:25-31.

56. Paladini D. Sonography in obese and overweight pregnant women; clinical, medicolegal and technical issues. Ultrasound Obstet Gynecol. 2009;33:720-9.
57. Rasmussen KM, Kjolhede CL. Pre-pregnant overweight and obesity diminish the prolactin response to suckling in the first week postpartum. Pediatrics. 2004;113:e465-71.
58. Perlow JH. Obesity in the obstetric intensive care patient. In: Foley N, Strong T (Eds). Obstetric Intensive Care: A Practical Manual. Philadelphia; WB Saunders;1997. pp. 77-90.
59. Simic BS. Childhood obesity as a risk factor in adulthood and its prevention. Prev Med. 1983;12:47-51.
60. O'Reilly JR, Reynolds RM. The risk of maternal obesity to the long-term health of the offspring. Clin Endocrinol (Oxf). 2013;78(1):9-16.
61. Briley AL, Barr S, Badger S, Bell R, Croker H, Godfrey KM, et al. A complex intervention to improve pregnancy outcome in obese women; the UPBEAT randomized controlled trial. BMC Pregnancy and Childbirth. 2014;14:74.
62. Mills HL, Patel N, White SL, Pasupathy D, Briley AL, Santos Ferreira DL, et al. The effect of a lifestyle intervention in obese pregnant women on gestational metabolic profiles: findings from the UK Pregnancies Better Eating and Activity Trial (UPBEAT) randomized controlled trial. BMC Medicine. 2019;17:15.
63. Morin KH. Obese and nonobese postpartum women: complications, body image, and perceptions of the intrapartal experience. Appl Nurs Res. 1995;8:81-7.
64. Linne Y, Dye L, Barkeling B, Rossner S. Long-term weight development in women: a 15-year follow-up of the effects of pregnancy. Obes Res. 2004;12(7):1166-78.
65. Kim C, Newton KM, Knopp RH. Gestational diabetes and the incidence of type 2 diabetes: a systematic review. Diabetes Care. 2002;25:1862-8.
66. Rasmussen KL, Krue S, Johansson LE, et al. Obesity as a predictor of postpartum urinary symptoms. Acta Obstet Gynecol Scand. 1997;76:359-62.
67. Kehoe S. Obesity and female malignancies. In: Baker P, Balen AH, Poston L, Sattar N (Eds). Obesity and Reproductive Health. London: RCOG Press; 2007. pp. 221-9.
68. Kral JG, Hould FS, Marceau S, et al. Anti-obesity surgery for women planning pregnancy. In: Baker P, Balen AH, Poston L, Sattar N (Eds). Obesity and Reproductive Health. London: RCOG Press; 2007. pp. 181-95.
69. Sheiner E, Levy A, Silverberg D, Menes TS, Levy I, Katz M, et al. Pregnancy after bariatric surgery is not associated with adverse perinatal outcome. Am J Obstet Gynecol. 2004;190:1335-40.
70. Johannson KCS, Naslund I, Roos N, Roos N, Trolle Lagerros Y, Granath F, et al. Outcomes of pregnancy after bariatric surgery. New Engl J Med. 2015;372(9):814-24.
71. Weiss HG, Nehoda H, Labeck B, Hourmont K, Marth C, Aigner F. Pregnancies after adjustable gastric banding. Obes Surg. 2001;11:303-6.
72. Maggard MA, Yermilov I, Li Z, Maglione M, Newberry S, Suttorp M, et al. Pregnancy and fertility following bariatric surgery: a systematic review. JAMA. 2008;300:2286-96.
73. Furber CM, McGowan L. A qualitative study of the experiences of women who are obese and pregnant in the UK. Midwifery. 2011;27(4):437-44.
74. The American College of Obstetricians and Gynecologists. ACOG Committee Opinion No. 763: Ethical considerations for the care of patients with obesity. Obstet Gynecol. 2019;133(1):e90-e96.
75. Davies GAL, Maxwell C, McLeod L. Reaffirmed SOGC Clinical Practice Guideline No. 239-Obesity in pregnancy. J Obstet Gynaecol Can. 2018;40(8):E630-639.
76. Maxwell C, Gaudet L, Cassir G, Nowik C, McLeod NL, Jacob CÉ, et al. SOGC Clinical Practice Guideline No. 391-Pregnancy and maternal obesity Part 1: Pre-conception and prenatal care. J Obstet Gynaecol Can. 2019;41(11):1623-1640.
77. Maxwell C, Gaudet L, Cassir G, Nowik C, McLeod NL, Jacob CÉ, et al. SOGC Clinical Practice Guideline No. 392-Pregnancy and maternal obesity Part 2: Team planning for delivery and postpartum care. J Obstet Gynaecol Can. 2019;41(11):1660-75.
78. The American College of Obstetricians and Gynecologists. Indications for outpatient antenatal fetal surveillance. ACOG Committee Opinion No. 828, Obstet Gynecol. 2021;137(6):e177-97.
79. Institute of Medicine (US) and National Research Council (US) Committee to Reexamine IOM Pregnancy Weight Guidelines. Weight Gain During Pregnancy: Reexamining the Guidelines. Washington DC: National Academy of Sciences; 2009.
80. Institute of Obstetricians and Gynaecologists, Royal College of Physicians of Ireland. Obesity and Pregnancy. Clinical Practice Guideline. June 2011.
81. Royal College of Obstetricians and Gynaecologists. Reducing the risk of venous thromboembolism during pregnancy and the puerperium. Green-top Guideline No. 37a, April 2015.

# Gynecological Diseases in Pregnancy

*Smiti Nanda, Vani Malhotra*

## INTRODUCTION

There are various gynecological conditions, which can coexist with pregnancy and may affect the pregnancy outcome. Most common condition found during pregnancy is uterine leiomyoma followed by ovarian mass. Other less common conditions are retroversion of uterus, genital prolapse, preinvasive lesions of the cervix, and rarely cervical cancer. These conditions may remain asymptomatic and may get diagnosed during pregnancy. It is essential to understand these conditions so that pregnancy can be optimally managed in their presence with a good fetomaternal outcome.

## LEIOMYOMA AND PREGNANCY

The incidence of uterine myomas during pregnancy ranges from 0.09 to 3.9%.[1,2] The reason for this low incidence is that the majority of pregnancies occur within the age group below that of the development of fibroids. However, recently, as more and more women are delaying child bearing, with a resultant increase in incidence of fibroids.

The clinical diagnosis of uterine myoma in pregnancy is not always easy unless the myoma is discrete. During early pregnancy, the apparent asymmetrical enlargement of the uterus may be the only noticeable finding. Later on, uterus may appear larger than period of gestation.

Ultrasound establishes the diagnosis more accurately. Ultrasound criteria for diagnosis of myoma in pregnancy are as follows:[3]

- Size >3 cm
- Spherical shape
- Distortion of myometrial contour
- Different acoustic structure from myometrium
- Speckled pattern of internal echoes
- No enhancement of echoes behind the mass
- Color-flow Doppler showing splaying of blood vessels around the mass.

The ability of sonography for detection is limited due to difficulty in differentiating them from physiological thickening of the myometrium.

### Effect of Pregnancy on Myoma

Until recently, it was believed that fibroids increase in size during pregnancy in response to hormonal stimulation. Recent studies have demonstrated that approximately 80% of fibroids remain of the same size or even decrease during the course of pregnancy. The fibroids that increase during pregnancy mostly grow in first trimester. Growth of fibroids during pregnancy is not directly related to only increase in estrogen levels as evidenced by doubling in size of fibroid within 6-7 weeks of gestation when hormone levels are still low. Certain cytokines and growth factors produced by fetoplacental unit are also implicated for their growth.[4]

Red degeneration or carneous degeneration occurs in 5-8% of myomas and is mostly seen during the second half of pregnancy. The pathophysiology is unclear; however the rupture and obstruction of vessels in the periphery of tumor causes necrosis and infarction with release of prostaglandins that is responsible for the symptoms.

A study was conducted on 113 pregnant women presenting with fibroid in pregnancy. 9% of fibroids were associated with cystic changes on sonography. Of these, 70% (7 out of 10) had severe abdominal pain compared with 11.7% (12 of 103) women with no cystic changes on sonography.[5]

The signs and symptoms are variable and include localized pain, tenderness, low grade fever, premature labor, moderate leukocytosis, and peritoneal friction rub. Other causes of abdominal pain such as abruption, pyelonephritis, ureteric calculus, appendicitis, and adnexal torsion must be ruled out.[1] The treatment is conservative, i.e., rest, hydration, and analgesics.

### Effect of Myoma on Pregnancy

The impact of myoma on pregnancy depends on the size, number, and location of myoma. Most of the fibroids are asymptomatic and most (60-78%) do not demonstrate any change in volume during pregnancy. The overall risk of complication is 10-30%.

#### Pregnancy Loss

Uterine fibroids increase the risk of miscarriage and are a cause of recurrent pregnancy loss; however, not all fibroids pose equal risk. Large submucosal fibroids are consistently associated with recurrent pregnancy loss. Several mechanisms that have been suggested are distortion of cavity, compression of underlying endometrium leading to its dysfunction, distortion of its vascular architecture, failure of development of uteroplacental circulation, increased uterine contractility, and altered placental oxytocinase activity with the latter two causing disruption of placenta.[6]

### Preterm Labor

Increased risk of preterm labor has been reported with fibroids > 3 cm. Uteri with fibroids are suggested to be less distensible, which leads to preterm labor in a way similar to congenital mullerian abnormality of the uterus. Also, decreased oxytocinase activity in the gravid uterus with fibroid may result in a localized increase in oxytocin levels and predisposition to premature contractions.[6]

### Premature Rupture of Membranes

The association between premature rupture of membranes (PROM) and fibroids is not well established. The greater risk of PROM seems to be in women having retroplacental fibroid, however some studies have reported no increase in risk.

### Placental Abruption

Submucosal and retroplacental fibroids with volumes >200 mL (corresponding to 7-8 cm diameter) have the highest risk of abruption. The explanation for increased risk for abruption in the setting of uterine fibroids is likely related to placental and decidual necrosis.[6]

### Pain

It is the most frequent complication of fibroid in pregnancy with 5-15% of women requiring hospitalization at some point during antenatal period. This risk for pain increases with size and is especially high in fibroids > 5 cm in diameter.

Pain is likely to result from ischemia and necrosis with release of prostaglandins. Most patients are admitted for pain in the relative absence of symptoms such as nausea and vomiting, leukocytosis and pyrexia.

The management of pain due to fibroid includes rest, hydration, and analgesics. Although, ibuprofen is reported to be very effective, it is not recommended beyond 32 weeks because of the possibility of premature closure of ductus arterisous, neonatal pulmonary hypertension, oligohydramnios, and platelet dysfunction.[1,6]

### Placenta Previa

The presence of fibroid was thought to predispose to placenta previa, however, no such relation has been proved.[3]

### Preeclampsia

No significant increase was noted in prevalence of preeclampsia in association with fibroids but women having multiple fibroids are more likely to develop preeclampsia than those with single fibroid. The increased risk is due to disruption of trophoblastic invasion, which leads to inadequate uteroplacental vascular remodeling.

### Fetal Anomalies

The fetal anomalies reported with fibroid uterus are caudal dysplasia limb reduction defects, congenital torticollis, and head deformities. The risk is found to be two times greater than normal patients.[7]

### Malpresentations

Increased risk of malpresentation has been reported in pregnancies with fibroid uterus (odds ratio, 2.9; 2.6-3.2).[8] Large submucosal fibroids by distorting the shape of the cavity, have been consistently associated with malpresentations. However, increased prevalence is also noted with multiple fibroids, retroplacental fibroids or lower segment fibroids.[2-6]

### Dysfunctional Labor

The disruption in the coordinated spread of contractile wave leads in dysfunctional and prolonged labor.[9]

### Obstructed Labor

Cervical fibroid or fibroid very low in the uterus may, however, remain below the presenting part and may threaten to obstruct labor. The anterior fibroid has a far better opportunity of being drawn up out of the pelvis after the onset of labor than a posterior tumor which tends to get trapped within the pelvis.

### Cesarean Delivery

Cesarean delivery rates are increased due to factors such as an increased risk of malpresentations, dysfunctional labor, and placental abruption.

### Postpartum Hemorrhage

Pathophysiologically, uterine fibroids may predispose to postpartum hemorrhage by decreasing force and coordination of uterine contractions which leads to uterine atony. When the placenta happens to be situated over fibroid, there is often a defective decidual reaction so that it is liable to be morbidly adherent placenta. Very rarely, a fibroid situated at the fundus of the uterus may, for mechanical reason, precipitate uterine inversion.

*Retained Placenta*

An increased incidence of retained placenta in pregnant women with fibroid as compared to controls is observed regardless of location of the fibroids.

*Infection in the Postpartum Period*

Submucosal fibroids or fibroids lying adjacent to uterine incision may get infected in the postpartum period.

*Other Complications*

Less common complications such as spontaneous hemoperitoneum, disseminated intravascular coagulopathy (DIC), incarceration of uterus behind sacral promontory leading to urinary retention and rarely acute renal failure is also seen.[2]

## Myomectomy during Pregnancy

Every effort should be made to avoid surgery during pregnancy. It may be performed for intractable pain due to fibroids that is refractory to rest, hydration, and nonsteroidal anti-inflammatory drugs (NSAIDs) or narcotic analgesia. Other indications may include torsion of pedunculated fibroid causing necrosis resulting in peritoneal reaction, spontaneous rupture of degenerated fibroid, and hemorrhage. Sometimes, torsion of pedunculated fibroid can cause axial torsion of uterus leading to massive abruption and shock. Complications associated with antenatal removal of fibroid are injury to major vessels causing intractable hemorrhage, uterine atony, pregnancy loss, intestinal adhesions, and recurrence. The optimal technique is the open approach. Several studies have analyzed obstetric and neonatal outcomes after antenatal myomectomy and found comparable outcomes in both the groups except for slight increase in incidence of operative delivery due to fear of uterine rupture after myomectomy.[10]

## Myomectomy during Cesarean Section

Since a term uterus receives about 17% of the cardiac output, myomectomy at the time of cesarean section is associated with significant hemorrhage and has been discouraged traditionally. A few cases of myomectomy at the time of cesarean section have been reported in the recent literature. Myomectomy for nonpedunculated fibroids may be associated with severe hemorrhage. The decision to proceed with myomectomy should be approached with caution. It is especially indicated to gain access to the baby in patients in whom fibroids are obstructing the lower uterine segment, with pedunculated and anterior uterine fibroids, and when the fibroids cause difficulty with uterine wound closure thereby causing significant blood loss. Hassiakos et al. concluded that intramural myomas in the fundus, myomas located proximal to the fallopian tubes, and in cornua should be avoided.[11]

*Advantages of Cesarean Myomectomy*

There are many advantages of cesarean myomectomy if it can be safely done during cesarean delivery. Advantages include the following:

- It prevents the added morbidity of a separate procedure (laparotomy to remove fibroids, anesthesia, and its possible complications) in the future, justifying the cost effectiveness of the approach.
- Puerperal uterine subinvolution and other known complications of fibroids such as menorrhagia, anemia, and pain can be prevented.
- Fibroids are sometimes located in the lower uterine segment, their nonremoval will only leave the surgeon with one alternative: a "classical" incision on the uterus with all of its associated complications.
- It increases the chances of vaginal delivery in subsequent pregnancies when removed from the lower uterine segment.
- The scar integrity following cesarean myomectomy has been shown to be better than that following interval myomectomy, when assessed with serial ultrasound scans in subsequent pregnancies and at subsequent cesarean section.
- Enucleation of the fibroid is technically easier in gravid uterus owing to greater looseness of the capsule.[12]

Several recent studies have described techniques which can minimize blood loss at cesarean myomectomy. These include the application of a tourniquet to encompass and compress both uterine arteries at the base of the broad ligament and the vessels in the infundibulopelvic ligament after lifting away the fallopian tubes, thus creating a relatively bloodless operating field, bilateral uterine artery ligation, use of electrocautery for uterine incision over the myoma, and coagulation of vessels supplying it, high-dose oxytocin infusion during (i.e., after the delivery of the baby and placenta) and after the surgery and a combination of uterine tourniquet and high-dose oxytocin infusion. **Figures 1A to C** show the removal of a subserous fibroid during cesarean section.

## CERVICAL CANCER IN PREGNANCY

The incidence of invasive cervical cancer ranges from 1.5 to 12/10,000 pregnancies, the incidence of abnormal Pap smear ranges from 2 to 7%.[12] However, cervical cancer remains the most common malignancy diagnosed during pregnancy. Approximately 30% cervical cancers are diagnosed during child-bearing age with 3% of cervical cancers diagnosed during pregnancy and 0.05% of all pregnancies are complicated by cervical cancers.[13]

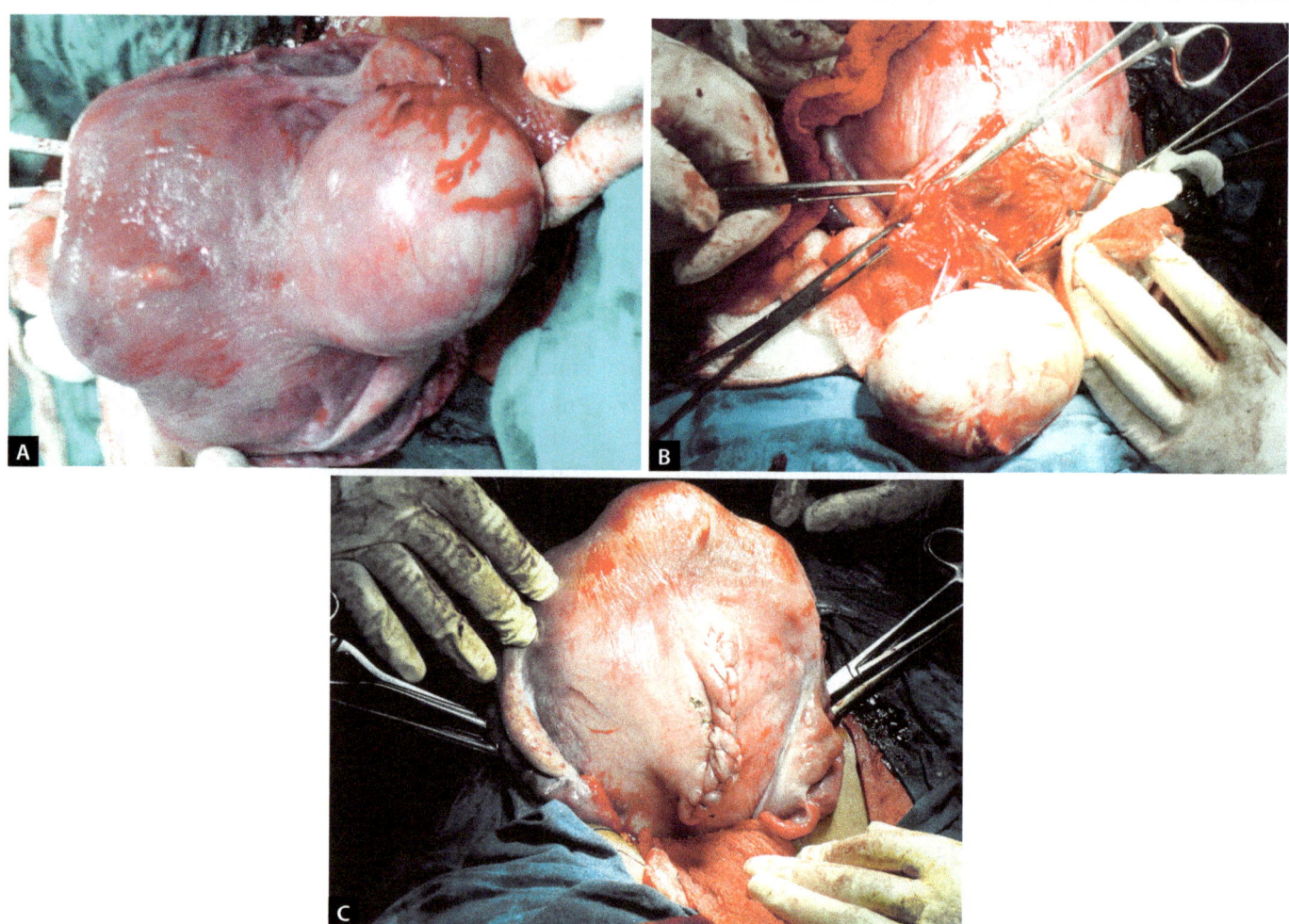

**Figs. 1A to C:** Steps of cesarean myomectomy.

## Screening during Pregnancy

Pregnancy and prenatal care offer an excellent opportunity to implement screening for premalignant disease, especially in women who do not seek routine health care.

The physiological changes in the lower genital tract secondary to pregnancy may cause specific alterations that may make screening a challenge; but the effectiveness of Papanicolaou smear and colposcopy in the detection of preinvasive and early invasive disease is well proven. Pregnancy does not alter the rates of false, negative results significantly; however, diagnostic difficulties in interpretation of a smear do occur. Recommendation for Pap smear screening includes screening at first prenatal visit and again at 6 weeks postpartum.[14]

## Diagnostic Pitfalls Associated with Pap Smear in Pregnancy

- The exaggerated ectropion in pregnancy exposes the glandular epithelium to the harsh vaginal environment, making inflammatory changes more common on smear. *Candida* and trichomonas are the most common organisms in the smear.
- The exposure of endocervical epithelium to acidic pH increases the number of foci of squamous metaplasia, giving an erroneous impression of dysplasia.
- Decidualization of the cervix and endocervix has been reported. Cytologically, the decidual cells can be confused with normal parabasal cells and high-grade dysplastic cells. Decidual cells tend to be polygonal to round with sharp cytoplasmic borders having vacuolated, basophilic cytoplasm, and large hypochromatic centrally placed nuclei with prominent nucleoli. Dysplastic cells rarely have nucleoli and have clumped chromatin.
- Trophoblast cells, typically seen as multinucleated giant cells, can be shed and picked up by Pap smear which should be differentiated by the presence of beta human chorionic gonadotropin (ßhCG) on immunohistochemistry from low-grade dysplasia, viral infection [human papillomavirus (HPV) or herpes simplex virus (HSV)] or granulomatous condition (tuberculosis).
- Arias-Stella reaction related cells (9% of pregnancies) are seen as small loosely cohesive cells in a clean (nondesmoplastic) background and exhibit high nuclear-to-cytoplasmic ratio with eccentric nuclei and

prominent cherry red nucleoli. These mimic high-grade adenocarcinoma, which is verified on biopsy.
- Due to immunosuppression, the prevalence of HPV and its sequelae may increase during pregnancy. Studies suggest increased incidence of high cancer risk viruses— HPV type 16, 18, 31, 35, 45, 51, 52, and 56 as compared with nonpregnant women.

## Preinvasive Lesions of Cervix

The main treatment of preinvasive disease during pregnancy is observation. Pregnancy does not influence cervical lesions and progression to invasive disease is rare. Colposcopy and directed biopsy are safe in pregnancy but endocervical curettage is contraindicated.

The American Society for Colposcopy and Cervical Pathology (ASCCP) states that rate of finding cervical intraepithelial neoplasia (CIN) 2-3 on postpartum follow-up is only 3.7% in case of atypical squamous cells of undetermined significance (ASC-US) or low-grade squamous intraepithelial lesions (LSILs) so, colposcopy can be deferred to 6 weeks postpartum while in patients with high-grade squamous cell intraepithelial lesions (HSILs), it is recommended to perform colposcopy (with directed biopsy). When CIN 2-3 is biopsy proven or absence of invasion is certain, repeat cytology and colposcopy is performed every 12 weeks. Postpartum regression of CIN 2-3 is fairly common.

The diagnostic accuracy of colposcopy is 99% and complication rate <1%. During pregnancy it is easy to perform as the transformation zone is better exposed due to physiological eversion. Colposcopy is a safe and reliable method for evaluating pregnant patients with abnormal cervical cytological findings.

### Colposcopy in Pregnancy

The challenges of performing an adequate colposcopic examination in pregnancy are increased friability caused by relative eversion of the columnar epithelium, cervical distortion from a low riding fetal head, early effacement, and obstruction of visualization by the mucus plug.[12,13] Special considerations for colposcopy in pregnancy are as follows:[15]
- Expert colposcopist should perform the evaluation.
- Unsatisfactory examinations may be satisfactory in 6-12 weeks or by 20 weeks.
- Limit biopsy to worst area.
- Be prepared for increased biopsy site bleeding.
- Re-evaluate lesion with Pap smear or colposcopy every 8-12 weeks.
- Perform repeat biopsy only if lesion worsens.
- Recommend excision biopsy only if concerned about invasive cancer.

It is important, however, not to treat or perform a diagnostic excisional procedure on women who are pregnant unless invasive cancer is present or of significant concern (high-risk). Unless invasive cancer cannot be ruled out, high-grade disease detected during pregnancy is generally followed until postpartum because of the low-risk of progression to invasion and the potential to regress postdelivery. Follow-up is generally by cytology and colposcopy every 8-12 weeks and 6 weeks postpartum. The relative increase in immune response postpartum and the decrease in hormonal influences that promote progression, result in regression in 69% cases.

### Conization in Pregnancy

Conization is only indicated if uncertainty persists, suspicion of microinvasive disease is high, colposcopy is unsatisfactory or cytology and colposcopy do not correlate.

It is reserved only for case with high suspicion of invasive cancer.[15] Classical conization in pregnancy can be disastrous, resulting in significant hemorrhage (>500 mL) necessitating vaginal packing, transfusion, hospitalization, miscarriage, fetal loss, and increased perinatal death rates. If absolutely indicated, a flat cone biopsy is best performed between 14 and 20 weeks with or without cervical cerclage.[14] Management of preinvasive lesions during pregnancy is depicted in **Flowchart 1**.

### Invasive Cervical Cancer

Among patients with the diseases approximately 1-3% are pregnant at the time of diagnosis. The diagnosis of cancer evokes a multitude of feelings ranging from denial and disbelief to anxiety and anger. The management of such

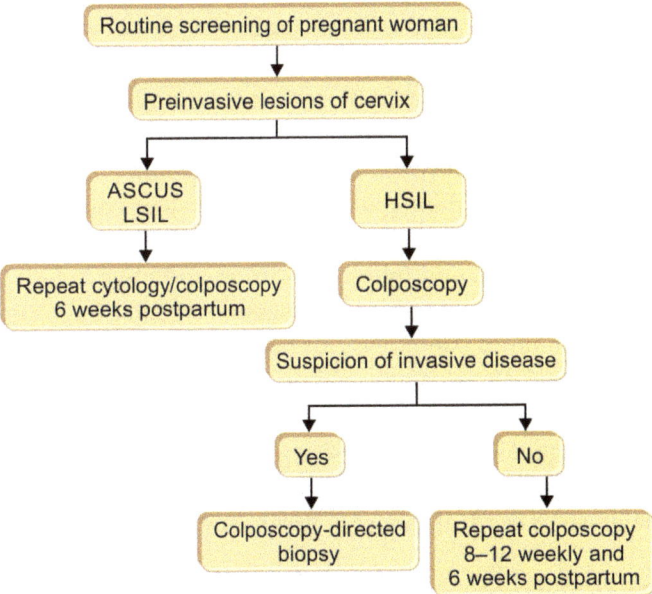

**Flowchart 1:** Management of preinvasive lesions of cervix during pregnancy.

(ASCUS: atypical squamous cells of undetermined significance; HSIL: high-grade squamous intraepithelial lesion; LSIL: low-grade squamous intraepithelial lesion)

patients can present difficult ethical, emotional, and social considerations for the patient, fetus, and healthcare team.

## Diagnosis and Evaluation

Pregnancy represents an ideal time for cervical cancer screening. Preinvasive or invasive disease may be picked up on routine screening. Symptoms are variable and pregnancy can mask some of the common symptoms. More than 70% are asymptomatic during presentation. The recognition of the cancer cervix in pregnancy may be missed through attributing vaginal bleeding directly to pregnancy-threatened abortion in early pregnancy, and placenta previa or accidental hemorrhage in the later months. Vaginal discharge and pain are some nonspecific and less common symptoms.[16]

A pelvic examination including visual inspection of the cervix, cervical cytology from the ectocervix, and bimanual examination is a routine part of prenatal care. Accurate determination of the extent of cancer is more difficult during pregnancy because induration of parametrium may be less prominent during pregnancy. Such induration in nonpregnant women characterizes tumor spread beyond the cervix.

The initial step in the evaluation of the cancer cervix is Pap smear.

When there is a lesion, biopsy should be performed. FIGO staging of cancer cervix has been clinical till now with addition of certain procedures that were allowed by FIGO to change the staging. In 2018, this has been revised by the FIGO Gynecologic Oncology Committee to allow imaging and pathological findings, where available, to assign the stage.[17] Staging of cancer cervix involves general physical examination, systemic examination, per speculum examination, and per rectal examination. Other diagnostic modality such as magnetic resonance imaging (MRI), a noninvasive modality is useful in assessing tumor volume and the extent of disease, stromal, vaginal and parametrial invasion in pregnant patients with cervical cancer.[18] In addition, it may be used to monitor lymph node infiltration, tumor response, and follow-up during and after radiation treatment. Pelvic lymph node assessment either by MRI or surgical removal should be part of assessment. Zemlickis et al. analyzed 40 pregnant women presenting with cervical cancer and found early disease as compared to their nonpregnant counterparts because of regular obstetric examinations.[19] The role of tumor markers is questionable in diagnosis of cervical cancer in pregnancy.

## Management

Treatment varies for each patient depending on the stage of disease, duration of pregnancy, and the woman's desire to continue the pregnancy. Counseling and treatment include a multidisciplinary approach.

Broadly, the management of cervical cancer in pregnancy follows the same principles as in the nonpregnant state.[17]

### Pregnancy Preserving Management

*Microinvasive Disease[20]*

In stage IA1 tumors, that is, where depth of stromal invasion is ≤3 mm, and there is no lymphovascular space invasion, cone biopsy may be the treatment.

For stage IA1 with lymphovascular space invasion and stage IA2 (depth of invasion > 3 mm but ≤5 mm), staging lymphadenectomy should be performed as a first step. Individualized treatment of pregnant patients with cervical cancer can be planned depending on the lymph nodes status. Pelvic lymphadenectomy can be done by laparoscopy or by laparotomy usually up to 20–22 weeks of gestation.

If pelvic lymph nodes are negative, chances of parametrial involvement is negligible; delayed definitive treatment postdelivery in cases with early-stage disease can be advised.

In case of negative nodes, simple trachelectomy or delayed treatment after delivery may be done. Termination of pregnancy is recommended in case of positive lymph nodes and definitive treatment is given on the same principles as in nonpregnant women.

Beyond 22 weeks of gestation, the treatment may be delayed till after delivery or neoadjuvant chemotherapy (NACT) may be initiated.

*Invasive Disease*

As per the recent guidelines (2019), based on a third international consensus meeting on gynecologic cancers in pregnancy, pregnancy-preserving management with regular follow-up should be considered initially in early disease, as no negative impact of pregnancy has been observed on prognosis of cancer cervix.[20]

Stage IB1 can be managed in the same way as IA2 cancer cervix as described above, under the management of microinvasive lesions.

In stage IB2 (tumor 2 cm to 4 cm) with pregnancy < 22 weeks, one option is to perform pelvic lymphadenectomy as a first step followed by either chemotherapy or follow-up. Second option is to give NACT followed by surgical staging of the disease. If lymph nodes are negative delayed treatment after delivery is given. In case lymph nodes are found to be positive (including micrometastases) termination of pregnancy with definitive treatment is to be given.

In stage IB2, with pregnancy >22 weeks NACT is given during pregnancy followed by radical hysterectomy after delivery. NACT during pregnancy helps to stabilize or reduce the size of cervical cancer.

In stage IB3 [cervical growth >4 cm—(according to the new FIGO 2018 classification)] pregnancy-preserving option is not advisable, but if woman does not want termination of pregnancy NACT can be given to control the disease followed by definitive treatment after delivery. Management of early stage invasive cancer cervix is summarized in **Flowchart 2**.

## Pregnancy Non-preserving Management

In case patient diagnosed with carcinoma cervix chooses not to continue pregnancy or if cancer is in advanced stage or if lymph nodes are positive, immediate treatment is advisable in cases with pregnancy < 20 weeks.

During the latter half of pregnancy, a reasonable option is to wait for not only the fetal viability but also fetal maturity. There are issues regarding the safety of a planned delay in treatment. With recent advances in neonatal care the definition of fetal viability has been lowered. The survival of neonates born at earlier gestations has improved with steroids, surfactant, and contemporary neonatal intensive care. Antepartum steroids should be given to enhance fetal lung maturity. Accurate dating of pregnancy is important to determine the timings of delivery. Delivery should be considered as soon as fetal viability can be expected with minimal anticipated neonatal morbidity.[18]

### Mode of Delivery

Cesarean section is the recommended mode of delivery although studies suggest that survival after vaginal delivery is not significantly different from after abdominal delivery.

Other concerns include hemorrhage and obstructed labor associated with vaginal delivery in pregnant patients with cervical cancer. Episiotomy site recurrences may be associated with high mortality. Recurrences at the episiotomy site most likely occur from direct tumor spillage and implantation during vaginal delivery. Owing to these concerns, cesarean delivery should be the mode of delivery.

Pregnant women diagnosed with cervical cancer in the first or second trimester who require immediate treatment with radiation should be allowed to abort or deliver vaginally. Hysterotomy during the second trimester usually requires a vertical uterine incision and can result in large blood loss. Thus, in patients in whom a planned delay in treatment is not possible, radiation should be given without exposing the patient to the high morbidity associated with hysterotomy.[18]

### Surgical Treatment

Radical hysterectomy and lymphadenectomy are widely accepted as the preferred therapy for early stage cervical cancer (Stage I and IIA) in pregnant and nonpregnant women. Radical hysterectomy can be performed along with cesarean section (CS-RH) or 6 weeks postpartum. It is a rare surgical procedure associated with high blood loss. Pregnant women are most likely to benefit from surgical treatment as the ovarian function can be preserved.[17]

Except for the increased blood loss in conjunction with cesarean section, the studies have reported that the outcome of radical hysterectomy with the fetus in situ or after cesarean delivery did not differ significantly from that of radical hysterectomy in the nonpregnant state. There were also no differences in operative morbidity and major complication

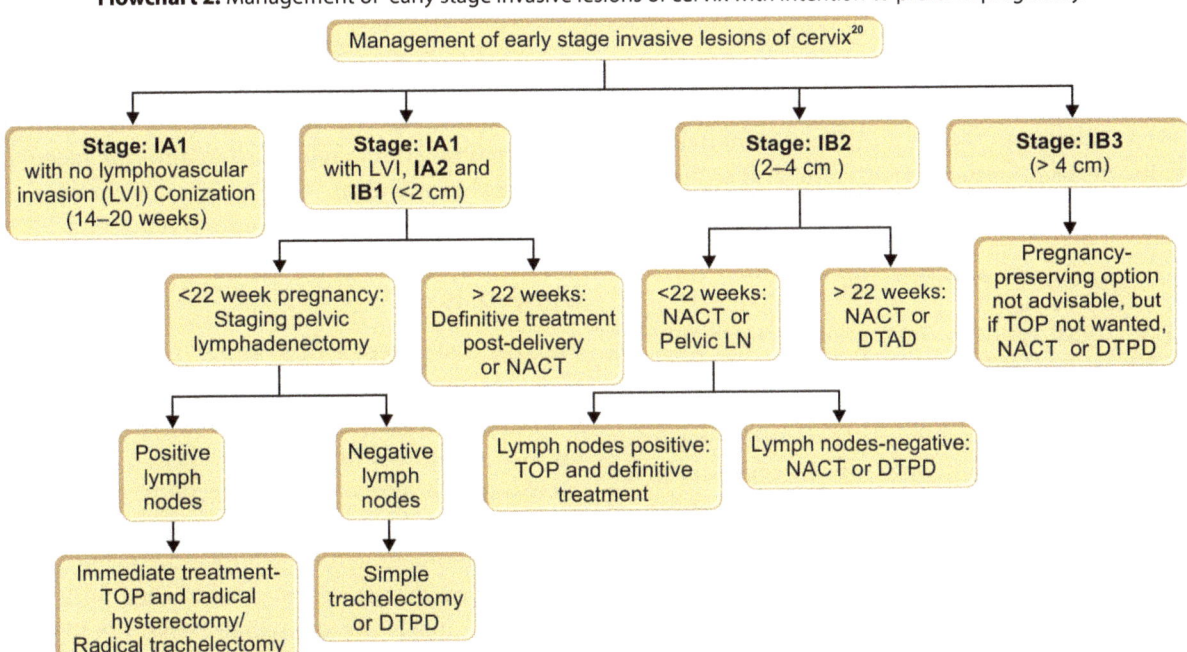

**Flowchart 2:** Management of early stage invasive lesions of cervix with intention to preserve pregnancy.*

*If patient chooses not to continue pregnancy; or cancer is in advanced stage; or if lymph nodes are positive, termination of pregnancy and immediate treatment is advisable if pregnancy < 20–22 weeks.
(LVI: lympho-vascular invasion; LN: lymphadenectomy; NACT: neoadjuvant chemotherapy; TOP: termination of pregnancy; DTPD: delayed treatment post-delivery)

rates. Thus, the surgical management of cervical cancer complicating pregnancy seems to be safe and effective, with morbidity rates comparable with those for nonpregnant patients.[18] Some authors, however, report more blood loss, longer hospital stay, postoperative ileus/small bowel obstruction, and pyelonephritis; and recommend performing radical hysterectomy 4–6 weeks postpartum.[21]

Before 20 weeks gestation, radical hysterectomy can usually be performed with the fetus in situ. If the fetal age is >20 weeks or if better visualization is needed, the fetus can be delivered via hysterotomy through a fundal incision or classic cesarean section prior to hysterectomy. The lower uterine segment and the cervix should be avoided during fetal delivery.[17]

Intraoperatively, surgery should not be abandoned on the basis of enlarged pelvic and para-aortic lymph nodes because node hypertrophy can occur with pregnancy alone. Physiologic decidual cell reactions in lymph nodes, as a result of pregnancy can be confusing, and histological evaluation should be carefully performed.[18]

### Chemoradiation

In stage IB3 or higher stage, chemoradiation is usually given with the fetus in utero in the first trimester, while initial hysterotomy is advised in second trimester.[20]

### Radiation Treatment

Treatment for stage IIB and higher stages cervical cancer is usually limited to radiation therapy. In addition, woman at high-risk for surgical morbidity and mortality should also be treated primarily with radiotherapy. When the fetus is viable, delivery should be performed via cesarean section prior to radiation. The mean radiation dose at which abortion occurs in 34 Gy. Teletherapy is safe and effective modality for evacuating the uterus prior to brachytherapy. If spontaneous abortion does not occur, evacuation is performed.[17]

### Role of Neoadjuvant Chemotherapy

Neoadjuvant chemotherapy during pregnancy can be used to stabilize or reduce the size of cervical cancer.[22] Chemotherapy for cervical cancer should be platinum based but the addition of paclitaxel will increase the response rates. Paclitaxel-carboplatin regime may be considered as an alternative to cisplatin based regimens because of its favorable toxicity profile.

## ■ RETROVERSION OF THE GRAVID UTERUS

Of all the displacements of gravid uterus, retroversion is the most important, for the reason that certain serious complications can occur if spontaneous correction does not occur. One in every ten women has a retroverted uterus.

Though, it is not uncommon for a normally placed uterus to become retroverted during early pregnancy by mechanical reasons, i.e., increased weight of the uterus, however, in majority of cases, this condition results from occurrence of conception in a uterus which is already retroverted or retroflexed.

### Clinical Features

In majority of women with uterine retroversion, no symptoms occur because spontaneous correction takes place soon after the 12th week of pregnancy when gravid uterus grows out of pelvis. Only if this rectification fails to occur, symptoms are produced due to incarceration of uterus.

There is pelvic discomfort and low sacral pain. The prominent symptom is retention of urine. Usually, the onset is gradual. The initial symptom is frequency of micturition progressing to retention of urine and then overflow incontinence. Mechanical pressure upon the bladder neck and elongation of the urethra resulting from upward displacement of the cervix and stretching of the anterior vaginal wall are the obvious reasons for the retention. Edema in the region of bladder neck adds its effect to those of mechanical compression and neuromuscular incoordination. Usually, isolated case reports are published but a study has described colonoscopic assisted reposition of incarcerated uterus in four patients.[23]

Consequent to urinary retention, the bladder may become enormously distended and its wall thickens leading to true hypertrophy and edema. Rupture of bladder either spontaneously or following manual rectification is extremely rare. Overdistention of bladder predisposes to cystitis, pyelitis, and pyelonephritis.

Bowel disturbance may occur with persistent constipation. Rarely, uterus continues its development in abnormal position, giving rise to anterior sacculation. This may persist until term. More commonly abortion takes place if the displacement remains uncorrected.

### Diagnosis

Marked disturbance of bladder function in association with 3 or 4 months of pregnancy should raise the suspicion of retroverted gravid uterus. On abdominal examination, an over distended bladder reveals itself as a soft swelling, reaching well above the umbilicus in extreme cases. Any doubt can be dispelled by passing the catheter. On per vaginal examination, there is forward bulging of the posterior vaginal wall due to retroverted uterus and the direction of vaginal canal is altered so that it passes from below upward and a little forward instead of upward and backward. Secondly, cervix is felt high up behind the public symphysis. Diagnosis can be confirmed with ultrasound which helps exclude extrauterine pregnancy, ovarian cyst or a posterior wall fibroid.

## Differential Diagnosis

Extrauterine pregnancy can be confused with retroverted gravid uterus especially if the sac has ruptured and there is pelvic hematocele. But in this condition one usually gets a history of acute abdominal pain and blood-stained vaginal discharge; the retention of urine is rare, there is often rectal tenesmus, adnexa is tender on palpation, and the cervix is seldom displaced upward so much. An ovarian cyst, or more commonly a posterior wall fibroid, may cause trouble in diagnosis.

## Treatment

In the absence of symptoms, no attempt should be made to correct the retroversion discovered on routine vaginal examination in early pregnancy. Because uterus as a rule correct itself in majority of cases and secondly manipulation especially a difficult one may induce abortion. Postural treatments by exaggerated Sim's position is encouraged. Frequent bladder evacuation and abstinence from intercourse to avoid risk of miscarriage is advocated.

In cases presenting with bladder symptoms, treatment must not be delayed. Best method of treatment is bed rest in semi prone or exaggerated Sim's position and indwelling catheter to keep the bladder empty. In most of cases, uterus undergoes spontaneous correction within 24–48 hours. Very rarely, if it fails, manual reposition should be tried by pushing the fundus upwards and forwards with two fingers in the vagina. Manipulation is done in genupectoral (knee-chest) or Sim's position. The advantage of Sim's position is that it does not preclude the administration of anesthesia should this be necessary. While pushing the fundus, pressure should be made more to one side to avoid sacral promontory. A finger in the rectum usually succeeds where vaginal manipulation fails. If an anesthetic is administered, manipulation will often succeed after being employed unsuccessfully without it. Even when manipulation fails initially, it may succeed after a few days of bed rest.

## ADNEXAL MASS IN PREGNANCY

Adnexal mass of any type can complicate pregnancy. The incidence of adnexal mass varies depending on the age group studied and frequency with which prenatal sonography is used. With the widespread use of routine prenatal ultrasound, the finding of an adnexal mass in pregnancy is becoming increasing common. The reported incidence of adnexal mass in pregnancy varies from 1 in 80 to 1 in 8,000 pregnancies.

Most of the adnexal masses are ovarian in origin.

Most common adnexal mass in pregnancy is functional cyst followed by persistent corpus luteum cyst which accounts for 13–17% of all cystic adnexal masses. Other benign masses such as dermoid cyst (7–37% incidence), serous cystadenoma (5–28%), mucinous cystadenoma, endometrioma, hydrosalpinx, heterotropic pregnancy, and leiomyoma may be associated with pregnancy. The incidence of malignancy in an adnexal mass varies from 1 to 8%.[24]

## Clinical Features

Symptoms of adnexal mass are variable. They are often discovered incidentally during routine ultrasound examinations and are usually asymptomatic, but sometimes these can be responsible for abdominal or pelvic pain.[25]

The most common adnexal masses are ovarian cysts. Sometimes, it is possible to discern a groove between the fundus of gravid uterus and an ovarian cyst if the patient is placed in head down Trendelenberg's position (Hingorani' sign). The most common presenting complaint is pain due to torsion, rupture or intracystic hemorrhage. Torsion occurs mostly during the puerperium when rapid changes in the anatomical relations of the pelvic viscera combined with lax abdominal musculature favors twisting. Second trimester is another period during which the chances of torsion are increased as uterus becomes an abdominal organ and intestinal peristalsis can initiate torsion. Large cysts can lead to malpresentation, obstructed labor, and increased risk of cesarean delivery.[26] They can also cause pressure symptoms. The most important risk is miscarriage and premature delivery which may be induced by surgical removal of these masses.

## Diagnosis

Ultrasound is the preferred radiological modality in determining the malignant potential of an adnexal mass. Characteristics suggestive of malignancy are septations, solid components, nodules, papillary excrescences or a size of >5 cm diameter. Lerner et al. characterized 350 ovarian and adnexal masses in pregnant patients with a modified ultrasound scoring system and demonstrated that a score of 3 or greater had 96.8% sensitivity and 77% specificity for predicting malignancy. They also concluded that the more complex a mass looks, the higher the risk for malignancy.[26]

Computed tomography (CT) exposes the mother and fetus to at least 2–4 rads and contrast materials can pass the placental barrier but it is better than ultrasound in resolution of an adnexal mass.[27] MRI is generally considered safe in pregnancy and may help when the sonographic appearance is nonspecific. It is better than ultrasound at distinguishing paraovarian cystic lesions, determines the extent of possible malignancy and tissue characterization, and differentiating from acute bowel pathologies such as appendicitis and inflammatory bowel disease better than ultrasound.[28]

## Management

Management depends upon symptoms, gestational age, size, and characteristics of the mass. Small simple ovarian cysts < 6 cm are managed conservatively.

*Surgery is usually indicated if:*

- Malignancy is suspected (complex masses with increased flow on Doppler ultrasound or ascites).
- Acute complications such as torsion, rupture or intracystic hemorrhage develop.
- Size of mass likely to cause difficulty such as obstruction, malpresentation or preterm delivery.
- A size > 6 cm persists during second trimester.

Elective surgery is delayed until the second trimester, a time associated with reduced risk of spontaneous abortion, hormonal independence of the corpus luteum of pregnancy, and resolution of functional cysts. The procedure should ideally be performed at 18–20 weeks of gestation preferably under general anesthesia. Once the neoplasm is identified at surgery, the other adnexa should be examined for pathology. In the majority of cases the adnexal mass is benign. A simple cystectomy should be attempted as primary therapy.

If malignancy is suspected, it can be managed in different ways such as primary cytoreductive surgery with termination, surgery during pregnancy followed by chemotherapy after delivery, debulking surgery during pregnancy and chemotherapy followed by complete surgery after delivery, and expectant management. Staging laparotomy is advocated after first trimester including washing cytology, ipsilateral salpingo-oophorectomy, peritoneal biopsies, omentectomy, and even lymphadenectomy in case of palpable lymph nodes. Fertility sparing surgery is recommended in germ cell malignancies if contralateral ovary is normal while only advocated in stage IA/IB, grade 1 epithelial ovarian cancer. A frozen section should be obtained and decision is taken accordingly. Elective surgery for an adnexal mass any time during pregnancy increases the risk of pregnancy loss and the likelihood of intrauterine growth restriction and preterm delivery.

Adjuvant chemotherapy is not needed in FIGO stage I dysgerminoma and immature teratoma. Chemotherapy with paclitaxel-carboplatin is advocated and etoposide should be avoided in germ cell malignancy as it lead to increased fetal risk and leukemia if used in pregnancy. Bleomycin, etoposide, and cisplatin (BEP) should be replaced by carboplatin-paclitaxel or cisplatin-vinblastin-bleomycin.

While performing a laparotomy for an adnexal mass, the surgeon must take into account a number of variables when selecting the type of incision (i.e., vertical vs. transverse). In general, if malignancy is suspected, or if uterine manipulation is to be minimized, a vertical incision is best. Other considerations include a prior scar, body habitus, obstetric issues, and the patient's wishes.

## Laparoscopy or Laparotomy?

The data on laparoscopy during the first and second trimesters of pregnancy indicates that it is as safe as laparotomy. The choice of surgery depends on the surgeon's experience, the type of procedure, and the gestational age. Laparoscopy is considered "minimally invasive" because it reduces manipulation of the pregnant uterus during adnexal surgery. Yuen et al. reported a series of 67 patients undergoing laparoscopic surgery for an adnexal mass in pregnancy over a period of 10 years. No maternal and fetal complication was noted.[29]

A recent, large retrospective cohort study has compared outcomes in pregnant women undergoing laparoscopy versus laparotomy. The authors concluded that laparoscopy was associated with shorter operative time, duration of hospital stay, and less adverse effects on the fetus.[30]

As per Society of American gastrointestinal and endoscopic surgeons (SAGES) recent guidelines, laparoscopy can be safely performed during any trimester of pregnancy when operation is indicated and it offers similar benefits to pregnant and nonpregnant patients compared to laparotomy.[31] Some of these guidelines are as follows:

- After first trimester of pregnancy, woman should be placed in the left lateral or partial left lateral decubitus position to minimize compression of the vena cava.
- Open (Hasson), veress needle, or optical trocar technique can be used for initial abdominal access and entry point should be adjusted according to the uterine height.
- $CO_2$ insufflation of 10–13 mm Hg can be safely used and $CO_2$ monitoring should be done by capnography.
- Intraoperative and postoperative pneumatic compression devices and early postoperative ambulation are recommended as prophylaxis for deep venous thrombosis.
- The procedure should ideally not be longer than 90–120 minutes.
- Prophylactic tocolytics are not recommended but are to be considered perioperatively if signs of preterm labor are present.[31]

## Follow-up with Tumor Markers

Several researchers have reported elevations of maternal serum CA 125 values during normal pregnancy. Serum CA 125 values are highest during the first trimester, levels as high as 1,250 U/mL have been reported. Serum CA 125 values decrease during the late first trimester and remain below 35 U/mL until delivery. However, within 1 hour after a term delivery the CA 125 values transiently rise and decrease rapidly thereafter.

Serum alpha-fetoprotein (AFP) levels have been used as a tumor marker for the follow-up of patients with germ cell malignancies. It is routinely measured at approximately 16–20 weeks of gestation to screen for neural tube defects. Marked elevations of maternal AFP levels have resulted in the antenatal diagnosis of germ cell tumors in asymptomatic pregnant women.

Lactic dehydrogenase (LDH) has been used as a marker for gonadal and extragonadal dysgerminomas. With the exception of pre-eclampsia, LDH values change little with pregnancy and the puerperium. In both cases, the LDH values closely correlate with the clinical activity of diseases.

More recently, human epididymis protein 4 (HE4) and OVA 1 are used in diagnosis and treatment of ovarian cancer in pregnancy.

## MALIGNANCY AND PREGNANCY

- Multidisciplinary approach should be utilized for optimal maternal and neonatal outcomes.
- Fertility sparing should always kept in mind especially in those who wishes to conceive further. Advanced assisted reproductive technology (ART) techniques can be used for oocyte freezing for future fertility.
- Sonographic evaluation of fetus should be done prior to any mode of treatment.
- Surgical procedures should be preferred in second trimester followed by continuous maternal and fetal surveillance.
- Chemotherapy should not be administered beyond 35 weeks or 3 weeks prior to anticipated delivery.
- Maximum efforts to defer the radiation after delivery.
- Placenta should be examined for metastatic disease.
- Breastfeeding is contraindicated with chemotherapy.
- Avoidance of pregnancy by appropriate contraceptive methods should be advised when there is active disease or ongoing treatment. Estrogen containing contraceptives should be avoided because of risk of thromboembolism.

## GENITAL PROLAPSE AND PREGNANCY

Genital prolapse also referred as uterocervical prolapse is not uncommon in pregnancy with an estimated prevalence of 1 in 547 pregnancies in India.[32] Slight degree of displacement of cervix that is first degree uterine prolapse with mild cystocele and rectocele may be seen in many parous women but pregnancy is uncommon with second degree prolapse and very rare in third degree prolapse.

This risk of prolapse is higher with increasing parity and the prevalence is 7 times higher in those who have 7 children or more as compared to one.

Increased levels of cortisol and progesterone, tearing of supporting structures of uterus, and alteration in collagen strength may be predisposing factors for prolapse during pregnancy.

Prolapse that exist before pregnancy usually present in first and second trimester and usually corrects itself by the end of second trimester and recurs after delivery. Prolapse that develops during pregnancy presents itself at third trimester and managed conservatively during pregnancy.

## Effect of Pregnancy on Prolapse

Due to pregnancy related anatomical changes there is aggravation of prolapse and stress urinary incontinence, marked hypertrophy and edema of the cervix, and excessive vaginal discharge. The discharge may be blood stained if decubitus ulcer develops on prolapsed part. Rarely, the uterus may become incarcerated in pelvis if it fails to rise above pelvis by second trimester. Stress urinary incontinence is increased as a result of imbalance of elastic fibers homeostasis and urethral hypermobility.

## Effect of Prolapse on Pregnancy

During pregnancy prolapse is associated with an increase in the incidence of abortions and urinary tract infection. PROM, intrauterine infection, and preterm birth. Preterm labor is the most common antepartum complication. Cervical edema as a result of venous obstruction and stasis and impaired arterial blood flow leads to increased chances of abortion and preterm labor.

There is increased incidence of early rupture of membranes, cervical dystocia resulting in prolonged and obstructed labor and operative interventions in labor. Rarely, uterine rupture is also reported as a result of obstructed labor.

In puerperium, there is an increase in subinvolution of uterus and puerperal sepsis.

## Management

### During Pregnancy

No special treatment is required for first and second degree prolapse. The woman is reassured and explained that prolapse will reduce itself by second trimester.

In cases of third degree prolapse with edema and congestion of prolapsed part, the prolapse should be covered by gauze soaked with glycerine and acriflavine till edema subsides after which it should be replaced inside the vagina and kept in with a ring pessary. The pessary is kept till such time the enlarged uterus grows out of the pelvis and rests on pelvic rim (usually 20 weeks).

Usually, Hodge Smith pessaries are used. Pessaries prevent preterm labor and PROM by preventing shortening and dilatation of cervix. Disadvantages of its use are undue manipulation of cervix leading to preterm labor. Pessaries if inserted are kept throughout pregnancy and these patients should be followed up closely.

An unusual case of breech stillbirth was reported that was caused by forgotten pessary around fetal abdomen and umbilical cord. The patient reported in labor and was delivered after cutting the pessary.[33]

The management of prolapse during pregnancy should be individualized. When conservative approach fails, minimally invasive procedures during pregnancy may also be considered but only with experienced hands. Laparoscopic directed suspension may be tried when conservative procedures fail or patient denies prolonged bed rest or experiences recurrent attacks of urinary infections and retention.

### During Labor

Pregnant woman should be confined to bed as it will prevent early rupture of membranes and also facilitate reposition of uterus into vagina. Vaginal packing with acriflavine glycerine packing is effective in relieving the edema of cervix facilitating cervical dilatation. Prophylactic antibiotics should be administered. Manual stretching of cervix may facilitate the process of delivery when the woman is bearing down with head lying low in the pelvis and fundal pressure to facilitate should be avoided. If cervix is thick, edematous, and head is high up, cesarean section may be preferred to prevent uterine rupture or annular detachment of cervix.[34] However, Duhrssen's incision at 2 and 10 o'clock position may be given in case the head is low down in the pelvis with a thin incompletely dilated cervix. Magnesium solution or ointment can be used also to relieve the edema.

### During Puerperium

Prophylactic antibiotics are continued. The prolapsed part should be reposited back in the vagina. If the woman was using pessary it can be reinserted to support the uterus during puerperium. In case the prolapse cannot be reduced, it should be covered with gauze soaked in glycerine and acriflavine. The woman is asked to rest and avoid straining.

## KEY POINTS

- The various gynecological conditions existing with pregnancy are uterine leiomyoma, ovarian mass, retroversion of uterus, genital prolapse, preinvasive lesions of the cervix, and rarely cervical cancer.
- The incidence of uterine leiomyoma in pregnancy is about 0.09–3.9% and most myomas remain asymptomatic during pregnancy with an overall complication rate of 10–30%.
- Complications include recurrent pregnancy loss, preterm labor, PROM, abruption, pain due to ischemia and necrosis, malpresentations, dysfunctional labor, and postpartum hemorrhage.
- All uterine myomas complicating pregnancies should be managed conservatively and myomectomy is reserved only for subserosal or pedunculated fibroids in cases refractory to medical management.
- Myomectomy during cesarean section should be approached with caution.
- The incidence of invasive cervical cancer in pregnancy ranges from 1.5 to 12/100,000 pregnancies and the incidence of abnormal Pap smear ranges from 2 to 7%.
- Therapy for preinvasive carcinoma of cervix can usually be postponed to postpartum period due to the low-risk of progression to invasion and the potential to regress postdelivery.
- In case of invasive cervical cancer, immediate treatment is commenced if diagnosed in the first half of pregnancy. However, a planned delay in treatment, to allow fetal maturity, may be considered in case of the disease diagnosed in the latter half of the pregnancy.
- Cesarean is the recommended mode of delivery in pregnancies with invasive cervical cancer.
- Uterine retroversion associated with pregnancy usually corrects itself in majority of cases.
- Postural treatment with exaggerated Sim's position and frequent bladder evacuation may help in symptomatic cases. If it fails, manual reposition may be done through the vaginal or rectal route.
- Most adnexal masses in pregnancy are benign and may be observed expectantly during pregnancy.
- Surgery is indicated for persistent adnexal masses > 6 cm in size, if there is suspicion of malignancy, or if there are acute complications such as torsion or rupture and in presence of pressure symptoms.
- Laparoscopy is as safe as laparotomy in pregnancy and is considered minimally invasive.
- Genital prolapse during pregnancy has an estimated prevalence of 1 in 547 pregnancies in India.
- Prolapse with pregnancy increases the incidence of preterm labor, PROM, urinary tract infection, cervical dystocia, operative interference, subinvolution, and puerperal sepsis.
- No specific management is required for first and second degree prolapse.
- In cases of third degree prolapse with edema and congestion of the prolapsed part, the prolapse is covered by gauze soaked with glycerine and acriflavine till edema subsides, after which it is replaced inside the vagina with a pessary which is usually required till 20 weeks.

## REFERENCES

1. Phelan JP. Myomas and pregnancy. Obstet Gynecol Clin North Am. 1995;22(4):801-5.
2. Coronado GD, Marshall LM, Schwartz SM. Complications in pregnancy, labor and delivery with uterine leiomyomas: a population based study. Obstet Gynecol. 2000;95(5):764-9.
3. Kessler A, Mitchell DG, Kuhlman K, Goldberg BB. Myomas vs. contraction in pregnancy: differentiation with color Doppler imaging. J Clin Ultrasound. 1993;21(4):241-4.

4. Benaglia L, Cardellicchio L, Filippi F, Paffoni A, Vercellini P, Somigliana E, et al. The rapid growth of fibroids during early pregnancy. PloS One. 2014;9(1):e85933.
5. Lev-Toaff AS, Coleman BG, Arger PH, Mintz MC, Arenson RL, Toaff ME. Leiomyomas in pregnancy: sonographic study. Radiology. 1987;164(2):375-80.
6. Ouyang DW, Economy KE, Norwitz ER. Obstetric complication of fibroids. Obstet Gynecol Clin North Am. 2006;33:153-69.
7. Graham JM, Miller ME, Stephen MJ, Smith DW. Limb reduction anomalies and early in utero limb compression. J Pediatr. 1980;96(6):1052-6.
8. Klatsky PC, Tran ND, Caughey AB, Fujimoto VY. Fibroids and reproductive outcomes: a systematic literature review from conception to delivery. Am J Obstet Gynecol. 2008;198(4):357-66.
9. Szamatowicz J, Laudanski T, Bulkszas B, Akerlund M. Fibromyomas and uterine contractions. Acta Obstet Gynecol Scand. 1997;76(10):973-6.
10. Rothmund R, Taran FA, Boeer B, Wallwiener M, Abele H, Campo R, et al. Surgical and conservative management of symptomatic leiomyoma during pregnancy: a retrospective Pilot study. Geburtshilfe Frauenheilkd. 2013;73(4):330-4.
11. Hassiakos D, Christopoulos P, Vitoratos N, Xarchoulakou E, Vaggos G, Papadias K. Myomectomy during cesarean section: a safe procedure? Ann N Y Acad Sci. 2006;1092:408-13.
12. Kwawukume EY. Myomectomy during cesarean section. Int J Gynaecol Obstet. 2002;76(2):183-4.
13. Nguyen C, Montz FJ, Bristow RE. Management of stage I cervical cancer in pregnancy. Obstet Gynecol Surv. 2000;55(10):633-43.
14. Muller CY, Smith HO. Cervical neoplasia complicating pregnancy. Obstet Gynecol Clin North Am. 2005;32(4):533-46.
15. Wright TC Jr, Cox JT, Massad LS, Twiggs LB, Wilkinson EJ. 2001 consensus guidelines for the management of women with cervical cytological abnormalities. JAMA. 2002;287(16):2120-9.
16. Sood AK, Sorosky JI, Krogman S, Anderson B, Benda J, Buller RE. Surgical management of cervical cancer complicating pregnancy: a case control study. Gynecol Oncol. 1996;63(3):294-8.
17. Bhatla N, Aoki D, Sharma DN, Sankaranarayanan R. Cancer of the cervix uteri. Int J Gynaecol Obstet. 2018;143(Suppl 2):22-36.
18. Sood AK, Sorosky JI. Invasive cervical cancer complicating pregnancy. How to manage the dilemma. Obstet Gynecol Clin North Am. 1998;25(2):343-52.
19. Zemlickis D, Lischner M, Degendorfer P, Panzarella T, Sutcliffe SB, Koren G. Maternal and fetal outcome after invasive cervical cancer in pregnancy. J Clin Oncol. 1991;9(11):1956-61.
20. Amant F, Berveiller P, Boere IA, Cardonick E, Fruscio R, Fumagalli M, et al. Gynecologic cancers in pregnancy: guidelines based on a third international consensus meeting. Ann Oncol. 2019;30(10):1601-12.
21. Matsuo K, Mandelbaum RS, Matsuzaki S, Licon E, Roman LD, Klar M, et al. Cesarean radical hysterectomy for cervical cancer in the United States: a national study of surgical outcomes. Am J Obstet Gynecol. 2020;222(5):507-11.e2.
22. Marana HR, de Andrade JM, Silva Mathews AC, Duarte G, da Cunha SP, Bighetti S. Chemotherapy in the treatment of locally advanced cervical cancer and pregnancy. Gynecol Oncol. 2007;4:269-72.
23. Dierickx I, Van Holsbeke C, Mesens T, Gevers A, Meylaerts L, Voets W, et al. Colonoscopy-assisted reposition of the incarcerated uterus in mid-pregnancy: a report of four cases and literature review. Eur J Obstet Gynecol Reprod Biol. 2011;158(2):153-8.
24. Yakasai IA, Bappa LA. Diagnosis and management of adnexal masses in pregnancy. J Surg Tech Case Rep. 2012;4(2):79-85.
25. D'Ambrosio V, Brunelli R, Musacchio L, Del Negro V, Vena F, Boccuzzi G, et al. Adnexal masses in pregnancy: an updated review on diagnosis and treatment. Tumori. 2021;107(1):12-16.
26. Lerner JP, Timor-Tritsch IE, Federman A, Abramovich G. Transvaginal characterization of ovarian masses with an improved, weighted scoring system. Am J Obstet Gynecol. 1994;170(1 Pt 1):81-5.
27. Giuntoli RL, Vang RS, Bristow RE. Evaluation and management of adnexal masses during pregnancy. Clin Obstet Gynecol. 2006;49(3):492-505.
28. Chiang G, Levine D. Imaging of adnexal masses in pregnancy. J Ultrasound Med. 2004;23(6):805-19.
29. Yuen PM, Ng PS, Leung PL, Rogers MS. Outcome in laparoscopic management of persistent adnexal mass during the second trimester of pregnancy. Surg Endosc. 2004;18(9):1354-7.
30. Shigemi D, Aso S, Matsui H, Fushimi K, Yasunaga H. Safety of laparoscopic surgery for benign diseases during pregnancy: a nationwide retrospective cohort study. J Minim Invasive Gynecol. 2019;26(3):501-6.
31. Pearl JP, Price RR, Tonkin AE, Richardson WS, Stefanidis D. SAGES guidelines for the use of laparoscopy during pregnancy. Surg Endosc. 2017;31(10):3767-82.
32. Gupta R, Tickoo G. Persistent uterine prolapse during pregnancy and labour. J Obstet Gynaecol India. 2012;62(5):568-70.
33. Gupta A, Hooda R, Nanda S. Perinatal loss: a rare complication of vaginal ring pessary used for prolapse in in pregnancy. J Gynecol Surg. 2013;29(5):260-1.
34. Chandru S, Srinivasan J, Roberts ADG. Acute uterine cervical prolapse in pregnancy. J Obstet Gynaecol. 2007;27(4):423-4.

# Critical Care in Obstetrics

*Nidhi Bhatia, Satinder Gombar, Kanti Gombar*

## INTRODUCTION

The management of critically ill pregnant and early postpartum patient presents challenges to the intensive care team due to disease states unique to pregnancy, concurrent anatomic changes, altered cardiopulmonary physiology of mother and the concerns for the second patient, the fetus. Less than 1% of all intensive care unit (ICU) admissions are obstetric admissions. The mortality rate in obstetrics ICU admissions is 2–3%.[1] The profile of patients admitted to ICU in developed and developing countries are the same, however, significantly higher maternal mortality rate has been seen in developing countries, (median 3.3% vs. 14.0% $p< 0.002$).[2]

The obstetric patients are young, usually without any pre-existing morbidity, their recovery is rapid following rectification of acute insult. Majority are admitted to an ICU for <48 hours unlike their nonpregnant counterparts. Outcome is influenced by the precipitous deterioration which can occur and an equally rapid recovery which may follow appropriate and prompt management. Pregnant and postpartum patients requiring invasive hemodynamic monitoring, intensive respiratory care, and an increased level of nursing care need transfer to ICU. Once the patient is in ICU, the critical care should focus on various aspects of disease processes and the effect of treatment on mother and fetus.

Of all obstetric ICU admissions, 71% are due to obstetrical complications and 29% are due to medical conditions unrelated but aggravated by pregnancy. Severe pre-eclampsia and postpartum hemorrhage are the common obstetrical indications for ICU admission. Pre-eclampsia and its complications, account for 40% of all ICU transfers.[3] Peripartum cardiomyopathy, pulmonary thromboembolism, acute respiratory distress syndrome (ARDS), disseminated intravascular coagulopathy (DIC), hepatic encephalopathy, neurologic complications, status asthmaticus, and other medical disorders associated with pregnancy are other indications for ICU admission.

## PHYSIOLOGICAL CHANGES IN PREGNANCY[4,5]

During pregnancy, significant anatomical and physiological changes occur. The understanding of these changes is important to differentiate normal adaptations of pregnancy from abnormal changes (**Box 1**).

### Cardiovascular System

Circulatory changes during pregnancy include an increase in maternal blood volume which is almost 40% above baseline by 30th week. This increase is due to 20–40% increase in the red cell mass and 40–50% increase in plasma volume, with resultant dilutional anemia. Cardiac output is increased by 30–40% due to an increase in both stroke volume and heart rate, and reaches its maximum by 32 weeks after which there is only a slight increase. The increase in stroke volume is due to an increase in preload secondary to an increased venous return and to a decrease in after load secondary to fall in systemic vascular resistance (SVR). The fall in SVR is

---

**BOX 1:** Cardiopulmonary and other changes during pregnancy.

*Cardiovascular changes*
- Increased heart rate by 15–20 beats/min and increased cardiac output by 40%
- Decreased blood pressure and decreased systemic and pulmonary vascular resistance
- Decreased colloid oncotic pressure

*Respiratory changes*
- Decreased functional residual capacity and increased minute ventilation

*Laboratory variables*
- Increased $PaO_2$, decreased $PaCO_2$, and serum bicarbonate ($HCO_3$)
- Decreased hemoglobin and hematocrit levels; increased white blood cell count and ESR
- Decreased serum protein levels and coagulation factors XI and XIII levels
- Increased level of coagulation factors VII, VIII, IX, X, levels and fibrinogen
- Increased level of D-dimer
- Decreased levels of serum creatinine, blood urea nitrogen (BUN), and uric acid
- Increased level of alkaline phosphatase
- Increased serum total cortisol, free cortisol, and cortisol-binding globulin
- Increased level of insulin and decreased level of fasting blood glucose
- Increased levels of triglyceride, cholesterol, low-density lipoprotein, and high-density lipoprotein

(ESR: erythrocyte sedimentation rate)

attributable to increased synthesis of prostacyclin and to arteriovenous shunting to the low resistance placental bed which lacks autoregulation. Aortocaval compression by the gravid uterus in supine position is extremely important especially in late pregnancy. It may result in nearly complete obstruction of inferior vena cava (with venous return occurring through azygos, lumbar, and paraspinal veins) and supine hypotension.

## Clinical Implications

When the maternal circulation is compromised, compensatory vasoconstriction occurs, and uteroplacental perfusion is reduced, leading to rapid fetal hypoxia and acidosis. For this reason, evidence of fetal distress such as fetal bradycardia may be a sign of maternal deterioration. For the team of intensivist and obstetrician, fetal heart monitoring provides crucial information about both the maternal and fetal conditions. Secondly, because of the cardiovascular changes, patient can bleed extensively and lose almost 35% of her blood volume before the normally recognizable physical signs of hemodynamic instability, such as tachycardia and or hypotension can be identified.

## Respiratory System

Significant changes occur in lung volume and capacity. Elevation of the hemidiaphragm occurs due to enlarging uterus especially during the last trimester, leading to decrease in functional residual capacity (FRC) by as much as 20% of prepregnant values. Total lung capacity remains unchanged, but minute ventilation increases by 45% primarily due to increase in tidal volume (VT) thus, decreasing the expiratory reserve volume and FRC. As such these changes make critical closing capacity (CC) come very near to FRC. There is no change in lung compliance, but chest wall compliance is reduced. Reduction in FRC leads to increase in ventilation perfusion mismatch resulting in hypoxemia. There is an increase in minute ventilation through an increase in VT and generally unchanged respiratory rate. Consequently, arterial blood gas (ABG) analysis typically shows respiratory alkalosis with $PaCO_2$ in the range of 28–32 mm Hg.

## Clinical Implications

The reserve of respiratory system in a pregnant woman is reduced consequent to increased maternal and uteroplacental demand of oxygen. In situations, where FRC is further decreased with procedures such as mechanical ventilation, supine positioning, and obesity, CC is increased and airway closure may occur during tidal breathing. Events such as apnea make the pregnant woman and fetus more susceptible to hypoxia due to decreased FRC and increased oxygen consumption. Hence, in serious illness, swift and severe respiratory decompensation may occur.

## Gastrointestinal System

The pregnant woman is at an increased risk of gastric aspiration due to progesterone induced decreased tone of lower esophageal sphincter and reduced gastric motility.

## Renal System

Serum creatinine levels are lower than the baseline, usually at the lower limit of normal range. This is due to an increase in glomerular filtration rate (GFR) and renal blood flow.

## Clinical Implications

Creatinine levels that may be considered normal in nonpregnant patients may indicate renal dysfunction in pregnant patients. Glycosuria is a common finding attributable to increase in GFR and reduced renal tubular resorption capacity.

## EARLY WARNING SIGNS IN OBSTETRICS

Several early warning systems (EWS) are used in obstetrics for early detection and timely intervention to avert morbidity and mortality. EWS combine clinical observations such as vital signs, clinical examination findings, and laboratory tests to identify a pattern that is consistent with an increased risk of clinical deterioration. These have been modified for the obstetric population [modified early obstetric warning system (MEOWS)].[6,7] Both, the Saving Mothers' Lives report, a comprehensive review of maternal deaths in the United Kingdom, and the National Partnership for maternal safety, a multistakeholder leadership organization in the United States, have advocated the use of EWS.[8,9] These include MEOWS, maternal early warning criteria (MEWC), and maternal early warning trigger (MEWT).[10]

## FINDINGS IN AN OBSTETRIC PATIENT INDICATING NEED FOR INTENSIVE CARE UNIT

Patients in need of circulatory or pulmonary support should be transferred to an ICU. This need is evident by various signs, symptoms, and laboratory parameters as described here.[11,12]

## General Physical Examination

Assess for level of consciousness; an altered sensorium or decreased level of consciousness is suggestive of decreased cerebral oxygenation or perfusion. Presence of tachycardia, tachypnea, labored breathing, cyanosis, airway obstruction, sweating, and oliguria or anuria indicates a sick patient.

### Vital Signs

- *Blood pressure:* A fall in arterial blood pressure to <80 mm Hg systolic or mean arterial pressure of <60 mm Hg is suggestive of decreased intravascular volume, increased venous capacitance or myocardial depression. Severe hypotension occurs after compensatory mechanisms are exhausted. Increased pressures of ≥160 mm Hg systolic and or ≥110 mm Hg diastolic may indicate acute hypertensive crisis, stress response, anxiety, or excessive vasopressor therapy.

- *Heart rate:* Patient may have tachycardia (rate >100 beats/min) or bradycardia (rate <50 beats/min), or rhythm disturbances.
- *Respiratory rate:* A rate of >35 breaths/minute is suggestive of respiratory insufficiency.
- *Temperature:* Temperature elevation is present in infections. However, patients in septic shock may be hypothermic.
- *Pupils:* Unequal pupils in an unconscious patient could be due to some intracranial pathology.
- *Oxygen saturation:* Normally, arterial oxygen saturation while breathing room air is 95–100%. Levels between 91 and 94% are average or may indicate mild hypoxia and require close monitoring. Levels that are below 90% indicate need for intervention for hypoxemia.
- *Central venous pressure (CVP):* A low CVP indicates hypovolemia, normal range is 5–10 mm Hg.
- *Urine output:* Hourly urine output is a rough approximation of renal perfusion, provided that the patient has adequate blood volume, is well hydrated and has no pre-existing renal disease. Urine output <400 mL in 24 hours, or <160 mL in 8 hours and no response to simple routine measures indicates need for intensive care.
- *Laboratory values* such as ABG analysis, serum electrolytes, hematocrit, coagulation profile, and blood glucose should be measured. Values are considered grossly abnormal if:
  - Serum sodium level is <120 mEq/L or >160 mEq/L
  - Serum potassium level is <3 mEq/L or >5.5 mEq/L
  - *Arterial blood gas:* PaO$_2$ of <60 mm Hg; pH level of <7.1 or >7.6.

*Other investigations:* Electrocardiographic findings that indicate ICU admission in women include myocardial infarction and complex arrhythmia, hemodynamic instability or congestive heart failure, ventricular tachycardia or fibrillation, and complete heart block with hemodynamic instability.

Imaging studies such as chest radiography or computerized tomography (CT) scan are helpful in supporting the diagnosis of conditions like pulmonary edema, cardiac enlargement suggestive of cardiomyopathy.

Echocardiography may be useful in diagnosing, and guiding therapy of massive pulmonary embolism. The findings suggestive of massive embolism are right ventricular dilation and hypokinesis, paradoxical septal motion, and compression of the left ventricle.

> **BOX 2:** Maternal parameters suggesting need for ICU admission.[13]
> - Respiratory rate <8 and >35 breaths/min
> - Heart rate <50 and >140 beats/min
> - Systolic BP <80 mm Hg, or 30 mm Hg below patient's usual BP
> - Urine output <400 mL in 24 hours, or <160 mL in 8 hours and no response to simple routine measures
> - Glasgow coma score (GCS) <8 in the context of nontraumatic coma
> - Any unarousable patient
> - Serum sodium outside the range 110–160 mmol/L
> - Serum potassium outside the range 2.0–7.0 mmol/L
> - pH outside the range 7.1–7.7
> - PaO$_2$ <6.6 kPa and/or PaCO$_2$ >8.0 kPa
> - SaO$_2$ <90% on supplemental oxygen
> - Need for advanced respiratory support
> - Need for inotropic support
> - Cases with disseminated intravascular coagulation (DIC)
> - Adult respiratory distress syndrome (ARDS) cases
> - Cases with multiorgan failure
>
> (ICU: intensive care unit)

As per ministry of health and family welfare, Government of India guidelines (MoH, GoI)[13] maternal parameters suggesting need for admission to ICU are given in **Box 2**.

## Identification and Management of an Unstable Pregnant Patient[14]

It is essential to diligently monitor pregnant and immediate postpartum patients who are at high-risk of potentially life-threatening conditions. Woman's condition can rapidly deteriorate, and timely institution of appropriate treatment can avert adverse outcome including a sudden cardiac arrest. Recommendation for a hemodynamically unstable, hypoxic woman includes placing the woman immediately in left lateral position, administration of 100% oxygen by face mask, and establishing an intravenous (IV) access above the diaphragm. Complete and thorough evaluation of the woman including relevant investigations should be carried out to find the cause of instability and all efforts should be made to promptly treat it.

### Transfer of Patient to Intensive Care Unit (Modified from MoH, GoI, Guidelines)[13]

- Inform the family/attendants about the condition and need for the pregnant woman to be shifted to ICU, and take consent and document it.
- ICU staff should be informed.
- Patient should be escorted by doctor/staff and treatment should be continued during transfer, including maintenance of patient IV line and oxygen administration, if required.
- Prevent supine hypotension in the pregnant woman by performing lateral tilt of 15–20 degree or keeping her in left lateral position.
- Ensure patent airway.
- Keep monitoring the vitals of the patient.

- Pulse oximetry and electrocardiography, arterial or central lines or other invasive monitoring devices if any, should be monitored.
- In an intubated patient, position of endotracheal tube should be confirmed, and adequacy of oxygenation and ventilation should be checked before transportation.
- Medical record containing history, examination, investigations, and management given till the time of transfer should be maintained and handed over to ICU staff.
- If possible, treating obstetrician should continue to be part of management team of ICU.

## GENERAL CONSIDERATIONS

### Scoring Systems for Critically Ill Obstetric Patients

Several disease-severity-scoring systems have evolved for predicting mortality in ICU patients. Acute physiology and chronic health evaluation (APACHE), simplified acute physiology score (SAPS), and mortality probability models (MPMs) are some of the scoring systems that are commonly used for objectively assessing the clinical status and severity of disease of critically ill patients in general.[15]

Knaus et al.[16] devised APACHE II score in 1985 with the aim to stratify prognostic groups of critically ill patients and to find out the success of different forms of treatment. Various clinical and physiologic parameters such as temperature, mean arterial pressure, heart and respiratory rates, oxygen saturation, pH, serum bicarbonate and electrolyte levels, serum creatinine, hematocrit, and white blood cell (WBC) counts are scored. This reasonably predicts the mortality on admission to the ICU. It is a general measure of disease severity based on current physiologic measurements, age, and previous health condition. Scores range from 0 to 71; increasing score is associated with an increasing risk of hospital death.

APACHE II score = (acute physiology score) + (age points) + (chronic health points)

There is paucity of literature on prediction of outcomes in obstetric patients. There are no models particularly designed for obstetric patients. A range of scoring tools derived from nonobstetric populations, such as the APACHE II, and the SAPS II, has been applied to obstetric populations to predict the probability of mortality. However, the results are conflicting, and these scores tend to overestimate mortality in obstetric patients. This is due to normal physiologic changes in obstetric patients such as the lower serum creatinine, blood urea nitrogen, hematocrit, increased respiratory rate, and heart rate of pregnancy. In obstetric patients with hypertensive disorders, tests of liver function and platelet count are important in the assessment. These variables are not accounted for in available scoring systems for critical illness.[17] Given this scenario, the study by Tempe et al.[18] is unique in that it attempts to provide a retrospective review of the utility of SAPS II for predicting maternal mortality in obstetric patients admitted to a multidisciplinary ICU at a tertiary care center in a teaching hospital in New Delhi, India. They have observed that maternal mortality in obstetric ICU admissions was 1.15/1,000 deliveries and the mean SAPS II was significantly higher (40.04 ± 12.97 vs. 22.6 ± 7.31; $p < 0.001$) in those patients who died compared to survivors. The authors suggest that computation of SAPS II score as a routine in obstetric patients admitted to the ICU may help in identifying those at high risk of mortality so that an attempt may be made to reduce this risk.

### The "FAST HUG" Approach

The "FAST HUG" approach[19] should be considered for every intensive care patient at least once a day. **(Table 1)** "FAST HUG" is a mnemonic proposed by Jean-Louis Vincent as a way of assisting healthcare workers looking after critically ill patients. "FAST HUG" mnemonic has seven basic components.

### Monitoring[20]

#### Routine Noninvasive Monitoring

- Continuous noninvasive blood pressure monitoring is used to measure systolic, diastolic, and mean arterial pressure (One-third of the sum of systolic pressure and twice diastolic pressure).
- Heart rate may be measured electronically from the electrocardiogram (ECG) or the arterial pulse wave. When premature ventricular contractions or other rhythm abnormalities are present, the true heart rate may be determined by auscultation at the cardiac apex.
- *Electrocardiographic monitoring*: Continuous ECG monitoring is essential while caring for critically ill patients.

**TABLE 1:** FAST HUG approach.

| Component | Consideration for intensive care unit (ICU) team |
|---|---|
| Feeding | Can the patient be fed orally, if not enterally? If not, should we start parenteral feeding? |
| Analgesia | The patient should not suffer pain, but excessive analgesia should be avoided |
| Sedation | The patient should not experience discomfort, but excessive sedation should be avoided; patient should be "calm, comfortable, and collaborative" |
| Thromboembolic prevention | Should we give low-molecular-weight heparin or use mechanical adjuncts? |
| Head of the bed elevated | Optimally, 30–45°, unless contraindications (threatened cerebral perfusion pressure) |
| Stress ulcer prophylaxis | Usually $H_2$ antagonists; sometimes proton pump inhibitors |
| Glucose control | Within limits defined in each ICU |

(FAST HUG: Feeding, Analgesia, Sedation, Thromboembolic prophylaxis, Head-of-bed elevation, stress Ulcer prevention, and Glucose control)

| TABLE 2: Showing $SpO_2$ and $PO_2$ levels at normal pH. | |
| --- | --- |
| $SpO_2$ | $PO_2$ (mm Hg) |
| • 50% | • 27 |
| • 75% | • 40 |
| • 90% | • 60 |
| • 97% | • 80–100 (normal arterial values) |

ECG changes during normal pregnancy include a right axis deviation, right bundle branch block, and ST segment depression of 1 mm on left precordial leads. Ectopic beats, and bouts of supraventricular tachycardia (SVT) are frequent, T wave negativity in Lead III, V2 and V3 and "Positional" Q waves in Lead III.

- *Temperature*: The central core temperature may be measured at the nasopharynx, tympanic membrane or at the mid esophagus for greater accuracy.
- *Pulse oximetry*: Pulse oximeter is used to measure arterial oxygen saturation, which is an indirect measure of arterial $PO_2$ at normal pH **(Table 2)**.
- *Capnography*: It measures and displays exhaled $CO_2$ throughout the respiratory cycle. During expiration, the capnogram initially reads no $CO_2$, but as the anatomical dead space and alveolar gas is exhaled there is a rise in exhaled $CO_2$ to a plateau which falls to zero with onset of inspiration. End-tidal $CO_2$ is the value at the end of the plateau and is only slightly less (4–6 mm Hg) than $PaCO_2$ (normal value: 36–44 mm Hg). During pregnancy, the normal values of $PaCO_2$ are 32–34 mm Hg.
- *Urine output*: In the absence of renal disorders, urine output may reflect intravascular volume status. Minimal to acceptable values within the normal range are 0.5–1.0 mL/kg/h.
- Thromboelastography is a useful investigation in an obstetric patient with suspected coagulopathy/bleeding/DIC.

### Point-of-care Ultrasonography

Point-of-care ultrasonography (PoCUS) can be invaluable in management of a critically ill pregnant woman, both as a diagnostic as well as therapeutic tool. Multiorgan PoCUS allows early diagnosis of the main causes of circulatory failure and cardiac arrest at the patient's bedside.

It can quickly detect sudden causes of hemodynamic instability and shock such as hemoperitoneum, concealed placental abruption. Echocardiography and lung ultrasound can be combined with ultrasound of the leg veins to differentiate between the various causes of acute respiratory failure such as pulmonary embolism. Lung ultrasound can help in diagnosing pneumothorax, pleural effusion, pulmonary edema, and pulmonary consolidation. There are specific ultrasound patterns seen for a normal lung, a pneumothorax, interstitial edema, and pneumonia.

Combined cardiac and lung ultrasound can determine the potential risk:benefit of fluid administration. Such prediction is of critical importance in an obstetric patient, because of the tendency of pregnant women to develop pulmonary edema.[21]

Instead of using invasive CVP monitoring, PoCUS can be used to predict fluid responsiveness by measuring the diameter or collapsibility of the inferior vena cava.[11.]

PoCUS can be especially useful in the management of pre-eclampsia, pulmonary arterial hypertension, and peripartum cardiomyopathy.[22]

### Invasive Monitoring

- Intra-arterial blood pressure measured via the radial, ulnar, femoral, or axillary artery, provides continuous display of the arterial waveform along with measurements of systolic, diastolic, and mean pressures. Under normal conditions, pressures obtained from intra-arterial catheters are about 2–8 mm Hg greater than cuff-measured pressures. In critically ill patient, intra-arterial pressures may be 10–30 mm Hg greater than cuff-measured pressures.
- *Central venous pressure*: This is used to guide fluid therapy in conditions with suspected blood volume deficits or excesses. Catheter insertion sites are subclavian, internal jugular or femoral vein. The catheter is simple to place and pressures easy to read. The zero-reference point for venous pressures in the thorax is a point on external thorax where the fourth intercostal space intersects the mid-axillary line (phlebostatic axis). CVP values in healthy persons range from –2 to +6 mm Hg during normal inspiration and expiration, respectively. On assuming the supine position, healthy, ambulatory individuals have CVP values that average 6–8 mm Hg. A value of 10 mm Hg is commonly used as the upper limit of normal for acutely ill patients. Critically ill patients receiving mechanical ventilation and PEEP (positive end-expiratory pressure) who require fluid to maintain arterial pressure may develop a CVP value 20 mm Hg, however, when CVP values exceed 15–18 mm Hg, a pulmonary artery (PA) catheter may be used to measure the PA wedge pressure for more precise titration of fluids. Despite the normally elevated cardiac output during pregnancy, filling pressures are usually in the range seen in the nonpregnant state, and left ventricular function is well preserved in most obstetric patients. In pre-eclamptic women or in cases of simple blood loss, a CVP line provides adequate monitoring of intravascular volume. However, in patients with cardiac failure, refractory pulmonary edema, or nonhemorrhagic shock, PA catheterization may be quite beneficial.
- Mixed venous $SvO_2$ (oxygen saturation of mixed venous blood) represents product of $O_2$ delivery and

consumption. It is affected by Hb, $FiO_2$ (fraction of inspired air), cardiac output, and oxygen consumption. It is the earliest indicator of patient compromise. Normal value is 75–85%. It is considered abnormal if it decreases 5–10% over 5 minutes (very concerning if <60%).

- *Pulmonary artery occlusion pressure (PAOP)*: The PA catheter is commonly used to measure PA pressure and PA occlusion pressure to assess left ventricular filling pressure. The PAOP closely parallels left atrial and left ventricular end-diastolic pressures unless significant mitral valve stenosis or pulmonary venous resistance exists. In normal conditions, left atrial pressure is within 2- or 3-mm Hg of the PAOP.
- Transesophageal echocardiography is not a routine investigation but is indicated when cardiac wall motion abnormalities are suspected.

## Arterial Blood Gases

The analysis of ABG provides valuable information about the patient's oxygenation, ventilation, and acid-base status.

Normal ABG values in obstetric patient are given in **Table 3**.

**Table 4** lists values indicating tissue hypoxia with anaerobic metabolism consequent to inadequate tissue perfusion.

Sodium bicarbonate is given in the setting of severe acidosis only (pH <7.2), in the dose calculated as; dose (mEq) = 0.3 × Weight (kg) × Base excess (mEq/L). Bicarbonate therapy should be reserved for emergencies and situations in which indications are compelling. It is usual to give a reduced dose (about one-half) for several reasons.

- After administration, most bicarbonate is converted to $CO_2$. For each 100 mEq of $NaHCO_3$, about 2.24 L of $CO_2$ must be exhaled, equivalent to 10 minutes of normal production.
- The $CO_2$ enters the cells and lowers intracellular pH.
- It is accompanied by $Na^+$ load which may lead on to increased osmolarity that may be critical.
- A residual metabolic alkalosis may lead to shift of oxygen dissociation curve to left resulting in poor oxygen delivery in an already compromised patient.

### Ventilatory Monitoring

Ventilation is assessed by VT (6–12 mL/kg), minute volume (100 mL/kg), and respiratory rate (10–15 breaths/min).

Airway pressures are displayed by ventilators and from this display, mean airway pressure, peak airway pressure, and plateau pressure (should be <30 cm of $H_2O$) may be derived.

### Fetal Monitoring

Continuous fetal monitoring is valuable especially in later part of pregnancy when early delivery may yield a potentially viable fetus. Tocographic monitoring is helpful after trauma or surgery to demonstrate premature uterine contractions.

## Respiratory Care in Pregnancy

Intervention is generally required in cases of failure of adequate oxygenation or ventilation.[23,24]

### Oxygen Therapy

There are numerous methods available for delivering supplemental oxygen **(Table 5)**.

The minimal acceptable level of oxygenation is suggested to be a $PaO_2$ of 60 mm Hg ($SaO_2$ of 90%) when patient breathes a fraction of inspired oxygen ($FiO_2$) of 0.6. Any obstetric patient who requires $FiO_2$ > 0.6 with a mask to achieve a $SaO_2$ of 90% is at constant risk of significant hypoxemia. Should the mask be removed for a short period of time, an obstetric patient with pregnancy induced reduction in FRC will desaturate faster than a nonpregnant patient, causing all possible catastrophic results due to maternal and fetal hypoxia. In pregnancy, normal $PaCO_2$ is 30–34 mm Hg. This respiratory alkalosis begins during the first trimester. Thus, a seemingly normal $PaCO_2$ of 40 mm Hg in a pregnant patient is elevated and must be thoroughly assessed as a possible indication of acute respiratory failure.

**TABLE 3:** Normal arterial blood gases values (ABG) in pregnant and nonpregnant women.

|  | Pregnant | Nonpregnant |
|---|---|---|
| pH | 7.42–7.46 | 7.35–7.45 |
| $PaCO_2$ | 28–32 mm Hg | 35–45 mm Hg |
| $PaO_2$ | 95–105 mm Hg | 80–100 mm Hg |
| $HCO_3$ | 18–22 mEq/L | 22–26 mEq/L |

**TABLE 4:** Values indicating tissue hypoxia with anaerobic metabolism consequent to inadequate tissue perfusion.

| Metabolic disorder | Values |
|---|---|
| • Acidosis | pH < 7.35 |
| • Base deficit | > -5 mEq/L and bicarbonate < 18 mmol/L |
| • Blood lactate levels | > 2 mEq/L |

**TABLE 5:** Methods of delivering oxygen therapy.

| Methods | Maximum $FiO_2$ (fraction of inspired air) |
|---|---|
| • Nasal cannulas | • 0.40 |
| • Simple mask | • 0.60 |
| • Partial rebreathing mask | • 0.8 |
| • Nonrebreathing mask | • 0.9 |
| • Venturi mask | • 0.60 |
| • Continuous positive airway pressure (CPAP) | • 1.0 |
| • Tracheal intubation | • 1.0 |

## Continuous Positive Airway Pressure

For patients requiring respiratory support beyond supplemental oxygen, continuous positive airway pressure (CPAP) delivered by well-fitting face mask may be sufficient in obstetric patient who can protect her own airway. It helps to maintain FRC, reduces alveolar flooding, decreases work of breathing, improves ventilation, and avoids tracheal intubation with its attendant hazards. However, one must watch out for any evidence of gastric insufflation because these patients are already at increased risk of pulmonary aspiration.

*Technique:* Start with a CPAP of 5 cmH$_2$O with FiO$_2$ of 0.40. Gradually, increase the pressure/FiO$_2$ depending on patients' tolerability and requirement.

## Tracheal Intubation and Mechanical Ventilation

The guidelines for intubation and mechanical ventilation are essentially the same for pregnant patients as for nonpregnant patients:

- Inability to maintain a minimal PaO$_2$ of 60-65 mm Hg with supplemental oxygen with FiO$_2$ of 0.6.
- Uncompensated respiratory acidosis.
- Inability to clear secretions.
- Need to protect the airway because of altered mental status.

Intubation in pregnant patients differs from that in nonpregnant patients in the following aspects:

- Hyperemia associated with pregnancy can narrow the upper airway, increasing risk of upper airway trauma.
- Edema of the upper airway, increased breast size, and generalized weight gain can delay the establishment of adequate ventilation and intubation. Therefore, it is essential that oxygenation and ventilation be restored expeditiously while maintaining cricoid pressure.
- Nasotracheal intubation is relatively contraindicated in pregnancy due to engorged, hyperemic and friable nasal mucosa.
- Decreased FRC in pregnancy may lower the oxygen reserve such that, at time of intubation, even a short-period of apnea may be associated with precipitous decrease in PaO$_2$.
- Severe hypertension may result from laryngoscopy especially in patients with hypertensive disorders of pregnancy.

*Mechanical ventilation:* General principles in obstetric patients.

- *Conventional mechanical ventilation*: 8-12 mL/kg VT at rates of 10-12/min results in acceptable alveolar ventilation.
- Minute ventilation should be adjusted to aim for PaCO$_2$ of 30-34 mm Hg, the normal level in pregnancy.
- If possible, maternal PaO$_2$ should be maintained above 75-85 mm Hg to maximize oxygen delivery to the fetus.
- Respiratory rate and VT may be increased when maintaining oxygenation is a problem but marked respiratory alkalosis should be avoided because of resultant decrease in uterine blood flow.
- The use of low VT, volume cycled, pressure-controlled ventilation PEEP, and inverse ratio ventilation (IRV) may be considered in pregnant and early postpartum patients but use of permissive hypercapnia should be avoided as it results in fetal respiratory acidosis.
- Plateau pressure, which reflects transalveolar pressure, should be kept under 30 cmH$_2$O to minimize risk of volutrauma.
- In obstetric patients, there is a natural occurrence of reduction in FRC. When the physiological phenomenon is further compromised by an additional superimposed reduction in FRC in acute respiratory failure, profound increases in intrapulmonary shunting and reductions of PaO$_2$ will occur. PEEP and CPAP are used to increase FRC, reduce shunting, and improve oxygenation.
- Mechanical ventilation during pregnancy should include consideration of physiological changes present during pregnancy. Thus, the adverse effects of reduction in cardiac output due to mechanical ventilation on the uteroplacental circulation cannot be overlooked which maybe further compounded by uterine compression of maternal vena cava while the mother is in supine position.

## Nutrition

In critically ill obstetric patients, nutritional support is important for both maternal and fetal outcome as maternal malnutrition may result in fetal growth restriction. In obstetric patients, enteral nutrition is preferred over parenteral nutrition as in nonobstetric patients. The aim is to avoid the risk of complications associated with central venous catheters for administering parenteral nutrition, to reduce the cost, and to minimize gastric mucosal atrophy. Pregnancy is associated with decreased lower esophageal sphincter tone and decreased gastric motility; therefore, nasoduodenal tubes are preferred over nasogastric tube to decrease the likelihood of reflux and aspiration. Total parenteral nutrition (TPN) can provide complete nutritional support during pregnancy in patients who are unable to eat for more than a couple of days and whose gastrointestinal system must be rested. A balanced daily energy supply of fat and glucose is commonly used for TPN **(Table 6)**. This approach may decrease the problems in hepatic and pulmonary function that occur with high glucose loads. All solutions should contain the daily requirement of essential electrolytes and vitamin supplementation. Role of immune-nutritional support remains controversial. Due to concerns over macrosomia and other adverse effects of hyperglycemia,

| TABLE 6: Composition of a standard TPN formula (per liter). | |
| --- | --- |
| Amino acids | 50 g |
| Dextrose | 600 kcal (17.5%) |
| Fat 20% | 250 kcal (125 mL) |
| Standard electrolytes* | |
| Trace elements | 1 mL/day |
| Multivitamins | 10 mL/day |

*Standard electrolytes: Na 37 mEq, K 30 mEq, Ca 5 mEq, Cl 30 mEq, acetate 35 mEq, and phosphate 9 mM
(TPN: total parenteral nutrition)

glucose levels should be maintained at <120 mg/dL. Large quantities of IV lipids (>40% of calories) should be avoided because of experimental evidence showing fatty infiltration of the placenta.[25,26]

### Creating a Total Parenteral Nutrition Regime[25]

*Step 1:* Estimate daily protein and calorie requirement:
- *Calorie requirement*: 25 kcal/kg/day
- *Protein requirement*: 1.4 g/kg/day.

*Step 2:* The next step is to take a standard mixture of 10% amino acids (500 mL) and 50% dextrose (500 mL) and determine the volume of this mixture that is needed to deliver the estimated daily protein requirement.

*Step 3:* Using the total daily volume of dextrose-amino acid mixture determined in step 2, the next step is to determine the total calories that will be provided by dextrose in the mixture. (Each gram of dextrose provides 3.4 kcal, and each gram of amino acid provides 4 kcal).

*Step 4:* The remaining calories are provided by IV lipid emulsion. A 10% lipid emulsion (1 kcal/mL) is used to provide these calories.

### Complications of Total Parenteral Nutrition
- *Carbohydrate infusions*: Hyperglycemia, fatty liver, and hypercapnia resulting in delayed or difficult weaning from mechanical ventilation.
- *Lipid infusions*: Increased risk of oxidation induced cell injury.
- *Gastrointestinal complications*: Mucosal atrophy and acalculous cholecystitis.

## Medications

Numerous medications may be used in caring for the critically ill obstetric patient in the ICU.[7,26]

### Analgesics and Anxiolytics

Morphine and related opiates have not been associated with fetal malformations. Transfer across the placenta is rapid and prolonged use may lead to fetal withdrawal, which is usually seen only in mothers addicted to these drugs. Large doses of morphine or other opiates given near delivery may cause respiratory depression in newborn. Their use is also associated with decreased FHR variability. Diazepam, once thought to be associated with cleft lip, seems to be free of teratogenic effects. However, neonatal depression at delivery may be seen if large doses are given.[7]

### Vasoconstrictor and Inotropic Agents

Hypotension refractory to fluids and postural changes may require vasoconstrictor and inotropic therapy. Of the agents with alpha agonistic activity, ephedrine seems to best preserve uterine blood flow. Use of phenylephrine in treating hypotension due to spinal or epidural anesthesia seems safe, but its excessive alpha agonistic activity makes it less attractive in critically ill patients. Beta-agonists such as isoproterenol may diminish uterine blood flow if maternal hypotension ensues. Dopamine and dobutamine are not known to have any significant adverse effects on the fetus.

## Radiation Exposure

Radiography is often essential in diagnosis and management of critically ill patient, but in a pregnant patient one must be concerned about radiation exposure to the fetus. The risks to fetus of death, malformation, or childhood cancers in later life depend upon gestational age at the time of exposure and the amount of radiation delivered. In the first few weeks of pregnancy radiation doses of 10 centigray (cGy) may cause fetal death. The risk of malformations is much increased at doses above 15 cGy. A chest roentgenogram exposes the maternal lungs to approximately 0.5 cGy and the shielded fetus to much less ionizing radiation. Abdominopelvic CT scans deliver a larger radiation dose, between 5 and 10 cGy, to the fetus. Therefore, plain films necessary for diagnosis and safe care of the pregnant patient should be obtained without undue concern over fetal exposure.[26]

## DIAGNOSIS AND MANAGEMENT OF SOME CRITICAL CONDITIONS IN OBSTETRIC PATIENTS

### Maternal Hemorrhage[2,7,27]

Hemorrhage during pregnancy may be massive and is frequently associated with coagulation failure. Most often initial care is provided in the labor and delivery suite, but continued bleeding and resuscitation may require ICU.

### Management of Maternal Hemorrhage
- All efforts should be made to prevent and manage hemorrhage promptly and appropriately. Extra help and senior obstetrician should be available to provide medical and surgical treatment of obstetric conditions causing excessive and uncontrolled bleeding such as severe antepartum or postpartum hemorrhage due to

placenta accreta spectrum (PAS), rupture uterus, atonic uterus, traumatic delivery or DIC.
- Maternal monitoring should include arterial pressure, ECG, urinary output, arterial oxygen saturation, blood gas analysis, serum chemistry, and coagulation profile.
- The establishment of appropriate venous access, immediate volume resuscitation with crystalloid or colloid should be undertaken to restore the circulating blood volume until blood is available.
- Evidence for coagulopathy should be identified early and appropriate blood component therapy be instituted.
- Recombinant activated factor VII has recently shown to be an adjunctive hemostatic measure for the treatment of severe obstetric hemorrhage. Based on the mechanisms of action, circulating factor VII is active after it binds to tissue factor, which is exposed at sites of vessel injury. This complex initiate coagulation on activated platelet surfaces adhering to the site of injury and resulting into formation of a localized fibrin clot. The drug can be administered in obstetric cases with life-threatening hemorrhage, even in the presence of DIC. A dose of 90–200 µg/kg seems to be appropriate. However, it is important that the fibrinogen levels are ≥50 mg/dL preferably 100 mg/dL and platelet count is ≥50,000/dL.[2,27]
- In antepartum hemorrhagic shock, it is essential to position the patient in left lateral position to ensure that vena caval obstruction does not worsen already diminished venous return. In undelivered patients, immediate correction of fetal distress is mandatory. Fetal distress correction should be achieved by placing the mother in left lateral position, increasing the inspired concentration of oxygen, using intermittent positive pressure breathing, correcting maternal hypotension, and discontinuing oxytocin.

### Hemorrhagic Shock

Massive obstetric hemorrhage (MOH) is defined as a loss of over 1,500 mL of blood and is associated with significant morbidity and mortality. It can also be defined as a drop in hemoglobin concentration of ≥4 g/dL, or the need for transfusion of ≥5 red cell concentrate units.[28-30] Hemorrhagic shock is the inadequate perfusion of the tissues, as a result of massive blood loss, leading to imbalance between oxygen demand of tissues and the body's ability to supply it. As a result, mitochondria switch from aerobic metabolism to the less efficient anaerobic metabolism, thus leading to increased lactic acid production and worsening acidosis. The first step in managing hemorrhagic shock is its early recognition. Initial resuscitation requires prompt and effective teamwork. The correction of hypovolemia by means of IV administration of crystalloids and/or colloids is a priority. Resuscitation with IV fluids should begin immediately, without relying on hemoglobin test results.

Infusion of large volume of crystalloids and colloids can cause dilutional coagulopathy, metabolic acidosis, tissue edema, and tissue hypoxia. Thus, IV fluids should be limited to 1.5–2 L of warm crystalloids and 1–1.5 L of colloids till the arrival of blood and blood products.[29] Obstetric units should have massive transfusion protocols in place to deal with these emergencies. Such protocols enable rapid transfusion of sufficient volume of blood products. On activation of massive transfusion protocol, the blood bank should respond within minutes by delivering adequate amounts of blood products, including red cell concentrates, fresh frozen plasma, and apheresis platelet units. It is essential that all obstetric units should have immediate access to a "massive transfusion "pack" consisting of four units of O-negative blood, four units of fresh frozen plasma, and one apheresis pack of platelets. The recommendations are to use packed cells and fresh frozen plasma in the ratio of 1:1 with early use of platelets.[31] In addition, fibrinogen concentrates, and prothrombin complex concentrates should also be available. Further, the cause of hemorrhage should be identified and treated.

## Sepsis

Sepsis is currently defined as a "life-threatening organ dysfunction caused by a dysregulated host response to infection".[32] In the Third International Consensus Definitions for Sepsis and Septic Shock (Sepsis-3) from the Society of Critical Care Medicine and the Society of European Intensive Care Medicine, the terms systemic inflammatory response syndrome (SIRS) and severe sepsis were removed and terms infection, sepsis, and septic shock are being used.[11] In the consensus statement, patients without organ dysfunction are classified as having an infection, infection with organ dysfunction is sepsis, and septic-shock is a subset of sepsis in which patients require vasopressor support to maintain a mean arterial pressure > 65 mm Hg and have a serum lactate level >2 mmol/L after adequate fluid resuscitation.[11]

Sepsis-induced organ dysfunction is defined by "an acute change in total SOFA (sequential organ failure assessment) score of two points or more, consequent to infection, reflecting an overall mortality rate of approximately 10%". Q SOFA (quick SOFA) is a bedside scoring tool. It incorporates hypotension (systolic blood pressure ≤100 mm Hg), altered mental status, and tachypnea (respiratory rate > 22 breaths/min): the presence of at least two of these criteria indicates organ dysfunction and predicts poor outcome in patients with clinical suspicion of sepsis.

### Septic Shock

Septic shock is an important cause of hypoperfusion in obstetrics and accounts for 15% of all maternal deaths. Septic shock is defined as a "subset of sepsis where underlying circulatory and cellular or metabolic abnormalities are profound enough to substantially increase mortality". The common causes of sepsis in obstetrics include septic abortion, puerperal sepsis, chorioamnionitis, etc. Diagnosis of septic shock may be obscured by the normal hemodynamic changes seen during pregnancy. The most useful clinical signs of sepsis such as tachycardia, hypotension, and low SVR are present in both pregnant and septic states. The extreme values and or rapid changes in hemodynamic parameters usually point toward infection. Untreated and unresolved sepsis may progress to adult respiratory distress syndrome and DIC due to uncontrolled pulmonary capillary leak and derangement in the coagulation cascade.[1,2]

The immediate management of critically ill septic patient involves:
- Restoration of intravascular volume
- Restoration of tissue perfusion
- Restoration of oxygen delivery.

### General Considerations

- Early goal-directed therapy for sepsis should not be delayed until the admission to the ICU but should begin as soon as septic shock is diagnosed.
- All relevant cultures blood, urine, throat, high vaginal swab, wound swab, etc., should be drawn prior to initiating antibiotic therapy.
- Broad spectrum antibiotics covering likely pathogens based on site of infection, host factors, and culture sensitivity should be started, preferably within 1 hour of the diagnosis of severe sepsis or septic shock.
- Multiple-organ failure is a strong predictor of mortality in patients with sepsis with ARDS.
- Oxygen and mechanical ventilation should be instituted early for successful outcome.
- For associated hypotension, use crystalloid fluid within 3 hours and further fluid as indicated by dynamic measures of fluid responsiveness
- Target mean arterial pressure of 65 mm Hg using noradrenaline as first-line vasopressor.
- Target a VT in ventilated patients of 6 mL/kg (predicted body weight) and plateau pressure of <30 cm of $H_2O$.
- Metabolic acidosis, if severe (pH <7.2), must be corrected to achieve desired results with inotropes and vasopressors.
- There is no definitive role of corticosteroids in the management of septic shock.
- Activated protein C (Drotrecogin), a circulating anticoagulant with anti-inflammatory properties, has been shown to reduce mortality rate in patients with severe sepsis with high APACHE II score and high risk of death, but this has not been studied specifically in pregnancy.[1,33]
- Strict glycemic control is recommended in critically ill patients, particularly in patients with sepsis. Blood glucose levels should be maintained below 150 mg/dL. The goals of tighter control may be especially prudent in obstetric patients.
- Early goal directed therapy:[34]
  Goals during first 6 hours are to maintain:
  - *Central venous pressure:* 8–12 mm Hg
  - Mean arterial pressure > 65 mm Hg
  - Urine output > 0.5–1 mL/kg/h
  - Central venous (superior vena cava) or mixed venous oxygen ($SvO_2$) saturation >70%
  - If central venous or mixed venous $O_2$ saturation <70% after CVP of 8–12 mm Hg then transfuse packed RBCs to increase hematocrit to 30% and give dobutamine to maximum 20 µg/kg/min
  - Begin IV antibiotics within first hour of recognition of severe sepsis.

### Sepsis Bundle: Recent Guidelines

The "sepsis bundle" has been central to the implementation of the surviving sepsis campaign (SSC). In response to the publication of "SSC: International Guidelines for Management of Sepsis and Septic Shock: 2016", a revised "hour-1 bundle" has been developed and includes:[35]

- Measure lactate level [repeat lactate if initial lactate elevated (>2 mmol/L)].
- Obtain blood cultures before administering antibiotics.
- Administer broad-spectrum antibiotics.
- Begin rapid administration of 30 mL/kg crystalloid for hypotension or lactate >4 mmol/L.
- Start vasopressors if hypotensive during or after fluid resuscitation to maintain mean arterial pressure ≥ 65 mm Hg.

## Acute Respiratory Distress Syndrome

Acute respiratory distress syndrome can occur in obstetric patients as a complication of pneumonia, aspiration, sepsis, and amniotic fluid embolism. ARDS during pregnancy is often initiated by potentially reversible or self-limiting disease processes. Thus, it potentially carries a greater chance of recovery if the underlying disease resolves. Physiological consequences are hypoxemia, decreased compliance, and pulmonary hypertension.

The most recent definition of ARDS, the Berlin definition, was proposed by a working group under the aegis of the European Society of Intensive Care Medicine.[36] It defines ARDS by the presence within 7 days of a known clinical insult or new or worsening respiratory symptoms of a combination of acute hypoxemia ($PaO_2/FiO_2$ ≤ 300 mm Hg), in a ventilated patient with a PEEP of at least 5 $cmH_2O$, and bilateral opacities not fully explained by heart failure or volume overload. The Berlin definition uses the $PaO_2/FiO_2$ ratio to distinguish mild ARDS (200 mm Hg < $PaO_2/FiO_2$ ≤ 300 mm Hg), moderate ARDS (100 mm Hg< $PaO_2/FiO_2 \leq 200$ mm Hg), and severe ARDS ($PaO_2/FiO_2 \leq 100$ mm Hg)

Respiratory system compliance may already be compromised in pregnant women near term because of upward displacement of the diaphragm, so end-inspiratory (plateau) pressure may be elevated even without severe ARDS. The management of pregnant patients is like nonpregnant population with ARDS. The essential support in patients with ARDS is mechanical ventilation using low VTs (6 mL/kg), limited maximum plateau pressures to 30 cm-$H_2O$ to minimize ventilator induced lung injury (VILI), with PEEP. Additional strategies like prone positioning are not feasible in pregnancy. The utilization of low VTs in treatment of pregnant patients with acute lung injury, is based on studies proving the efficacy of this mode of ventilation in nonpregnant patients with ARDS. The goal of low VT therapy is to avoid overdistention of the lung. As the total lung capacity is comparable between the pregnant and nonpregnant women, it is logical to use this method of determining VT. It is important to maintain maternal arterial $PCO_2$ in its usual range of 28–32 mm Hg. Transfer of $CO_2$ across the placenta is dependent on a $PCO_2$ difference of approximately 10 mm Hg between fetal and maternal umbilical veins. This difference remains constant over a wide range of $CO_2$ tensions. Permissive hypercapnia is not advisable for ventilating the pregnant patient as maternal hypercapnia quickly results in fetal respiratory acidosis.[37] In addition, it is also essential to avoid volume overload that would exacerbate capillary leak, pulmonary edema, and ventilation perfusion mismatching. Nitric oxide (NO) has been utilized in the treatment of ARDS in nonpregnant patients, but there is still no consensus on whether inhaled NO improves clinical outcome as defined by oxygen requirements, ventilator days, or mortality.[37]

## Trauma

Trauma in pregnancy is common and complicates 6–7% of pregnancies. Maternal injury has been associated with an increased incidence of spontaneous abortion, premature labor, abruptio placentae, fetomaternal hemorrhage, and intrauterine fetal demise.

The physiologic and anatomic changes that occur during pregnancy alter the type of injuries seen and the maternal response to accompanying blood loss. The increase in blood volume that accompanies gestation may improve tolerance for hemorrhage but may significantly delay the appearance of signs until severe shock is manifested. As fetal well-being depends on uterine blood flow, moderate decreases in maternal cardiac output and blood pressure, which are insufficient to cause maternal shock, may be detrimental to the fetus. As the uterus grows and becomes an abdominal organ, it becomes more vulnerable to direct trauma. The initial concerns in the management of these patients are establishment of a patent airway, functional breathing, and adequate circulation. Standard fluid and blood resuscitation should be used to restore circulating blood volume, keeping in mind the requirement of an increased blood volume in pregnancy. If possible, the pregnant patient should be transported and cared for lying on the left side, to improve venous return to the heart. Mother and fetus should have continuous monitoring. It is important that the fetus has cardiotocographic monitoring because fetal demise is much more common than maternal death.[1,2,7]

The definitive therapy rendered to the pregnant trauma victim should mirror that given to those who are not pregnant. Because of increased vascularity around the uterus, pelvic fractures should be aggressively stabilized. Special consideration should be given to cesarean section in situations of fetal distress and in states of refractory maternal shock. Removal of the fetus may be lifesaving to the child and to the mother and the increase in venous return after delivery may improve resuscitative efforts.

## Obstetrician's Role in a Critical Care Unit

Multidisciplinary team approach is essential for the critically ill obstetric patient. In ICU, patient care decisions must be made jointly by intensivist, obstetrician, and neonatologist and should involve the patient, her family, or both. Obstetrician's inputs include evaluation of vaginal or intra-abdominal bleeding, obstetric sources of infection, and duration of specific therapies such as magnesium sulfate for eclampsia. There may be issues related to surgical interventions, including re-exploration of the abdomen or reclosure of abdominal or vaginal incisions. In postpartum ICU patients, feasibility of breastfeeding in view of the safety of various medications to the neonate, needs to be considered. When a pregnant patient is transferred to the ICU, members of the care team should assess the anticipated course of her condition or disease, including possible complications and set parameters for delivery, if appropriate. The plan should be clear to the medical team and to the patient's family and patient herself if she is able to understand.[11]

# CARDIOPULMONARY RESUSCITATION IN OBSTETRIC PATIENT[14]

Knowledge, preparedness, and good resuscitation skills can avoid a maternal and perinatal mortality. A rate of 58.9% survival after maternal cardiac arrest has been reported, which is better than those of most arrest populations.[38]

Hence, the hospital staff should be trained to provide prompt and good quality resuscitation in event of a cardiac arrest in a pregnant woman. Following resuscitation measures should be started immediately and simultaneously for which help of at least four personnel, trained in basic life support (BLS), is required.[14]

- Placement of the backboard (it makes the cardiac compressions effective by preventing the sagging of mattress or bed)
- Provision of chest compressions
- Manual left uterine displacement (LUD)
- Appropriate airway management
- Defibrillation when appropriate.

## Chest Compressions

For chest compressions it is recommended to place the hands in the same way as in nonpregnant woman because as per recent American Heart Association (AHA) statement, there is no scientific data to support the placing of hands slightly higher on the sternum in the pregnant patient, as was stated in previous AHA guidelines.[14] Heel of one hand should be placed on the middle of woman's chest, that is, on the lower half of the sternum and the heel of the other hand is put on top of the first so that the hands overlap and are parallel. Give 100 compressions per minute, compress to a depth of 5 cm, allow complete chest recoil and minimize interruptions.

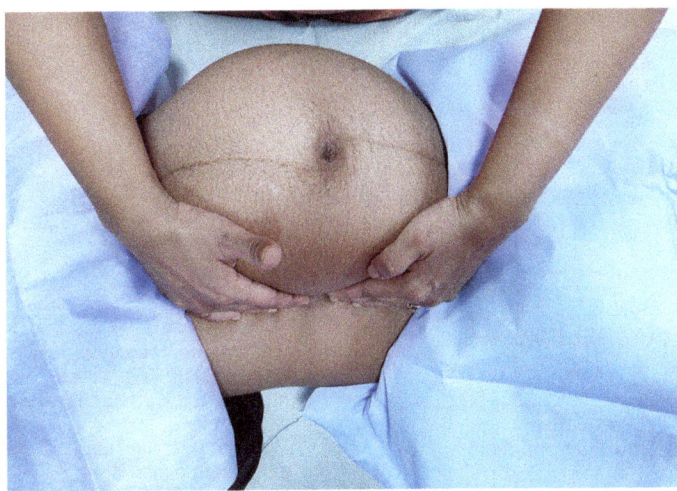

**Fig. 1:** Manual left uterine displacement from patient's left side.

## Manual Left Uterine Displacement

The uterus, if it is bigger than 20 weeks size gestation, causes aortocaval compression leading to cardiovascular compromise and therefore, needs to be "lifted off" the abdominal vessels. As per latest AHA recommendations manual LUD should be done and it is preferred over the 15-degree tilt.

As compared to 15° tilt, LUD has many advantages:
- It is more effective in reducing aortocaval compression
- Patient can remain supine which allows more effective chest compressions, and
- Airway management and defibrillation can be carried out more easily.

Left uterine displacement can be performed from the left of the patient **(Fig. 1)**, where the uterus is lifted up and toward left, or from the right of the patient **(Fig. 2)**, where the uterus is pushed upward and to the left of the maternal vessels.

## Airway and Ventilation

Head tilt-chin up maneuver is used to keep the airway open. Bag and mask ventilation with 100% oxygen at a rate of 15 L/min is considered the most effective, noninvasive way to start ventilation. To maintain airway patency, oral airway can be used. Compression-ventilation ratio of 30:2 is recommended as it reduces interruptions in chest compressions and avoids hyperventilation.[14]

## Defibrillation

Defibrillation protocol in pregnant woman is same as in nonpregnant woman and is indicated for ventricular

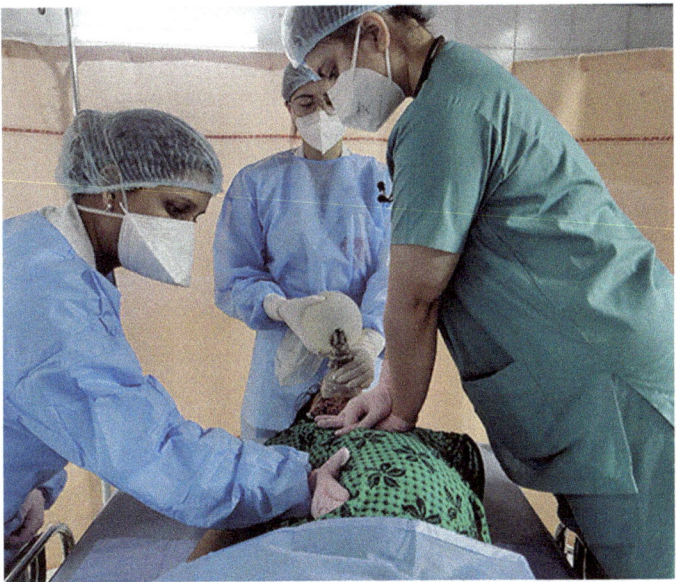

**Fig. 2:** Manual left uterine displacement from patient's right side.

fibrillation and pulseless ventricular tachycardia. An automated external defibrillator may be considered.[14] It is important to resume compressions immediately after the electric shock.[14]

**Flowchart 1** shows resuscitation steps in obstetric patient.

## Resuscitative Hysterotomy[11]

If initial efforts to resuscitate a pregnant woman do not lead to return of circulation within 4–5 minutes and pregnancy is >20 weeks duration, immediate cesarean delivery is recommended. Emptying the uterus improves the cardiac output by removing the aortocaval compression and makes cardiopulmonary resuscitation (CPR) more effective and resuscitation more likely to succeed. Chances of survival of the mother and fetus are better if cesarean is carried out early, that is, soon after 4–5 minutes of cardiac arrest. Cesarean can be performed even after this time limit as 50% injury-free

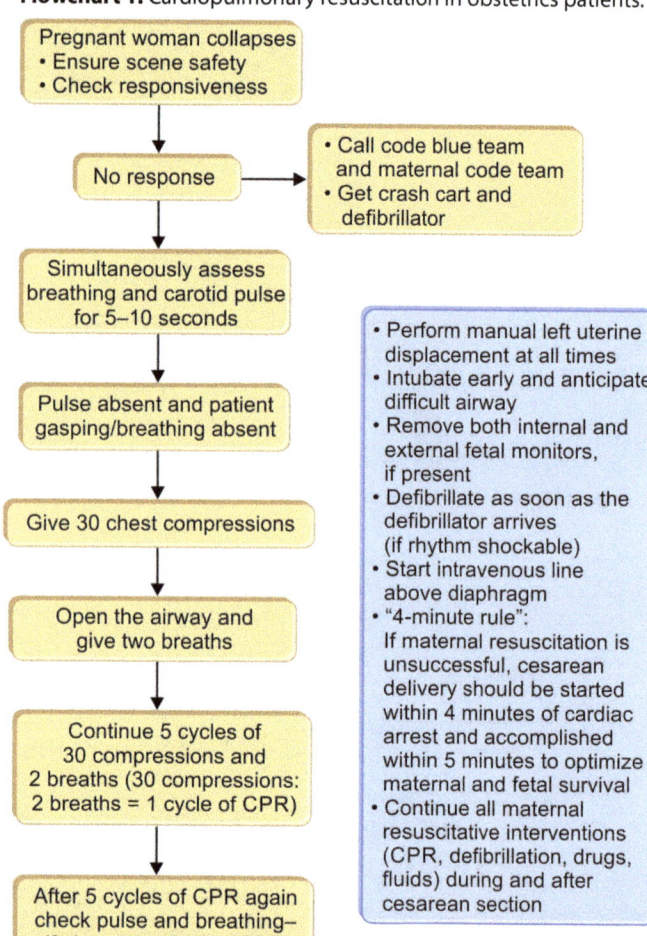

**Flowchart 1:** Cardiopulmonary resuscitation in obstetrics patients.

(CPR: cardiopulmonary resuscitation)

maternal and neonatal survival rates have been reported with perimortem cesarean delivery even at 25 minutes after maternal cardiac arrest.[39] But it has also been advocated that during maternal cardiac arrest in third trimester one should proceed directly to cesarean rather than wait for 4 minutes for pulse to return.

A Cardiac Arrest in Pregnancy Study (CAPS) from UK found that 25% of cardiac arrest in pregnancy were caused by anesthesia and rapid perimortem cesarean improved survival. It was found that the time from collapse to perimortem cesarean section (PMCS) was significantly shorter in women who survived (median interval 3 vs. 12 minutes, $p = 0.001$). Maternal survival rates of 58% were achieved with timely resuscitation, including PMCS.[40]

Hence, once a decision to deliver is made, one should proceed directly to cesarean delivery during maternal cardiac arrest in the third trimester rather than waiting for 4 minutes for restoration of the maternal pulse.[39]

## Cardiopulmonary Resuscitation in Coronavirus Disease-19 Positive Mother

The expanding coronavirus disease-19 (COVID-19) outbreak has created important challenges to resuscitation efforts and requires potential modifications of established processes and practices. The challenge is to ensure that COVID-19 patients who experience cardiac arrest get the best possible chance of survival without compromising the safety of rescuers. BLS and advanced cardiac life support (ACLS) recommendations remain the same, but all rescuers should don personal protective equipment (PPE) to guard against contact with both airborne and droplet particles. Oxygenation and ventilation strategies with low aerosolization risk should be prioritized:

- Attach a high efficiency particulate air (HEPA)/heat and moisture exchanger (HME) filter securely to any manual or mechanical ventilation device in the path of exhaled gas before administering any positive pressure breaths
- Bag mask ventilation should be minimized
- Patients in cardiac arrest should be intubated with a cuffed tube at the earliest feasible opportunity and attached to a closed-circuit ventilation.
- Minimize the likelihood of failed intubation attempts by the following:
  - Assigning the provider and approach with the best chance of first-pass success to intubate
  - Pausing chest compressions to intubate
  - Video laryngoscopy may reduce the exposure of the person intubating to aerosolized particles and should be considered, if available
  - Once on a closed circuit, minimize disconnections to reduce aerosolization
  - Suctioning through an endotracheal tube should occur through a closed inline system.

The cardiopulmonary physiological changes of pregnancy may increase the risk of acute decompensation in critically ill pregnant patients with COVID-19. In addition, preparation for perimortem delivery, to occur after 4 minutes of failed resuscitation, should be initiated early in the resuscitation algorithm to allow the assembly of obstetric and neonatal teams with PPE.

## CRITICALLY ILL CORONAVIRUS DISEASE-19 POSITIVE OBSTETRIC PATIENTS

Critical care management of covid-19 positive obstetric patient should be based on the same principles as that of nonpregnant adult population. Management of these patients involves multidisciplinary care by an expert team consisting of intensivists, obstetricians, neonatologists, nursing staff, critical care experts, infectious disease, and infection control experts. Important considerations include:[41]

- Pregnant women, especially those with associated medical diseases (diabetes, asthma, etc.) may present with pneumonia and marked hypoxia.
- Immunocompromised and elderly pregnant women may present with atypical features such as fatigue, malaise, body ache and/or gastrointestinal symptoms such as nausea and diarrhea.

- Based on their clinical signs and symptoms, COVID-19 positive pregnant patients may be classified as having mild (clinical symptoms are mild and no evidence of pneumonia on imaging), moderate (fever, respiratory distress, and radiological evidence of pneumonia) or severe disease (respiratory rate > 30 breaths/min, oxygen saturation < 93% at rest, $PaO_2/FiO_2$ ratio of <300 mm Hg, and >50% lesion progression on lung imaging within 24–48 hours).
- Pregnant patients are known to have a low FRC and increased oxygen consumption. Thus, they are known to develop hypoxemia rapidly. So, consider early oxygen therapy in these patients and target oxygen saturations ≥ 95% and/or partial pressure of oxygen ≥ 70 mm Hg.
- Patients with respiratory failure requiring mechanical ventilation, presence of shock, or other organ failure that requires intensive care management are critically ill.
- Early detection of severe illness and individualized decisions regarding the use of adjunctive medications is warranted because pregnant women are not included in many of the current clinical trials that are exploring treatment options for COVID-19.
- There is evidence that awake prone position, which can be achieved with pillows under the chest and pelvis, relieves both, aorta caval and diaphragmatic compression.
- The incidence of thrombotic complications in these patients is high. In addition to this, as pregnancy is a hypercoagulable state, the use of high-dose prophylactic and therapeutic anticoagulation treatment should be strongly considered in critically ill, COVID-19 positive pregnant patients.
- Unique challenges that are limited to pregnant patients include decisions about fetal monitoring, administration of antenatal corticosteroids, and delivery, all of which should be individualized because data guiding specific management strategies in this disease are lacking.

## KEY POINTS

- The obstetric patient poses exceptional challenges in the ICU. Knowledge of the physiologic changes of pregnancy and specific pregnancy-related disorders is necessary for optimal management.
- Obstetric ICU admissions include pre-eclampsia, including the hemolysis, elevated liver enzymes, and low platelet count (HELLP) syndrome, maternal hemorrhage, pulmonary embolic disease, amniotic fluid embolism, respiratory infection, ARDS, and sepsis. Hemorrhage and hypertension are the most common causes of admission from obstetric services to intensive care.
- Timely recognition of pregnant women at risk of potentially life-threatening conditions and institution of prompt and appropriate treatment can reduce maternal and perinatal morbidity and mortality.
- Hemodynamically unstable, hypoxic pregnant woman should be managed promptly by placing her in left lateral position, administering 100% oxygen by mask, and establishing an IV line and treating the cause.
- Scoring systems such as the APACHE II or the SAPS score accurately predict hospital mortality among obstetric patients admitted to the ICU for medical reasons but perform poorly in predicting deaths from patients admitted purely for obstetric reasons.
- Treatment of sepsis should not await admission to an ICU but should begin as soon as septic shock is diagnosed.
- Decisions about care for a pregnant patient in the ICU should be made collaboratively with the intensivist, obstetrician, and neonatologist.
- Necessary medications and radiological studies should not be withheld because of fetal concerns but if possible, fetal exposure to radiation and teratogenic medication should be minimized.
- Cardiac arrest in pregnancy is managed with the same ratio of chest compressions to breaths (30:2), respiratory support, drugs, and defibrillation as for a nonpregnant woman. If the uterus is bigger than 20 weeks size, continuous manual left uterine displacement during CPR is done to prevent aortocaval compression.
- After an unsuccessful attempt at CPR, cesarean delivery should be considered for both maternal and fetal benefit approximately 4 minutes after or even earlier, if a woman has experienced cardiopulmonary arrest in the third trimester. Survival benefit for both mother and fetus has been reported with cesarean delivery even if it was performed 25 minutes after cardiac arrest.
- Critical care management of COVID-19 positive obstetric patient should be based on the same principles as that of nonpregnant adult population. Decisions about medication, fetal monitoring, administration of antenatal corticosteroids, and delivery needs to be individualized because data guiding specific management strategies in this disease are lacking.

## REFERENCES

1. Shapiro JM. Critical care of the obstetric patient. J Intensive Care Med. 2006;21(5):278-86.
2. Pollock W, Rose L, Dennis CL. Pregnant and postpartum admissions to the intensive care unit: a systematic review. Intensive Care Med. 2010;36(9):1465-74.
3. Lapinsky SE, Kruczynski K, Seaward GR, Farine D, Grossman RF. Critical care management of obstetric patient. Can J Anaesth. 1997;44(3):325-9.
4. Vincent LJ, Frise CJ. Management of the critically ill obstetric patient. Obstet Gynaecol Reprod Med. 2018;28(8):243-52.
5. Ross A. Physiological changes of pregnancy. In: Birnbach DJ, Gatt SP, Datta S, (Eds). Textbook of Obstetric Anaesthesia. New York: Churchill Livingstone; 2000. pp. 31-45.
6. Birnbach DJ, Browne IM. Anesthesia for Obstetrics. In: Miller RD (Ed). Miller's Anesthesia, 6th edition. Philadelphia: Elsevier; 2005. pp. 2307-42.

7. Singh S, McGlennan A, England A, Simons R. A validation study of the CEMACH recommended modified early obstetric warning system (MEOWS). Anaesthesia. 2012;67(1):12-8.
8. McClure JH, Cooper GM, Clutton-Brock TH. Saving mothers' lives: reviewing maternal deaths to make motherhood safer: 2006-8: a review. Br J Anaesth. 2011;107(2):127-32.
9. Cantwell R, Clutton-Brock T, Cooper G, Dawson A, Drife J, Garrod D, et al. Saving Mothers' Lives: reviewing maternal deaths to make motherhood safer: 2006-2008. The Eighth Report of the Confidential Enquiries into Maternal Deaths in the United Kingdom. BJOG. 2011;118(Suppl 1):1-203.
10. Mhyre JM, D'Oria R, Hameed AB, Lappen JR, Holley SL, Hunter SK, et al. The maternal early warning criteria: a proposal from the national partnership for maternal safety. Obstet Gynecol. 2014;124(4):782-6.
11. ACOG Practice Bulletin No. 211: Critical care in pregnancy. Obstet Gynecol. 2019;133(5):e303-19.
12. Nates JL, Nunnally M, Kleinpell R, Blosser S, Goldner J, Birriel B, et al. ICU admission, discharge, and triage guidelines: a framework to enhance clinical operations, development of institutional policies, and further research. Crit Care Med. 2016;44(8):1553-602.
13. Maternal Health Division Ministry of Health and Family Welfare, Government of India. (2016). Guidelines for Obstetric ICU and HDU [online]. Available from: http://nhm.gov.in/images/pdf/programmes/maternal-health/guidelines/Guidelines_for_Obstetric_HDU_and_ICU.pdf [Last accessed July, 2021].
14. Jeejeebhoy FM, Zelop CM, Lipman S, Carvalho B, Joglar J, Mhyre JM, et al. Cardiac Arrest in Pregnancy: A Scientific Statement from the American Heart Association. Circulation. 2015;132(18):1747-73.
15. Aggarwal AN, Sarkar P, Gupta D, Jindal SK. Performance of standard severity scoring systems for outcome prediction in patients admitted to a respiratory intensive care unit in North India. Respirology. 2006;11(12)):196-204.
16. Knaus WA, Draper EA, Wagner DP, Zimmerman JE. APACHE II: a severity of disease classification system. Crit Care Med. 1985;13(10):818-29.
17. Vasquez DN, Estenssoro E, Canales HS, Reina R, Saenz MG, Das Neves AV, et al. Clinical characteristics and outcomes of obstetric patients requiring ICU admission. Chest. 2007;131(3):718-24.
18. Tempe A, Wadhwa L, Gupta S, Bansal S, Satyanarayana L. Prediction of mortality and morbidity by simplified acute physiology score (SAPS II) in obstetric ICU admissions. Indian J Med Sci. 2007;61(4):179-85.
19. Vincent JL. Give your patient a fast hug (at least) once a day. Crit Care Med. 2005;33(6):1225-9.
20. Shoemaker WC. Routine clinical monitoring in acute illnesses. In: Shoemaker WC, Velmahos GC, Demetriades D, (Eds). Procedures and monitoring for the critically ill. Philadelphia: Saunders Elsevier; 2002. pp. 155-66.
21. Zieleskiewicz L, Bouvet L, Einav S, Duclos G, Leone M. Diagnostic point-of-care ultrasound: applications in obstetric anaesthetic management. Anaesthesia. 2018;73(10):1265-79.
22. Van de Putte P, Vernieuwe L, Bouchez S. Point-of-care ultrasound in pregnancy: gastric, airway, neuraxial, cardiorespiratory. Curr Opin Anaesthesiol. 2020;33(3):277-83.
23. Santos AC, Braveman FR, Finster M. Obstetric anesthesia. In: Barash PG, Cullen B F, Stoelting RK, (Eds). Clinical Anesthesia, 5th edition. Philadelphia: Lippincott Williams & Wilkins; 2006. pp. 1153-80.
24. Pilbeam SP. Oxygenation and acid-base evaluation. In: Pilbeam SP, Cairo JM, (Eds). Mechanical Ventilation: Physiological and Clinical Applications, 4th edition. Philadelphia (PA): Churchill Livingstone Elsevier; 2006. pp. 1-11.
25. Marino PL. Parenteral Nutrition. In: Zinner R (Ed). The ICU Book, 3rd edition. Pennysylvania: Williams & Wilkins; 2004. pp. 754-65.
26. Critchlow JF. Obstetric Problems in the Intensive Care Unit. In: Irwin RS, Cerra FB, Rippe JM (Eds). Irwin and Rippe's Intensive Care Medicine, 4th edition. Philadelphia: Raven; 1999. pp. 1950-57.
27. Kjaer K, Cappielo E. Peripartum hemorrhage. In: Yao FF (Ed). Yao & Artusio's Anesthesiology: Problem-oriented Management, 6th edition. Philadelphia: Lippincott Williams & Wilkins; 2008. pp. 881-903.
28. Marr L, Lennox C, McFadyen AK. Quantifying severe maternal morbidity in Scotland: a continuous audit since 2003. Curr Opin Anaesthesiol. 2014;27(3):275-81.
29. Girard T, Mörtl M, Schlembach D. New approaches to obstetric hemorrhage: the postpartum hemorrhage consensus algorithm. Curr Opin Anaesthesiol. 2014;27(3):267-74.
30. Collis RE, Collins PW. Haemostatic management of obstetric haemorrhage. Anaesthesia. 2015;70 Suppl 1:78-86.
31. Trikha A, Singh PM. Management of major obstetric haemorrhage. Indian J Anaesth 2018;62(9):698-703.
32. Singer M, Deutschman CS, Seymour CW, Shankar-Hari M, Annane D, Bauer M, et al. The Third International Consensus Definitions for Sepsis and Septic Shock (Sepsis-3). JAMA. 2016;315(8):801-10.
33. Dellinger RP, Carlet JM, Masur H, Gerlach H, Calandra T, Cohen J, et al. Surviving sepsis campaign guidelines for management of severe sepsis and septic shock. Crit Care Med. 2004;32(3):858-73.
34. Rivers E, Nguyen B, Havstad S, Ressler J, Muzzin A, Knoblich B, et al. Early goal-directed therapy in the treatment of severe sepsis and septic shock. N Engl J Med. 2001;345(19):1368-77.
35. Levy MM, Evans LE, Rhodes A. The surviving sepsis campaign bundle: 2018 update. Crit Care Med. 2018;46(6):997-1000.
36. Ranieri VM, Rubenfeld GD, Thompson BT, Ferguson ND, Caldwell E, Fan E, et al. Acute respiratory distress syndrome: the Berlin Definition. JAMA. 2012;307(23):2526-33.
37. Campbell LA, Klocke RA. Implications for the pregnant patient. Am J Respir Crit Care Med. 2001;163(5):1051-4.
38. Mhyre JM, Tsen LC, Einav S, Kuklina EV, Leffert LR, Bateman BT. Cardiac arrest during hospitalization for delivery in the United States, 1998-2011. Anesthesiology. 2014;120(4):810-8.
39. Benson MD, Padovano A, Bourjeily G, Zhou Y. Maternal collapse: challenging the four-minute rule. EBioMedicine 2016;6:253-7.
40. Beckett VA, Knight M, Sharpe P. The CAPS Study: incidence, management and outcomes of cardiac arrest in pregnancy in the UK: a prospective, descriptive study. BJOG. 2017;124(9):1374-81.
41. NIH. (2021). COVID-19 treatment guidelines [online]. Available from: https://covid19treatmentguidelines.nih.gov/introduction/ [Last accessed July, 2021].

# Drugs in Pregnancy

*Pikee Saxena, Manju Saini*

## INTRODUCTION

The use of drugs in pregnancy requires special attention. There are many issues which must be considered prior to the administration of a drug during pregnancy. It is clear that any drug or chemical substance administered to the mother may cross the placenta unless it is destroyed or altered during this process. Transplacental transport is established at about 8th week of gestation and is dependent on molecular weight and lipid solubility of the substance. It is, therefore, important to determine the rate and extent of transfer sufficient to result in significant concentration within the fetus.

Number of drugs prescribed during pregnancy should be restricted to a minimum, with the lowest effective dose given for the shortest time. Drugs should be prescribed in pregnancy only if the benefits outweigh the risks.[1-3] Drugs should be given after enquiring about the last menstrual period and should be avoided especially in the first trimester of pregnancy as this is a critical period when the drugs have the greatest potential to cause gross malformations during organogenesis. The time period between day 35 and day 55 from last menstrual period is most crucial because prior to day 35 all cells are totipotent, so any insult before day 35 will result in either a missed abortion or has no effect on the growing embryo. Most women who become pregnant do not consult a doctor until 6 weeks of gestation, by which time organogenesis is well under way for the central nervous system (CNS), ears, and eyes. This must be taken into account when prescribing drugs to any woman of childbearing age, many of whom may be unaware that drugs may harm the fetus even before pregnancy has been diagnosed and some of whom will have unplanned pregnancies. These women should also be targeted to ensure that the beneficial effects of folate supplements in reducing fetal abnormalities are fully realized.

The effects of the drugs on fetal development are not only an issue for the mother but sometimes drug intake by sexually active men, is excreted in their semen and may cause fetal problems. Low doses of 5-alpha reductase inhibitors such as finasteride[4] given to husbands of sexually active women during pregnancy can cause abnormalities of the external genitalia of the male offspring. Griseofulvin also appears in the semen, and men should be advised not to try to father a child within 6 months of treatment.

There is another concern that relates to unknowns. Many pregnant women are turning to herbal remedies and dietary supplements, believing that they might be safer than synthetic drugs. But since there is often even less safety information about the effects of these remedies in general and especially in pregnant women, this represents a risk of unknown magnitude.

Concern related to the effect of a drug on both mother and fetus used by pregnant women is not new. In 1979, the United States Food and Drug Administration (FDA)[5] introduced a classification of fetal risks due to pharmaceuticals **(Table 1)**.

**TABLE 1:** United States FDA pregnancy letter categories.

| | |
|---|---|
| Pregnancy category A | Well-controlled studies have failed to demonstrate a risk to the fetus in the first trimester of pregnancy (and there is no evidence of risk in later trimesters), e.g., multivitamins |
| Pregnancy category B | Animal reproduction studies have failed to demonstrate a risk to the fetus and there are no adequate and well-controlled studies in pregnant women; or animal studies which have shown an adverse effect, but adequate and well-controlled studies in pregnant women have failed to demonstrate a risk to the fetus in any trimester, e.g., penicillins |
| Pregnancy category C | Animal reproduction studies have shown an adverse effect on the fetus and there are no adequate and well-controlled studies in humans, but potential benefits may warrant use of the drug in pregnant women despite potential risks, e.g., aminoglycosides and trimethoprim |
| Pregnancy category D | There is positive evidence of human fetal risk based on adverse reaction data from investigational or marketing experience or studies in humans, but potential benefits may warrant use of the drug in pregnant women despite potential risks, e.g., carbamazepine and phenytoin |
| Pregnancy category X | Animal or human studies have demonstrated fetal abnormalities and/or there is positive evidence of human fetal risk based on adverse reaction data from investigational or marketing experience, and the risks involved in use of the drug in pregnant women clearly outweigh potential benefits, e.g., thalidomide and methotrexate |

(FDA: Food and Drug Administration)

The United States FDA has the following definitions for the pregnancy categories.

## TERATOGENICITY

Teratogens are agents which act during embryonic and fetal development and result in permanent alteration of form or function. Teratogenic drugs[6,7] are drugs which have potential to develop congenital anomalies in the fetus when administered to a pregnant woman.

Now in 2015, FDA replaced the above pregnancy risk letter categories on prescription and biological drug and pregnancy and lactation labeling rule (PLLR) came into effect on 30th June 2015.

This PLLR has replaced the A, B, C, D, and X categories with narrative sections and subsections:[8] This rule helps the physicians regarding the risk-benefit ratio so that they may counsel the pregnant women and lactating mothers who need to take medication, thus enabling them to make informed and educated decisions for themselves and their children. PLLR needs to be updated as and when new evidence is available. It has the following three categories:

1. *Pregnancy (including labor and delivery):*
   - Pregnancy exposure registry available
   - Risk summary
   - Clinical consideration
   - Data
2. *Lactation (includes nursing mothers):*
   - Risk summary
   - Clinical consideration
   - Data
3. *Females and males of reproductive potential (New category):*
   - Pregnancy testing
   - Contraception
   - Infertility

It is not possible to study medication safety or teratogenicity in pregnant women through a well-planned prospective study as pregnant women belong to vulnerable or special group for ethical reasons. Due to this limitation, the only medication approved from 1996 to 2011, specifically for pregnancy was "hydroxyprogesterone caproate" for recurrent preterm birth. Therefore, drug safety data is collected through the following study types:

- *Case reports and case series:* Congenital rubella syndrome was identified by Gregg (1941), an Australian ophthalmologist who challenged the view that the uterine environment was impervious to noxious agents. A major limitation of case series is the lack of control group.
- *Pregnancy registries:* Potentially harmful agents may be monitored by clinicians who prospectively enroll exposed pregnancies in a registry. The prevalence of an abnormality is identified among exposed infants and compared with prevalence in the general population.

**TABLE 2:** Mechanism of teratogenicity.[5-7]

| | |
|---|---|
| Disruption of folic acid metabolism | Hydantoin and valproic acid |
| Formation of oxidative intermediates | Carbamazepine and phenobarbitone |
| Fetal genetic composition or genetic mutation | Thalidomide and methotrexate |
| Chaotic gene expression due to homeobox regulatory genes | Retinoic acid and valproic acid |

For example, metropolitan Atlanta congenital defects program is an active surveillance program ongoing since 1967 for fetuses and infants with birth defects.

- *Case control studies:* In this, investigators retrospectively assess prenatal exposure to particular substance between affected infants and controls. The only limitation is recall of bias. Moreover, the studies can only evaluate associations, rather than causality and are thus, hypothesis generating.

The mechanism of teratogenicity is as described in **Table 2**.

### Criteria for Establishing Teratogenicity

- The defect must be completely characterized
- The agent must cross placenta
- Exposure must occur during the critical period
- Cause and effect must be biologically plausible
- Epidemiological studies must be consistent.

Some drugs have effects even after they are discontinued. For example, isotretinoin used to treat skin disorder is stored in fat beneath the skin and is released slowly. This can cause birth defect if the woman becomes pregnant within 2 weeks after the drug is stopped. Therefore, women are advised to wait for at least 3–4 weeks after the drug is stopped, before they conceive.

### Drugs with Proven Teratogenic Potential

Some of the drugs with proven teratogenic potential and their effects on the developing fetus include:[6-10]

- *Angiotensin converting enzyme inhibitors:* Renal damage in the fetus especially during second and third trimester.
- *Carbamazepine:* Neural tube defects if administered during the first trimester.
- *Cocaine:* Contraindicated in all trimesters. Can lead to various congenital anomalies.
- *Anticancer drugs:* With cyclophosphamide, cytarabine, methotrexate, etc. various congenital malformations can result if given during the first trimester.
- *Diethylstilbestrol:* Vaginal adenosis and clear cell vaginal adenocarcinoma in pubertal girls exposed to diethylstilbestrol during pregnancy.
- *Ethanol:* Fetal alcohol syndrome.

- *Etretinate and isotretinoin*: High-risk of multiple congenital anomalies especially of CNS, face, ear, and other organs.
- *Iodide*: Congenital goiter and hypothyroidism.
- *Lithium*: Ebstein's anomaly.
- *Phenytoin*: Fetal hydantoin syndrome.
- *Tetracycline*: Discoloration and defects of teeth and altered bone growth.
- *Thalidomide*: Phocomelia.
- *Valproic acid*: Neural tube defects.
- *Warfarin*: CNS and facial abnormalities.

## TOCOLYTICS

These are drugs which are used to suppress premature labor when delivery would result in premature birth. Consideration should be given for the administration of tocolytics[11-14] to women experiencing preterm labor when there is a need to delay delivery in order to:

- Permit in-utero transfer to a tertiary perinatal center for multidisciplinary management (obstetrician, neonatologist, and anesthetist); and/or
- Gain up to 48 hours to allow for the administration and effect of corticosteroids to enhance pulmonary maturity.

Several factors may contraindicate delaying birth with the use of tocolytic medications:[12]

- Fetus is older than 36 weeks gestation.
- Fetus is in acute distress or has died (or has a fatal anomaly).
- Cervical dilation is ≥4 cm.
- Presence of chorioamnionitis or intrauterine infection.
- Mother has severe pregnancy-induced hypertension (PIH), eclampsia, and active vaginal bleeding, is having cardiac disease or any other condition which warrants termination of pregnancy.
- Heavy vaginal bleeding during pregnancy which may cause risk to mother or fetus.

Commonly used tocolytic drugs, their mechanism of action and their doses:[13,14]

- *Beta*-agonists: These agents act on adrenergic receptors to cause smooth muscle relaxation.
  - *Ritodrine*: It is phenylethylamine derivative with plasma half-life of 2–2.5 hours. Loading dose 30–350 µg/min intravenous (IV) or 10 mg, 2 hourly to 10–20 mg, 4–6 hourly orally.
  - *Salbutamol*: Dose 10–50 µg/min.
  - *Terbutaline*: Dose 250 µg S/C every 1–6 hours or by IV infusion started at 2.5–5 µg/min and increased every 20 minutes by increments of 5 µg/min to a maximum of 25 µg/min.
  - *Isoxsuprine*: Dose 0.5–1 µg/min IV infusion to 10 mg IM 8 hourly followed by 10–20 mg orally 8 hourly.
- *Magnesium sulfate*: Magnesium ions reduce uterine contractility by displacing calcium ions, thus reducing excitation of the muscle.
  - Dose 4 g IV over 5–10 minutes or in 200 mL of normal saline to be given slowly over 20 minutes followed by 1–2 g/h intravenously as infusion.
  - Now, it has been reviewed that $MgSO_4$ has both tocolytic and neuroprotective role. When given between 24 and 32 weeks for at least 12 hours.
  - Magnesium sulfate should not be combined with nifedipine as nifedipine enhances neuromuscular blocking effects of magnesium interfering with pulmonary and cardiac function.
- *Calcium channel blockers (CCBs)*: These are the first line tocolytic agent in developing countries.
  - *Nifedipine*: Inhibits both prostaglandin and oxytocin induced contractions resulting in uterine relaxation.
  - Dose 20 mg oral (not sublingual) stat followed by 10–20 mg, 6–8 hourly. A total dose of 60 mg or more is associated with a three-to-four-fold increase in adverse events, such as headache and hypotension.
- *Atosiban*: It is an oxytocin antagonist and thus inhibits uterine contractions. It has lesser side effects compared to Beta-agonist.
  - *Dose*: One bolus dose 0.9 mL (6.75 mg) is given IV over 1 minute, high dose infusion 24 mL/h (300 µg/min) during the first 3 hours, and low-dose infusion 8 mL/h (100 µg/min) up to 45 hours.
- *Indomethacin*: It blocks the pathway for stimulation of uterine muscle contractions as it is a prostaglandin inhibitor.
  - *Dose:* 100 mg loading dose per rectum followed by 50 mg orally 6 hourly.
- *Glyceryl trinitrate*: It is a nitric oxide (NO) donor and causes smooth muscle relaxation via the metabolite NO which acts as a second messenger to increase calcium ion uptake. Dose 5–10 mg transdermal patch is applied to abdominal skin and repeat dose in 1 hour if contractions persist (maximum dose 20 mg in 24 hours).

### Adverse Effects[13,14]

*Salbutamol:*
- *Maternal side effects*: Tremor, anxiety, nausea, palpitations, chest pain, and dyspnea or vomiting.
- *Fetal and neonatal side effects*: Fetal tachycardia, respiratory distress syndrome (RDS), and intracranial hemorrhage.

*Terbutaline:*
- *Maternal side effects*: Pulmonary edema, cardiac or cardiopulmonary arrhythmias, myocardial ischemia, hypotension, and tachycardia.

- *Fetal and neonatal side effects*: Fetal hyperinsulinemia, hyperglycemia, myocardial and septal hypertrophy, myocardial ischemia, and tachycardia.

*Ritodrine:*
- *Maternal side effects*: Metabolic hyperinsulinemia, hyperglycemia, hypokalemia, antidiuresis, altered thyroid function, physiologic tremors, palpitations, nervousness, nausea or vomiting, fever, and hallucinations.
- *Fetal and neonatal side effects*: Neonatal tachycardia, hypoglycemia, hypocalcemia, hyperbilirubinemia, hypotension, and intraventricular hemorrhage.

*Isoxsuprine:*
- *Maternal side effects*: Severe allergic reactions (rash, hives, difficulty in breathing, tightness in the chest, and swelling of the mouth, face, lips, or tongue), chest pain, fast or irregular heartbeat, and severe or persistent dizziness.
- *Fetal and neonatal side effects*: Fetal tachycardia, hypocalcemia, hypoglycemia, ileus, and hypotension at high doses.

*Magnesium sulfate:*
- *Maternal side effects*: Flushing, lethargy, headache, muscle weakness, diplopia, dry mouth, pulmonary edema, and cardiac arrest.
- *Fetal and neonatal side effects*: Lethargy, hypotonia, respiratory depression, and demineralization with prolonged use.
- Prolonged use of $MgSO_4$ may cause fetal and neonatal bone demineralization and fractures. So, US FDA has advised not to use $MgSO_4$ > 5-7 days.[15]

*Calcium channel blockers:*
- *Maternal side effects*: Flushing, headache, dizziness, nausea, and transient hypotension. Caution should be used in patients with hypotension. In addition, concomitant use of CCBs and magnesium sulfate is potentially harmful and can result in cardiovascular collapse.
- *Fetal and neonatal side effects*: None noted as yet.

*Atosiban:*
- *Maternal side effects*: Cardiac arrhythmias, muscular paralysis, CNS, and respiratory depression in mother.
- *Fetal and neonatal side effects*: Cardiac arrhythmias, muscular paralysis, CNS, and respiratory depression.

*Indomethacin:*
- *Maternal side effects*: Nausea and heartburn.
- *Fetal and neonatal side effects*: Constriction of ductus arteriosus, pulmonary hypertension, and reversible decrease in renal function with oligohydramnios, intraventricular hemorrhage, hyperbilirubinemia, and necrotizing enterocolitis.

*Glyceryl trinitrate:*
- *Maternal side effects*: Headache, flushing, hypotension, and tachycardia.
- *Fetal and neonatal side effects*: Tachycardia and asphyxia.

Combining tocolytic drugs potentially increases maternal morbidity and should be used with caution.

## CORTICOSTEROIDS

- Both topical and systemic corticosteroids are used for a variety of autoimmune and inflammatory conditions such as eczema, psoriasis, and asthma. Topical and inhaled steroid therapy during pregnancy for other diseases is not associated with any risks for the child even though small amounts of the steroids are absorbed. Recent meta-analysis suggests a small but significant association between use of systemic corticosteroids during the first trimester and oral clefts. This is consistent with results of animal studies. No similar evidence exists for topical or inhaled corticosteroids, probably because of much lower systemic exposure.
- Liggins and Howie[16] were the first to describe the beneficial effects of antenatal corticosteroids (ANCS) on lung maturity in preterm neonates. Use of ANCS has been associated with a decrease in RDS related mortality and morbidity in infants <34 weeks of gestation. Additionally, long-term follow-up studies have ruled out any harmful effect on the lungs, growth, and development.[16,17] The national institute of health consensus statement (1995) endorsed the use of ANCS and since then, this has become standard practice in the management of preterm labor (<34 weeks of gestation).
- Beta-agonists should be used to delay delivery for 24–48 hours in order to administer corticosteroids to promote fetal lung maturation. Maternal corticosteroid is administered by giving two doses of 12 mg betamethasone 24 hours apart or four doses of 6 mg dexamethasone intramuscularly 12 hours apart. The effect of treatment is optimal if the baby is delivered between 24 hours and 7 days after the start of treatment. Although it seems that the effect on lung maturity can be sustained effectively by repeated courses of ANCS, use of multiple courses may cause potential side effects of steroids on the fetal hypothalamic-pituitary-adrenal (HPA) axis, future growth, and development. A retrospective analysis of 710 infants enrolled in the North American Thyrotropin-releasing hormone trial,[18] has shown that >2 courses of ANCS was associated with a small decrease in fetal growth and lower plasma cortisol levels at 2 hours of age but no change in head circumference or neonatal mortality. Therefore, more than one course of ANCS is not recommended.[19]
- Cochrane database systematic review, 2008 compared different corticosteroids and regimens for accelerating

fetal lung maturation for women at risk of preterm birth. They concluded that dexamethasone has some benefits compared with betamethasone such as less intraventricular hemorrhage, although perhaps a higher rate of neonatal intensive care unit (NICU) admission (seen in only one trial). Apart from a suggestion from another small trial that the intramuscular route may have advantages over an oral route for dexamethasone, few other conclusions about optimal ANCS regimens were made.

- Royal College of Obstetricians and Gynecologists (RCOG) (2017a) recommended a single dose of betamethasone for women at risk for late preterm delivery as respiratory complications were lesser with use of ANCS between 34 and 36 weeks. Although repeat course of corticosteroid (rescue therapy) is not recommended [American College of Obstetricians and Gynecologists (ACOG 2017)] because of more side effects such as maternal and neonatal sepsis, etc.[20,21]
- Injection dexamethasone sodium phosphate and injection betamethasone acetate + phosphate are the two corticosteroids which are effective and safe in pregnancy. In India, betamethasone phosphate is available but the recommended betamethasone acetate + phosphate is not available. This salt is short acting and requires frequent dosing like injection dexamethasone so there is no advantage of injection betamethasone phosphate as far as frequency of administration is concerned. In addition, it is also more expensive and less stable than injection dexamethasone sodium phosphate at higher temperatures. Hence, injection dexamethasone is preferred drug for administration for fetal lung maturity in India. However, injection betamethasone phosphate may be administered when injection dexamethasone phosphate is not available.

## ANTIEMETICS

### Antiemetic Drugs used in Pregnancy[1,3]

Nausea and vomiting in pregnancy (NVP) is a common complaint especially during the first trimester. It generally subsides after first trimester and does not require any medication. Sometimes, it becomes excessive and may cause dehydration and electrolyte imbalance which is known as hyperemesis gravidarum (HG). In such cases it becomes essential to treat the condition vigorously. **Table 3** gives the doses and safety profile of commonly used antiemetics in pregnancy.

In extreme cases, hydrocortisone 100 mg daily IV till condition improve and then prednisolone 40–50 mg daily with gradually tapered dose until the lowest maintenance dose that control symptoms is reached. (RCOG 2017). Steroids have teratogenic potential like cleft lip and avoid to use in pregnancy.

**TABLE 3:** List of commonly used antiemetics.[22]

| Drugs | Dose | Maximum dose | Adverse effects | Safety in pregnancy |
|---|---|---|---|---|
| Antihistamines | | | | |
| Doxylamine + pyridoxine (B6) | 10 mg (+10 mg vitamin $B_6$)<br>• 1 BD during day and 2 HS | -<br>40 mg | Sedation<br>— | Safe and first line |
| Antihistamines | | | | |
| Promethazine | 25 mg PO TDS | 100 mg | Sedation | • Use with caution<br>• First line drug |
| Pheniramine | 43.5 mg ½ tablet PO TDS | 130 mg | Sedation | Use with caution |
| Dimenhydrinate | 50 mg PO TDS | 150 mg | Sedation | Use with caution |
| Dopaminergic antagonists | | | | |
| Metoclopramide | 10 mg PO or IV TDS (maximum 5 days duration) | 30 mg | Dystonia, extrapyramidal effects, and sedation | Risk of EPS so used as second line drug |
| Prochlorperazine | 5 mg PO/PR TDS or 12.5 mg IM/IV TDS | 35–50 mg | Dystonia, extrapyramidal effect, and sedation | • Use with caution<br>• First line drug |
| Domperidone | 25 mg PR, 10–20 mg PO TDS | 60 mg | Extrapyramidal reactions rare | • Use with caution<br>• Second line drug |
| 5 HT3 receptor antagonists | | | | |
| Ondansetron | 2–8 mg PO/IV TDS, 8 mg over 15 minutes IV then BD | 32 mg | Sedation, prolonged QT-interval, and serotonin syndrome | Data are limited so used as second line drug |
| Granisetron | 2 mg daily | | Serotonin syndrome and prolonged QT interval | |

(EPS: extrapyramidal symptoms; IV: intravenous; IM: intramuscular)

## DRUGS FOR BRONCHIAL ASTHMA

A joint committee of the ACOG and the American College of Allergy, Asthma, and Immunology (ACAAI)[23] was recently convened to provide guidance for physicians on asthma management of pregnant patients, particularly with regard to the use of newer asthma and allergy medications. The committee's recommendations included:

- A stepped approach, beginning with inhaled β2-agonists for mild, intermittent asthma and including inhaled cromolyn for mild persistent asthma; inhaled corticosteroids for moderate persistent asthma, and inhaled plus oral corticosteroids for severe persistent asthma **(Table 4)**.
- Use of either beclomethasone or budesonide if inhaled corticosteroids are initiated during pregnancy.
- Consideration of inhaled salmeterol instead of or in addition to, theophylline for asthma that is not controlled by inhaled corticosteroids.
- Avoidance of oral decongestants during the first trimester.

In general, the committee preferred inhaled medications (because they have fewer systemic effects) and time-tested drugs (because of greater experience with their use during pregnancy). Physicians are advised to limit the use of medication as much as possible during the first trimester, although birth defects related to most asthma drugs are uncommon.

### Safety in Pregnancy[3,5,23]

#### Inhaled Steroids

Beclomethasone, 2–5 puffs 6–12 hourly for asthma and/or two sprays in each nostril 12 hourly to control allergic rhinitis. It may be used safely during pregnancy and lactation in usual doses.

#### Oral Steroids

Prednisone, short courses of 40 mg/day in single or divided doses for 1 week and then taper over 1 week. If prolonged therapy is necessary, a single morning dose of prednisone on alternate days may help to minimize side effects. Intake of steroid tablets for a long time may increase the risk of cleft palate in the baby.

#### Cromolyn Sodium

Mast cell stabilizer, 2 puffs 6 hourly for asthma and/or two sprays in each nostril 6–12 hourly to control allergic rhinitis. It may be used safely during pregnancy and lactation in usual doses.

#### Inhaled Beta-Agonists

Two puffs every 4 hours as needed. No adverse effect has been seen in the fetus during pregnancy and lactation in usual doses.

#### Theophylline

Oral sustained-release preparations to reach serum concentrations of 8–12 μg/mL. Despite widespread use no harmful effects on unborn fetus have been described.

#### Decongestants

Pseudoephedrine, phenylephrine, phenylpropanolamine and oxymetazoline, intranasal spray for rhinosinusitis can be used in pregnancy. No adverse effect has been seen in

**TABLE 4:** Step therapy for chronic asthma during pregnancy.

| Category | Frequency/severity of symptoms | Pulmonary function (untreated) | Step therapy |
| --- | --- | --- | --- |
| Mild intermittent | • Symptoms not > twice/week<br>• Nocturnal symptoms < twice/month brief exacerbations<br>• Asymptomatic between episodes | • Normal > 80%<br>• Pulmonary function between episodes | Inhaled β2-agonists as needed |
| Mild persistent | • Symptoms > twice/week but persistent not daily<br>• Nocturnal symptoms > twice/month<br>• Exacerbations affect activity | 80% | Inhaled cromolyn; continue inhaled nedocromil; substitute inhaled beclomethasone/budesonide if not adequate |
| Moderate persistent | Daily symptoms:<br>• Nocturnal symptoms > once/week<br>• Exacerbations affect activity | 60–80% | • Inhaled beclomethasone or budesonide continue<br>• Inhaled salmeterol, add oral theophylline and/or inhaled salmeterol for patients inadequately controlled by medium-dose inhaled corticosteroids |
| Severe persistent | • Continual symptoms<br>• Limited activity<br>• Frequent nocturnal symptoms<br>• Frequent acute exacerbations | <60% | Treatment as described above, plus oral corticosteroids |

the fetus during pregnancy and lactation in usual doses with these medicines.

## Antihistaminics[24]

Chlorpheniramine, brompheniramine, and triprolidine are first generation antihistamines and can be safely used in pregnancy. Diphenhydramine is safe in pregnancy but may exert oxytocic action. Terfenadine is also not associated with increased risk to fetus. But these agents have more sedation and anticholinergic side effects.

Second generation agents such as loratadine, cetirizine, fexofenadine, astemizole, and cromolyn sodium do not have increased risk of congenital anomalies in the fetus. They are long acting but poorly lipophilic. Hence, have no entry to CNS and no sedation occurs.

## Expectorants

With use of guaifenesin with or without dextromethorphan, no adverse effect has been seen in the fetus during pregnancy and lactation. Other mucolytics or expectorants containing potassium iodide should be avoided after 10 weeks as iodide can cross the placenta and may cause fetal goiter.

## Antitussives

Dextromethorphan is safe in pregnancy. Alcohol containing preparations should be avoided for long-term use.

# ANTIHISTAMINICS

## Antitussives

*Opium alkaloids and derivatives:* codeine, dextromethorphan, dihydrocodeine, and pholcodine are safe for use in pregnancy. Nasal drops such as xylometazoline, oxymetazoline, budesonide, and cromoglycate are safer alternatives in pregnancy.

# EXPECTORANTS AND MUCOLYTICS

Codeine, dextromethorphan, ammonium chloride, bromhexine, guaifenesin, ipecacuanha, and saponins may be used in pregnancy.

## Decongestants

Phenylephrine, phenylpropanolamine, and pseudoephedrine may be used in pregnancy.

# GASTROINTESTINAL DRUGS

## Antacids

Antacids containing aluminum, calcium, magnesium, magaldrate, sodium bicarbonate, and combinations of these are associated with minimal risk to fetus when used in moderate doses.

**TABLE 5:** Oral option for gastroesophageal reflux.

| | |
|---|---|
| *H2 receptor antagonists* | |
| Ranitidine | 150 mg twice daily |
| Cimetidine | 400 mg 4 times daily up to 12 weeks |
| Nizatidine | 150 mg twice daily |
| Famotidine | 20 mg twice daily up to 6 weeks |
| *Proton pump inhibitors* | |
| Pantoprazole | 40 mg daily up to 8 weeks |
| Lansoprazole | 15 mg daily up to 8 weeks |
| Omeprazole | 20 mg daily for 4–8 weeks |
| Dexlansoprazole | 30 mg daily for up to 4 weeks |

## Proton Pump Inhibitors

Omeprazole and pantoprazole are used to treat hyperacidity during pregnancy and have not shown to increase adverse effects on the fetus.

## H2 Receptor Antagonist

Ranitidine has been the preferred antacid and was considered safe in pregnancy. However, many drug regulators across the globe have banned ranitidine until its safety profile is verified and assured.[25a]

Commonly used drugs which are given in gastroesophageal reflux disease (GERD) are mentioned with doses in **Table 5**.[25b]

## Laxatives

Dietary fibers, ispaghula, and lactulose are safer alternatives in pregnancy. Senna, bisacodyl, docusates, and saline purgatives are unsafe in pregnancy.

# ANTIDOPAMINERGIC DRUGS IN PREGNANCY

Issues surrounding the treatment of hyperprolactinemia in pregnancy are mainly concerned with the effects of dopamine agonists on the fetus and the possible stimulatory effect of the increased estrogen levels of pregnancy on tumor size.

The safety of bromocriptine exposure in utero has been evaluated by extensive monitoring including a multicentric study of 2,587 pregnancies in 2,437 women exposed to bromocriptine during part or all of gestation, with examinations of offspring up to the age of 9 years. The drug does not appear to be associated with any increase in the risk of spontaneous abortion, congenital abnormalities, multiple pregnancies, and no adverse effects on postnatal development have been detected. However, it is advised that fetal exposure to bromocriptine should be limited to as short a period as possible by discontinuing the drug as soon as pregnancy is confirmed.

Data on the safety of use in pregnancy of cabergoline and quinagolide is limited compared with bromocriptine. Over 300 pregnancies have been recorded in women taking cabergoline and almost 200 in women taking quinagolide and no apparent adverse effects on the pregnancy or fetal development have been detected.[26,27]

For women with microadenomas, the subsequent risk of adenoma growth during pregnancy appears to be 1% after discontinuing the drug and symptomatic follow-up in each trimester appears to be reasonable in such patients. For women with macroadenomas, prepregnancy debulking of the tumor may be undertaken with appropriate follow-up (2.8% risk of tumor enlargement).

## Dose

Bromocriptine is started at 1.25 mg orally at bedtime for a week after which it is gradually increased up to 5 mg 12 hourly.

Cabergoline is started at 0.25 mg twice a week or 0.5 mg once a week for 4 weeks. The dose can be increased stepwise in 0.5 mg increments until reaching lowest maximally effective and tolerated dose. Consensus has not been reached regarding maximum safe dose during pregnancy. For suppressing lactation, 0.25 mg is given 12 hourly for 2 days or 1 mg stat may be given.

## ANTIEPILEPTICS IN PREGNANCY[1-6]

Approximately 0.5–2% of pregnant women are on antiepileptic medication. A benefit-risk assessment is important for the mother and child and usually there is more risk for both mother and the child if the mother's seizures are not controlled during pregnancy. It is best that women with epilepsy who are wishing to get pregnant should have their epilepsy properly controlled before conceiving and have higher doses of folic acid supplements. Pregnancy seems to affect different epileptic women in different ways. There is no change in the status of 50%, about 40% show improvement and remaining 10% get worse.

Single drug therapy at the lowest effective dose should be aimed for. Women should be offered a detailed level II ultrasound examination and their levels of maternal serum alpha-fetoproteins should be monitored. With proper prenatal and postpartum management, up to 95% of pregnancies in which women took antiepileptics are reported to have favorable outcome.

Although most first-line antiepileptic drugs have been associated with some degree of fetal risk, the vast majority of exposed fetuses are not affected. Dose of antiepileptic drug may have to be increased with advancing period of gestation especially if other high-risk factors such as hypertension, hyponatremia, and hypoalbuminemia are associated **(Table 6)**.

**TABLE 6:** Antiepileptics in pregnancy.

| Drug | Fetal risk | Effect on fetus | Acts by |
|---|---|---|---|
| Phenytoin: 100 mg, 12 hourly to a maximum of 400 mg/day | 10% (highest risk) | Fetal hydantoin syndrome | Prolonged inactivation of sodium channels, increasing GABA |
| Valproic acid: 200 mg TDS, maximum of 800 mg, 8 hourly | 5–9% risk | Neural tube and limb defect | As above |
| Carbamazepine: 200–400 mg, TDS | 1% lowest risk | Neural tube and limb defect | Prolonged inactivation of sodium channels |
| Phenobarbital: 60 mg, 1–3 times a day | Risk not high | Studies claim that it lowers IQ | GABA receptor mediated synaptic inhibition |
| Levetiracetam | 2% | Neural tube defects | |
| Newer antiepileptics lamotrigine, gabapentin, topiramate, and oxcarbazepine | 0–2.4% | Neural tube defects | |

(GABA: gamma-aminobutyric acid)

All three first-line drugs for treating epilepsy—carbamazepine (Tegretol), valproic acid (Depakote), and phenytoin (Dilantin) have been associated with some fetal risks[28-34] **(Table 6)**.

Patients on carbamazepine, valproic acid, and phenytoin can breastfeed their infants because a very small amount of these drugs is excreted into breast milk. These have no apparent effect on the baby. Phenobarbital, however, is excreted in large amounts into breast milk and is not compatible with breastfeeding, because it may cause sedation and CNS depression in the baby.

The babies of women treated with enzyme inducing anticonvulsants (carbamazepine, phenytoin, primidone, and phenobarbitone) are at increased risk of hemorrhagic disease of the newborn caused by deficiency of vitamin K-dependent clotting factors. Women on these drugs should be treated prophylactically with vitamin K daily from 36 weeks gestation at a dose of 10 mg/day oral × 1 month prepartum until delivery and their babies should receive vitamin K 1 mg, IM at birth.

Some newer agents such as lamotrigine, levetiracetam, and topiramate appear safe but the number of reported pregnancies to date is smaller. First trimester exposure of these medications compared with no exposure was not associated with increased risk of major birth defect (1–2%)

(Molagarrd et al.). The mother risk was also reviewed by eight studies of levetiracetam and concluded that monotherapy was not associated with a 2% major malformation rate, which is similar to general population risk.[34]

Data regarding safety of antiepileptics in breastfeeding women are limited. No gross harmful effects have been reported (Brigg 2015).[6]

## ANTIHYPERTENSIVES IN PREGNANCY

Hypertensive disorders during pregnancy are classified into four categories, as recommended by the National High Blood Pressure Education Program. Working group on high blood pressure (BP) in pregnancy: Chronic hypertension, preeclampsia-eclampsia, preeclampsia superimposed on chronic hypertension, and gestational hypertension (transient hypertension of pregnancy or chronic hypertension identified in later half of pregnancy). This terminology is preferred over the older but widely used term PIH because it is more precise.

Antihypertensive drugs should be used in pregnancy if conservative therapy including optimum bed rest and diet control fails.[35-41] Recent National Institute for Health and Care Excellence (NICE) guidelines 2019 recommend starting antihypertensive if BP ≥ 140/90 mm Hg keeping the target BP below 135/85 mm Hg. The purpose of giving treatment is to prevent maternal complications and if possible, to prolong pregnancy till the fetal maturity is achieved.

*The commonly used drugs can be classified as:*
- *Sympatholytics*
    - *Central sympatholytics*: Methyldopa, clonidine, Beta-adrenergic blockers, propranolol, metoprolol, and atenolol
    - *Alpha adrenergic blockers*: Prazosin, and phentolamine
    - *Alpha and beta adrenergic blockers*: Labetalol
- *Vasodilators:* Arteriolar: Hydralazine, diazoxide arteriolar + venous, and sodium nitroprusside
- *Diuretics*: Not used in pregnancy as antihypertensives but is used selectively in some patients with pulmonary edema or congestive heart failure
- *Calcium channel blockers*: Nifedipine and verapamil
- *Angiotensin-converting enzyme (ACE) inhibitors*: Contraindicated in pregnancy.

## Labetalol

It is a reasonably safe first-line medication with combined alpha and beta adrenergic blocking action. It is widely used in treating hypertension during pregnancy. Unlike some other beta-blockers, it is not associated with fetal growth restriction. IV and oral forms are used as an alternative to hydralazine in severe preeclampsia/eclampsia. It is contraindicated in patients with hypersensitivity, cardiogenic shock, pulmonary edema, bradycardia, atrioventricular block, uncompensated congestive heart failure, and asthma. Dose: Labetalol—400-800 mg/day in divided doses to a maximum of 2,400 mg/day. If BP ≥ 160/110 mm Hg: 20 mg IV bolus; subsequent doses of 40 mg followed by 80 mg, IV may be administered at 10 minutes intervals to achieve BP control or up to a total of 220 mg. If hypertension persists hydralazine is given (ACOG 2017a).[42] Labetalol frequently causes maternal hypotension and bradycardia. It is also associated with reduced frequency of fetal heart rate acceleration (Cahill 2013).[43] It may also be administered as continuous infusion of 1 mg/kg/h.

## Alpha-methyldopa (Aldomet)

Alpha methyldopa is a safe antihypertensive drug. It acts on central alpha 2 receptors to decrease efferent sympathetic activity. It reduces the peripheral vascular resistance with minimal effect on cardiac output. Aldomet leads to dilatation of both arteries and veins which increases intravascular volume. It also maintains renal blood flow. After oral administration, less than one-third of the dose is absorbed. It is partly metabolized and is partly excreted in urine. The onset of its antihypertensive effect is over 4-6 hours and lasts for 12-24 hours. Aldomet crosses the placenta and is excreted at low concentration in human breast milk, but no neonatal side effect has been associated with its use. Side effects associated with this drug occur in about 22% of patients who may suffer from mild depression, sedation, postural hypotension, and hepatitis. It might lead to a problem during cross matching of blood, as methyldopa treatment causes a positive direct Coomb's test. Dose: 250 mg BD or TDS, gradually increasing as required over a period of 2 days to a maximum of 3 g/day. Contraindications to methyldopa are hepatic disorders, psychiatric patients, and congestive cardiac failure.

## Atenolol

It is not safe for use in pregnancy as it is associated with intrauterine growth restriction when used in randomized trials focusing on the treatment of chronic hypertension during pregnancy. Selectively blocks beta-1 receptors with little or no effect on beta-2 receptors.

## Vasodilators

### Hydralazine

It acts on the smooth muscles of arterial vasculature leading to vasodilatation. Hydralazine increases cardiac output by vasodilatation. It also increases plasma volume by reflex stimulation of the renin-angiotensin system. If administered orally, peak action occurs by 3-4 hours. Action of hydralazine lasts for 6-12 hours. Its side effects include headache, anxiety, nausea, flushing, epigastric pain, and lupus like syndrome.

It may be given IV during hypertensive crisis starting with a 5-mg initial dose, followed by 5-10-mg doses at 15-20-minute intervals until a satisfactory response is achieved or up to a maximum of 30 mg, per cycle. Oral dose is 40-200 mg twice a day.

### Nitroprusside

Reduces peripheral resistance by acting directly on arteriolar and venous smooth muscle. This is a rapid-acting parenteral antihypertensive of short duration of action. Its use is restricted to cases of severe hypertension not responsive to other drugs. Its safety for use during pregnancy has not been established. It is contraindicated in documented hypersensitivity; subaortic stenosis, idiopathic hypertrophic cardiomyopathy, and atrial fibrillation or flutter. If BP ≥ 160/110 mm Hg it is given in the dose of 0.25 µg/kg/min continuous IV infusion, titrate to BP with maximum dose of 5 µg/kg/min. Infusion rates >10 µg/kg/min IV may lead to cyanide toxicity.

## Calcium Channel Blockers

### Nifedipine

Acts by decreasing peripheral resistance without compromising cardiac output. Their onset of action is fast without any sedative effect. These agents prevent influx of calcium in vascular smooth muscle cells leading to vascular relaxation. They also relax the uterus and can be used for tocolysis. It causes no major side effect on the mother or the fetus. It can also be used in cases of fulminating pre-eclampsia by oral route to obtain a quick reduction in BP levels. Sublingual administration should be avoided as it may lead to unpredictable absorption resulting in sudden fall in maternal BP which might compromise the maternal cerebral circulation and decrease the uteroplacental blood flow with consequent fetal distress. Avoid concurrent use with magnesium sulfate because of risk of profound hypotension. Side effects are mild in the form of flushes, headache, gastrointestinal (GI) upset, and ischemic pain. *Dose:* Nifedipine 5-30 mg, 2-3 times/day, maximum dose 80-120 mg/day.

## Diuretics

Hypertension in pregnancy is accompanied by depletion of the central intravascular volume which is worsened by diuretics. So diuretic use in PIH should be avoided. However, it may be used with caution in cases of pregnancy-induced hypertensive disorder with pulmonary edema or with congestive heart failure. Diuretics causes hyperuricemia and hinders the use of serum uric acid as a sensitive indicator of disease process in PIH. It increases excretion of water by interfering with chloride-binding cotransport system, which in turn inhibits sodium and chloride reabsorption in ascending loop of Henle and distal renal tubule. Dose: 10 mg IV initial dose of furosemide increased to 20-80 mg/day PO/IV/IM.

### Angiotensin Converting Enzyme Inhibitor

These agents are strictly contraindicated in pregnancy as they might cause renal failure in the fetus. Skeletal abnormalities such as deficient skull ossification and limb reduction defects are drugs specific abnormalities.

## ANTICONVULSANTS

Convulsions in a pregnant patient may endanger life of both mother and fetus.

### Magnesium Sulfate

Magnesium sulfate is the drug of choice for prophylaxis and treatment of eclamptic fits. Compared with the traditional drugs used to terminate seizures (e.g., diazepam and dilantin), magnesium sulfate has a lower-risk of recurrent seizures with lower perinatal morbidity and mortality and avoids CNS depression. Women with severe preeclampsia and eclampsia are usually given $MgSO_4$ during labor or 24 hours after delivery as this is the most likely time to develop convulsion. Both IM and IV routes are equally effective.

$MgSO_4$ acts on cerebral cortex and exerts its anticonvulsion action by following methods:
- Blocking neuromuscular transmission by reducing presynaptic release of neurotransmitter glutamate
- Blocking N-methyl-d-aspartate (NMDA) receptors
- Enhancement of adenosine action
- Blockage of calcium entry via voltage gated channel.

Seizures usually terminate after the loading dose of magnesium and after few hours patients regain consciousness and oriented to time, place, and person. Once the seizures terminate, most patients have an improved BP control. Benzodiazepine or phenytoin (Dilantin) can be used for seizures that are not responsive to magnesium sulfate. After the initial loading dose of magnesium, significant hypertension continues in approximately 10-15% of eclamptic patients. It can be given by IV/IM route for seizure prophylaxis in preeclampsia but for treating true eclampsia, IV route is preferred for a quicker action although both routes are equally effective.

*Pritchard regimen:* On admission 4 g (8 mL; 50% weight per volume ampoules) is diluted with 12 mL of distilled water (20% solution) and injected IV over 5-10 minutes followed by 10 mL of 50% solution (5 g) IM in each buttock. Subsequent dose of 10 mL 50% solution (5 g) of magnesium sulfate IM is given in alternate buttock every 4 hours. In cases of eclampsia, $MgSO_4$ is continued for 24 hours after delivery.

*Zuspan regimen:* Loading dose of magnesium sulfate for an active/recent seizure is 4–6 g IV over 20 minutes (dilute the 50% solution with normal saline and administer the 20% solution using an infusion pump) followed by a maintenance dose of magnesium sulfate 1–2 g/h as IV infusion. This regimen requires continuous maternal electrocardiographic (ECG) monitoring and regular serum Mg levels. But now ACOG 2013 has recommended IV regimen for management of pre-eclampsia with severe features.

$MgSO_4$ may cause hyporeflexia, respiratory depression, and bradycardia. Patient's reflexes should be monitored and infusion should be discontinued if reflexes are absent or if serum magnesium level exceeds 7 mEq/L. Levels of 8–12 mEq/dL may cause loss of reflexes, diplopia, flushing or slurring of speech; levels >12 mEq/dL may cause muscular paralysis, ventilatory failure, and circulatory collapse; patients should have frequent neurological evaluation. Presence of patellar reflex, adequate respiratory function respiratory rate (RR) > 14 breaths/min, and urinary output >25 mL/h is ensured before administering each dose. Loss of deep tendon reflex indicates that the magnesium level may be toxic, some clinicians follow serum magnesium levels 6 hourly along with neurological examination. But routine $MgSO_4$ levels are not recommended (ACOG 2017). Magnesium may alter cardiac conduction, leading to heart block in digitalized patients.

Magnesium is cleared by renal excretion, in case of impaired renal function (serum creatinine > 1.0 mg/mL), maintenance dose should be altered. To monitor toxicity, Mg levels should be done. Calcium gluconate 10% solution 10–20 mL slow IV can be given as an antidote for clinically significant hypermagnesemia.

Recently, it has been studied that $MgSO_4$ has neuroprotective role in very low birth weight neonates (BEAM study).[44]

## Phenytoin

It is used if the patient has recurrent seizures despite optimum magnesium sulfate therapy. May also be used in cases of renal failure, serious magnesium-related toxicity or when seizures occur due to causes other than eclampsia. Phenytoin acts on motor cortex where it inhibits spread of seizure activity. Activity of brain stem centers responsible for tonic phase of grand mal seizures also may be inhibited. Dose of phenytoin is 20 mg/kg loading by infusion at a maximum rate of 50 mg/min IV followed by maintenance dose of 200 mg, 8 hourly.

## Diazepam

It is useful for treatment of seizures resistant to magnesium sulfate. It depresses all levels of CNS, possibly by increasing activity of gamma-aminobutyric acid (GABA). Dose is 10 mg, slow IV at a rate of 1 mg/min.

## ■ INSULIN THERAPY IN PREGNANCY

Insulin is the preferred first line agent for persistent hyperglycemia in women with gestational diabetes (ACOG 2017).[45] Women suffering from preexisting type 1 diabetes require constant adjustment in the insulin regimen due to continuous fluctuations in the body. Insulin requirement lessens during the first trimester due to increased insulin sensitivity. However, insulin requirement increases in the later stages due to increased circulating placental hormones.

Women suffering with type 2 diabetes usually require higher insulin doses for each trimester as compared to type 1 patients. The insulin requirements in both conditions are comparable during the first trimester which increases in the second trimester for patients with type 1 diabetes.

A mixed regimen (intermediate-acting and short-acting) may be used twice daily and dose adjustments are based on glucose levels at particular times of the day. Short acting insulin is given 30 minutes before meal while rapid acting insulin is administered right before meals. Nowadays, a bolus regimen thrice a day before the meals to control postprandial glycemia along with a shot of basal or intermediate insulin to normalize the fasting glucose are recommended. In special conditions where control of diabetes is difficult, a continuous subcutaneous insulin infusion (CSII) pump can be used.

### Human Insulin

- *Regular insulin*: FDA has received enough data regarding the use of regular insulin in management of diabetes during pregnancy. It is a drug with low-risk for the mother as well as the fetus. However, there are chances of occurrence of hypoglycemic events.
- *Neutral Protamine Hagedorn insulin*: Neutral Protamine Hagedorn (NPH) has a pronounced peak effect. It has onset of action in 1 hour and lasts 16–18 hours. However, it is incapable to provide once-daily basal insulin. Moreover, the uncontrollable pharmacokinetics may sometimes make glycemic control difficult.

### Rapid-acting Analogs

Rapid-acting analogs of insulin have a rapid onset of action and are helpful in reducing the postprandial hyperglycemia. The efficiency of these analogs in reducing the postprandial hyperglycemia is due to their faster actions immediately after administration. Lispro and aspart belong to category "B" and have demonstrated clinical effectiveness.

- *Lispro:* Produced by recombinant deoxyribonucleic acid (DNA) technology, it has an onset of about 10–15 minutes and requires 30–60 minutes to reach the peak concentration. It can produce its actions for up to 3–4 hours. The shortened onset, allows more flexibility than regular insulin. Several studies have indicated that insulin lispro is as effective as regular insulin in achieving adequate glycemic controls in type 1 diabetic pregnancies. Thus, lispro may be considered as a safe alternative to human insulin in controlling diabetes.

- *Aspart*: It is a recombinant, rapid-acting analog with an onset of 10–20 minutes. Moreover, it takes 40–50 minutes to reach its peak concentration and has duration of action of 3–5 hours. Insulin aspart has not shown any significantly different adverse effects from that of regular insulin and is therefore considered to be reasonably safe for administration in pregnancy.
- *Glulisine:* Recombinant insulin analog produced in a laboratory strain of *Escherichia coli*. Glulisine takes about 20 minutes to initiate its action and about 55 minutes to reach the peak concentration. This analog does not have any remarkable toxic effects on the fetus. However, no significant clinical data is available for using insulin glulisine in pregnancy.

### Long-acting Analogs

Among the long-acting analogs, insulin glargine has been assigned category "C" while insulin detemir has been shifted to category "B".

- *Glargine*: It is a long-acting basal insulin analog with onset of action after 60–120 minutes. The maximum duration of action is 24 hours. Pharmacokinetically, insulin glargine has a steady action and usually does not cross the placenta. Current clinical data shows comparable fetal outcomes between regular insulin and glargine. However, to further justify its safety and efficacy in pregnancy large randomized trials are required to be conducted.
- *Detemir:* Long-acting human insulin analog for maintaining basal level of insulin. It has its onset in 60–120 minutes after administration. The maximum duration of action is 20 hours.
- *Degludec:* It is an ultra-long-acting basal insulin analog with its onset 30–90 minutes after administration. The duration of action is reported to be >24 hours. There is no significant clinical data available to justify the use and safety of insulin degludec in pregnancy. Thus, it is not yet recommended to be used in pregnancy.

*Description of various types of insulin available is given in* **Table 3** *of Chapter 18 (in chapter on Diabetes Mellitus in Pregnancy) (Page 225).*

### ORAL ANTIDIABETIC AGENTS IN PREGNANCY

Oral hypoglycemic agents are being increasingly used for gestational diabetes. Metformin and glyburide are the two oral hypoglycemic agents commonly used in pregnancy. FDA has not approved them for this indication but ACOG (2017a) recommends both agents as a second line agents.[46]

*Metformin:* Serves as a second line approach and ACOG recommends that metformin may be used as an alternative to insulin during pregnancy in women who are not willing for insulin injections and are not able to monitor their plasma glucose levels. Its use in pregnant patients alone or with insulin supplements is not associated with increased perinatal complications. The advantages of metformin use in pregnancy are low-cost, ease of administration, requires less stringent monitoring, decreased weight gain during pregnancy, and has a comparable efficacy to insulin for achieving normoglycemia. However, its administration should still be accompanied with counseling about chances of preterm birth, placental transfer of the drug, and lack of approval from regulatory authorities in absence of long-term data in exposed offspring. Although high proportion of women (30–45%) required supplementary insulin but at lower doses.[46] In women requiring high dose of insulin, metformin may be added to control plasma glucose levels. Side effects such as nausea, vomiting, and diarrhea. Other rare complications such as lactic acidosis and hypersensitivity reactions. *Dose:* 500 mg OD to 2 g/day.

*Glyburide:* It belongs to sulfonylurea group and acts by releasing insulin from pancreas. It should not be used if insulin or metformin can be administered to the patients (ACOG 2017).[45] Although it has comparable effects as that of metformin, glyburide treatment is associated with increased risks of neonatal hypoglycemia, high maternal weight gain, and macrosomia. Common side effects are nausea, vomiting, diarrhea, muscle pain, and allergic reactions. Dose 2.5–20 mg/day.

### ANTITHROMBOTIC THERAPY

Use of antithrombotic drugs is required during pregnancy for prevention of venous thromboembolism (VTE) in high-risk patients, treatment of VTE and prevention of arterial emboli in patients with mechanical heart valve prostheses.[47-49] However, there are several problems with use of antithrombotic drugs during pregnancy.

### Warfarin

Warfarin, as well as the other coumarin compounds, cross the placenta and have the potential to cause both bleeding in the fetus and teratogenicity. Warfarin embryopathy may occur in 4–10% of patients if it is given during the first trimester. The daily maintenance dose of warfarin differs greatly between individuals, commonly between 0.5 and 15 mg/day, and often fluctuates.

The drug is rapidly and completely absorbed and immediately blocks further hepatic synthesis of the functional vitamin K-dependent procoagulants (II, VII, IX, and X). However, its impact on the INR (international normalized ratio) is delayed until preformed coagulation factors are removed, so dose adjustment must allow for these delayed effects. INR is a good indicator of effectiveness and risk of bleeding during warfarin therapy and is best kept at about 2.5, with a target range of 2.0–3.0. Maternal effects of warfarin sodium can be reversed by giving fresh frozen plasma but the fetus requires 1–2 weeks after discontinuation of treatment to reverse anticoagulant effect. A pregnant woman on warfarin therapy is switched over to heparin during the first 12 weeks to avoid teratogenic effects and last 4 weeks of pregnancy to avoid fetal maternal complications during delivery.

## Unfractionated Heparin and Low-molecular-weight-heparin

These do not cross the placenta and are safe for the fetus, but long-term treatment with unfractionated heparin (UFH) is problematic because of its inconvenient route of administration, need to continuously monitor anticoagulant activity, and its potential side effects, such as heparin-induced thrombocytopenia and osteoporosis.

The low-molecular-weight-heparin (LMWH) is the drug of choice in the prevention and treatment of VTE during pregnancy because of the ease of administration, monitoring, and lower risk of side effects. Patients with mechanical heart valve prostheses represent a major clinical challenge. Warfarin, the drug of choice in nonpregnant women, can be administered between the 12th and 36th week. Full-dose UFH is recommended in the first trimester and after week 36. The patient on heparin will have normal clotting 4–6 hours after discontinuing the medication.[41] *Table 4 of Chapter 25 depicts anticoagulants dose, side effects, and monitoring in chapter on Thromboembolism in Pregnancy (Page 313).*

Monitoring of a patient on UFH is done by activated partial thromboplastin time (aPTT). Routine monitoring with LMWH is controversial in pregnant patients, however, if needed, may be done with anti-Xa levels. The effects of heparin may be reversed by protamine sulfate.

## ANTITUBERCULAR DRUGS IN PREGNANCY

Pregnancy with tuberculosis presents a therapeutic challenge. Snider et al.[50] reviewed all available literature on pregnant women treated with isoniazid (INH), ethambutol (EMB), rifampicin (RMP) or streptomycin (SM) and reported on the relative safety of these drugs and whether risk of teratogenesis justifies abortion on medical grounds. Other than the ototoxicity of SM, none of these drugs in normal dosages are proved teratogens to human fetuses. The use of INH in combination with EMB for a pregnant woman with tuberculosis is recommended, if the disease is not extensive. If a third drug is warranted, then RMP could be added. Because of its ototoxicity, SM should not be used, unless RMP is contraindicated or proves unsatisfactory. Routine therapeutic abortion is not indicated for a pregnant woman who is taking first-line antituberculosis drugs.

As per World Health Organization (WHO) 2018 recommendation which are adopted by Revised National Tuberculosis Control Program (RNTCP) are that all new patients whether smear positive or negative, pulmonary or extrapulmonary should be given category 1. In case of treatment failure and defaulter, category 1 should be advised after ruling out drug resistance.[51]

## VACCINES

Vaccination of a pregnant woman with inactivated vaccines has not been shown to cause an increase risk to the fetus. Live vaccines are usually contraindicated in pregnancy because pregnancy is an immunocompromised state and there is a potential risk of causing the disease in the mother and the fetus.

### Vaccines that should be avoided during Pregnancy

- *Live, attenuated influenza vaccine:* While a woman is recommended to receive the influenza vaccine while pregnant, she should not receive the live version of the vaccine.
- *Measles, mumps, and rubella*: Women who are pregnant should not receive live, weakened viral vaccines, including the ones for measles, mumps, and rubella (MMR). A woman should avoid becoming pregnant for 4 weeks after receiving this vaccine.
- *Varicella*: As with MMR, this vaccine contains a live, weakened virus and should not be given to pregnant women. Additionally, women should avoid becoming pregnant for at least 1 month after receiving this vaccine.
- *Tetanus toxoid, reduced diphtheria toxoid, and acellular pertussis vaccine (Tdap):* This vaccine is administered once in pregnancy between 27 and 36 weeks gestation for prevention of pertussis in the newborn during first few weeks of life.
- Rabies vaccine contains inactivated rabies virus and can be given to pregnant woman in case of exposure.
- *Coronavirus disease (COVID-19) vaccine*: Development and regular approval of this vaccine is rapidly progressing. The FDA has issued an emergency use authorization (EUA) for the following vaccine:
  - *Pfizer-Bio-N-tech messenger ribonucleic acid (mRNA) vaccine (BNT162B2)*: ≥16 years and older as a 2-dose regimen given 3 weeks (21 days) apart.
  - *Moderna mRNA-1,273 vaccine*: ≥18 years and older as a 2-dose regimen given 1 month (28 days) apart.

Advisory Committee on Immunization Practices (ACIP) also issued recommendations for use of these vaccine.

American College of Obstetricians and Gynecologists recommends that COVID-19 vaccine should not be withheld from pregnant individual who meet criteria for vaccination based on ACIP recommended priority groups.[52]

Ministry of Health and Family Welfare, Government of India, has approved vaccination of pregnant women against COVID-19. Expected side effects should be explained as part of counseling patients including that they are a normal part of body's reaction to the vaccines and developing antibodies to protect against COVID-19 illness.

## ANTIDEPRESSANT DRUGS

- Selective serotonin reuptake inhibitors are good therapeutic choices during pregnancy except paroxetine which has been associated with a higher risk for cardiac anomalies, particularly atrial and ventricular septal defects.[53]
- Lithium salts should be discontinued till 8 weeks as it may cause Ebstein anomaly. Neonatal lithium toxicity occurs from exposure near delivery which may include neonatal hypothyroidism, diabetes insipidus, cardiomegaly, bradycardia, electrocardiogram abnormalities, cyanosis, and hypotonia (ACOG 2016).
- Monoamine oxidase (MAO) inhibitors should be avoided as threatening hyperthermic crisis may be precipitated.
- Antipsychotic medications are safe in pregnancy but exposed neonates can manifest abnormal extrapyramidal muscle movements and withdrawal symptoms.[54]

## ANALGESICS DURING PREGNANCY

- *Salicylates:*[55] They pose theoretical risk of closure of ductus arteriosus and associated cardiac and pulmonary abnormality.
- No adverse outcome with low dose aspirin and paracetamol intake.
- Ketorolac and pentazocine should be used cautiously during pregnancy and safety has not been established during lactation.
- *Tramadol*: Safety has not been established during pregnancy or lactation.
- Analgin and nimesulide are contraindicated during pregnancy.
- *Indomethacin*: Its effects are reversible as long as drug is not given after 34 weeks. It causes oligohydramnios, constriction of ductus arteriosus, intraventricular hemorrhage, and necrotizing enterocolitis.
- *Narcotic analgesic (meperidine and morphine)*: It causes neonatal withdrawal syndrome.

## IMMUNOSUPPRESSIVE DRUGS

- Used in patients with organ transplants.
- Corticosteroids therapy is associated with cleft lip and cleft palate in animal studies.
- Azathioprine is safe for use in human pregnancy.
- Cyclosporine has significant maternal toxicity especially nephrotoxicity and should be given only if benefits outweigh risks.
- Cyclophosphamide is a suspected teratogen and should be avoided in early pregnancy.

## ANTINEOPLASTICS

The use of antineoplastic agents in pregnant women poses obvious risks to both the woman and the developing fetus, particularly during organogenesis.

### Antimetabolites

Folate antagonists (aminopterin and methotrexate) cause fetal aminopterin syndrome and should be avoided during pregnancy.

### Alkylating Agents

Busulfan causes fetal growth retardation, cleft palate, and eye defects in the fetus. Use of cyclophosphamide during pregnancy is associated with major congenital anomalies in 14% while 86% fetuses were normal. It causes cleft palate, absence of digits, imperforate anus, and fetal growth retardation. It should be avoided during first trimester but can be given later.

### Plant Alkaloids

Vincristine and vinblastine have shown to slightly increase the risk of developing congenital anomalies during first trimester but can be given to treat life-threatening malignancies like acute leukemias.

### Antibiotics

Use of daunorubicin, doxorubicin, and bleomycin should be guarded especially during the first trimester but they may be administered later in pregnancy. No reports linking the use of bleomycin with congenital defects in humans have been seen. These drugs may be used during first trimester to treat acute leukemias or lymphomas as life-saving therapy, although adverse effects on the fetus cannot be ruled out.

### Alcohol

- Causes growth restriction and behavioral disturbances in the fetus.
- Brain, cardiac, and spinal defects in the baby has been noted.
- Craniofacial abnormalities are associated.
- Even low levels of alcohol cannot be recommended during pregnancy.

## ANTI-INFECTIVE AGENTS (TABLE 7)

### Antiretroviral Agents

These are the drugs active against human immunodeficiency virus (HIV) which is a retrovirus. They help in prolonging and improving the quality of life and postponing complications

**TABLE 7:** Anti-infective agents.[3,4]

| Category A | Category B | Category C | Category D |
|---|---|---|---|
| Nystatin vaginal tablets | • Amoxicillin, ampicillin, amoxicillin-clavulanate, nitrofurantoin, metronidazole (although there is some controversy about oral intake in the first trimester), cephalosporins, clindamycin, erythromycin, azithromycin, sulfa drugs (except near term), and famciclovir valacyclovir<br>• Clotrimazole-vaginal | Septran, trimethoprim, clarithromycin, ciprofloxacin, fluconazole, miconazole, isoniazid, rifampin, mebendazole, albendazole zidovudine, chloroquine, acyclovir, pyrantel ganciclovir, and oseltamivir (Tamiflu) | Tetracycline derivatives, which can cause discoloration of teeth: Tetracycline, doxycycline, minocycline, sulfa drugs—if near delivery (because they can increase the chance of serious newborn jaundice), quinine, aminoglycosides (cause ototoxicity in 1–2%), and chloramphenicol (Gray baby syndrome) |

of acquired immunodeficiency syndrome (AIDS) or AIDS related complex (ARC) but do not cure the infection.

## Classification of Antiretroviral Drugs

- *Nucleoside reverse transcriptase inhibitors (NRTIs)*: Zidovudine (AZT), didanosine, zalcitabine, stavudine, lamivudine, and abacavir.
- *Non-nucleoside reverse transcriptase inhibitors (NNRTIs)*: Nevirapine, efavirenz, and delavirdine.
- *Protease inhibitor*: Ritonavir, indinavir, nelfinavir, saquinavir, amprenavir, and lopinavir. Safety in pregnancy and side effects of ARV agents are given in **Table 8**.

# DRUGS FOR URINARY TRACT INFECTION IN PREGNANCY (TABLE 9)

Urinary tract infection (UTI) is one of the most common infections occurring during pregnancy. *Escherichia coli* (90–95%), *Klebsiella pneumoniae*, Enterococci, *Proteus mirabilis*, and *Pseudomonas aeruginosa* are the most common organism found in UTI.

# ANTIAMOEBICS

Diloxanide furoate is a safer alternative in pregnancy. Metronidazole, tinidazole, and quiniodochlor should be used with caution in pregnancy.

# ANTIHELMINTICS

Piperazine and niclosamide are safer alternatives in pregnancy. Albendazole, mebendazole, ivermectin, pyrantel pamoate, praziquantel, and diethylcarbamazine may be used with caution in pregnancy.

# ANTIFUNGALS

Topical antifungal agents such as clotrimazole, nystatin, and tolnaftate are safer alternatives in pregnancy.

Amphotericin B, fluconazole, itraconazole, ketoconazole, griseofulvin, and terbinafine are unsafe in pregnancy.

Fluconazole—single dose therapy (150 mg) does not appear to cause adverse pregnancy effects. Repeated doses of fluconazole (400–800 mg daily) have been associated with

**TABLE 8:** Anti-retroviral agents in pregnancy.

| S. no. | Drug | Safety in pregnancy | Adverse effect |
|---|---|---|---|
| 1. | Didanosine | Unsafe | Peripheral neuropathy, rarely pancreatitis, diarrhea, abdomen pain, and nausea |
| 2. | Zidovudine | Safe | Anemia, neutropenia, nausea, anorexia, abdominal pain, headache, insomnia, and myalgia |
| 3. | Lamivudine | Safe | Headache, fatigue, nausea, anorexia, abdominal pain, pancreatitis, and neuropathy |
| 4. | Nevirapine | Safe | Rashes, nausea, headache, fever, rise in liver enzymes, and hepatotoxicity |
| 5. | Nelfinavir | Safe | Diarrhea and flatulence |
| 6. | Saquinavir | Safe | Photosensitivity can occur |
| 7. | Abacavir | Unsafe | Rashes, fever, and flu-like symptoms |
| 8. | Indinavir | Unsafe | Gastrointestinal intolerance, excess of fluids must be consumed to avoid nephrolithiasis |
| 9. | Ritonavir | Unsafe | Nausea, diarrhea, paresthesias, fatigue, and lipid abnormalities |
| 10. | Efavirenz | Unsafe | Rashes, dizziness, headache, insomnia, and variety of neuropsychiatric symptoms |

**TABLE 9:** Common antibiotics for urinary tract infection.

| S. no. | Drug | Dose | Frequency |
|---|---|---|---|
| 1. | *Oral antibiotics* | | |
| | Nitrofurantoin | 100 mg | QID |
| | Ampicillin | 500 mg | QID |
| | Amoxicillin | 500 mg | TDS |
| | Cephalexin | 250 mg | TDS |
| 2. | *Intravenous antibiotics (for pyelonephritis)* | | |
| | Cefuroxime | 750 mg | TDS |
| | Co-amoxiclav | 1.2 g | TDS |
| | Gentamicin | 2–5 mg/kg/day | 8 hourly divided dose |

a consistent pattern of birth defects similar to those seen in animal studies.

## ANTIVIRALS

None of the drugs are safe in pregnancy.

Acyclovir, ganciclovir, foscarnet, amantadine, vidarabine, α-interferon, ribavirin, and zalcitabine are unsafe in pregnancy.

## DRUGS FOR VAGINAL INFECTIONS

Topical vaginal medication such as clindamycin, clotrimazole, econazole, miconazole, and nystatin are safe in pregnancy. Dienestrol and isoconazole are unsafe in pregnancy.

## ANESTHETIC DRUGS

### General Anesthesia

No report of teratogenicity in humans has been associated with the use of thiopental, curare, and succinylcholine.

Inhalational anesthesia including nitrous oxide and halothane have not been reported to increase risk to fetus.

### Local Anesthesia

Use of lidocaine and bupivacaine is not associated with any major or minor malformations of the fetus.

## ORAL CONTRACEPTIVES

Accidental use of oral contraceptives during pregnancy has not been reported to be associated with congenital anomalies.

## ESTABLISHING PREGNANCY EXPOSURE REGISTRIES[56]

In spite of the lack of data on the safety of drug use in human pregnancies, pregnant women are exposed to drugs either as prescribed therapy or inadvertently before pregnancy is known (over one-half of pregnancies are unplanned). Because little is known about the teratogenic potential of a drug in humans before marketing, epidemiologically sound, written study protocols for postmarketing surveillance of drug use in pregnancy is critical for the detection of drug-induced fetal effects.

The FDA defines a pregnancy exposure registry as a prospective observational study that collects information on women who take medicines and vaccines during pregnancy. FDA (2017b) maintain an active list on their webpage titled pregnancy Registries. As of 2017, this included registries for 100 individual medications and for medication groups used to treat asthma, autoimmune disease, cancer, epilepsy, HIV infection, and transplant rejection.[57]

Enrolment requires that the health of the baby be unknown to reduce bias. Data collected on babies born to women taking a particular medicine are compared with babies of women not taking the medicine. Thus, these studies are being increasingly used to proactively monitor for major fetal effects and to describe margins of safety associated with drug exposure during pregnancy. These will provide vital information to the clinicians regarding counseling of a patient on medication as to the actual risk involved to the fetus at different periods of gestation.

While sufficient data is not available to give definitive recommendations regarding the ideal therapy for most of the disorders during pregnancy, this chapter attempts to outline the broadly acceptable clinical therapeutic guidelines and other suitable options available. This chapter is not exhaustive and the reader is encouraged to refer to package inserts and evolving management options appearing from time-to-time in recent journals.

## KEY POINTS

- The use of drugs in pregnancy should be done with caution as any drug or chemical substance administered to the mother may cross the placenta.
- Number of drugs prescribed during pregnancy should be restricted to a minimum, with the lowest effective dose given for the shortest time.
- Drugs should be prescribed in pregnancy only if the benefits outweigh the risks.
- The time period between 35 and 55 days from last menstrual period is most crucial because prior to day 35 all cells are totipotent, so any insult before day 35 will result in either a missed abortion or has no effect on the growing embryo.
- Drugs taken by sexually active men may be excreted in their semen and cause fetal problems.
- Teratogenic drugs are drugs which have potential to develop congenital anomalies in the fetus when administered to a pregnant woman and may cause teratogenicity by disruption of folic acid metabolism, formation of oxidative intermediates, fetal genetic mutations or chaotic gene expression.
- There is paucity of data on the safety of drug use in human pregnancies.
- Epidemiologically sound study protocols for surveillance of drug use and setting up of pregnancy exposure registries is critical for the detection of drug induced fetal effects.

## REFERENCES

1. Young LY, Koda-Kimble MA. Applied Therapeutics: The Clinical Use of Drugs. 6th edition. Vancouver, WA: Applied Therapeutics, Inc.; 1995.
2. DiPiro JT, Talbert RL, Yee GC, Matzke GR, Wells BG, Posey LM. Pharmacotherapy: A Pathophysiologic Approach, 3rd edition. Stamford, CT: Appleton and Lange; 1997. pp. 1565-84.

3. Berkow R. The Merck Manual of Diagnosis and Therapy, 16th edition. In: Rahway NJ (Ed). Boston: Merck Research Laboratories; 1992. pp. 1857-62.
4. Finasteride for benign prostatic hyperplasia. Drug Ther Bull. 1995;33(3):19-21.
5. FDA. Federal Register. 1980;44:37434-67.
6. Briggs GG, Freeman, Roger K. Drugs in Pregnancy and Lactation. A Reference Guide to Fetal and Neonatal Risk, 10th edition. Baltimore, MD: Lippincott Williams & Wilkins; 2015.
7. McQueen KD. Drugs in Pregnancy and Lactation. In: Herfindal T, Gourley DR (Eds). Textbook of Therapeutics: Drug and Disease Management, 6th edition. Baltimore MD: Lippincott Williams & Wilkins; 1996.
8. Food and drug administration, HHS. Content and format of labeling for human prescription drug and biological products; requirements for pregnancy and lactation labeling. Final rule Fed Regist. 2014;79(233):72063-103.
9. Koren G, Pastuszak A, Ito S. Drugs in pregnancy. N Engl J Med. 1998;338(16):1128-37.
10. Koren G, Bologa M, Long D, Feldman Y, Shear NH. Perception of teratogenic risk by pregnant women exposed to drugs and chemicals during the first trimester. Am J Obstet Gynecol. 1989;160(5 Pt 1):1190-4.
11. Saxena P, Salhan S, Sarda N, Nandan D. A randomized comparison between sublingual, oral and vaginal route of misoprostol for pre-abortion cervical ripening in first-trimester pregnancy termination under local anaesthesia. Aust N Z J Obstet Gynaecol. 2008;48(1):101-6.
12. King JF, Grant A, Keirse MJ, Chalmers I. Beta-mimetics in preterm labour: an overview of the randomized controlled trials. Br J Obstet Gynaecol. 1988;95(3):211-22.
13. Goodwin TM, Zograbyan A. Oxtocin receptor antagonists. Update. Clin Perinatol 1998;25(4):859-71.
14. Slattery MM, Morrison JJ. Preterm delivery. Lancet 2002;360(9344):1489-97.
15. Food and drug administration. FDA recommends against prolonged use of Mgso4 to stop preterm labour due to bone changes in exposed babies. Silver Spring: FDA drug safety communication; 2013.
16. King J, Flenady V. Prophylactic antibiotics for inhibiting preterm labor with intact membranes. Cochrane Database Syst Rev. 2002;(4):CD000246.
17. Effect of corticosteroids for fetal maturation on perinatal outcomes. NIH Consensus Development Panel on the effects of cortiocosteroids for fetal maturation on perinatal outcomes. JAMA. 1995;273(5):413-8.
18. Doyle LW, Ford GW, Richards AL, Kelly EA, Davis NM, Callanan C, et al. Antenatal corticosteroids and outcome at 14 years of age in children with birth weight less than 1501 grams. Pediatrics. 2000;106(1):E2.
19. Banks BA, Cnaan A, Morgan MA, Parer JT, Merrill JD, Ballard PL, et al. Multiple courses of antenatal corticosteroids and outcome of premature neonates. North American Thyrotrophin-Releasing Hormone Study Group. Am J Obstet Gynecol. 1999;181(3):709-17.
20. Committee on Obstetric Practice. Committee Opinion No. 713: Antenatal corticosteroid therapy for fetal maturation. Obstet Gynecol. 2017;130(2):e102-9.
21. Gyamfi-Bannerman C, Thom EA, Blackwell SC, Tita AT, Reddy UM, Saade GR, et al. Antenatal betamethasone for women at risk for late preterm delivery. N Engl J Med. 2016;374(14):1311-20.
22. Royal College of Obstetricians & Gynaecologists. The Management of Nausea and Vomiting of Pregnancy and Hyperemesis Gravidarum. Green Top Guidline No. 69. 2016. pp. 25.
23. The use of newer asthma and allergy medications during pregnancy. The American College of Obstetricians and Gynecologists (ACOG) and The American College of Allergy, Asthma and Immunology (ACAAI). Ann Allergy Asthma Immunol. 2000;84(5):475-80.
24. Kar S, Krishnan A, Preetha K, Mohankar A. A review of antihistamines used during pregnancy. J Pharmacol pharmacother. 2012;3(2):105-8.
25a. FDA. (2020). Ranitidine products have been withdrawn from the (Zantac) from the market [news release] [online]. Available from: https://www.fda.gov/news-events/press-announcements/fda-requests-removal-all-ranitidine-products-zantac-market [Last accessed July, 2021].
25b. Mahadevan U, Kane S. American Gastroenterological Association Institute technical review on the use of gastrointestinal medication in pregnancy. Gastroenterology. 2006;131(1):283-311.
26. Webster J. A comparative review of the tolerability profiles of dopamine agonists in the treatment of hyperprolactinaemia and inhibition of lactation. Drug Saf. 1996;14(4):228-38.
27. Webster J. Clinical management of prolactinomas. Baillieres Best Pract Res Clin Endocrinol Metab. 1999;13(3):395-408.
28. Fried S, Kozer E, Nulman I, Einarson TR, Koren G. Malformation rates in children of women with untreated epilepsy: a meta-analysis. Drug Saf. 2004;27(3):197-202.
29. Wyszynski DF, Nambisan M, Surve T, Alsdorf RM, Smith CR, Holmes LB. Increased rate of major malformations in offspring exposed to valproate during pregnancy. Neurology. 2005;64(6):961-5.
30. Cunnington M, Tennis P. Lamotrigine and the risk of malformations in pregnancy. Neurology. 2005;64(6):955-60.
31. Holmes LB. Increased risk for non-syndromic cleft palate among infants exposed to lamotrigine during pregnancy. Teratology. 2006;76(5):318.
32. Montouris G. Gabapentin exposure in human pregnancy: results from the Gabapentin Pregnancy Registry. Epilepsy Behav. 2003;4(3):310-7.
33. Montouris G. Safety of the newer antiepileptic drug oxcarbazepine during pregnancy. Curr Med Res Opin. 2005;21(5):693-701.
34. Molgaard-Nielsen D, Hviid A. Newer generation antiepileptics drugs and the risk of major birth defects. JAMA. 2011;305(19):1996-2002.
35. Askie LM, Duley L, Henderson-Smart DJ, Stewart L. Antiplatelet agents for prevention of pre-eclampsia: a meta-analysis of individual patient data. Lancet. 2007;369(9575):1791-8.
36. National High Blood Pressure Education Working Group Report on high blood pressure in pregnancy. Am J Obstet Gynecol. 1990;163(5 Pt 1):1691-712.
37. Sibai BM, Caritis SM, Thom E, Klebanoff M, McNellis D, Rocco L, et al. Prevention of preeclampsia with low-dose aspirin in healthy, nulliparous pregnant women. The National Institute of Child Health and Human Development Network of Maternal-Fetal Medicine Units. N Engl J Med. 1993;329(17):1213-8.

38. Hauth JC, Goldenberg RL, Parker CR, Philips JB 3rd, Copper RL, DuBard MB, et al. Low-dose aspirin therapy to prevent preeclampsia. Am J Obstet Gynecol. 1993;168(4):1083-91.
39. Kyle PM, Redman CW. Comparative risk-benefit assessment of drugs used in the management of hypertension in pregnancy. Drug Saf. 1992;7(3):223-34.
40. Pangle BL. Drugs in pregnancy and lactation. In: Herfindal ET, Gourley DR (Eds). Textbook of Therapeutics: Drugs and Disease Management, 7th edition. Baltimore: Lippincott Williams and Wilkins; 2000. pp. 2037-50.
41. Horvath JS, Phippard A, Korda A. Clonidine hydrochloride—a safe and effective antihypertensive agent in pregnancy. Obstet Gynecol. 1985;66(5):634-8.
42. Committee on Obstetric Practice. Committee opinion No. 692: Emergent therapy for acute onset, severe hypertension during pregnancy and the postpartum period. Obstet Gynecol. 2017;129(4):e90-5.
43. Cahill A, Odibo AO, Roehl KA, Macones G. 615: Impact of intrapartum antihypertensive on electronic fetal heart rate (EFM) pattern in labor. Am J obstet Gynecol. 2013;208(1):S262.
44. Rouse DJ, Hirtz DG, Thom E, Varner MW, Spong CY, Mercer BM, et al. A randomized controlled trial of magnesium sulphate for the prevention of cerebral palsy (BEAM study). N Engl J Med. 2008;359(9):895-905.
45. OBG Project. (2017). Updated ACOG guidance on gestational diabetes [online]. Available from: https://www.obgproject.com/2017/06/25/acog-releases-updated-guidance-gestational-diabetes/ [Last accessed July, 2021].
46. Rowan JA, Hague WM, Gao W, Battin MR, Moore MP. Metformin versus insulin for the treatment of gestational diabetes. N Engl J Med. 2008;358(19):2003-15.
47. Evans W, Laifer SA, McNanley TJ, Ruzycky A. Management of thromboembolic disease associated with pregnancy. J Matern Fetal Med. 1997;6(1):21-7.
48. Vitale N, de Feo M, de Santo LS, Pollice A, Tedesco N, Cotrufo M. Dose-dependent fetal complications of warfarin in pregnant women with mechanical heart valve. J Am Coll Cardiol. 1999;33(6):1637-41.
49. Practice bulletin No. 123: thromboembolism in pregnancy. Obstet Gynecol. 2011;118(3):718-29.
50. Snider DE Jr, Layde PM, Johnson MW, Lyle MA. Treatment of tuberculosis during pregnancy. Am Rev Respir Dis. 1980;122(1):65-79.
51. RNCT. (2018). Revised National Tuberculosis control Programme (RNTCP) Status Report. Central TB Division, Directorate General of Health Services, Ministry of Health and Family Welfare [online]. Available from: http://www.tbcindia.org [Last accessed July, 2021].
52. American Colleges of Obstetricians & Gynaecologists. (2020). Vaccinating pregnant and Lactating patients against COVID-19 [online]. Available from: http://www.aofog.net/pdf/Vaccinating%20Pregnant%20and%20Lactating%20Patients%20Against%20COVID-19%20_%20ACOG.pdf [Last accessed July, 2021].
53. Bar-Oz B, Einarson T, Einarson A, Boskovic R, O'Brien L, Malm H, et al. Paroxetine and congenital malformations: meta-analysis and consideration of potential confounding factors. Clin Ther. 2007;29(5):918-26.
54. American College of Obstetricians and Gynecologists. Practice Bulletin No. 92: Use of psychiatric medications during pregnancy and lactation. 2008.
55. Livshits A, Seidman DS. Role of NSAIDS in gynecology drugs. Pharmaceuticals (Basel). 2010;3(7):2082-9.
56. Kennedy DL, Uhl K, Kweder SL. Pregnancy Exposure Registries. Drug Saf. 2004;27(4):215-28.
57. Food and drug administration. (2017). Pregnancy registry information for health professional 2017b [online]. Available from: https://www.fda.gov/science-research/womens-health-research/pregnancy-registry-information-health-professionals [Last accessed July, 2021].

# Index

*Page numbers followed by b refer to box, f refer to figure, fc refer to flowchart, and t refer to table.*

## A

Abacavir 407
Abdomen 28
　palpation of 167
Abdominal wall defect 26, 27, 35, 37f
Aberrant right subclavian artery 14, 27
Ablatio placenta 58
ABO incompatibility 150
Abortion 67, 243, 285
Abruptio placentae 51, 58, 170, 210
　diagnosis of 59
　management of 59, 60fc
　types of 58f
Abruption, risk of 366
Acardiac twin 69f
Acellular pertussis vaccine 405
Acetaminophen 277
Achondrogenesis 37
Achondroplasia 11, 37
Acidemia 90
Acid-fast bacilli 329
Acidic glycoprotein 286
Acidosis 254
Acriflavine glycerine 376
Actim® premature rupture of membranes test 127
Activated partial thromboplastin time 311
Activated protein C 387
Acupuncture 140
Acute respiratory distress syndrome 378, 387
Acyclovir 353
Adenosine
　deaminase 330
　monophosphate 116
Adnexa 373
Adnexal mass 373, 374
　symptoms of 373
Adrenoreceptor blockers 207
Adult polycystic disease 34
Advanced cardiac life support 390
Airway 389
　obstruction 379
Alanine
　aminotransferase 311
　transaminase 264, 311
Alcohol 4, 406
　consumption 48
Alkaline phosphatase 264, 266
Alloimmune hemolytic disease 143
Alloimmunization 90
Alpha-adrenergic blockers 401
Alpha-fetoprotein 293, 374
Alpha-methyldopa 277, 282, 401
Alpha-thalassemia 195
　trait 195, 197
Alprazolam 322, 326
American College of Medical Genetics 12
American College of Obstetricians and Gynecologists 7, 12, 80, 93, 108, 114, 136, 139, 154, 169, 172, 188
American Diabetes Association 7, 221
American Institute of Ultrasound in Medicine Practice Guideline 13
American Society for Reproductive Medicine 43
Amniocentesis 11, 18, 19, 19f, 22, 44, 71, 142, 348, 350
Amnioinfusion 108
Amnioreduction 105
Amniosense 127
Amniotic fluid 102, 126, 147, 349, 350
　abnormalities 90, 349
　changes 137
　derangements 102
　disorders of 102
　embolism 387
　index 84, 95, 102-104, 107, 128, 130, 207
　spectrophotometry 147
　volume 91, 94
　　assessment of 102
AmniSure 127
　test 127
Amodiaquine 336
Amoxicillin 407
Amphotericin B 407
Ampicillin 407
Analgesia 381
　epidural 253, 256
Analgesics 385, 406
Anemia 2, 66, 186, 186t, 189t, 190fc, 243, 252, 263
　causes of 188, 189
　classification of 186t, 187t
　clinical features of 187
　congenital 354
　dilutional 378
　etiopathogenesis of 186
　hemolytic 143, 353
　high-risk of 187b
　megaloblastic 194
　severe 90, 199, 335
　treatment for 282
　types of 188, 189, 189t
Anencephaly 30, 137
Anesthesia 359
　general 208, 210, 374
　regional 210
Anesthetic drugs 408
Aneuploidy, invasive prenatal testing for 22
Aneurysm, rupture of cerebral 211
Angiotensin II infusion test 205
Angiotensin receptor blockers 5
Angiotensin-converting enzyme inhibitor 5, 49, 107, 282, 394, 402
*Anopheles culicifacies* 334
Anophthalmia 16
Antacids 399
Antara 200
Antenatal
　care 260
　complications 152
　corticosteroid 54, 62
　　treatment 131
　counseling 159
　factors 154
　fetal compromise, evidence of 171
　management 72, 341
　period 180
Antepartum 361
　aortic balloon valvuloplasty 254
　fetal surveillance 90, 231
　　indications for 90b
　　objectives of 90
　　physiological basis of 90
　　techniques 91
　hemorrhage 51, 62, 64, 66, 187, 188, 385
　　causes of 51, 51fc, 61
　　history of 169
　management, principles of 282
Antiamoebics 407
Antibiotics 116, 142, 406
　indications of 260b
　parenteral 284
Anticancer drugs 394
Anticentromere antibody 190
Anticoagulants, classification of 309
Anticoagulation 302, 313
Anticonvulsants 209, 402
Anti-D immunoglobulin 145
Antidepressants 277, 323, 324, 326
　drugs 406
Antidopaminergic drugs 399
Antiemetics 277, 397
　drugs 397
Antiepileptics 400, 400t
　drugs 290, 291, 292b, 400
　　teratogenic side effects of 292t
　lamotrigine 400
Antifungals 407
　agents 277
Antigens 142t
Antihelmintics 407
Antihistamines 397

Antihypertensive 207, 214, 216, 401
    drugs 208f, 401
        therapy 207, 216
            parenteral 208
Anti-infective agents 406, 407t
Anti-Kell alloimmunization 147
Antimetabolites 406
Antineoplastics 406
Antinuclear antibody 46, 190
Antiobesity surgery 360
Anti-obsessive medication 322
Antiphospholipid syndrome 45, 205, 300
        diagnostic criteria 300
        epidemiology 300
        fetal risks 301
        management 301
        maternal risks 301
        pathogenesis 300
        preconception counseling 301
Antipsychotics 323, 324, 326
Antiretroviral agents 406, 407t
Antiretroviral drugs 342
    classification of 407
Antiretroviral therapy 331, 342
Anti-Sjögren syndrome 190
Antithrombotic agents, dose of 301
Antithrombotic therapy 404
Antithyroid
    antibodies 238
    drugs 239, 241
    medication, high doses of 241
Antitubercular drugs 405
Antitubercular treatment 331
Antitussives 399
Antivirals 408
Anuria 335
Anxiety 5, 327
    antenatal 357
    disorder 293, 320
        generalized 319
        perinatal 319
    symptoms 319
Anxiolytics 385
Aorta, coarctation of 16, 30, 256
Aortic coarctation 214
Aortic dissection 257, 312
Aortic stenosis 30, 254
Aortic valve 254
Appendicitis 213, 373
Arachnoid cyst 33
Aripiprazole 322
Array-based comparative genome
    hybridization 20, 44
Arrhythmias 249, 252, 259, 259b
    cardiac 259
    supraventricular 255
Artemisia annua 336
Arterial blood gas 383
    analysis 311
    values 383t
Arteriography 312
Artery
    peak systolic velocity 146
    pulmonary 258, 382
Arthralgia 349
Arthritis 349

Artificial larynx 94
Ascites 265
Aspartate transaminase 311
Asphyxia 138
Aspiration 387
Aspirin 258
    low-dose 214, 298
Assisted breech delivery 173, 174f
Assisted reproductive technique 2, 52, 64,
    65, 302
Asthma 4, 5, 390, 396, 398t
Atelectasis 138
Atenolol 401
Atosiban 395, 396
Atrial flutter 29
Atrial septal defect 16, 29, 255
Attenuated influenza vaccine 405
Augmentation 160
Autoimmune diseases 297, 303
Autoimmune disorders 297, 298
Autonomic dysfunction 230
Autosomal dominant polycystic kidney
    disease 286
Azathioprine 299
Azygos 379

## B

Bacteriuria 281
    asymptomatic 113, 284
Balloon mitral valvotomy 254
Banana sign 31
Bariatric surgery 360
Barker hypothesis 7
Beclomethasone 398
Behavioral disorders 318
Behçet's disease 302, 303
Benzodiazepine 322, 323, 326
Beta-adrenergic blockers 401
Beta-agonists 395, 396
Beta-blockers 239, 240, 258, 282
Betadine 344
Betamethasone acetate 397
Betamimetics 116
Beta-thalassemia 11, 195
    major 195, 198
    minor 195, 197
    pathophysiology of 196fc
Bicarbonaturia 281
Bicuspid aortic valve 257
Biochemical serum markers 13, 14, 112
Biometry 82
Biophysical profile 84, 86, 91, 94, 139, 206,
    300
    interpretation of 95
    modified 91, 95
    physiologic basis for 94
    score 94t, 131
Biophysical tests 205
Birth
    asphyxia 179
    defects, majority of 25
    preterm 2, 5, 7, 110, 158, 207, 358
    trauma 225
        injury 227
Bladder 26
    function, disturbance of 372

Blake's pouch cyst 32
Blastomere biopsy 22
Bleomycin 374, 406
Blood
    count, complete 129, 211
    glucose 220
        control 222
    pressure 188, 202, 275, 282, 379
        high 401
        measurement of 202
    sugar
        estimation 104
        level 225
        monitoring of 222, 230
    tests 39
    transfusion 159, 200
        indications of 199t
Body mass index 64, 87, 154, 218, 220
    abnormal 48
Bone
    fracture 138
    length abnormalities 37
    marrow
        activity 188
        aspiration 190
Bradycardia 29
Brain 204
Breast abscess 340
Breastfeeding 1, 241, 260, 340, 345
Breech
    complete 167
    delivery 174
        conduct of 173
        perinatal outcome in 179
        spontaneous 173
    extraction 178
    incomplete 167
    presentation 166, 166f, 167, 167f, 168
        management of 169
    types of 167
    vaginal delivery 169
Bromocriptine 400
Brompheniramine 399
Bronchial asthma, drugs for 398
Bronchocele, congenital 182
Brow presentation 183
Budd-Chiari syndrome 277
Burn Marshall's technique 173,
    176, 177f
Buspirone 322

## B

Cabergoline 257, 400
Calcium 360
    channel blockers 116-118, 208, 258,
        395, 396, 401, 402
Canadian Early and Mid-Trimester
    Amniocentesis Trial 19
Cancer
    cervix 6, 370, 371
    extent of 370
Candida 368
Cannabis 4
Capnography 382
Carbamazepine 292, 293, 322, 394, 400

Carbimazole 240
Carbohydrate
 infusions 385
 metabolism 218, 219, 219*fc*
Carcinoma, hepatocellular 274
Cardiac arrest 389
Cardiac decompensation 199
Cardiac defects 16, 29, 252
 structural 29
Cardiac disease 357
 congenital 5
Cardiac dysfunction 6
Cardiac failure 239
 congestive 196
Cardiac involvement 214
Cardiac lesions, risk categories of 250*b*
Cardiac output 249
Cardiomyopathy
 hypertrophic 7, 258
 peripartum 257
Cardiotocography 84, 86, 115, 130, 131, 150
 computerized 84, 86
 continuous 160
Cardiovascular defects 25
Cardiovascular disease 80, 228, 293
Cardiovascular system 205, 230, 378
Cartridge based nucleic acid amplification technology 331
Cataracts 353
Catheter embolectomy 314
Caudal dysplasia limb reduction defects 366
Caudal regression syndrome 228
Cavum septum pellucidum 27
Cefuroxime 407
Centchroman 200
Central nervous system 17, 25, 92, 393
 malformations 16
Central venous pressure 61, 380, 382
Cephalexin 407
Cephalopelvic disproportion 225
Cerebral artery, middle 83, 83*f*, 85, 86, 95, 96, 97*f*, 104, 146, 147, 354
Cerebral venous sinus thrombosis 291
Cerebroplacental ratio 80, 85, 86, 97
Cerebrospinal fluid 330, 335
Cervical
 assessment 112
 cancer 367, 370-372
  diagnosis of 370
  invasive 369
  management of 370
 cerclage 113
 distortion 369
 edema 375
 fibroid 366
 function, abnormal 111
 incompetency 45
 weakness 45
Cervicovaginal discharge, microscopic examination of 126*f*
Cervicovaginal fibronectin 112
Cervix 181
 detachment of 376
 dilated 376
 early stage invasive lesions of 371*fc*

 local lesions of 61
 manual stretching of 376
 preinvasive lesions of 369, 369*fc*
Cesarean delivery 66, 75, 153*t*, 169, 366
 previous 52, 153*f*
Cesarean myomectomy
 advantages of 367
 steps of 368*f*
Cesarean scar pregnancy 152
Cesarean section 56, 60-62, 128, 145, 152, 179, 181, 225, 367
 multiple 152
 primary 183
Chayya 200
Chemoprophylaxis 336
Chemoradiation 372
Chemotherapy 372
 adjuvant 374
Chest
 compressions 389
 X-ray 331
Childhood infection, mild 353
Chills 352
Chlamydia trachomatis 339, 341
Chlordiazepoxide 322, 326
Chlorhexidine 344
Chlorothiazides 277
Chlorpheniramine 399
Chlorproguanil 336
Chlorpromazine 322
Cholangitis, primary sclerosing 269
Cholesterol 282
Cholestyramine 270
Chondrodysplasia punctata 37
Chorioamnionitis 128, 149, 339, 344
 signs of 131*b*
 symptoms of 131*b*
Chorioangioma 80
Chorionic villus sampling 11, 20, 20*f*, 44, 71, 144, 348, 349
 transabdominal 20
 transcervical 20
Chorionicity, determination of 77
Chorioretinitis 353
Choroid plexus cyst 27
Chromosomal study 40
Chromosomal trisomies 27
Churg-Strauss syndrome 302
Cimetidine 399
Circumvallate placenta 80
Cirrhosis 276
 diagnosis of 276
 primary biliary 269
Cisplatin 374
Cisterna magna, obliteration of 31
Cleft lip 16
Cleft palate 16
Clomipramine 322
Clonazepam 322
Clozapine 322
Clubfoot 16
Coagulation
 abnormal 203
 disorder 62
 failure 62
Coagulopathy, management of 61

Co-amoxiclav 407
Cocaine 394
Coeliac disease 231
Collagen vascular
 disease 205
 disorders 90, 319
Colposcopy 369
Computed tomography 168
 pulmonary angiography 312
Congenital defects 249
Congenital disorder 10
Conjunctivitis 349
Connective tissue disorders 29, 214
Conservative surgery 161
Continuous electronic fetal heart monitoring 150
Continuous intravenous infusion 212
Continuous positive airway pressure 384
Contraception 1, 200, 226, 261, 294, 295, 332, 345
Contraceptives
 effect of 326
 emergency 345
 metabolism of 327
Contraction stress test 91
Coombs' test, indirect 144, 145
Copper intrauterine contraceptive device 200
Cord
 blood sampling 348, 350
 compression 128
 examination of 40
 multiple loops of 182
 prolapse 3, 128, 178
 round neck, tight loop of 182
Cordocentesis 21, 21*f*, 147
 intrahepatic 21*f*
Coronavirus disease-19 (COVID-19) 390, 391
 vaccine 405
Corpus callosum, agenesis of 16
Cortical necrosis 214
Corticosteroids 73, 86, 115, 270, 299, 302, 303, 396
 therapy 299
Corticotropin releasing hormone 110, 112
Coryza, mild 349
Cotrimoxazole prophylactic therapy 343, 344
Cough, nocturnal 251
Cranial abnormalities 349
C-reactive protein 131, 190
Creatinine 202
Crepitations 187
Cromolyn sodium 398
Crown-rump length 12
 measurement 25
Cushing's syndrome 214
Cyanosis 311, 379
Cyclooxygenase 119, 299
Cyclophosphamide 298
Cyclopia 16
Cyclosporine 299
 metabolism 260
Cyclovir 354

Cystadenoma
- mucinous 373
- serous 373

Cystic fibrosis 11, 15
Cystic hygroma 27, 33, 33*f*, 34*f*
- detection of 12

Cytokines 365
Cytomegalovirus 85, 347-349
- infection 15
  - management of 352
  - prevention of 352
  - primary maternal 351

Cytotrophoblast 20
- invasion, abnormal 203

# D

Daily fetal movement count 131
Dalteparin 310
Danaparoid 309, 310
Dandy-Walker malformation 32, 33, 33*f*
Dapsone 336
Daunorubicin 406
Deaf mutism 243
Death, perinatal 159
Debulking surgery 374
Decidual cell reactions 372
Deep vein thrombosis 307, 308, 309*fc*, 313
- management of 309
- prevention of 307
- signs 307
- symptoms 307

Defibrillation 389
Degludec 404
Dehydration 3
Delivering oxygen therapy, methods of 383*t*
Delivery 1, 56, 209, 215, 343
- conduct of 120
- indications of 86*b*, 86*t*
- mode of 85, 132, 153, 209, 225
- morbidity 228
- preterm 111*b*, 228
- route of 54, 74
- timing of 54, 57, 73, 85, 86*t*, 132, 150, 224

Deoxyribonucleic acid 15
Depot medroxyprogesterone acetate 200, 345
Depression 3, 4, 5, 327
- antenatal 357
- perinatal 318
- postnatal 2
- postpartum 66, 226, 357

Depressive disorder 320
Detemir 404
Dexamethasone sodium phosphate 397
Dexlansoprazole 399
Diabetes in Pregnancy Study Group 221
Diabetes insipidus 213
Diabetes mellitus 4, 5, 90, 205, 214, 218, 219, 220*b*, 229*b*, 390
- classification of 218
- effect of 228
- epidemic of 218
- gestational 2, 5-7, 66, 138, 219, 220, 221*t*, 222, 323, 357, 360, 404
- glycemic management of 225
- pathophysiology of 218
- pregestational 80, 218, 227, 229, 230
- prevalence of 218
- signs of 229
- symptoms of 229
- type 1 226
- type 2 231

Diabetic ketoacidosis 226, 232
- treatment of 232

Dialysis 287
Diaphragmatic hernia 16, 17, 300
- prognosis of 37*b*

Diazepam 322, 326, 402, 403
Dichorionic twin pregnancy 25*f*
Didanosine 407
Dietary therapy 231
Diethylstilbestrol 111, 394
Differential leukocyte count 129, 130
Dimenhydrinate 397
Direct antiglobulin test 150
Direct thrombin inhibitors 310
Direct-acting antiviral drugs 274
Discordant fetal growth 72
Disseminated intravascular coagulation 59, 204, 213, 265
Diuretics 402
Dizygotic twins 64
Domestic abuse 4, 319
Domperidone 397
Dopaminergic antagonists 397
Doppler
- assessment 82
- sonography 12
- ultrasonography 95
- velocimetry 91, 131
- venous ultrasound 308, 308*f*

Double outlet right ventricle 16, 30
Double vessel umbilical cord 17
Down syndrome 11, 13-15, 17, 19, 232
Doxorubicin 406
Doxylamine 397
Drugs 393
- number of 393
- resistant tuberculosis, programmatic management of 331
- treatment 131, 191
- use of 393

Duchenne muscular dystrophy 11
Ductus venosus 12, 83, 84*f*, 85, 95
- Doppler 98*f*
- sonography of 12
- normal 84*f*

Duodenal atresia 16, 36
Dye dilution method 102
Dye test, negative 126
Dyselectrolytemia 232, 291
Dysfunctional labor 128, 366
Dysgerminomas, extragonadal 375
Dyslipidemia 359
Dysplasia
- chondroectodermal 37
- low-grade 368
- lymphatic 38
- multicystic 34
- skeletal 37

Dyspnea
- progressive 251
- sudden 311

# E

Echogenic bowel 15, 27
Eclampsia 210, 211, 213, 216, 293, 294
Eczema 314, 396
Edema 203
- cerebral 278
- interstitial 382
- pulmonary 210, 249, 252, 253, 312

Edward syndrome 11, 17
Efavirenz 407
Ehlers-Danlos syndrome 125
Eisenmenger syndrome 256
Elective repeat cesarean delivery 157
Electrocardiogram 311
Electroconvulsive therapy 325
- modified 325

Electrolytes 225, 282, 310
Elemental iron content 193*t*
Embolism, pulmonary 311, 313*fc*
Emphasis 342
Encephalitis 211, 293
Encephalocele 30, 30*f*, 40*f*
Encephalopathy 265
- hepatic 278, 378
- hypoxic ischemic 143, 157, 159

End-diastolic
- flow 82
- velocity 82*f*-84*f*

Endocardial cushion defects 16
Endocarditis, infective 249, 253
Endocrine disorders 214
Endometrioma 373
Endometritis 48
- postpartum 128

Endothelial cell injury 203
Endothelial dysfunction 358
Endotoxemia 284
Endotracheal intubations 207
Enoxaparin 301, 310
Enterocolitis, necrotizing 131
Enzyme-linked immunosorbent assay 112
Epilepsy 4, 211, 290, 291
- effect of 291
- management of 294*b*, 295
- uncontrolled 293

Episodes 321
Epithelium, columnar 369
Ergometrine 258
Erythema 308
- infectiosum 353

Erythroblast precursors 353
Erythrocyte sedimentation rate 378
Erythropoiesis 143
*Escherichia coli* 407
Escitalopram 322
Esophageal atresia 16, 36
Estriol, unconjugated 14
Ethambutol 405
Ethanol 394
Ethionamide 332

Etoposide 374
Etretinate 395
European Society of Human Reproduction 43
Euthyroid 47
Expectorants 399
External cephalic version 74, 169, 170, 170f, 181
    complications of 170
    timing of 169
Extrahepatic biliary obstruction 277
Ex-utero intrapartum treatment 39
Eyes 205

## F

Face 27
    presentation 182
Facial anomalies 16
Facial cleft 33
Famotidine 399
Fast hug approach 381, 381t
Fatty liver
    acute 213, 263, 265, 267, 267b, 267t, 271, 275
    disease, non-alcoholic 276
Federation of Obstetric and Gynaecological Societies of India 43, 47
Feeding 381
Femur 15
    length 83f
Fern test 126
Ferrous
    ascorbate 192
    fumarate 192
    gluconate 192
    glycine sulfate 192
    salts 277
    succinate 192
    sulfate 192
Fertility 356
    sparing surgery 374
Fetal
    abdomen, transverse scan of 36f, 38f
    acidosis 159
    affection 350, 352
    alcohol syndrome 4
    anemia, estimate severity of 148f
    aneuploidy 11
        high-risk of 19
    anomaly 64, 366
        detection of 84
    arterial Doppler 95
    asphyxia 293
    autopsy 40
    blood 20, 339
        sampling 21, 147, 149
        vessels 20
    breathing movements 94
    cardiac
        arrhythmia 29
        blood sampling 21
    cells 17, 19
    chromosomal abnormalities 18, 28
    complications 103, 189, 357, 358

    compromise 98f
        Doppler in 98
    cystoscopy 108
    death 27, 90, 210
        unexplained 145
    deoxyribonucleic acid, detection of 17
    distress 170
    ductus venosus 97
    dysrhythmias 28
    echocardiography 29
        indications for 28b
    evaluation 206
    extracardiac abnormalities 28
    extremity 29
    factors 91
    fibronectin 112, 115fc
        assay 114
    growth restriction 3, 7, 17, 64, 80, 81, 85, 87t, 90, 96f, 97, 106, 169, 186, 205, 224, 229, 306, 329
        early-onset of 80, 85fc
        etiology of 80t
        late onset 81, 86
        management of 85
        prevention of 86
        risk of 282
        screening of 86
    heart 28f, 55
        rate 29, 90, 92f, 129
        sound 60, 173
        tracing 137
    hematopoiesis 143
    hemoglobin, hereditary persistence of 196
    hypothyroidism, treatment for 241
    hypoxia 103, 138
    imaging 16
    implications 359
    infection 85, 353, 354
        diagnosis of 347
    intrahepatic vessel sampling 21
    kick count 91
    macrosomia 137, 225
    membranes 124
        rupture of 124
        status of 339
    monitoring 131, 138, 383
    movement assessment 91
    nasal bone 26
    neuroprotection 73, 115, 132
    nonstress test 224
    outcome 137
    presentation, abnormal 3
    risks 66, 67, 157, 214
    structural malformation 16
    surgery, role of 39
    surveillance 207, 283
        indications of 90
    thyroid
        function 241
        gland 237
        physiology 237
    thyrotoxicosis 241, 242
    tissue biopsy 21
    tone 94

    transfusion therapy 149
    triploidy 205
    venous Doppler 97
        basis of 97
        evaluation of 97
    weight, estimated 80, 85, 171
Fetomaternal
    monitoring 129
    factors 137
Fetoscopy 22
Fetus
    assessment of 90
    congenital
        anomaly of 169
        malformations of 182
    papyraceus 67f
    transverse scan of 34f, 35f
    upper abdomen of 37f
Fever 391
Fibroids 366
    nonpedunculated 367
First trimester screening 12, 25
    objectives of 25
Flexed breech 166f, 167
Fluconazole 407
Fluid management 254
Fluorescent in situ hybridization 19, 44
Fluoxetine 322
Fluvoxamine 322
Folic acid 32, 187, 193
    deficiency 58, 193
    high dose 229, 321, 323
    supplementation 230, 292
    tablet 343
Fondaparinux 309, 310
Footling breech 167, 167f, 171
Frank breech 167
Fresh frozen plasma 60
Furosemide 285
Fusobacterium 111

## G

Gabapentin 292, 400
Gallbladder
    disease 213
    function 268
Gamma-aminobutyric acid 400
    activity of 403
Gamma-glutamyltransferase 266
Gastroenteritis 213
Gastroesophageal reflux, oral option for 399t
Gastrointestinal
    anomalies 17
    complications 385
    drugs 399
    malformations 16
    symptoms 241
    system 35, 379
    tract 104
Gastroschisis 35, 37f
Genetic sonography 16
Genital
    infection 357
    prolapse 375

tract 358
    viral load in 340
  ulcers 303
Genitourinary
  anomalies 17
  injury 159
  system 33
  tract 28
Gentamicin 407
German measles 348
Gestation, multiple 90, 120, 205
Gestational age 25, 54, 80, 83f, 86, 181
  small for 2, 87, 291
Gilbert's disease 277
Girth, abdominal 81, 82
Glargine 404
Glomerular capillary endotheliosis 283
Glomerular filtration rate 227, 236, 281
Glomerulonephritis 213, 214, 284
  mesangiocapillary 281
  primary 284
Glucocorticoids 108
  therapy, antenatal 115
Glucose
  control 381
  level, abnormal 222
  tolerance test 104
Glulisine 404
Glyburide 223, 404
  dose of 223
Glycemic control 225, 230
Glyceryl trinitrate 395, 396
Gonadotropin-releasing hormone 6
Granisetron 397
Granuloma, caseating 330
Grave's disease 5, 238, 240, 242, 245
Gravid uterus
  displacements of 372
  retroversion of 372
Great vessels, transposition of 30
Griseofulvin 393, 407
Growth
  abnormalities 67
  fetal assessment of 252
Gynecological diseases 365

## H

Halofantrine 336
Haloperidol 322
Hashimoto's thyroiditis 242
Hb Bart's disease 195
HbH disease 195, 197
Head 30
  delivery of 176
Headache 212, 352
  persistent severe 210
Hearing loss, sensorineural 352
Heart 25, 28
  block 259
  burn 223
  defects 357
  disease 249, 251, 253b
    antenatal 252
    congenital 28, 249, 251, 255
    diagnosis and workup 251

history 251
  ischemic 5
  management 252
  maternal complications of 252
  physical examination 251
  preconception counseling 250
  preconception risk assessment 250
  rheumatic 249, 253, 255
  types of 249
failure 258
  congestive 252, 256, 354
lesions, cyanotic 257
rate 380
  baseline 93f
  irregular 29
transplant 259
valves, prosthetic 255
*Helicobacter pylori* infection 272
Hemodialysis 287
Hemodynamic instability, causes of 382
Hemolysis, elevated liver enzymes and low
    platelets syndrome 210-212, 216,
    263, 265-268, 270, 271, 275
  clinical features 270
  course 271
  diagnosis of 212
  differential diagnosis of 213, 271
  laboratory changes 270
  management of 271
  mode of delivery 271
  pathogenesis 270
  prognosis 272
Hemolytic disease 142t
Hemolytic-uremic syndrome 213, 271, 283,
    285, 286
Hemoptysis 251
Hemorrhage 66, 228, 371
  accidental 51, 58
  antepartum 51, 62, 64, 66,
    187, 188, 385
  causes of 386
  cerebral 213, 257
  decidual 111
  fetomaternal 142, 143, 144b
  gastric 263
  intracerebral 213
  intracranial 211, 294
  intraventricular 87, 129
  maternal 385
  postpartum 3, 67, 187, 188, 263,
    366, 385
  severe 62
Heparin 310
  unfractionated 46, 309, 311, 405
Hepatic dysfunction, acute 275t
Hepatic failure, acute 275, 277
Hepatic injury, drug-induced 277
Hepatic microsomal enzymes 295
Hepatitis 275
  A virus 267, 273
  acute viral 263, 272, 275
  autoimmune 276
  B 341
    infection 273
    surface antigen 267
    virus 273, 343

  C 339, 341
    virus 273, 274, 343
  chronic 269
  E 274
    virus 267, 273, 274
  viral 213, 271, 273t
Hepatorenal failure 263
Hepatorenal syndrome 286
Hepatotoxins 276
Hernia
  congenital diaphragmatic 36
  physiologic 26
Herpes simplex 348
  hepatitis 274
  virus 339, 347, 349, 368
    infection, recurrent 352
High-grade squamous intraepithelial
    lesion 369
High-performance liquid chromatography
    196
Histopathology 40
Holoprosencephaly 16, 32
Homan's sign 308
Home uterine activity monitoring 111
Homocysteine, serum 194
Hookworm 339
Hormone, luteinizing 47
Horseshoe kidney 16, 17
Human chorionic gonadotropin 43, 86,
    236, 368
  free beta-subunit of 12
Human epididymis protein 375
Human fetal brain 237
Human fetus 90
Human immunodeficiency virus
    329, 334, 338, 338t, 339b,
    345, 406
  cesarean section 344
  effect of 345
  factors affecting 338
  infections 338
    management 341
  management of 341
  maternal factors 339
  postpartum care 345
  steady decline of 338t
  transmission of 341
  viral load 339
Human insulin 403
Human leukocyte antigen 46, 143, 260
Human papillomavirus 368
Human parvovirus B19 353
Human placental lactogen 219
Hyaline membrane disease 227
Hydralazine 209, 401
Hydramnios 66, 103
  mild 103
  moderate 103
  severe 103
  types of 103t
Hydration 115
Hydrocephalus 32
Hydrocortisone 397
Hydronephrosis 16, 17, 35
Hydrops fetalis 38, 39b
Hydrosalpinx 373

Hydroxychloroquine 298, 299
Hydroxyprogesterone caproate 394
Hyperaldosteronism, primary 214
Hyperandrogenism 47
Hyperbilirubinemia 143, 227, 229, 276
    congenital 277, 277*fc*
Hypercalcemia 272
Hypercalciuria 286
Hypercapnia, permissive 384
Hypercarbia 254
Hypercoagulability 306
Hyperemesis gravidarum 66, 213, 260, 266, 272, 397
    clinical features 272
    differential diagnosis 272
    liver involvement 272
Hyperglycemia 218, 224, 226, 232
    classification of 219*fc*
    maternal 232
Hyperinsulinemia 47
Hyperparathyroidism 214
Hyperprolactinemia 47
Hyperpyrexia, maternal 336
Hypersecretion 47
Hyperstimulation 92
Hypertension 4, 5, 58, 66, 138, 169, 202, 213, 228, 252, 282, 357, 400
    acute severe 208, 209*t*, 216
    chronic 7, 80, 202, 203, 205, 214, 214*b*, 216, 282, 401
    classification of 203, 203*b*
    control severe 211
    essential 214
    gestational 202, 203, 209, 243
    noncirrhotic portal 276
    portal 276
    portopulmonary 87
    pregnancy-induced 2, 3, 108, 187
    pulmonary 254, 256, 387
        artery 256
    renovascular 214
    severe 303
    uncontrolled severe 210
Hypertensive disorders 7, 90, 202, 357
Hyperthyroid disease 239
Hyperthyroidism 29, 214, 238, 252
    antenatal management of 239
    diagnosis of 239
    effect of 239
    fetal effects of 241
    gestational transient 238
    management of 241*b*
    medical therapy 239
    surgical treatment 240
    treatment of 239*b*
Hypoalbuminemia 400
Hypocalcemia 7, 227, 229
Hypoglycemia 138, 224, 227, 229, 265, 291, 335
    detection of 225
    hypoketonemic 227
    neonatal 223, 240
    risk of 218, 230
    symptomatic 227
Hypomagnesemia 227, 229

Hyponatremia 400
Hypoperfusion 285
Hypoplasia
    adrenal 137
    muscular 353
    pulmonary 106, 128
Hypoplastic nasal bone 14, 27
Hypospadias 291
Hypotension 311, 387
Hypothalamic-pituitary axis
    activation of 110
    dysfunction 6, 110
Hypothyroid, subclinical 47
Hypothyroidism 242, 243
    antenatal management 243
    clinical features 242
    diagnosis 242
    fetal concerns 243
    intrapartum management 243
    management of 243, 244*b*
    maternal concerns 243
    postnatal management 243
    subclinical 46, 242, 244
Hypovolemia 285
Hypoxemia 90, 249
Hypoxia 90, 254
    maternal 241
    monitoring for 85
Hysterectomy 58, 159, 161
Hysterosalpingography 44
Hysterotomy, resuscitative 389

# I

Immunofluorescence
    assay 340
    test 354
Immunoglobulin
    G 298, 351
    intravenous 302
    M 267, 350
Immunosuppressive
    agents 302
    drugs 406
    therapy 257
Immunotherapy 46
Imperforate anus 16
In vitro fertilization 6, 64, 87, 302, 307
    conceptions 356
Indigo carmine test 126
Indinavir 407
Indirect thrombin inhibitors 309
Indomethacin 105, 395, 396, 406
Induction 160
Indwelling catheter 373
Infarctions 47, 80, 128, 228, 358, 367
Infections 111
    congenital 347, 348, 354
    opportunistic 341
    potential routes of 340
    signs of 354
    symptoms of 354
    treatment of 113
    viral 275, 368
Inferior vena cava 97, 249, 314
Inflammation 111

Inflammatory bowel disease 4, 5, 373
Infliximab 299
Injury
    avoidance of 211
    endothelial 306
Insulin 223, 403
    analogs 224
    detemir 223
    glargine 223, 224
    like growth factor binding protein-1 126
    metabolism 47
    pump therapy 231
    rapid-acting analogs of 403
    regimens 224
    resistance, development of 219
    sensitizing agents 359
    therapy 223, 231, 403
    types of 223, 404
Intensive care unit 130, 378, 380
Interferon 274
    gamma release assays 330
Intermittent intramuscular injections 212
Internal podalic version 179*f*
International Association of Diabetes and Pregnancy Study Group 221
International Normalized Ratio 266, 311
Intra-amniotic thyroxine 241
Intracranial damage 138
Intracytoplasmic sperm injection 64
Intrahepatic cholestasis 90, 263, 268
    clinical course 269
    diagnosis 269
    etiology 268
    incidence 268
    management 270
    symptoms of 269
Intrapartum
    care 150, 260
    considerations 225
    issues 359
    management 74, 105, 210, 314, 326
    period 180
Intrauterine
    contraceptive device 188, 226
    death 138, 169, 205, 293
    devices 261
    fetal death 229
    growth restriction 69
        symmetrical 28
    transfusion 142, 146, 149
Intravascular intrauterine transfusion 149*b*
Invasive amnioreduction 105
Invasive disease 370
Invasive obstetric procedures 142
Iodides 240, 395
Iodine
    deficiency
        chronic 237
        maternal 237
        severe 237
    nutrition 237
    requirements 236
Iron 360
    deficiency 190
        anemia 186, 189, 191, 191*t*
    dextran 192

prophylaxis 191
sucrose 192
supplementation 191
therapy 193
Irritable bowel syndrome 277
Isolated mild renal dysfunction 281
Isometric exercise 205
Isoniazid 330, 405
Isotretinoin 395
Isoxsuprine 395, 396
Itraconazole 407

## J

Jaundice 263, 264, 265, 267*fc*, 335
   causes of 264, 264*t*
   hemolytic 276
   history of 264
   prevalence of 263
Joint pain 223
Joubert syndrome 33, 33*f*
Jugular venous pressure 187, 188

## K

Kanamycin 332
Ketoconazole 407
Kidney 26, 205
   abnormalities 33
   disease, multicystic 34*f*
   dysfunction 283
   function test 211
   injury, acute 61
   stones 283
   transplant recipients 288
*Klebsiella pneumoniae* 407
Kleihauer screening test 145
Kleihauer-Betke test 145
Koplik's spots 349

## L

Labetalol 208, 209, 282, 401
Labor
   after cesarean delivery, trial of 154, 157
   and delivery 32, 35, 36, 252
   augmentation of 161
   conduct of 120
   induction of 136, 138, 139, 357
   management of 160, 199
   mechanism of 168, 183
   monitoring progress of 173
   obstructed 366
   spontaneous 210, 256
      onset of 139
   third stage of 61, 161
Lactate dehydrogenase 190, 194, 266, 271
Lactational amenorrhea method 200
Lactic acid dehydrogenase 204, 375
Lamivudine 407
Lamotrigine 292, 293, 295, 322
Lansoprazole 399
Laparoscopy 374
Laparotomy 374
Last menstrual period 81, 136, 139
Laxatives 399

Leflunomide 298
Left ventricular hypertrophy 214
Leiomyoma 365
Lemon sign 31, 31*f*
Leopold's maneuvers 167
Lepirudin 309
Leukocytosis 366
Leukomalacia, periventricular 87
Levetiracetam 292, 400
Levonorgestrel intrauterine system 282
Levothyroxine 242
   trial 47
Lewis antibodies 150
Limbs
   defects, risk of 228
   shortening of 37*t*
Line probe assay 331
Lipid infusions 385
Lithium 322, 323, 324, 395
Liver 204
   biopsy 271
   disease 266*t*
      causes of 263
      chronic 267
      end-stage 278
      pregnancy-related 265
   enzymes 343
   failure, acute 275
   function 263
      test 211, 263-265, 275, 277
   hematoma, subcapsular 213
   injury, drug-induced 277
   support 278
   transplantation 278
Lorazepam 322, 326
Lovset's maneuver 175, 175*f*
Low-birth weight 1, 5, 6, 67
   babies 2
   breech 171
Low-dose dopamine infusion 285
Lower segment cesarean section 31, 56, 139, 153, 171, 181
Lower urinary tract obstruction 35, 107
Low-grade squamous intraepithelial lesion 369
Low-molecular weight heparin 46, 283, 309, 311, 405
Lumefantrine 336
Lupus
   anticoagulant 190, 298
   antibody 108
   favor of 284
   neonatal 298
   nephritis 283
Luteal phase defect 47
Lymph nodes 330, 370
   infiltration 370
Lymphadenectomy 371
Lymphovascular invasion 371

## M

Macroglossia 16
Macrosomia 3, 138, 158, 227, 229, 357, 358
Magaldrate 399

Magnesium sulfate 73, 86, 115, 117, 118, 132, 209, 212, 216, 395, 396, 402
Major depression 318
   diagnosis of 318
Malaria 85, 334, 349
   clinical features 335
   complete 335
   complicated 337
   congenital 336
   diagnosis 335
   pathogenesis 334
   severe 335
   signs 335
   symptoms 335
   treatment 335
Malarial parasite, life cycle of 334
Malformation
   congenital 25*t*, 29, 68, 228
   conotruncal 30
Malpresentation 52, 67, 128, 166, 366
   risk of 366
   types of 166
Mantoux test 330
Manual left uterine displacement 389
Marfan's syndrome 250
Maternal
   antithyroid drugs, fetal effects of 241
   benefits 157
   blood 339
   complications 103, 189, 357
   consequences 359
   death 159
      causes of 263
   deterioration, signs of 379
   diabetes 28
   factors 91
   fetal surveillance 130*t*
   hemoglobin disorder 90
   hemorrhage 385
      management of 385
   infection 348, 350
      diagnosis of 347
   morbidity 156
   mortality 156
      high risk of 251*b*
   neutralizing antibody status 339
   risks 66, 214
   serum alpha-fetoprotein 14, 26
   surveillance 207, 282
   systemic lupus erythematosus 28
   transmission 297
   uterine circulation 98
   weight 3
Mauriceau-Smellie-Viet maneuver 176, 178*f*
Measles 405
Mechanical ventilation 384
   conventional 384
Meckel-Gruber syndrome 40*f*, 41*f*
Meconium 137
   aspiration syndrome 137, 138
   stained liquor 268
Medical nutrition therapy 222
Mefloquine 336
Mega cisterna magna 32, 33*f*

Megaloblastic anemia
    diagnosis of 194
    etiopathogenesis of 193
Membranes 129
    artificial rupture of 56, 60
    prelabor rupture of 124
    preterm prelabor rupture of 110, 131*b*, 132, 149
    rupture of 210
    sweeping of 139
Meningitis 211
Meningomyelocele 16
Mental
    disorder 318, 323, 324*fc*, 326
        conceives 324
        screening for 327
    health, perinatal 326
    illness 318, 325*fc*, 326
Meperidine 406
Mesenchyme 20
Metabolic disorder 19
Metabolic syndrome 6, 357
Metalloproteinase, tissue inhibitor of 112
Metformin 222, 359, 404
Methergine 56
Methimazole 239
Methotrexate 300
Methyldopa 208
Methylene tetrahydrofolate reductase 49
Methylmalonic acid 194
Methylprednisolone 284
Metoclopramide 397
Metroplasty 45
Microadenomas 400
Microalbuminuria 286
Microcephaly 16, 291
Microinvasive disease 370
Microophthalmia 16, 353
Minor blood group antigens 150
Mirtazapine 322
Miscarriage 229, 398
    recurrent 48, 357
    risk of 43, 365
    spontaneous 357, 358
Misoprostol 140
Mitochondrial trifunctional protein 265
Mitral regurgitation 254, 255
Mitral stenosis 253
Mitral valve 254, 255
    prolapse 255
Monoamniotic twins 68, 75
Monochorionic diamniotic
    gestation 70
    placenta 65*f*
Monochorionic multiple gestations 69
Monochorionic twin pregnancy 26*f*
Monozygotic pregnancy 64
    types of 64
Monozygotic twins 65*f*
    incidence of 64
Mood stabilizers 323, 324, 325, 326
Morphine 406
Mucolytics 399
Mullerian abnormality, congenital 366
Multifetal gestation 27, 64, 72
Multifetal pregnancy 64, 72

frequency of 64
Multiparity 52, 182
Mumps 405
Muscle pain 223
Muscular tone 90
Myalgia 352
Mycobacteria growth indicator tube 330
*Mycobacterium tuberculosis* 331
Mycophenolate 300
    mofetil 298
*Mycoplasma hominis* 111
Myocardial infarction 258
    causes of 258
    complications 259
    diagnosis 258
    management 258
    prognosis 259
Myoma
    effect of 365
    intramural 367
    location of 365
Myomectomy 367

# N

Nadroparin 310
Naegele's formula 136
Narcotic analgesic 406
Nasal bone 26*f*
    sonography 12
Natural killer cells 46
Nausea 212, 223
Neck 30
    congenital tumors of 182
*Neisseria gonorrhoeae* 341
Nelfinavir 407
Neoadjuvant chemotherapy 370, 371
    role of 372
Neonatal
    intensive care unit 207, 358
    management 227
    morbidities 87
    outcome 138
Nephropathy 227, 229
    diabetic 214, 230, 286
Nephrotic syndrome 214, 283
Neural tube defect 5, 11, 26, 27*t*, 30, 31*f*
    risk of 358
Neurological disorder 290
Neuropathy 228
Neutral Protamine Hagedorn insulin 403
Neutrophil collagenase 112
Nevirapine 342, 344, 407
    cimetidine 277
Newborn intensive care unit 103
Nifedipine 118, 208, 209, 226, 282, 395, 402
Nipple stimulation 140
Nitrates 258
Nitrazine test 126
Nitric oxide
    donor 117, 119
    endothelial 249
    levels 203
Nitrofurantoin 407
Nitroglycerin 209
Nitroprusside 402

Nizatidine 399
Nonimmune hydrops 28
    etiology of 38*t*
Noninvasive methods 22
Noninvasive prenatal test 13, 144
Noninvasive procedures 11
Noniron deficiency anemia 193
Non-prostaglandin induction 161
Nonsteroidal anti-inflammatory drugs 193, 277, 282, 299, 367
Nonstress test 84, 91, 92, 105, 130, 139, 206
Nuchal fold 27
    thickness 15
Nuchal translucency 12, 13, 25, 26, 26*f*, 71
    sonography 12
Nucleic acid amplification technology 330
Nulliparity 205
Nutrition 384
Nutritional deficiencies 3
Nystatin vaginal tablets 407

# O

Obesity 47, 205, 252, 356, 359
    maternal 149
    related adverse pregnancy 357
Obsessive-compulsive disorder 319
Obstetric
    complications 228, 357, 358
    management 224
Obstruction
    partial 286
    renovascular 285
Obstructive sleep apnea 358
Olanzapine 322
Oligohydramnios 27, 70, 106, 137, 138
    diagnosis of 107
    etiology of 106, 107*fc*
    evaluation of 106, 107*fc*
    late onset 106
    severe 106
    subsequent 90
Oliguria 379
    persistent 210
Omeprazole 399
Omphalocele 16, 17, 35, 36*f*, 357
    typical 36*f*
Ondansetron 397
Operative vaginal delivery 343
Opium alkaloids 399
Oral antidiabetic agents 222, 404
Oral antihyperglycemic agents 222, 231
Oral contraceptive 408
    interaction 327*t*
    pills 263
Oral dydrogesterone 48
Oral glucose tolerance test 221
Oral hematinic therapy 200
Oral iron
    intake 192
    therapy 191
Oral labetalol 208
Oral levothyroxine 243

Orofacial clefts 357
Orthopnea 251
Osteogenesis imperfecta 37
Osteoporosis 255, 301
Ovarian cancer 6
Ovarian cyst 372, 373
Ovarian function, loss of 6
Ovarian hyperstimulation syndrome 302
Overt hypothyroid 47
Ovulation induction drugs 65
Oxcarbazepine 292, 293, 400
Oxygen
    consumption 379
    saturation 380
    therapy 383
Oxymetazoline 398
Oxytocin
    antagonist 117
    challenge test 91
    infusion 258
    receptor antagonists 116, 118, 119

## P

Pain 366
Palpation, abdominal 183
Pancreas, annular 16
Pancreatitis 213, 265
Panic disorder, diagnostic criteria for 319
Panniculus adiposus 359
Pantoprazole 399
Papanicolaou smear 368
Paradoxical emboli 255
Paramethadione 292
Paraovarian cystic lesions 373
Parasite 335
Parasitemia, peripheral 334
Paraspinal veins 379
Parenteral iron therapy 192, 192b
Parity 3
Paroxetine 322
Partial thromboplastin time 61, 275
Parvovirus 347, 349, 353
    fetal infection 354
    treatment 354
Patau syndrome 11
Patent ductus arteriosus 256
Peak systolic velocity 82f-84f, 104, 146, 147
Pelvic
    contraction 169
    deformity 169
    examination 370
    inflammatory disease, risk of 261
    lymph node 370
    lymphadenectomy, laparoscopic 6
Pelvi-femoral grip 174f
Pelvis, contracted 182
Perfusion scan 312, 312f
Perinatal mental disorders 318, 321
    classification of 318
    intrapartum management of 326
    management of 323
    postnatal management of 326
Perinatal morbidity
    causes of 179

Perinatal obsessive-compulsive disorder 319
Peripheral nerve paralysis 138
Personal protective equipment 390
Pheniramine 397
Phenobarbitone 292, 400
Phenylephrine 398
Phenylketonuria, maternal 28
Phenylpropanolamine 398
Phenytoin 292, 395, 400, 403
Pheochromocytoma 214
Pigmentation 314
Pinard's maneuver 174f
Piperaquine 336
Placenta 335, 358
    accreta 56, 153t
        spectrum 52, 56, 57, 62, 153
    adherent 366
    chorioangioma of 27
    disruption of 366
    examination of 40
    increta 53, 56f
    percreta 53
    posterior 149
    previa 51-53, 56, 62, 153, 153t, 366
        accreta 153f
        active management of 55b
        chances of 66
        incidence of 51
        management of 53, 53fc
        previous history of 52
Placental abruption 58, 128, 153, 243, 285, 366
    history of 205
    risk of 66
Placental alpha microglobulin-1 126
Placental mosaicism 80
Placental oxytocinase 366
Placentation, abnormal 52
Plant alkaloids 406
Plasma protein A, pregnancy associated 87
*Plasmodium*
    *falciparum* 198, 334
    *vivax* 337
Platelet
    count 210
    dysfunction 366
Pneumatic compression 314
*Pneumocystis jiroveci* pneumonia 341
Pneumonia 312, 353, 382, 387
    radiological evidence of 391
Pneumothorax 312, 382
Polyangiitis, microscopic 303
Polyarteritis nodosa 281, 303
Polycystic kidney
    bilateral 40f
    disease 16, 27, 34, 35f, 107, 214
Polycystic ovarian syndrome 47, 220
Polycythemia 7, 227
Polydactyly 16, 40f, 41f
Polydipsia 265
Polyhydramnios 28, 103, 105, 228, 229
    acute 103
    chronic 103
    etiology of 104fc
    evaluation of 104fc

    idiopathic 106
    mild 105
    moderate-to-severe 105
    oligohydramnios 102
    recurrent 10
    treatment of 104
Polymerase chain reaction 329, 335, 349
Porcine tissue valves 255
Posterior fossa defects 16
Postmaturity syndrome 137
Postnatal
    advice 226
    care 200
Postpartum 362
    care 260
    hemorrhage 3, 67, 187, 188, 263, 366, 385
    risk of 57
    issues 359
    management 75, 106, 314
    period 367
    thyroiditis 239, 245
        management 245
        neonatal concerns 245
Post-renal
    failure 285
    transplant 283
Post-thrombotic syndrome 306, 314
Preconception 19, 259
    and Prenatal Diagnostic Techniques Act 19
    care 282
    counseling 250, 260, 297
    risk assessment 250, 259
Prednisolone 288
Preeclampsia 64, 80, 169, 202, 203, 205, 209, 228, 229, 283, 297, 357, 366
    classification of 203t
    favor of 284
    mild 203, 211fc
    pathogenesis of 204fc
    risk of 228, 357
    severe 210b, 211fc
    superimposed 203, 215
Pregnancy 1, 7, 393
    acute fatty liver of 213, 263, 267, 267b, 267t, 275
    ectopic 142, 152
    extrauterine 372, 373
    heterotropic 373
    high-risk 1, 6, 323
    hypertensive disorders of 7, 202
    intrahepatic cholestasis of 90
    loss 297, 365
        previous 44
        recurrent 43, 47
    management of 138, 139fc, 197, 222, 230, 276
    medical termination of 41, 113, 332
    morbidity 300
    multiple 169
    nonalloimmunized 144
    non-preserving management 371
    postdated 171
    post-term 139

preserving management 370
prolonged 136
registries 394
termination of 86, 371
Premature rupture of membranes 107, 124, 125*f*, 125*t*, 126*f*, 127, 128, 128*t*, 129, 211, 366
etiopathogenesis of 124*fc*
management of 129, 133*fc*
Prenatal screening procedures 22
Prepregnancy 113, 360
Preterm labor 67, 103, 110, 366
etiopathogenesis of 110
management of 72, 121*b*, 226
prediction of 72
symptoms of 114
Primidone 400
Primigravida 335
Pritchard regimen 402
Prochlorperazine 397
Progesterone 48, 249, 268
role of 48
therapy 113
Prolactin disorder 47
Prolapse
management of 375
risk of 375
Promethazine 397
Prophylactic antibiotic 129, 132, 288, 376
therapy 131
Prophylactic cervical cerclage 73
Prophylaxis 145, 340
Propylthiouracil 239, 277
Prostacyclin 204
Prostaglandin 204
concentration 140
induction 160
synthetase inhibitor 117, 119
Protease inhibitors 341, 407
Protein 202
Proteinuria 202, 281
abnormal 202
*Proteus mirabilis* 407
Prothrombin time 275
Proton pump inhibitors 399
Pruritus 269
Pseudoephedrine 398
*Pseudomonas aeruginosa* 407
Psoriasis 396
Psychiatric disorders 318
risk factors 320
Psychosis, perinatal 319
Psychotropics 326
drugs, safety of 321
metabolism of 326
Pulmonary artery 258, 382
hypertension 256
occlusion pressure 383
Pulmonary embolism 311, 313*fc*
clinical features 311
diagnosis of 312
diagnostic tests 311
management of 313
pulmonary hypertension 257
Pulsatility index 80, 82*f*-84*f*, 96, 96*f*-98*f*
Pupils 380

Pyelectasis 15, 27
Pyelonephritis 213
acute 284
chronic 214
Pylectasis 35
Pyrazinamide 330, 332
Pyrexia 366
Pyridoxine 397
deficiency 193
supplementation 330
Pyrimethamine 336

## Q

Quadruple test 14, 232
Queenan curve 148*f*
Quetiapine 322

## R

Radiation
exposure 385
treatment 372
Radical trachelectomy 6
Radioactive iodine 244
Randomized controlled trials 39, 45, 86
Ranitidine 277, 399
Rapid-acting insulin 223
Reactive nonstress test, trace of 93*f*
Rectal tenesmus 373
Red blood cell 21, 188, 190, 196
Reflux nephropathy 285
Refractory pulmonary edema 382
Regurgitation 254
aortic 254
Renal agenesis 33
bilateral 33
Renal anomalies 27
Renal calculi 286
Renal cortical necrosis 283, 285
Renal disease 205, 281
effect of 281
Renal disorders 214
Renal dysfunction, acute 283
Renal failure 59, 285, 286*t*
acute 214, 265, 278, 285
chronic 214
Renal function, abnormal 214
Renal impairment 281
Renal malformations 16
Renal pelvic anteroposterior
diameter 35*t*
Renal system 379
clinical implications 379
Reproductive tract infections 341
Rescue cervical cerclage 120
Resistance index 82*f*-84*f*
Respiratory 5
care 383
complications 358
distress syndrome 129, 157, 229
rate 380
system 379, 388
reserve of 379
Resuscitation, cardiopulmonary 388-390, 390*fc*

Reticulocyte hemoglobin 190
Retinopathy 214, 227
diabetic 230
Reverse end-diastolic
flow 82
velocity 85, 86
Reviparin 310
Rhesus
alloimmunization 142, 150
pathophysiology of 142
antibodies 146
Rheumatic disease 298
Rheumatoid arthritis 298
epidemiology 299
fetal risks 299
management 299
maternal risks 299
pathophysiology 299
preconception counseling 299
Ribavirin 274
Ribonucleic acid 405
Rifampicin 331, 405
Right ventricular
failure 257
hypertrophy 254
Risperidone 322
Ritodrine 117, 395, 396
Ritonavir 407
Rituximab 300
Robert syndrome 37
Rocker bottom feet 16
Roll over test 205
Rubella 347-349, 405
congenital 347
prevention of 350

## S

Sacrococcygeal teratoma 27
S-adenosyl methionine 270
Salbutamol 395
Salicylates 406
Saline infusion sonohysterography 44
Salivary estriol 112
Salt iodization 238
Saquinavir 407
Scar thickness 160
Schizophrenia 320
Scleroderma, renal 281
Second trimester screening 13, 26
Sedation 115, 381
Sedative 325, 326
Seizures
control of 294
disorders 5
focal 290, 291
unknown onset 291
Sepsis 386, 387
bundle 387
Septal defects 29
Sertraline 322
Serum glutamic
oxaloacetic transaminase 204
pyruvic transaminase 204
Sexually transmitted infections 2, 339

Shock 62
    hemorrhagic 386
    hypovolemic 59
    septic 386
Short long bones 27
Short rib polydactyly 37
Shoulder dystocia 225, 357
Sickle cell 5
    anemia 2, 198
    disease 11, 198
Sildenafil 86
    therapy 86
Sim's position 373
Single drug therapy 400
Single gene disorder 11, 22
Single umbilical artery 27
Skeletal deformities 106
Skeletal malformations 16
Skeletal system 37
Skeleton 26
Skin edema 38$f$
Sodium
    bicarbonate 383, 399
    nitroprusside 209
Soft tissue swelling 33$f$
Solitary toxic nodule 238
Sonography 168
Spastic motor disorder 243
Sperm sorting techniques 22
Spina bifida 31, 31$f$, 228, 357
    risk of 292
Spinal abnormality 10
Spinal muscular atrophy 11
Spine 27, 30
Spiramycin 354
Spondylocostal dysplasia 10
Sporozoites 334
Squamous cells, atypical 369
Status asthmaticus 378
Status epilepticus 293
Stenosis, pulmonary 30
Steroids
    antenatal 132, 207, 224
    antepartum 371
    inhaled 398
Stillbirth 138, 145, 153, 358
    antepartum 157
Stomach 26
Streptokinase 314
Streptomycin 330, 405
Stress 48
    ulcer prevention 381
Substance abuse 4, 80
Sudden cardiac death 249
Sulfadoxine 336
Sulfasalazine 299
Supine hypotension syndrome 249
Sweating 379
Sympatholytics, central 401
Symphysio-fundal height 81, 99, 102
Symphysis pubis 179$f$
Syncope 291
Syphilis 85
Systemic arterial pressure 249
Systemic inflammatory response syndrome 386

Systemic lupus erythematosus 5, 213, 214, 283, 297
    diagnosis 297
    epidemiology 297
    fetal risks 297
    management of 298
    maternal risks 297
    pathophysiology 297

## T

Tachycardia 29, 187, 311, 387
    supraventricular 29, 257, 259
Tachypnea 187
    transient 157
Takayasu's arteritis 303
Teenage pregnancy 1
    risk of 2$b$
Telangiectasis 314
Temazepam 326
Tender loving care 48
Tenofovir 342
Teratogenicity 291, 394
    mechanism of 394$t$
Terbinafine 407
Terbutaline 117, 395
Tetanus toxoid 405
Tetracycline 395
Tetralogy of Fallot 16, 30, 257
Thalassemia 5, 193, 195-197
Thalidomide 395
Thanatophoric dysplasia 37, 40$f$
Theophylline 398
Thionamides 239
Thrombin inhibitors 309
Thrombocytopenia 242, 301
    heparin-induced 310
    idiopathic 213
    neonatal 297
Thrombocytopenic purpura 286
Thromboembolic disease, chronic 256
Thromboembolic prophylaxis 381
Thromboembolism 249, 306, 357, 358
    pathophysiology 306
Thrombolytic therapy 313
Thrombophilia 45, 47, 203, 205, 213, 306, 307
    acquired 45
    hereditary 45, 46
Thromboprophylaxis 307
    antepartum 361
Thrombosis 211
Thrombotic thrombocytopenic purpura 213, 271, 283
Thyroid
    antibodies 47
    autoantibodies 238
    binding globulin 236
    carcinoma 244
    disease 205, 236, 243
    disorders 5, 46, 236
    dysfunction 236, 242
        screening for 245
    function 236
        assessment of 237
        measurement of 242
    hormone 237-239
    insufficiency 242
    nodules 244
    peroxidase
        antibody 245
        autoantibodies 46
    physiology 236, 236$t$
    stimulating hormone 46, 236
    storm 241
        management of 241
Thyroidectomy, subtotal 240
Thyroiditis
    acute 238
    postpartum 239, 245
    subacute 238
Thyrotoxicosis 239
    maternal 90
Thyroxine 245
    supplementation 243
Tinzaparin 310
Titrate insulin 224
Tocolysis 116
Tocolytics 120, 132, 395
    medications 395
    role of 120
    therapy 73, 116$t$, 120
Topiramate 292, 400
Torticollis, congenital 366
Total body irradiation 6
Total iron-binding capacity 190, 191
Total leukocyte count 130
Total parenteral nutrition 384, 385
    complications of 385
Toxic multinodular goiter 238
Toxic side effects 354
*Toxoplasma* 348, 354
    *gondii* 347, 348
Toxoplasma, rubella, cytomegalovirus, herpes infections 47, 104, 347, 354
    fetal and neonatal features of 348$t$
    fetal effects of 347
    prenatal diagnosis of 349$t$
    serology, interpretations of 348$t$
Toxoplasmosis 85, 349
    acute 350, 351$f$, 351$b$
    congenital 351$t$
Tracheal intubation 384
Tracheoesophageal fistula 16, 36
Tramadol 406
Transverse lie 180, 180$f$
Trauma 388
    abdominal 145
    external 58
Tricuspid regurgitation 13
Trimethadione 292
Triprolidine 399
Trisomy 11, 17, 18
Trophoblast cells 368
Trophoblastic disease 205
    gestational 27
Truncus arteriosus 30
Tuberculin skin test 330
Tuberculosis 188, 329, 343, 368
    abdominal 329
    clinical features 329
    diagnosis of 329

extrapulmonary 331*fc*
growth of 330
histopathology 330
management 330
pulmonary 331*fc*
radiology 330
treatment 330
Tubular necrosis 214, 285
Tumor
  cerebral 211
  extrathoracic 38
  markers 374
  necrosis factor-alpha 46
    antagonists 299
Turner's syndrome 256
Twins
  conjoined 68, 68*f*
  delivery 145
  gestation 158
  intrapartum management of 74
  locking of 76, 76*f*
  peak sign 70*f*
  reversed arterial perfusion 68
  to-twin transfusion syndrome 38, 68, 69, 103, 104, 107

## U

Ultrasonography 12, 14-16, 25, 67, 70, 82, 102, 104, 105, 107, 126, 128, 130, 146, 147, 211, 277
  point-of-care 382
Ultrasound 14, 104, 349
Umbilical artery 80, 95, 96*f*
  Doppler 82, 83*f*, 85, 86, 92, 96*f*, 97*f*
    normal 83*f*
Umbilical cord 174*f*
  blood 241
  cysts 17
Umbilical vein 83
*Ureaplasma urealyticum* 111
Uremia 282
Uric acid
  levels 282
  serum 402
Urinary obstruction 27
Urinary stasis 286
Urinary tract
  infection 187, 188, 357, 407*t*
    asymptomatic 260
    drugs for 407
  malformations 38
  obstruction, upper 285

Urine 13
  output 380, 382
  protein 282
Urokinase 314
Uropathy, obstructive 35
Ursodeoxycholic acid 270
Urticaria 240
Uterine
  anomalies, congenital 44
  artery 80, 95
    Doppler 82, 82*f*, 205
    pulsatility index 205
  contractions 74
  factors 91
  fibroids 365
  imaging 44
  malformations 169
  overdistention, pathologic 111
  reconstruction 45
  rupture 52, 159, 162
    rates of 161*t*
    risk of 156
Uteroplacental circulation 205
Uterus, scarred 169

## V

Vaccination, types of 261
Vaccines 405
Vaginal birth after cesarean section 152, 154, 155*f*, 155*t*, 159, 225, 357
Vaginal bleeding 59
  third-trimester 90
Vaginal canal, direction of 372
Vaginal delivery 62, 74, 171, 172, 212, 216, 253, 271, 288, 343
Vaginal infections, drugs for 408
Vaginal wet mount preparation 114
Valaciclovir 353
Valproate 291, 292, 322
Valproic acid 292, 395, 400
Valsalva maneuver 259
Valve disease 5
Valvular defects 16
Varicella 405
  pneumonitis 353
  syndrome, congenital 353
  zoster virus 347, 349, 353
    infection 353
Vasa previa 51, 54, 61
Vascular disorders 214
Vascular thrombosis 300
Vasculitis 302

Vasodilation 204
Vasodilators 257, 401
Venlafaxine 322
Venous thromboembolism 302, 306, 358
  anticoagulants for 310
  risk factors for 306, 307*t*
Ventilation 312, 389
Ventricular septal defect 16, 29, 256
Ventriculomegaly 15, 16, 27
Vermian hypoplasia 33
Vibroacoustic stimulation 94
Vinblastine 374, 406
Viral hepatitis 213, 271
Virus
  phenotype of 339
  types of 339
Vitamin
  A 186
  B12 193, 194, 360
    deficiency 193
  C 206
  D 299, 360
  E 206
  K 309, 344, 400, 404
    antagonists 309
  supplementation 384
Vomiting 212, 366

## W

Warfarin 314, 395, 404
Wegener granulomatosis 302, 303
Weight gain, gestational 361*t*
Wernicke's encephalopathy 272
White blood cell 190, 266
World Health Organization 186
Wound infection 357

## X

X-linked
  disorder, diagnosis of 22
  placental sulfatase deficiency 137

## Z

Zatuchni-Andros breech scoring index 172, 172*t*
Zidovudine 342, 407
Zona pellucida, micromanipulation of 64
Zonisamide 292
Zuspan regimen 403

EU GSPR Authorised Reprsentative
Logos Europe, 9 rue Nicolas Poussin
1700, La Rochelle, France
Phone: +33 (0) 6 67 93 73 78
E-mail: contact@logoseurope.eu

www.ingramcontent.com/pod-product-compliance
Ingram Content Group UK Ltd.
Pitfield, Milton Keynes, MK11 3LW, UK
UKHW051847210426

5322IPUK00019B/289